HEAD
and NECK
IMAGING

Volume One

HEAD
and NECK
IMAGING

Third Edition

Edited by

PETER M. SOM, M.D.
Professor of Radiology and Otolaryngology,
Mount Sanai School of Medicine of the City University of
    New York;
Chief of Head and Neck Radiology,
Mount Sinai Hospital,
New York, New York

HUGH D. CURTIN, M.D.
Professor of Radiology and
    Otolaryngology,
University of Pittsburgh School of Medicine;
Director of Radiology,
Eye and Ear Hospital,
Pittsburgh, Pennsylvania

Chief of Radiology,
Department of Radiology,
Massachusetts Eye and Ear Infirmary,
Boston, Massachusetts

with 3822 illustrations and 27 color plates

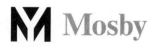

St. Louis Baltimore Boston Carlsbad Chicago Naples New York Philadelphia Portland
London Madrid Mexico City Singapore Sydney Tokyo Toronto Wiesbaden

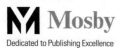

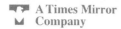

Vice President and Publisher: Anne S. Patterson
Senior Developmental Editor: Sandra Clark Brown
Project Manager: Carol Sullivan Weis
Senior Production Editor: Christine Carroll
Manufacturing Supervisor: David Graybill

THIRD EDITION

Printed in the United States of America
Composition by NuComp
Illustration preparation by Accu-Color, Inc.
Printing/binding by Maple Vail Book Mfg. Group

Mosby–Year Book, Inc.
11830 Westline Industrial Drive
St. Louis, MO 63146

Library of Congress Cataloging in Publication Data
Head and neck imaging / edited by Peter M. Som, Hugh D. Curtin.—3rd
ed.
           p.   cm.
Includes bibliographical references and index.
ISBN 0-8151-7718-6 (hardcover)
1. Head—Imaging. 2. Neck—Imaging. I. Som, Peter M. II. Curtin, Hugh D.
[DNLM: 1. Head—radiography. 2. Neck—radiography. 3. Magnetic Resonance
Imaging. 4. Tomography, X-Rayed Computed. WE 705 H43031 1996]
RC936.H43 1996
617.5' 10754—dc20
DNLM/DLC
for Library of Congress   95-25522
                                                               CIP

95 96 97 98 99 / 9 8 7 6 5 4 3 2 1

Contributors

JAMES J. ABRAHAMS, M.D.
Associate Professor and Director of Medical Studies,
Department of Diagnostic Radiology,
Section of Neuroradiology,
Yale University School of Medicine,
New Haven, Connecticut

NOLAN R. ALTMAN, M.D.
Chief, Department of Neuroradiology,
Miami Children's Hospital,
Miami, Florida

WILLIAM G. ARMINGTON, M.D.
Neuroradiologist,
Mercy Baptist Medical Center;
Assistant Clinical Professor of Radiology,
Tulane University School of Medicine,
New Orleans, Louisiana

BRUCE S. BAUER, M.D., F.A.C.S.
Head, Division of Plastic Surgery,
Children's Memorial Hospital;
Associate Professor of Surgery,
Northwestern University Medical School,
Chicago, Illinois

MANFERD T. BENSON, M.D.
Staff Radiologist,
Department of Diagnostic Radiology,
Macomb Hospital Center,
Warren, Michigan

MARK L. BENSON, M.D.
Clinical Assistant Professor,
Russell H. Morgan Department of Radiology and
  Radiological Sciences,
The John Hopkins Medical Institutions,
Baltimore, Maryland;
Department of Radiology,
Wheeling Hospital,
Wheeling, West Virginia

R. THOMAS BERGERON, M.D.
Professor of Clinical Radiology,
State University of New York Health Science Center
  at Brooklyn;
Chairman and Attending Radiologist,
Long Island College Hospital,
Brooklyn, New York

LARISSA T. BILANIUK, M.D.
Professor of Radiology,
University of Pennsylvania School of Medicine;
Staff Radiologist,
Children's Hospital of Philadelphia,
Philadelphia, Pennsylvania

MARGARET BRANDWEIN, M.D.
Department of Radiology,
Mount Sinai Medical Center of the City University of
  New York,
New York, New York

IRA F. BRAUN, M.D
Clinical Professor of Radiology,
University of Miami School of Medicine;
Director, Interventional Neuroradiology,
Miami Vascular Institute - Department of Radiology, Baptist
Hospital of Miami,
Miami, Florida

RONALD A. BROADWELL, M.D.
Assistant Professor of Radiology,
Department of Radiology,
University of North Carolina at Chapel Hill,
Chapel Hill, North Carolina

JAN W. CASSELMAN, M.D., PH.D.
Director of MRI and Head and Neck Radiology,
Department of Radiology and Medical Imaging,
A.Z. Sint-Jan Brugge,
Bruges, Belgium

MAURICIO CASTILLO, M.D.
Chief of Neuroradiology,
Associate Professor of Radiology,
University of North Carolina School of Medicine,
Chapel Hill, North Carolina

DONALD W. CHAKERES, M.D.
Professor of Radiology,
Director of Magnetic Resonance Imaging,
Section Head of Neuroradiology,
Ohio State University, College of Medicine,
Columbus, Ohio

HUGH D. CURTIN, M.D.
Formerly, Professor of Radiology and Otolaryngology, University of Pittsburgh School of Medicine;
Director of Radiology,
Eye and Ear Hospital,
Pittsburgh, Pennsylvania;
Currently, Chief of Radiology,
Department of Radiology,
Massachusetts Eye and Ear Infirmary,
Boston, Massachusetts

ANTON N. HASSO, M.D.
Professor of Radiology and Otolaryngology/Head and
    Neck Surgery,
Loma Linda University School of Medicine;
Director of Neuroradiology, Department of Radiology,
Associate Director for Research,
Section of Magnetic Resonance Imaging,
Loma Linda University Medical Center,
Loma Linda, California

ROY A. HOLLIDAY, M.D.
Assistant Professor of Radiology and Otolaryngology,
Department of Radiology,
New York University Medical Center,
New York, New York

PATRICIA A. HUDGINS, M.D.
Associate Professor of Radiology and Otolaryngology,
Emory University School of Medicine,
Atlanta, Georgia

IAN N. JACOBS, M.D.
Assistant Professor of Surgery,
Division of Otolaryngology,
Emory University School of Medicine,
Atlanta, Georgia

EDWARD E. KASSEL, D.D.S., M.D.
Chief, Department of Medical Imaging,
Mount Sinai Hospital;
Associate Professor, Department of Medical Imaging,
University of Toronto,
Toronto, Canada

RICHARD WIER KATZBERG, M.D.
Professor and Chairman, Department of Radiology,
University of California at Davis,
Sacramento, California

WILLIAM W.M. LO, M.D., F.A.C.R.
Clinical Professor of Radiology,
University of Southern California School of Medicine;
Section Chief of Neuroradiology,
St. Vincent Medical Center,
Los Angeles, California

MAHMOOD F. MAFEE, M.D.
Professor of Radiology,
Director, MRI Center,
Director, Radiology Section, Eye and Ear Infirmary,
University of Illinois at Chicago Medical Center,
Chicago, Illinois

SURESH K. MUKHERJI, M.D.
Director of Head and Neck Radiology,
Neuroradiology Section,
Assistant Professor of Radiology and Surgery,
School of Medicine,
University of North Carolina at Chapel Hill,
Chapel Hill, North Carolina

LYN NADEL, M.D.
Attending Radiologist,
Deering Hospital,
Miami, Flordia

THOMAS P. NAIDICH, M.D., F.A.C.R.
Director of Neuroradiology, MR and CT,
Department of Radiology,
Baptist Hospital of Miami,
Miami, Florida

MARY OEHLER, M.D.
Assistant Professor, Division of Neuroradiology,
Department of Radiology,
Ohio State University College of Medicine,
Columbus, Ohio

PATRICK J. OLIVERIO, M.D.
Clinical Assistant Professor,
Russell H. Morgan Department of Radiology and
    Radiological Sciences,
The Johns Hopkins Medical Institutions,
Baltimore, Maryland;
Radiological Consultants Associated, Inc.,
Fairmont, West Virginia

RANDON L. OPP, M.D.
Clinical Assistant,
Department of Radiology,
Loma Linda University Medical Center,
Loma Linda, California

DEBORAH L. REEDE, M.D.
Associate Professor of Clinical Radiology,
SUNY Health Science Center at Brooklyn;
Adjunct Professor of Radiology,
New York University School of Medicine,
Brooklyn, New York

CHARLES J. SCHATZ, M.D.
Clinical Professor of Radiology and Otolaryngology,
University of Southern California;
Director, Head and Neck Imaging,
St. John's Hospital and Health Center,
Santa Monica, California

ALICE M. SCHEFF, M.D.
Assistant Professor of Radiology,
Hospital of the University of Pennsylvania,
Philadelphia, Pennsylvania

PETRA SCHMALBROCK, Ph.D.
Research Scientist, Division of Magnetic Resonance
  Imaging,
Department of Radiology,
Ohio State University College of Medicine,
Columbus, Ohio

STEVEN J. SCRIVANI, D.D.S., M.D.
Department of Oral and Maxillofacial Surgery,
Massachusetts General Hospital,
Boston, Massachusetts

WAYNE SLONE, M.D.
Assistant Professor, Division of Neuroradiology,
Department of Radiology,
Ohio State University College of Medicine,
Columbus, Ohio

WENDY R.K. SMOKER, M.D., F.A.C.R.
Professor of Radiology,
Director of Neuroradiology,
Department of Radiology,
Medical College of Virginia,
Richmond, Virginia

LIVIA G. SOLTI-BOHMAN, M.D., F.A.C.R.
Clinical Assistant Professor of Radiology,
University of Southern California at Los Angeles;
Radiologist,
St. Vincent Medical Center,
Los Angeles, California

PETER M. SOM, M.D.
Professor of Radiology and Otolaryngology,
Mount Sinai School of Medicine of the City
  University of New York;
Chief of Head and Neck Radiology,
Mount Sinai Hospital,
New York, New York

JOEL D. SWARTZ, M.D.
Chairman, Department of Radiology,
The Germantown Hospital and Medical Center;
Professor of Radiology, Department of Radiologic
  Sciences,
The Medical College of Pennsylvania,
Philadelphia, Pennsylvania

ALFRED L. WEBER, M.D.
Professor of Radiology,
Harvard Medical School;
Chief of Radiology,
Massachusetts Eye and Ear Infirmary,
Boston, Massachusetts

JANE L. WEISSMAN, M.D.
Department of Radiology and Otolaryngology,
Director of Head and Neck Imaging,
University of Pittsburgh Medical Center,
Pittsburgh, Pennsylvania

PER-LENNART WESTESSON, D.D.S., PH.D.
Professor of Radiology and Chief of Head and Neck
  Imaging,
Department of Radiology;
Professor of Clinical Dentistry,
University of Rochester School of Medicine and Dentistry;
Professor of Orthodontics,
Eastman Dental Center,
Rochester, New York;
Adjunct Professor of Oral Medicine,
State University of New York at Buffalo,
Buffalo, New York;
Associate Professor (Docent) of Oral Radiology,
  University of Lund,
Sweden

DAVID M. YOUSEM, M.D.
Associate Professor of Radiology, Otolarynogology-
  Head and Neck Surgery,
University of Pennsylvania Medical Center,
Philadelphia, Pennsylvania

DAVID P. ZADVINSKIS, M.D.
Staff Radiologist,
Macomb Hospital Center,
Department of Diagnostic Radiology,
Warren, Michigan

ROBERT A. ZIMMERMAN, M.D.
Chief, Pediatric Neuroradiology,
Professor of Radiology,
University of Pennsylvania School of Medicine;
Department of Radiology,
Children's Hospital of Philadelphia,
Philadelphia, Pennsylvania

S. JAMES ZINREICH, M.D.
Department of Neuroradiolgy,
Johns Hopkins Hospital,
Baltimore, Maryland

We dedicate this book to our wives, who stood by us and gave us encouragement and understanding when it was most needed. You have our love.

To Judy and Carole

P.M.S. and H.D.C

Preface

Since publication of the second edition of this book, the field of head and neck imaging has continued to mature as a subspecialty of radiology. Today, more radiologists are aware of the excitement generated by this case material and the often pivotal role head and neck imaging plays in the management of patients with these diseases. There also has been a continued diversification of the head and neck imaging audience. Although the majority of radiologists who read this case material are still classic neuroradiologists, there are increasing numbers of body imagers and growing numbers of clinicians who want to better understand the imaging of their patients. Finally, the field itself has continued to develop, and as clinicians have placed greater demands on the radiologist, the imaging community has responded with greater interest and knowledge regarding the clinical problems and new innovative ideas of how to attain information.

In the past few years, to answer the demands of radiologists to learn about head and neck imaging, a number of excellent books have appeared that address the problems of either introducing the new reader to the field or providing an overview of the topic for the more experienced reader. However, the readers of the second edition of *Head and Neck Imaging* created a special niche for the book, distinguishing it from these other books. Specifically, it became the reference text on the field, and it was with this mission in mind that the third edition was created.

The new table of contents shows that there is a newly organized, more thorough treatment of the field. The book is now divided into six anatomic sections, each subdivided into the areas that the editors felt best provided complete coverage of the topic. Of those chapters retained from the second edition, each was thoroughly updated and expanded. In addition, there are completely new chapters included in the third edition that address the osteomeatal complex and endoscopic surgery, oral implants and DentaScanning, pediatric airway disease, thyroid and parathyroid diseases, and the postoperative neck. There are also more thorough treatments of the fascia and spaces of the neck, the embryology of the neck and congenital neck lesions, the cervical lymph nodes, the lacrimal system, and, in response to the growing demands of the skull base surgeon, a new, more thorough chapter on the skull base. There are a few chapters that have retained some material from the previous edition. However, such material was purposely kept because the third edition of *Head and Neck Imaging* is now one of the few new references in which the reader can learn about these topics.

In addition to discussing imaging, emphasis has been placed on embryology, anatomy, clinical material, and histopathology, which are discussed in each chapter as they pertain to the subject matter. However, there are several chapters that specifically discuss pathology in great detail, and the reader is encouraged to use these chapters as a pathology resource for the head and neck in general. Although kept to a minimum, there are a number of lesions that are discussed in several different chapters. Each discussion relates to the specific chapter topic, and the reader is encouraged to examine the various treatments of such subjects to obtain the most thorough understanding of the topic as expressed by different authors.

The references in each chapter are as detailed and current as possible, and the index to the book has been made as thorough as possible, with extensive cross-referencing to ease the reader's search for a specific detail.

Although no book can be thoroughly complete or totally current, the editors have tried to achieve these goals to the best of their abilities. When readers brought to our attention omissions or incompletely treated subjects in the second edition, we specifically addressed each of these areas in this third edition.

The effectiveness of a book as a teaching tool and as a resource of current information is a direct result of the quality of the material submitted by the contributors. The editors feel that we have assembled a knowledgeable and renowned group of contributors, who number among them some of the most internationally and nationally established names in the field, as well as some new head and neck imagers. It is the presence of these new radiologists that testifies to the growing pool of talented physicians who are involved in the field of head and neck imaging. Together, these radiologists, in this pressing period of limited academic time, have provided excellent, thorough chapters with high-quality images. We want to thank and commend each of them for their efforts and the time spent helping create this third edition.

The editors also want to thank the staff of Mosby–Year Book, who showed great interest and concern for this project and shared the editors' wishes to produce a book of the highest quality. It was their attention to detail, thoroughness, and experience that allowed this ever-enlarging book to be tightly compact and presented in a readable format. In particular, we want to thank Anne Patterson, Sandy Clark Brown, and Christine Carroll for their contributions and guidance.

Finally, the editors hope that the readers of this book will enjoy learning about the field of head and neck imaging, will find this book the reference that we hope it is, and will grow to love the field as we do.

P.M.S and H.D.C

Contents

HEAD
and NECK
IMAGING

PART I

Midface and Sinonasal Cavities

1

Midface: Embryology and Congenital Lesions

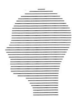

THOMAS P. NAIDICH
ROBERT A. ZIMMERMAN
BRUCE S. BAUER
NOLAN R. ALTMAN
LARISSA T. BILANIUK

BASIC EMBRYOLOGY OF THE FACE, EYE, AND CORPUS CALLOSUM

The embryogenesis of the midface and upper lip, the optic nerve and globe, and the corpus callosum share many spatial, temporal, and histologic features that appear to explain the frequency of concurrent anomalies of these structures.

Face

The face has a dual embryonic origin.[1] The median facial structures, bones and soft tissues, derive from the frontonasal prominence. The lateral facial structures, bones and soft tissues, arise from the branchial arches. For this reason, anomalies tend to affect either median or lateral structures separately or their lines of junction.

The major features of the face develop in the fourth to eighth week of gestation by growth, migration, and merging of a number of processes bordering the stomodeum, which is a slitlike invagination of the ectoderm that marks the location of the mouth.[2] At 4 weeks of gestation (Fig. 1-1, *A*), the stomodeum is bordered superiorly by the unpaired, median frontal prominence, laterally by the paired maxillary processes, and inferiorly by the paired mandibular processes. The frontal prominence is composed of surface ectoderm and a thin layer of mesenchyme overlying the developing forebrain. This mesenchyme derives principally from neural crest cells, not mesoderm per se.[3] The maxillary and the mandibular processes derive from the first branchial arch. The nasal placodes are paired epithelial thickenings that arise near the lateral margins of the overhanging frontal prominence.

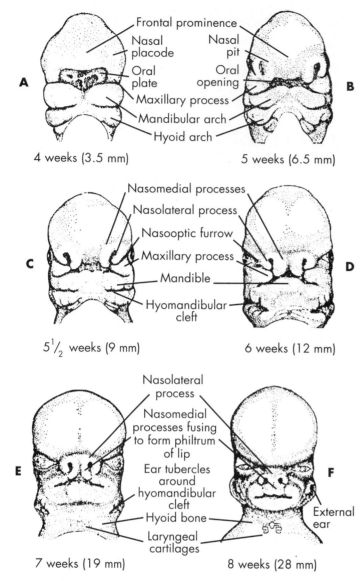

4 weeks (3.5 mm)   5 weeks (6.5 mm)

5½ weeks (9 mm)   6 weeks (12 mm)

7 weeks (19 mm)   8 weeks (28 mm)

FIG. 1-1 **A** through **F,** Embryogenesis of face from 4 to 8 weeks of gestation. (From Patten BM. The normal development of the facial region. In: Pruzansky S. Congenital anomalies of the face and associated structures. Springfield, Ill: Charles C Thomas, Publisher, 1985.)

By 5 weeks of gestation (Fig. 1-1, *B, C*), horseshoe-shaped elevations have appeared around the nasal placodes, so the placodes seem recessed beneath the surface. These recesses are called the nasal pits. The longer medial limbs of the horseshoes are designated the nasomedial processes, and the shorter lateral limbs of the horseshoes are designated the nasolateral processes. The lowermost portions of the nasomedial limbs are designated the globular processes.[4] At this time the nasomedial and the nasolateral processes lie adjacent to, but appear separated from, the now larger maxillary processes. The mandibular arches have enlarged. These merge together during the fifth week to form the lower lip and underlying structures.

During the sixth week (Fig. 1-1, *D, E*), the nasomedial

processes increase in size and become displaced toward each other by marked enlargement of the two maxillary processes lateral to them. They merge with the frontal prominence to form the frontonasal prominence. From this key frontonasal prominence will come the nasal bones, the frontal bones, the cartilaginous nasal capsule, the central one third of the upper lip, the central one third of the superior alveolar ridge including the incisors, and the primary palate. At each side a groove called the *nasooptic furrow* extends from the medial canthus of the orbit toward the developing nose along the line between the nasolateral and the maxillary processes. The nasolacrimal duct will develop along this line. It is not known whether the deep portion of the furrow becomes the nasolacrimal duct or whether a separate epithelial tube grows down from the orbit to the nasal cavity along the course of the furrow.[2] By the seventh week, the nasolateral processes merge with the maxillary processes to complete the ala nasi of each side. The nasomedial processes still remain separate.

By the eighth week (Fig. 1-1, *F*), the upper lip is formed by the merging of each nasomedial process with the ipsilateral maxillary process, followed by the merging of the two nasomedial processes in the midline. This merging completes formation of the columella and the philtrum (Fig. 1-1, *E*), and merging of the maxillary and mandibular processes forms the cheeks and the corners of the mouth. During this time, there is also descent of the nose and medial migration of the orbits above the nose.

The frontonasal process (including the merged nasomedial processes) may be considered to constitute an intermaxillary segment. The superficial portion of this segment, termed the prolabium, forms the medial portion of the upper lip. The deeper gnathogingival segment will develop into the premaxillary portion of the upper jaw, containing the four upper incisors. The palatal component will form a triangular midline wedge of palate designated the primary palate. This becomes continuous with the rostralmost portion of the nasal septum.

The maxillary processes form the lateral portions of the upper jaw and contribute all of the upper teeth behind the incisors. During the sixth to eighth weeks, the maxillary processes also give rise medially to paired palatal shelves. Initially these shelves curve ventrally alongside the tongue (Fig 1-2, *A, B*). When growth of the mandible permits descent of the tongue, these shelves swing medially toward each other above the tongue (Fig. 1-2, *C, D*). The shelves then merge (1) with each other in the midline and (2) with the primary palate anteriorly to form the definitive palate (Fig. 1-2, *E, F*). That portion of the definitive palate contributed by the maxillary processes is designated the secondary palate. The secondary palate is far larger than the primary palate. The lines of fusion of the palate appear Y-shaped. The incisive foramina lie at the midpoint of the Y, marking the junction between the V-shaped primary palate anteriorly and the paired halves of the secondary palate more posteriorly. While the palate is forming, the nasal septum grows downward and fuses with its cephalic surface.

Formation of the Mouth, Nostrils, and Posterior Choanae

The ectoderm overlying the early forebrain extends into the stomodeum. At this site it lies adjacent to the developing foregut. The junctional zone between the surface ectoderm and the subjacent endoderm is called the buccopharyngeal membrane.

The line of attachment of the buccopharyngeal membrane corresponds to Waldeyer's ring, connecting the nasopharyngeal adenoids, the palatine tonsils, and the lingual tonsils.[5] Dissolution of the buccopharyngeal membrane in the early somite stage permits communication between the mouth and the foregut regions. The position of Waldeyer's ring in the postnatal human, deep to a well-developed mouth, indicates the extent to which formation of the face arises by the thickening of the tissues external to the original surface level, represented by the stomodeum.

By a similar thickening of surrounding surface tissues, the nasal pits become progressively recessed. The ectoderm overlying the nasal pits fuses with the ectoderm overlying the stomodeum to form the bucconasal (oronasal) membrane. Eventual disappearance of this membrane establishes communication between the nose and the upper part of the stomodeal cavity. The external openings of the nasal pits are designated the nostrils (external nares). The new, more dorsal openings into the stomodeal cavity are called the *posterior nares,* or *primitive choanae.* The paired nostrils and primitive choanae gradually become separated by the developing nasal septum. By the middle of the second month of gestation, the secondary palate subdivides the more rostral portion of the original stomodeal chamber into separate nasal and oral cavities. The palatal shelves elongate the nasal cavities, so that the new posterior openings—the secondary, or permanent, choanae—now are located at the junction of the nasal cavity and nasopharynx.

The fusion of the palatal processes of the maxillary swellings with the septum occurs along the anterior or ventral three quarters of the nasal septum by the ninth week. Thus the left and right nasal chambers become separated about the same time that the nasal chambers separate from the oral cavity. Posteriorly or dorsally the palatal shelves fail to fuse with the nasal septum and instead form the soft palate.[5-9] Development of the nasal cavity is complete by the second month of fetal life. From the second to the sixth month of prenatal life, the nostrils are closed by epithelial plugs that then recanalize to reestablish a patent nasal cavity.[5]

The exact origin and development of the nasal septum are poorly understood. It is known that the septum is originally thicker and then narrows progressively. The septum may arise by fusion of the mesenchymal cores of the nasomedial and frontal processes to form the frontonasal processes. The core would then gradually thin out, atrophy, and disappear. Badrawy, however, suggests that the narrowing of the frontonasal process could arise by an inward folding of the cartilage of the nasofrontal prominence (Fig. 1-3). This action would simultaneously cause approximation of the sides of the nose, deepening of the nasal fossae, and creation of the intervening septum.[10]

At the sixth fetal week the nasal capsule consists of one continuum of hyaline cartilage. The lower part of the nasal capsule ossifies in membrane from various centers outside the perichondrium. The membranous bone of the vomer is ossified at birth.[11] The upper part of the nasal capsule, like the neighboring base of the cranium, ossifies in cartilage. At birth the ethmoidal plate is still cartilage; it commences to ossify postnatally *(vide infra).* The anterior portion of the cartilaginous nasal septum is never enclosed by bone. The hyaline cartilage grows and persists as the cartilaginous part of the septum and the cartilage of the external nose. More posteriorly the original cartilage of the septum remains sandwiched for a time between two laminae of membranous bone before it finally atrophies and disappears.[11] Processes develop along the lateral nasal walls, which eventually give rise to the turbinates.

During the fifth and sixth weeks of gestation, the earliest evidence of the cranium is found when several dense mesenchymal masses migrate to regions that correspond to the primitive ethmoid, auditory, nasal, and optic centers. The first evidence of intracartilaginous skull formation arises in the basisphenoid, basiocciput, and around the auditory vesi-

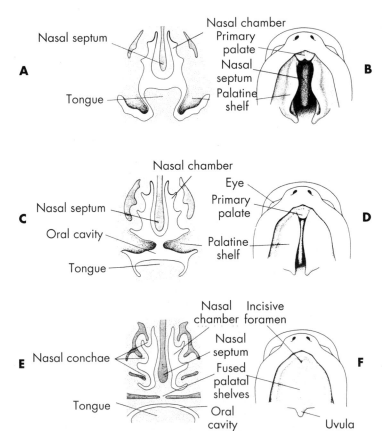

FIG. 1-2 **A** through **F,** Embryogenesis of the palate from 6½ to 10 weeks of gestation. (From Langman J. Medical embryology: human development, normal and abnormal. 2nd Edition. Baltimore, Md: Williams & Wilkins, 1969.)

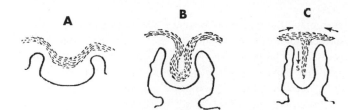

FIG. 1-3 Embryogenesis of nasal septum. Diagram of coronal section of the frontonasal process above the stomodeum (proposed theory). **A,** Early embryo. Dashed lines represent cartilage. **B,** Folding of frontonasal process narrows its transverse dimension and begins formation of the nasal septum. **C,** Continued medial migration further reduces the transverse dimension and merges the originally bilaminar folded cartilage to a single layer.

cles. The developing brain is enveloped by a membranous cranium, and the primitive cranial foramina remain when the developing cranial membrane grows around the cranial nerves. At this time the sides and roof of the calvarium are a connective tissue capsule in which membranous bones are destined to appear.[6,12-14]

At about the second fetal month, fusion of the mesenchymous elements occurs, followed by cartilage formation. This action results in the formation of the primitive base of the cranium. Cartilage also forms around the auditory and olfactory primary centers. Initially these cartilage centers are widely separated from that of the primitive base of the cranium. However, by day 45 of gestation the auditory capsule has fused with the basal cartilage. Concurrently a broad, thin cartilage plate grows anteriorly from the lateral aspects of the occipital cartilage around the lower portion of the brain to form the early foramen magnum.[12,13]

The entire fused cartilaginous area is called the *chondrocranium*. Within it various ossification centers appear, and from them the chondrocranium is almost entirely converted into bone. The chondrocranium is continuous with the remaining cranial vault; consequently, some of the skull bones are of both cartilaginous and intramembranous origin. The bones of the cranial vault, face, and vomer are entirely of intramembranous origin with ossification occurring directly in the membrane; more specifically they are the parietal, frontal, nasal, lacrimal, zygomatic, vomer, inferior concha, maxilla, and palatal bones. Bones formed chiefly in cartilage but partly in membrane are the occipital, sphenoid, and temporal bones. The ethmoid bone is the only craniofacial bone to be entirely of cartilaginous origin.[6,12-14]

Eye

During the fourth week of gestation, the optic vesicle begins to invaginate to form the optic cup. This invagination extends along the inferolateral border of the optic cup and the optic stalk to form the fetal choroidal fissure. The lips of the fissure begin to close together during the sixth week and then fuse together, obliterating the choroidal fissure by the end of the seventh week.[15] The fissure begins to close near the equator of the future globe and continues to close in two

directions, both proximally and distally. The anterior end of the optic cup forms the pupil. Defective closure of the anterior end of the ocular choroidal fissure bordering the pupil produces colobomas of the iris (and perhaps adjacent choroid). Defective closure of the midportion of the fissure produces colobomas of the choroid. Defective closure of the fissure where the cup joins the optic stalk (future optic nerve) produces papillary and peripapillary colobomas and pits of the optic disc.[2,15-18] Large papillary colobomas are associated with microphthalmos.

During the fifth week of gestation, mesenchyme invades the then open choroidal fissure and contributes to the formation of the hyaloid vasculature, which nourishes the developing eye. The developing hyaloid artery enters the choroidal fissure along the optic stalk and then becomes enclosed within the globe and the optic nerve as the choroidal fissure closes. The hyaloid artery grows anteriorly to reach the posterior surface of the developing lens where it ramifies on its posterior surface. Glial cells derived from Bergmeister's papilla proliferate to form the sheath of the hyaloid artery. This artery and sheath later undergo regression. By term, the portion of the hyaloid artery within the globe has atrophied almost completely. The residual anteriormost segment forms a characteristic, clinically insignificant opacity on the posterior surface of the lens, the Mittendorf dot. The residual portion of the hyaloid artery within the optic nerve forms the central artery of the retina. Atrophy of Bergmeister's papilla forms the physiologic optic cup. Incomplete regression of the hyaloid vessels and their sheath may be associated with remnant vessels in the persistent primary vitreous of the posterior chamber. There also may be proliferation of fibroglial tissue just anterior to the papilla. Excess regression of the artery and sheath may produce a deepened physiologic cup; this process has been proposed as another mechanism for the development of papillary colobomas.[2,15-19] The diverse anomalies of the papilla discussed here may be designated generically as optic nerve dysplasia.

Corpus Callosum

The nature and sequences of events leading to the formation of the corpus callosum are poorly understood. It is widely accepted, however, that the corpus callosum forms by a series of stages during the period from 3 weeks of gestation (closure of the anterior neuropore) to approximately 8 weeks of gestation. The anterior commissure may be recognized at about 7 to 8 weeks, the hippocampal commissure slightly thereafter, and the earliest definite corpus callosal fibers by the tenth week of gestation. The genu and splenium are recognizable by 20 weeks of gestation and have adult shape (not size) by 22 weeks.[20,21]

COMMON FACIAL CLEFTS

Failure of the proper development of the frontonasal process or failure of its merging with adjacent processes results in a

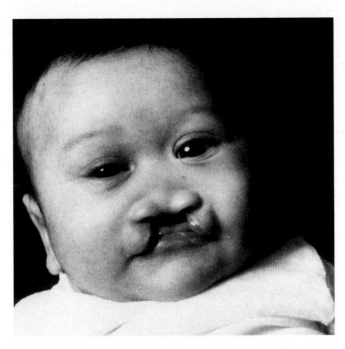

FIG. 1-4 Facies. Absence of intermaxillary segment with hypotelorism. Holoprosencephaly not detectable by axial CT. The maxillary processes formed normal lateral thirds of the upper lips. Midline rectangular defects indicate the site of deficient intermaxillary segment with absent prolabium, incisors, and primary palate. There was consequent cleft of the secondary palate.

coherent series of malformations. Thus insufficiency of the frontonasal process may result in absence of the intermaxillary segment with a roughly rectangular defect in the middle one third of the upper lip, absence of the incisors, absence of the primary palate with a cleft in the secondary palate, and hypotelorism. The resultant facies is one common manifestation of holoprosencephaly (Fig. 1-4).

Failure of the nasomedial processes to merge with the maxillary processes on one or both sides produces the typical unilateral or bilateral common (lateral) cleft lip (Figs. 1-5 to 1-7). Posterior extension of the cleft between the primary and secondary palates and then further backward between the left and right halves of the secondary palate produces the typical unilateral or bilateral common (lateral) cleft palate (Fig. 1-8). Because the two processes fail to merge, they may grow discordantly, resulting in malposition of the premaxillary segment. Widened nostril, depressed ala nasi, and anomalous nasal septum commonly concur.

Failure to merge the nasolateral process with the maxillary process results in an oblique cleft extending from the inner canthus to the nose. This cleft may occur in association with bilateral common cleft lip and palate (Fig. 1-9).

Failure to merge the maxillary with the mandibular process, unilaterally or bilaterally, results in a transverse facial cleft, also designated as *Wolf mouth* or *macrostomia* (Fig. 1-10).

Failure of the two nasomedial processes to merge in the midline produces the rarer true midline cleft lip. Posterior

extension of this cleft may result in a cleft superior alveolar ridge, diastasis of the medial incisors, double frenulum of the upper lip, and a cleft primary palate. Such a cleft palate may continue posteriorly as a midline cleft of the secondary palate or uvula (see following discussion of midline cleft lip).

In some patients, bands of amnion constrict the amniotic cavity. They mold the developing embryo, sometimes pressing deeply into tissue to amputate digits or produce long linear scars that may contain amnion at birth. Such bands can lead to nonanatomic facial clefts and encephaloceles (Fig. 1-11).

MIDLINE CLEFT LIP AND MEDIAN CLEFT FACE SYNDROME

The diverse midline craniofacial dysraphisms fall naturally into two groups: an inferior group (A), in which the clefting primarily involves the upper lip (with or without the nose), and a superior group (B), in which the clefting primarily affects the nose (with or without the forehead and upper lip). Group A is associated with basal encephaloceles (i.e., sphenoidal, sphenoethmoidal, and ethmoidal encephaloceles) with callosal agenesis (rarely lipoma) and with optic nerve dysplasias such as optic pits, colobomata, megalopapilla, persistent hyperplastic primary vitreous with hyaloid artery and morning glory syndrome. Group B consists of those patients with the median cleft face syndrome. This group is characterized by hypertelorism, a broad nasal root, and a median cleft nose, (with or without median cleft upper lip, median cleft premaxilla, and cranium bifidum occultum frontalis).[22,23] Group B patients manifest an increased incidence of frontonasal and intraorbital encephaloceles, anophthalmos or microphthalmos, and callosal lipomas (less frequently, callosal agenesis). Group B has only a weak association with basal encephaloceles or with optic nerve dysplasia.

Group A (Inferior Group)

True clefting of the upper lip is typically associated with hypertelorism and is a clear stigma of the likely concurrence of basal encephalocele, callosal agenesis or lipoma, and any of the diverse forms of optic nerve dysplasia (Figs. 1-12 to 1-14). The labial defect observed varies from a small notch, to a vertical linear cleft, to a small triangular deficiency of the midline upper lip vermilion (with or without the philtrum) with absence of the labial tubercle. This defect is designated true midline cleft upper lip. Rarely this defect may also occur as an isolated finding or as part of the orofacial digital syndromes I and II (Fig. 1-15).[24-27]

Median cleft lip is a rare anomaly. In Fogh-Andersen's series of 3988 craniofacial clefts collected over 30 years, median clefts of the upper lip were observed in only 15 cases (0.38%).[28] Five (0.13%) were true median cleft lips (as considered here); three more (0.08%) were true median cleft lips occurring as part of the orofacial digital syndrome, and

Text continued on p. 14.

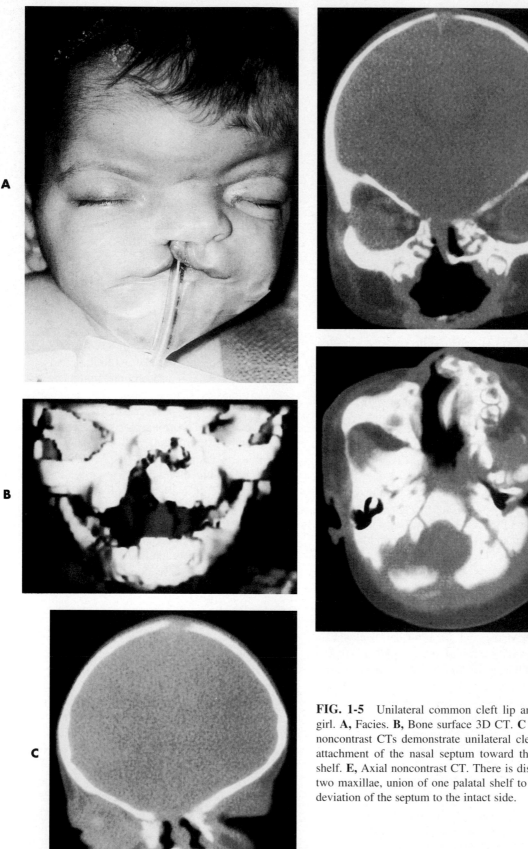

FIG. 1-5 Unilateral common cleft lip and palate in 4-day-old girl. **A,** Facies. **B,** Bone surface 3D CT. **C** and **D,** Direct coronal noncontrast CTs demonstrate unilateral cleft lip and palate with attachment of the nasal septum toward the contralateral palatal shelf. **E,** Axial noncontrast CT. There is discordant growth of the two maxillae, union of one palatal shelf to the bony septum, and deviation of the septum to the intact side.

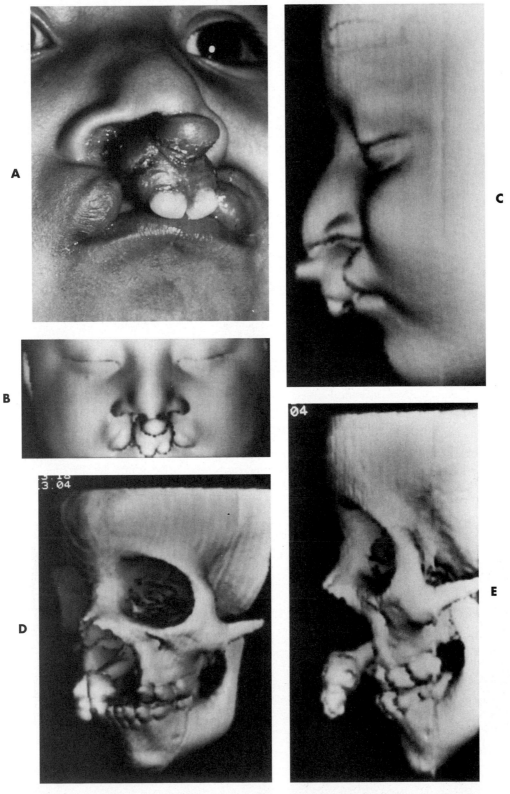

FIG. 1-6 Bilateral common cleft lip and cleft palate with discordant growth of the intermaxillary segment in a 4-year-old boy. **A,** Facies. Skin surface 3D CT. **B,** Frontal view. **C,** Lateral view. Bone surface 3D CT. **D,** Oblique view. **E,** Lateral view. Normal canthi, alae nasi, and lateral thirds of the lip and jaw indicate normal formation and merging of the maxillary and nasolateral processes. The abortive prolabium, central incisors, and central third of the superior alveolar ridge are supported on the vomer, well anterior to expected position, because failure to merge led to discordant growth of the maxillary and intermaxillary segments.

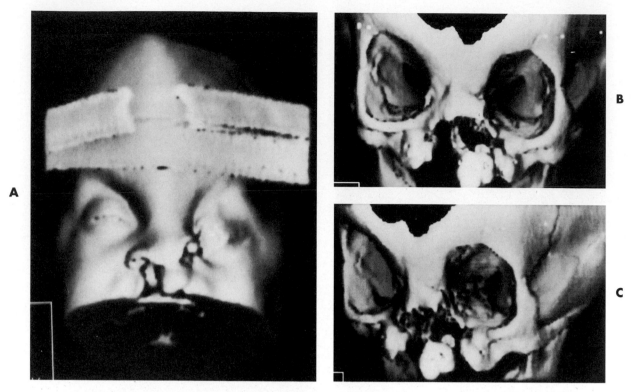

FIG. 1-7 Substantially asymmetrical bilateral common cleft lip and palate. Note partial clefting along the nasooptic furrow. **A,** Three-dimensional CT of air–soft-tissue surface displays the wide right cleft lip, the incomplete merging of the left lip, and distortion of the prolabium, the nostrils, and the alae nasi. The left orbit is asymmetrically lower than the right with lower palpebral fissure. **B** and **C,** Three-dimensional CTs of the bone surface show the wide cleft of the superior alveolar ridge on the right, substantial deviation of the vomer and the central incisors to the left, narrow left cleft superior alveolar ridge seen best in oblique view **(C)** and deficiency in the orbital floor anteromedially.

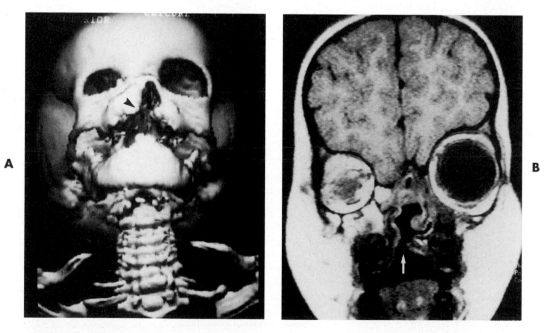

FIG. 1-8 Common cleft lip, cleft palate, and right microphthalmia. **A,** Bone surface 3D CT shows clefting of the superior alveolar ridge *(arrowhead)* and a small right orbit. **B,** Coronal T1W MRI shows cleft palate *(white arrow),* small right orbit and globe, and asymmetrically lower right frontal fossa.

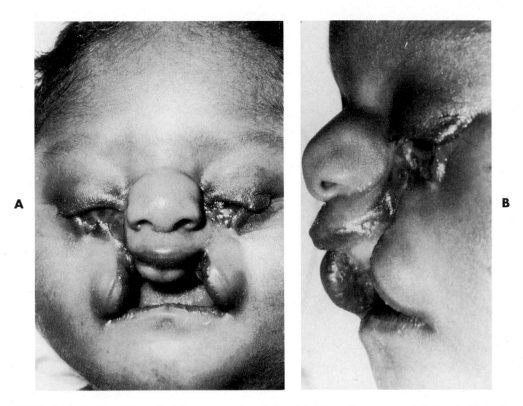

FIG. 1-9 Facies. Bilateral oblique oroocular clefts with bilateral common cleft lip. **A,** Frontal view. **B,** Lateral view.

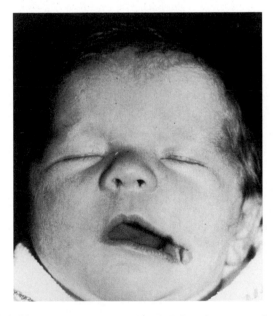

FIG. 1-10 Facies. Transverse facial cleft and macrostomia. Unilateral, infant girl. (From Bauer BS, Wilkes GH, Kernahan DA. Incorporation of the W-plasty in repair of macrostomia. Plast Reconstr Surg 1963; 31:507.)

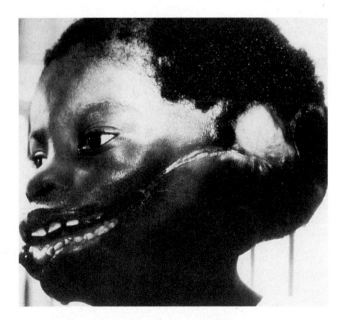

FIG. 1-11 Facies. Nonanatomic clefts occurring with syndrome of amnionic bands in 12-year-old mentally retarded girl. Lateral view. A long, thin, bandlike scar extends across the scalp and face from the temporoparietal region through cheek and corner of mouth to lower lip. The large posterior zone of atrophic skin and absent hair is associated with a bulge that displaces the ear inferiorly. This is the site of a temporoparietal encephalocele. On CT the alveolar ridge showed notching and separation of teeth where it was crossed by the band.

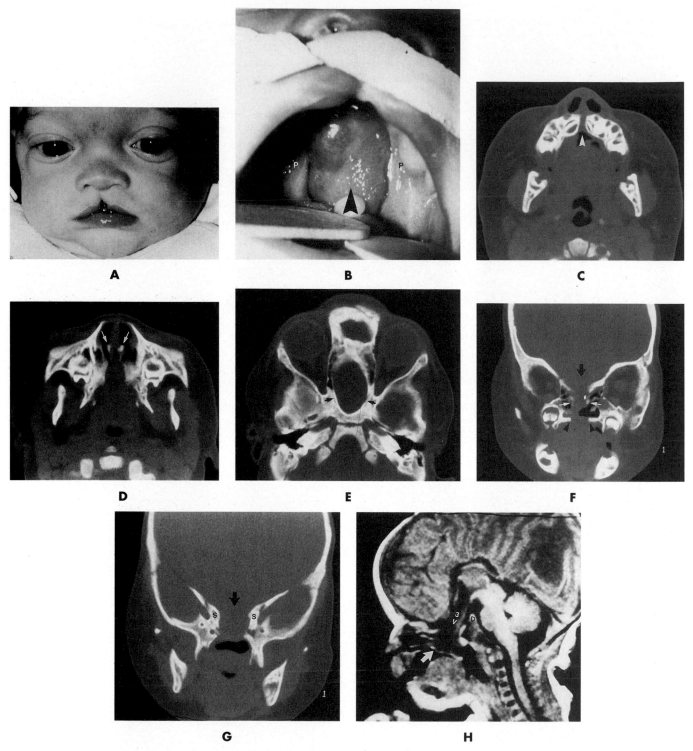

FIG. 1-12 Craniofacial cerebral dysraphism. True midline cleft vermilion and philtrum with hypertelorism. Four-month-old boy with progressive compromise of the airway. **A,** Facies. **B,** View through the open mouth toward the palate demonstrates cleft palate with wide separation of the palatal shelves *(P)* and downward protrusion of a soft-tissue mass *(arrowhead)* into the oral cavity. CT in axial (**C** through **E**) and coronal (**F** through **G**) planes demonstrates midline clefting in the superior alveolar ridge *(arrowhead* in **C**), abnormally wide nasal septum with cleft ethmoids *(white arrows* in **D** and **F**), cleft palate *(black arrowheads* in **F**) and a soft tissue mass *(black arrow* in **F** and **G**) that bulges inferiorly through the sharply marginated ovoid canal *(black arrows* in **E**) in the cleft sphenoid *(S)* and ethmoid bones. **H,** T1W MRI in sagittal plane demonstrates callosal agenesis and a transphenoidal-ethmoidal cephalocele *(white arrows)* containing third ventricle *(3V),* hypothalamus, and portions of the frontal lobes. The cephalocele extends downward into the oral cavity through the cleft sphenoid just anterior to the dorsum sellae *(D).* (Courtesy Dr. Sharon Byrd, Chicago.)

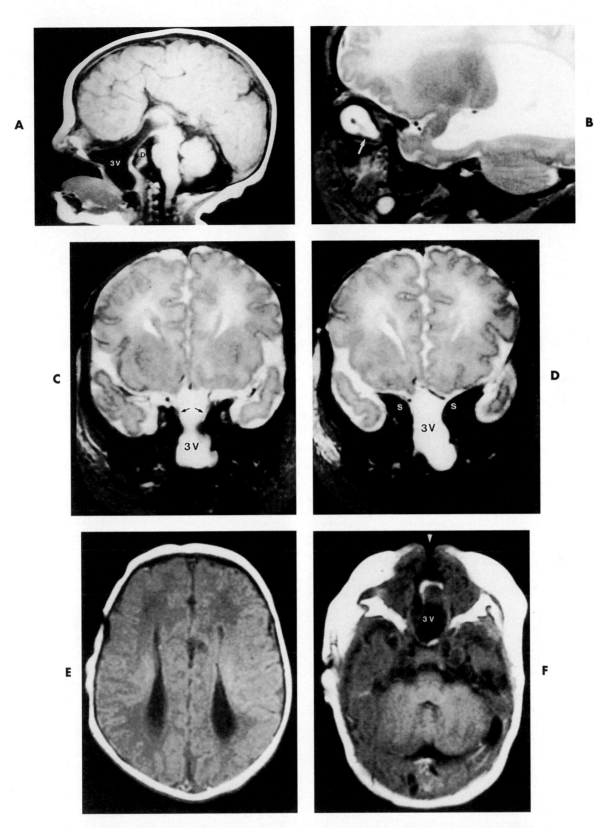

FIG. 1-13 Craniofacial cerebral dysraphism. True midline cleft upper lip. **A,** Midsagittal MR with T1W image shows a transsphenoidal-ethmoidal cephalocele with the third ventricle *(3V)* and optic apparatus protruding downward through the defect in the sphenoid bone immediately anterior to the dorsum sellae *(D)* to rest on the tongue. The corpus callosum is absent. **B,** Sagittal T2W MR through the ocular globe demonstrates microphthalmia with coloboma *(arrow).* **C** and **D,** Coronal T2W images through the cleft in the sphenoid *(S).* The cavernous sinuses *(arrows)* form the lateral walls of the hernia ostium. **E** and **F,** Axial T1W images display the callosal agenesis **(E),** ovoid contour of the third ventricle *(3V)* within the midline defect in the sphenoid, and the midline cleft upper lip *(arrowheads)* **(F).**

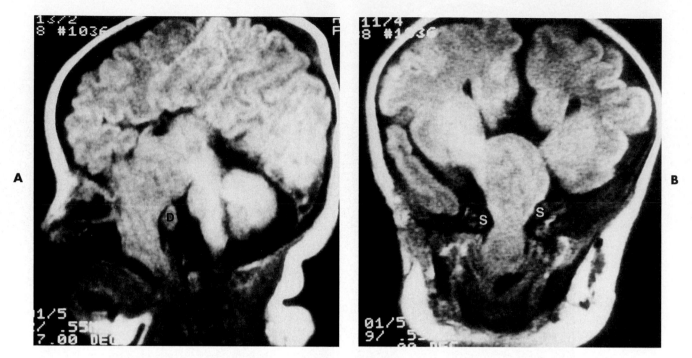

FIG. 1-14   Transphenoidal cephalocele in an 11-day-old boy. **A** and **B,** T1W midsagittal **(A)** and rotated coronal **(B)** MRI demonstrate callosal agenesis, neuronal migration disorder with malformed gyri, and solid possibly hypothalamic tissue protruding through the cleft sphenoid *(S)* anterior to the dorsum sellae *(D)* and then through the cleft palate into the oral cavity.

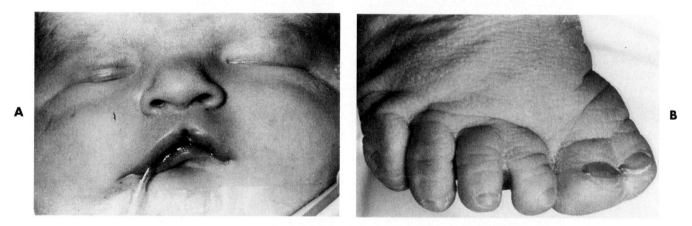

FIG. 1-15   Orofacial digital syndrome II (Mohr syndrome). **A,** Facies with true midline cleft lip. **B,** Duplication of hallux.

seven (0.17%) were pseudomedian cleft lips. An additional four cases (0.10%) were cases of median cleft nose.

Basal encephaloceles are also rare anomalies, estimated to constitute 1.2% of all encephaloceles (Figs. 1-12 to 1-14).[29] Table 1-1 summarizes the findings in a total of 30 cases collected from the literature and personal material. In this series, 50% manifested midline cleft lip (but not nose), an additional 13% manifested midline cleft lip plus nose, 40% to 43% manifested callosal agenesis, and 40% manifested optic nerve dysplasia (i.e., any of the spectrum of optic pit, optic or perioptic coloboma, morning glory disc, or megalopapilla).

Because the reports are incomplete in many cases, the true concurrence of these anomalies is likely to be even higher.[30-51]

To date, no report details the true incidence of encephalocele, callosal agenesis, and facial clefting in patients with optic nerve dysplasias; however, Beyer et al found one sphenoidal encephalocele in eight patients with ten morning glory discs, a single series incidence of 10% to 15%.[52-58]

Lipoma of the corpus callosum is observed in approximately 0.06% of all patients in both in vivo and necropsy studies.[53] Agenesis of the corpus callosum is present in 35% to 50% of such cases.[59] The lipoma may be associated with

TABLE 1-1
Anomalies Associated with 30 Basal Encephaloceles*

Anomaly	Manifestation	Number	%
Encephalocele site[†]	Sphenoidal	18	60.0
	Sphenoethmoidal	10	33.3
	Ethmoidal	2	0.7
	Hypothalamus, third ventricle or pituitary in cephalocele	15	50.0
Endocrine dysfunction	Hypothalmic/pituitary	6	20.0
	Diabetes insipidus with normal anterior pituitary	1	0.3
Corpus callosum	Agenesis	12(+1?)	40.0(43.0?)
	Median cleft lip but not nose	15	50.0
	Median cleft lip and median cleft nose	4	13.3
	"Fissure lip"[‡]	1	0.3
	"Harelip"[‡]	1	0.3
	Cleft palate[‡] (of any type)	14	47.0
Eye anomalies	Hypertelorism	22	73.0
	Optic nerve dysplasia[§]	12	40.0
	Persistent fetal ocular vasculature	1	0.3
	Microphthalmos	2	0.7
Other pathology	Absent optic chiasm	1	0.3
	Absent chiasm and tracts	1	0.3
	Polymicrogyria	1	0.3
	Preauricular skin tags	1	0.3
	Hypospadias, chordee lumbar dimple plus hemangioma	1	0.3

*Includes data from references 22 (patient 13), 30, 31 (case 1), 32, 33 (case 3), 34, 35 (cases 1 and 2), 36, 37 (cases 1 and 2), 38 (case7), 39, 40, 41, 42, 43, 44, 45, 46, 47 (cases 1 through 5), 48, 49, 50, and 51. Series with no contributory data on eye or on facial changes excluded (34 and 46).
[†]In many cases this is the best guess from the limited data available.
[‡]In these cases the exact nature of the cleft is uncertain.
[§]Any of the spectrum: optic pit, optic coloboma, megalopapilla, morning glory disc.

midline subcutaneous lipomas with cranium bifidum and with frontonasal encephaloceles.[22,60,61]

Group B (Superior Group)

Median cleft face syndrome (also called *frontonasal dysplasia*) is a rare form of dysraphism that affects the midface (Fig. 1-16). The characteristic physical findings in median cleft face syndrome include hypertelorism, cranium bifidum occultum frontalis, widow's peak hairline, and midline clefting of the nose (may involve upper lip, premaxilla, and palate).[22,23,62-65] There may also be common clefts of the upper lip and palate, primary telecanthus, ocular colobomas, microphthalmia, and notching of the alae nasae. Hypertelorism is present in all cases of median cleft face syndrome and is the one obligatory finding.[23] The next most constant finding is true midline bony clefting of the nose. The other facial deformities may be present or not present in varying degrees.

The types of facial clefting seen in this syndrome have been classified differently by different authors.[22,23,,64,65] DeMyer classified the median cleft face syndrome into four classic facies that represent the most frequently encountered combinations of the major and minor defects (Table 1-2).[1] Sedano et al proposed an alternate classification of median cleft face syndrome (Table 1-3).[23] These systems differ in part in the importance attributed to notching of the alae nasae; however, the Sedano classification appears to correlate best with the intracranial pathology and may be the most useful system (Table 1-4). Tessier proposed another system for classifying the craniofacial skeletal clefts and their associated soft-tissue counterparts.[64] In his system the clefts most frequently associated with the median cleft face syndrome are found along the Tessier number 0 to 14 and 1 to 13 meridians. Some patients with median cleft face syndrome appear to have a furrowing of their nose rather than a "clefting." Such cases support Badrawy's theory that the nasal septum forms as a folding of the frontonasal process with subsequent resorption and thinning because improper folding and resorption could lead to the facies observed.

Nearly all cases of median cleft face syndrome occur sporadically with no evidence for a genetic basis.[3] Only a few familial cases have been reported.[22,62,66,67] An unexpect-

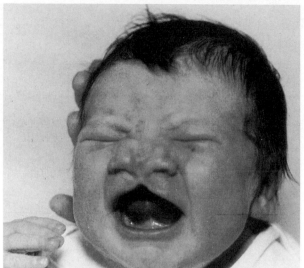

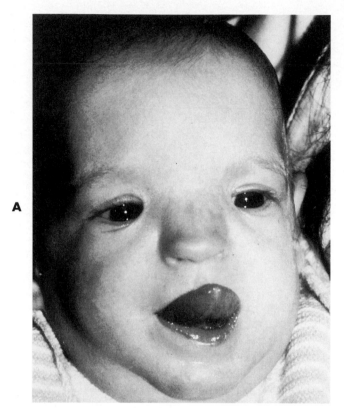

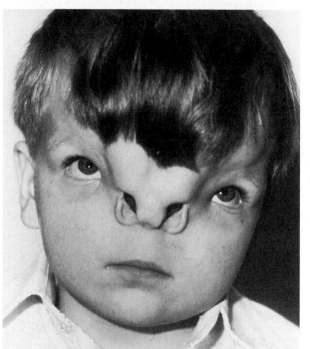

FIG. 1-16 Median cleft face syndrome, typical facies. **A,** Sedano Facies Type A in 3-month-old boy. **B,** Sedano facies type B in 4-day-old boy. **C,** Sedano Facies Type D in 3½-year-old boy. (From Naidich TP et al. J Comput Assist Tomogr 1988; 12:57.)

edly high 12% to 18% of patients with median cleft face syndrome are the products of twin gestation, but the other twin is usually normal.[22,62,66]

Focal neurologic deficits are not reported with median cleft face syndrome and do not appear to form a part of the disease.[22,23,66,68-76] These patients have variable intellectual development, and patient IQ does not appear to be related to the severity of facial clefting.

Median cleft face syndrome has been found to coexist with a variety of other syndromes or syndrome-like sequences, including the Goldenhar-Gorlin syndrome (oculoauricular-vertebral dysplasia), characterized by hypopla-

sia of the soft tissue and bony structures of the face resulting in (1) ocular anomalies such as upper lid colobomas, epibulbar dermoids and lipomas, microphthalmia, and anophthalmia; (2) auricular anomalies such as deformity, hypoplasia, or aplasia of the external ear, preauricular skin tags, and preauricular sinuses; and (3) vertebral anomalies such as block vertebra, hemivertebra, spina bifida, and associated rib anomalies.[77-79] Pituitary gland duplication and a triad of cleft mandible, bifid dens, and absent anterior arch of C1 may be seen with the median cleft face syndrome.[80,81]

In one review of 11 cases of median cleft face syndrome, there were three type A facies, four type B, four type D, and

TABLE 1-2
DeMyer Classification

Facies	Characteristics
I	Hypertelorism
	Median complete cleft nose
	Absence, hypoplasia, or median clefting of upper lip and premaxilla
	Cranium bifidum
II	Hypertelorism
	Median cleft nose
	A. Nose completely cleft
	B. Cleft nose with divided nasal septum
	C. Slight hypertelorism
	No median cleft of upper lip, premaxilla or palate
	Cranium bifidum present or not
III	Hypertelorism
	Median cleft nose and upper lip with or without median cleft premaxilla
	No median cleft palate
	No cranium bifidum
IV	Hypertelorism
	Median cleft nose
	No median cleft of upper lip, premaxilla or palate
	No cranium bifidum

From DeMyer W. Neurology 1967; 17:961.

TABLE 1-3
Sedano Classification*

Facies	Characteristics
A	Hypertelorism
	Broad nasal root
	Median nasal groove with absence of nasal tip
	No true clefting of the facial midline
	Anterior cranium bifidum present or not
B	Hypertelorism
	Broad nasal root
	Deep medial facial groove or true cleft of the nose or nose and the upper lip
	Cleft palate present or not
	Anterior cranium bifidum present or not
C	Hypertelorism
	Broad nasal root
	Nasal alar notching (unilateral or bilateral)
	Anterior cranium bifidum present or not
D	B and C

From Sedano HO et al. J Pediatr 1970; 76:906.
*Anterior cranium bifidum may be present or not in all four facies, A through D.

TABLE 1-4
Correlation of Sedano and DeMyer Classifications

Sedano Classification	Corresponding DeMyer Classification (Per Sedano)	Corresponding DeMyer Classification (Observed in this Series)
Type A	IV	IIB, IV
Type B	IA,* IIB, III	I, IIA, IIB
Type C	IIC	—
Type D	IA,* IB, IIA	I, IIA, IIC

Modied from Sedano HO et al. J Pediatr 1970; 76:906.
*Patients who would be classified into DeMyer's Group IA may be classified as either Sedano facies type B or Sedano facies type D.

no type C. Of these 11 patients, hypertelorism and broad nasal root were found in 100% (by definition), true midline bony cleft of the nose in eight (all cases except type A facies), median cleft upper lip in three, common cleft lip in three, common cleft palate in three, cranium bifidum in six, calcified falx in six, interhemispheric lipoma in five, Goldenhar-Gorlin-syndrome in two, and twinning in two of the patients.[62]

The imaging features of median cleft face syndrome include hypertelorism, cranium bifidum, facial clefting, and intracranial calcifications, related to either interhemispheric lipoma and/or calcification of the anterior aspect of the falx (Fig. 1-17).[63,82,83] The calcification of the falx produces a thick frontal crest. The crest is found most commonly when a lipoma is present but may be present without associated lipoma.[63]

NORMAL DEVELOPMENT OF THE NASAL SEPTUM AND FRONTONASAL JUNCTION

The normal nasal septum and skull base form in a predictable fashion. Knowledge of this pattern is necessary for interpreting imaging studies of this region without serious error. In brief the cartilage of the nasal capsule is the foundation of the upper part of the face (Figs. 1-18, 1-19).[84] The bony elements of the facial skeleton appear around it and replace it in part (Figs. 1-20, 1-21). The lateral masses of the ethmoid form by enchondral ossification of the nasal capsule. The frontal processes of the maxillary bones, premaxillary bone, nasal bones, lacrimal bones, and palatine bones all form in membrane in close relationship with the roof and lateral walls of the cartilaginous nasal capsule.[84] The vomer develops in membrane in relation to the perichondrium of the septal process.[84] Eventually, nearly all the nasal capsule becomes ossified or atrophied. All that remains of the cartilage of the nasal capsule in adults is the anterior part of the nasal septum and the alar cartilages that surround the nostrils.

More specifically the midline septal cartilage is directly continuous with the cartilaginous skull base. At birth the skull base has three major ossification centers: the basioccipital center, the basisphenoid center, and the presphenoid center. The septal cartilage has not yet ossified. The lateral masses of the ethmoid have ossified, forming paired paramedian bones, but the cribriform plate is still cartilaginous or fibrous.[84] At birth therefore on imaging, the entire midline of the face may be a lucent stripe of cartilage situated between the paired ossifications in the lateral masses of the ethmoids, and this may simulate a midline cleft. The septal cartilage extends along the midline from the nares to the presphenoid bone.[84] Anteriorly and inferiorly the septal cartilage attaches to the premaxillary bone by fibrous tissue.[84] Posteriorly the septal cartilage is continuous with the carti-

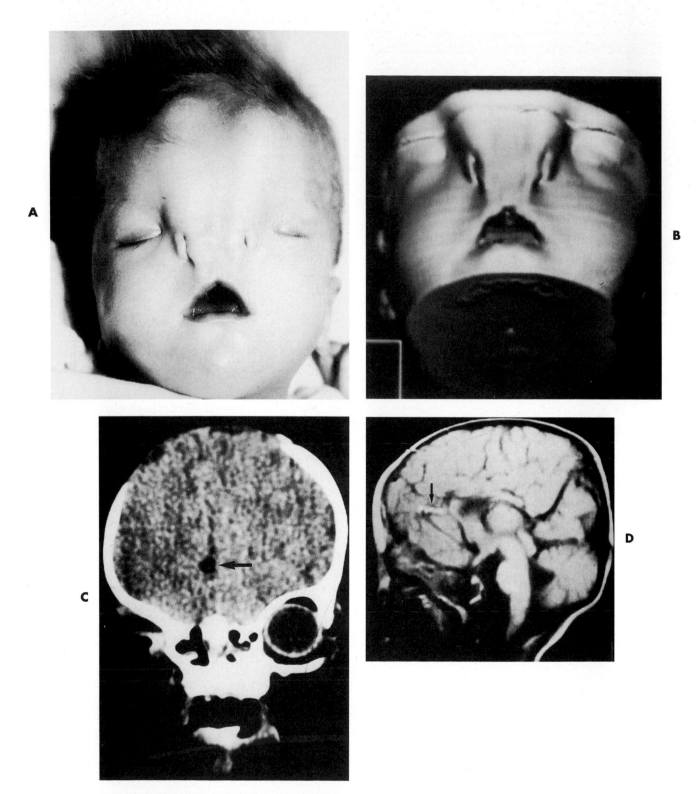

FIG. 1-17   Median cleft face syndrome. Nasal dermal sinus and interhemispheric lipoma in a 3½-year-old girl. **A,** Sedano facies type D. **B,** 3D CT skin surface. **C,** Coronal plane image displays a midline tubular lipoma *(arrow)* with low density on CT. **D,** Midsagittal T1W MR shows a flat forehead, dysplastic corpus callosum, anomalous high course of the vein of Galen toward the vertex, and the high signal tubular lipoma *(arrow).*

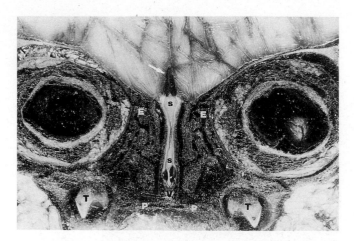

FIG. 1-18   Coronal cryomicrotome section through the nasal cavity of a full-term stillborn at the level of the optic globes. The lateral ethmoid centers *(E)*, the midline vomer *(V)*, and the palatal shelves *(P)* of the maxillae are well ossified. The unossified septal cartilage *(S)* slots into the vomerine groove in the upper surface of the Y-shaped vomer. The crista galli *(arrow)* is beginning to ossify, forming a pointed "cap." The cribriform plates have not ossified. Note the normal position of the floor of the anterior fossa with respect to the two orbits and optic globes. *T,* Unerupted teeth.

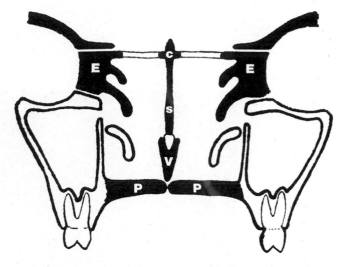

FIG. 1-19   Diagram of the pattern of ossification around the nasal cavity. The ossified crista *(C)* and septal cartilage *(S)* form a "cristal" cross that is isolated from the lateral ethmoid centers *(E)* by the unossified cribriform plates and from the vomer *(V)* by the sphenoidal tail. Although the maxillae are ossified, only the palatal shelves *(P)* have been inked in to emphasize their relationships to the vomer. (Modified from Scott JH. Br Dent J 1953; 95:37.)

lage of the cranial base. Inferiorly the lower edge of the septal cartilage is slotted into a U- or V-shaped groove that runs along the entire upper edge of the vomer (Figs. 1-19, 1-22).[84] This groove is designated the vomerine groove and should not be mistaken for a midline cleft in the septum.

At about the time of birth or during the first year, a fourth mesethmoid center appears in the septal cartilage anterior to the cranial base. This center will form the perpendicular plate of the ethmoid.[84] The residual portion of still-unossified septal cartilage that extends posterosuperiorly toward the cranial base between the perpendicular plate and the vomer is designated the sphenoidal tail of the septal cartilage.[84]

Initially the ossifying perpendicular plate is separated from the rest of the facial skeleton by (1) the unossified cartilage or fibrous tissue of the cribriform plates and (2) the sphenoidal tail (Figs. 1-18, 1-19, 1-22). In about the third to sixth year the lateral masses of the ethmoid and the perpendicular plate of the ethmoid become united across the roof of the nasal cavity by ossification of the cribriform plate.[84,85]

Somewhat later the perpendicular plate unites with the vomer below.[84] As the two bones approach, the vomerine groove may become converted into a vomerine tunnel. It should not be mistaken for a bony canal around a dermal sinus or cephalocele. Growth of the septal cartilage continues for a short period after craniofacial union is complete, which probably explains the common deflection of the nasal septum away from the midline.[84]

Because the appearance of the nasal septum varies with patient age, one must interpret computed tomography (CT) "evidence" of midline defects and sinus tracts carefully. Review of the CT appearance of the midline anterior fossa

and nasal septum in 100 children age 2 days to 18 years by Naidich, Takahashi, and Towbin revealed the following normal patterns (Figs. 1-20, 1-21)[86]:

1. The lateral ethmoid centers were ossified in all subjects.
2. No midline ossifications of the anterior fossa or septum were present in 14% of patients less than 1 year of age.
3. The cribriform plate was not ossified in patients under 2 months of age. It could be ossified from 2 to 8 months of age. It was fused across the midline from 8 months onward. This ossification occurred earlier than is stated elsewhere in the literature.[84]
4. The tip of the crista could be ossified from 2 days onward. It was invariably ossified from 2½ years onward.
5. The crista and the cribriform plate formed a __/__-ossification with no ossification of the perpendicular plate in patients from 2 months to 5 months of age.
6. The ossified crista, cribriform plate, and perpendicular plate could form a bony "cristal cross" from 4 months onward. These ossifications invariably formed a cross from 11 months onward.
7. A zone of unossified tissue was seen within the crista in 60% of those with a cristal cross. Such ostia could be present at any age from 4 months onward.
8. The perpendicular plate of the ethmoid could be ossified as a single plate in patients aged 11 months to 18 years. It was ossified in the vast majority of patients older than 2 years.
9. The perpendicular plate ossified as 2 parallel laminae in 15% of patients.
10. The nasal septum was widest at the midpoint of its ver-

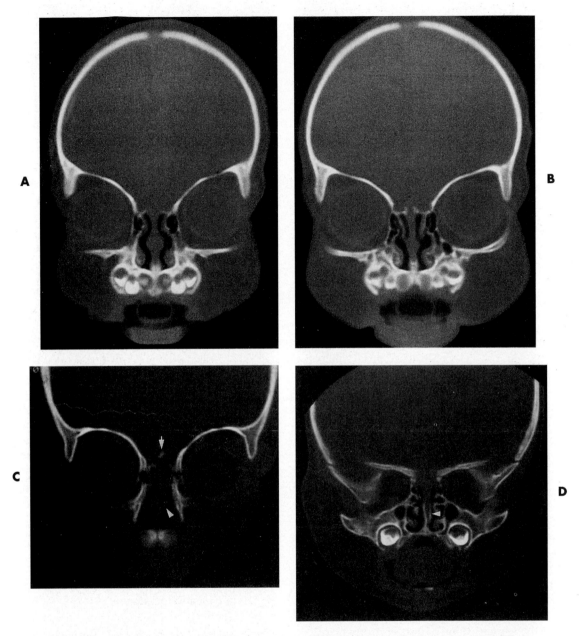

FIG. 1-20 Normal patterns of ossification of the nasal capsule as shown by direct coronal CTs in progressively older patients. **A** and **B,** Four-month old girl. The lateral ethmoid centers and a small segment of vomer are ossified. The midline septal cartilage is entirely unossified. **C** and **D,** Five-month-old boy. The lateral ethmoid centers, the palatal shelves, the vomer, and the tip *(white arrow)* of the crista galli are ossified. The widened midportion of the septum *(white arrowhead* in **C**) is designated the septal diamond. The two sides of the vomerine groove give the posterior septum a bilaminar appearance *(white arrowhead* in **D**).

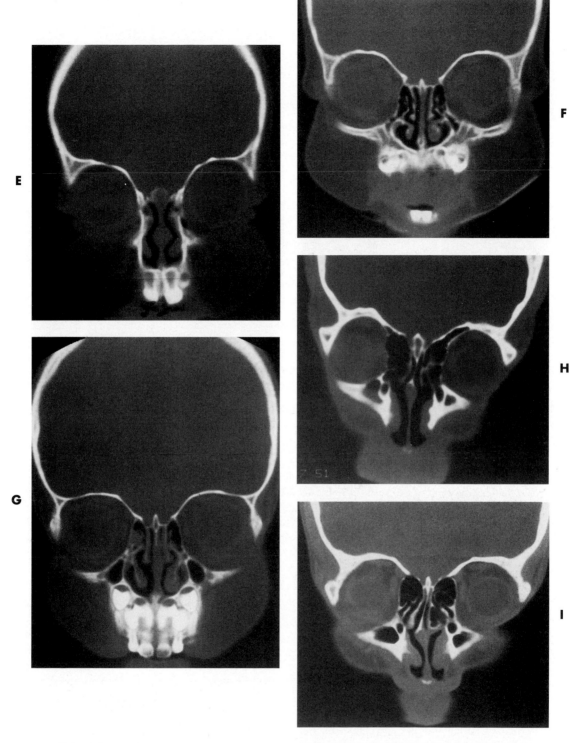

FIG. 1-20, cont'd   **E,** Eight-month-old boy. Anteriorly the crista galli is incompletely ossified, forming a hollow cap. **F,** Further posteriorly the crista and the cribriform plates have ossified together, roofing over the nasal cavity. The perpendicular plate of ethmoid is beginning to ossify as a bilaminar plate. The Y-shaped vomer is larger. **G,** Nine-month-old girl. The ossified perpendicular plate has enlarged and extended inferiorly toward the septal diamond. The ossified crista resembles a hollow diamond **H,** A 17-year old boy. The ossified perpendicular plate reaches the top of the septal diamond where it widens into a knob or it forks. **I,** Eleven-month-old boy. The nasal septum frequently buckles at the septal diamond.

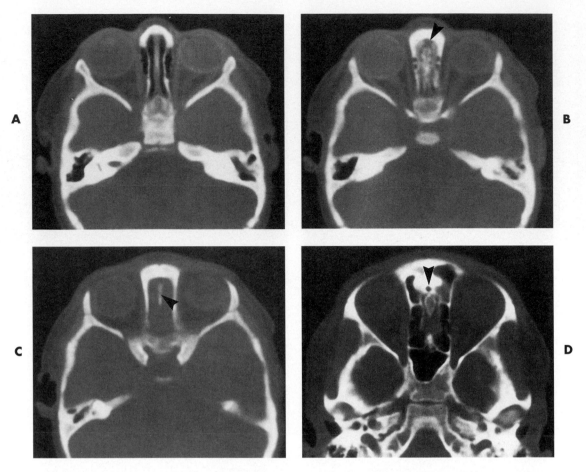

FIG. 1-21   Normal pattern of ossification as shown on axial noncontrast CTs. In the eleven-month old girl shown in **A** through **C,** serial axial images display the following: **(A)** The normal, thin nasal septum with faint parallel ossifications representing the vomer, **(B)** the normal midline defect *(black arrowhead)* anterior to the normal parallel ossification within the closing cribriform plates and crista, **(C)** the upper portion of the crista *(arrowhead)* with a small fossa anterior to it. Comparing these images with the coronal sections in Figs. 1-18 through 1-20 aids understanding of how the parallel ossifications arise. **D,** Twelve-year-old boy. The foramen cecum *(black arrowhead)* is a well-defined ostium situated just anterior to the diamond shaped ossified crista galli.

tical dimension in nearly all subjects of all ages. This widening was designated the septal diamond.

11.   The ossified perpendicular plate widened inferiorly or split to form an inverted Y at the septal diamond in 30% of patients, all older than 6 years.

12.   The ossified perpendicular plate reached as far inferiorly as the septal diamond in 32% of all patients, 92% after age 6, and 100% after age 13.

13.   The ossified vomer exhibited a V- or Y-shaped superior border in 80% of patients at any age. The vomerine ossification appeared as a single point anteriorly and a *V* or *Y* posteriorly in 21%. In 8%, it was seen only as a single point.

In a normal situation then, one may expect to see no ossification in the midline of children under 1 year of age, an unossified zone within 60% of the cristal crosses, a "bilaminar" perpendicular plate of the ethmoid in 15%, and a V- or Y-shaped upper surface of the vomer in at least 80% of

patients (Figs. 1-20, 1-21). These should not be overinterpreted as indications of pathologic conditions.

In the early embryo the developing frontal bones are separated from the developing nasal bones by a small fontanelle called the fonticulus nasofrontalis.[87] The nasal bones are separated from the subjacent cartilaginous nasal capsule by the prenasal space (Fig. 1-23). This space extends from the base of the brain to the nasal tip.[88] Midline diverticula of dura normally project anteriorly into the fonticulus nasofrontalis and anteroinferiorly into the prenasal space. These diverticula may touch the ectoderm. Normally the diverticula regress before the closure of the bony plates of the anterior skull base. The fonticulus nasofrontalis is closed by the nasal processes of the frontal bone to make the frontonasal suture.[79] The prenasal space becomes obliterated.[89] The cartilaginous nasal capsule develops into the upper lateral nasal cartilages and the ethmoid bone, including the crista galli, cribriform plates, and perpendicular plate of the

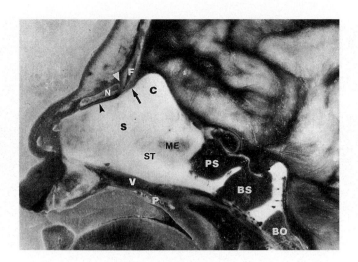

FIG. 1-22 Midsagittal cryomicrotome section of a full-term newborn demonstrates the normal relationships at birth among the ossified frontal bone *(F)*; the ossified nasal bone *(N)*; the nasofrontal suture *(white arrowhead)*; and the cartilaginous nasal capsule *(large white structure)* that forms the yet unossified nasal septum *(S)* and crista galli *(C)*. The ossified hard palate *(P)* and ossified vomer *(V)* lie below the septal cartilage. Note the direct line from the prenasal space *(black arrowhead)* through the foramen cecum *(black arrow)* to the normal depression or "fossa" just anterior to the crista galli. The midline septal cartilage is directly continuous with the cartilaginous skull base. The basioccipital *(BO)*, the basisphenoidal *(BS)*, and the presphenoidal *(PS)* ossification centers are well formed. The mesethmoidal *(ME)* ossification center is just beginning to form. When the vomer and mesethmoid enlarge, the residual cartilage between them is designated the sphenoidal tail *(ST)*.

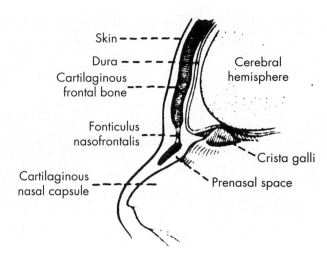

FIG. 1-23 Diagram of the normal embryonic relationships among the dura, fonticulus nasofrontalis, prenasal space, and surrounding structures. (From Gorenstein A et al. Arch Otolaryngol 1980; 106:536.)

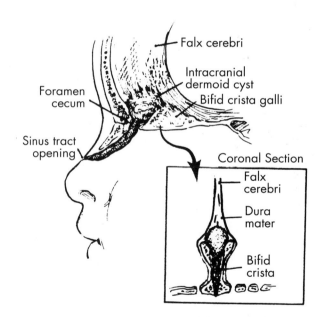

FIG. 1-24 Diagram of a typical nasal dermal sinus and cyst traversing the prenasal space and the enlarged foramen cecum to form a mass anterior to and within a grooved, bifid crista galli. Inset, The anatomic relationships of the leaves of the falx to the sides of the crista galli direct upward extension of the mass into the interdural space between the leaves of the falx. (From Gorenstein A et al. Arch Otolaryngol 1980; 106:536.)

septum.[87] The two leaves of the falx insert into the crista galli, one leaf passing to each side of the crista.

At the skull base the frontal and ethmoid bones close together around a strand of dura, leaving a small ostium designated the foramen cecum. Normally this transmits a small vein. This foramen is easily seen at the bottom of a small depression that lies just in front of the crista galli. Whether the foramen is situated exactly at the frontoethmoidal junction or between the nasal processes of the frontal bones is not certain.[87]

If the diverticula of dura become adherent to the superficial ectoderm, they may not regress normally. Instead they may pull ectoderm with them as they retreat, creating an ectodermal tract that extends from the glabella through a canal at the nasofrontal suture to the crista galli or beyond the crista to the interdural space between the two leaves of the falx.[87,90,91] A similar persistent tract may pass from the external surface of the nose, under or through the nasal bones, and ascend through the prenasal space to enter the cranial cavity at the foramen cecum just anterior to the crista galli (Fig. 1-24). Such a tract would be associated with a widened foramen cecum, distortion and grooving of the crista galli, and extension into the interdural space between the two leaves of the falx. Depending on the precise histology of the portions of the tract that persist, these tracts could

develop into superficial glabellar and nasal pits, fully patent glabellar and nasal dermal sinuses, or one or several epidermoid cysts or fibrous cords, exactly as the analogous remnants of the vitelline duct and neurenteric canal do. Rarely the sinus tracts, cysts, and cords may extend into or become adherent to the brain itself.[92]

Nasal cephaloceles and gliomas may arise by an analogous mechanism. If the same dural diverticula were to persist as patent communications that contained leptomeninges,

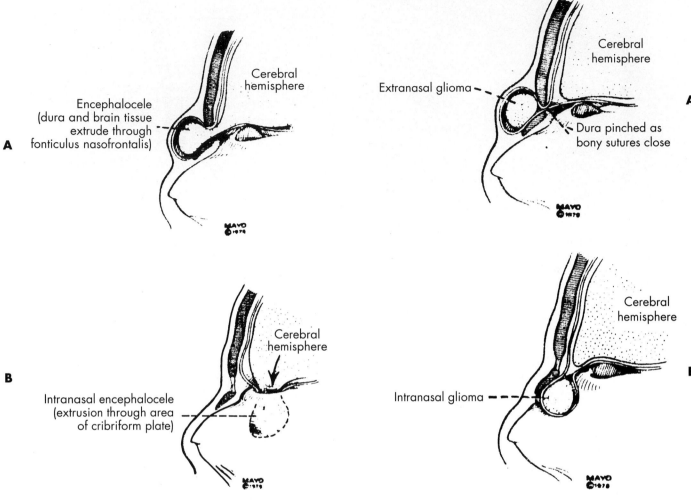

FIG. 1-25   Schematic representation of the origin of extranasal (glabellar) **(A)** cephaloceles and, intranasal transethmoidal cephaloceles **(B)**. (From Gorenstein A et al: Arch Otolaryngol 106:536, 1980.)

FIG. 1-26   Schematic representation of the origin of extranasal gliomas **(A)** and nasal gliomas **(B)**. (From Gorenstein A et al. Arch Otolaryngol 1980; 106:536.)

cerebrospinal fluid (CSF), and neural tissue, they would constitute glabellar and nasal meningoencephaloceles (Fig. 1-25). Were such developing meningoencephaloceles to become pinched off and (nearly) isolated from the cranial cavity by subsequent constriction of the dura and bone, they would then constitute heterotopic foci of meninges and neural tissue at the glabella and nose. These benign nonneoplastic heterotopias are given the dreadful name of glabellar and nasal gliomas (Fig. 1-26).

Nasal Dermal Sinuses and Dermoids

Dermoids of the skull occur at diverse locations believed to be related to the sites of closure of the neural tube, the sites of diverticulation of the cerebral hemispheres, and the lines of closure of the cranial sutures. In Pannell's series of 94 dermoids of the skull, 43% were midline, 45% were frontotemporal, and 13% were parietal.[93] The midline dermoids affected the anterior fontanelle (25), glabella (1), nasion (2),

vertex (1), and occipital-suboccipital region (11). The frontotemporal dermoids affected the sphenofrontal (15), frontozygomatic (16), and sphenosquamosal (11) sutures. The parietal dermoids affected the squamosal (8), coronal (1), lambdoid (1), and parietomastoid (2) sutures.

A nasal dermal sinus is a thin epithelial-lined tube that arises at an external ostium situated along the midline of the nose and extends deeply for a variable distance, sometimes reaching the intradural intracranial space. A nasal dermal cyst is a midline epithelial-lined cyst that arises along the expected course of the dermal sinus. It may exist as an isolated mass, or it may coexist with a dermal sinus (Fig. 1-27). Histologically, nasal dermal sinuses may be true dermoids containing skin adnexae or pure epidermoids devoid of such adnexae.[94] Dermoids and epidermoids are equally common. However, dermoid cysts and sinuses are found more commonly along the bridge of the nose. Pure epidermoids are more common at the glabella-nasion and have a sevenfold increased incidence of associated infection.[94]

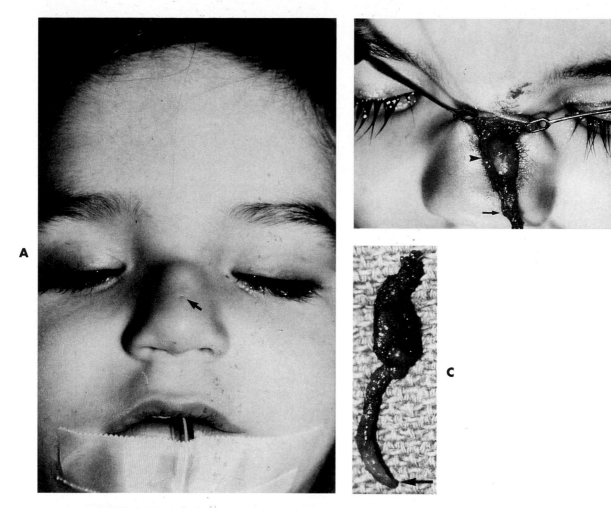

FIG. 1-27 Nasal dermal sinus in 10-month-old boy with increasing swelling of the nose. **A,** Swelling and a pinpoint ostium *(arrow)* on the dorsum of the nose. **B,** Surgical dissection traces the sinus tract *(black arrow)* inward from the ostium to a well-defined ovoid dermoid cyst *(black arrowhead)* within the septum. The cyst reached just to the cribriform plate. **C,** Operative specimen demonstrates the proportions and contours of the dermal sinus and cyst. Arrow indicates the superficial cutaneous end of the tract.

Nasal dermal sinuses and cysts constitute 3.7% to 12.6% of all dermal cysts of the head and neck and 1.1% of all such cysts throughout the body.[87] They may be detected at any age, but most appear early (mean age 3 years).[95] There is no sex predilection.[87,95,96] Most cases arise sporadically, though kindreds with nasal dermal sinus have been reported.[97,98]

The lesions may appear at any site from the glabella downward along the bridge (dorsum) of the nose to the base of the columella (Fig 1-28). Approximately 56% of lesions appear as midline cysts (Fig. 1-29). The other 44% present as midline sinus ostia. The external ostium of the sinus lies at the glabella-nasion in 29%, the bridge of the nose in 21%, the nasal tip in 21%, and the base of the columella in 29%.[95] Rarely, multiple sinus ostia are present, or sinuses and cysts coexist at both the glabella and nasal bridge.[87]

Nasal epidermoid cysts are usually found in one of the following three areas: in the midline just superior to the nasal tip, at the junction of the upper and lower lateral carti-

lages, or in the medial canthal area. Glabellar cysts external to the frontal bone are less common. The cysts may be soft and discrete or indurated. They may erode through the overlying skin to form secondary pits.

Clinically these lesions appear as midline pits or fenestra, occasionally containing sparse wiry hairs (Fig. 1-30), as intermittent discharge of sebaceous material or pus, as intermittent inflammation, as increasing size of the mass with variable degrees of broadening of the nasal root and bridge, as intermittent episodes of meningitis; or as a behavioral change secondary to a frontal lobe abscess. At times the ostium is tiny and undetectable until pressure is applied against the adjacent tissue to express cheesy material from the ostium (Fig. 1-31).[87]

The deep extension of nasal dermal sinuses and cysts is variable. They can be shallow pits that end blindly in the superficial tissues. They can wander extensively intracranially and extracranially.[87] In Bradley's review of 67 children with nasal dermoids, the lesion was confined to the

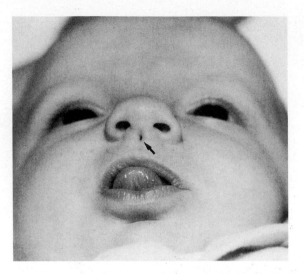

FIG. 1-28   Nasal dermal sinus in a 3-month-old girl. When the sinus ostium *(arrow)* lies at the base of the columella, extension to the intracranial space is uncommon.

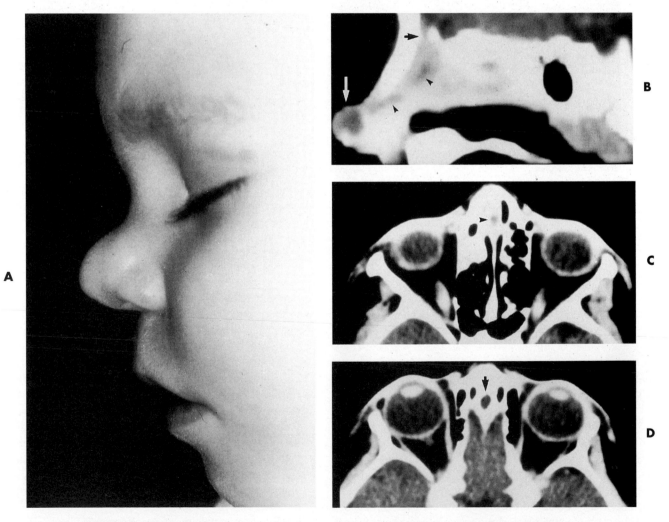

FIG. 1-29   Dermoid cysts at the nasal tip in two patients. **A,** Lateral view of the face shows bulbous expansion of the nasal tip. **B,** Sagittal reformatted CT shows that the lucent dermoid cyst *(white arrow)* at the nasal tip leads by a lucent track *(black arrowheads)* toward an expanded foramen cecum *(black arrow)*. **C** and **D,** Axial CTs confirm the lucent track *(arrow in C)* and expansion of the foramen cecum *(arrowhead in D)*.

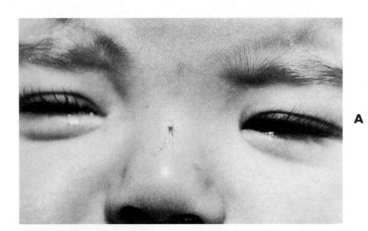

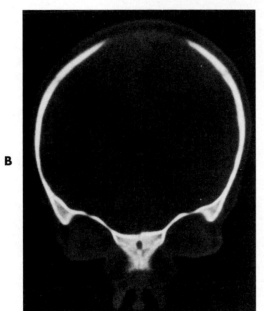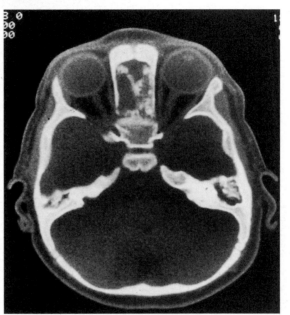

FIG. 1-30   Nasal dermal sinus with intracranial extension in a 1-year-old girl with clinically evident sinus. **A,** A small tuft of hairs protrudes from a midline dermal sinus on the dorsum of the nose. **B,** Direct coronal CT. A well-marginated canal penetrates between the nasal processes of the frontal bones. **C,** Axial CT scan reveals a large foramen cecum and bifid crista galli. At surgery the dermal sinus tract and extranasal dermoid were traced upward through the foramen cecum into a 2 to 3 cm intracranial dermoid. This extended intradurally but did not attach to brain. A second "arm" of the intranasal dermoid passed posteriorly toward the sphenoid bone.

skin in 61% and extended deeply to invade the nasal bones in 10%.[94] The lesion extended into the septal cartilage in 10%, the nasal bones and cartilage in 6%, and the cribriform plate in 12% of the cases. Rare sinuses traverse the entire anteroposterior extent of the nasal septum to end at the basisphenoid where they attach to the dura just anterior to the sella.[87] The frequency of intracranial extension varies widely from 57% to 0%.[88]

Intracranial extension can be associated with cysts and sinuses at any site. Sinuses at the base of the columella are least likely to extend intracranially (Fig. 1-28). Thus in Pensler's series, each of four sinuses situated at the base of the columella passed directly to the nasal spine of the maxilla with no intracranial extension.[95] However, Mühlbauer

and Dittmar reported a similar sinus that ascended to end in the ethmoid air cells; it did not enter the cranial cavity.[97]

True intracranial extension of the epidermoid usually affects the epidural space of the anterior fossa near the crista galli and may continue deeper, between the two leaves of the falx as an interdural mass (Fig. 1-32).[95] Rarely the lesions also extend into the brain.[92] An additional 31% of cases have intracranial extension of a fibrous cord devoid of epidermoid elements.[95] At present, intracranial extension of a fibrous cord is not considered significant and has not been associated with sequelae on follow-up examinations.[95]

Nasal dermal sinuses are resected for cosmetic reasons, to avoid or treat the complications of local infection, and to prevent or treat secondary meningitis and cerebral abscess

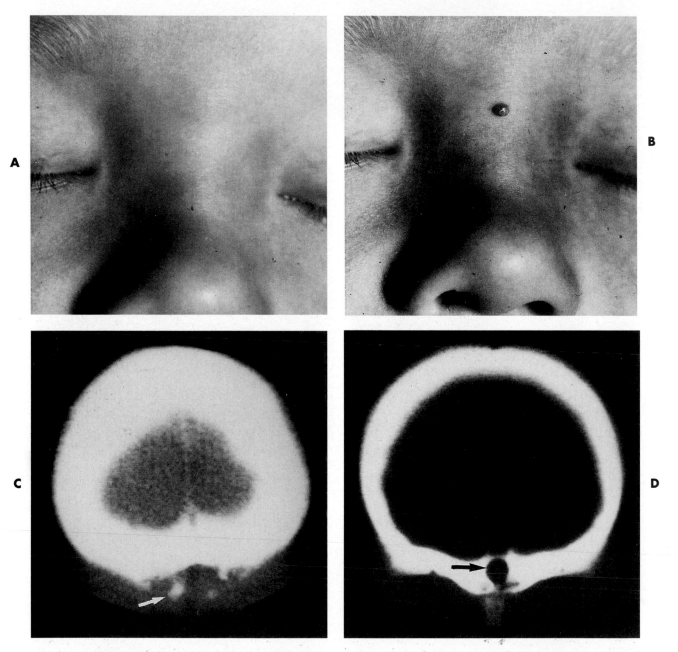

FIG. 1-31 Infected dermal sinus in a 16-month-old boy with intermittent painful swelling, redness, and discharge at the glabella. **A,** Frontal view of the glabella shows swelling of the nasal root but no ostium or discharge. **B,** Immediately thereafter, pressure applied at both sides of the nasal root expresses pus. **C,** Coronal CT demonstrates cellulitis and secondary osteomyelitis with multiple sequestra *(white arrow)*. **D,** A well-defined midline canal *(black arrow)* extends through the frontal bones just superior to the frontonasal suture. At surgery this led toward an intracranial epidural mass situated between the leaves of the falx anterosuperior to the crista galli.

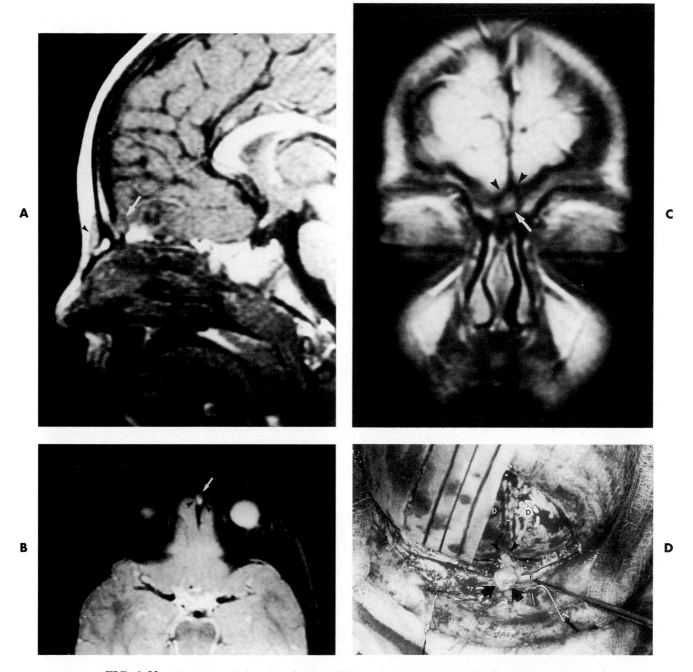

FIG. 1-32 Nasal dermal sinus in a 3½-year-old boy. **A,** Midsagittal T1W MR shows prominent subcutaneous tissue *(arrowhead)* extending along the dorsum of the nose in relation to a midline interdural dermoid *(white arrow)* situated just anterior to the crista galli. **B,** T2W image shows that the interdural dermoid *(white arrow)* is enclosed between the two reflections of low signal dura *(arrowheads)* that form the falx. **C,** Coronal proton density MR displays the characteristic midline spade-shaped mass *(white arrow)* situated immediately superior to the foramen cecum, between the dural reflections *(arrowheads)*. **D,** Surgical exposure of a second patient with a dermoid cyst. The dermoid *(black arrows)* extends from the glabella through a defect in the frontal bones *(F)* into the anterior falx where it is enclosed between the converging reflections *(arrowheads)* of the dura *(D)* overlying the two frontal poles.

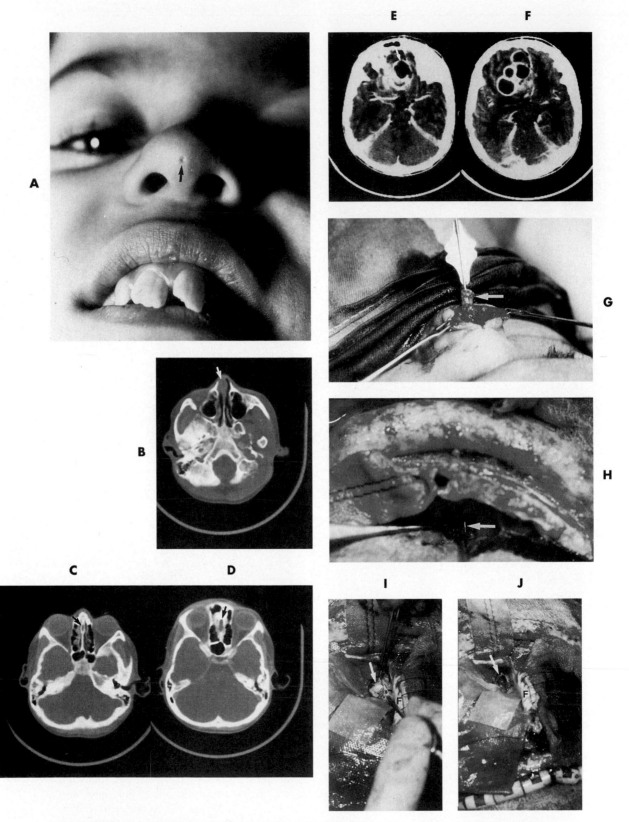

FIG. 1-33 Nasal dermal sinus, intranasal dermoid, intracranial dermoid, and multilocular cerebral abscesses in 10-year-old boy. **A,** Dermal sinus *(arrow)* at the nasal tip. **B** through **D,** Serial axial CTs demonstrate a bony canal (**C** and **D**), *(black arrows)* through the nasal septum into the skull base. **E** and **F,** Contrast-enhanced axial CT scans demonstrate the multilocular right frontal abscesses extending upward from the skull base. The very lucent right paramedian cyst *(arrow)* is the intracranial dermoid itself. **G** through **J,** At surgery a probe was passed through the dissected dermal sinus tract *(white arrow* in **G**) into the extradural intracranial space *(white arrow* in **H**). Dissection downward along the falx *(F)* revealed the intradural dermoid *(white arrow* in **I**) that was debrided to display the cyst wall *(white arrow* in **J**).

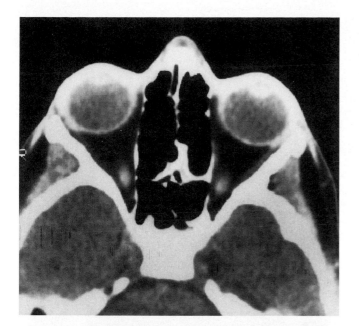

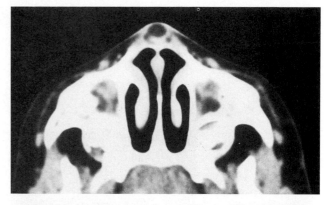

A

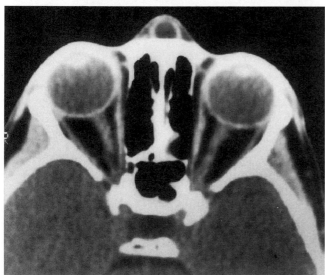

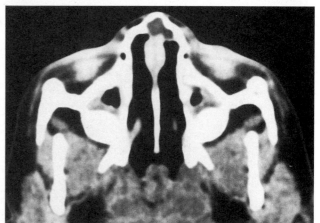

B

FIG. 1-34 Extranasal epidermoid cyst with no infection in a 4-year-old boy. Axial noncontrast CTs. The well-defined isodense cyst wall and lucent center are clearly separable from adjoining soft tissues. The nasal bones are flattened. No intracranial component is present.

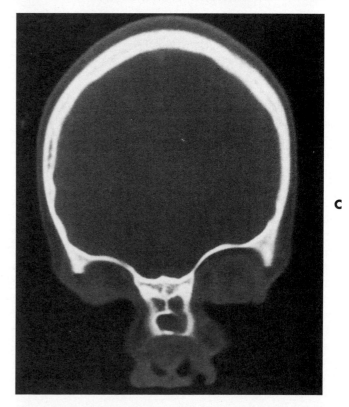

C

(Fig. 1-33). Late development of squamous cell carcinoma is a theoretical rationale for resection, but such carcinoma has not been observed with nasal dermal sinuses to date.

In patients with dermal sinuses and cysts, CT successfully displays the course of the tract and any sequelae of infection. The ostium and tract usually appear as an isodense fibrous channel or as a lucent dermoid channel that extends inward for a variable distance. Bony canals indicate the course of the sinus through the nasal bones, ossified nasal septum, and skull base. An uncomplicated dermoid cyst appears as a well-defined lucency with an isodense capsule (Fig. 1-34). Swelling and edema around the cyst suggest secondary inflammation (Fig. 1-35).[99] The intracranial ends

FIG. 1-35 Mixed extranasal-intranasal dermoid with infection. **A** and **B,** Axial noncontrast CTs demonstrate, extranasal (**A**) and intranasal (**B**) mass, scalloped erosion of the nasal bones, and edema of the fat planes surrounding the cyst. **C,** Direct coronal CT shows the broadening and erosion of the nasal bridge.

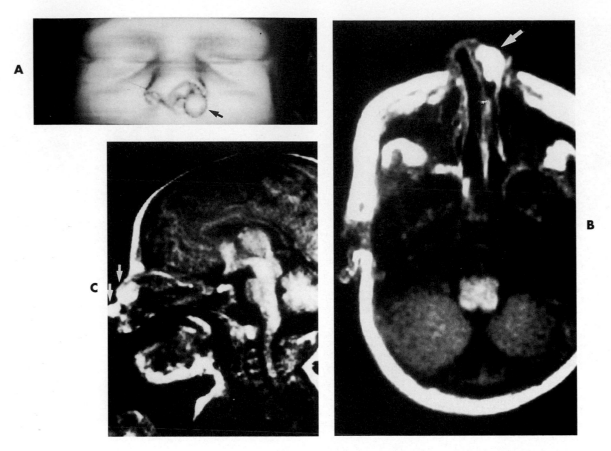

FIG. 1-36 Protruding nasal dermoid. **A,** 3D CT skin surface image shows asymmetric enlargement of the left nostril and left nasal passage by an intranasal mass. A pedunculated exophytic extension *(arrow)* protrudes anterior to the nostril. **B** and **C,** T1W MR in axial **(B)** and sagittal **(C)** planes. The mass is a lobulated, high signal intranasal dermoid *(white arrows)*.

of dermoid cysts typically lie in a hollowed-out gully along the anterior surface of a thickened enlarged crista, and this hollow may give a false impression of a "bifid" crista.[79,87] The intracranial portion of the dermoid may be lucent or dense. Occasional lesions protrude externally at the nostril (Fig. 1-36).

On MR, dermoids may show high signal intensity on T1-weighted (T1W) and low signal intensity on T2W images. Epidermoids usually exhibit low signal intensity on T1W and increased signal intensity on proton density and T2W images. However, the specific appearance is variable from patient to patient.[100] Unfortunately, the only sure proof of an intracranial extension is the actual demonstration of an intracranial mass. CT and MR demonstration of an enlarged foramen cecum and distorted crista galli is suggestive but not proof of an intracranial extension. Foraminal enlargement and distortion of the crista seem to form part of this malformation and may be present (1) with intracranial extension, (2) without intracranial extension, or (3) with intracranial extension of a fibrous cord rather than a dermoid.[49] To avoid unnecessary craniotomies therefore surgical studies suggest that the best approach is to dissect the extracranial portion of the tract along its entire length from the superficial ostium to the extracranial surface of the enlarged foramen cecum.[87,95] The tract is then severed, and the severed end is sent for pathology. If the cephalic end has dermal elements, the dissection is then extended intracranially. If no dermal elements are found and if no mass was shown by CT, the procedure is concluded at that point.

NASAL GLIOMAS

Nasal gliomas are benign masses of glial tissue of congenital origin that occur intranasally or extranasally at or near the root of the nose. They may or may not be connected to the brain by a pedicle of glial tissue. By definition they do not contain any CSF-filled space that is connected with either the ventricles or the subarachnoid space of the head.[101,102]

Nasal gliomas and cephaloceles form a spectrum of related diseases (Figs. 1-23 to 1-26).[65] Characteristic encephaloceles contain ependyma-lined ventricles filled with CSF. Prototypical nasal gliomas consist of solid masses of glial tissue, which are entirely separate from the brain.[101] Transitional forms include solid lesions with microscopic ependyma-lined canals, solid lesions intimately attached to the brain by glial pedicles with no ependyma-lined spaces,

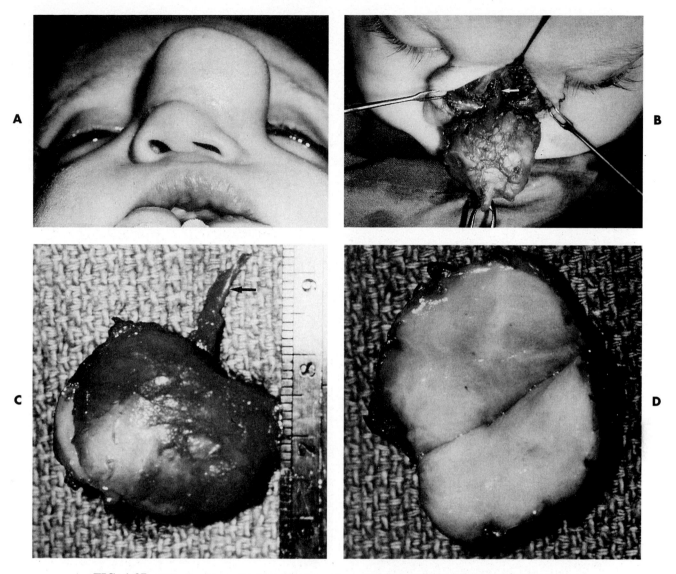

FIG. 1-37 Mixed extranasal-intranasal glioma in an 8-month-old boy with nasal mass that was present at birth and grew in proportion with the child. **A,** View of the face demonstrate a 3 × 3 cm, firm left paramedian subcutaneous mass that displaces the septal and alar cartilage, narrowing the nostril. The mass did not pulsate or change size with crying. **B** and **C,** At surgery the mass was not bound to the subcutaneous tissue. It lay nearly entirely external to the nasal bones, to the left of midline. A narrow stalk *(arrows)* passed directly through the left nasal bone and extended upward to the left cribriform plate. **D,** Bisecting the specimen revealed a homogeneous mass of smooth grayish-white shiny tissue. Histological examination revealed brain and fibrous tissue consistent with nasal glioma.

and solid lesions attached to the dura by fibrous bands with no glial pedicles.[101] Analysis of cases reveals that the presence or absence of a pedicle and thin ependyma-lined channel is not helpful in making surgically and radiologically useful distinctions among these lesions. Thus the medically significant differential diagnosis between nasal gliomas and encephaloceles depends on the presence (encephalocele) or absence (nasal glioma) of communication between the intracranial CSF and any fluid spaces within or surrounding the mass.[103] Indeed, nasal gliomas remain connected with

intracranial structures in 15% of cases, usually through a defect in or near the cribriform plate.[91]

Nasal gliomas are uncommon lesions, with perhaps 100 cases now reported. They occur sporadically with no familial tendency and no sex predilection.[91] They are rarely associated with other congenital malformations of the brain or body.

Nasal gliomas are subdivided into extranasal (60%), intranasal (30%), and mixed (10%) forms (Figs. 1-37, 1-38).[91] The extranasal gliomas lie external to the nasal bones and nasal cavities. Most frequently these occur at the bridge

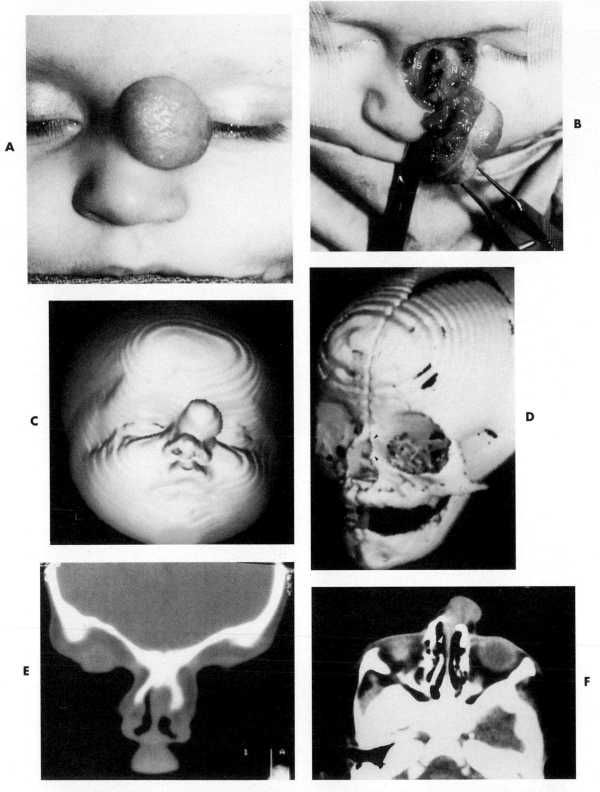

FIG. 1-38 Mixed extranasal-intranasal glioma in a 6-month-old boy. **A,** Facies. The globular mass overlies the dorsum of the nose on the left. **B,** At surgery the lesion extended through the left nasal bones, bowed the septum *(S)* rightward and bowed the residual left nasal bones *(N)* leftward. It was attached by a pedicle to the foramen cecum. **C** and **D,** 3D surface CT for skin **(C)** and bone **(D).** The predominantly extranasal mass molds (*black arrowheads* in **D**) the left nasal bone and bows it outward. **E** and **F,** Coronal and axial CT show that the mass extends through the resultant defect into the thickened nasal septum (*white arrowhead* in **F**). The crista galli and brain were normal. (Courtesy Dr. Sharon Byrd, Chicago).

of the nose, to the left or right of the midline, but curiously not in the midline itself. Extranasal gliomas may also be found near the inner canthus, at the junction of the bony and cartilaginous portions of the nose, or between the frontal, nasal, ethmoid, and lacrimal bones.

Intranasal gliomas lie within the nasal or nasopharyngeal cavities, within the mouth, or rarely within the pterygopalatine fossa (Figs. 1-39, 1-40).[104] They may protrude anteriorly through the nostril.[105] In mixed nasal gliomas the extranasal and intranasal components communicate via a defect in the nasal bones (Fig. 1-41) or around the lateral edges of the nasal bones. Rarely the two portions communicate through defects in the orbital plate of the frontal bone or the frontal sinus. When extranasal gliomas lie to both sides of the nasal bridge, the two components communicate with each other via a defect in the nasal bones, constituting a mixed nasal glioma.[103]

Clinically, extranasal gliomas usually appear in early infancy or childhood as firm, slightly elastic, reddish to bluish, skin-covered masses. Capillary telangiectasias may cover the lesion. They exhibit no pulsations, do not increase in size with Valsalva maneuver (crying), and do not pulsate or swell following compression of the ipsilateral jugular vein (negative Fürstenburg sign).[91,101,106,107] These lesions usually grow slowly in proportion to adjacent tissue but may grow more or less rapidly.[91] They can cause severe deformity by displacing the nasal skeleton, the adjoining maxilla, and the orbital walls, and hypertelorism may result.[91]

Intranasal gliomas usually appear as large, firm, polypoid submucosal masses that may extend inferiorly toward or nearly to the nostril.[91,107] They commonly attach to the turbinates and lie medial to the middle turbinate, between the middle turbinate and the nasal septum.[91] Rarely they attach to the septum itself. These intranasal masses expand the nasal fossa, widen the nasal bridge, and deviate the septum contralaterally. Obstruction of the nasal passage may lead to respiratory distress, especially in infants, and blockage of the nasolacrimal duct may cause epiphora on the affected side. CSF rhinorrhea, meningitis, or epistaxis may be the presenting complaint.

Intranasal gliomas are commonly confused with inflammatory polyps. However, nasal gliomas usually have a firmer consistency and appear less translucent than inflammatory polyps.[101,108] Intranasal gliomas typically lie medial to the middle turbinate, whereas inflammatory polyps typically lie inferolateral to the middle turbinate. Only posterior ethmoid polyps project into the same space as the nasal glioma. Most important, nasal gliomas usually occur in infancy, whereas ordinary nasal polyps are almost unheard of under 5 years of age.[109]

Pathologically, nasal gliomas resemble reactive gliosis rather than neoplasia.[109] No invasion of surrounding tissue has ever been observed; no metastases have been reported.[110] Thus they are classified as heterotopias, not neoplasias.

Histologic studies show that the nasal glioma consists of small or large aggregates of fibrous or gemistocytic astro-

cytes. The cells may be multinuclear, but they exhibit no mitotic figures and no bizarre nuclear forms.[107] Fibrous connective tissue enwraps the blood vessels and extends outward to form collagenous septa that partially subdivide the mass.[107] Prominent zones of granulation tissue may be present.[107] The lesion is usually not encapsulated.[3,91] However, astrocytic processes, fibroblasts, and collagen may form a loose or dense connective tissue capsule.[107] Extranasal gliomas are then surrounded by dermis with dermal appendages.[91] Intranasal gliomas are surrounded by minor salivary glands, fibrovascular tissue, and nasal mucosa.[91]

Only 10% of reported nasal gliomas contain neurons.[107] This lack of neurons in 90% has been attributed to insufficient supply of oxygen to support them or to failure of neurons to differentiate from the embryonic neuroectoderm within the isolated glioma.[107]

Imaging studies display the nasal glioma as an isodense soft-tissue mass that deforms the nasal fossa with or without evidence of extension through the glabella, nasal bones, cribriform plate, or foramen cecum (Fig. 1-39). Calcification may be present in rare cases.[101] Nasal gliomas tend to show nonspecific soft-tissue density on CT. On MR they are often isointense or hyperintense to gray matter on T1W and T2W images. Imaging studies may fail to differentiate between nasal glioma and encephalocele unless a large, communicating CSF space is present to suggest a diagnosis of cephalocele. MRI or positive contrast CT cisternography may be necessary to document the presence or absence of CSF communication.

CEPHALOCELES

Cephaloceles are congenital herniations of intracranial contents through a cranial defect. When the herniation contains brain, it is a meningoencephalocele. If the herniation contains only meninges, it is a cranial meningocele. As a group, the cephaloceles are characterized by heterogeneous mixed density or signal on CT and MR, corresponding to the herniating brain and CSF spaces. Cephaloceles are classified by the site of the cranial defect through which the brain and meninges protrude (see box on p. 37), and the size of the fluid spaces does not determine patient prognosis.[65,111-113]

Cephaloceles situated in the anterior part of the skull are often designated sincipital cephaloceles and include the frontoethmoidal cephaloceles and the interfrontal subtype of cranial cephaloceles.[65,109] Basal cephaloceles include intranasal, nasopharyngeal, and posterior orbital cephaloceles classified as transethmoidal, sphenoethmoidal, transsphenoidal, and frontosphenoidal cephaloceles. The fundamental difference between sincipital and basal cephaloceles is that sincipital cephaloceles always appear as external masses along the nose, orbital margin, or forehead; whereas basal cephaloceles are not visible externally, unless they grow large enough to protrude secondarily through the nostril or mouth.[85]

Cephaloceles are common lesions, with an incidence of 1 per 4000 live births.[114] Overall, occipital cephaloceles are

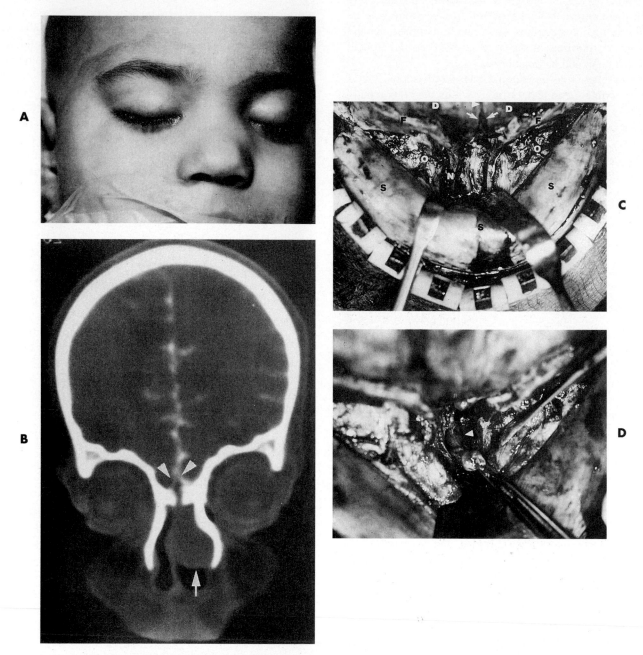

FIG. 1-39   Intranasal glioma with intracranial attachments. **A,** Widening of the nasal bridge and the left nostril (present before intubation). **B,** Water-soluble positive contrast cisternography. Direct coronal and reformatted sagittal CT sections demonstrate a large left unilateral intranasal mass *(arrows)* that deviates the nasal septum rightward, bows the left nasal bone outward, and extends superiorly through a widened foramen cecum into the interdural space between the leaves *(white arrowheads)* of the falx. Opacified CSF outlines the intracranial portion of the mass but does not extend extracranially into or around the intranasal portion of the mass. **C and D,** Frontal intraoperative photographs oriented like **A** and **B**. **C,** The scalp *(S)* has been reflected over the orbits *(O)*. Keyhole resection of the frontonasal junction exposes the frontal dura *(D)* and nasal cavity, bounded by remnant frontal bone *(F)* at the supraorbital ridges and remnant nasal bone *(N)* laterally. The frontal dura of each side is reflected inward in the midline *(white arrowhead)* to form the falx. The interdural space *(white arrows)* is widened inferiorly. **D,** Further dissection frees the interdural portion (between forceps) of the nasal glioma and proves it is directly continuous with the intranasal portion *(white arrowhead)* of the mass.

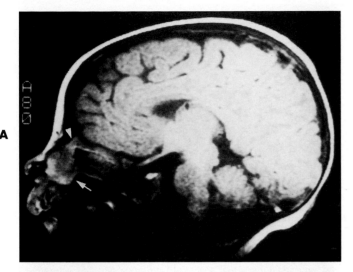

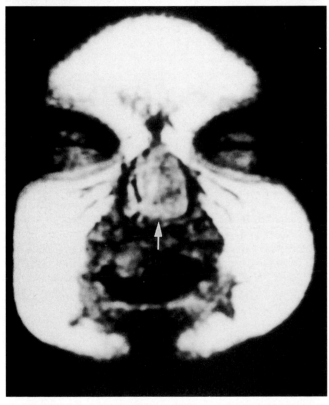

A

B

FIG. 1-40 Intranasal glioma. **A,** Midsagittal T1W MR. **B,** Coronal T1W MR. The mass *(white arrows)* protrudes inferiorly through an enlarged foramen cecum *(white arrowhead)* to expand the left nasal passage. The nasal septum and left nasal bones are bowed outward.

the most frequent type (67% to 80%). Sincipital cephaloceles (15%) and basal cephaloceles (10%) are less common.[111,114] The occipital and the sincipital cephaloceles appear to be distinctly different diseases. Occipital cephaloceles are linked with neural tube defects such as myelomeningocele; sincipital cephaloceles are not.[115] Occipital cephaloceles are the most frequent type among people of European descent, and sincipital cephaloceles are

CLASSIFICATION OF CEPHALOCELES

I. Occipital cephaloceles
    A. Cervico-occipital (continuous with cervical rachischisis)
    B. Low occipital (involving foramen magnum)
    C. High occipital (above intact rim of foramen magnum)

II. Cephaloceles of the cranial vault
    A. Temporal
    B. Posterior Fontanelle
    C. Interparietal
    D. Anterior fontanelle
    E. Interfrontal

III. Frontoethmoidal cephaloceles *(sincipital cephaloceles)*
    A. Nasofrontal
    B. Nasoethmoidal
    C. Nasoorbital

IV. Basal cephaloceles
    A. Transethmoidal
    B. Sphenoethmoidal
    C. Transsphenoidal
    D. Frontosphenoidal

V. Cephaloceles associated with cranioschisis
    A. Cranial-upper facial cleft
    B. Basal-lower facial cleft
    C. Acrania and anencephaly

Modified from Suwanwela C, Suwanwela N. J Neurosurg 1972; 36:201.

the most frequent type among Malaysians and certain other Southeast Asian groups. Thus among Australian aborigines (nearly) all cephaloceles are sincipital, whereas among Australians of European descent 67% are occipital and 2% are sincipital.[111,115]

Frontoethmoidal cephaloceles are characterized by a cranial defect at the junction of the frontal and ethmoid bones.[113,116-120] In 90% of these cephaloceles the intracranial end of the defect is a single midline ostium that corresponds to the foramen cecum. In 10% of these cephaloceles an intact midline bridge of bone divides the defect into bilateral, paired ostia situated at the anterior ends of the cribriform plates.

The frontoethmoidal cephaloceles are subdivided into three types in accord with the position of the facial end of the cranial defect (Fig. 1-42).[113] In the nasofrontal form (50% to 61%), the facial end of the defect lies between the frontal and the nasal bones so the ostium presents at the nasion between deformed orbits (Figs. 1-43, 1-44).[121,122] Specifically, in this type the frontal bones are displaced superiorly. The nasal bones, frontal processes of maxillae, and nasal cartilage are all displaced inferiorly, away from the frontal bone, but they retain a normal relationship to each other. The ethmoid bone is displaced inferiorly so that

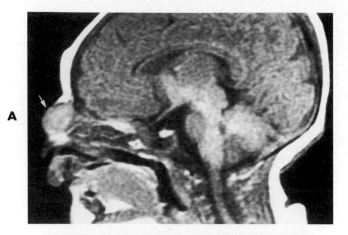

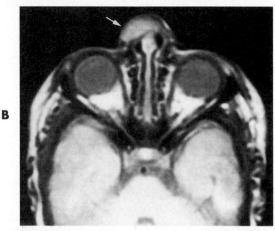

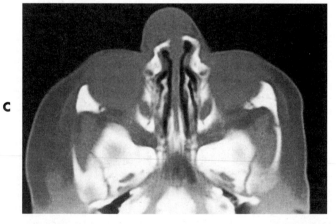

FIG. 1-41   Mixed intranasal-extranasal glioma in a 1-day-old boy. **A,** Midsagittal T1W MR. **B,** Axial proton density MR. **C,** Axial CT scan. The large, sharply marginated eccentric predominantly extranasal mass *(arrows)* connects through a defect in the deformed nasal bones with a smaller intranasal intraseptal component.

the midline portion of the anterior fossa is very deep, and the crista projects into the defect from its inferior rim. The anterior portions of the medial orbital walls are displaced laterally. The bone canal is short because the intracranial (frontoethmoidal) and the extracranial (nasofrontal) ends of the defect lie close together.[113]

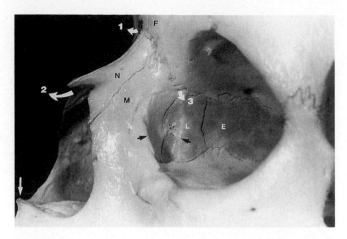

FIG. 1-42   Sites of the anterior ostia of frontoethmoidal cephaloceles. Dried adult skull displays the contours and relationships of the individual bones of the skull and face and the intervening sutures. Ethmoid bone or lamina papyracea *(E)*; frontal bone *(F)*; lacrimal bone *(L)*; frontal process of the maxilla *(M)*; and nasal bones *(N)*. Note the interfrontal, internasal, frontonasal, and frontomaxillary sutures; the nasal spines *(arrow)* of the maxillae; and the lacrimal sac fossa (between *black arrows*). The anterior crest of the lacrimal sac fossa is formed by the frontal process of maxilla. The posterior crest is formed by the lacrimal bone. Cartilaginous structures are not displayed. The sites through which the three subtypes of the frontoethmoidal cephaloceles protrude are indicated by the numbered arrows. *1,* Nasofrontal cephalocele. The nasofrontal forms emerge at the nasofrontal junction. The frontal bones form the superior margin of the defect. The nasal bones, frontal processes of the maxillae, and nasal cartilage form the inferior margin of the defect. *2,* Nasoethmoidal cephalocele. The nasoethmoidal forms emerge beneath the nasal bones superior to the cartilaginous nasal capsule. The nasal bones and the frontal processes of the maxillae form the superior margin of the defect. The nasal cartilage and nasal septum form the inferior margin of the defect. *3,* Nasoorbital cephalocele. The nasoorbital forms emerge along the medial wall of the orbit between the frontal processes of maxilla and the lacrimal-ethmoid bones. The frontal process of maxilla forms the anterior margin of the defect. The lacrimal bone and lamina papyracea of the ethmoid form the posterior wall of the defect.

The associated soft-tissue mass lies at the glabella or nasal root.[113] The mass may be small (1 to 2 cm), or it may be larger than the infant's head. Most of the nasofrontal cephaloceles are firm, solid masses and exhibit no transmitted pulsations. Some are cystic, compressible, pulsatile and increase in size with Valsalva maneuver (crying).[100] The mass usually grows as the child grows. Cystic masses may increase in size disproportionately rapidly as CSF pools within the sac. The cephalocele may be covered by intact skin, thin skin that ruptures to leak CSF, or no skin at all, exposing brain to the environment. The falx frequently extends into the sac, partially subdividing it. The herniated brain may be well preserved with recognizable gyri and sulci that converge toward the hernia ostium, or the herniated brain may be reduced to a mass of distorted gliotic tis-

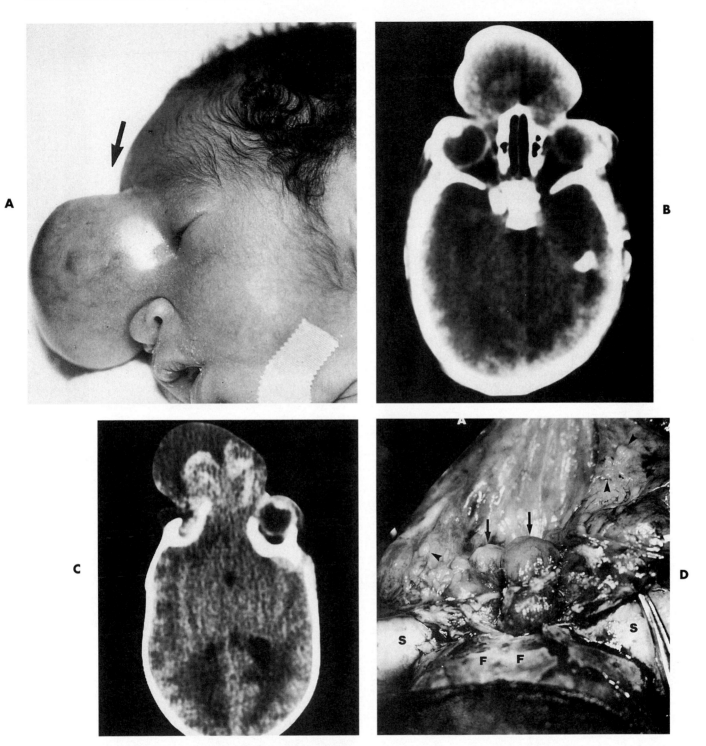

FIG. 1-43 Nasofrontal form of frontoethmoidal cephalocele in newborn girl. **A,** Lateral view of the face. A large skin-covered midline mass protrudes between the two orbits, overlies the nasal bones and nasal cartilage, and compresses the nostrils. Arrow indicates the angle of observation for the surgical photographs. **B,** Noncontrast CT. **C,** Contrast-enhanced CT on two different days, oriented as in **D,** the surgical specimen. The ostium of the cephalocele lies above the ethmoid and nasal bones but below the frontal bones, so the lesion is a frontonasal type of frontoethmoidal cephalocele. The mass is predominantly cystic. The inferior portions of both frontal lobes protrude directly into the sac to different degrees, greater on the left. **D,** Surgical photograph. Anterior *(A)* view of the frontal bone *(F)* after reflection of the scalp *(S)* anteriorly and opening of the upper wall of the cephalocele to expose its contents. Most of the sac was filled by CSF. Portions of both frontal lobes *(arrows)* protrude into the sac, separated by the interhemispheric fissure. Multiple glial nodules *(black arrowheads)* stud the meninges that form the inner lining of the sac.

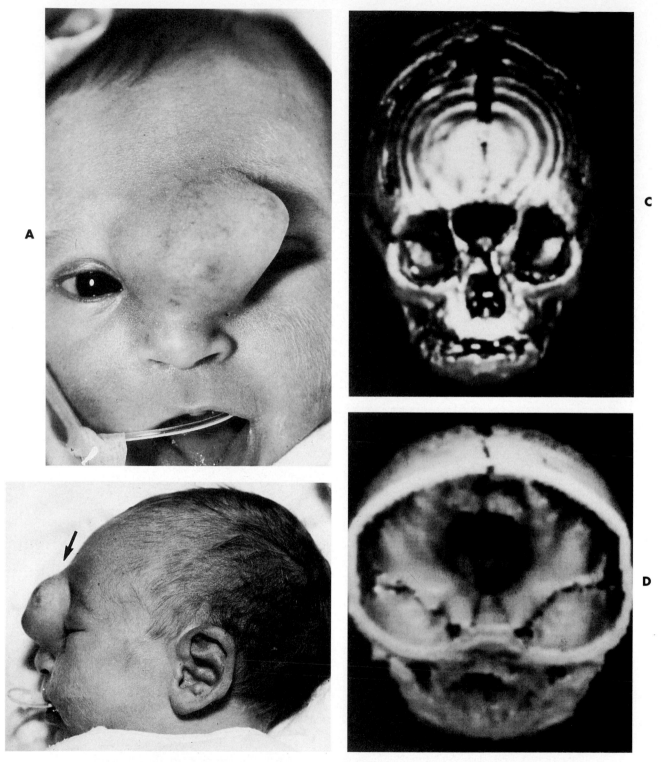

FIG. 1-44 Nasofrontal form of frontoethmoidal cephalocele in 1-week-old girl. **A** and **B,** Lobulated 3 × 3 cm skin-covered mass that protrudes between the orbits over the nasal bones and nasal cartilage. Arrow indicates the angle of observation for the surgical photographs. **C** and **D,** 3D CT of bone surface viewed from **(C),** anterior and **(D),** posterior (intracranial) show the characteristic deformities of the frontal bones superolateral to the ostium and the characteristic position of the nasofrontal sutures, nasal bones, and crista galli inferior to the ostium.

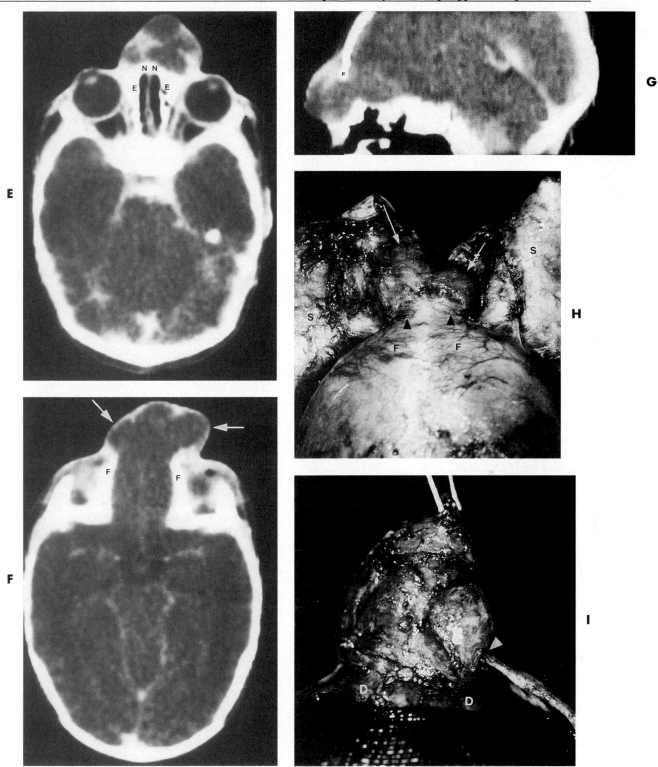

FIG. 1-44, cont'd **E** and **F,** Axial noncontrast CTs. **G,** Sagittal reformatted CT. Portions of both frontal lobes *(arrows)* protrude anteriorly through a defect in the frontal bones to form a lobulated mass anterior to the nasal bones. Because the superior margin of the ostium is frontal bone *(F)* and the inferior margin is nasal bones *(N),* this is a nasofrontal cephalocele. Note the larger size of the defect on the left and the crista galli at the floor of the intracranial end of the canal. **H** and **I,** Surgical exposure seen from above after bifrontal craniotomy and scalp dissection. The superior margin of the ostium was formed by frontal bones. The sac contained distorted, lobulated neural tissue that protruded through the defect. A small dermoid is seen at the tip of the mass (between forceps). The whole lesion was resected. Histological examination revealed that the sac contents were glial tissue containing numerous blood vessels.

sue. Typically the brain is not adherent to the base of the sac at the ostium, but it may be adherent to the meninges at the dome of the sac (60%).[121]

The tips of the frontal lobes usually protrude into the defect, symmetrically or asymmetrically. The olfactory bulbs may herniate with the brain; the olfactory tracts are stretched. The optic nerves enter the skull normally, but they may then recurve sharply anteriorly toward the hernia orifice, and the internal carotid arteries course with the optic nerves. The anterior communicating artery may lie near the ostium, and concurrent anomalies such as holoprosencephaly and hydrocephalus may be present.

In the nasoethmoidal form (30% to 33%) of frontoethmoidal cephaloceles, the facial end of the defect lies between the nasal bones and the nasal cartilage so the ostium is situated at the widened dorsum of the nose. Specifically, in the nasoethmoidal form the nasal bones and the frontal processes of the maxillae remain attached to the frontal bones above the sac, forming the anterosuperior wall of the canal. The nasal cartilage, nasal septum, and ethmoid bone are displaced posteroinferiorly, forming the posteroinferior wall of the canal. The crista projects upward into the canal from the depths of the floor. The medial walls of the orbit form the lateral borders of the defect and may be bony or membranous. In this group, because the canal is long, a greater distance exists between the intracranial (frontoethmoid) and extracranial (nasoethmoid) ends of the defect.

Clinically, nasoethmoidal cephaloceles are similar to nasofrontal cephaloceles except that the defect and soft-tissue mass lie more inferiorly along the dorsum of the nose and often extend to the inner canthus. Cystic swellings may be present on both sides of the nose. Hydrocephalus is common. In Suwanwela's series, one of three patients had concurrent agenesis of the corpus callosum with an interhemispheric cyst.[89,113]

Harverson et al detailed the radiologic differences between the nasofrontal and nasoethmoidal cephaloceles.[105] In the nasofrontal form the defect in the frontal bone is V-shaped. The superior aspects of the medial orbital walls are bowed and displaced laterally. The nasal bones remain attached to the cribriform plate at the lower margin of the ostium. Thus the cribriform plate and nasal bones are seen lying unusually low between the orbits. A large gap exists between the frontal and ethmoidal bones. The soft-tissue mass lies directly in front of the bone defect, usually in the midline, and it is often spherical. Conversely, in the nasoethmoidal form the bone defect is usually circular and is situated between the orbits, causing increased interorbital distance. The nasal bones remain attached to the frontal bones along the upper margins of the ostium, and the cribriform plate lies at a normal height with respect to the orbits. The soft-tissue mass lies to one side of the midline, beside the nasal cartilage. It may be bilateral.[123]

In the nasoorbital form of frontoethmoidal cephalocele (6% to 10%), the facial end of the defect lies at the medial wall of the orbit, so the ostium shows at the inner canthus

and nasolabial folds (Figs. 1-45, 1-46). Specifically the frontal process of the maxilla is separated from the lacrimal and ethmoid bones. The abnormal frontal process of the maxilla forms the anterior margin of the defect. The lacrimal bone and lamina papyracea of the ethmoid form the posterior edge of the defect.[113] The frontal bones, nasal bones, and nasal cartilage retain their normal relationship to one another. In this type of cephalocele the intracranial (frontoethmoid) and extracranial (medial orbital) ends of the defect are widely separated, so the canal is very long.

Patients with nasoorbital cephalocele may have cystic soft-tissue masses at the nasolabial folds between the nose and the lower eyelid. These masses may contain nubbins of brain.[113] The orbital fat, muscle cones, and globes are displaced laterally by the medial intraorbital component of the cephalocele. The nasal mucosa is displaced inferomedially. Arachnoid cysts of the temporal fossa are common in these patients and may protrude into the orbit with the cephalocele.[121,124-126]

Suwanwela and Hongsaprabhas reviewed the clinical findings in 25 patients with frontoethmoidal cephaloceles.[109] Microcephaly was present in 24%, unilateral or bilateral microphthalmos in 16%, hydrocephalus in 12%, and seizures in 4%. Mental retardation was present in 43% of those old enough to test. CSF leakage and continuous bleeding from the exposed brain were major problems in those cephaloceles that lacked a skin cover or those in which the thin skin cover ruptured. Rappoport, Dunn, and Alhady found significant associated congenital anomalies such as microphthalmos, mental retardation, and syndactyly with appendicular constriction bands in 33% of these patients.[121]

The anterior basal cephaloceles tend to occur in patients with more generalized craniofacial-cerebral dysraphism manifested in part as a midline cleft upper lip, optic nerve dysplasias, and callosal dysgenesis.[19,127] The two major types are transethmoidal and transsphenoidal cephaloceles. The transethmoidal defects lie anteriorly, either along the midline or along the cribriform plate and do not involve the sella turcica. The hernia sac extends inferiorly into the sinuses or the nasal cavity and typically contains portions of the frontal lobes and olfactory apparatus.

The transsphenoidal cephaloceles extend downward through a defect in the floor of the sella turcica to reach the nasal cavity (Figs. 1-12 to 1-14). If the palate is cleft, they may also extend further inferiorly into the oral cavity. The posterior margin of these defects is always the dorsum sellae. The lateral walls are the cavernous sinuses and the widely separated halves of the sphenoid bone. The anterior extent is very variable. The defect may involve the sella only, sella and planum, or the sphenoid and part of the posterior ethmoid bone. The latter form is sometimes designated sphenoethmoidal cephalocele.

Transsphenoidal cephaloceles typically contain the pituitary gland and the hypothalamus, the anterior recesses of the third ventricle, and the optic apparatus. Symptoms vary. In neonates and infants, the intranasal-pharyngeal soft-tissue

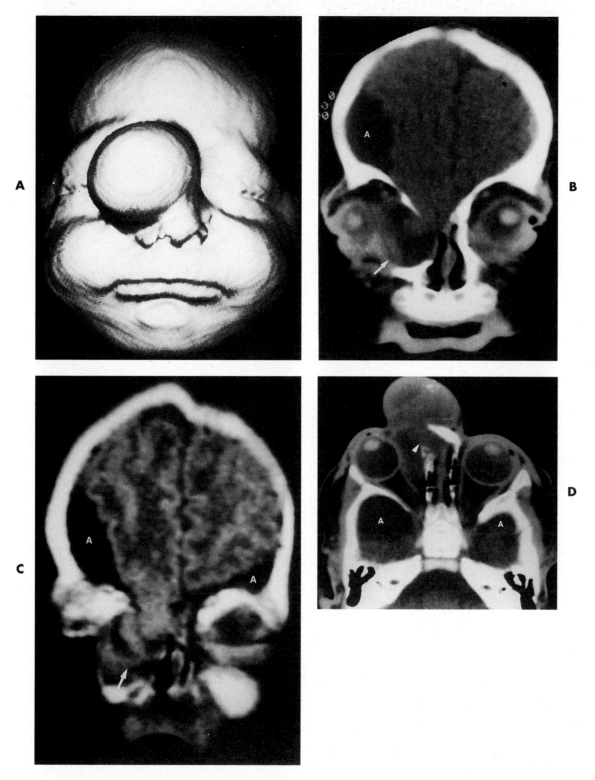

FIG. 1-45   Unilateral nasoorbital cephalocele. **A,** Skin surface 3D CT shows a large, eccentric, skin-covered mass at the medial right canthus. The cartilaginous nose is deviated inferiorly and leftward. **B,** Coronal CT. **C,** Coronal T1W MR. **B** and **C** show lateral deviation of the right globe and muscle cone by inferior protrusion of a unilateral cephalocele *(white arrows)* containing brain and meninges. The cephalocele displaces the nasal mucosa medially and the orbital contents laterally. Bilateral anterior temporal fossa CSF spaces suggest concurrent arachnoid cysts *(A)*. **D,** Axial CT demonstrates the defect *(arrowhead)* in the medial wall of the right orbit, the characteristic displacement of the muscle cone, and the narrowing of the ipsilateral nasal passage.

Continued

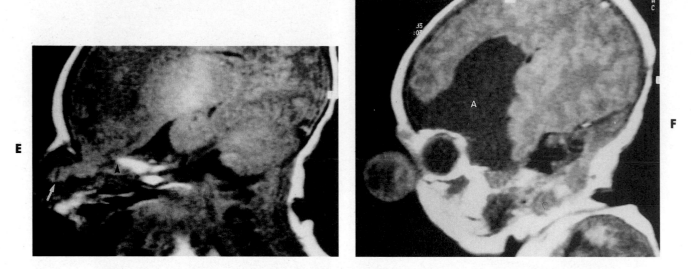

FIG. 1-45, cont'd   **E** and **F,** Sagittal T1W MR. **F,** Paramedian section demonstrates the intracranial end *(black arrowhead)* of the osseous canal and direct extension of brain tissue *(white arrow)* into the medial orbit. **F,** Lateral section demonstrates the prominent arachnoid cyst commonly found in these lesions.

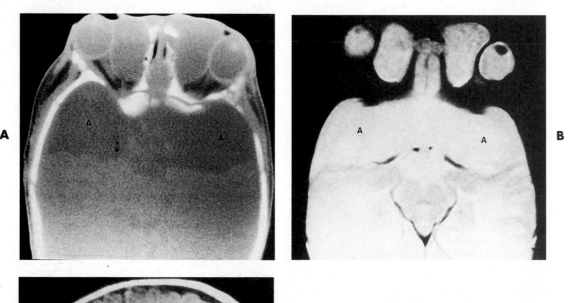

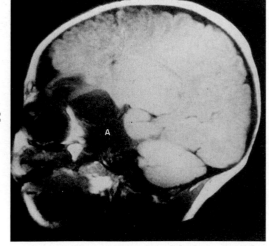

FIG. 1-46   Bilateral nasoorbital cephaloceles in a 5-week-old boy. **A** and **B,** Axial plane CT and T2W MRI demonstrate lateral displacement of the globes and muscle cones by large, predominantly cystic cephaloceles that extend into the orbit via bilateral defects in the medial walls of the orbits. There are prominent bilateral temporal fossa arachnoid cysts. **C,** Paramedian sagittal T1W MR shows direct connection between the brain and the intraorbital sac indicating cephalocele. (Courtesy Dr. Robert Dorwart, Indianapolis.)

mass usually causes a runny nose, nasal obstruction, mouth breathing, or snoring. Frequently these symptoms are ignored.[128] If noted, the intranasal lesions then discovered may be mistaken for nasal polyps exactly as is true for nasal gliomas.[89,129] If the early signs are not appreciated, the basal cephaloceles may not be detected until adulthood, when they tend to appear as visual disturbance, pituitary-hypothalamic dysfunction, or CSF rhinorrhea.[128]

Clinical diagnosis of basal cephalocele is achieved most easily by appreciating that cleft hypertelorism, median cleft upper lip with or without cleft nose, and optic nerve dysplasias are highly significant stigmata. They suggest the presence of basal cephaloceles, especially the transsphenoidal cephaloceles (Table 1-2).[19,61]

PREMATURE CRANIAL SYNOSTOSIS
Primary Cranial Synostosis

Virchow (1852) first recognized that fusion of a calvarial suture distorted and redirected skull growth by (1) restricting growth in the direction perpendicular to the suture and (2) initiating compensatory enlargement of the calvarium in the direction parallel to the suture (Fig. 1-47).[130] Virchow suspected that the primary disease process occurred where the sutures abutted. Moss (1950s) demonstrated that premature closure of sutures at the skull base influenced growth of the sutures in the vault.[131] Cohen (1977) later hypothesized that changes in the mesenchymal blastema affected the sutures of both the skull base and the vault.[132]

Cranial synostoses may be classified into three broad categories: primary cranial synostosis, secondary cranial synostosis, and metabolic craniosynostosis. This classification focuses medical attention on the major source of disease. Primary cranial synostoses are those in which the suture synostosis occurs in the absence of underlying brain disease or metabolic impairment. Primary synostoses may be simple, isolated synostoses that affect one or two adjacent sutures with no associated genetic abnormality (for example, sagittal synostosis), or primary synostoses may form one part of a multifocal, heritable syndrome affecting the calvarium, the facial skeleton and ears, the extremities and other organs such as the heart *(vide infra)*.

Secondary cranial synostosis occurs as an indirect consequence of primary intracranial disease. Normally, increasing intracranial volume is the stimulus for the expansion of the vault and continued growth at the sutures. If the intracranial volume stops increasing for any reason, for example, anoxic infarction of the brain or shunting of hydrocephalus with reduced ventricular volume, then there is no further stimulus for continued calvarial expansion. The sutures stop growing and may fuse secondarily. Metabolic synostoses are those that arise from metabolic disorders such as hypophosphatasia; these affect multiple bones, not just the calvarium.

Early descriptions of craniosynostosis were based on the cosmetic appearance of the patient.[133] The term *scaphocephaly* (dolichocephaly, boat head, or canoe head) was

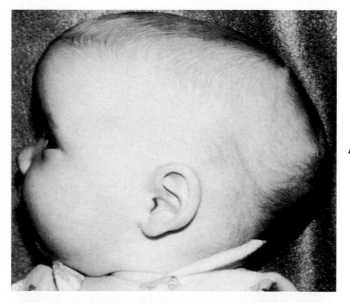

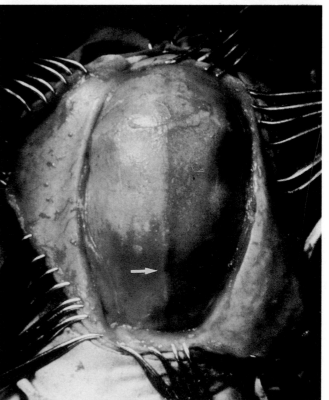

FIG. 1-47 Sagittal synostosis in two patients. **A,** Lateral view of the head shows scaphocephaly with slight ridging near to vertex. **B,** Surgical exposure, vertex view, shows scaphocephaly with prominent ridging *(arrow)* along the synostosed sagittal suture.

used to signify elongation of the calvarium in the anteroposterior (A-P) direction (Fig. 1-47). In this condition, premature closure of the sagittal suture reduced the transverse (biparietal) diameter of the head and led to an elongated A-P dimension, parallel to the sagittal suture (Fig. 1-48). Premature sagittal synostosis with scaphocephaly is the most common form of craniosynostosis. It accounts for

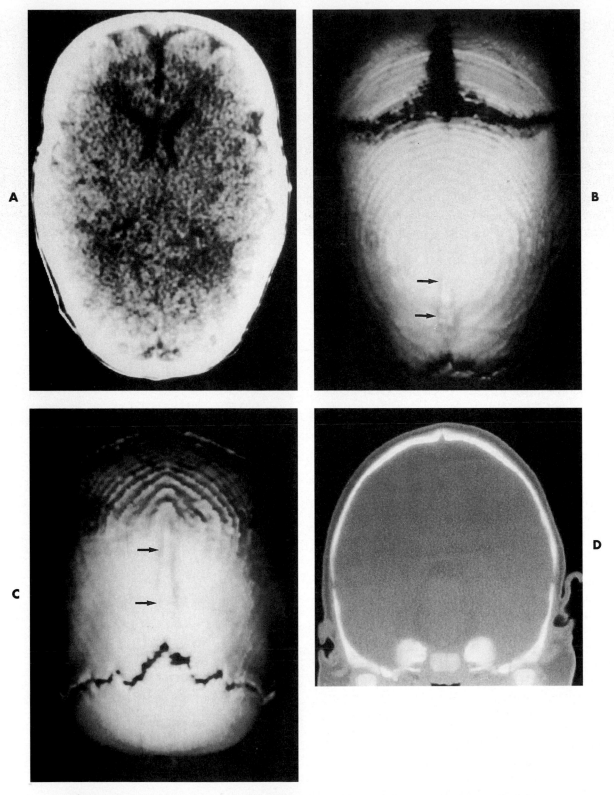

FIG. 1-48   Sagittal synostosis in a 2-month-old boy. **A,** Axial CT shows scaphocephaly, narrow posterior calvarial contour, and compression of sulci, ventricles, and brain where posterior sagittal synostosis has restricted transverse growth. **B** and **C,** 3D bone surface CTs of the skull from above (**B**) and behind (**C**) show narrowed transverse calvarial dimensions, especially posteriorly; marked ridging *(arrows)* of the posterior sagittal suture; closure of the whole sagittal suture; elongation of the AP dimension of the skull; marked widening of the metopic and both coronal sutures; and slight widening of both lambdoid sutures. **D,** Coronal bone algorithm CT shows "pile up" of bone at the synostosing suture.

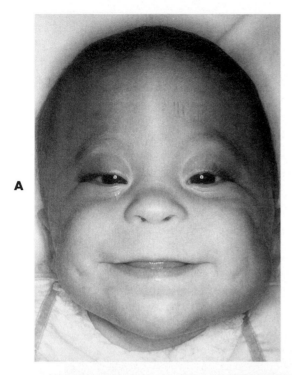

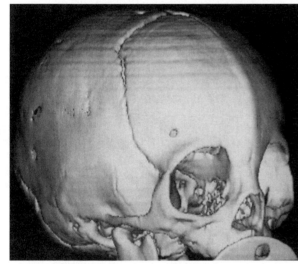

FIG. 1-49 Trigonocephaly. Metopic synostosis **A,** Facies. Note hypotelorism, anteromedial inclination of the orbits, and prominent midline ridge. **B,** Oblique 3D bone surface CT shows marked ridging along the expected position of the metopic suture and superomedial "pointing" of the orbital rims.

approximately 50% of all cases of synostosis and usually is an isolated condition with no syndromic associations. In contrast to other synostoses, sagittal synostosis causes remarkably little deformity of the face. The sphenoid wings and orbits are not affected.

Trigonocephaly signifies an ax head or keel-shaped deformity with sharp anteriorly directed ridging of the midline frontal contour, orbital hypotelorism, and ethmoid hypoplasia (Fig. 1-49).[133] The crista galli remains intact. In this condition, premature synostosis of the metopic suture is believed to restrict frontal growth, leading to symmetrical lateral sloping of the forehead, short anterior fossa, and forward bowing of the coronal sutures.[134] The nasal septum and facial midline are usually straight. The medial walls of the orbits are thickened and rise unusually high, so the bony orbits appear pointed superomedially and fall away laterally (Figs. 1-50, 1-51). The two frontal lobes, the frontal sulci, and the ventricles are usually compressed. Less commonly, hydrocephalus causes ventriculomegaly.

Brachycephaly signifies an abnormally wide transverse (bicoronal or biparietal) diameter of the calvarium with a shortened A-P dimension. It typically results from coronal or lambdoidal synostoses that limit growth in the A-P direction (Figs. 1-52, 1-53). Oxycephaly (turricephaly) indicates a towering calvarium. This is usually associated with bilateral coronal or bilateral lambdoid synostosis and may represent growth redirected anteriorly toward the anterior fontanelle-metopic suture complex or posteriorly toward the posterior fontanelle and lambdoid sutures. Plagiocephaly signifies an asymmetrically deformed calvarium presumed to result from unilateral synostosis or from asynchronous asymmetrical bilateral synostoses of multiple sutures.

Kleeblattschädel (cloverleaf skull) signifies a severe deformity with an apparent circumferential constriction of calvarial growth.[133] It appears to result from multiple bilateral premature synostoses in the calvarium and skull base. The coronal and lambdoid sutures are markedly thickened into dense bony struts, restricting A-P growth and leading to shallow orbits and anterior fossa (Fig. 1-54). Redirected growth at the sagittal sutures or the fontanelles leads to turricephaly, and redirected growth at the squamosal sutures leads to lateral bulging and brachycephaly. The floor of the middle fossa is nearly flat. The anterior temporal fossae expand inferior to the orbits. Severe growth constriction and any concurrent hydrocephalus cause marked scalloped erosions along the inner margins of the calvarium.[135]

Unfortunately, descriptive terms and patient appearances are not specific. They do not necessarily predict the skull radiographs, the CT appearance, or the specific sutures that are or are not fused.

Craniofacial Dysostosis

Recent work indicates that the syndromic primary craniosynostoses may be related to each other. As a group they tend to be autosomal, dominant traits that affect the coronal sutures, more than other sutures and they tend to affect the distal extremities. These conditions may all have genetic defects that lead to impaired fibroblast growth factor receptors (FGFR). Thus far four FGFR have been identified, designated FGFR 1, 2, 3, and 4. All four FGFRs encode transmembrane tyrosine kinase receptors, which regulate (signal) cell functions such as cell proliferation, cell migration, and cell differentiation.

Mutations affecting FGFR receptors have been identified in the Crouzon, Pfeiffer, and possibly Apert syndromes.[136-138] In Crouzon's syndrome the extremities are not affected. In Pfeiffer's and Apert's syndrome they are, affected. In Pfeif-

Text continued on p. 52.

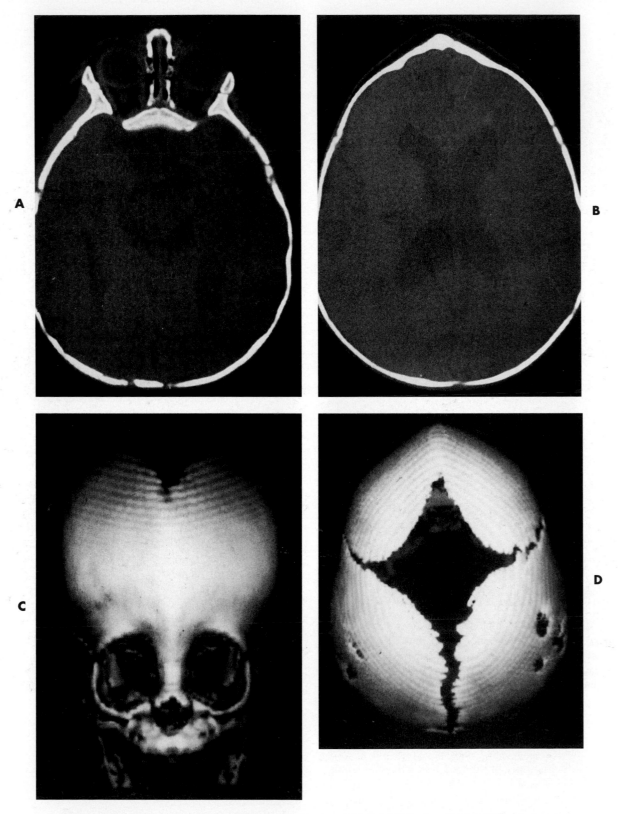

FIG. 1-50   Trigonocephaly. Metopic synostosis. **A** and **B,** Axial CTs show marked hypotelorism (**A**) and sharp ax-head pointing of the midfrontal contour. The ventricles are dilated. **C** and **D,** 3D bone surface CTs from anterior (**C**) and above (**D**) show hypotelorism, superomedial pointing of the orbital rims, and metopic suture synostosis with marked thickening and buttressing of bone along the midline. The coronal sutures, sagittal suture, and anterior fontanelle are widely patent.

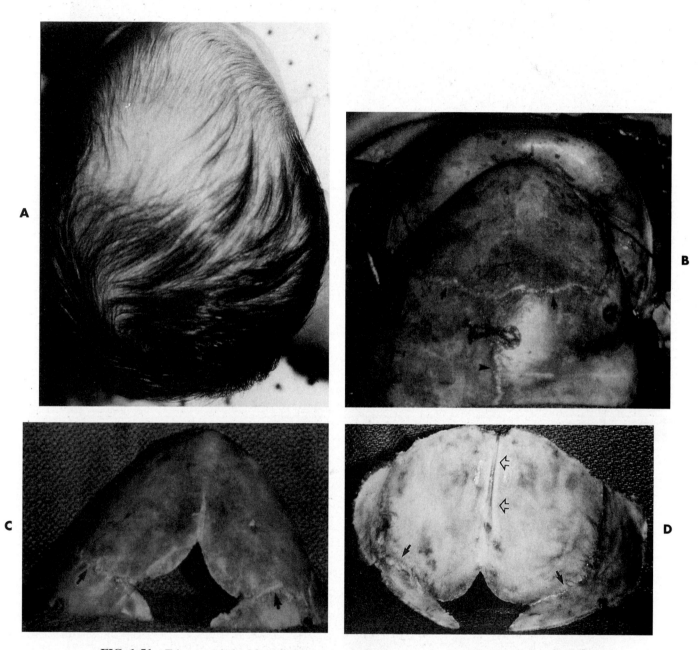

FIG. 1-51 Trigonocephaly. Metopic synostoses. **A,** Vertex view. Ax-head deformity. **B,** Exposed calvarium. Note the patent coronal sutures *(arrows),* sagittal suture *(arrowhead)* and anterior fontanelle with no patent metopic suture. **C** and **D,** Resected anterior calvarium during repair, seen from above **(C)** and "inside" **(D).** Note the marked buttressing *(open black arrows)* of bone along the metopic suture.

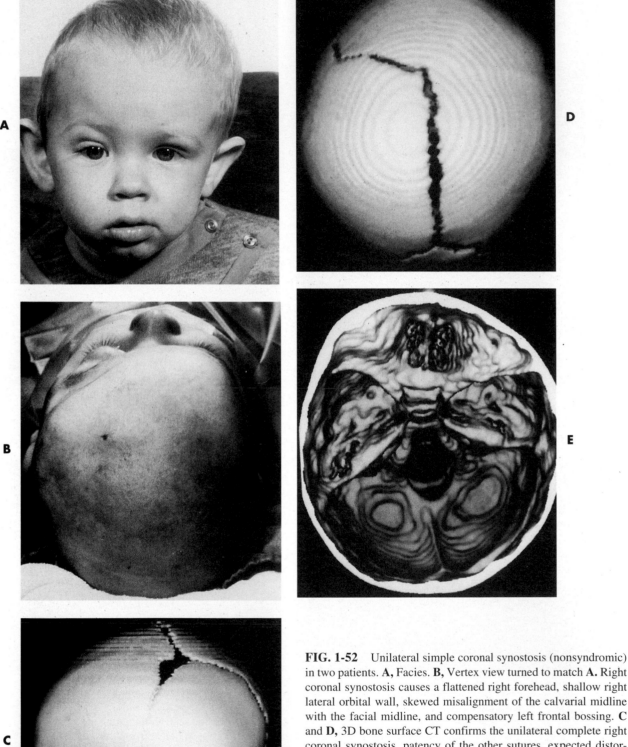

FIG. 1-52 Unilateral simple coronal synostosis (nonsyndromic) in two patients. **A,** Facies. **B,** Vertex view turned to match **A.** Right coronal synostosis causes a flattened right forehead, shallow right lateral orbital wall, skewed misalignment of the calvarial midline with the facial midline, and compensatory left frontal bossing. **C** and **D,** 3D bone surface CT confirms the unilateral complete right coronal synostosis, patency of the other sutures, expected distortion of the orbits and frontal contour, and skewed craniofacial midline with oblique nasofrontal sutures. **E,** 3D bone surface CT of the inside of the skull base as seen from above. Note the shallow anterior and middle fossae and skew deviation of the anterior and posterior cranial midlines.

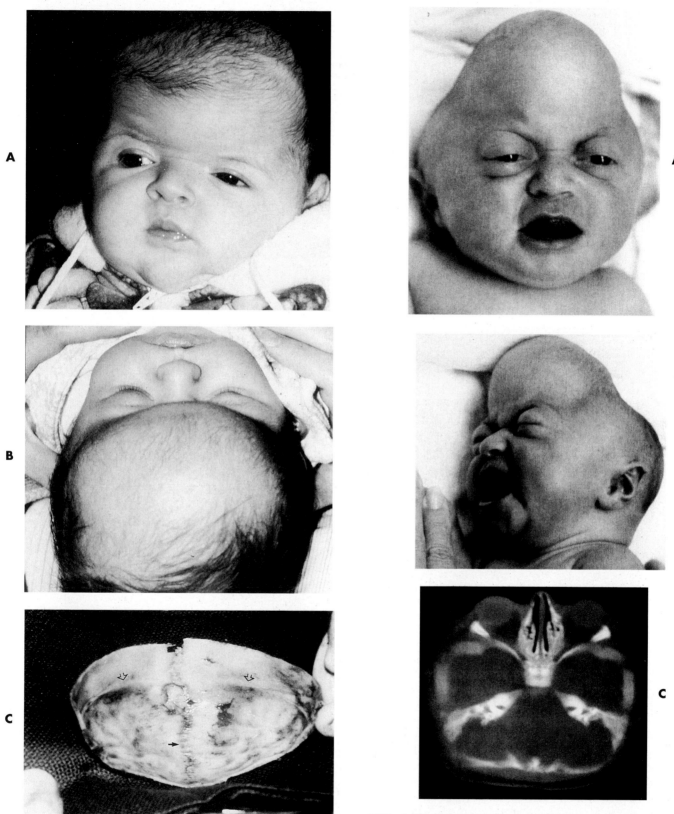

FIG. 1-53 Simple bicoronal synostosis. Nonsyndromic. **A,** Facies. **B,** Vertex view. **C,** Intraoperative specimen (different patient) during repair. The sagittal suture *(arrow)* is patent. Bilateral ridges *(open arrows)* replace the lengths of the coronal sutures.

FIG. 1-54 Kleeblattschädel (clover-leaf skull) in a newborn male. **A,** Frontal facies. **B,** Oblique view of head. **C,** Axial CT demonstrates the short AP dimension, wide transverse dimension at the temporal fossae, shallow lateral orbital walls with exorbitism, and scalloped erosions of the internal margin of the calvarium where the brain grows against the restricting calvarium and base.

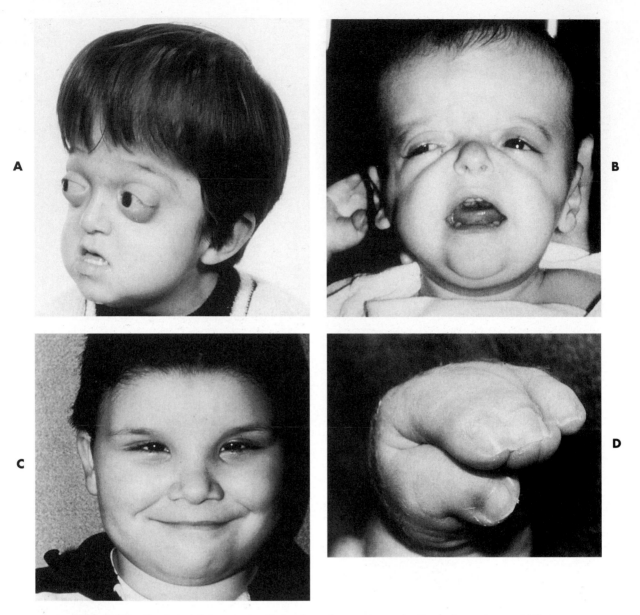

FIG. 1-55   Craniofacial dysostosis. Facies from three patients. **A,** Cruzon's syndrome. Oblique view shows turricephaly, midface hypoplasia, hypertelorism, shallow bony orbits, marked bilateral exorbitism, and partial surgical closure of the eyelids to protect the globe. **B,** Apert's syndrome (acrocephalosyndactylism type I). Frontal view shows similar facies with bilateral syndactylism. **C** and **D,** Saethre-Chotzen syndrome (acrocephalosyndactylism type II). **C,** Frontal view shows relatively mild facial asymmetry, mild midface hypoplasia and ptosis of the eyelids. **D,** The hand shows cutaneous syndactyly of the index and middle fingers.

fer's syndrome the abnormal gene maps to chromosome 8p11.2-p12 and has been found to affect FGFR 1.[137] In Apert's syndrome the genetic abnormaity appears to lie at 10q25-q26 and cause problems with FGFR 2.[138] In Crouzon's syndrome the affected gene lies on the distal long arm of chromosome 10.[139] Interestingly, abnormalities of FGFR 3 receptors have now been found to be involved in achondroplasia, a disease process without craniosynostosis.[140,141] Other syndromes with craniosynostosis are now being mapped genetically, including Saethre-Chotzen's syndrome, to 7p21-p22,[142] and Greig cephalopolysyndactyly syndrome, to 7p13.[143,144]

Cruzon's syndrome, Apert's syndrome, and Saethre-Chotzen's syndrome are considered related forms of craniofacial dysostosis (Fig. 1-55). Crouzon syndrome is the most frequent form of craniofacial dysostosis with an incidence of 1 in 25,000 in the general population. It is an autosomal dominant trait with variable expressivity. Crouzon's first family (1912) exhibited characteristic exorbitism, paradoxical retrogenia, retromaxillism, and inframaxillism (Fig. 1-56, *A*). In this condition, bilateral coronal synostosis causes a brachycephalic or oxycephalic cranial vault with shallow orbits and ocular proptosis. The mid-face is flat, and the

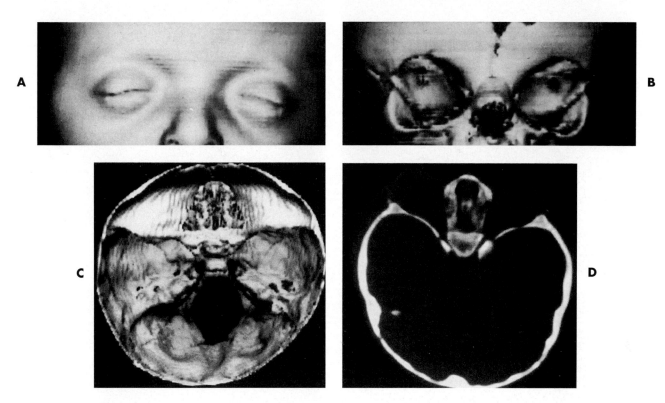

FIG. 1-56 Cruzon's syndrome. **A,** 3D skin surface CT. **B,** Frontal 3D bone surface CT. **C,** 3D bone surface CT of the skull base as seen from above. **D,** Axial CT through the orbits. There are bilaterally symmetrical hypertelorism, shallow bony orbits, exorbitism, and a short anterior fossa.

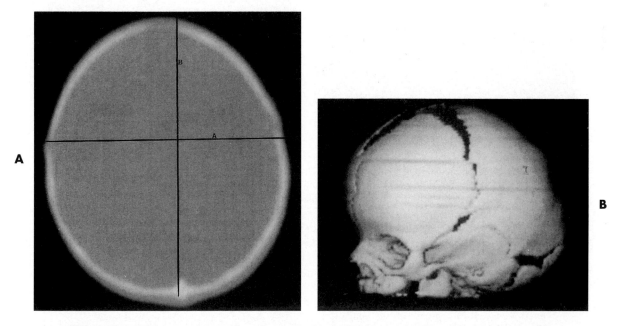

FIG. 1-57 Crouzon's syndrome in a 11-month-old. **A,** Axial bone algorithm CT at the level of the anterior horns of the lateral ventricles demonstrates an increased intercoronal distance *(A)*, defined as the distance between the outer tables of the skull at the level of the anterolateral extent of the lateral ventricles (normal range is 93.4 to 97.1 mm). There is a reduction in the cephalic length *(B)*, defined as the distance between the anterior and posterior points of the outer table of the skull at the level of the anterior horns of the lateral ventricles (normal range is 143.4 to 149.3 mm). **B,** The 3D bone surface CT shows narrowed but patent inferior coronal sutures.

(Continued)

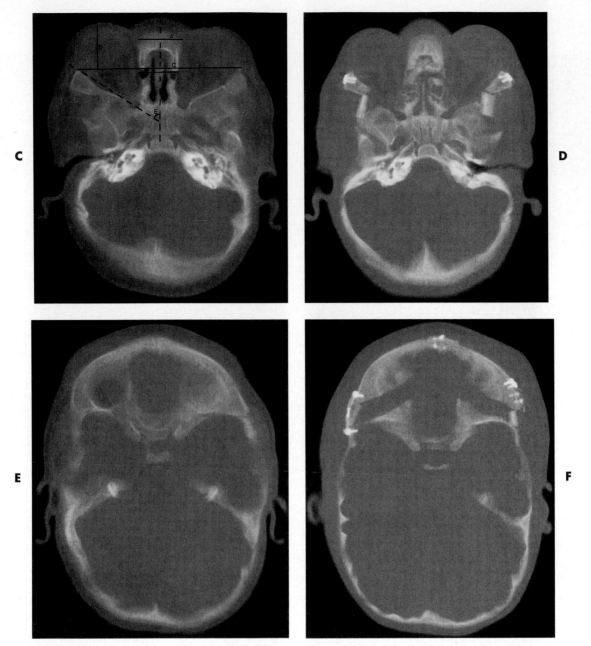

FIG. 1-57, cont'd   **C,** Axial bone algorithm CT at the level of the mid-orbit and orbital roof, before **(C)** and after **(D)** surgery. **C,** Preoperatively the mid-orbit axial bone algorithm image *(C)* demonstrates hypertelorism with widened anterior interorbital distance, mid-orbital distance and lateral orbital distances. The anterior interorbital distance *(A)* is measured between points on the anteriormost aspect on each lacrimal bone along the anterior end of the medial orbital wall (normal range is 17.5 to 18.5 mm). The mid intraorbital distance *(B)* is measured between two points situated midway along the medial orbital wall between the lacrimal bone and the orbital strut (normal range is 16.2 to 17.4 mm). The lateral orbital distance *(C)* is measured between the anterior edges of the lateral orbital walls (normal range is 68.9 to 71.7 mm). Ocular proptosis (exorbitism) is indicated by an increase in the globe proptosis and lateral orbital wall angle. Globe proptosis *(D)* is defined as an increase in the perpendicular distance between the anterior tip of the lateral orbital wall and the most anterior aspect of the globe (normal range is 13.3 to 14.2 mm). The lateral orbital wall angle *(E)* is formed by a line joining the anterior and posterior ends of the lateral orbital wall and the midsagittal axis (normal range is 42.3 to 43.9 degrees). The shallowness of the orbits is also indicated by reduced lateral orbital wall length (normal range is 36.2 to 37.9 mm) and reduced medial orbital wall length (normal range is 31.9 to 33.8 mm). **D,** Postoperative axial bone algorithm CT demonstrates the placement of spit-thickness calvarial grafts along the lateral orbital walls and the cribriform plate to increase the lengths of the lateral and medial orbital walls. **E,** Preoperative axial bone algorithm CT demonstrates a shallow anterior cranial fossa floor and narrow optic canals. **F,** Postoperative axial bone algorithm CT through the floor of the anterior cranial fossa shows osteotomies through the orbital roofs and placement of nail-and-plate fixation devices.

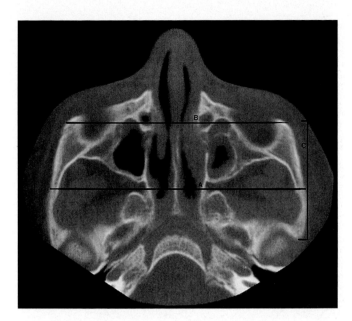

FIG. 1-58 Crouzon's syndrome. Maxillary hypoplasia. Axial bone algorithm CT through the zygomatic arches demonstrates low to normal range measurements of the interzygomatic arch distance, interzygomatic buttress distance, and zygomatic arch length. The interzygomatic arch distance *(A)* is defined as the distance between the most lateral aspect of each zygomatic arch (normal range is 79.1 to 82.8 mm). The interzygomatic buttress distance *(B)* is the distance between the anterolateral extent of each zygomatic buttress (normal range is 65.5 mm to 69.2 mm). Zygomatic arch length *(C)* is the distance from the base of the zygomatic arch to the insertion into the zygomatic buttress (normal range is 37.6 to 40.4 mm).

nasal passages are partially obstructed, causing mouth breathing. The extremities are spared. Tessier (1971) performed the first definitive repair of Crouzon's syndrome in adults.[145]

Apert's syndrome (acrocephalosyndactyly type 1) is a second, less common form of craniofacial dysostosis with an incidence of 1 in 100,000 in the general population (Fig. 1-56, *B*). It is also an autosomal dominant trait, but most cases are sporadic, indicating new mutations. First reported in 1894 and later by Apert in 1906, this condition is characterized by bilateral coronal synostoses, deformity of the cranial vault, syndactylism, and mental retardation associated with blindness. Hydrocephalus may require shunt decompression before craniofacial surgery is performed. The cranial changes appear to be more severe in Apert's syndrome than in Crouzon's syndrome, causing more severe redirection of the anterior cranial base and orbits with greater brain compression and more prominent bulging eyes.[146] Orbital hypertelorism is usually present. Midface hypoplasia, class III malocclusion and anterior open-bite deformities are more severe than those seen in Crouzon patients.[146] The incidence of cleft palate is 30%. Other associated abnormalities include ankylosis of the elbows, hips, and shoulders and associated cardiovascular, gastrointestinal, and genitourinary problems.

Saethre-Chotzen syndrome (acrocephalosyndactyly type II) was first described by Saethre in 1931 and then Chotzen in 1932. These children have multiple synostoses of the cranial sutures, facial asymmetry, mild midface hypoplasia, ptosis of the eyelids, anti-mongoloid slant of the palpebral fissures, beaked noses, and low-set frontal hairlines (Fig. 1-56, *C*). The cutaneous syndactyly typically involves the second and third fingers (Fig. 1-56, *D*).[147]

Surgical repair of these craniofacial syndromes is usually performed as a staged reconstruction consisting of three to four major types of craniomaxillofacial procedures.[146] These include cranial vault reconstruction in infancy, further revision with cranioorbital reshaping in later infancy or early childhood, and total mid-face osteotomy and advancement in later childhood around 5 to 7 years of age. LeFort III osteotomy or monobloc osteotomies are usually performed. Maxillary repositioning (LeFort I osteotomy) with genioplasty in adolescence may also be required. Recent work has shown that despite early surgical attempts at craniofacial correction, little long-term improvement of the craniofacial dysmorphology of these children results. These efforts, however, do limit the effect of increased intracranial pressure on the brain and orbit.[148-150]

Imaging procedures in patients with craniofacial dysostosis are directed at quantifying the severity of pathology in the craniofacial region and documenting the response to surgical intervention. To this end, cephalometric radiography utilizes plain skull radiographs obtained at predetermined distances and angles to compare the preoperative and postoperative changes and improvements.[151] Digital cephalometric procedures now allow on-line computer analysis of these data.[152] Roentgen stereometry assesses motion between skull bones in three dimensions (3D) to monitor postoperative resolution of the synostoses and associated facial hypoplasia.[153]

Presently CT and 3D CT surface renderings are the paramount diagnostic tool for craniofacial dysostosis (Figs. 1-57, 1-58). Children with craniofacial dysostosis exhibit a widened anterior intercoronal distance and a slightly reduced cranial length corresponding to the clinical findings of brachycephaly (Fig. 1-57, *A-D*). The orbits reveal widened anterior and mid-interorbital distances, which confirm the clinical observation of hypertelorism. The lateral and medial orbital walls are short and the globe protrudes anterior to a coronal plane through the two lateral orbital walls. The two lateral orbital walls form a more obtuse angle in relation to each other, and these findings account for the clinically noted proptosis (Fig. 1-57, *E-H*). In the upper midface region the width of the zygomatic arch distances is reduced, and the lengths of the zygomatic arches are usually shortened and identified as clinical maxillary hypoplasia (Fig. 1-58).[154,155]

To study these patients, the patient is positioned in the scanner as evenly as possible, using scout views in both the A-P and sagittal planes to help with alignment. This may

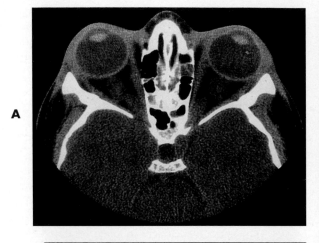

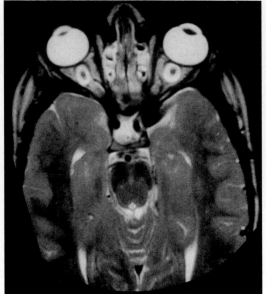

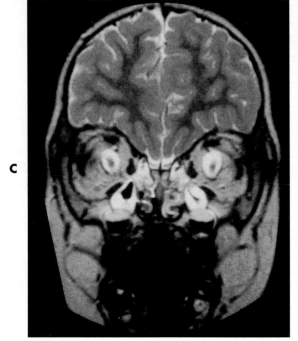

FIG. 1-59 *(right)* Untreated Crouzon's syndrome in a 3-year-old. **A,** Axial CT demonstrates orbital hypertelorism, bilateral shallow orbits, and ocular exorbitism. Increased thickness along the optic sheaths could be enlarged optic nerves, sheaths, or neoplasm. **B** and **C,** Axial and coronal T2W MR demonstrate bilateral prominent perineural subarachnoid space and normal optic nerves. The optic canals appear small. There is a mild harlequin shape to the orbit.

prove difficult when there is marked calvarial asymmetry. Routine axial sections are then performed along the canthomeatal line. Spiral CT is performed in axial and coronal planes with 3 mm interval and a pitch of 1 to 1. Three dimensional reformation is performed utilizing 1 mm interpolated images, and the 3D images are displayed at 15° intervals.

Quantitative orbital measurements are obtained from an axial scan through the ocular globe, optic nerve, ethmoid air cells, nasal bones, and superior aspect of the frontal processes of the zygomatic bones. Measured distances consist of lateral orbital distance, globe protrusion, medial orbital wall length, lateral orbital wall length, lateral orbital wall angle, and anterior and mid-interorbital distances (Fig. 1-57, *E*)

Measurements of the upper midface (zygomatic) region are performed on an axial scan transecting the zygomatic arches. The interzygomatic arch distances, interzygomatic buttress distance, and zygomatic arch lengths are recorded (Fig. 1-58).

The calvarium is measured on an axial scan through the anterior horns of the lateral ventricles. Distances measured are the intercoronal distance and cephalic length (Fig. 1-57, *C*). These measurements assist the craniofacial surgeons in following the disease, planning surgical correction, and assessing operative results.

MR may also be performed in these patients to evaluate the optic nerve and to distinguish it from the optic sheath and perineural space, which may become enlarged secondary to hydrocephalus and small optic canals (Fig. 1-59). MR is also useful in following the extent of any concurrent hydrocephalus and in evaluating concurrent anomalies of the craniovertebral junction.

References

1. DeMyer W. Median facial malformations and their implications for brain malformations. Birth defects (Orig Article Ser) 1975; 11:155.

2. Patten BM. The normal development of the facial region. In: Pruzansky S, ed. Congenital anomalies of the face and associated structures. Springfield, Ill: Thomas Publishing Co, 1985.

3. Johnston MC, Hassell JR, Brown KS. The embryology of cleft lip and cleft palate. Clin Plast Surg 1975; 2:195-203.

4. Kawamoto HK Jr. The kaleidoscopic world of rare craniofacial clefts: order out of chaos (Tessier classification). Clin Plast Surg 1976; 3:529.

5. Davies J. Embryology and anatomy of the face, palate, nose and paranasal sinuses. In: Paparella MM, Shumrick DA, eds. Otolaryngology. Vol 1. Philadelphia, Pa: W B Saunders Co, 1973.

6. Arey LB. Developmental anatomy. Philadelphia, Pa: W B Saunders Co, 1962.

7. Corliss CE. Patten's human embryology. New York, NY: McGraw-Hill Inc, 1976.

8. Moore KL. The developing human. Philadelphia, Pa: W B Saunders Co, 1977.

9. Wilson DB. Embryonic development of the head and neck. III. The face. Head Neck Surg 1979; 2:145.

10. Badrawy R. Midline congenital anomalies of the nose. J Laryngol Otol 1967; 81:419-429.

11. Last RJ. Anatomy regional and applied. 6th Edition. London, England: Churchill Livingstone Inc, 1978; 398.

12. Etter LE. Atlas of roentgen anatomy of the skull. 3rd Edition. Springfield, Ill: Thomas Publishing Co, 1970.

13. Henderson SG, Sherman LS. The roentgen anatomy of the skull in the newborn infant. Radiology 1946; 2:107-118.

14. Streeter GL. Developmental horizons in human embryo, 1948. In: Paparella MM, Shumrick DA, eds. Otolaryngology. Vol 1. Philadelphia, Pa: W B Saunders Co, 1973.

15. Langman J. Medical embryology: human development, normal and abnormal. 2nd Edition. Baltimore, Md: Williams & Wilkins, 1969.

16. Apple DJ, Rabb MF, Walsh PM. Congenital anomalies of the optic disc. Surv Ophthal 1982; 27:3-41.

17. Steinkuller PG. The morning glory disk anomaly: case report and literature review. J Pediatr Ophthal Strabismus 1980; 17:81-87.

18. Yanoff M, Fine BS. Ocular pathology: a text and atlas. 2nd Edition. Philadelphia, Pa: Harper & Row, Publishers Inc, 1982; 608.

19. Naidich TP, et al. Midline craniofacial dysraphism: midline cleft upper lip, basal encephalocele, callosal agenesis, and optic nerve dysplasia. Concepts Pediatr Neurosurg 1977; 4:186.

20. Probst FP. Congenital defects of the corpus callosum: morphology and encephalographic appearances. Acta Radiol 1973; 331 (suppl):1-152.

21. Rakic P, Yakovlev P. Development of the corpus callosum and cavum septi in man. J Comp Neurol 1968; 132:45-72.

22. DeMyer W. The median cleft face syndrome: differential diagnosis of cranium bifidum occultum, hypertelorism, and median cleft nose, lip and palate. Neurology 1967; 17:961-971.

23. Sedano HO, Cohen MM Jr, Jirasek J, et al. Frontonasal dysplasia. J Pediatr 1970; 76:906-913.

24. Gorlin RJ, Anderson VE, Scott CR. Hypertrophied frenuli, oligophrenia, familial trembling and anomalies of the hand: report of four cases in one family and a forme fruste in another. N Engl J Med 1961; 264:486-489.

25. Townes PL, Wood BP, McDonald JV. Further heterogeneity of the oral-facial-digital syndromes. Am J Dis Child 1976; 130:548-554.

26. Goodman RM, Gorlin RJ. Atlas of the face in genetic disorders. 2nd Edition. St. Louis, Mo: CV Mosby Co, 1975.

27. Starck WJ, Epker BN. Surgical repair of a median cleft of the upper lip. J Oral Maxillofac Surg 1994; 52:1217-1219.

28. Fogh-Anderson P. Rare clefts of the face. Acta Chir Scand 1965; 129:275-281.

29. Ingraham RD, Matson DD. Spina bifida and cranium bifidum. IV. An unusual nasopharyngeal encephalocele. N Engl J Med 1943; 228:815-820.

30. Avanzini G, Crivelli G. A case of sphenopharyngeal encephalocele. Acta Neurochir 1970; 22:205-212.

31. Baraton J, Ernest C, Poree C, et al. The neuroradiological examination of endocrine disorders of central origin in the child (precocious puberty, hypopituitarism). Pediatr Radiol 1976; 4:69-478.

32. Byrd SE, Harwood-Nash DC, Fitz CR, et al. Computed tomography in the evaluation of encephaloceles in infants and children. J Comput Assist Tomogr 1978; 2:81-87.

33. Corbett JJ, Savino PJ, Schatz NJ, et al. Cavitary developmental defects of the optic disc: visual loss associated with optic pits and colobomas. Arch Neurol 1980; 37:210-213.

34. Danoff D, Serbu J, French LA. Encephalocoele extending into the sphenoid sinus. J Neurosurg 1966; 24:684-686.

35. Ellyin F, Khatir AH, Singh SP. Hypothalamic-pituitary functions in patients with transsphenoidal encephalocele and midfacial anomalies. J Clin Endocr Metab 1980; 51:854-856.

36. Exner A. Uber basale Cephalocelen. Dt Z Chir 1907; 908:23-41.

37. Goldhammer Y, Smith JL. Optic nerve anomalies in basal encephalocele. Arch Opthal 1975; 93:115-118.

38. Jacob JB. Les Menigo-encephaloceles anterieures de la base du crane, Maroc Med 1961; 40:73-104.

39. Koenig SB, Naidich TP, Lissner G. The morning glory syndrome associated with sphenoidal encephalocele. Ophthalmology 1982; 89:1368-1373.

40. Larsen JL, Bassoe HH. Transsphenoidal meningocele with hypothalamic insufficiency. Neuroradiology 1979; 18:205-209.

41. Lewin ML, Shuster MM. Transpalatal correction of basilar meningocele with cleft palate. Arch Surg 1965; 90:687-693.

42. Lichtenberg G. Congenital tumour of the mouth involving the brain and connected with other malforma-

tions. Trans London Soc Pathol 1867; 18:250.

43. Manelfe C, Starling-Jardin D, Toubi S, et al. Transsphenoidal encephalocele associated with agenesis of corpus callosum: value of metrizamide computed cisternography. J Comput Assist Tomogr 1978; 2:356.

44. Modesti LM, Glasauer FE, Terplan KL. Sphenoethmoidal encephalocele: a case report with review of the literature. Child's Brain 1977; 3:140-153.

45. Oldfield MC. An encephalocele associated with hypertelorism and cleft palate. Brit J Surg 1938; 25:757-764.

46. Pinto RS, George AE, Koslow M, et al. Neuroradiology basal anterior fossa (transethmoidal) encephaloceles. Radiology 1975; 117:79-85.

47. Pollock JA, Newton TH, Hoyt WF. Trans-sphenoidal and transethmoidal encephaloceles: a review of clinical and roentgen features in 8 cases. Radiology 1968; 90:442-453.

48. Sadeh M, Goldhammer Y, Shacked I, et al. Basal encephalocele associated with suprasellar epidermoid cyst. Arch Neurol 1982; 39:250-252.

49. Sakoda K, Ishikawa S, Uozumil T, et al. Sphenoethmoidal meningoencephalocele associated with agenesis of corpus callosum and median cleft lip and palate: case report. J Neurosurg 1979; 51:397-401.

50. Van Nouhuys JM, Bruyn GW. Nasopharyngeal transsphenoidal encephalocele, crater-like hole in the optic disc and agenesis of the corpus callosum: pneumoencephalographic visualization in a case. Psychiatria Neur Neurochir 1964; 67:243-258.

51. Weise GM, Kempe LG, Hammon WM. Transsphenoidal meningohydroencephalocele: case report. J Neurosurg 1972; 37:475.

52. Collier M, Adias L. Les anomalies congenitales des dimensions papillaires. Cliniq Ophtal 1960; 2:1.

53. Kindler P. Morning glory syndrome: unusual congenital optic disk anomaly. Am J Ophthal 1970; 69:376-384.

54. Krause U. Three cases of the morning glory syndrome. Acta Ophthal 1972; 50:188.

55. Malbran JL, Maria-Roveda J. Megalopapila. Archos Oftal B Aires 1951; 26:331-335.

56. Itakura T, Miyamoto K, Uematsu Y, et al. Bilateral morning glory syndrome associated with sphenoid encephalocele: case report. J Neurosurg 1992; 77:949-951.

57. Wexler MR, Benmeir P, Umansky F, et al. Midline cleft syndrome with sphenoethmoidal encephalocele: a case report. J Craniofac Surg 1991; 2:38-41.

58. Beyer WB, Quencer RM, Osher RH. Morning glory syndrome: a functional analysis including fluorescein angiography, ultrasonography, and computerized tomography. Ophthalmology 1982; 89:1362-1367.

59. Yock DH Jr. Choroid plexus lipomas associated with lipoma of the corpus callosum. J Comput Assist Tomogr 1980; 4:678-682.

60. Suemitsu T, Nakajima SI, Kuwajimak, et al. Lipoma of the corpus callosum: report of a case and review of the literature. Child's Brain 1979; 5:476-483.

61. Zee CS, McComb JG, Segall HD, et al. Lipomas of the corpus callosum associated with frontal dysraphism. J Comput Assist Tomogr 1981; 5:201-205.

62. Naidich TP, Osborn RE, Bauer B, et al. Median cleft face syndrome: MR and CT data from 11 children. J Comput Assist Tomogr 1988; 12:57-64.

63. Pascual-Castroviejo I, Pascual-Pascual SI, Perez-Higueras A. Fronto-nasal dysplasia and lipoma of the corpus callosum. Euro J Pediatr 1985; 144:66-71.

64. Tessier P. Anatomical classification of facial, craniofacial, and lateral facial clefts. J Maxillofacial Surg 1976; 4:69-92.

65. Naidich TP, Braffman BH, Altman N, et al. Congenital malformations involving the anterior cranial fossa. Riv Neuroradiologica 1994; 7:359-576.

66. Cohen MM, et al. Frontonasal dysplasia (median cleft face syndrome): comments on etiology and pathogenesis. Birth Defects 1971; 7:117.

67. Warkany J, Bofinger MK, Benton C. Median facial cleft syndrome in half-sisters: dilemmas in genetic counseling. Teratology 1973; 8:273-285.

68. Bakken AF, Aabyholm G. Frontonasal dysplasia: possible hereditary connection with other congenital defects.

Clin Genet 1976; 10:214-217.

69. Fontaine G, Walbaum R, Poupard B, et al. La dysplasie frontonasale. J Genet Hum 1983; 31:351-365.

70. Fragoso R, Cid-Garcia A, Hernandez A, et al. Frontonasal dysplasia in the Klippel-Feil syndrome: a new associated malformation. Clin Genet 1982; 22:270-273.

71. Francois J, Eggermont E, Evens L, et al. Agenesis of the corpus callosum in the median facial cleft syndrome and associated ocular malformations. Am J Ophthalmol 1973; 76:241-245.

72. Fuenmayor HM. The spectrum of frontonasal dysplasia in an inbred pedigree. Clin Genet 1980; 17:137.

73. Hori A. A brain with two hypophyses in median cleft face syndrome. Acta Neuropathol 1983; 59:150-154.

74. Ide CH, Holt JE. Median cleft face syndrome associated with orbital hypertelorism and polysyndactyly. Eye Ear Nose Throat Monthly 1975; 54:150-151.

75. Kinsey JA, Streeten BW. Ocular abnormalities in the median cleft face syndrome. Am J Ophthalmol 1977; 83:261-266.

76. Roizenblatt J, Wajntal A, Diament AJ. Median cleft face syndrome or frontonasal dysplasia: a case report with associated kidney malformation. J Pediatr Ophthalmol Strabis 1979; 16:16.

77. Aleksic S, et al. Intracranial lipomas, hydrocephalus, and other CNS anomalies in oculoaricularvertebral dysplasia (Goldenhar-Gorlin syndrome). Child's Brain 1984; 11:285-297.

78. Gorlin RJ, Pindborg JJ, Cohen MM Jr. Syndromes of the head and neck, New York, NY: McGraw-Hill Inc, 1964; 10.

79. Shokeir MHK. The Goldenhar syndrome: a natural history. Birth Defects 1977; 13:67-83.

80. Ryals BD, Brown DC, Levin SW. Duplication of the pituitary gland as shown by MR. AJNR 1993; 14:137-139.

81. Chapman S, Goldin JH, Hendel RG, et al. The median cleft face syndrome with associated cleft mandible, bifid odontoid peg and agenesis of the anterior arch of atlas. Br J Oral Maxillofac Surg 1991; 29:279-281.

82. Kurlander GJ, DeMyer W, Campbell JA. Roentgenology of the median

cleft face syndrome, Radiology 1967; 88:473-478.

83. de Villiers JC, Cluver PF, Pter JC. Lipoma of the corpus callosum associated with frontal and facial anomalies. Acta Neurochir Suppl (Wien) 1991; 53:1-6.

84. Scott JH. The cartilage of the nasal septum (a contribution to the study of facial growth). Br Dent J 1953; 95:37-43.

85. Mood GF. Congenital anterior herniations of brain. Ann Otol Rhinol Laryngol 1938; 47:391-401.

86. Naidich TP, Takahashi S, Towbin RB. Normal patterns of ossification of the skull base: ages 0-16 years. Paper presented at the 71st Scientific Assembly and Annual Meeting, Chicago, Ill: Radiological Society of North America, Nov 19, 1985.

87. Sessions RB. Nasal dermal sinuses— new concepts and explanations. II. Laryngoscope 1982; 92(suppl 29).

88. McQuown SA, Smith JD, Gallo AE Jr. Intracranial extension of asal dermoids. Neurosurgery 1983; 12:531-535.

89. Chaudhari AB, Ladapo F, Mordi VP, et al. Congenital inclusion cyst of the subgaleal space. J Neurosurg 1982; 56:540-544.

90. Choudhury AR, Taylor JC. Primary intranasal encephalocele: report of four cases. J Neurosurg 1982; 57:552-555.

91. Gorenstein A, Kern EB, Facer GW, et al. Nasal gliomas. Arch Otolaryngol 1980; 106:536-540.

92. Card GG. Dermoid cyst of nose with intracranial extension. Arch Otolaryngol 1978; 104:301-302.

93. Pannell BW, Hendrick EG, Hoffman JH, et al. Dermoid cysts of the anterior fontanelle. Neurosurgery 1982; 10:317-323.

94. Bradley PK. Nasal dermoids in children. Int J Pediatr Otorhinolaryngol 1981; 3:63.

95. Pensler JM, Bauer BS, Naidich TP. Craniofacial dermoids. Plast Reconstr Surg 1988; 82:953-958.

96. Griffith BH. Frontonasal tumors: their diagnosis and management. Plast Reconstr Surg 1976; 57:692-699.

97. Muhlbauer WD, Dittmar W. Hereditary median dermoid cysts of the nose. Br J Plast Surg 1976; 29:334-340.

98. Plewes JL, Jacobson I. Familial frontonasal dermoid cysts: report of four cases. J Neurosurg 1971; 34:683-686.

99. Johnson GF, Weisman PA. Radiological features of dermoid cysts of the nose. Radiology 1964; 82:1016-1021.

100. Barkovich AJ, Vandermarck P, Edwards MSB, et al. Congenital-nasal masses: CT and MR imaging features in 16 cases. AJNR 1991; 12:105-116.

101. Black BK, Smith DE. Nasal glioma: two cases with recurrence. Arch Neurol Psychiatr 1950; 64:614-630.

102. Harley EH. Pediatric congenital nasal masses. Ear Nose Throat J 1991; 70:28-32.

103. Walker EA Jr, Resler DR. Nasal glioma. Laryngoscope 1963; 73:93-107.

104. Derkay CS, Tunnessen WW Jr. Pictures of the month case 1 nasal glioma. Arch Pediatr Adolesc Med 1994; 148:953-954.

105. Braun M, Boman F, Hascoet JM, et al. Brain tissue heterotopia in the nasopharynx: contribution of MRI to assment of extension. J Neuroradiol 1992; 19:68-74.

106. Christianson HB. Nasal glioma: report of a case. Arch Derm 1966; 93:68-70.

107. Smith KR Jr, Schwartz HG, Luse SA, et al. Nasal gliomas: a report of five cases with electron microscopy of one. J Neurosurg 1963; 20:968-982.

108. Witrak BJ, Davis PC, Hoffman JC Jr. Sinus pericranii: a case report. Pediatr Radiol 1986; 16:55-56.

109. Suwanwela C, Hongsaprabhas C. Frontoethmoidal encephalomeningocele. J Neurosurg 1966; 25:172-182.

110. Kurzer A, Arbelaez N, Cassiano G. Gliomas of the face: case report. Plast Reconstr Surg 1982; 69:678-682.

111. Naidich TP, Altman NR, Braffman BH, et al. Cephaloceles and related malformations. AJNR 1992; 13:655-690.

112. Finerman WB, Pick EI. Intranasal encephalo-meningocele. Ann Otol Rhinol Laryngol 1953; 62:114-120.

113. Suwanwela C, Suwanwela N. A morphological classification of sincipital encephalomeningoceles. J Neurosurg 1972; 36:201-211.

114. Blumenfeld R, Skolnik EM. Intranasal encephaloceles. Arch Otolaryng 1965; 82:527-531.

115. Simpson DA, David DJ, White J. Cephaloceles: treatment, outcome and antenatal diagnosis. Neurosurgery 1984; 15:14-20.

116. Mahatumarat C, Taecholarn C, Charoonsmith T. One-stage extracranial repair and reconstruction for frontoethmoidal encephalomeningocele: a new simple technique. J Craniofac Surg 1991; 2:127-134.

117. Clauser L, Baciliero U, Nordera P, et al. Frontoethmoidal meningoencephalocele: a one-stage correction, reconstruction, and plating by means of the micro system. J Craniofac Surg 1991; 2:2-8.

118. Willner A, Kantrowitz AB, Cohen AF. Intrasphenoidal encephalocele: diagnosis and management. Otolaryngol Head Neck Surg 1994; 111:8348-837.

119. Jacob OJ, Rosenfeld JV, Watters DA. The repair of frontal encephaloceles in Papua New Guinea. Aust N Z J Surg 1994; 64:8568-8600.

120. Smit CS, Zeeman BJ, Smith RM, et al. Frontoethmoidal meningoencephaloceles: a review of 14 consecutive patients. J Craniofac Surg 1993; 4:210-214.

121. Rappoport RL II, Dunn RC, Alhady F. Anterior encephalocele. J Neurosurg 1981; 54:213.

122. Wakisaka S, Okuda S, Soejima T, et al. Sinus pericranii. Surg Neurol 1983; 19:291.

123. Harverson G, Bailey IC, Kiryabwire JWM. The radiological diagnosis of anterior encephalocoeles. Clin Radiol 1974; 25:317-322.

124. Levy RA, Wald SL, Aitken PA, et al. Bilateral intraorbital meningoencephaloceles and associated midline craniofacial anomalies: MR and three-dimensional CT imaging. AJNR 1989; 10:1272-1274.

125. Naidich TP, Bauer B. Infected dermal sinus. Case 11, set 28: Neuroradiology test and syllabus part 1. Reston, American College of Radiology, 1990; 242-304.

126. Naidich TP, Osborn RE, Bauer BS, et al. Embryology and congenital lesions of the midface. In: Som PE, Bergeron RT eds. Head and neck imaging. St. Louis, Mo: Mosby–Year Book, 1991; 1-50.

127. Cohen MM Jr, Lemire RJ. Syndromes with cephaloceles. Teratology 1982; 26:161-172.

128. Yokota A, Matsukado Y, Fuwa I, et al.

Anterior basal encephalocele of the neonatal and infantile period. Neurosurgery 1986; 19:468-478.

129. Schmidt PH, Luyendijk W. Intranasal meningoencephalocele. Arch Otolaryngol 1974; 99:402-405.

130. Virchow HR. Ueber den Cretinismus, namentlich in Franken, und uber pathologische Schadelforamen. Ver Phys Med Ges Wurzburg 1852; 2:230-241.

131. Moss ML. Functional anatomy of cranial synostosis. Childs Brain 1975; 1:22-33.

132. Cohen MM Jr. Genetic perspectives on craniosynostosis and syndromes with craniosynostosis. J Neurosurg 1977; 47:886-898.

133. Fernbach SK, Naidich TP. Radiological evaluation of craniosynostosis. In: Cohen MM Jr. Craniosynostosis, diagnosis, evaluation and management. New York, NY: Raven Press, 1986; 191-214.

134. Posnick JC, Lin KY, Chen P, et al. Metopic synostosis: quantitative assessment of presenting defority and surgical results based on CT scans. Plast Reconstr Surg 1994; 93:16-24.

135. Gault DT, Renier D, Marchac D et al. Intracranial pressure and intracranial volume in children with craniosynostosis. Plast Reconstructr Surg 1992; 90:377-381.

136. Reardon W, Winter RM, Rutland P, et al. Mutations in the fibroblast growth receptor 2 gene cause Crouzon syndrome. Nature Genet 1994; 8:98-103.

137. Muenke M, Schell U, Hehr A, et al. A common mutation in the fibroblast growth factor receptor 1 gene in Pfeiffer syndrome. Nature Genet 1994; 8:269-274.

138. Wilkie AOM, Slaney SF, Oldridge M, et al. Apert syndrome results from localized mutations of FGFR2 and is allelic with Crouzon syndrome. Nature Genet 1995; 9:165-172.

139. Preston RA, Post JC, Keats BJ et al: A gene for Crouzon craniofacial dysostosis maps to the long arm of chromosome 10. Nature Genet 1994; 7:149-153.

140. Shiang R, Thompson LM, Zhu YZ, et al. Mutations in the transmembrane domain of FGFR3 cause the most common genetic form of dwarfism, achondroplasia. Cell 1994; 78:335-342.

141. Rousseau F, Bonaventure J, Legeai-Mallet L, et al. Mutations in the gene encoding fibroblast growth factor receptor-3 in achondroplasia. Nature 1994; 371:252-254.

142. Brueton LA, van Herwerden L, Chotai KA, et al. The mapping of a gene for craniosynostosis: evidence for linkage of the Saethre-Chotzen syndrome to distal chromosome 7p. J Med Genet 1992; 29:681-685.

143. Vortkamp A, Gessler M, Grzeschik KH. GLI3 zinc-finger gene interrupted by translocations in Greig syndrome families. Nature 1991; 352:539-540.

144. Hui CC, Joyner AL. A mouse model of Greig cephalopolysyndactyly syndrome: the extra-toes mutation contains an intragenic deletion of the Gli3 gene. Nature Genet 1993; 3:241-246.

145. Tessier P. The definitive plastic surgical treatment of the severe facial deformities of craniofacial dysostosis: crouzon's and apert's diseases. Plastic Reconstructive Surgery 1971; 48:419-422.

146. Posnick JC. Craniofacial dysostosis: staging of reconstruction and management of the midface deformity. Neurosurgical Clinics of North 1991; America 2(3).

147. Som PM, Bergeron RT, eds. Head and neck imaging. 2nd Edition. St. Louis, Mo: Mosby–Year Book, 1991; 771-776.

148. Posnick JC, Lin KY, Jhawar BJ, et al. Crouzon syndrome: quantitative assessment of presenting deformity and surgical results based on CT scans. Plastic Reconstructive Surgery 92: 1991; 1027-1037.

149. Machado HR, Hoffman, HJ. Long-term results after lateral canthal advancement for unilateral coronal synostosis. J Neurosurg 1992; 76:401-407.

150. Marchac D, Renier D, Broumand S. Timing of treatment for craniosynostosis and faciocraniosynostosis: a 20-year experience. Br J Plast Surg 1994; 47:211-222.

151. Kreiborg S, Aduss H. Pre- and post-surgical facial growth in patients with Crouzon and Apert syndromes. Cleft Palate Jour. 1986; 23(suppl. 1):78.

152. Friede H, Lilja J, Lauritzen L, et al. Skull morphology after early craniotomy in patients with premature synostosis of the coronal suture. Cleft Palate Jour 1986; (suppl. 1): 1-8.

153. Rune B, Selvik G, Kreiborg S, et al. Motion of bones and volume changes in the neurocranium after craniectomy in Crouzon's disease: A roentgen stereometric study. J Neurosurgery 1979; 50:494-498.

154. Waitzman AA, Posnick JC, Pron GE, et al. Craniofacial skeletal measurements based on computed tomography: part II. Normal values and growth trends. Cleft Palate Craniofacial Jour 1992; 29:118-128.

155. Carr M, Posnick JC, Pron G, et al. Cranio-orbito-aygomatic measurements from standard CT scans in unoperated crouzon and apert infants: comparison with normal controls. Cleft Palate Craniofacial Jour 1992; 29:129-136.

2

Sinonasal Cavities: Anatomy, Physiology, and Plain Film Normal Anatomy

PETER M. SOM
MARGARET BRANDWEIN

SECTION ONE
INTRODUCTION TO
THE SINONASAL CAVITY

To many physicians, the nasal cavity and paranasal sinuses represent the centerpiece of the head and neck region. The common nature of sinonasal allergic or infectious disease renders it the most often imaged and therefore the best known of the areas of the head and neck. Facial fractures are also common, ranging from the broken nose to the more severe fractures associated with automobile accidents. Lastly the disfiguring tumors of the sinonasal cavities earn their fearsome reputation because of their poor prognosis and the facial carnage they wreak. It thus seems reasonable to start the discussion of head and neck imaging with the sinonasal region.

ANATOMY AND PHYSIOLOGY

The anatomy of the nose, the paranasal sinuses in general, and the osteomeatal complex in specific are discussed. The imaging appearances of these regions are then presented.

The Nose and Nasal Fossae

The external nose has an overall pyramidal shape.[1-4] The cranial portion of the nose that joins the forehead is called the root. The lower, or caudal free margin, is known as the apex, or tip. The upper midline margin near the root that is supported by the nasal bones is called the bridge, and the more caudal midline, slightly curved ridge is referred to as the dorsum. The lateral nasal margins or sides have expanded, rounded lower aspects called the alae, which unite with the upper lip at the nasolabial sulcus. The caudal aspect of the midline nasal septum and the nasal alae form the boundaries of the nostrils, or nares, which are the external openings of the nose that provide entrance into the nasal fossa, or nasal vault. The lower aspect of the nasal septum that borders the nostrils and merges with the nasolabial sulcus is called the columella (Fig. 2-1).

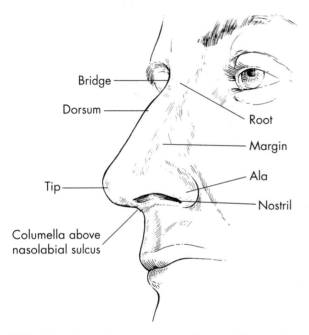

FIG. 2-1   The surface anatomy of the nose illustrated in a left anterior oblique view.

The two nasal bones are usually narrower and thicker on their cranial margins and wider and thinner on their caudal aspects. The medial articular surfaces are broader than the lateral margins. The posterior aspects of the nasal bones in the midline project backward and downward to form a small crest that contributes to the nasal septum. The nasal bones articulate with the nasal process of the frontal bone, the perpendicular plate of the ethmoid bone, and the septal cartilage of the nose (Fig. 2-2). The midline point at which the nasal bones meet the frontal bone is called the nasion. The inferior or caudal midline point where the suture between the nasal bones meets the upper nasal cartilages is referred to as the rhinion. Rarely the nasal bones are fused in the midline or are absent and replaced by an elongated frontal process of the maxilla. The nasal bones are very infrequently multiple.

The osseous opening of the nose is called the pyriform aperture. The lateral nasal cartilages attach to the upper edges of this aperture. There are five major nasal cartilages that form the main support of the lateral and lower nose. There are two lateral, or upper, nasal cartilages; two greater alar, or lower, nasal cartilages; and a median, septal, or quadrangular cartilage. Frequently the lateral nasal and septal cartilages are fused into a single cartilage, the nasoseptal cartilage. There are also a variable number of minor cartilages, including two or three lesser alar cartilages and one or more accessory cartilages (Fig. 2-3). The alar cartilages are formed from elastic cartilage, and the remaining nasal cartilages are formed from hyaline cartilage. Both the bony bridge of the nose and the portion of the nasal dorsum formed by the lateral nasal cartilages have an intrinsic physical strength because these structures on each side are supported and fused in the midline, thus forming an archlike system. These structures are additionally supported in the midline by the septal cartilage. The greater alar cartilages have slender medial crura and broader lateral crura. The lateral crura are curved

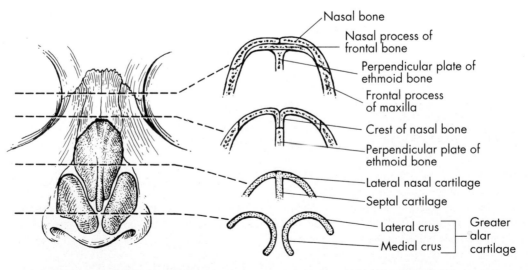

FIG. 2-2   Frontal view of the nose with cross-sectional diagrams at various levels illustrating the support structure of the nasal pyramid. (Modified from Anatomy for Surgeons. Vol 1. The head and neck. New York, NY: Hoeber-Harper, 1954.

plates that form the boundaries of the lateral aspects of the nostrils. In supporting the alae of the nose, the greater alar cartilages are assisted by the lesser alar cartilages. The medial crura join to form the mobile portion of the nasal septum and the support of the columella.[1-5]

The nasal muscles refer to the procerus, nasalis (compressor naris), levator labii superioris alaeque nasi, and the anterior and posterior dilator naris. The procerus and the forehead muscles elevate the skin over the dorsum of the nose. The nasalis (both the transverse and the alar portions) compresses the naris, and the dilators and the levator superioris alaeque nasi dilate the nostrils (Fig. 2-4).

The nasal cavities, or nasal fossae, are separated in the midline by the nasal septum. Each cavity is roughly pear-shaped, being narrow above (cranially) and wide below (caudally) (Fig. 2-5). The roof is formed by the thin cribriform plate of the ethmoid. It is only 5 mm across at its widest posterior margin. The floor is formed by the hard palate. Anteriorly the hard palate is formed by the palatine processes of the maxillae (the anterior two thirds of the hard palate) and posteriorly by the horizontal portions of the palatine bones (the posterior one third of the hard palate) (Fig. 2-6).

The anterior portion of the nasal fossa that corresponds to the alar region of the nose is called the vestibule. It is lined

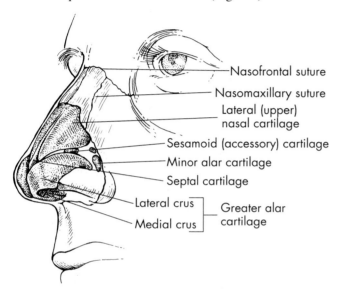

FIG. 2-3 Left anterior oblique view of the nasal skeleton indicating the osseous and cartilagenous anatomy.

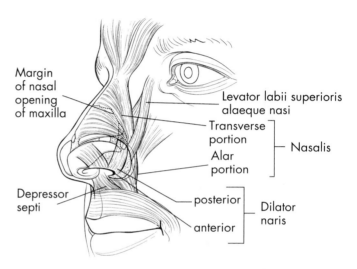

FIG. 2-4 Left anterior oblique veiw of the nose illustrating the nasal musculature.

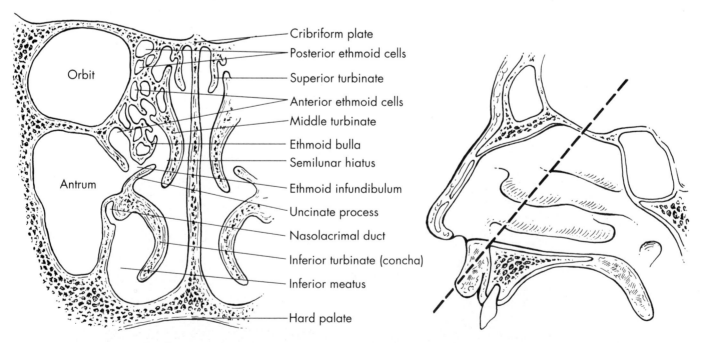

FIG. 2-5 Diagram of a composite oblique section through the nasal fossae structures in the plane depicted in the smaller diagram. Some of the more important anatomic landmarks are identified.

with hair-bearing skin and sebaceous glands. Along the nasal septum there is no demarcation between the vestibule and the remaining nasal fossa. However, along the lateral wall there is a ridge, the limen vestibuli, that corresponds to the lower margin of the lateral nasal cartilage and marks the line of change from the skin of the vestibule into the mucous membrane of the remaining nasal fossa (Fig. 2-7).

The mucosa of the nasal fossa is a reddish, vascular, pseudostratified columnar ciliated epithelium that contains both serous and mucinous glands. The term Schneiderian membrane is given to this mucosa, which is derived embryologically from the invaginating nasal placodes. In the upper margins of the nasal fossa, in a region bounded laterally by the superior nasal concha and the lateral nasal wall above this level and medially by a corresponding portion of the nasal septum, there is a yellowish epithelium with decreased vascularity that is the olfactory mucosa. It contains the bipolar olfactory nerve fibers that transform physical and chemical stimuli into a nerve impulse, which is then transmitted cranially via nerve fibers through the cribriform plate into the olfactory bulbs.[1-4] This mucosa secretes a "mucus" lipolipid material that spreads evenly over the surface of the olfactory epithelium, keeping it moist. The odor that one perceives is the result of the input from the olfactory, trigeminal, glossopharyngeal, and vagus nerves. The properties of a partic-ular odorant appear to determine the particular mix of these neural inputs. Olfactory nerve stimulation, which is necessary to identify most odorants, depends on the odorant molecules reaching the olfactory mucosa. Although diffusion of odorants can provide such access to the olfactory mucosa, the transport is facilitated by normal inhalation. However, because there is no ciliary action on the olfactory mucosa, sniffing appears to be the most efficient way of transporting, via the olfactory recess, the odorant to the olfactory mucosa. The absorption of molecules to the

mucus-lined mucosal passages of the nasal fossa may separate the odorants before they reach the olfactory mucosa, with highly absorbable chemicals possibly having little or no odor because they are absorbed by the nasal wall mucosa before they reach the olfactory mucosa. It appears that the odorant molecules must interact with the olfactory mucus, overlying the receptor cells, because odor apparently is not perceived unless it is in solution. With a dried olfactory mucosa, therefore, there is no perception of smell.[2] In fact, the odors perceived may be the resulting changed molecules. Thus the olfactory mucosa presents the odorant molecules with certain constraints of absorption, solubility, and chemical reactivity.

Once the odorant molecule reaches the receptor cell membrane, this molecule must alter the membrane potential of the olfactory receptor cell. The exact manner in which this is accomplished is not fully understood.[6] Clinically, olfactory cognition appears to develop between the ages of 3 and 5 years. Somewhere between the ages of 3 and 7 years, odor preferences are identified, and these are similar to those of adults living in the same area. Odors appear to be appreciated based upon individual experience and cultural restraints.

The mucosa lining the paranasal sinuses is very similar to that of the nonolfactory portion of the nasal fossa except that it is less vascular, thinner, and more loosely attached to the bone.

The major portion of the nasal septum is formed by the perpendicular plate of the ethmoid bone posteriorly and the septal cartilage anteriorly. The vomer completes the posteroinferior portion of the septum. The medial crura of the greater alar cartilages form the anteroinferior septal margin, or mobile septum. Nasal crests from the maxilla and palatine bones complete the inferior nasal septal margin (Fig. 2-6). The proportionate size of the septal cartilage and the perpendicular plate of the ethmoid bone varies from patient to patient. The septum provides the major support for the dor-

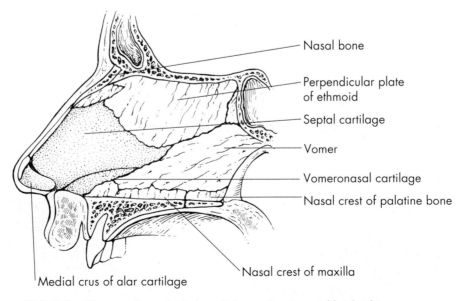

Nasal bone

Perpendicular plate
of ethmoid

Septal cartilage

Vomer

Vomeronasal cartilage

Nasal crest of palatine bone

Nasal crest of maxilla

Medial crus of alar cartilage

FIG. 2-6   Diagram of a sagittal view of the nasal septum and hard palate.

sum of the nose and the region below this, extending to the tip. Damage to the septal cartilage can result in a depressed, "saddle nose" deformity.

The septal cartilage has an unusual mobile articulation with the surrounding bones. The perichondrium of the septal cartilage and the periostium of the perpendicular plate of the ethmoid bone meet in an end-to-end relationship. There is a tongue and groove relationship between the septal cartilage and the vomer, with the thin edge of the cartilage fitting into a groove on the edge of the vomer. Only connective tissue stabilizes this junction. These relationships allow a mobility that minimizes the chance of fracture and allows considerable septal deviation without dislocation.

When compared with the medial septal wall, the lateral nasal wall, which is discussed in detail in Chapter 3, is more intricate (Fig. 2-8). The paranasal sinuses open into the lateral nasal wall, and three or four nasal turbinates, or conchae, project from it. These conchae are delicate, scroll-like projections of bone that are named from below to upward as inferior, middle, superior, and supreme turbinates, respectively. These structures become smaller as they ascend the nasal cavity.

The air space beneath and lateral to each concha is called the meatus. The inferior meatus thus lies beneath and lateral to the inferior turbinate. The middle and superior meati have similar relationships to their respective conchae (Fig. 2-5). The supreme concha is present in only 60% of patients; the supreme meatus is usually only a small furrow beneath it.[1] The dominant structures of the lateral nasal wall are the inferior and middle turbinates.

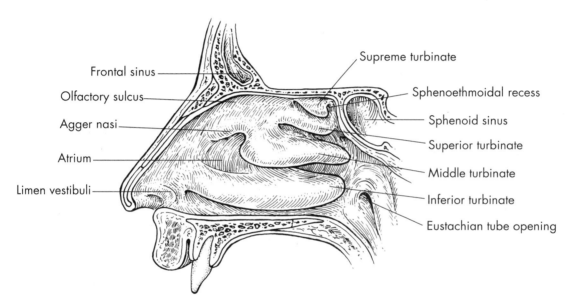

FIG. 2-7 Diagram of a sagittal view of the lateral nasal fossa wall. The midline nasal septum has been removed.

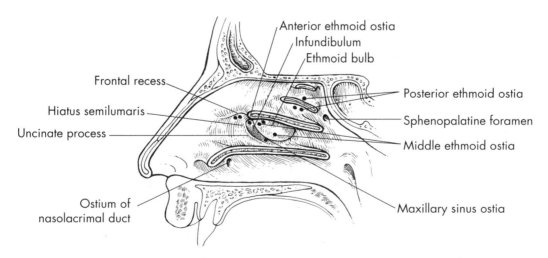

FIG. 2-8 Diagram of a sagittal view of the lateral nasal fossa wall with the turbinates removed. The most common locations of the sinus ostia are indicated.

The inferior turbinate is an independent bone that is covered by a thick mucous membrane, which contains a dense venous plexus, large vascular spaces, and erectile tissue. The nasolacrimal duct is the only major ostium that opens into the inferior meatus. This ostium usually lies high and anteriorly in the lateral nasal wall under the attachment of the inferior turbinate, approximately 2 cm posterior to the nostril. When the nasolacrimal duct opening is high in the inferior meatus, it tends to be wide. When it is located lower in the lateral nasal wall, it tends to be slitlike. As it runs obliquely through the mucosa, it is protected by a fold of this mucous membrane known as the plica lacrimalis, or valve of Hasner. The middle turbinate is part of the ethmoid bone and, like the inferior concha, is also covered with some erectile tissue and a thick, vascular mucous membrane.

The nose functions in breathing, warming, moisturizing, and cleaning inspired air. The teleologic explanation for the division of the nasal fossa by the nasal septum is that one nasal chamber can rest while the other carries on the functions of the nose.[4] This alternation of nasal function is referred to as a nasal cycle, and it is present in about 80% of patients. In a normal nose, one side of the nasal fossa opens with an outpouring of serous and mucinous secretions, while the opposite airway closes with almost complete cessation of such secretory activity. The passage of respiratory air is carried on almost entirely through the open nasal chamber. As the functioning side pours out serous and mucinous secretion, its mucosa shrinks. In addition, there is concurrent shunting of blood to the contralateral highly vascular mucosa, primarily over the inferior and middle turbinates. The nonfunctioning side thus retains secretions and becomes vascularly congested and engorged. This nasal cycle constantly changes the internal dimensions of the nose every 30 minutes to 3 to 7 hours. The total nasal resistance, or conductance, tends to remain constant throughout the cycle. This nasal cycle is most common in the second through fourth decades of life and gradually decreases with progressive age. This cycle can be documented by sectional imaging.[5]

The effect of gravity on the pooling of blood in the excessively vascular tissues over the turbinates is commonly demonstrated by the observation that in many patients, when they lie on one side, the dependent nasal chamber becomes progressively obstructed over a 15- to 20-minute period. When the patient turns to the opposite side, the clogged nasal fossa opens, and the dependent chamber becomes congested within 10 to 15 minutes.[5]

Because there is both a superficial mucosal vascular plexus and a deep erectile vascular zone, there are four major responses that the nasal tissue can give, depending on the nature of the inspired air: (1) hyperemia of surface vessels and filling of the erectile, cavernous tissue in response to cold, dry air, (2) ischemia of the surface vessels and shrinkage of the erectile, cavernous tissue in response to warm, moist air, (3) ischemia of the surface vessels and filling of the erectile, cavernous tissue in response to warm air of average relative humidity, and (4) hyperemia of the surface vessels and shrinkage of the erectile, cavernous tissue in response to superficial irritation.[2]

Under normal conditions, the major air pathway is through the middle meatus. There is less airflow through the inferior meatus, and the least airflow is in the superior recesses of the nose.

Between 1 and 2 L of serous, watery secretions are produced daily by the serous glands, half of which are used to warm and humidify inspired air.[7] Thus air entering the nose is efficiently warmed and humidified before reaching the lungs; the average air temperature before entering the pharynx is 31° to 37° C, and the air humidity is 100%. To perform this function, the average nose has about 160 cm^2 of mucous membrane.[6]

The nose also cleanses inspired air before the air reaches the lungs. A surface film of mucus traps more than 95% of particulate matter larger than 4.5μm. There is a coordinated ciliary action of the nasal mucosa that propels mucus backward and downward into the nasopharynx at the rate of about 6.7 to 10 mm per minute. The cilia beat at a rate of 160 to 1500 beats per minute. The cilia function normally under most circumstances unless the mucous blanket is removed and drying occurs. In this circumstance, cilial function ceases.[6] This movement of mucus is also affected by gravity and the traction that results from swallowing. It has been estimated that three fourths of the bacteria entering the nose are trapped by the mucus and that this nasal mucous blanket is renewed about every 10 to 20 minutes.[7] The normal nasal mucosa resists infection because the mucous blanket removes bacteria and some viruses before they can penetrate the mucosa. In addition, the nasal mucus contains antibodies against both bacteria and viruses.

The motor supply to the nasal respiratory muscles (the procerus, the nasalis, and the depressor septi nasi) is mediated through the seventh cranial nerve. The integration of their contraction with the respiratory cycle is carried to the seventh cranial nerve via the tenth cranial nerve. The physiologically important control of the circulation and secretomotor function to the normal airway is mediated by the autonomic system, primarily via the sphenopalatine ganglion. Sympathetic stimulation results in a pale, dry, shrunken mucosa, and parasympathetic stimulation causes a hypersecreting, hyperemic, swollen mucosa. Pain, temperature, and touch are mediated by branches of the first division of the fifth cranial nerve.[7,8]

Anatomically the vascular and nerve supplies of the nasal fossa almost coincide. One difference is that the nerves tend to pass out of the nose, and the arteries are reinforced by vessels that pass into the nose.[2] The lymphatic drainage follows the veins rather than the arteries. The lymphatics of the anterior half of the nose drain across the face to enter into the submandibular lymph nodes. The lymphatics of the posterior half of the nose and nasopharynx drain into the retropharyngeal and internal jugular chain of nodes.

The venous drainage of the nose is via the anterior facial

vein, then via the common facial vein to the internal jugular vein. The anterior facial vein also communicates with the ophthalmic veins, which drain either directly or via the pterygoid venous plexus into the cavernous sinus. Thus infection of the nose may rapidly spread into the cavernous sinus.[7]

The vascular anatomy of the nasal fossa is complex, involving both external and internal carotid arterial supplies. Of the five arteries that supply the mucoperiosteum of the nasal cavity, the sphenopalatine artery is the most important.[9]

The sphenopalatine artery originates from the third, or pterygopalatine, segment of the maxillary artery. Before it exits the pterygopalatine fossa, the sphenopalatine artery occasionally gives rise to a posterior nasal branch. More commonly, it first exits the superomedial aspect of the pterygopalatine fossa by way of the sphenopalatine foramen. The sphenopalatine artery then enters the nasal fossa behind and slightly above the middle concha.

The sphenopalatine artery has two major groups of branches—the posterior lateral nasal branches and the posterior septal branches. The posterior lateral nasal arteries ramify over the nasal conchae, first giving off branches that supply the inferior turbinate and then giving rise to superior branches that supply the middle and superior turbinates. These lateral nasal branches also assist in supplying the maxillary, ethmoid, and sphenoid sinuses.

After giving origin to the posterolateral nasal branches, the main trunk of the sphenopalatine artery continues medially along the roof of the nasal cavity. When it reaches the nasal septum, the sphenopalatine artery gives off its medial branches, the posterior septal arteries. These branches course anteriorly along the nasal septum. The most

inferior of these branches becomes the nasopalatine artery. This vessel runs through the incisive canal to become continuous with the greater palatine artery (Fig. 2-9).

The anterior and posterior ethmoid arteries originate from the ophthalmic artery and send numerous small branches through the cribriform plate to anastomose with nasal branches of the sphenopalatine artery. This rich anastomotic network provides an important potential collateral pathway between the internal and external carotid circulations.

There are two other arteries that also provide some blood supply to the nasal fossa. The terminal branch of the greater palatine artery enters the incisive foramen, where it anastomoses with the nasopalatine artery (a septal branch of the sphenopalatine artery). The final artery supplying the nasal fossa is the septal branch of the superior labial artery. It originates from the facial artery and supplies the medial wall of the nasal vestibule.

Little's, or Kiesselbach's, area is a localized region of the anteroinferior nasal septum (Fig. 2-9). It is supplied by branches of the facial, sphenopalatine, and greater palatine arteries. This is often referred to as Kiesselbach's plexus and is the site of 90% of the cases of epistaxis.[1]

The Paranasal Sinuses

All of the paranasal sinuses originate as evaginations from the nasal fossae.[10] As such, they are lined by a mucosa similar to that found in the nasal cavity. It is a pseudostratified columnar ciliated epithelium that contains both mucinous and serous glands. The nasal septum by contrast is lined by squamous mucosa with a paucity of minor salivary glands and a thinner, tightly tethered lamina propria.

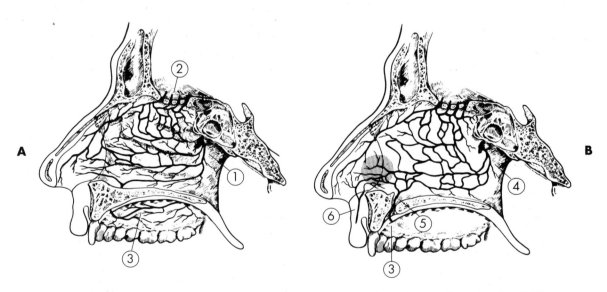

FIG. 2-9 Diagrams of a sagittal view of the vascular supply of the (**A**) lateral nasal wall and (**B**) the nasal septum. *1,* The posterior lateral nasal branches of the sphenopalatine artery; *2,* the anterior and posterior ethmoidal arteries; *3,* the greater palatine artery; *4,* the posterior septal branches of the sphenopalatine artery; *5,* the nasopalatine artery; and *6,* the septal branch of the superior labial artery. The area of Kiesselbach's plexus is in dots on **B**. (From Osborn AG. The nasal arteries. AJR 1978; 130:89-97. Copyright 1978, American Roentgen Ray Society.)

Frontal Sinus

The frontal sinuses arise from one of several outgrowths originating in the region of the frontal recess of the nose. Their site of origin can be identified on the mucosa as early as 3 to 4 months in utero. The frontal sinuses are in effect displaced anterior ethmoid cells, and because they develop from a variable site along the lateral nasal fossa wall, depending on the precise site of origin, their drainage will be either via a nasofrontal duct into the frontal recess or more directly into the anterior infundibulum.[10,11] Less often, the frontal sinus drains directly into the anterior ethmoid cells, which in turn opens into the infundibulum or the bulla ethmoidalis. Because the frontal sinuses do not reach up into the frontal bone until around the age of 6 years, these sinuses are essentially the only paranasal sinuses that are absent at birth. Their development is quite variable but appears to effectively start only after the second year of life.[12] In otherwise normal patients, both frontal sinuses fail to develop in only 4% of the population. If there is persistence of a metopic suture, the frontal sinuses are small or absent. On the average, by the age of 4 years the cranial extent of the frontal sinus reaches half the height of the orbit, extending just above the top of the most anterior ethmoid cells. By the age of 8 years the top of the frontal sinuses is at the level of the orbital roof, and by the age of 10 years the sinuses extend into the vertical portion of the frontal bone. The final adult proportions are reached only after puberty.[1,12]

Based on a study of 100 normal frontal sinuses, the area of a patient's frontal sinuses correlates well with two lines that can be drawn on either a plain film or a coronal CT scan. One line extends vertically from the level of the highest point of the orbital roof to the most cranial margin of the sinus. The other line extends from the base of the crista galli obliquely to the most lateral margin of the sinus. On a Franklin type head unit or on CT, the maximum length for each line is 63 and 74.5 mm, respectively. If either of these lengths is exceeded, the sinus is larger than the 99th percentile of the normal population and is considered abnormally enlarged.[13] The average frontal sinus has been described as being 28 mm high, 24 mm wide, and 20 mm deep. However, there is a wide range in frontal sinus size, and the frontal pneumatization may involve the vertical plate (squamousal portion) of the frontal bone, the horizontal plate (orbital roof) of the frontal bone, or both of these areas. Recognition of an orbital recess to the frontal sinus is particularly important if frontal sinus obliterative surgery is to be performed. If only the vertical portion of the sinus is obliterated because an orbital recess was not preoperatively identified, a mucocele eventually develops in the obstructed orbital recess.

Because the frontal sinuses develop from a variable site, in approximately 50% of cases the ethmoidal infundibulum acts as a channel for carrying the secretions (and infection) from the frontal sinus to anterior ethmoid cells and the maxillary sinus. It is only in the patient whose nasofrontal duct opens directly in the frontal recess or above the infundibulum (85% of cases) that the frontal sinus is accessible to intranasal cannulation.

The factors responsible for determining the extent of frontal sinus growth are poorly understood. Some of the factors implicated in influencing frontal sinus growth include a relationship between the cessation of frontal lobe growth and the development of the frontal sinus. Frontal lobe expansion normally ceases its anterior growth by 7 years of age, at which time the inner table of the frontal bone stops its forward migration. Any further development of the frontal bone occurs secondary to anterior growth of the outer frontal table and sinus pneumatization. The ipsilateral frontal sinus is abnormally enlarged in patients with the Dyke-Davidoff-Masson syndrome with an underdeveloped hemicerebrum, and in cases of early childhood damage to the frontal lobe.[14,15] In addition, a direct relationship between the mechanical stresses of mastication and frontal sinus enlargement has been demonstrated, as has a direct relationship with growth hormone.[15,16]

In some patients a frontal bulla develops. This is an upward displacement of the frontal sinus floor caused either by encroachment from the opposite frontal sinus or more frequently by an underlying ethmoid cell. This bulla may influence frontal sinus drainage, and it has been implicated as a cause of chronic frontal sinusitis in some patients.[1]

Each frontal sinus is a single cavity, although rare duplication of a sinus has been reported.[1] Usually the frontal sinuses are asymmetric in size. Often the larger sinus extends across the midsagittal plane so that a midline incision may inadvertently enter this sinus rather than the intended opposite smaller sinus.[1] The normal sinus contour tends to be slightly scalloped, and intrasinus septa may extend into the sinus from one half to one third the height of the sinus cavity. Such septations can create recesses of the sinus that can be overlooked at surgery if preoperative imaging was not performed. The larger the sinus cavity, the better the septations are developed. Conversely, in a hypoplastic frontal sinus the sinus is usually a single, smoothly contoured cavity devoid of septations (Fig. 2-10). As mentioned the frontal sinus can pneumatize both the vertical and the horizontal (orbital) plates of the frontal bone. The deepest area of the vertical portion of the sinus is near the midline at the level of the supraorbital ridge, and the medial sinus floor and the caudal anterior sinus wall are thinnest in this area. As a result the sinus is best approached for a trephination at this level. This thin anterior wall also permits the controlled fracture that is necessary in creating an osteoplastic flap of the frontal sinus.[17]

The intersinus septum is in reality the remaining frontal bone between the two frontal sinuses. It is usually in the midline at its base or lower portion; however, it may then deviate far to one side, depending on the differential growth rates of the frontal sinuses (Fig. 2-11). Although the septum is almost always complete, focal areas of acquired or congenital dehiscence do occur, allowing intercommunication between the two frontal sinuses or herniation of the mucosa of one sinus into the contralateral sinus.[10] The normal well-developed frontal sinus abuts the superomedial orbital margin, but it does not encroach on the orbit and remodel it. Any

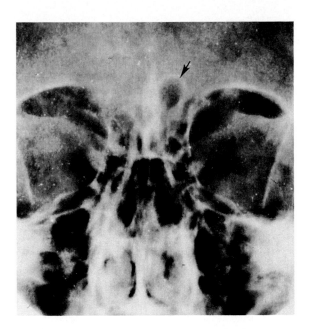

FIG. 2-10 Caldwell view shows an aplastic right frontal sinus and a hypoplastic left frontal sinus *(arrow)*. Note the smooth rounded contour of the hypoplastic sinus.

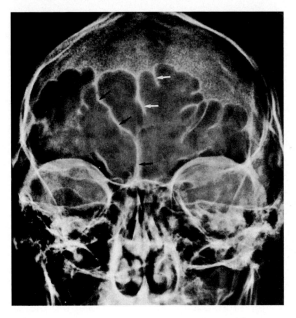

FIG. 2-11 Caldwell view shows a well-developed frontal sinus. Note the scalloped contour and the thin white mucoperiosteal line. Normal septations project into the sinus cavity *(white arrows)*. The intersinus septum is to the right of the midline cranially but is near the midline caudally *(black arrows)*. Despite the large size of the frontal sinuses, the orbital contours remain normal and are not encroached upon.

flattening of this orbital margin should suggest the presence of an expanding frontal sinus process (mucocele, pneumocele, etc.).

Occasionally a central frontal sinus cavity is encountered, in the midline, just above the level of the nasion. This presumably is the result of a displaced ethmoid cell.

There is a rich venous plexus (Breschet's canals) that communicates with both the diploic veins and the dural spaces. The main arterial supply is via the supraorbital and supratrochlear arteries derived from the ophthalmic artery. The venous drainage is primarily through the superior ophthalmic vein, and the sinus lymphatics drain across the face to the submandibular lymph nodes. The sensory innervation of the sinus mucosa is via the supraorbital and supratrochlear branches of the frontal nerve, which is a branch of the first division of the trigeminal nerve.

Ethmoid Complex

The ethmoid sinuses begin formation in the third to fifth fetal month when numerous separate evaginations arise from the nasal cavity. The anterior and middle cells are the first to evaginate; the posterior cell evaginations follow. The cells progressively enlarge during fetal life. There is great variation in the location of the ethmoid cell openings because they arise from various possible diverticulae, for example, those situated above, on, or below the ethmoid bulla, those that arise from any portion of the middle meatus, the frontal recess, the superior meatus, or above and behind the superior nasal concha.[1] These cells are present at birth and continue to grow and honeycomb the ethmoid bone until either late puberty or until the sinus walls reach a layer of compact bone. The adult ethmoid has 3 to 18 cells, and these cells are grouped as anterior, middle, or posterior,

according to the location of their ostia.[17] In general the anterior ethmoid cells are defined as those cells that have their ostia in relationship to the infundibulum. The middle cells have their ostia either above, on, or under the bulla, and the posterior cells have their ostia in the superior meatus. At birth the anteromiddle ethmoid complex is about 5 mm high, 2 mm long, and 2 mm wide. The posterior cell group is 5 × 4 × 2 mm. In the adult the anteromiddle ethmoid group averages 24 mm high, 23 mm long, and 11 mm wide, and the posterior group is 21 × 21 × 12 mm. The total number and size of the ethmoid cells are inversely related. In general the posterior cells are both larger and fewer than the anterior cells.

The ostia of the ethmoid sinuses are the smallest of any paranasal sinus. They measure only 1 to 2 mm in diameter.[17] The anterior ethmoid cells have smaller ostia than the posterior cells, a factor probably contributing to the higher incidence of anterior ethmoid mucoceles.[17]

The fetal support of the middle and superior turbinates is a partition of bone, the basal lamella, that continues from the base of each turbinate laterally through the mass of ethmoid cells to attach to the medial side of the lamina papyracea. In the case of the middle turbinate, the basal lamella only extends from its more posterior portion where it is attached to the lateral nasal wall. No basal lamella is present along the anterior portion of the middle turbinate where it attaches to the lateral cribriform plate. The basal lamella for the superior turbinate is along the most posterior aspect of the lateral nasal vault. These two lamella thus divide the ethmoid cells into anterior, posterior, and postreme groups. In the adult the lamella is not a straight dividing plate because the developing air cells have pushed and distorted the original straight partition that was present in the fetal ethmoid bone.[17] Usually the actual lamellar bone cannot be distinguished from the adjacent ethmoid septa. This subject is discussed in more detail in the section on the osteomeatal complex.

Each ethmoidal labyrinth lies between the orbit and the upper nasal fossa. The left and right groups of ethmoid cells are connected in the midline by the cribriform plate (nasal roof) of the ethmoid bone. The crista galli extends from the midline upward into the floor of the anterior cranial fossa. The perpendicular plate of the ethmoid bone extends downward from the cribriform plate to contribute to the nasal septum. The medial wall of each ethmoid labyrinth is formed by a thin lamella of bone from which arises the middle, superior, and supreme turbinates. The lateral ethmoid wall is formed by the thin lamina papyracea, which separates the ethmoid cells from the orbit. Dehiscences can occur in the lamina papyracea, and mild degrees of hypoplasia can result in a lateral concavity to the lamina papyracea. This also occasionally results in a wide beveled opening in the lamina papyracea where the anterior and posterior ethmoidal canals are located. The lateral caudal margin of the ethmoid cell complex articulates with the maxilla, forming the ethmoidomaxillary plate.

The roof of the ethmoid complex is formed by a medial extension of the orbital plate of the frontal bone, which projects to articulate with the cribriform plate. This is often referred to as the fovea ethmoidalis. The ethmoidal vessels and nerves pass into the ethmoid complex via the anterior and posterior ethmoidal canals. The upper portion of these canals is formed by the frontal bone, and the lower margins are formed by the ethmoid bone. Thus a line connecting these canals identifies the frontoethmoid junction and is just below the dural line.

The ethmoid sinuses receive their blood supply from nasal branches of the sphenopalatine artery and the anterior and posterior ethmoidal arteries, which are branches of the ophthalmic artery. Thus the ethmoid sinuses receive blood from both the internal and external carotid arteries. The venous drainage is into the nose via the nasal veins or via the ethmoidal veins, which drain into the ophthalmic veins. This latter pathway is responsible for cavernous sinus thrombosis after ethmoid sinusitis. The sensory innervation of the ethmoid mucosa is via the ophthalmic and maxillary divisions of the trigeminal nerve. The nasociliary branch of the ophthalmic division supplies the anterior cells via the anterior ethmoidal nerve. The posterior ethmoid cells are supplied by the posterior ethmoidal nerve from the ophthalmic division and the posterolateral nasal branches of the sphenopalatine nerve from the maxillary division of the trigeminal nerve. The lymphatics drain into the submandibular lymph nodes.[17,18] The proximity of the posterior ethmoid cells to the orbital apex, optic canal, and optic nerve can lead to loss of vision as a complication of benign or malignant disease or surgery on these sinuses.

Sphenoid Sinus

The sphenoid sinuses emerge in the fourth fetal month as evaginations from the posterior nasal capsule into the sphenoid bone. This occurs just above a small crescent-shaped ridge of bone, the sphenoidal conchae, that projects from the undersurface of the body of the sphenoid bone. These conchae grow forward, fusing with the posterior ethmoid labyrinth. Complete absence of the sphenoid sinus is rare. The degree of pneumatization, however, varies considerably. The sinus starts its major growth in the third year of life, and by age 10 to 12 years the sinus usually has obtained its adult configuration.[11] The lack of any sinus pneumatization by the age of 10 years should suggest the possibility of "occult" sphenoid pathology.[19] The average adult sphenoid sinus measures 20 mm high, 23 mm long, and 17 mm wide. The posterior sinus development is variable. In 60% of pneumatized sinuses the sinus cavity extends posteriorly to the anterior sella wall and lies under the sella floor. In 40% of sinuses the sinus cavity extends only to the anterior wall of the sella turcica. In fewer than 1% of cases the sphenoid sinuses do not develop posteriorly enough to reach the anterior sella wall. In this latter group of patients the thick, bony posterior sinus wall is a contraindication to transsphenoidal hypophysectomy.[20]

The sphenoid sinus septum is usually in the midline anteriorly, aligned with the nasal septum. However, from this point it can deviate far to one side, creating two unequal sinus cavities. With the exception of the sinus roof, the other sinus walls are of variable thickness, depending on the degree of pneumatization. However, even in poorly developed sinuses the roof is thin, often measuring only 1 mm (planum sphenoidale). This wall is thus consistently vulnerable to perforation during surgery.

The anatomic relationships of the sphenoidal sinus are important because of the symptoms that can arise from sinus disease and the complications that can arise during sinus surgery. Anteriorly to posteriorly, the sinus roof is in relationship to the floor of the anterior cranial fossa, the optic chiasm, and the sella turcica. The lateral wall is related to the orbital apex, the optic canal, the optic nerve, and the cavernous sinus (the internal carotid artery). Situated posteriorly are the clivus, prepontine cistern, pons, and basilar artery. The sinus floor is the roof of the nasopharynx, and the anterior sinus wall is the back of the nasal fossa. In well-pneumatized sinuses, ridges or indentations may project into the sinus wall, corresponding to the location of the internal carotid artery, the maxillary nerve, the vidian nerve, the optic nerve, and the sphenopalatine ganglion.[21] These relationships can present potential surgical hazards because fracture and removal of these septa can damage the adjacent vessel or nerve. In addition, surgery in the sphenoid sinus can perforate the sinus walls. This is especially relevant because regions of anatomic bony dehiscence have been reported along the walls.[22]

In 48% of people there are lateral recesses from the main sphenoid sinus cavity that extend into the greater sphenoid wing where it forms the floor of the middle cranial fossa and the posterior orbital wall, the lesser sphenoid wing, or the pterygoid process. The pterygoid process is pneumatized in 25% of patients and is extensively pneumatized in 8% of patients.[23] There is great variability between the degree of pneumatization on the left and right sides.

The normal drainage of each sphenoid sinus in the erect posture is achieved entirely through ciliary action because the ostium is typically located 1.5 cm above the sinus floor. The ostium is usually 2 to 3 mm in diameter and 2 to 5 mm from the midline.

The sphenoid sinus has arterial supply from branches of both the internal and external carotid arteries. The posterior ethmoidal branch of the ophthalmic artery may contribute vessels to the roof of the sphenoid sinus, and the floor of the sinus receives blood from the sphenopalatine branch of the maxillary artery. The venous drainage flows into the maxillary vein and the pterygoid venous plexus.

The sphenoid sinus is innervated from both the second and third divisions of the trigeminal nerve. The posterior ethmoid nerve from the nasociliary branch of the ophthalmic division supplies the roof of the sinus, and the sphenopalatine branches of the maxillary division supply the sinus floor.[22] The lymphatics drain into the retropharyngeal lymph nodes.[2]

Maxillary Sinus

The maxillary sinus is the first of the paranasal sinuses to form. At approximately the seventieth day of gestation, after each nasal fossa and its turbinates are established, a small ridge develops just above the inferior turbinate, marking the future uncinate process. Shortly after this, an evagination starts just above this ridge and enlarges laterally from the nasal cavity. By birth a rudimentary sinus, measuring approximately 7 × 4 × 4 mm, is present with its longest dimension in the anteroposterior axis.[15] The developing maxillary sinus initially lies medial to the orbit. The annual growth rate of the maxillary sinus is estimated to be 2 mm vertically and 3 mm anteroposteriorly.[24] By the end of the first year the lateral margin of the sinus extends under the medial portion of the orbit. The sinus reaches the infraorbital canal by the second year and passes inferolaterally to it during the third and fourth years. By the ninth year the lateral sinus margin extends to the malar bone. Lateral growth ceases by the fifthteenth year.

In infancy the maxillary sinus floor lies at the level of the middle meatus. By the eighth to ninth year the sinus floor is near the level of the nasal fossa floor.[25] From this point there is considerable variation in the further growth of the lower recess of the sinus. If the sinus continues to grow downward, it reaches the actual plane of the hard palate by age 12 years. The final descent of the sinus, signaling the cessation of sinus growth, is not complete until the third molar has erupted. In 20% of adults the most dependent portion of the maxillary sinus is above the nasal cavity floor; it lies at the same level as the nasal floor in 15% of adults and below this level in 65% of adults.[25] The mean dimensions of the adult maxillary sinus are 34 mm deep, 33 mm high, and 25 mm wide. The average volume of the adult maxillary sinus is 14.75 ml.

For the most part the maxillary sinuses develop symmetrically with only minor, common variations. Unilateral hypoplasia and bilateral hypoplasia occur in 1.7% and 7.2% of people, respectively.[26,27] Hypoplasia of the maxilla results from trauma, infection, surgical intervention, or irradiation that occurs during the development of this bone. These conditions can damage the maxillary growth center and produce a small maxilla and thus a hypoplastic sinus. Underdevelopment also occurs in first and second branchial arch anomalies such as Treacher Collins syndrome, mandibulofacial dysostosis, and thalassemia major when the demand for marrow prohibits sinus pneumatization.

The maxillary sinus lies within the body of the maxillary bone. Behind the orbital rims, each sinus roof, or orbital floor, slants obliquely upward so that the highest point of the sinus is in the posteromedial portion, lying directly beneath the orbital apex. The groove and canal for the maxillary nerve lie in the middle third of the sinus roof. The medial antral wall is the inferolateral wall of the nasal cavity. The curved posterolateral wall separates the sinus from the infratemporal fossa. The anterior sinus wall is the facial surface of the maxilla, and it is perforated about 1 cm below the orbital rim by the infraorbital foramen. Each sinus has four recesses: the zygomatic recess, extending into the malar eminence or body of the zygoma; the palatine recess, which is small and variable, extending into the hard palate; the tuberosity recess, extending downward above and behind the third upper molar; and the alveolar recess, extending into the alveolar process of the maxilla.

The floor of the sinus is lowest near the second premolar and first molar teeth and usually lies 3 to 5 mm below the nasal floor. The roots of the three molar teeth often form conical elevations that project into the sinus floor. Less often the roots of the premolar and, even more rarely, the canine teeth project into the antrum. Occasionally there is dehiscent bone over the tooth roots so that only sinus mucosa covers these roots and separates them from the main sinus cavity.[17] The lower expansion of the antrum is intimately related to dentition; when a tooth erupts, the vacated space becomes pneumatized, thus expanding the sinus lumen.

For the maxillary sinus, as well as for all of the other paranasal sinuses, the ostium is always located at the site of the initial embryonic evagination from the nasal chamber. In the case of the antrum the ostium is on the highest part of the medial wall and is approximately 4 mm in diameter. It does not open directly into the nasal fossa but rather into the ethmoidal infundibulum, which, via the hiatus semilunaris, opens into the nasal cavity. The channel of the infundibulum is approximately 5 mm long and is directed upward and medially into the nasal fossa. The sinus ostial location dictates that sinus drainage in the erect position is accomplished by intact ciliary action. A narrow infundibulum can further interfere with sinus drainage, as can intraantral septations that can compartmentalize portions of the maxillary sinus. These uncommon septa usually divide the antrum into anterior and posterior sections, each of which may drain via accessory ostia into the nasal fossa. Rarely a horizontal septum can divide the antrum into superior and inferior, or medial and lateral, portions.

In the adult skull the medial wall of the maxillary bone has a large hole, the maxillary hiatus, that exposes the interior of the maxillary sinus. This hole is covered in part by portions of four bones. The perpendicular plate of the palatine bone lies posteriorly, and the lacrimal bone is situated anterosuperiorly. The inferior turbinate covers the inferior portion of the maxillary hiatus, and resting above the line of attachment of this turbinate is the uncinate process of the ethmoid bone. Above the uncinate process the medial maxillary hiatus is covered by the redundant nasal and sinus mucosa. This membranous area is important in efforts to irrigate the antrum. When the natural maxillary ostium cannot be clinically canulated, primarily because of a large uncinate process, the thin membranous area of the middle meatus can be penetrated.[17]

The maxillary sinus is vascularized via branches of the maxillary artery, and the supply is essentially topographic. Thus the infraorbital, greater palatine, posterosuperior alveolar, and anterosuperior alveolar arteries all contribute blood supply. In addition, there are lateral nasal branches of the sphenopalatine artery and a small contribution from the facial artery. The venous drainage anteriorly is via the anterior facial vein and posteriorly via the maxillary vein. The maxillary vein joins the superficial temporal vein to form the retromandibular (posterior facial) vein, which drains into the jugular vein. However, the maxillary vein also communicates with the pterygoid venous plexus that anastomoses with the dural sinuses through the skull base. It is through this latter pathway that maxillary sinusitis can lead to a meningitis.[22]

The nerve supply to the antrum is via branches of the second division of the trigeminal nerve, namely the superior alveolar nerves (posterior, middle, anterior), the anterior palatine nerve, and the infraorbital nerve. Of these the posterior superior alveolar nerve pierces the posterior antral wall and runs forward and downward in a small canal to supply the molar teeth. The lymphatics of the main sinus drain into the lateral retropharyngeal and internal jugular nodes, and those of the lateral portion of the antrum drain into the submandibular nodes.

References

1. Hollinshead WH. The nose and paranasal sinuses. In: Anatomy for surgeons. Vol 1. The head and neck. New York, Ny: Hoeber-Harper Book, 1954; 229-281.
2. Last RJ. Anatomy: regional and applied. Ed 6. London, England: Churchill Livingstone Inc, 1978; 398-406.
3. Goss CM, ed. Gray's anatomy of the human body. Ed 27. Philadelphia, Pa: Lea & Febiger, 1963; 1167-1176.
4. Williams HL. Nasal physiology. In: Paparella MM, Shumrick DA. Otolaryngology. Vol 1. Basic science and related disciplines. Philadelphia, Pa: WB Saunders Co, 1973; 329-346.
5. Zinreich SJ, Kennedy DW, Kuman AJ, et al. MR imaging of normal nasal cycle: comparison with sinus pathology. J Comput Assist Tomogr 1988; 12:1014-1019.
6. Leopold DA. Physiology of olfaction. In: Cummings CW, Fredrickson JM, Harker LA, et al, eds. Otolaryngology: head and neck surgery. Vol 1. St. Louis, Mo: The CV Mosby Co, 1986; 527-545.
7. Paff GH. Anatomy of the head and neck. Philadelphia, Pa: WB Saunders Co, 1973; 183-203.
8. Fried R. The hyperventilation syndrome: research and clinical treatment. Baltimore, Md: The Johns Hopkins University Press, 1987.
9. Osborn AG. The nasal arteries. AJR 1978; 130:89-97.
10. Schaeffer JP. The embryology, development and anatomy of the nose, paranasal sinuses, nasolacrimal passageways and olfactory organs in man. Philadelphia, Pa: P Blakiston's Son & Co, 1920.
11. Van Alyea OE. Nasal sinuses: anatomic and clinical considerations. Baltimore, Md: Williams & Wilkins, 1942.
12. Dodd GD, Jing BS. Radiology of the nose, paranasal sinuses and nasopharynx. Baltimore, Md: Williams & Wilkins, 1977; 3-8, 59-65.
13. Urken ML, Som PM, Lawson W, et al. The abnormally large frontal sinus. I. a practical method for its determination based upon an analysis of 100 normal patients. Laryngoscope 1987; 97:602-605.
14. Enlow DH. Handbook of facial growth. Philadelphia, Pa: WB Saunders Co, 1975; 120-121.
15. Shapiro R, Schorr S. A consideration of the systemic factors that influence frontal sinus pneumatization. Invest Radiol 1980; 15:191-202.
16. Clementine C, ed. Gray's anatomy of the human body. Ed 30. Philadelphia, Pa: Lea & Febiger, 1985; 299.
17. Ritter RN. The paranasal sinuses: anatomy and surgical technique. Ed 2. St. Louis, Mo: The CV Mosby Co, 1978.
18. Zinreich SJ, Mattox DE, Kennedy DW, et al. Concha bullosa: CT evaluation. J Comput Assist Tomogr 1988; 12:7787-84.
19. Fujioka M, Young LW: The sphenoidal sinuses: radiographic pattern of normal development and abnormal findings in infants and children. Radiology 1978; 129:133-136.
20. Yanagisawa E, Smith AW: Normal radiographic anatomy of the paranasal sinuses. Otolaryngol Clin North Am 1973; 6:429-457.
21. Graney DO. Anatomy. In: Cummings CW, Fredrickson JM, Harker LA, et al, eds. Otolaryngology: head and neck surgery. Vol 1. St. Louis, Mo: The CV Mosby Co, 1986; 845-850.
22. Pandolfo I, Gaeta M, Blandino A, et al. The radiology of the pterygoid canal: normal and pathologic findings. AJNR 1987; 8:479-483.
23. Etter LE. Atlas of roentgen anatomy of the skull. Springfield, Ill: Charles C Thomas, 1955.
24. Proetz AW. Essays on the applied physiology of the nose. Ed 2. St. Louis, Mo: Annals Publishing Co, 1953.
25. Alberti PW. Applied surgical anatomy of the maxillary sinus. Otolaryngol

Clin North Am 1976; 9:3-20.

26. Karmody CS, Carter B, Vincent ME: Developmental anomalies of the maxillary sinus. Trans Am Acad Ophthalmol Otolaryngol 1977; 84(4, Part 1):723-728.

27. Sperber GH. Craniofacial embryology. Ed. 4. London, England: Wright, 1989; 144-146.

Section Two
IMAGING

Radiographic Technique
Plain Films

Although computed tomography (CT) and magnetic resonance imaging (MRI) have for the most part replaced routine plain film examination of the paranasal sinuses, these plain film studies are still often performed as the first roentgen examination. There are numerous radiographic views available for evaluating the paranasal sinuses. However, only four of these projections are normally employed in the routine examination. These consist of two frontal projections—the Caldwell view and the Waters view—a base (submentovertex) view, and a lateral view. Supplemental studies occasionally are employed. These other views include the oblique projection (Rhese view), other craniocaudal angulations of the frontal projection (transorbital, posteroanterior projections), the Towne views, the Granger view, and the modified Waters view.[1,2]

If possible the paranasal sinus radiographic examination ought to be obtained with the patient in the erect position. Such erect filming allows clear identification of an air-fluid level. If the patient cannot tolerate erect positioning, a cross-table lateral film with a horizontal beam should be obtained. If neither of these approaches is used, any free sinus fluid layers on the dependent sinus wall are not seen as an air-fluid level.

Horizontal Beam 5 Degrees Off-Lateral View

To achieve the horizontal beam 5 degrees off-lateral view, the patient's head is positioned laterally relative to the cassette, the nose is then rotated 5 degrees toward the cassette from the true lateral position. If the patient is seated, the cassette is usually placed in the vertical position. If the patient is lying down in either the semiprone or the prone position, the cassette is positioned horizontally. The central ray enters perpendicular to the cassette and is centered at the outer canthus of the eye in the middle of the film. The orbitomeatal line is parallel to the base of the film (Fig. 2-12). The purpose of using the 5 degrees off-lateral view rather than the true lateral view is to rotate the posterior walls of the maxillary antra slightly so that they do not superimpose on one another. This permits individual evaluation of the integrity of the posterior antral bony margins.

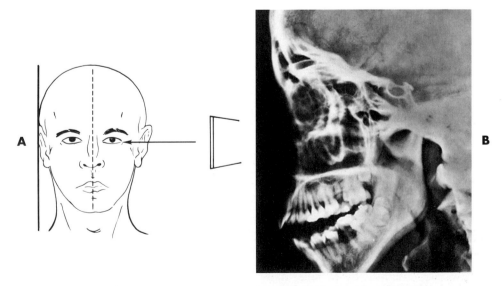

FIG. 2-12   Lateral view. **A,** Positioning diagram. **B,** Sample radiograph.

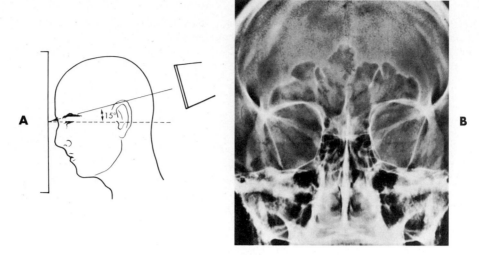

FIG. 2-13   Modified Caldwell view. **A,** Positioning diagram. **B,** Sample radiograph.

Modified Caldwell View

For the modified Caldwell view, the patient is positioned directly facing the cassette in either the sitting or the prone position. The midsagittal plane is perpendicular to the film. The orbitomeatal line is perpendicular to the cassette, and the central ray is angled 15° caudally as it enters the posterior skull. The central ray also serves as the centering point of the skull on the cassette. If the patient is properly positioned, this view projects the petrous pyramids in the lower third of the orbits (Fig. 2-13). The Caldwell view is the best projection for examining the frontal and ethmoid sinuses in the frontal projection.

Modified Waters View

For the modified Waters view, the patient is positioned facing the cassette in either the erect or the prone position. The orbitomeatal line is angled 37° to the plane of the cassette. The central ray is centered on the film perpendicular to the cassette, emerging at the anterior nasal spine of the patient (Fig. 2-14, *A, B*).

Variations in the positioning angle may be required to give the "perfect" Waters view. On one hand, if the head is not sufficiently extended, the petrous pyramids are projected over the maxillary sinuses, thereby obscuring sinus detail. On the other hand, if the head is hyperextended, the maxillary sinuses become distorted and foreshortened, thus obscuring sinus disease. The "perfect" Waters view has the petrous pyramids projected just below the floor of the sinus cavities. This is the best single view for the evaluation of the maxillary antra in the frontal projection. Another variation is to use the Mahoney modification with the mouth open.[2] The open-mouth Waters view normally allows good visualization of the lower posterior sphenoid sinus margins (Fig. 2-14, *C*).

Modified Base (Submentovertical or Submentovertex) View

The modified base view was described by Schuller and Pfeiffer.[2] The reference line used is the infraorbital line,

which runs from the infraorbital margin to the center of the external auditory meatus. The goal of the positioning is to have the infraorbitomeatal line parallel to the film plane. This projection is considerably easier to obtain with the patient in either the sitting (erect) or the prone position. Patients with cervical or thoracic degenerative disease, those with a short neck, or those who are obese have difficulty extending the head sufficiently, if the examination is attempted with the patient supine. The central ray is directed perpendicular to the infraorbitomeatal line and centered ¾ inch anteriorly to the plane of the external auditory meatus (Fig. 2-15). A modification, with the centering 1½ inches in front of the external auditory meatus, has also been suggested.

A variation of the traditional submentovertex view is the Welin, or overangulated base, view. This view results in an average angle of 120° open posteriorly between the infraorbitomeatal line and the cassette. This overangulation is accomplished by tilting the top of the cassette toward the patient while the patient's head is fully extended as in the modified base projection. The central ray is directed to the level of the frontal sinus. This position is a useful adjunct view for evaluation of the anterior and posterior walls of the frontal sinuses (Fig. 2-16). It is also a good view for evaluating the lateral and, to a lesser extent, medial walls of the maxillary antra. The sphenoid and ethmoid sinuses, with the nasal cavity superimposed, are thrown into relief with this projection.

Rhese or Oblique View

The Rhese view is excellent for studying the posterior ethmoid air cells, which are otherwise obscured by superimposition of the anterior cells in the frontal views. Superimposition of the anterior right and left ethmoid cells in the Rhese view, however, tends to limit its usefulness in paranasal sinus examination. Correct positioning places the optic canal just off the midorbit in the lower outer quadrant. Each side is taken separately and then compared. The patient is placed in either a seated erect position or the prone position. Then the median sagittal plane of the body is cen-

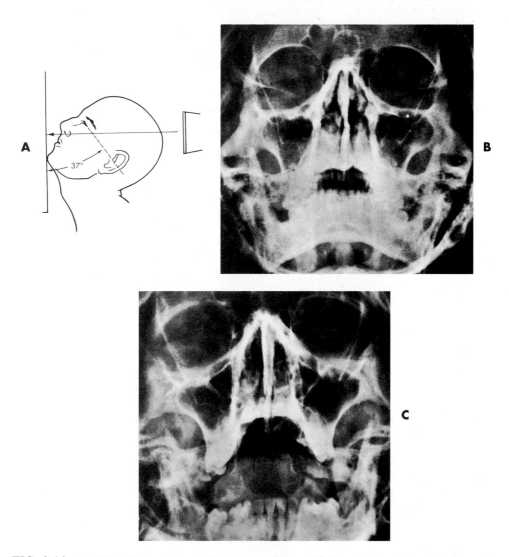

FIG. 2-14   Modified Waters view. **A,** Positioning diagram. **B,** Sample closed-mouth radiograph. **C,** Sample open-mouth radiograph.

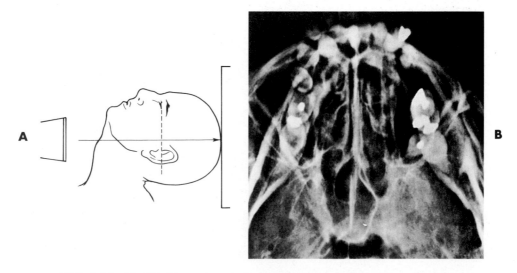

FIG. 2-15   Modified base view. **A,** Positioning diagram. **B,** Sample radiograph.

tered with the midline of the cassette. With the orbit centered in the portion of the cassette to be used, the flexion of the head is adjusted so that the canthomeatal line is perpendicular to the film. The patient's head is rotated so that the median sagittal plane forms an angle of 53° with the plane of the film. The central ray enters the skull posteriorly at an angle of 15° with the canthomeatal line and emerges at the midorbit (Fig. 2-17).[2] Short of sectional imaging, the oblique views coupled with a Caldwell view provide the least obscured images of the ethmoid cells.

Nasal Bone Lateral View

To achieve the nasal bone lateral view, the patient is usually placed in a semiprone position, with the body rotated so that the median sagittal plane of the head is horizontal and parallel to the plane of the tabletop. The interpupillary line is also perpendicular to this plane. The flexion of the head ought to be such that the orbitomeatal line is parallel with the transverse axis at the tabletop. The jaw should be supported with a sandbag to prevent rotation. The film is placed under the frontonasal region and centered at the nasion. The focal-film distance should be 36 inches (Fig. 2-18).

Nasal Bone Axial View

The success of the nasal bone axial projection depends on either having the patient hold the occlusal film correctly between the front teeth or placing the larger film cassette under the patient's chin so that the plane of the film is at right angles to the glabelloalveolar line. The central ray should be directed along this line at right angles to the plane of the film (Fig. 2-19).

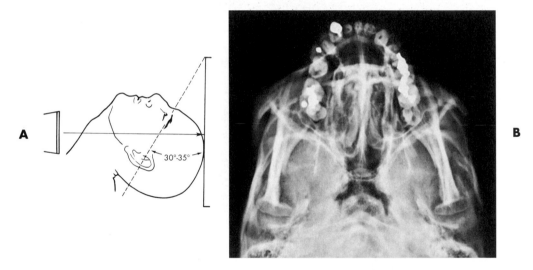

FIG. 2-16 Overangulated base view. **A,** Positioning diagram. **B,** Sample radiograph.

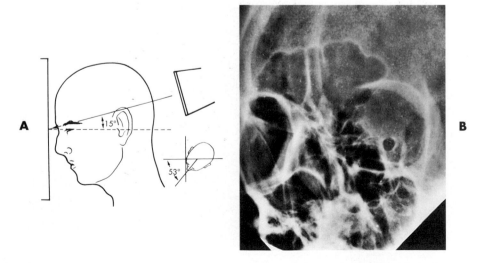

FIG. 2-17 Rhese (oblique) view. **A,** Positioning diagram. **B,** Sample radiograph.

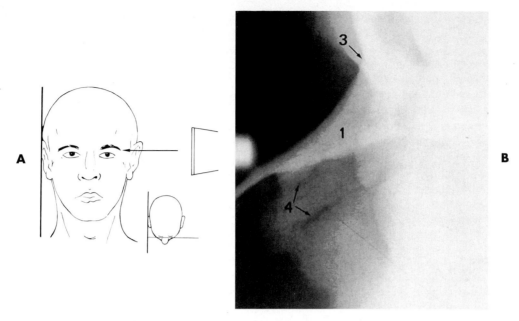

FIG. 2-18 Lateral nasal bone view. **A,** Positioning diagram. **B,** Sample radiograph.

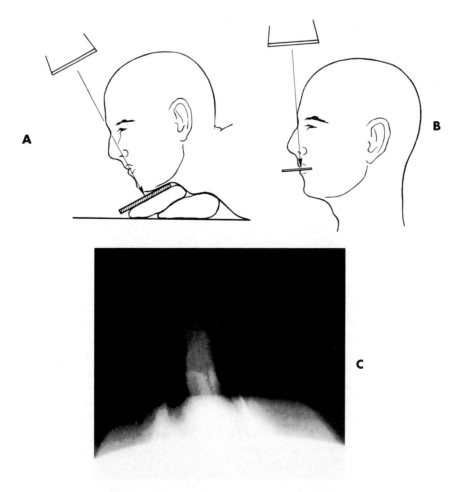

FIG. 2-19 Axial nasal bone view. **A,** Positioning diagram with film under chin. **B,** Positioning diagram with film in teeth. **C,** Sample radiograph.

SECTIONAL IMAGING TECHNIQUES
Computed Tomography

The mucosal surfaces and the bony framework of the sinonasal cavities are well suited for investigation by CT. Because the radiologist and clinician are as interested in soft tissue disease as they are in bony changes, in theory each scan should be photographed at an appropriate window and center level that optimizes both subtle soft tissue differences in attenuation and fine bony detail. Unfortunately, there is no one combination of window and center (level) settings that optimally accomplishes both of these aims. The soft tissues are best shown at narrow windows that allow easy discrimination between the attenuation values of muscle, fat and tumor, as well as some distinction between entrapped secretions and cellular soft tissues. In addition, narrow windows allow prompt detection of any enhancement differences on postcontrast CT scans. Such soft tissue settings have window values in the range of 150 to 400 HU.

Conversely, bone detail is best shown at wide window settings in the range of 2000 to 4000 HU. In addition, these wide window settings allow the most accurate evaluation of the air–soft-tissue interfaces. This reflects the fact that the algorithms in use by virtually every CT manufacturer have difficulty handling abrupt transitions in attenuation values from very low (air) to very high (bone) attenuation regions. This is easily noticeable when the same images are viewed side-by-side at both narrow and wide window settings. At narrow settings the air spaces and bone appear larger than they do when they are viewed at the wide window settings. In fact the wide window appearance correlates very accurately with the true measurements of the air spaces and the bone. At narrow window settings, this same phenomenon leads to volume-averaging errors that allow a small soft-tissue mass to be obscured by surrounding sinus air and allow focal areas of abnormal bone to be obscured by adjacent normal bone. Because of this, the most accurate assessment of mucosal soft-tissue disease and bone changes is accomplished at wide window settings. However, the best distinction of watery sinonasal secretions from more viscous or desiccated secretions or a tumor requires narrow window settings.

In the last decade the definition of what constitutes an adequate CT examination of the sinonasal cavities has become a topic of some controversy. Because of the popularity of endoscopic sinus surgery and its focus on the osteomeatal complex, limited coronal studies have become the most requested examination of this area. In part driven by the changing medical economic picture, low mAs—low-cost limited coronal CT studies—have become the examination most requested. Such an examination is designed to limit patient radiation dose and to sufficiently limit the CT study to allow the radiologist to charge a price comparable to that of a plain film study. Although this approach may be adequate for most patients, there are some pitfalls to interpreting such a limited study. The anterior and posterior walls of the frontal, maxillary, and sphenoid sinuses are not well imaged in the coronal view. Any abnormality or violation of these walls is most often overlooked or underestimated if only coronal views are available. In addition, because of varying patient compliance with the degree of neck extension, the coronal scan angle varies from patient to patient, and often from examination to examination on the same patient. This alters the appearance of some anatomic landmarks and may make precise localization of ethmoid disease difficult. However, axial studies complement the coronal views by showing the various anterior and posterior sinus walls and allowing precise mapping of ethmoid disease. Thus for a patient with suspected inflammatory sinus disease, an adequate CT examination may be a limited coronal study; however, the complete CT examination is an axial and coronal study. If the patient has a suspected neoplasm, the complete examination ought to be performed to provide the most detailed analysis of the sinonasal cavities and the adjacent skull base.[3-6]

The axial examination is most often performed with the patient supine and the scanning plane parallel to the inferior orbitomeatal (IOM) line. The IOM line is readily identified on a lateral scout film. In addition, the cranial (the level just above the top of the frontal sinuses) and caudal (the maxillary teeth) limits of the average examination can be localized off the lateral scout view. The routine study should be obtained with 3 to 5 mm thick, contiguous scans throughout the scan volume. Narrower slice thicknesses are usually unnecessary unless there is a specific region of interest.

Just as volume averaging may cause diagnostic difficulties in the coronal view, there are three levels in the axial view that may cause interpretive difficulty. These levels correspond to three bony planes, all of which are nearly parallel to the axial scan plane: the floor of the anterior cranial fossa, portions of the orbital floor, and the hard palate. Because knowledge of extension of disease across these bony planes is critical for the surgeon in determining some surgical procedures (for example, an antral tumor growing into the orbit, or a nasoethmoid or sphenoid tumor extending into the anterior cranial fossa), a coronal study must also be obtained when the imaging of these bony planes is essential.

Because most adult patients have dental amalgams or metal bridges that cause considerable degradation of the CT images, direct 90° coronal scans (to the IOM plane) are usually of little diagnostic value because the involved teeth lie immediately below the sinonasal areas of interest. In addition, many patients cannot sufficiently extend their neck (because of pain, vertigo, arthritis, etc.) in either the supine or prone position to obtain such 90° coronal studies. In general a scan plane is chosen that extends from a caudad margin just anterior to the dental fillings to a cranial point just posterior to the area of greatest interest (osteomeatal unit, orbit, sphenoid, etc.). These coronal studies are routinely obtained as 3 to 5 mm thick, contiguous slices.[7,8] (See Chapter 3).

For the routine CT study performed to evaluate inflammatory disease, contrast is usually not necessary. However, if it is necessary to determine whether a nasal mass extends into an adjacent sinus or whether it simply obstructs the sinus or if there is suspected intracranial extension of disease, contrast should be given. There are a variety of methods for administering the contrast. Today, commonly a power injector is used and a small volume (10 to 20 ml) is given as a bolus to "load" the patient. The remaining contrast is then given at a slow rate throughout the examination. If spiral CT is used, the rapid scanning time allows the delivery of a larger effective bolus throughout the examination. Although the resolution of a spiral CT study of the paranasal sinuses is not as good as that of a conventional CT examination, the spiral technology allows better coronal (or other projection) reconstruction in those patients who cannot manage positioning for direct coronal studies.

Magnetic Resonance Imaging (MRI)

As the era of MRI procedes, new approaches as to how to best image the sinuses are born almost monthly. However, these approaches are primarily variations of facilitating the acquisition of basic T1-weighted (T1W) and T2-weighted (T2W) information. MRI in general provides better soft-tissue discrimination than does CT, and MR also offers true multiplanar image acquisition. The advantage of not having ionizing radiation is occassionally outweighed by a patient's claustraphobic rejection of the procedure (about 10% of cases), or metal hardware or a pacemaker abrogating the examination. However, during the past decade, industry has responded by producing nonmagnetic materials that are implanted in the patient and nonparamagnetic support equipment for the more critically ill patient. Although bone is not directly imaged on MRI, invasion of bone marrow and gross bone erosion can be identified.[9,10] However, fine bone alterations are difficult to see on MRI and are far better demonstrated on CT.

The indications for the use of contrast material, though still somewhat debatable, are being resolved. Below the skull base, contrast enhancement occurs in most tumors, in inflammatory tissue, and in some normal mucosa. Thus if contrast material is utilized, the pathology often appears larger than it is. Nonetheless, some authors recommend the use of double and triple dose MR contrast agents to better visually assess the pathology. However, no new pathology was identified in such high-dose studies.[11] In day-to-day practice, pathology is usually better mapped on noncontrast T1W and T2W images than on enhanced studies. If intracranial extension has occurred, contrast MRI has been reported to be better than noncontrast MRI in demonstrating the intracranial tumor margin and any intracranial complications of sinusitis such as meningitis, cerebritis, intracranial abscess, thrombophlebitis, and orbital complications.[11,12] An additional use of MR contrast occurs when a mass of indeterminate etiology is visualized on noncontrast studies. Further distinction can be made between entrapped secretions and a solid mass because enhancement occurs peripherally in inflamed mucosa around secretions, whereas

tumors usually enhance more solidly and centrally.[13,14]

The basic MRI examination usually includes axial (transverse) and coronal images. The scan thickness should be no more than 5 mm, and a narrow interslice distance (1 mm) is suggested. Basic or equivalent T1W and T2W information should be obtained whether by conventional spin echo or fast scan imaging. Fat suppression can be used in selected cases but is rarely necessary. The best study for an individual patient is often the one that is most confidently read by the radiologist. Thus sagittal images, though not necessary in the routine case, may help, especially if evaluating the cribriform plate region or the orbital floor. Because there is no uniformity in the literature regarding the optimal TR and TE, these parameters can be varied to some degree to limit the total duration of the MRI study, alter the resolution, or produce more scan slices in a single scan sequence. The greatest challenge for the imager is to tailor the examination to each patient so that all of the necessary information is gathered without unduly lengthening the examination and thereby limiting the number of patients examined.

PLAIN FILM AND SECTIONAL IMAGING ANATOMY

Despite the most careful and meticulous attention to technical detail, plain film examinations have substantial limitations. Even if interpreted by a knowledgeable radiologist, the degree of soft-tissue disease and bone destruction may be consistently underestimated. However, because of their comparatively low cost, low radiation dose, and ready availability, plain film studies are still the most frequent initial study. Today, limited, low-cost, low-dose, coronal CT studies, which are being performed as an alternative to the plain film examination are growing in popularity. Despite having a radiation dose lower than the routine CT examination, the associated radiation dose with these limited CT studies is usually higher than the dose of a plain film series. This fact, plus the frequency of these examinations, represents a net radiation risk to the population. Thus the clinical setting for performing these studies should be carefully monitored so that patient dose and examination cost are balanced by the radiologists choice of the best study to provide the information needed by the clinician determining patient management.

Patients who have signs and symptoms of acute sinonasal disease usually do not require any radiologic study. Most often the acute disease responds to conservative medical management. If the clinician is concerned that the maxillary sinus may require washing, the plain film study, performed with the patient in the erect position, allows good visualization of an air-fluid level. The plain film examination also provides a gross assessment of sinus disease, usually all the information that is needed by the clinician at this initial stage of the disease. If the patient has unusual signs or symptoms such as headache, retroorbital pain, orbital pain, suboccipital pain, or facial swelling, axial and coronal CT scans provide better disease mapping, and in these circum-

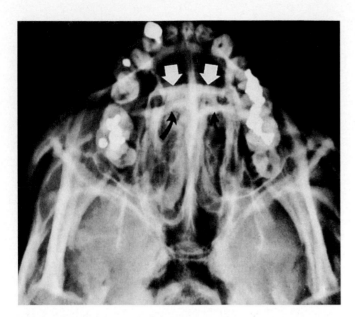

FIG. 2-20   Overangulated base view with the anterior table of the frontal sinus *(large arrows)* and the posterior table *(curved arrows)* projected over the mid-palate and nasal structures.

stances a contrast study should be performed to better image any intacranial disease component.

It is estimated that between one third and one half of patients with acute sinonasal inflammatory disease will progress to chronic disease. In such cases, it is probable that some type of surgical intervention will be a part of further treatment, and a preoperative CT scan ought to be obtained. Not only is disease mapping more complete on CT scans than on plain films, but normal anatomic variants can be identified that may influence surgery or aid the surgeon in avoiding an operative complication. Thus if surgery is planned, a plain film examination can be avoided. CT, not MRI, is suggested as the first examination because air and desiccated secretions can be distinguished from one another on CT but may be indistinguishable on MRI. However, if the clinician suspects that a sinonasal tumor is present, the examination of choice is MRI because of its better soft-tissue resolution and its ability to better distinguish between tumor and adjacent obstructed secretions or inflammatory disease.

To identify the early manifestations of sinonasal disease, it behooves the radiologist to become fluent in sinonasal anatomy as it appears on plain films, CT, and MRI. Before mastery in the analysis of pathologic cases is possible, the radiologist must be able to move confidently through the visual thicket of normal radiographic anatomy and its variants. The important role of the radiologist in evaluating disease in the sinonasal cavities is better appreciated when it is considered that the clinician can directly observe only a small portion of the volume of interest. Clearly, radiography provides the most thorough noninvasive evaluation of the nasal cavity and paranasal sinuses.

The following section addresses the normal sinonasal anatomy as seen on plain films and CT scans. The common denominator leading to the successful interpretation of these examinations is the anatomy itself, and once this is learned, its depiction as rendered by any specific modality will be clearly and easily approached. Technology per se is irrelevant as long as it meets the final test of delineation of structure.

The normal sinonasal anatomy is presented in two sections. The first discusses the normal anatomy as seen on plain films and contains a presentation of anatomic variants and potential problems that are created by overlying soft-tissue structures and bones.[15-20] The second section, which is in Chapter 3, presents sectional anatomy and is illustrated with CT images.[21-26]

Plain Film Anatomy
The Frontal Sinuses

The main or vertical portion of the frontal sinuses is best visualized in the Caldwell and Waters projections (Figs. 2-13, 2-14). On occasion the Rhese view can better display some of the sinus contours, particularly in the smaller sinuses (Fig. 2-17). The anterior and posterior sinus walls are best evaluated in the lateral and base (submentovertex) views (Figs. 2-12, *B,* 2-20). However, in these projections, only those portions of the sinus walls that are parallel to the incident beam (perpendicular to the film plane) are visualized. The adjacent curvilinear surfaces are obliquely oriented to the incident x-ray beam and only contribute to the perceived density of the adjacent calvarium. Thus on the lateral view, only the midsagittal anterior and posterior frontal sinus tables are visualized, and on the base view (depending on the angulation and the particular curvature of the skull), it is usually the caudal portions of the sinus walls that are identified. It is important to remember that only these limited areas of the frontal sinus anterior and posterior walls are seen routinely on these projections. One may not assume that the entire sinus table is normal simply because it appears intact on the lateral or base views. This is especially true in suspected fractures of the posterior table or if an erosion of this bone is in question. Sectional imaging clarifies this issue.

The horizontal portion of the frontal sinus is best seen in Caldwell and lateral views (Fig. 2-21). The depth of this recess can be best assessed by evaluating the posterior extent of pneumatization in the bony roof of the orbit as shown on these projections.

Because the frontal sinuses develop independently from anterior ethmoid cells, asymmetry is the rule. Differential sinus growth is responsible for displacement of the intersinus septum to one side. However, this septum is usually near the midline at its caudal extreme, near the level of the glabella (Figs. 2-11, 2-13). If the intersinus septum is displaced far to one side at this lower margin, an expansile process such as a mucocele within a frontal sinus should be suspected.

Unilateral or bilateral sinus aplasia or hypoplasia can occur. The smaller sinuses usually consist of a single, centrally concave recess (Fig. 2-10). Because of their small size, there is little sinus air compared with the amount of overlying bone, and these sinuses almost always appear somewhat "clouded" on plain films, even if they are disease free. As such, they are difficult to evaluate. Rhese and Waters views may help to evaluate these small sinuses (Fig. 2-22).

The normally developed frontal sinus is always less dense than the adjacent frontal bone. The frontal bone, as part of the calvarium, is composed of cortical bone that forms both its inner and outer tables, and interposed between the two is its middle table, or diploic space. The diploic space is made up of a bony latticework that is less dense than cortical bone but osseous nonetheless. Frontal sinus development proceeds by invagination of an air-containing mucosal sac into the diploic space, thus displacing the osseous latticework otherwise sandwiched between the inner and outer tables of the skull. Therefore, despite the cortical nature of the bone comprising their inner and outer walls, the sinuses invariably appear less dense than the adjacent frontal bone. In general the density of the normal frontal sinus is comparable to that of the superior orbital fissure as seen on the Caldwell view.

The larger sinuses have scalloped margins with septations that can project well into the sinus cavity (Figs. 2-11, 2-21). If this scalloping is lost and instead a smoothly ovoid shape is seen, an expansile process such as a mucocele should be considered. In a well-developed sinus in the presence of an expansile process, this smooth appearance is created by the slow, progressive erosion of the septa and the bone between the scallops.

Normally the frontal sinuses never violate the orbital contour, no matter how large they become (Fig. 2-11). If there is a downward and lateral flattening of the superomedial orbital rim, a mucocele should be suspected.

The normal superomedial orbital margin often appears unsharp on Caldwell or Waters views. This is because this area curves not only from medially to laterally in the orbital rim, but it also curves from vertically to horizontally as the bone of the forehead region merges into the bone of the orbital roof. Usually a repeat Caldwell view at a slightly different angulation or a Rhese view allows this orbital margin to be visualized intact so that erosion is not erroneously diagnosed.

The margins of each frontal sinus are outlined by a thin (1 mm), dense rim—the mucoperiosteal (white) line—that separates the sinus from the adjacent frontal bone (Figs. 2-11, 2-21, 2-22). If this line is not visualized, it could be because of active infection, which is common, or bone destruction from tumor, which is rare. In active inflammatory disease, there is increased vascularity, which results in increased mobilization of calcium and a loss of the mucoperiosteal white line. In chronic infection the thin, sharp, white line is replaced by an unsharp, thick zone of sclerosis or reactive bone. This thickened white zone indicates only that the frontal sinus was exposed to previous chronic infection and does not necessarily imply that there is currently active infection in the sinus.

In the Caldwell view, the lambdoidal perisutural sclerosis of the occiput, a normal finding, can be projected over the region of the frontal sinus and can mimic a chronically thickened reactive margin of an opacified sinus (Fig. 2-23).

Comparison of the Caldwell film to Waters or Rhese views permits correct interpretation.

On occasion, it is difficult to distinguish between a completely clouded (opacified) frontal sinus and an absent (aplastic) sinus. With good quality films, some frontal sinus margin can almost always be identified, albeit poorly, on at least one of the plain films in the sinus series. If no such margin is seen, an aplastic sinus is the probable diagnosis. Sectional imaging will resolve any remaining issue.

On the lateral view there usually is a bone density area seen at the base of the frontal sinuses anteriorly, near the nasion (Fig. 2-24). This represents the overlapping lower bony sinus walls and the superomedial orbital margins. The nasofrontal suture is usually just anteriorly situated. The dense bony area should not be confused with an osteoma. When seen from the front (Caldwell and Waters views), no "osteoma" is visualized and the bone in this region appears normal. Occasionally on the lateral view, small bony ridges also are seen projecting from the anterior or posterior sinus walls. These are the sinus septa seen from the side.

The Ethmoid Sinuses

The ethmoid sinuses are best evaluated on the Caldwell view. However, in every plain film projection, some ethmoid cells are superimposed on others. This reflects the fact that the ethmoid sinuses are not a single sinus cavity, as are the other paranasal sinuses, but rather are formed by 3 to 18 cells that are packed into the ethmoid bone. This superimposition can lead to confusion on the plain film examination when the patient has symptoms referable to these cells, and yet the ethmoid sinuses appear normal. This situation arises because an isolated group of cells can be totally opacified, while all of the adjacent cells remain normally aerated. The air in these normal cells nullifies the plain film "clouding" of the infected cells, and the net result is often a very unimpressive plain film appearance. In this clinical circumstance, sectional imaging identifies any localized ethmoid disease.

On the Caldwell view the normal density of the ethmoid sinuses can be judged by comparing it with the air density around the inferior turbinate of the nasal fossae. This reflects the fact that the ethmoid sinuses and the nasal fossae are of approximately the same anteroposterior depth, and thus the density of the air volume is about the same.

The thin lamina papyracea forms the lateral boundary of the ethmoid bone, separating it from the orbit. This medial orbital wall is oriented obliquely to an anteroposterior incident beam. Thus the majority of this oblique, thin bony plate is not visualized on routine plain film studies. The straight or slightly concave lateral line that appears to form the medial orbital wall on a Caldwell view is in reality only the posterior ethmoid margin near the sphenoid bone. The anterior margin abutting the lacrimal bone is more medially placed and often is poorly seen (Fig. 2-25). It can be best localized by following the outline of the orbital rim from the superior aspect around to the superomedial margin and then caudally to the medial contour.

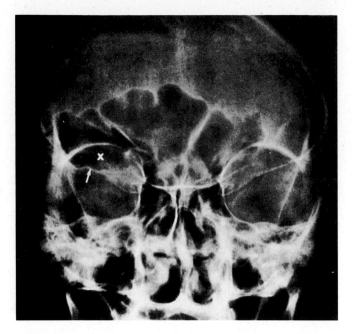

FIG. 2-21 Caldwell view shows well-developed frontal sinuses. On the right side the sinus pneumatizes the roof of the orbit and this is seen as air *(x)* contained within a thin white sinus margin *(arrow)* that is projected through the orbit.

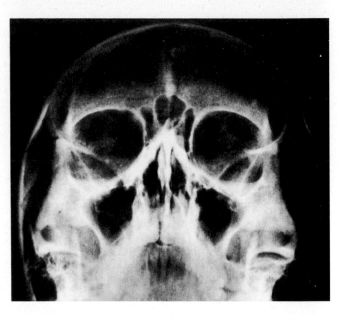

FIG. 2-22 Waters view shows hypoplastic frontal sinuses and small central sinus cell, not an uncommon finding. This Waters view compliments the Caldwell projection for evaluating the frontal sinuses.

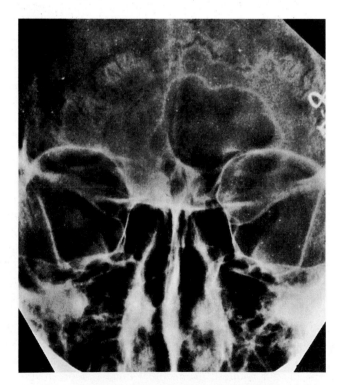

FIG. 2-23 Caldwell view shows a moderately well-developed left frontal sinus. The right frontal sinus is aplastic. The perisutural sclerosis of the lambdoid suture is projected over the right frontal area and may mimic a clouded sinus contour.

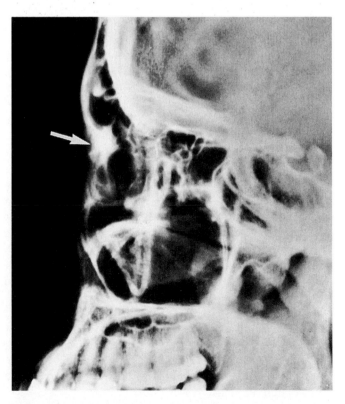

FIG. 2-24 Lateral view shows normal bone density near the anterior base of the frontal sinuses *(arrow)*. This "pseudo-osteoma" is not seen on either the Caldwell or Waters views.

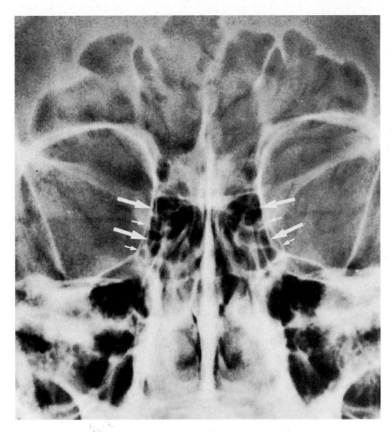

FIG. 2-25   Caldwell view shows the posterior ethmoid lamina papyracea *(small arrows)* is lateral to the more anterior lamina papyracea *(large arrows)*. The medial orbital wall extends obliquely between them, reflecting the conical shape of the orbit. Also note the horizontally oriented normal ethmoid septa.

On the Waters view, only the most anterior ethmoid cells can be visualized, with the lacrimal bone separating them from the orbit (Fig. 2-26). The middle and posterior ethmoid cells are hidden from view by the nasal fossae structures. Similarly the lateral and base views have so many overlapping structures that only gross localization of an ethmoid process can be achieved. On the base view the palate, nasal septum, turbinates, and anterior calvarium overlay the ethmoids, and on the lateral view the lateral orbital margins and even the frontal processes of the maxilla may project as vague dense zones overlying the ethmoid cells (Figs. 2-20, 2-24). These should not be misinterpreted as sites of pathology. Although some isolation of the posterior ethmoid cells can be obtained on a Rhese view, some overlapping of ethmoid cells still occurs. Sectional imaging is indicated for proper mapping.

On the Caldwell view a small indentation, or groove, is often seen along the upper medial orbital wall. This is the anterior ethmoidal canal, and it transmits the vessels of the same name along with the nasociliary nerve (Fig. 2-27). Because the canal is formed from the ethmoid bone below and the frontal bone above, it represents the level of the floor of the anterior cranial fossa. Less often seen on plain films are the posterior ethmoidal canals, which transmit the posterior ethmoidal nerve and vessels.

The ethmoidomaxillary plate is the posteroinferior boundary between the ethmoid and maxillary bones. It is best seen in the Caldwell view and is a useful plain film landmark for localizing the spread of tumors (Fig. 2-28).

Supraorbital ethmoid cells are ethmoid sinus extensions into the orbital plate of the frontal bone. Unlike the frontal sinuses, the supraorbital ethmoid cells tend to be symmetric. If such a cell is present on one side, it should be present on the opposite side. If one of these supraorbital cells is not seen, opacification or destruction should be suspected. Sectional imaging performed in the coronal plane resolves any questionable case. On the Caldwell view the supraorbital ethmoid cells appear as slightly curvilinear lucent zones in the superomedial orbital roof (Fig. 2-29). Their posterior extent is best evaluated on either a Waters or a lateral view. It is clinically important to ascertain whether a pathologic process is in a supraorbital ethmoid sinus or in the frontal sinus because the surgical approaches to these sinuses differ.

The Maxillary Sinuses

The maxillary sinuses are best evaluated by the Waters view. Unlike the frontal and sphenoid sinuses, the maxillary sinuses tend to be symmetric in size and configuration with only minor variations being common. When some degree of

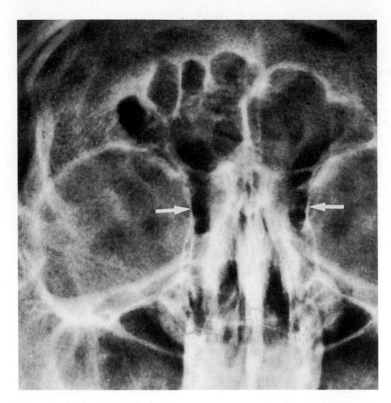

FIG. 2-26   Waters view isolates the anterior ethmoid cells and the overlying lacrimal bones *(arrows)*.

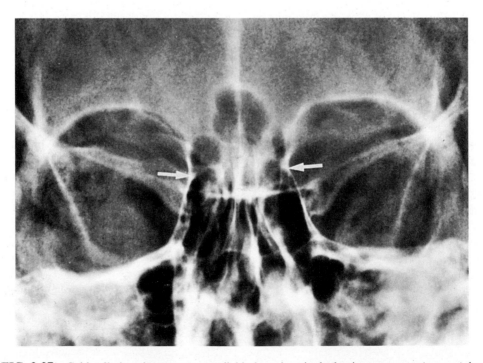

FIG. 2-27   Caldwell view demonstrates medial indentations in the lamina papyracea *(arrows)* that represent the anterior ethmoidal canals. These canals mark the level of the floor of the anterior cranial fossa.

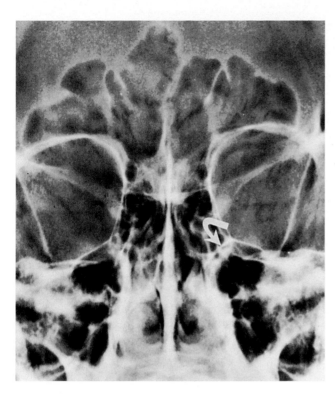

FIG. 2-28 Caldwell view shows ethmoidomaxillary plate (*curved arrow*). This is the boundary between the posteroinferior ethmoid bone and the maxillary bone.

hypoplasia is present, the roof of the smaller antrum has a greater downward slant on its lateral margin than does the larger sinus (Fig. 2-30). On plain films this may simulate a blowout-type orbital floor fracture. However, in the hypoplastic sinus there usually is an identifiably thicker lateral bony sinus wall that results from the poorer than normal pneumatization of the maxilla. Although this may be misdiagnosed as thickened sinus mucosa, this confusion is not likely to be made by the radiologist who is aware of the appearance of a hypoplastic antrum.

A small sinus can also result from diseases of the sinus wall that cause bone expansion with resultant encroachment into the antral cavity (Fig. 2-31). Such diseases include fibrous dysplasia, "brown" tumors of hyperparathyroidism, Paget's disease, and rare giant cell tumors. In these cases, at least one dimension of the original sinus may be identified as being fully developed, and the "bony changes" can be visualized bulging into the sinus, as well as being formed by abnormally textured bone. These changes differentiate these conditions from a simple hypoplastic antrum. Often sectional imaging may be necessary to resolve difficult cases.

Similarly, conditions that arrest the growth of the maxilla result in a hypoplastic antrum. These childhood conditions include severe infection, trauma, tumor, irradiation, and congenital first arch syndromes.

The most lateral extension of the maxillary sinus is the zygomatic recess. This portion of the sinus hollows out the body of the zygoma, and when compared with the main antral

cavity, it has less air and more surrounding bone. Because of this, the recess usually appears "clouded" on a Waters view and is often misinterpreted as representing mucosal thickening (Fig. 2-26). True mucosal changes are best seen extending along the adjacent lower lateral antral wall, and it is there that such mucosal disease is better evaluated.

On the lateral view, the anterior and posterior walls of the zygomatic recesses are seen as two overlapping *V*'s projected over the main maxillary sinuses. These should be evaluated routinely to assess the possibility of early bone destruction in these recesses (Fig. 2-32). Also seen on the lateral view is the cranial continuation of the posterior wall of the zygomatic recess, which is also the most anterior margin of the temporal fossa and represents that portion of the greater sphenoid wing that forms the oblique orbital line on the Waters and Caldwell views (Fig. 2-33).

The infratemporal maxillary sinus wall is a sigmoid-shaped, curved posterolateral surface. It is poorly seen on the Caldwell and Waters views. The most lateral extent (the back of the zygomatic recess) and the most medial margin (the anterior wall of the pterygopalatine fossa) can be identified on the lateral view (Fig. 2-33). The base view provides the best visualization of the curved nature of this wall, as well as an enface projection of portions of the pterygopalatine fossa and pterygoid plates (Figs. 2-34, 2-35).

The medial wall of the maxillary sinus is best seen on the Caldwell view. Unfortunately, the overlying nasal structures anteriorly and the sphenoid sinuses and skull base structures posteriorly obscure most detail. Only the inferior turbinates and the lower medial antral wall are identified consistently. The clinically important osteomeatal complex is well visualized only on coronal sectional imaging.

Slight asymmetry, minimal rotation, and the physiologic nasal cycle all contribute to making one nasal turbinate larger than the other. As long as some air can still be visualized around the contour of the turbinate, separating it from the lateral nasal fossa wall and the nasal septum, the turbinate is probably not pathologically enlarged. Asymmetry per se should not be overdiagnosed as pathology. On the lateral view, the posterior tips of the inferior conchae are often seen projecting over the posterior antra, and they should not be confused with a pathologic mass. Also on the lateral view, air trapped under or above the inferior turbinate can produce a linear lucency that may mimic a fracture (Fig. 2-36).

Little consistent detail about the middle turbinates is obtained from plain film studies, and sectional imaging is necessary to provide accurate information.

The anterior antral wall is not well seen on any view. Both the lateral and the overangulated base views reveal only limited portions of this wall (Fig. 2-35).

The lateral view best delineates the inferior extension of the maxillary sinus and its relationship to the hard palate and teeth roots (Fig. 2-37). The sinus cortex of this alveolar recess can be elevated normally by unerupted molar teeth. Although this is well seen on the lateral view, its often broad upper surface can simulate an air-fluid level or a localized

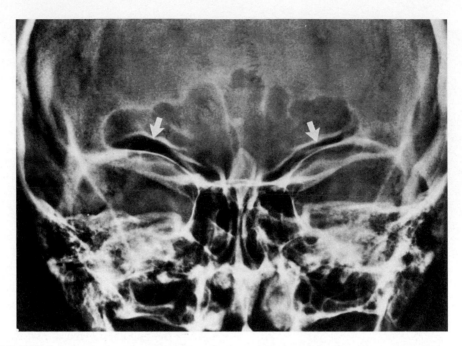

FIG. 2-29   Caldwell view shows curvilinear collection of air (*arrows*) just above each orbital margin. These areas appear darker than the frontal sinuses because the air in these supraorbital ethmoid cells is projected over the air in the frontal sinuses.

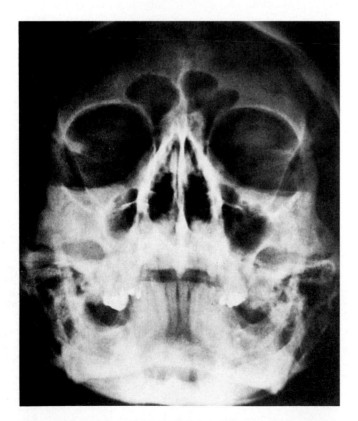

FIG. 2-30   Waters view shows the right maxillary sinus is smaller than the left. This hypoplasia is noted by the thicker lateral bony sinus wall and the more exaggerated downward slant of the sinus roof when compared with the left side. Also note that there is a suggestion of mucosal thickening in this normal hypoplastic right antrum due to its smaller sinus cavity and its thicker sinus walls when compared with the left side.

mass on a Waters view. This is especially notable in older children and teenagers.

The antral roof, or orbital floor, is flattest and lowest anterolaterally. It is also highest and most angulated posteromedially. The majority of the midportion of the antral roof is seen almost tangentially on a Caldwell view, and thus this large surface is usually seen as a single line in this projection. On the Caldwell view a second, smaller, more slanted line is seen superomedially in the orbital floor. This line represents the orbital apex floor; a notch at the lateral aspect of this line identifies the site of the infraorbital groove (Fig. 2-38).

On the lateral view the orbital floor is usually seen as two separate lines—one anteriorly, near the level of the inferior orbital rim, represents the lowest, most lateral, and flattest area of the floor; the second, located higher and more posteriorly, represents the medial, orbital apex region. The slanting floor joining these two areas is not normally seen on the lateral view (Fig. 2-37). However, on a nonconed Rhese view (or optic canal view), the contralateral orbital floor is often seen extending from the anterior orbital rim almost to the orbital apex.

The Waters projection gives a better view of the inferior orbital rim. However, much of the orbital floor is seen obliquely en face, and small fractures, depressions, or erosions may not be detected. Three roughly parallel lines are seen near the inferior orbital margin in the Waters view. The most superior of these is the soft-tissue skin margin, overlying the inferior orbital rim. The middle line is the actual bony inferior orbital rim, and the lowest line is the roof of the antrum located about 1 cm behind the rim, the lowest

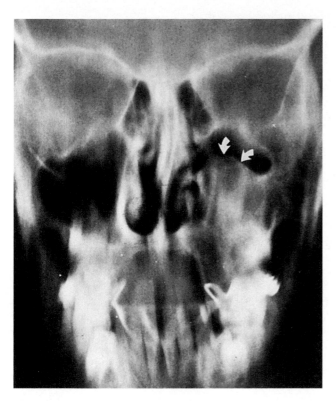

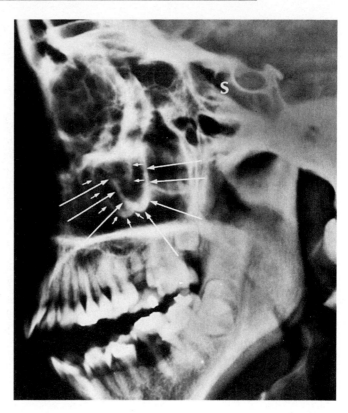

FIG. 2-31 Coronal tomogram of patient with ossifying fibroma of the lateral wall and floor of the left antrum. The arrows indicate the elevation of the sinus floor by this expansile mass. This may simulate the findings of a hypoplastic sinus, but it has a distinctly different appearance (compare with Fig. 2-30).

FIG. 2-32 Lateral view with large arrows pointing to the zygomatic recess of one maxillary sinus and small arrows outlining the opposite zygomatic recess. These recesses are routinely seen on lateral views as overlapping *V*s. The air around them is air in the main maxillary sinus cavities, which are located nearer the midline. The *S* is in the sphenoid sinus with its posterior and superior limits clearly visible on this lateral film.

point of the orbital floor. About 1 cm below the middle third of the inferior orbital rim, the infraorbital foramen is seen. It transmits the second division of the trigeminal nerve to the cheek and nasal region (Fig. 2-39).

On the Waters view a small lucency is occasionally seen in the lateral antral wall. This is the canal for the posterior superior alveolar nerve and should not be confused with a fracture (Fig. 2-40).

On the Caldwell view the foramen rotundum is projected through the superomedial portion of the antrum (Figs. 2-38, 2-41). The superior orbital fissure is easily identified and normally has a slightly concave lateral appearance (Figs. 2-39, 2-41). If the superior orbital fissure is followed inferiorly and slightly laterally, it points to the foramen rotundum. The maxillary nerve (V_2) runs through this foramen, crosses the pterygopalatine fossa and retromaxillary fissure, enters the infraorbital fissure, exits via the infraorbital canal, and supplies the cheek and nasal regions.

The two foramina rotunda are usually symmetric in size and configuration. The superior orbital fissures, on the other hand, need not be as symmetric. The most important observation is that the bony cortical rims on each side of each fissure are thin and sharply defined. These fissures are narrower superolaterally and wider inferomedially. It is through this

wider area that the veins and nerves traverse the fissure (Fig. 2-41). On the Waters view the lower portions of the superior orbital fissures are projected through the upper medial antra. These can simulate either a fracture of the inferior orbital rim or a septum of the antral roof (Fig. 2-39).

The infraorbital fissure can sometimes be seen on the Waters view as a pair of parallel thin cortical lines that are oriented anteroposteriorly. Their course is parallel, rather than divergent, and their configuration distinguishes them from the posteriorly located superior orbital fissure.

The inferior orbital fissure is poorly seen on the routine sinus views and can be best evaluated on the Towne view (Fig. 2-42).

The oblique orbital lines (linea innominata) are seen in both the Waters and the Caldwell views. They represent the most anterior portions of the medial temporal fossa and usually are formed by the greater sphenoid wings. At the lower margin of each innominate line a sharp medial turn is seen, indicating the lower margin of the temporal fossa and the beginning of the infratemporal fossa. Occasionally this line is seen to continue medially and then bend downward, outlining the lateral pterygoid plate (Figs. 2-43, 2-44).

The superior bony margin of the middle cranial fossa is a concave posterior ridge that is formed medially by the lesser

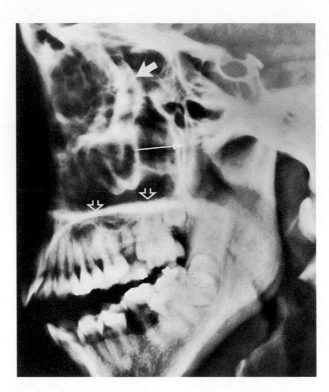

FIG. 2-33 Lateral view with long arrows pointing to one posterior antral wall, which also forms the anterior margin of the pterygomaxillary fissure near the midline. The short arrow indicates the upward continuation of the posterior portion of one *V* that forms the zygomatic recess of one antrum (Fig. 2-32). The short arrow points to the bone just behind the orbit, which forms the anterior border of the temporal fossa. Open arrows indicate the upper, flat nasal fossa surface of the hard palate. The lower oral surface is slightly concave downward in configuration.

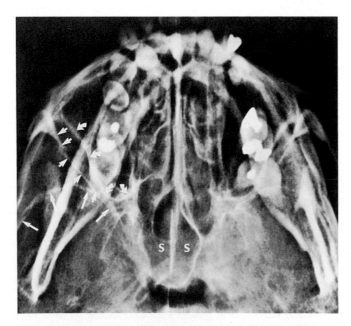

FIG. 2-34 Base view with large arrows pointing to the curved anterior margin of the right middle cranial fossa (greater sphenoid wing). The small, straight arrows indicate the straighter posterior wall of the right orbit. The lateral margin is formed by the zygoma; the medial portion is formed by the greater sphenoid wing. The curved arrows outline the "sigmoid-shaped" posterior wall of the maxillary sinus. Each sphenoid sinus cavity *(S)* is seen well.

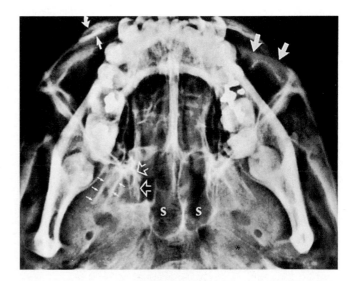

FIG. 2-35 Base view with open arrows pointing to the medial pterygoid plate. Because the lateral pterygoid plate curves laterally as it descends from the skull base, the two small arrows point to the line of the lateral pterygoid plate near the skull base, and the three small arrows indicate the lateral pterygoid plate near the level of the hard palate. The large arrows point to the anterior wall of the left zygoma and maxilla. The frontal bone's anterior table *(curved arrow)* and posterior table *(small, straight arrow)* are also indicated on the right side. Each sphenoid sinus cavity *(S)* is seen well.

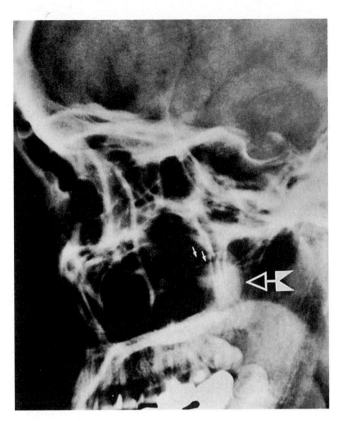

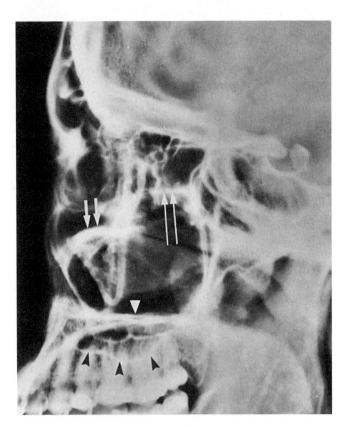

FIG. 2-36 Lateral view with large arrow pointing to posterior tip of normal inferior turbinate. Normal air just above turbintes *(small arrows)* may mimic a fracture line.

FIG. 2-37 Lateral view demonstrates maxillary sinus extension *(black arrowheads)* below the level of the hard palate *(white arrowhead)*. The smaller arrows point to the anterolateral and most inferior orbital floor on one side, and the longer arrows point to the posteromedial and most superior orbital floor near the orbital apex.

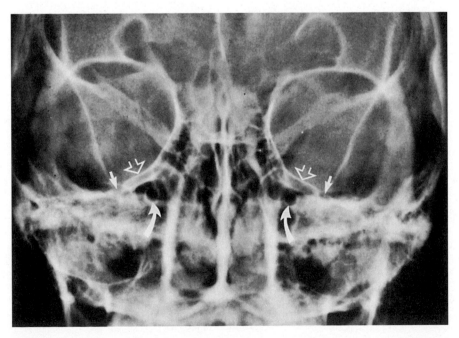

FIG. 2-38 Caldwell view with open arrowheads indicating posteromedial orbital floors. The straight arrows point to the posterior margin of infraorbital canals. The curved arrows point to each foramen rotundum.

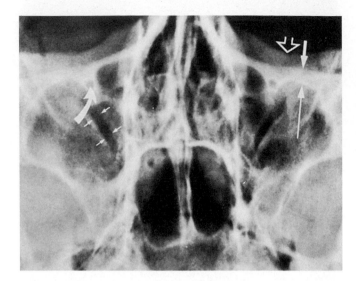

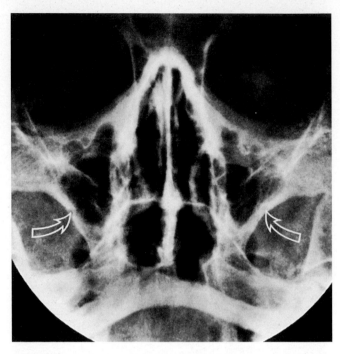

FIG. 2-39 Waters view with curved arrow pointing to infraorbital foramen. The open arrow indicates soft tissue line over inferior orbital rim. The short arrow points to the bony inferior orbital rim, while the long arrow indicates the lowest point of the orbital floor, which is about 1 cm posterior to the orbital rim. The small arrows outline the margins of the superior orbital fissue projected through the right antrum.

FIG. 2-40 Waters view with arrows indicating the canals for the posterior and superior alveolar nerves.

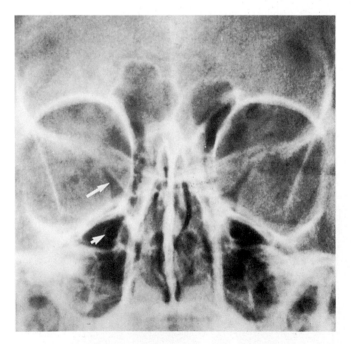

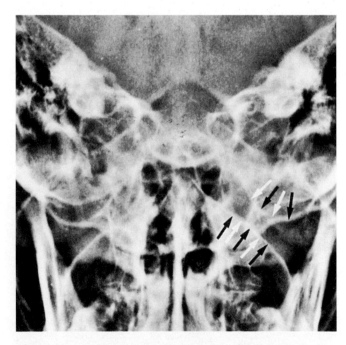

FIG. 2-41 Caldwell view shows superior orbital fissure *(large arrow)* and foramen rotundum *(short arrow)*, which is at the lower lateral margin of the superior orbital fissure.

FIG. 2-42 Towne view with arrows outlining the margins of the inferior orbital fissure. The superior line is formed by the sphenoid bone, and the inferior line is formed by the maxilla.

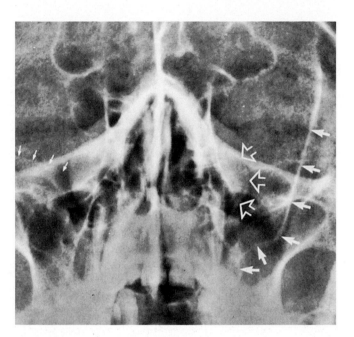 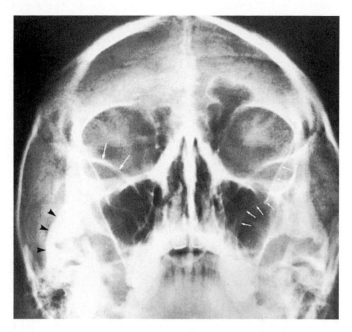

FIG. 2-43 Waters view with arrows pointing to left oblique orbital line. At its lower margin the line bends medially at the level of the infratemporal fossa. The line then bends downward at the level of the lateral pterygoid plate. The small, white arrows point to the upper rim of the right middle cranial fossa. The open arrows indicate the left nasal margin, which can mimic a cyst or polyp in the medial antrum.

FIG. 2-44 Waters view with smaller arrows outlining the left oblique orbital line and its inferior extension to the infratemporal fossa and finally the lateral pterygoid plate. The larger arrows point to the upper anterior margin of the right middle cranial fossa. The arrowheads outline the right zygomatic arch.

sphenoid wing and laterally by the posterior edge of the orbital plate of the frontal bone. The curved margin can be seen projected through the orbit and upper antrum on the Waters view (Figs. 2-43, 2-44).

The body of the zygoma and the zygomatic arches are well seen in the Waters and base views (Figs. 2-20, 2-44). Alternate views for this arch are the underpenetrated base view and the "jug handle," or oblique zygomatic projection. The posterior portions of the arch are best seen on a Towne view. The zygomaticotemporal suture in the zygomatic arch is an obliquely oriented line that is seen routinely and should not be confused with a fracture. Occasionally the zygomaticofacial canal can be seen in the lateral body of the zygoma. It transmits the zygomaticofacial nerve.

On the Waters view the soft tissue shadow of the upper lip is often seen traversing the lower antrum (Fig. 2-45). This shadow usually extends laterally to the lower maxillary sinus margin. Similarly a mustache also can produce such a shadow. These soft tissue densities should not be confused with true retention cysts of the lower antrum, which unlike the shadows just described can be identified as cysts on a lateral view. Similarly the nasal alae can mimic cysts of the medial antral wall in the Waters view (Fig. 2-43).

Soft tissue swelling of the cheek can mimic clouding of the antrum on a Waters view. This usually can be identified by elevation of the superior skin line over the inferior orbital rim. However, sectional imaging may be necessary in some

cases to isolate the maxillary sinus from the overlying swollen skin and subcutaneous tissues.

In the lateral view the coronoid processes of the mandible project over the inferoposterior maxillary sinuses. This is especially noted if the mouth is closed. If these coronoid processes are blunt or rounded, they may simulate retention cysts (Fig. 2-46). If the coronoid processes are sharply pointed, they may simulate a fractured bone segment or an unerupted tooth.

The Sphenoid Sinuses

The sphenoid sinuses are probably the most difficult sinuses to evaluate by routine films because they are buried deep in the skull base and are surrounded by the facial bones, nasal cavity structures, and occiput on the frontal views; the mastoids and lateral skull base structures on the lateral view; and the calvarium and pharynx on the base views. The sphenoid sinuses are extremely variable in their configuration. About one half of the population has only a central sinus cavity, and the other half has, in addition, lateral recesses. These recesses can extend into the greater wings of the sphenoid, lesser wings, and pterygoid processes.

The central, or main, sphenoid sinus cavity is best evaluated on the lateral, base, and open mouth Waters views (Figs. 2-14, 2-32, 2-35). The sinus roof (planum sphenoidale), the sella floor (lamina dura), and the posterior development of the sinus cavity are all well seen on the lateral view; the floor and anterior sinus walls, however, are

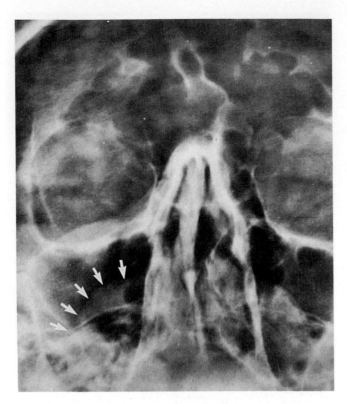

FIG. 2-45 Waters view with arrows outlining the shadow of the upper lip, which is projected over the lower maxillary sinus.

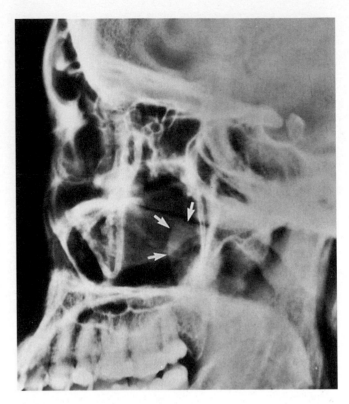

FIG. 2-46 Lateral view with arrows pointing to the coronoid process of the mandible, which is projected over the lower posterior antrum in this closed-mouth view.

partially obscured by the overlapping lateral skull base. The base view provides a means of evaluating the sinus depth and lateral extension. The open mouth Waters view allows evaluation of the lower posterior sinus wall as it is projected through the mouth.

The lateral sinus extensions into the greater wing of the sphenoid can go into the floor of the middle cranial fossa and up into the posterior orbital wall. These extensions are seen best on the Caldwell and Waters views. On the Caldwell view the "orbital recess" is seen as a "lytic" area in the lower lateral orbit. There is a thin, cortical white line outlining its contour except in its lower, medial portion. It is at this margin that this sphenoid recess communicates with the main sinus cavity (Fig. 2-47). On the Waters views the lateral sphenoid sinus recesses in the floor of the middle cranial fossae are projected through the maxillary sinuses. They have a variable shape, depending on the configuration of the recess. They can appear as "dog ears" or can simulate compartments of the maxillary sinus (Fig. 2-48). Regardless of their shape they always join the central sphenoid sinus medially and, when normal, are always rimmed by a thin, white cortical line.

Pterygoid pneumatization results in a triangular lucency in the pterygoid plates in the lateral view and a round or oval lucency in the pterygoid process in the base view (Fig. 2-49). These recesses, when normal, are again outlined by a thin, white cortical line.

The plain film appearances of all of these recesses are classic. Once mastered, the interpreter should not confuse them with pathologic processes.

In patients with a pituitary mass who may require a transpsphenoidal surgical approach, special attention should be given to evaluating the posterior extent of the main sphenoid sinus cavity. If more than 1 or 2 mm of bone remain between the posterior margin of the pneumatized sinus and the anterior sella wall (less than 1% of the cases), most surgeons avoid a transsphenoidal hypophysectomy. This relationship is most easily seen in the lateral view.

Associated Structures Surrounding the Paranasal Sinuses

There are a number of important structures that surround the paranasal sinuses and project over them on the plain film examinations.

On the lateral view the anterior walls of the middle cranial fossa are seen as paired curvilinear lines that project over the sphenoid sinus cavities and merge posteroinferiorly with the bone density of the skull base. The planum sphenoidale is clearly identified as a straight bony line. The cribriform plate is not visualized as well; it continues anteriorly from the planum sphenoidale. However, a line drawn, connecting the nasion and anterior planum, very closely approximates the level of the cribriform plate. The fovea ethmoidalis (ethmoid sinus roofs) lie just lateral to and above

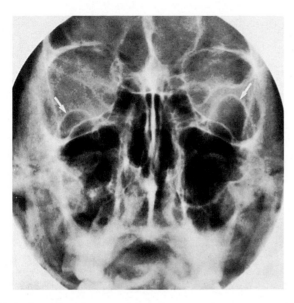

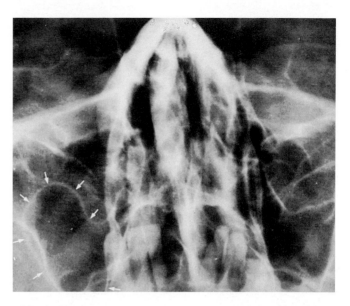

FIG. 2-47 Caldwell view shows lateral sphenoid sinus pneumatization of the greater sphenoid wings as they form the posterior orbital walls *(arrows)*. They are limited on all but their inferomedial margins (where they join the main sinus cavity) by the thin white mucoperiosteal line of the sinus margin.

FIG. 2-48 Waters view shows lateral recesses of sphenoid sinuses extending into the greater sphenoid wings in the floor of the middle cranial fossa. The arrows outline the right "dog-ear–shaped" recess projected through the maxillary sinus. There is also a recess on the left side.

the cribriform plates. They usually are identified as slightly concave, downward, thin, bony lines positioned just above the plane of the cribriform plates. The orbital roofs are situated higher and more laterally than the fovea ethmoidalis. Thus one can roughly localize a lytic process on a lateral film by evaluating which of these lines is eroded. The more superior the line, the more lateral the process (Fig. 2-50). The midline crista galli is best seen on the Caldwell view. This intracranial structure rests on the midline upper surface of cribriform plates.

The bony nasal septum is not seen optimally on any plain film projection, but it is best evaluated on the Caldwell view. Only gross deviation of the bony septum can be appreciated. The cartilaginous septum is poorly seen on plain films and is well visualized only on sectional imaging.

In the lateral view the anterior nasal spine usually has a sharply triangular appearance. The film must often be "bright lighted" to properly evaluate the spine. Destruction of the anterior nasal spine should raise the question of prior surgery or trauma. Midfacial anomalies, Hansen's disease (leprosy), other infectious processes, and carcinomas can also result in nonvisualization of this spine.

The hard palate is best evaluated in the lateral view. Its upper nasal surface is flat and usually has a clear cortical margin. The lower oral surface is slightly concave downward, and it also has a good cortical margin (Fig. 2-33).

In the base view, three paired lines are consistently seen. The most posterior of these is concave posteriorly and represents the greater wings of the sphenoid bone as they form the anterior margin of the middle cranial fossae. Most often the anterior pair of lines is relatively straight, being obliquely oriented to the midsagittal plane and openfaced

anteriorly. Each line is composed medially by the sphenoid bone as it forms the posterior orbital wall and laterally by the orbital surface of the zygoma. The suture between these bones often can be identified clearly. Medially these two sets of paired lines (each primarily formed by the sphenoid bone) join at the pterygoid processes. The third pair of lines are sigmoid (S-shaped) and represent the infratemporal or posterolateral antral walls. Depending on the angulation used to make the base view, the sigmoid line can be anterior to, overlapping and crossing, or posterior to the orbital lines (Figs. 2-34, 2-35).

In the base view the pterygoid fossa is seen as a V-shaped space with its apex placed anteriorly. The pterygoid plates are usually seen as three thin bony lines. The medial pterygoid plate is seen as a single line. However, the lateral pterygoid plate is seen as two separate lines—a lateral line that represents the most caudal end of the lateral pterygoid plate at the level of the hard palate and a central or medial line that represents the lateral pterygoid plate near the skull base. The lateral pterygoid plate is seen as two lines because this plate has a curved, laterally tilted shape, which results in the main body of this plate being oblique to a craniocaudal incident beam and only the upper and lower bony margins being directly "on end" to the beam. Occasionally the hamulus of the medial pterygoid plate can be seen on the base view. The pterygoid fossa is thus the space, open posteriorly, between the medial and central pterygoid lines near the skull base and between the medial and lateral lines near the hard palate.

In the base view the frontal bone casts two transverse lines across the anterior portion of the ethmoid and maxillary sinuses. These lines correspond to the anterior and posterior cortices of the frontal bone. In addition, the anterior surface

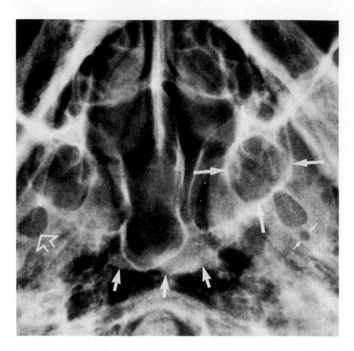

FIG. 2-49   Base view with large arrows outlining pneumatized pterygoid process. The small arrows point to the foramen spinosum, and the open arrow indicates the right foramen ovale. The medium, white arrows outline the posterior margin of the tongue.

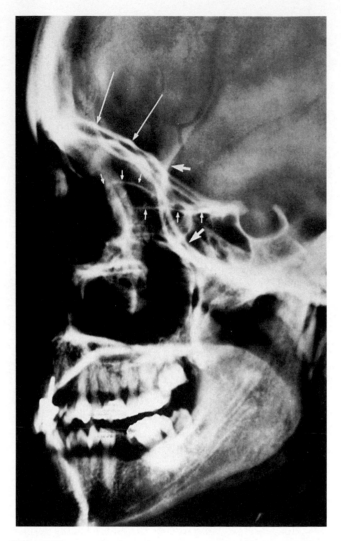

FIG. 2-50   Lateral view with small arrows pointing upward indicating the planum sphenoidale in the midline. The small arrows pointing downward outline the roof of the ethmoid sinuses (fovea ethmoidalis). The long arrows indicate the laterally positioned roofs of the orbit. The short arrows outline the curved anterior margins of the middle cranial fossa.

of the body of the zygoma and the anterior wall of the maxilla cast a transverse line across the anterolateral skull base. The relationship of the frontal table lines to the zygomatico-maxillary lines depends on the particular angulation used in the base view (Figs. 2-34, 2-35, 2-51). In the more markedly angulated base view, the lacrimal canals can also be seen projected through the medial antral walls and hard palate.

The nasopharyngeal soft tissues should be carefully and routinely examined because disease can spread from this area into the sinonasal cavities and vice versa. This evaluation is best accomplished on the lateral view. The presence of a soft tissue fullness in the roof and uppermost posterior wall of the nasopharynx may indicate adenoidal tissue, lymphoma, nasopharyngeal carcinoma, a Thornwalt cyst, or other lesion. If an " adenoidal" mass abuts on the upper surface of the soft palate, it may account for respiratory-related symptoms such as snoring or sleep apnea. Thus obliteration of the posterior nasal airway should always be noted in the radiologist's report.

On the base view the uvula, posterior surface of the soft palate, and the back of the tongue can all cast transverse soft tissue shadows across the skull base. In particular the tongue base is often visualized extending transversely across the sphenoid sinuses. This should not be confused with sinus clouding and should be correlated with the lateral and open mouth Waters views. The air in the nasopharynx and

oropharynx is routinely seen as a low-density region projected over the central skull base. The degree of tube angulation and neck extension determines if this air shadow primarily represents the nasopharynx or the oropharynx. Thus a rectangular shadow with its greatest dimension extending from side to side suggests the nasopharynx, while a more square-shaped shadow suggests the oropharynx. On the routine base view, fullness in the region of the palatine tonsils can produce lateral soft tissue masses that overlie the posterior nasal fossae and pharyngeal air way (Fig. 2-51).

On the lateral view the pinna of the ear occasionally is projected over the sphenoid sinus and nasopharynx. This

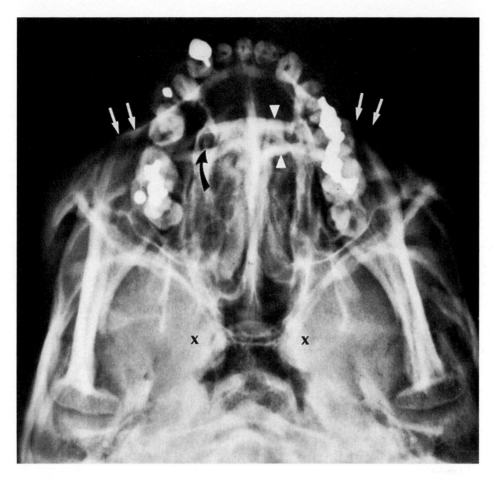

FIG. 2-51 Base view with arrows indicating the anterior wall margin of the maxilla and the zygoma. The curved arrow points to the nasolacrimal duct, which in this film is projected over the frontal bone's anterior and posterior margins *(arrowheads)*. The soft tissue shadows of the palatine tonsils *(Xs)* can also be seen.

may simulate a mass and is usually seen on slightly under-penetrated films. It can be identified as an artifact by tracing out the entire ear lobe.

The nasal bones are best evaluated in the lateral view (Fig. 2-18). The nasofrontal suture is identified easily at the level of the nasion. Also the nasomaxillary sutures can often be seen. There are no normal sutures or bone segments that routinely traverse the midline nasal bones. However, several radiolucent lines are usually present in the lateral aspect of the nasal bones. These lines, which are the normal grooves for the nasociliary nerves and vessels, roughly parallel the plane of the midline nasal bones, and they and should not be confused with fractures. As a general rule there should be no lucent lines that extend across the midline nasal bones, and any such line or lines must suggest the diagnosis of a fracture. Medial depression of the nasal bones is best evaluated

in the occlusal (axial) and Waters views. As mentioned, when evaluating the nasal bones, attention should also be paid to the anterior nasal spine.

In a patient with recent nasal trauma, clinical examination can usually determine whether or not a fracture is present. The examiner places thumb and index finger on either side of the bridge of the nose and gently rocks the fingers from side to side. In cases of fracture the patient has exquisite local pain. In cases of hemorrhage and edema (often markedly deforming the nasal contour) without fracture, the patient is only slightly tender. Thus in such cases, the x-ray request for nasal films should read, "Nasal fracture, please evaluate for the number of fractures and any displacement." The radiologist's report should include a comment on the number and location of the fractures and whether there is depression or elevation of the fracture segments.

References

1. Dodd GD, Jing BS. Radiology of the nose, paranasal sinuses and nasopharynx. Baltimore, Md: Williams & Wilkins, 1977.

2. Merrill V. Atlas of roentgenographic positions. 3rd Edition. St. Louis, Mo: The CV Mosby Co, 1967.

3. Hudgins PA. Complications of endoscopic sinus surgery: role of the radiologist in prevention. Radiol Clin North Am 1993; 31:21-32.

4. Mafee MF. Endoscopic sinus surgery: role of the radiologist. AJR 1991; 157:1099-1104.

5. Mafee MF, Chow JM, Meyers R. Functional endoscopic sinus surgery: Anatomy, CT screening, indications, and complications. AJR 1993; 160: 735-744.

6. Mafee MF. Preoperative imaging anatomy of nasal-ethmoid complex for functional endoscopic sinus surgery. Radiol Clin North Am 1993; 31:1-20.

7. Mancuso AA, Hanafee WN. Computed tomography and magnetic resonance imaging of the head and neck. 2nd Edition. Baltimore, Md: Williams & Wilkins, 1985; 1-19.

8. Som P. Paranasal sinuses and pterygopalatine fossa. In: Carter BL, ed. Computed tomography. New York, NY: Churchill Livingstone, 1985; 101-130.

9. Brant-Zawadzki M, Norman D. Magnetic resonance imaging of the central nervous system. New York, NY: Raven Press, 1987.

10. Lloyd GAS, Lund VJ, Phelps PD, et al. Magnetic resonance imaging in the evaluation of nose and paranasal sinus disease, Br J Radiol 1987; 60:957-968.

11. Vogl TJ, Mack MG, Juergens M, et al. MR diagnosis of head and neck tumors: comparison of contrast enhancement with triple-dose Gadodiamide and standard-dose Gadopentetate Dimeglumine in the same patients. AJR 1994; 163:425-432.

12. Youssem DM, Kennedy DW, Rosenberg S. Ostiomeatal complex risk factors for sinusitis: CT evaluation. J Otolaryng 1991; 20:419-424.

13. Yousem DM. Imaging of sinonasal inflammatory disease. Radiology 1993; 188:303-314.

14. Lanzieri CF, Shah M, Krauss D, et al. Use of Gadolinium-enhanced MR imaging for differentiating mucocele from neoplasms in the paranasal sinuses. Radiology 1991; 178:425-428.

15. Yanagisawa E, Smith HW. Radiographic anatomy of the paranasal sinuses IV: caldwell view. Arch Otolaryngol 1968; 87:311-322.

16. Yanagisawa E, Smith HW. Normal radiographic anatomy of the paranasal sinuses. Otolaryngol Clin North Am 1973; 6(2):429-457.

17. Yanagisawa E, Smith HW. Radiology of the normal maxillary sinus and related structures. Otolaryngol Clin North Am 1976; 9(1):55-81.

18. Yanagisawa E, Smith HW, Merrell RA. Radiographic anatomy of the paranasal sinuses III: submentovertical view. Arch Otolaryngol 1968; 87:299-310.

19. Yanagisawa E, Smith HW, Thaler S. Radiographic anatomy of the paranasal sinuses II: lateral view, Arch Otolaryngol 1968; 87:196-209.

20. Zizmor J, Noyek A. Radiology of the nose and paranasal sinuses. In: Paparella MM, Shumrick DA. Otolaryngology. Vol 1. Philadelphia, Pa: WB Saunders Co, 1973, 1043-1095.

21. Potter GD. Sectional anatomy and tomography of the head. New York, NY: Grune & Stratton Inc, 1971.

22. Gambarelli J, Gréinel G, Chevrot L, et al. Computerized axial tomography: an anatomic atlas of serial sections of the human body, anatomy-radiology-scanner. Berlin, Germany: Springer-Verlag, 1977.

23. Ferner H, ed. Pernkopf's atlas of topographical and applied human anatomy. Vol 1. Head and neck. Baltimore, Md: Urban and Schwarzenberg Inc, 1980.

24. Schatz CJ, Becken TS. Normal and CT anatomy of the paranasal sinuses. Radiol Clin North Am 1984; 22:107-118.

25. Terrier F, Weber W, Ruenfenacht D, et al. Anatomy of the ethmoid: CT, endoscopic and macroscopic, AJNR 1985; 6:77-84.

26. Daniels DL, Rauschning W, Lovas J, et al. Pterygopalatine fossa: computed tomography studies. Radiology 1983; 149:511-516.

3

Sinonasal Cavities: CT Normal Anatomy, Imaging of the Osteomeatal Complex, and Functional Endoscopic Surgery

S. James Zinreich
Mark L. Benson
Patrick J. Oliverio

HISTORIC PERSPECTIVE

Inflammatory sinus disease is a serious health problem, affecting an estimated 30 to 50 million people in the United States alone.[1] Because physical examination of these patients can be nonspecific, for many years, radiologic evaluation has been relied on to aid in confirming the diagnosis of paranasal sinus pathology. Traditionally, plain films were the modality of choice in the evaluation of the paranasal sinuses. Clinically and radiographically the emphasis was directed primarily to the maxillary and frontal sinuses. In recent years, however, because of technologic advancements in imaging and a change in therapeutic approach, computed tomography (CT) has supplanted conventional radiography as the primary diagnostic modality.

Although most patients with sinonasal inflammatory disease are initially treated medically, medical therapy alone often does not resolve the problem. The surgical treatment of refractory inflammatory sinus disease has undergone revolutionary change in the last decade. These advances are due to the combination of several factors: (1) an improved understanding of the mucociliary clearance pathways in the nasal cavity and paranasal sinuses, (2) improved endoscopes that afford direct access to nasal cavity and ethmoid sinus drainage portals, and (3) the availability of high-resolution coronal CT images that provide an accurate display of the regional anatomy.

Functional endoscopic sinus surgery (FESS) was first described independently by both Messerklinger in German literature and Wigand, Steiner, and Jaumann in English literature in 1978.[2,3,4] FESS was introduced in the United States in 1984 by Kennedy et al.[5] Subsequent advancement of the technique through innovations both in the surgical and radiologic fields has occurred.[6]

The objectives in this chapter are to discuss the available imaging modalities for patients with surgically amenable inflammatory sinus disease, describe the pertinent radiographic anatomy and anatomic variants of the paranasal sinuses and adjacent structures, review the radiographic appearance of inflammatory sinus disease, describe FESS procedures, and demonstrate the expected radiographic appearance in postoperative FESS patients, as well as the appearance of complications that can occur as a result of FESS.

TECHNIQUES OF EVALUATION
Conventional Radiography

The standard radiographic (plain film) sinus series usually consists of four views: lateral view, Caldwell view, Waters view, and submentovertex (SMV or base) view.[7] The anatomy displayed on each of these views is reviewed in Chapter 2.

Although the standard radiographs may be accurate in showing air-fluid levels, the degree of chronic inflammatory disease present is consistently and significantly underestimated. Furthermore, the superimposition of structures precludes the accurate evaluation of the anatomy of the osteomeatal channels with which the modern surgeon needs to be familiar.[6,8-11]

Computed Tomography (CT)
Rationale

CT is currently the modality of choice in the evaluation of the paranasal sinuses and adjacent structures.[6,8-11] Its ability to optimally display bone, soft tissue, and air facilitates accurate depiction of anatomy and extent of disease in and around the paranasal sinuses.[6,8-11] In contrast to standard radiographs, CT clearly depicts the fine bony anatomy of the osteomeatal channels.

Many authors stress the importance of performing the initial CT scan after a course of adequate medical therapy to eliminate reversible changes of mucosal inflammation and to better evaluate the underlying anatomic structures. Several authors also suggest routine pretreatment with a sympathomimetic nasal spray 15 minutes before scanning to reduce nasal congestion.[12] This minimizes the mucosal edema and allows an improved display of the fine bony architecture and any irreversible mucosal disease.

Positioning

Because the coronal plane optimally displays the osteomeatal unit (OMU) and the relationship of the brain and ethmoid roof, as well as depicts the relationship of the orbits to the paranasal sinuses, imaging in the coronal plane is recommended.[6,8-11] Because the coronal images closely correlate with the surgical approach, they should be obtained in all patients with inflammatory sinus disease who are endoscopic surgical candidates.[7]

Optimally the coronal study should be performed in the prone position, so that any remaining sinus secretions do not obscure the OMU. In patients who cannot tolerate prone positioning (children, patients of advanced age, etc.), the "hanging head" technique can sometimes be utilized. In this technique the patient is placed in the supine position, and the neck is maximally extended. A pillow placed under the patient's shoulders helps positioning. The CT gantry is angled as perpendicular as possible to the bony palate. It is not always possible to obtain direct coronal images with this technique.

In patients who are intubated or have tracheostomy sites, it is not technically feasible to position them for coronal scans. Also, young children, patients with severe cervical arthropathy, and patients who are otherwise debilitated usually cannot tolerate the examination. In such patients, thin section, contiguous axial CT images with coronal reconstructions are performed.

Direct axial images are recommended to compliment the coronal study when there is severe disease in the frontal, sphenoid, or posterior ethmoid sinuses and surgical treatment is contemplated. Spiral CT aids the evaluation of the pediatric or debilitated patient by allowing a rapid scan to be

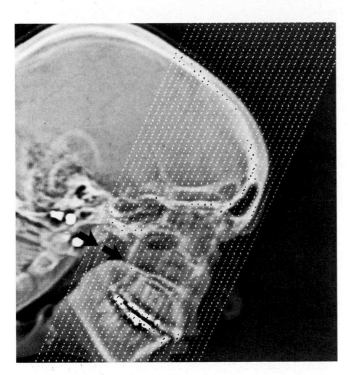

FIG. 3-1 CT lateral topogram shows the patient's position during the examination. Dotted lines represent the scanner gantry angulation, which should be as perpendicular as possible to the hard palate *(arrows)*.

<table>
<tr><td colspan="2" align="center">▼
BOX 3-1
PARAMETERS FOR SINUS CT</td></tr>
<tr><td>Patient position</td><td>Prone</td></tr>
<tr><td>Angulation</td><td>Perpendicular to hard palate</td></tr>
<tr><td>Field of View</td><td>14 cm</td></tr>
<tr><td>Thickness</td><td>3 mm, contiguous</td></tr>
<tr><td>Exposure</td><td>125 kVp and 80-160 mAs</td></tr>
</table>

TABLE 3-1
Relative Radiation Dose for Sinus CT (Utilizing 125 kVp)

mAs	Radiation Dose Equivalent
450	4.95-5.40 cSv (4.95 - 5.40 rem)
240	2.64 - 2.88 cSv (2.64 - 2.88 rem)
160	1.76 - 1.92 cSv (1.76 - 1.92 rem)
80	0.88 - 0.96 cSv (0.88 - 0.96 rem)

From Zinreich S. Imaging of inflammatory sinus disease. Otolaryngol Clin North Am 1993; 26(4):535-47.

performed and by providing improved quality multiplanar reconstructed images.

Examination Protocol

The patient is placed prone, with the chin hyperextended, on the bed of the CT scanner. The scanner gantry is angled as perpendicular as possible to the hard palate (Fig. 3-1). The angulation of the scan plane is very important. Melhem et al. showed that variations in scan angulation greater than 10° from the plane perpendicular to the hard palate result in significant loss of anatomic detail of the structures of the OMU.[13]

Scanning is performed as contiguous 3-mm thick images from the anterior wall of the frontal sinus through the posterior wall of the sphenoid sinus. Contiguous scans ought to be obtained to avoid loss of information through "skipped" areas.[13] The field of view should be adjusted to include only the areas of interest. This helps reduce artifact from the teeth and associated metallic restorations and magnifies the small anatomic structures of the nasal cavity and adjacent paranasal sinuses.[9]

Originally the exposure settings for sinus CT were kVp of 125 and mAs of 450 (5 second scan time). Babbel et al. showed that there is no compromise of the image's quality when the mAs is reduced to 200 (2 second scan time), and recent work of Melhem et al. showed no significant loss of diagnostic quality with mAs settings of 160 or even 80 (2

second scan times).[12,13] It is therefore recommended that the exposure settings be 125 kVp and 80 to 160 mAs.

Box 3-1 summarizes the sinus CT examination protocol.

Radiation Exposure

As a brief review, the radiation exposure (dose) that a patient receives is known as the radiation absorbed dose. This radiation absorbed dose is a measure of the total radiation energy absorbed by the tissues, and it is expressed in an SI unit known as the Gray (Gy). One Gy is the amount of radiation needed to deposit the energy of one joule (J) in one kg of tissue (Gy = 1 J/kg). Formerly the unit used to express radiation absorbed dose was the rad (1 rad = amount of radiation needed to deposit the energy of 100 ergs in 1 g tissue). The conversion of the rad to the Gy is: 1 Gy = 100 rad.[14,15]

A more useful term is "radiation dose equivalent," which takes into account the quality factor Q of the radiation (radiation dose equivalent = radiation dose absorbed × Q). This quality factor, accounts for the varying biologic effectiveness of different forms of ionizing radiation. For x-rays, Q = 1, and thus radiation absorbed dose is equivalent to the radiation dose equivalent. Currently the SI unit of radiation dose equivalent is the Sievert (Sv); the former unit was the rem. Therefore for diagnostic x-rays, 1 Gy = 1 Sv and 1 Sv = 100 rem.[14,15]

Radiation dose equivalent is dependant on the kVp and mAs. For a given kVp, radiation dose equivalent varies linearly with the mAs. At 125 kVp the radiation dose equivalent for a CT slice is approximately 1.1 to 1.2 cSv / 100 mAs (1.1 to 1.2 rem/ 100 mAs). The actual dose varies slightly from machine to machine. Table 3-1 shows that the radiation dose equivalent for a CT slice can be considerably reduced using a low mAs technique.

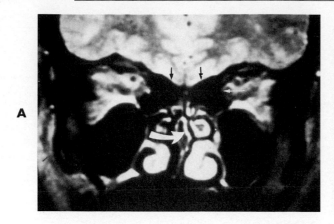 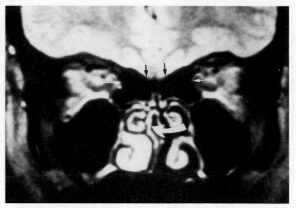

FIG. 3-2 **A** and **B,** Nasal cycle on MR imaging. Coronal T2W MR images of the anterior ethmoid sinuses show the changing edema of the nasal cavity *(curved arrow),* ethmoid sinus mucosa, and the changing size of the turbinates. Note the lack of signal for definition of the ethmoid sinus roof and lamina papyracea *(arrows).*

TABLE 3-2
Estimated Effective Dose Equivalent of Common Examinations

Examination	Effective Dose Equivalent
Sinus series, four views	7.0 mrem
Chest, PA and lateral	7.2 mrem
KUB	8.7 mrem
Lumbar spine, five views	125.1 mrem
CT, brain*	112.0 mrem
CT, sinus (160 mAs)†	51.2 mrem
CT, sinus (80 mAs)‡	25.6 mrem

From Zinreich S. Imaging of inflammatory sinus disease. Otolaryngol Clin North Am 1993; 26(4):535-47 and Zinreich S, Abidin M, Kennedy D. Cross-sectional imaging of the nasal cavity and paranasal sinuses. Operative Techniques in Otolaryngol Head Neck Surg 1990; 1(2):93-9.

*120 kVp, 240 mAs, 10 mm slice thickness, contiguous.
†125 kVp, 160 mAs, 3 mm slice thickness, contiguous.
‡125 kVp, 80 mAs, 3 mm slice thickness, contiguous.

In contiguous CT imaging the dose delivered to a particular region scanned (for example, the paranasal sinuses) is approximately equal to the per slice dose. The dose delivered to a region is less than the per slice dose if there is a gap between slices, and the delivered dose is higher if there is overlap between slices.

The *effective dose equivalent* was developed as a way of representing the fraction of the total stochastic risk of fatal cancers and chromosomal abnormalities resulting from the irradiation of a particular organ or tissue when the body is uniformly irradiated.[14,15] A system of weighting is used to take into account the individual sensitivity of the body's major tissues and organs.[14,15] A full discussion of effective dose is beyond the scope of this chapter. Suffice it to say that for a given examination, the effective dose to the patient is less than the dose (radiation dose equivalent) received by the area scanned. A list of effective dose equivalents for some common radiographic procedures is presented in Table 3-2.[14,16]

Image Display

Windows are chosen to highlight the air passages, the bony detail, and the soft tissues. Usually a window width of +2000 Houndsfield units (HU) with a level of −200 HU are good starting parameters. The window and level settings can then be manually manipulated to optimally display the anatomic detail of the uncinate process and ethmoid bulla, and once this is accomplished, these settings can be used to film the entire study.[6,8-11]

Sagittal reconstructions can be obtained for a morphologic orientation. Various distances and angles can be measured to aid in the passage of instruments during surgery. If only coronal scans are obtained, axial reconstructions can help display the position of the internal carotid arteries and optic nerves with respect to the bony margins of the posterior ethmoid and sphenoid sinuses.

Magnetic Resonance Imaging

Although magnetic resonance imaging (MRI) provides better visualization of soft tissue than CT, its disadvantage is its inability to optimally display the cortical bone-air interface.[9,10] Because both cortical bone and air have signal voids (no MR signal), at times, MR is unable to discern the intricate anatomic relationships of the sinuses and their drainage portals. Thus MRI cannot be reliably used as an operative "roadmap" to guide the surgeon during FESS.

There is a side-to-side cyclic variation in the thickness of the nasal mucosa known as the "nasal cycle" (see Chapter 2). The signal intensity of the mucosal lining of the nasal cavity and ethmoid sinuses varies in concert with the nasal cycle.[17,18] During the edematous phase of the nasal cycle, in both the ethmoid sinuses and the nasal cavity the mucosal signal intensity on T2-weighted (T2W) images is similar to the appearance of mucosal inflammation, which limits the usefulness of MRI (Fig. 3-2).[11,12] Interestingly there is no cyclic variation of the mucosal signal in the frontal, maxillary, or sphenoid sinuses, and increased mucosal thickness and increased signal on T2W images in these sinuses is always abnormal.[17,18] To date, with respect to sinus imaging, MRI has proven most helpful in the evaluation of regional and intracranial complications of inflammatory sinus disease and its surgical treatment, in the detection of neoplastic processes, and in providing an improved display of anatomic relationships between the intraorbital and extraorbital compartments.[19-23]

INTERPRETATION OF IMAGING STUDIES

In any radiologic study the radiologist must use a collection of skills to provide consistent, accurate interpretations of studies of the paranasal sinuses. These skills include the following:

1. A detailed knowledge of the anatomy of the paranasal sinuses.
2. A systematic reading pattern.
3. A detailed knowledge of the common pathologies affecting the region.
4. A working knowledge of the available surgical options and their radiographic appearance.
5. An awareness of common operative complications and their radiographic appearance.

NORMAL ANATOMY
Mucociliary Clearance

For a clear understanding of the regional anatomy and the importance of the anterior ethmoid sinus structures, it is critical that one understands the flow pattern of the mucous blanket coating the major sinuses (mucociliary clearance). Further, one must be acquainted with the concept that inflammatory sinus disease largely results from compromise of the drainage portals (osteomeatal channels) of the individual sinus cavities.

The mucosa of the paranasal sinuses is made up of a ciliated cuboidal epithelium, and a mucous blanket is secreted on its surface. The cilia are in constant motion and act in concert to propel the mucous in a specific direction. The pattern of flow is specific for each sinus and will persist even if alternative openings are surgically created in the sinus. [2-6,24,25] Therefore FESS has gained widespread acceptance because its goal is to restore drainage of the sinuses via their anatomic drainage pathways.

In the maxillary sinus the mucous flow originates in the antral floor, and it is then directed centripetally toward the primary ostium. The mucous is then transported through the infundibulum to the hiatus semilunaris, from where it is passed into the middle meatus and ultimately the nasopharynx. This pattern of mucous movement persists even after a nasal antrostomy is created.[2-6,24-26]

In the frontal sinus the mucous flow is up along the medial wall, laterally across the roof, and medially along the floor. As the flow approaches the medial aspect of the floor, some is directed into the primary ostium and the remainder

is recirculated. The cleared mucous travels down the frontal recess and then into the middle meatus where it joins the flow from the ipsilateral maxillary sinus.[2-6,24-26]

The posterior ethmoid and sphenoid sinuses clear their mucous into the sphenoethmoidal recess. The flow then enters the superior meatus and subsequently the nasopharynx.

Thus there are two main osteomeatal channels. The anterior OMU includes the frontal sinus ostium, frontal recess, maxillary sinus ostium, infundibulum, and middle meatus. These channels provide communication between the ipsilateral frontal, anterior ethmoid, and maxillary sinuses. The posterior OMU consists of the sphenoid sinus ostium, sphenoethmoidal recess, and the superior meatus. The radiologic representation of the anatomy should stress display of these osteomeatal channels.

Normal Anatomy (Osteomeatal Unit)

To correctly interpret imaging studies, it is essential to understand the anatomy of the lateral nasal wall and its relationship to adjacent structures (Fig. 3-3).[27,28] The lateral nasal wall contains three bulbous projections: the superior, middle, and inferior turbinates (conchae). The turbinates divide the nasal cavity into three distinct air passages: the superior, middle, and inferior meati. The superior meatus drains the posterior ethmoid air cells and, more posteriorly, the sphenoid sinus (via the sphenoethmoidal recess). The middle meatus receives drainage from the frontal sinus (via the nasofrontal recess), the maxillary sinus (via the maxillary ostium and subsequently the ethmoidal infundibulum), and the anterior ethmoid air cells (via the ethmoid cell ostia). The inferior meatus receives drainage from the nasolacrimal duct.

On CT scanning the first coronal images display the outline of the frontal sinuses (Fig. 3-4). The frontal sinuses are funnel shaped. Their aeration varies from patient to patient. They can be small and occupy only the diploic space of the medial frontal bone, or they can be large enough to extend through the floor of the entire anterior cranial fossa. In general a central septation separates the left and right sides, however, often there may be several septations. The floor of the frontal sinus slopes inferiorly toward the midline.

Close to the midline the primary ostium is located in a depression in the floor. The frontal recess is an hourglass-like narrowing between the frontal sinus and the anterior middle meatus through which the frontal sinus drains (Fig. 3-5).[8] It is not a tubular structure, as the term *nasofrontal duct* might imply, and therefore the term *recess* is preferred.

Anterior, lateral, and inferior to the frontal recess is the agger nasi cell. The agger nasi cell is a remnant ethmoturbinal, which is present in nearly all patients. It is aerated and represents the most anterior ethmoid air cell. It usually borders the primary ostium or floor of the frontal sinus, and thus its size may directly influence the patency of the frontal recess and the anterior middle meatus. The frontal recesses are the narrowest anterior air channels and are common sites of inflammation. Their obstruction subsequently results in loss of ventilation and mucociliary clearance of the frontal

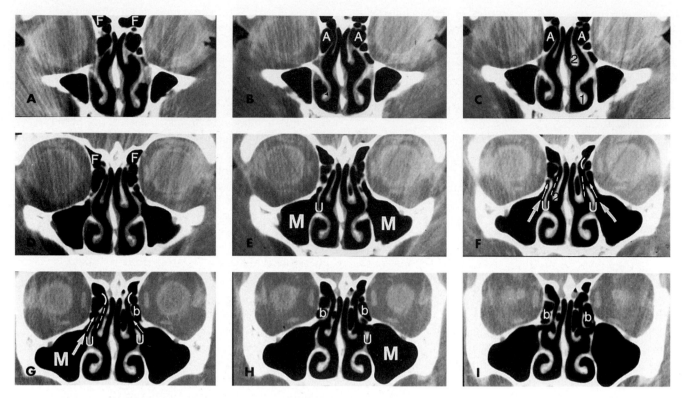

FIG. 3-3 **A** through **I,** Coronal CT display of paranasal sinus anatomy. Thin section coronal CT images of a cadaver specimen. Frontal sinus *(F),* agger nasi cell *(A),* ethmoid bulla *(b),* maxillary sinus *(M),* basal lamella *(black arrow),* sphenoid sinus *(S),* inferior turbinate *(1),* middle turbinate *(2),* superior turbinate *(3).* The anterior osteomeatal unit is displayed in images **F** through **H.** Frontal recess *(small curved lines),* middle meatus *(dashed lines),* infundibulum *(small arrows),* and primary ostium of the maxillary sinus *(large white arrows).*

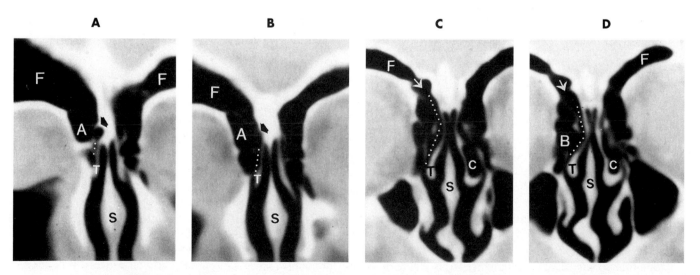

FIG. 3-4 Anatomy of the frontal sinus. Coronal CT images of the frontal sinuses from anterior **(A)** to posterior **(D)** show the relationship between the frontal sinus *(F)* and the middle meatus *(dotted line).* Note that there is a bony strut *(heavy black arrow* in **A** and **B),* separating the frontal sinus and the anterior middle meatus. This separation is lost on the more posterior images **(C** and **D)** revealing the position of the frontal recess *(white arrow).* Note the position of the agger nasi cell *(A)* and its relationship to the frontal recess. Nasal septum *(S),* ethmoid bulla *(B),* middle turbinate *(T),* and concha bullosa *(C).*

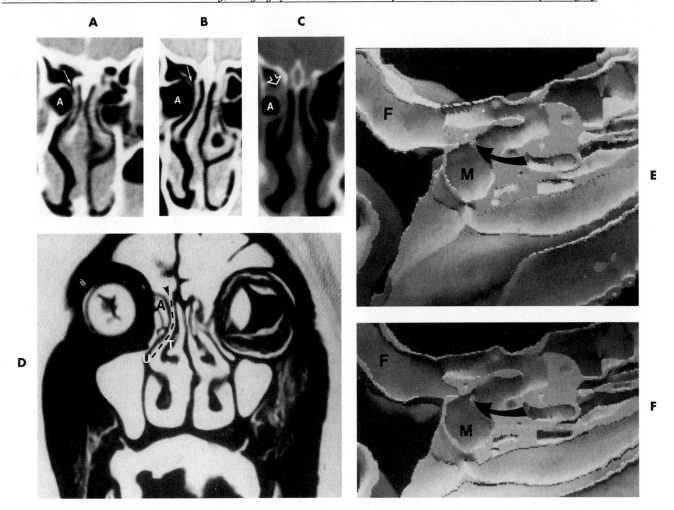

FIG. 3-5 Anatomy of the frontal recess. **A** and **B,** Coronal CT images reveal a patent frontal recess *(white arrow)* despite the presence of a large agger nasi cell *(A)*. **C,** Coronal CT in a different patient with an obstructed right frontal recess and mucoperiosteal thickening in the right frontal sinus *(open arrow)*. Agger nasi *(A)*. **D,** Density-reversed coronal CT image in a cadaveric specimen optimally demonstrates the position of the frontal recess *(arrowhead)*. Also note the relationship between the middle turbinate *(T)*, uncinate process *(U)*, agger nasi *(A)*, and middle meatus *(dashed line)*. **E** and **F,** Three-dimensional CT images with a sagittal cut–plane view of the paranasal sinuses show the position of the frontal recess *(curved arrow)* and show that its shape is that of an hourglass narrowing between the frontal sinus *(F)* and middle meatus *(M)*.

sinus. The uncinate process is a superior extension of the lateral nasal wall (medial wall of the maxillary sinus).[8,10] Anteriorly the uncinate process fuses with the posteromedial wall of the agger nasi cell and the posteromedial wall of the nasolacrimal duct. The uncinate process has a "free" (unattached) superoposterior edge. Laterally this free edge delimits the infundibulum (Fig. 3-6). The infundibulum is the air passage that connects the maxillary sinus ostium to the middle meatus. Posterior to the uncinate is the ethmoid bulla, usually the largest of the anterior ethmoid cells. The uncinate process usually courses medial and inferior to the ethmoid bulla. The ethmoid bulla is enclosed laterally by the lamina papyracea.

The gap between the ethmoid bulla and the free edge of the uncinate process defines the hiatus semilunaris. Medially the hiatus semilunaris communicates with the middle meatus, the air space lateral to the middle turbinate.[8,10] Lat-erally and inferiorly the hiatus semilunaris communicates with the infundibulum, the air channel between the uncinate process (caudal border) and the inferomedial margin of the orbit (cranial border). The infundibulum serves as the primary drainage pathway from the maxillary sinus.[10,11]

The structure medial to the ethmoid bulla and the uncinate process is the middle turbinate. Anteriorly it attaches to the medial wall of the agger nasi cell and the superior edge of the uncinate process. Superiorly the middle turbinate adheres to the cribriform plate. As it extends posteriorly, the middle turbinate emits a laterally coursing bony structure, the basal or ground lamella, that fuses with the lamina papyracea just posterior to the ethmoid bulla. The basal lamella demarcates the anterior ethmoid sinus from the posterior ethmoid sinus.

In most patients the posterior wall of the ethmoid bulla is

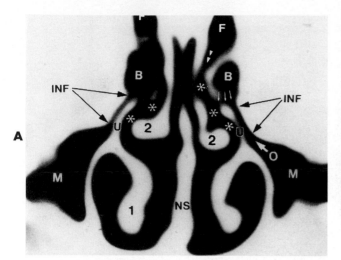
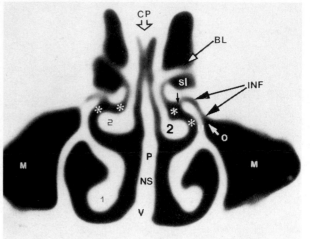

FIG. 3-6 Anterior osteomeatal channels. Coronal CT images through the anterior ethmoid sinuses show the air passages intercommunicating the frontal sinus *(F)*, anterior ethmoid sinus, and maxillary sinus *(M)*. The primary ostium *(O)* of the maxillary sinus communicates with the infundibulum *(INF)*. The infundibulum is bordered medially by the uncinate process *(U)* and laterally by the orbit. In turn the infundibulum communicates with the middle meatus *(asterisks)* through the hiatus semilunaris *(most medial white arrow* in **A**, *black arrow* in **B**). The frontal recess *(white arrowheads)* is patent. The ethmoid bulla *(B)* is usually the largest air cell in the anterior ethmoid sinus. Note the vertical attachment of the middle turbinate *(2)* to the cribriform plate *(CP)* and its lateral attachment to the lamina papyracea, the basal lamella *(BL)*. The air space between the basal lamella and the ethmoid bulla is the sinus lateralis *(sl)*. Inferior turbinate *(1)*, nasal septum *(NS)*, vomer *(V)*, and perpendicular plate of the ethmoid bone *(P)*.

intact, and an air space is usually found between the basal lamella and the posterior ethmoid bulla. This air space, the sinus lateralis, may extend superior to the ethmoid bulla and communicate with the frontal recess (Fig. 3-7). A dehiscence or total absence of the posterior wall of the ethmoid bulla is common and may provide communication between these two usually separated air spaces.

The posterior ethmoid sinus consists of air cells between the basal lamella and the sphenoid sinus. The number, shape, and size of these air cells vary significantly from person to person.[8,9,11,29]

The sphenoid sinus is the most posterior sinus. It is usually embedded in the clivus and is bordered superoposteriorly by the sella turcica. Its ostium is located medially in the anterosuperior portion of the anterior sinus wall and communicates with the sphenoethmoidal recess and posterior aspect of the superior meatus. The sphenoethmoidal recess lies just lateral to the nasal septum and can sometimes be seen on coronal images, but it is best displayed in the sagittal and axial planes (Fig. 3-8).[8-10]

The relationship between the aerated portion of the sphenoid sinus and the posterior ethmoid sinus must be accurately represented so the surgeon can avoid operative complications (Fig. 3-9). Usually, in the paramedian sagittal plane the sphenoid sinus is the most superior and posterior air space. More laterally (1 to 1.5 cm) the sphenoid sinus is located more inferiorly, and the posterior ethmoid air cells become the most superior and posterior air space. This

relationship is well demonstrated on axial and sagittal images. The number and position of the septations in the sphenoid sinus are quite variable. Of particular importance are septations that adhere to the bony canal wall, covering the internal carotid artery, which often projects into the posterolateral sphenoid sinus. Less often the canal of the Vidian nerve (pterygoid canal) and the canal of the second division of the trigeminal nerve can project into the floor of the sphenoid sinus.

Anatomically the paranasal sinuses are in close proximity to the anterior cranial fossa, the cribriform plate, the internal carotid arteries, the cavernous sinuses, the orbits and their contents, and the optic nerves as they exit the orbits.[30-34] The surgeon must be especially cautious when maneuvering instruments directed cranially and dorsally so that there is not inadvertent penetration and damage to these structures.[6,11,32,33]

ANATOMIC VARIATIONS AND CONGENITAL ABNORMALITIES

Even though nasal anatomy varies significantly from patient to patient, certain anatomic variations are observed nasal septum. However, its major curvature can project laterally, thus narrowing the middle meatus and infundibulum. Such a variant is called a paradoxical middle turbinate (Fig. 3-13). The inferior edge of the middle meatus may assume various shapes with excessive curvature,

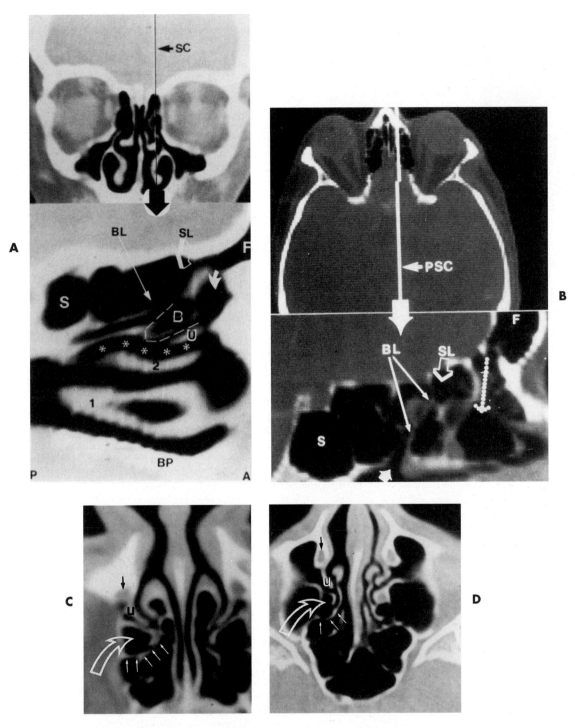

FIG. 3-7 Anatomy of the basal lamella and sinus lateralis. **A** and **B**, Sagittal reconstructed plane *(SC)* from direct coronal CT data **(A)** and sagittal reconstructed plane *(PSC)* from direct axial CT data **(B)** show the outline of the basal lamella *(BL)* and the position of the sinus lateralis *(SL)* in between the basal lamella and the ethmoid bulla *(B)*. The position of the hiatus semilunaris *(dashed U-shaped line* in **A**), the frontal recess, and the anterior middle meatus *(curved arrow* in **A** and *dotted line* in **B**) are noted. Frontal sinus *(F)*, sphenoid sinus *(S)*, uncinate process *(U)*, middle meatus *(asterisks)*, inferior turbinate *(1)*, middle turbinate *(2)*, bony palate *(BP)*, middle meatus-nasopharynx junction *(heavy white arrow* in **B**), anterior *(A)*, and posterior *(P)*. **C** and **D**. Axial CT images show the orientation of the uncinate process *(u)* and its association with nasolacrimal duct *(small black arrow)*. Note the attachment of the basal lamella *(small white arrows)* to the lamina papyracea. The ethmoid bulla *(curved arrow)* is the air cell anterior to the basal lamella, and in both of these patients the posterior wall of the air cell is incomplete, providing a direct communication between the ethmoid bulla and the sinus lateralis.

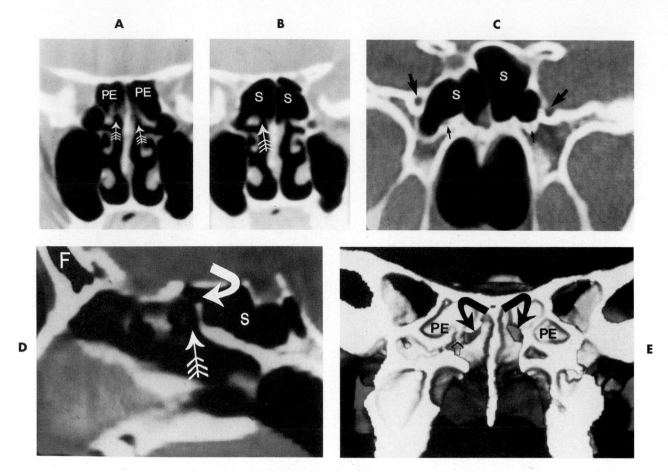

FIG. 3-8   Sphenoid sinus anatomy. **A** and **B,** Coronal CT images show the boundary between the posterior ethmoid sinus *(PE)* and the sphenoid sinus *(S).* This boundary is best recognized by the position of the sphenoethmoidal recess *(feathered arrows).* One is relatively sure that the coronal image is through the anterior sphenoid sinus when only the inferior edge of the sphenoethmoidal recess is identified (**B**). **C,** Coronal CT image through the sphenoid sinus *(S)* shows the number and orientation of septations within the sinus, as well as the relationship to the foramen rotundum *(heavy black arrow)* and vidian canal *(fine black arrow).* **D,** Paramedial sagittal CT image shows the position of the sphenoid sinus ostium *(curved arrow)* and the sphenoethmoidal recess *(feathered arrows).* Frontal sinus *(F),* and sphenoid sinus *(S).* **E,** Three-dimensional CT image with a coronal cut–plane view through the posterior aspect of the posterior ethmoid sinus *(PE)* reveals the orientation of the sphenoethmoidal recess *(open arrow)* and position of the sphenoid sinus ostia *(curved arrows).*

which in turn may obstruct the nasal cavity, infundibulum, and middle meatus (Fig. 3-14).

Concha Bullosa

A concha bullosa refers to an aerated middle turbinate and may be unilateral or bilateral (Fig. 3-10). Less frequently, aeration of the superior turbinate may occur; an aerated inferior turbinate is uncommon. A concha bullosa involving the middle turbinate may enlarge the turbinate so that it obstructs the middle meatus or the infundibulum. The air cavity in a concha bullosa is lined with the same epithelium as the rest of the sinonasal cavities, and thus these concha bullosa cells can experience the same inflammatory disorders that affect the paranasal sinuses. Obstruction of the drainage of a concha can lead to mucocele formation (Fig. 3-11).

Nasal Septal Deviation

This is an asymmetric bowing of the nasal septum that may compress the middle turbinate laterally, narrowing the middle meatus (Fig. 3-12). Bony spurs are often associated with septal deviation, and this may further compromise the OMU. Nasal septal deviation is usually congenital but may be posttraumatic in some patients.

Paradoxical Middle Turbinate

The middle turbinate usually curves medially toward the nasal septum. However, its major curvature can project laterally, thus narrowing the middle meatus and infundibulum. Such a variant is called a paradoxical middle turbinate (Fig. 3-13). The inferior edge of the middle meatus may assume various shapes with excessive curvature,

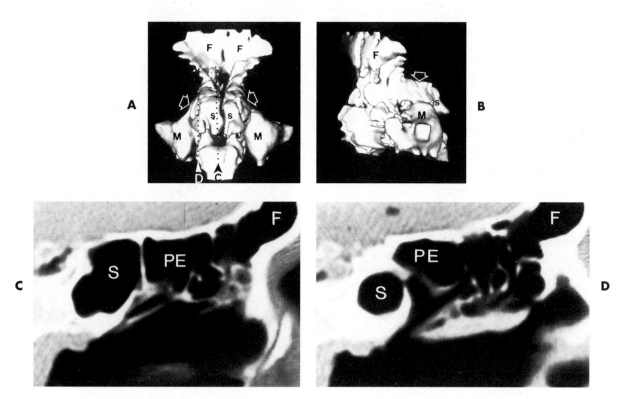

FIG. 3-9 Anatomic relationship of the posterior ethmoid and sphenoid sinuses. **A** and **B,** Posterior (A) and anterolateral (B) views from three-dimensional CT images of a "cast" of the aerated nasal cavity, nasopharynx, and paranasal sinuses viewed from behind **(A)** and the left side **(B)**. Note that the posterior ethmoid sinus *(open arrows)* is wider and positioned more superiorly than the sphenoid sinus *(S)*. The dotted lines denote the position of the sagittal planes displayed in **C** and **D**. Frontal sinus *(F),* and maxillary sinus *(M)*. **C,** Paraseptal CT image of a cadaver head shows that the sphenoid sinus *(S)* is the most posterior and superior air space and that it is accessible from the posterior ethmoid sinus *(PE)*. **D,** Sagittal CT image of a cadaver head performed approximately 1.5 cm lateral to the nasal septum shows that the sphenoid sinus *(S)* is inferior to the posterior ethmoid sinus *(PE)*. Frontal sinus *(F)*.

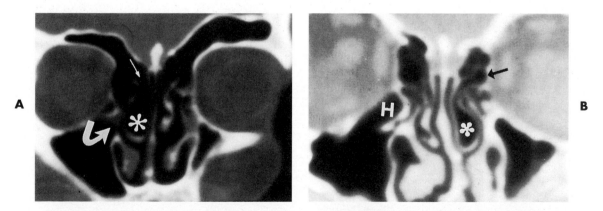

FIG. 3-10 Concha bullosa in two different patients. **A,** Coronal CT image demonstrates a prominent right concha bullosa *(asterisk)* with communication to the frontal recess *(small arrow)*. Note the obstruction of the right middle meatus *(curved arrow)*. **B,** Coronal CT image demonstrates a left-sided concha bullosa *(asterisk)* with communication to the sinus lateralis *(small arrow)*. Note the contralateral Haller cell *(H)*.

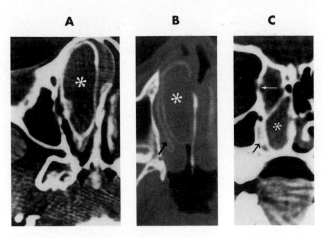

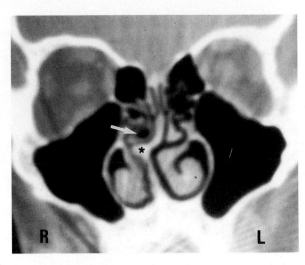

FIG. 3-11 Mucocele within a concha bullosa. Axial (**A** and **B**) and coronal (**C**) CT images show a prominent soft-tissue mass (*asterisk*) well circumscribed by a bony perimeter (the bony framework of the concha bullosa). The inferior turbinate is compressed against the medial wall of the maxillary sinus (*black arrow*). In the coronal image the extent of the obstruction of the nasal cavity is apparent as is the presence of a more superior mucocele, which erodes the lamina papyracea (*white arrow*).

FIG. 3-12 Nasal septal deviation with spurring. Coronal CT image demonstrates that there is deviation of the nasal septum toward the right side with a right-sided cartilaginous nasal "spur" (*asterisk*). Note the ipsilateral concha bullosa (*arrow*). Both of these anatomic variants contribute to marked narrowing of the right nasal cavity and ethmoid passages.

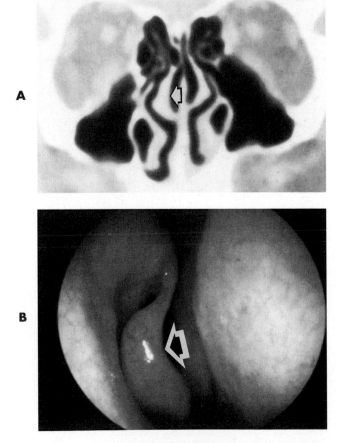

FIG. 3-13 Paradoxical middle turbinate. **A,** Coronal CT image demonstrates bilateral paradoxical middle turbinates. The right side is highlighted (*solid arrow*). **B,** Endoscopic view correlates with the CT findings (*arrow*).

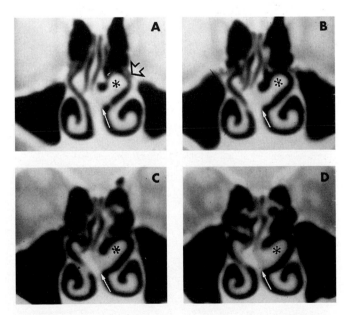

FIG. 3-14 **A** through **D,** Coronal CT scans. The free edge of the middle turbinate may also assume some other shapes. Note its prominent lateral curvature in this case (*asterisk*). It obstructs the nasal passage (*fine white arrows*) and contributes to the position of the uncinate process, and therefore, the prominent narrowing of the infundibulum (open arrow).

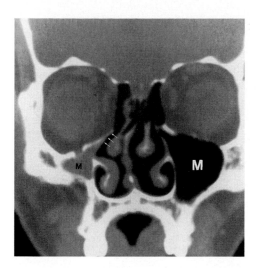

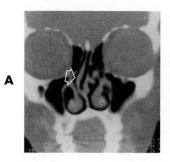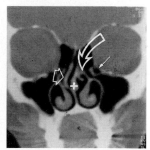

FIG. 3-16   **A** and **B,** Medially curved uncinate process. Coronal CT images through the ethmoid sinuses show a prominent right-sided deviation of the nasal septum *(straight open arrow)*. Note the medially curved left uncinate process *(curved open arrow)*, which is medially displacing the left middle turbinate (+) and obstructs the left middle meatus. A left-sided Haller cell is present *(small arrow).*

FIG. 3-15   Atelectatic uncinate process. Coronal CT scan shows that the right uncinate process is apposed to the inferomedial aspect of the orbit *(arrows)*. The resultant obstruction of the infundibulum is usually the cause of the prominent inflammatory process in the ipsilateral maxillary sinus *(small black M)*. Note that, in this case, as is often seen this is associated with hypoplasia of the ipsilateral maxillary sinus compared with its counterpart *(large white M).*

15). This variant is usually associated with a hypoplastic, and often opacified, ipsilateral maxillary sinus due to closure of the infundibulum. It is important to note this variant for surgical planning because as the ipsilateral orbital floor will be low-lying as a result of the hypoplastic maxillary sinus. This increases the risk of inadvertent penetration of the orbit during surgery. An additional variation of the uncinate is its extension superiorly to the roof of the anterior ethmoid sinus, causing the superior infundibulum to end as a "blind pouch." This is referred to as the lamina terminalis. Here the infundibulum drains via the posterior aspect of the middle meatus.

If the free edge of the uncinate deviates laterally, there can be obstruction of the infundibulum. Less frequently, "medial curling" of the uncinate is encountered which encroaches upon the middle meatus (Fig. 3-16).

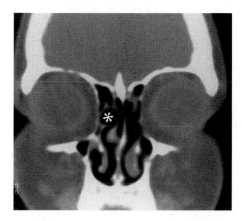

FIG. 3-17   Uncinate bulla. Coronal CT image demonstrates an air cell within the right uncinate process *(asterisk)*. The cell contributes to the narrowing of the right infundibulum and middle meatus.

which in turn may obstruct the nasal cavity, infundibulum, and middle meatus (Fig. 3-14).

Variations in the Uncinate Process

There are several variations for the course of the free edge of the uncinate process. In most cases, it either extends slightly obliquely toward the nasal septum with the free edge surrounding the inferoanterior surface of the ethmoid bulla, or it extends more medially to the medial surface of the ethmoid bulla.

Sometimes the free edge of the uncinate adheres to the orbital floor, or inferior aspect, of the lamina papyracea. This is referred to as an atelectatic uncinate process (Fig. 3-

Aeration of the Uncinate

This anomaly expands the width of the uncinate, thus potentially compromising the infundibulum (Fig. 3-17). Functionally, it acts like a concha bullosa or an enlarged ethmoid bulla. This is uncommon.

Haller Cells

Haller cells are ethmoid air cells that extend along the medial roof of the maxillary sinus (Fig. 3-18). They vary in appearance and size. When they are large, they may cause narrowing of the infundibulum. Haller cells may exist as discrete cells or they may open into the maxillary sinus or infundibulum.

Onodi Cells

Onodi cells are lateral and posterior extensions of the posterior ethmoid air cells. They effectively extend the paranasal sinus cavity and bring it in close proximity to the optic nerves as they exit the orbits. These "cells" may surround the optic nerve tract and put the nerve at risk during surgery. Onodi cells are rare.

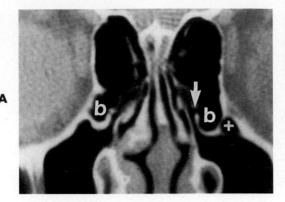
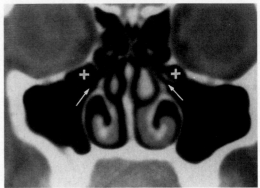

FIG. 3-18 Haller Cell. **A,** Note the left Haller cell (+) with ethmoid bulla ostia located medially *(b)*, opening into the infundibula. **B,** Bilateral Haller cells (+). Note their close proximity to the uncinate process and their influence on the infundibula *(small arrows).*

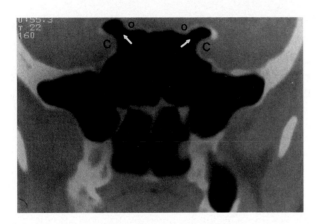

FIG. 3-19 Extensive pneumatization of the sphenoid sinus. Coronal CT image shows pneumatization of both anterior clinoid processes *(arrows)* and their relationship to the optic nerves *(o)* and internal carotid arteries *(C)*. The presence of anterior clinoid pneumatization is an important indicator of optic nerve vulnerability during FESS.

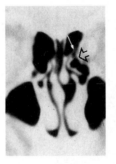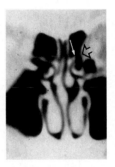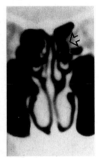

FIG. 3-20 Medial deviation of the left lamina papyracea. Coronal CT images optimally demonstrate the outline of the lamina papyracea in relationship to the anterior osteomeatal channels. Medial deviation *(open arrow)*, when present, should not be confused with an ethmoid bulla. Note that the medially deviated lamina papyracea lies in close proximity to the lateral attachment of the middle turbinate, the basal lamella *(white arrow).*

Giant Ethmoid Bulla

The largest of the ethmoid air cells, the ethmoid bulla may enlarge to narrow or obstruct the middle meatus and infundibulum.

Extensive Pneumatization of the Sphenoid Sinus

Pneumatization of the sphenoid sinus can extend into the anterior clinoids and clivus, surrounding the optic nerves. When this occurs, the optic nerves are at increased risk of being damaged during surgical exploration (Fig. 3-19).

Medial Deviation or Dehiscence of the Lamina Papyracea

This may be a congenital finding or it can be the result of prior facial trauma. In either case, the orbital contents are at risk during surgery because of the dehiscence in the medial orbital wall, as well as the ease of surgically confusing this "medial bulge" with the ethmoid bulla (Fig. 3-20). Both excessive medial deviation and bony dehiscence occur most often at the site of the insertion of the basal lamella into the lamina papyracea, thus rendering this portion of the lamina papyracea most delicate.

Aerated Crista Galli

Aeration of this normal bony structure can occur. When aerated, these cells may communicate with the frontal recess. Obstruction of this ostium can lead to chronic sinusitis and mucocoele formation within the crista galli. To avoid unnecessary extension of surgery into the anterior cranial vault, it is important to preoperatively recognize an aerated crista galli and differentiate it from an ethmoid air cell.

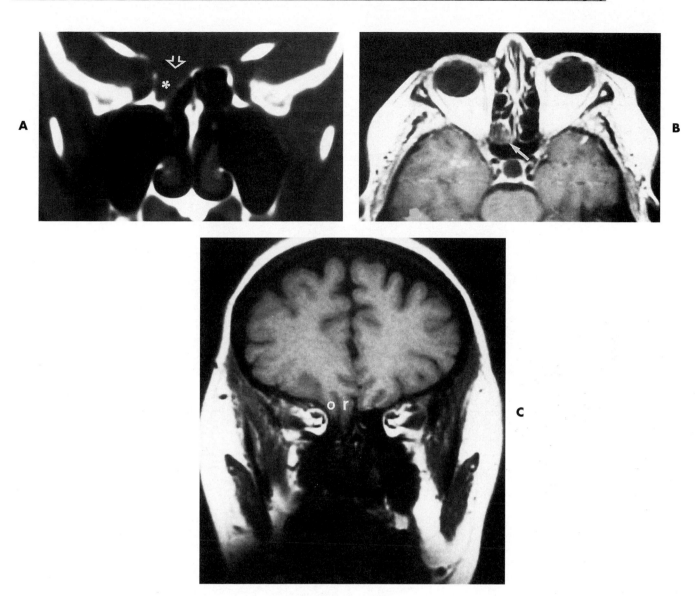

FIG. 3-21 A through **C,** CT and MR imaging display of an encephalocele. Coronal CT image **(A)** through the posterior ethmoid sinus shows erosion of the roof of the posterior ethmoid sinus (*open arrow*) and (*asterisk*). Axial T1W MRI **(B)** shows an isolated soft-tissue mass within the posterior ethmoid sinus (*arrow*), which on the coronal T1W MR image **(C)** is confirmed to be an encephalocele. Gyrus rectus *(r)* and Gyrus orbitales *(o)* are noted.

Cephalocele

Preoperative CT scanning is useful to assess congenital abnormalities, such as cephaloceles (Figs. 3-21, 3-22).[40] These may be congenital, may occur spontaneously, or may occur as a result of previous ethmoid or sphenoid sinus surgery. When diagnosing an isolated soft-tissue mass adjacent to the ethmoid or sphenoid roof, radiologists must consider a cephalocele, especially if there is adjacent bone erosion. The differential diagnosis includes mucocele, neoplasm, and less likely a polyp associated with an adjacent bony dehiscence. Coronal CT scanning best displays the extent of bony erosion, while sagittal and coronal MRI usually narrow the differential diagnosis.

Posterior Nasal Septal Air Cell

Air cells are commonly found within the posterosuperior portion of the nasal septum. When present, their communication is with the sphenoid sinus. They may be affected by any mucosal inflammatory disease that occurs within the paranasal sinuses (Fig. 3-23). Such disease may obliterate this cell, causing it to resemble a cephalocele. CT and MRI usually define the involved pathology and resolve any differential diagnostic problems.

Asymmetry in Ethmoid Roof Height

It is important to make note of any asymmetry in the height of the ethmoid roof. There is a higher incidence of intracra-

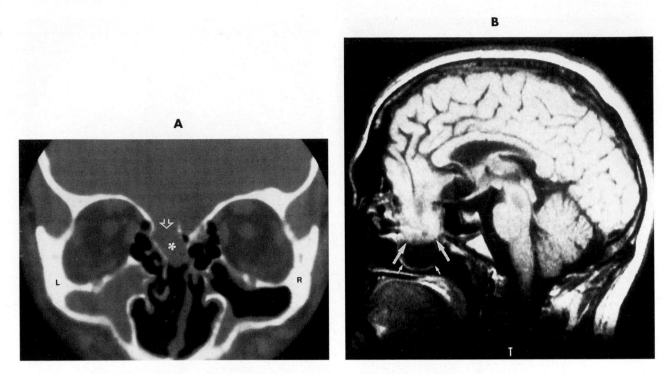

FIG. 3-22 CT and MR imaging appearance of an encephalocele. **A,** Coronal CT image through the posterior ethmoid sinus shows a wide erosion of the ethmoid sinus roof *(open arrow)* with a soft-tissue mass penetrating into the ethmoid sinus *(asterisk).* **B,** T1W sagittal MR image shows the outline of the brain tissue *(large arrows)* and meninges and cerebrospinal fluid *(small arrows).*

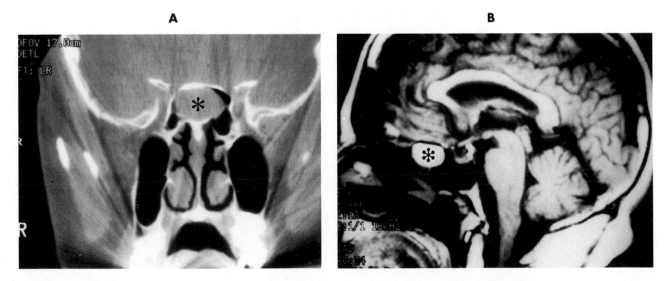

FIG. 3-23 Nasal septal air cell. **A,** Coronal CT image demonstrates an expansile mass in the anterior sphenoid sinus *(asterisk),* **B,** Sagittal T1W MR image displays the hyperintense inflammatory mass *(asterisk),* which is well separated from the intracranial compartment. This was proven to be a mucocele within a posterior nasal septal air cell.

nial penetration during FESS when this anatomic variation occurs. The intracranial penetration is more likely to occur on the side where the position of the roof is lower.[41]

ANATOMY ADJACENT TO THE SINONASAL CAVITIES
The Palate

Located far anteriorly in the hard palate is the anterior nasal spine and premaxilla. About 1 cm behind the anterior premaxilla is the incisive foramen. This foramen extends cranially as two separate incisive canals that open on either side of the base of the nasal septum. Together these canals and the foramen form a Y shape. These canals transmit the terminal branches of the sphenopalatine arteries and their anastomoses with the greater palatine arteries. The canals also transmit the nasopalatine nerves. The palatine spines are seen on the oral surface of the hard palate. Lateral to the spines are the palatine grooves in which run the palatine vessels and nerves. The greater palatine foramen can be seen posteriorly at the lateral junction of the hard palate and the maxillary alveolus. The anterior surface of this canal is formed by the maxilla, the posterior surface by the palatine bone. Thus posterior to this plane the hard palate is formed by the horizontal plates of the palatine bone. This is roughly the posterior third of the hard palate. At this level, most of the medial antral wall is now formed by the vertical plate of the palatine bone. The lower segment of the pterygopalatine canal extends upward from the greater palatine foramen toward the pterygopalatine fossa. The canal transmits the anterior palatine nerve and the descending palatine artery. Occasionally the lesser palatine foramen may be identified. It also extends to the pterygopalatine fossa and opens just posterior to the greater palatine foramen. The lesser palatine foramen transmits the posterior palatine nerve. The most posterior medial wall of the antrum is still formed by the vertical portion of the palatine bone.

The Pterygopalatine Fossa

The pterygopalatine fossa is a small space directly behind the palatine bone and in front of the pterygoid process of the sphenoid bone. The medial boundary of the fossa is formed by the sphenopalatine foramen, which is at the craniocaudal level of the posterior tip of the middle concha. This foramen may be seen connecting the nasal fossa with the pterygopalatine fossa. Within the pterygopalatine fossa are the sphenopalatine ganglion, portions of the maxillary nerve, and the internal maxillary artery. These structures are supported by fat, which fills the majority of the fossa. Posteriorly the pterygoid (Vidian) canal and the foramen rotundum may be seen in the skull base, extending into the middle cranial fossa. Inferiorly is the pterygopalatine canal, which communicates with the mouth. Laterally is the infratemporal fossa, and superiorly is the inferior orbital fissure, which in turn opens into the orbit.

The Pterygoid Plates

When the pterygoid plates are seen, the medial plate is almost vertically oriented. The lateral plate is tilted so that its lower end is lateral. The pterygoid fossa lies between these plates. The medial (internal) pterygoid muscle arises from the medial side of the lateral pterygoid plate within the pterygoid fossa, and the lateral (external) pterygoid muscle arises from the lateral side of the lateral plate. The tendon of the tensor veli palatini muscle passes around the laterally curved hamulus of the lower medial pterygoid plate.

The Nasal Septum

The nasal septum is formed anteriorly to posteriorly by the medial crura of the alar cartilages, the septal cartilage, the perpendicular plate of the ethmoid bone, and the vomer; below, the nasal crests of the maxilla and palatine bones contribute to the base of the septum. The posterior edge of the vomer joins the undersurface of the sphenoid bone at the sphenoid rostrum, a prominent triangular ridge on the underbody of the sphenoid bone that forms this articulation.

The Olfactory Recesses

The olfactory recess is the narrow channel-like portion of the nasal cavity on either side of the upper nasal septum. These spaces continue up to the cribriform plate. The olfactory recess on either side of the nasal septum widens posteriorly into the sphenoethmoidal recess. This marks the junction between the ethmoid and sphenoid bones. The nasal atrium refers to the anterolateral nasal cavity just below and medial to the agger nasi.

The Margins of the Orbit

When the superior orbital rims are visualized, a localized notch, or foramen, can be seen along the medial margin. This is the supraorbital notch (or foramen), and the supraorbital artery and nerve pass through it. Medial to the supraorbital notch is the frontal notch, which transmits the frontal artery and the frontal nerve. The roof of the orbit has bony ridges on its cranial aspect. These reflect, in a general way, the impressions of the gyri of the base of the frontal lobes.

Along the medial orbital walls are the anterior ethmoidal canals, which are seen as medial indentations in the upper lamina papyracea. They transmit the anterior ethmoidal nerves and vessels. The lower margins of these canals are formed by the ethmoid bones, and the upper margins are formed by the frontal bones. More posteriorly the similarly formed posterior ethmoidal canals are seen. They too transmit their respective vessels and nerves. In the middle third of the orbital floor is the infraorbital foramen and canal. The canal extends from the inferior orbital fissure posteriorly to the anterior maxilla. This canal runs parallel to the orbital floor except in its most anterior portion where it turns downward to exit in the infraorbital foramen, which is about 1 cm below the inferior orbital rim.

The inferior orbital fissure is about 2 cm long, and it is angled at about 45° (open anteriorly) with the midsagittal

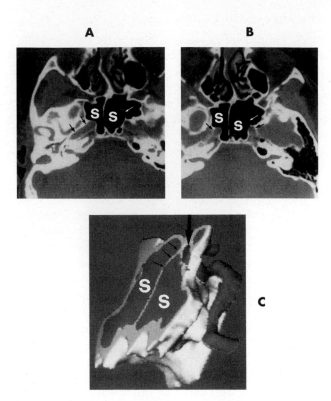

FIG. 3-24 Relationship of the carotid canal to the sphenoid sinus. **A** and **B,** Axial CT images through the sphenoid and ethmoid sinuses show that the carotid canals *(small black arrows)* penetrate into the sphenoid sinus *(S).* An incomplete sphenoid sinus septum *(white arrow)* connects to the bony covering of the carotid canal. **C,** Three-dimensional images of the sphenoid sinus *(S)* and presellar and juxtasellar portions of the internal carotid artery *(black arrow)* graphically display the close relationship between the internal carotid artery and the sphenoid sinus septation *(small black arrows).*

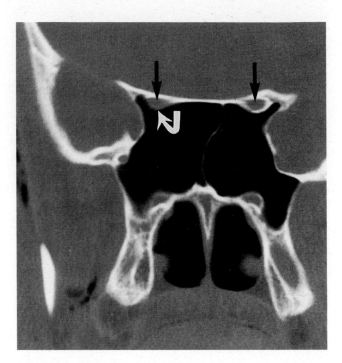

FIG. 3-25 Relationship of optic nerves to sphenoid sinus. Type three optic nerves *(black arrows)* course through the sphenoid sinus with greater than 50% of the nerves surrounded by air. Note that there is dehiscence of the bone covering the right optic nerve *(curved white arrow).* This increases the risk of optic nerve damage during FESS.

plane. This fissure is narrowest in its midportion and widens both at its medial and lateral margins. This fissure separates the lateral orbital wall from the orbital floor. At the level of the lateral margin of the inferior orbital fissure the temporal fossa becomes the infratemporal fossa. The circular configuration of the anterior orbit slowly changes to a more triangular shape in the posterior orbit. This change in shape occurs because the medial orbital floor elevates, and the lower lamina papyracea tilts laterally as the larger posterior ethmoid cells are encountered.

The Lacrimal Fossa and Nasolacrimal Duct

The medial wall of the lacrimal fossa is seen as a groove or defect in the medial orbital wall. The lacrimal fossa is anterior to the nasolacrimal canal in the medial antral wall. This reflects the anatomy of the nasolacrimal canal, which runs downward and posteriorly at about a 20° angle with the coronal plane. This normal dehiscence in the medial orbital floor for the lacrimal fossa and sac should not be confused

with a focal site of erosion. The lower opening of the nasolacrimal canal can be seen in the medial antral wall under the inferior turbinate (inferior meatus). The medial wall of the nasolacrimal canal is formed superiorly by the lacrimal bone and inferiorly by the lacrimal process of the inferior turbinate. The lateral wall is formed entirely by the maxilla. The thin lacrimal bone forms the anterior medial orbital wall, which overlies the anterior ethmoid cells. The lacrimal bone has a slightly concave lateral configuration. The ethmoid lamina papyracea, which lies just behind the lacrimal bone, tends to have a straighter configuration.

The Sphenoid Sinus Septum

The sphenoid intersinus septum is usually in the midline anteriorly but posteriorly may be angulated sharply to one side. This creates two unequally sized sinuses, and once the scan plane moves posterior to such an angled septum, it will appear as if there is only one sphenoid sinus cavity.

The Maxillary Sinus Walls

The medial wall of the maxillary sinus is partially bone and partially membrane. This membranous area forms a C shape, which is closed posteriorly and bridges the posterior attachment of the inferior turbinate. The anterior wall of the maxillary sinus has a slightly concave anterior configuration. This is the canine fossa, and it lies cranial to the lateral incisor and canine teeth and caudal to the infraorbital canal. The caninus muscle arises from this fossa. The infratemporal fossa fat is seen abutting the curved posterolateral antral walls. There is a thinning in this curved sinus wall that corresponds to the canal for the posterosuperior alveolar nerve. This should not be confused with a site of bone erosion.

SYSTEMATIC READING PATTERN
Routine Report

It is helpful to use a systematic approach when evaluating sinus CT studies. Most people use an anterior to posterior approach to interpretation. As one reads the study, a mental checklist should be made of important structures to evaluate and comment on.

The reporting system normally includes three steps.

Step One

Identify and describe the important structures of the paranasal sinuses (there are 14 such structures). The dictated report should mention the status of these structures on both the right and left sides. The structures to identify are as follows:

Frontal sinus	Uncinate process
Frontal recess	Infundibulum
Agger nasi cell and anterior ethmoid sinus	Maxillary sinus
Ethmoid roof	Middle meatus
Ethmoid bulla	Nasal septum and nasal turbinates
Basal lamella	Posterior ethmoid sinus
Sinus lateralis	Sphenoid sinus

Step Two

Evaluate the critical relationships. In addition to describing findings directly related to the diagnosis of inflammatory sinus disease, it is important for the radiologist to evaluate several critical areas that aid in surgical planning. The symmetry of the ethmoid roof should be noted. Discrepant heights of the ethmoid roof may lead to inadvertent penetration of the cranial vault if not recognized before FESS. Careful attention should be paid to the status of the lamina papyracea, and any dehiscence or excessive medial deviation of this bone should be reported. The relationship of the sphenoid sinus and posterior ethmoid air cells with the internal carotid artery and optic nerves should be clearly mentioned. Findings that put either of these structures at increased risk during endoscopic surgery should be conveyed to the referring surgeon. In particular, extensive expansion of the sinuses around the internal carotid artery or the optic nerve, as well as bony dehiscences adjacent to either structure, should be noted (Fig. 3-24). The incidence of bony dehiscence around the presellar and juxtasellar portions of the internal carotid artery ranges from 12% to 22%.[42-44] Quite frequently the carotid canal penetrates the aerated portion of the sphenoid sinus, and in many such cases the sphenoid sinus septations adhere to the bony covering of the carotid canal. The surgeon needs to be aware of this variation

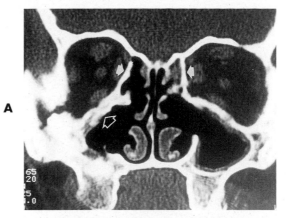

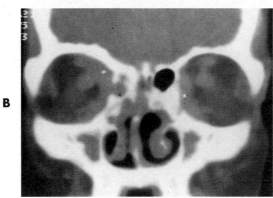

FIG. 3-26 Osteitis of the paranasal sinus walls. **A,** Coronal CT image through the ethmoid sinus shows that the patient has had bilateral antrostomies, uncinectomies, and partial anterior ethmoidectomies. Note the pronounced thickening of the orbital floors bilaterally but more severely on the right side *(open arrow)*. There is marked thickening of the lamina papyracea bilaterally *(solid arrows)*. These changes are occasionally seen in patients who have undergone multiple surgical procedures in this area. **B,** Coronal CT image through the anterior ethmoid sinus in a patient with Wegener's granulomatosis. Note the diffuse, pronounced bony thickening of the perimeter of the maxillary sinuses and lamina papyracea, as well as the presence of soft-tissue masses *(Asterisks)* within the orbits.

to prevent fracturing of the sphenoid sinus septum-carotid canal junction and puncturing the carotid artery.

The relationship between the posterior paranasal sinuses and the optic nerves is important to note so that operative complications can be avoided (Fig. 3-25). DeLano, Fun, and Zinreich classified this relationship in four discrete categories.[44] Type 1 includes those optic nerves coursing immediately adjacent to the sphenoid sinus without indentation of the wall or contact with the posterior ethmoid air cell. This is the most common type, occurring in 76% of patients. Type 2 nerves course adjacent to the sphenoid sinus, causing indentation of the sinus wall, without contact with the posterior ethmoid air cell. Type 3 nerves course through the sphenoid sinus with at least 50% surrounded by air. Type 4 nerves course immediately adjacent to the sphenoid sinus and posterior ethmoid sinus. The optic nerve is exposed

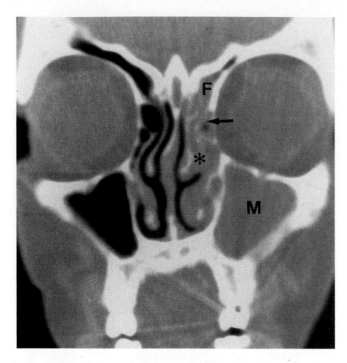

FIG. 3-27 OMU pattern of sinusitis. Inflammatory changes obstruct the left middle meatus *(asterisk)* with resulting opacification of the left maxillary *(M)*, frontal *(F)*, and anterior ethmoid *(arrow)* sinuses.

without a bony margin in all cases where it travels through the sphenoid sinus (Type 3) and in 82% of cases where the nerve impressed on the sphenoid sinus wall (Type 2). Delano et al. also found that 85% of optic nerves associated with a pneumatized anterior clinoid process were of Type 2 or 3 configuration, and 77% were dehiscent. Therefore the presence of anterior clinoid pneumatization is an important indicator of optic nerve vulnerability during FESS because of frequent associations with both bony dehiscence, as well as Type 2 and 3 configurations.[44]

Step Three

Evaluate the bony outline of the nasal cavity and para-nasal sinuses.

Bone Thickening. Lastly, but equally important to steps 1 and 2, is the evaluation of the "character" of the bony framework of the nasal vault and paranasal sinuses. It has been noted that a prominent thickening of the bone about a paranasal sinus may occur, especially in those patients who have had several surgical procedures and in those patients with repeated exacerbations of chronic inflammation (Fig. 3-26). Similar changes have been noted in patients with Wegener's granulomatosis and patients who suffer from a prolonged chronic inflammation and no previous surgery. Unfortunately, to date there is no good pathophysiologic explanation of this finding. However, it is felt that this change is directly related to the underlying inflammatory process and periosteal stimulation.

Bone Erosion. Bone may not be visualized on CT for several reasons. Bone may have been removed during a prior surgical procedure and, therefore, a defect is noted. Evidence of prior surgery should be looked for on the CT examination and established through a proper medical history. Bone may not be seen because it is deossified secondary to chronic pressure from a mucocele or because the bone is invaded and destroyed by tumor. The associated mass will suggest the etiology, and MRI may afford a distinction between these two processes. Lastly, bony dehiscences may also be developmental, and in the absence of prior surgery or associated pathology, this diagnostic possibility should be considered.

RADIOGRAPHIC APPEARANCES OF INFLAMMATORY SINUS DISEASE
Acute Sinusitis

Acute sinusitis usually is due to bacterial superinfection of an obstructed paranasal sinus. The obstruction is often the result of apposition of edematous mucosal surfaces from an antecedent viral upper respiratory tract infection. The edema disrupts the normal mucociliary drainage pattern of the sinus, and obstruction of the sinus ostium results. The accumulation of fluid within the sinus predisposes it to a bacterial superinfection. The bacterial pathogens most often responsible include *Streptococcus pneumoniae, Haemophilus influenzae,* beta hemolytic streptococcus, and *Moraxella catarrhalis.*[23,38,45] Acute sinusitis is only rarely the result of a pure viral infection. Acute sinusitis usually involves only a single sinus, with the ethmoid sinus being the most common location.[35,45] There is an increased risk of regional and intracranial complications with involvement of the frontal, ethmoid, and sphenoid sinuses.[35]

Radiographically the hallmark of acute sinusitis is an air-fluid level. However, the radiologic findings in acute sinusitis may be nonspecific with smooth or nodular mucosal thickening or complete opacification of the sinus. On MR imaging the findings are those of watery secretions with hypointense signal on T1W images and hyperintense signal on T2W images.

It should be noted that an air-fluid level is not a pathognomonic sign of acute sinusitis. This topic is discussed in detail in Chapter 4.

Chronic Sinusitis

Chronic sinusitis is diagnosed when the patient has repeated bouts of acute infection or persistent inflammation.[35,45] The responsible pathogens include staphylococcus, streptococcus, corynebacteria, bacteroides, fusobacteria, and other anaerobes.[38] Anaerobes are more commonly involved in chronic sinusitis than in acute sinusitis.[35,45] The radiographic findings are quite variable. Signs suggestive of chronic sinusitis include mucosal thickening or opacification, bone remodeling and thickening caused by osteitis from adjacent chronic mucosal inflammation, and polyposis.[23,45,46] The sinuses most commonly involved with chronic sinusitis are the anterior ethmoid air cells.

Opacification of the OMU has been found to predispose patients to the development of sinusitis. Zinreich et al. found middle meatus opacification in 72% of patients with chronic sinusitis. In this study, 65% of these patients had mucoperiosteal thickening of the maxillary sinus.[6,8,9] All of the patients with frontal sinus inflammatory disease had opacification of the frontoethmoidal recess.[6,8,9] Opacification of the OMU without frontal, maxillary, or anterior ethmoid sinus inflammatory disease was rare.[6,8,9] Yousem, Kennedy, and Rosenberg found that when the middle meatus was opacified, there were associated inflammatory changes in the ethmoid sinuses in 82% of patients and in the maxillary sinuses in 84% of patients.[39] Bolger, Butzin, and Parsons found that when the ethmoid infundibulum was free of disease, the maxillary and frontal sinuses were clear in 77% of patients.[38]

Babbel et al. reviewed 500 patients with screening sinus CT scans and defined five recurring patterns of inflammatory sinonasal disease.[47] The five anatomic patterns are as follows: infundibular, OMU, sphenoethmoidal recess, sinonasal polyposis, and sporadic or unclassifiable. The infundibular pattern (26% of patients) referred to focal obstruction within the maxillary sinus ostium and ethmoid infundibulum, which was associated with maxillary sinus disease. The OMU pattern (25% of patients) referred to ipsilateral maxillary, frontal, and anterior ethmoid sinus disease (Fig. 3-27). This pattern was due to obstruction of the middle meatus. Sparing of the frontal sinus was sometimes seen as a result of the variable location of the nasofrontal duct insertion in the middle meatus. The sphenoethmoidal recess pattern (6% of patients) resulted in sphenoid or posterior ethmoid sinus inflammation caused by sphenoethmoidal recess obstruction. The sinonasal polyposis pattern (10% of patients) was due to diffuse nasal and paranasal sinus polyps. Associated radiographic findings included infundibular enlargement, convexity (bulging) of the ethmoid sinus walls, and thinning of the bony nasal septum and ethmoid trabeculae.[27,47,48]

When sinus secretions are acute and of low viscosity, they are of intermediate attenuation on CT images (10 to 25 HU). In the more chronic state, sinus secretions become thickened and concentrated and the CT attenuation increases with density measurements of 30 to 60 H.U.[20] On MR imaging the appearance of chronic sinusitis is quite variable due to the changing concentrations of protein and free water protons.[20,21] This topic is discussed in detail in Chapter 4.

Certain anatomic variants, as described above, have been implicated as causative factors in the presence of chronic inflammatory disease. Stammberger and Wolfe[49] and Lidov and Som[50] found that a large concha bullosa produced signs and symptoms of sinusitis. However, Yousem[39] found that the presence of a concha bullosa did not increase the risk of sinusitis. This was corroborated by Bolger et al., who found that the presence of a concha bullosa, paradoxical turbinates, Haller cells, and uncinate pneumatization were not significantly more common in patients with chronic sinusitis than in asymptomatic patients.[38] Yousem et al. found the presence of nasal septal deviation and a horizontally oriented uncinate process was more common in patients with inflammatory sinusitis.[39] Although the presence of these variants may not necessarily predispose to sinusitis, it appears that the size of a given anatomic variant and its relationship to adjacent structures plays an important role in the development of sinusitis.[29]

Fungal Sinusitis

Fungal sinusitis may be suspected clinically when the patient fails to respond to standard antibiotic therapy.[29,35,39,51,52] This topic is discribed in detail in Chapter 4.

In general, on imaging the presence of an air-fluid level is uncommon. The maxillary and ethmoid sinuses are the most common sites of involvement.[20] The imaging findings are quite variable, depending on the aggressiveness of the fungus. Nonspecific mucosal thickening or sinus opacification may occur. The allergic form of aspergillus is associated with recurrent sinonasal polyps. With more invasive fungi, sinus opacification with a central mycetoma and associated bony thickening or erosion may occur.[20] With both mucormycosis and invasive aspergillus, vascular invasion may occur, which leads to intracranial and extracranial thrombosis and infarction. According to Som, two circumstances can be seen that suggest the presence of fungal infections: soft tissue changes in the sinus with thickened, reactive bone and localized areas of osteomyelitis,[20,21] and the association of inflammatory sinus disease with involvement of the adjacent nasal fossa and the soft tissues of the cheek. These signs of aggressive infection are atypical for bacterial pathogens.

Allergic Sinusitis

Allergic sinusitis occurs in 10% of the population.[27] It typically produces a pansinusitis with symmetrical involvement.[47] CT often shows a nodular mucosal thickening with thickened turbinates.[27] Air-fluid levels are rare unless bacterial superinfection occurs.[46] This topic is discussed in more detail in Chapter 4.

Orbital Complications of Sinusitis

The topics of retention cysts, mucoceles, and inflammatory polyps are discussed in Chapter 4.

About 3% of patients with sinusitis will have some form of orbital involvement. This complication is more common in children, and the orbital manifestations may be the first sign of sinus infection. Complicated sinusitis is the most common cause of orbital infection, accounting for 60% to 84% of cases.[30,53,54,55] The origin of the infection most commonly is in the ethmoid sinuses. In decreasing order of frequency, the sources of the infection are the frontal, sphenoid, and maxillary sinuses. The ethmoid and maxillary sinuses are present at birth and therefore are the source in

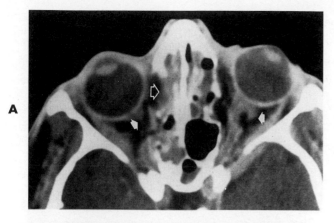

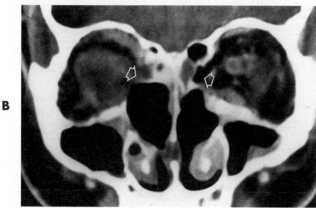

FIG. 3-28 Orbital complications from FESS. Axial **(A)** and coronal **(B)** CT images in a patient who was found to be blind after undergoing bilateral anterior ethmoidectomies, partial bilateral middle turbinectomies, and bilateral uncinate resections. Note the defects in the lamina papyracea bilaterally *(open arrows)* and severed bilateral optic nerves *(solid arrows)*.

younger children. The frontal sinuses are usually detectable radiographically after 6 years of age, but they are not usually significant sources of infection until after 10 years of age. The sphenoid sinuses likewise develop late and are rarely implicated in the pediatric age group.

In adults, most authors recommend obtaining a CT when there is clinical evidence of postseptal infection (i.e. when proptosis and limitation of eye movement are present) or when there is failure to improve with antibiotics.[27,47] Because the disease can be much more aggressive in the pediatric population, a CT should be considered when there is clinical evidence of preseptal inflammation.

Preseptal orbital edema is a common finding with sinusitis, especially in children. CT shows diffuse soft tissue density and thickening of the preseptal soft tissues. At this stage, clinically there is swelling and redness of the eyelids but no proptosis or limitation of eye movement. As infection spreads from the ethmoid sinus to the orbit, there is inflammation of the orbital periosteum (periorbita), which becomes thickened and elevated with accumulation of an inflammatory phlegmon. On CT this appears as an

ill-defined, slightly enhancing mass on the orbital side of the lamina papyracea. It is limited laterally by the periosteum; however, in more advanced cases, early orbital cellulitis is present with thickened and enhancing of the medial rectus muscle, which is displaced laterally. Subsequently, liquefaction may occur in the subperiosteal compartment to form an abscess. This will be evident on CT as a region of low density (which may have an enhancing rim) on the orbital side of the lamina papyracea.

Rare orbital complications of paranasal sinus infection include superior ophthalmic vein (SOV) thrombosis, cavernous sinus thrombosis, and blindness.[56] SOV thrombosis is suspected on CT scans when there is asymmetric enlargement of this vessel with relative lack of normal enhancement, though thrombus within the lumen can be hyperdense. MR may demonstrate these changes more accurately than CT. Magnetic resonance angiography (MRA), especially phase contrast techniques, can establish the presence of SOV thrombosis.

Cavernous sinus thrombosis may be evident as fullness of the affected cavernous sinus with lateral (rather than a medial) convexity of its lateral margin. Gadolinium-enhanced axial and coronal MR scans are usually better than CT for detecting the presence of cavernous sinus thrombosis.

Permanent loss of vision is a rare complication of sinusitis, although recent studies report about a 10% incidence in patients with postseptal infection.[51,53-55] The mechanism for loss of vision may be an optic neuritis, which is a reaction to adjacent infection. Ischemia, secondary to thrombophlebitis, arteritis, or pressure on the central retinal artery, also may result in blindness.

COMMON FESS TECHNIQUES

For inflammatory sinonasal disease, FESS has largely replaced the traditional techniques of sinus surgery. It is now believed that obstruction of the drainage portals of the sinuses, particularly the anterior ethmoids, is the primary cause of recurrent sinusitis. The rationale for FESS is that these techniques allow restoration of the flow of sinus secretions through their native drainage portals. Reestablishing the normal drainage pattern allows the inflamed sinus to return to a normal state, thus hopefully alleviating the patient's symptoms.[25,57,58]

Types of FESS

Panje and Anand have developed a classification system to standardize the type of FESS technique that is appropriate based on the preoperative extent of sinus disease as determined by CT imaging.[58]

The Anand and Panje Classification of types of FESS[58]

Type I
Uncinatectomy with or without agger nasi cell exenteration.

| **Indications** | 1. Isolated OMU thickening of mucous membrane |
| | 2. Infundibular disease |

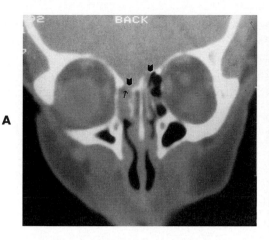 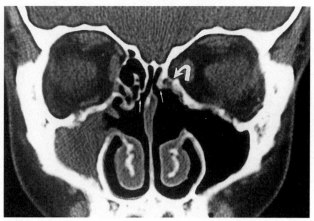

FIG. 3-29   Anatomic landmarks to be evaluated in patients after FESS. **A,** Coronal CT image through the anterior ethmoid sinuses shows a prominent asymmetry in the position of the roof of the ethmoid sinuses *(solid arrowheads)*. The intracranial penetration *(fine black arrow)* are usually on the side where the roof is lower in position. **B,** Coronal CT image through the anterior ethmoid sinus in a patient status post bilateral uncinatectomies and partial middle turbinectomies *(fine white arrows)*. If there is an intraorbital complication during such a surgical procedure, it usually involves the lamina papyracea at the attachment of the basal lamella *(curved arrow)*.

3. Patent maxillary sinus ostia without maxillary sinus membrane thickening or cysts
4. Unsuccessful prior inferior maxillary sinus antrostomy or antrotomy with irrigation
5. Prior septoplasty or adenoidectomy with continued paranasal sinus symptoms

Type II

Uncinatectomy, bulla ethmoidectomy, removal of sinus lateralis mucous membrane, and exposure of frontal recess or frontal sinus.

Indications   1. OMU thickening of mucous membrane
2. Evidence of anterior ethmoid sinus opacification, including obstruction of infundibulum
3. Limited frontal recess disease
4. Unsuccessful prior inferior maxillary sinus antrostomy or antrotomy with irrigation
5. Prior septoplasty or adenoidectomy with continued paranasal sinus symptoms

Type III

Type II plus maxillary sinus antrostomy through the natural sinus ostium.

Indications   Same as Type II with the following:
1. Maxillary sinusitis as evidenced by membrane thickening or sinus opacification
2. Stenotic or edematous maxillary sinus ostium

Type IV

Type III plus complete posterior ethmoidectomy.

Indications   Same as Type III with the following:
1. Total ethmoid involvement
2. Nasal polyposis with extensive ethmoidal and maxillary sinus disease
3. Prior Type I or Type II FESS without response, or with progression of sinus disease

Type V

Type IV plus sphenoidectomy and stripping of mucous membrane.

Indications   Same as Type IV with the following:
1. Evidence of sphenoid sinusitis
2. Pansinusitis and rhinitis

In practice, Types II and III are the most commonly performed FESS techniques.

RADIOGRAPHIC EVALUATION OF PATIENTS FOLLOWING FUNCTIONAL ENDOSCOPIC SINUS SURGERY
Expected Findings

The evaluation of the postoperative patient is similar to that of the preoperative patient. Ideally the CT should be performed in the coronal projection. Given the fact that a surgical procedure was performed, the type and extent of surgery must be established. Subsequently the emphasis is on the anatomy. The mental checklist should identify and mention the presence or absence of the 14 important structures discussed earlier in this chapter. A close look at the nasal cavity and paranasal sinus boundaries and the important relationships described previously should once again be looked for and commented on. Areas of bony thickening or dehiscence should be noted.

Areas that merit close scrutiny on follow-up CT scans are as follows:

1. Frontal recess

   The frontal recesses should be identified to determine their patency. Postoperatively, one often finds that recurrence of disease is due to persistent obstruction in this area. It is the narrowest channel within the anterior ethmoid complex, and it is a structure that is very difficult to access surgically. Therefore this is the area most likely to be affected with inflammatory disease in a patient

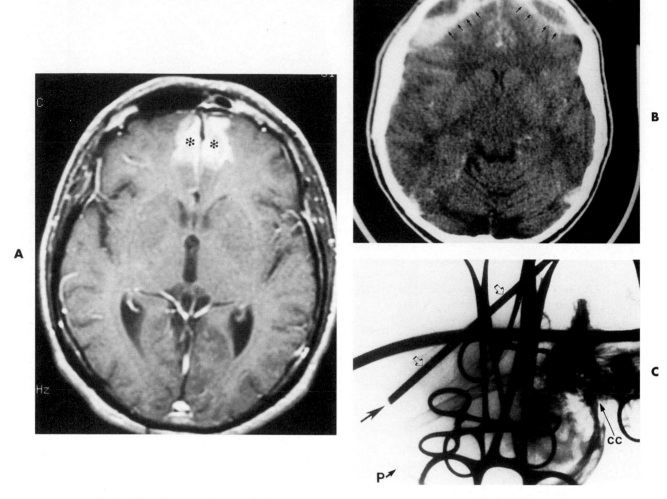

FIG. 3-30 Intracranial complications from FESS. **A,** Axial T1W MR image after gadolinium-DTPA administration shows abnormal bifrontal parenchymal enhancement *(asterisks)* caused by encephalitis from perforation through the cribriform plate. **B,** Axial CT image shows bilateral acute subdural hematomas *(arrows)* after FESS. **C,** Intraoperative cross-table lateral skull radiograph shows the intracranial extension of an endoscope *(open arrows)*. Note the position of the endoscope in the deep portion of the posterior frontal lobe *(solid black arrow)*. Overlying surgical instruments are noted. Craniocervical junction *(CC),* and parietal bone *(P).*

with a previous paranasal sinus surgical procedure. To this end, note should be made of the agger nasi cell (if it remains), because its persistence may continue to narrow the frontal recess.

2. OMU

Note should be made of the extent of the uncinatectomy and removal of the ethmoid bulla. The course of the infundibulum should be examined for persistent anatomic narrowing. The outline of the middle turbinate should be examined to determine whether a middle turbinectomy has been performed. If so, then careful attention should be paid to both the vertical attachment of the middle turbinate to the cribriform plate and the attachment of the basal lamella to the lamina papyracea. Traction applied on the vertical attachment and basal lamella of the middle turbinate, during the course of a middle

turbinectomy, can cause a fracture of the lamina papyracea or the cribiform plate. These breaks in the continuity of the laminal papyracea and ethmoid roof are easily demonstrated on coronal images (Figs. 3-29 to 3-32).

3. Lamina papyracea

Inspection of the entire course of the lamina papyracea should be carried out to evaluate the integrity of this structure. Postoperative dehiscences are commonly found just posterior to the nasolacrimal duct, and these may be caused by the uncinate resection (Figs. 3-8, 3-29).

4. Ethmoid roof

Asymmetry in position of the roofs (fovea ethmoidalis) of the ethmoid sinuses should be noted. Intracranial penetrations usually occur on the side where the position of the roof is lower. One should examine for a break in the continuity of this roof (Fig. 3-29).[41]

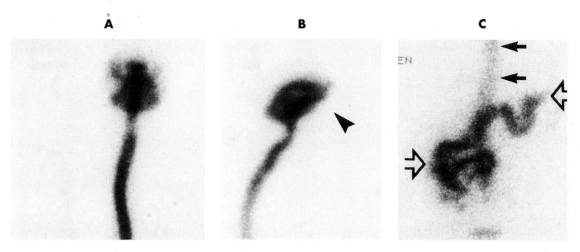

FIG. 3-31   Post FESS CSF leak. Indium-111 DTPA CSF study in the AP (**A**) and lateral projections (**B**) shows normal activity in the subarachnoid spaces. No activity is seen within the paranasal sinuses or nasal cavity (*black arrowhead*). Delayed AP image of the abdomen (**C**) shows abnormal bowel activity because of swallowed secretions from an occult CSF leakage *(open arrows)*. Residual activity within the subarachnoid space is noted *(black arrows)*.

5. Sphenoid sinus area

   The margins of the sphenoid sinus should be evaluated for bony dehiscence or cephalocele.

Operative Complications

The incidence of complications from FESS procedures is related to the instrumentation, the patient's underlying anatomy, the overall health of the patient, the extent of disease, and the experience of the surgeon.[31-34,59-61]

The field of view available to the surgeon during FESS is quite small, and variant anatomy can make surgical landmarks difficult to identify. The surgeon's view is limited to the surface mucosa; he or she cannot see beyond the mucosa directly in view. The presence of various anatomic variants can contribute to surgical complications if not noted prospectively.[32] As stated previously, because of the need for an accurate surgical road map, all patients scheduled to undergo FESS should have a preoperative coronal CT scan.

Brisk bleeding in the operative field and extensive nasal polyposis can hinder visibility and predispose the patient to operative complications.[32] Standard surgical techniques and microscope assisted surgery are adjuncts that can be used when the aforementioned problems arise. However, they are fraught with many of the same complications.

In general, complications are either minor or major.[31-33,60,61] Minor complications include periorbital emphysema, epistaxis, postoperative nasal synechiae, and tooth pain. Although these complications occur commonly, they are usually self-limited and do not require postoperative radiologic evaluation.

Major complications are rarer but can be devastating or fatal.[34] If there is preexisting or intraoperative disruption of the lamina papyracea, direct damage to the medial rectus muscle, superior oblique muscle, or other orbital contents can occur.[59] Injuries to the orbital contents may result in postoperative diplopia. The etiology of the diplopia can be from muscle entrapment among bone fragments or direct muscle laceration, or it can be secondary to nerve injury. Clinically, subconjunctival hemorrhage is often associated with extraocular muscle damage.[59] If intraorbital and intraocular pressure builds up because of an expanding hematoma or because of air being forced into the orbit from the nasal cavity (orbital emphysema via a dehiscent lamina papyracea), then visual impairment or blindness secondary to ischemia can result.[59]

Blindness, temporary or permanent, caused by injury of the optic nerve can occur during posterior ethmoidectomy, if the bony limit of the sinus is violated (Fig. 3-28).[31,34,59,61] Trauma to the vascular supply to the optic nerve can also result in visual loss.

Perforation of the cribiform plate can lead to intracranial hematoma or infection (see Fig. 3-30).

Massive hemorrhage from direct injury to major vessels can occur. Laceration of the internal carotid artery has been reported and is often a fatal complication.[31,32,34] Emergency angiography with balloon occlusion of the lacerated artery has been successfully performed in some patients. Patients who report severe postoperative headache, photophobia, or have signs that suggest subarachnoid hemorrhage should have a noncontrast head CT. If subarachnoid blood is found, cerebral angiography is recommended to detect vascular injury.[31,32,60]

Injury to the nasolacrimal duct can result during anterior enlargement of the maxillary ostium in the middle meatus. Injury to the membranous portion of the duct may be self-limited and remit by spontaneous fistulization into the middle meatus. Stenosis or total occlusion of the nasolacrimal duct can result from more severe injury.[59] Postoperative cerebrospinal fluid (CSF) leak is another major complication of FESS.[33,34,59,61] These leaks occur following inadvertent penetration of the dura via the cribriform plate,

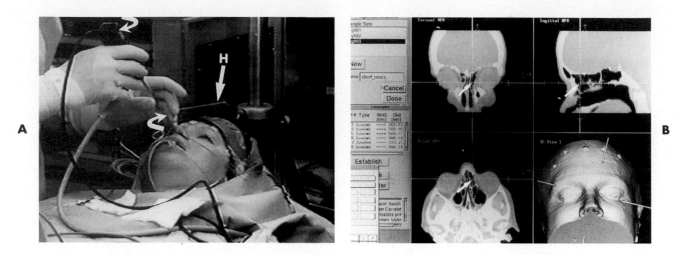

FIG. 3-32 Future developments. **A,** Patient under local anesthesia on the operating table. The endoscope *(curved arrows)* is in the patient's nasal cavity. The head follower *(H)* is affixed with three infrared sensors that provide an update to the computer with any of the patient's movements. Instruments outfitted with infrared sensors can be passed along the endoscope to pinpoint the location of specific anatomic structures (not shown in picture). **B,** Triplanar display and a three-dimensional CT display of the maxillofacial soft tissues are shown. The tip of the instrument outfitted with sensors is shown on the computer by the position of the "crosshairs" on the coronal, axial, and sagittal images *(arrows)*.

fovea ethmoidalis, anterior cranial fossa, or the middle cranial fossa skull base (refer to Fig. 3-9). Secondary nasal encephalocele or deep penetration of the cerebrum can also be seen following violation of the cranial vault.[23] A CSF leak may not become clinically apparent for up to 2 years after surgery.[31,32] CSF leaks will often close spontaneously with conservative measures.[31,32] However, if they persist, radiologic workup is indicated and reparative surgery may have to be performed.

In many institutions a radionuclide CSF study is utilized as the initial radiologic screening examination for such patients.[36,62] Before beginning the study, the otolaryngologist places absorbent pledgets in the nasal cavity. Usually, three to four are placed on each side, and note is made of their location within the nasal cavity. Subsequent to this, 400 to 500 Curie of Indium-III (In-111) labeled DTPA is

placed in the subarachnoid space by the neuroradiologist via a cervical or lumbar puncture. The patient is imaged with a gamma camera at multiple intervals for up to 24 hours. Any position or activity known to provoke the leak is encouraged. Even if the images of the head and neck do not show evidence of the leak, indirect scanning evidence may confirm the presence of a leak by showing activity in the bowel. Such activity indicates that the patient is swallowing CSF as it leaks into the nasal cavity (Fig. 3-31). At 24 hours the nasal pledgets are removed and assayed. The results are compared with In-111 activity in a serum sample drawn at the same time. A ratio of pledget activity to serum activity is determined and expressed in terms of counts per gram. Pledgets showing activity 1.5 times greater than serum activity are positive. It is then possible to predict the general area of the leak based on which pledgets show increased activity.

Even if none of the pledgets have increased activity, if there is increased activity over the abdomen, the radionuclide test is considered positive.

When the radionuclide test is positive (directly or indirectly), a contrast CT cisternogram in the coronal and axial planes is done to define the anatomy and to pinpoint the site of leakage. This CT scan can be of great help to the surgeon in planning further therapy to correct the leak.

COMPUTER ASSISTED SURGERY

A study performed by Kennedy for the American Academy of Otolaryngology and Head and Neck Surgery showed that there has been an increasing number of major surgical complications (i.e. death and orbital and intracranial damage) as the number of FESS procedures has increased.[63] Even though CT provides a "road map" for the surgeon, the information that is provided is remote. The surgeon must mentally transfer information from the image to the operative site.

Given the extreme variations in anatomy, extensive inflammatory disease, and the copious amount of intraoperative bleeding that can at times occur and make the anatomic landmarks difficult to identify, it is not surprising that inadvertent injuries to the orbital and intracranial compartments occur.

Thus there is a need for an objective and interactive correlation of the image data with the actual operative site in the patient. During the past 5 years, this goal has been achieved by using an ISG Allegro multimodality computer (manufactured by ISG Technologies in Mississauga, Ontario, Canada). At first this computer was attached to a mechanical sensor manufactured by Farro Medical Technologies; more recently the Pixys infrared sensor technology has been used.[64] The following technique is used. Before CT scanning, 5 to 10 external markers are placed on the patient's face. These are used to register the data in the computer so that they can be applied to the patient in vivo on the surgical table. With the registration complete and the patient immobilized, a mechanical arm holding a probe can be placed into the nasal cavity. The sensor is located in the tip of the probe. Axial, coronal, and sagittal reformatted images at the tip of the sensor are generated by the computer, and the location of the sensor in the patient is thus provided and shown by crosshairs on these images (Fig. 3-32). The Pixys sensors may be directly placed on the surgeon's instrument, and via a headband additional sensors may be directly placed on the patient's head. Thus two separate sets of sensors are available. One set is used to follow the position of the surgeon's instrument, and the other is used to update the computer with the patient's head motions. This new sensor technology allows the use of this instrumentation during surgery with either general or local anesthesia. In this manner the probe can be used to confirm the location of specific anatomic structures and to avoid penetration of the ethmoid roof and lamina papyracea. It can be used to easily identify the relationship of the sphenoid sinus to the optic nerves and carotid canals. The accuracy of this device has been shown to be approximately 2 mm.[64] There has been continuing improvement in sensor technology, and it is anticipated that in the near future this technology will gain widespread use. FESS has become the surgical treatment of choice for many patients with inflammatory sinus disease refractory to medical treatment. Coronal CT scanning is the imaging modality of choice for these patients. CT scanning provides an initial screening of these patients and can display anatomic causes of recurrent sinusitis when they exist. CT is essential in surgical planning, and it provides an operative "roadmap". Interactive image guided–computer assisted surgery now exists and holds great promise in objectively and directly integrating the imaging information with the endoscopic view, and thus improving the accuracy and safety of the operative management of patients undergoing FESS. Clearly, close cooperation between the radiologist and otolaryngologist-head and neck surgeon before surgery may bring to light imaging findings that may predispose the patient to operative complications.

References

1. Moss A, Parsons V. Current estimates from the National Health Interview Survey, United States, 1985. Hyattsville, Md: National Center for Health Statistics, 1986.

2. Messerklinger W. Endoscopy of the nose. Baltimore, Md: Urban & Schwartzenberg, Inc, 1978.

3. Messerklinger W. Zur Endoskopietchnik des mittleren Nassenganges. Arch Otorhinolaryngol 1978; 221:297-305.

4. Wigand ME, Steiner W, Jaumann MP. Endonasal sinus surgery with endoscopic control: from radical operation to rehabilitation of the mucosa. Endoscopy 1978; 10:255-260.

5. Kennedy DW, Zinreich SJ, Rosenbaum AE, et al. Functional endoscopic surgery: theory and diagnostic evaluation. Arch Otolaryngol 1985; 111:576-582.

6. Zinreich S, Kennedy D, Rosenbaum A, et al. Paranasal sinuses: CT imaging requirements for endoscopic surgery. Radiology 1987; 163(3):769-775.

7. Som P. Sinonasal cavity. In: Som P, Bergeron T, eds. Head and neck imaging. St. Louis, Mo: Mosby–Year Book Inc, 1991; 51-168.

8. Zinreich S. Paranasal sinus imaging. Otolaryngol Head Neck Surg 1990; 103(5/2):863-868.

9. Zinreich S. Imaging of chronic sinusitis in adults: x-ray, computed tomography, and magnetic resonance imaging. J Allergy Clin Immunol 1992; 90(3/2):445-451.

10. Zinreich S. Imaging of inflammatory sinus disease. Otolaryngol Clin North Am 1993; 26(4):535-547.

11. Zinreich S, Abidin M, Kennedy D. Cross-sectional imaging of the nasal cavity and paranasal sinuses. Operative Techniques in Otolaryngol Head Neck Surg 1990; 1(2):93-99.

12. Babbel R, Harnsberger HR, Nelson B, et al. Optimatization of techniques in screening CT of the sinuses. AJR 1991; 157:1093-1098.

13. Melhem ER, Oliverio PJ, Benson ML, et al. Optimal CT screening for functional endoscopic sinus surgery. (In press.)

14. Beck, DSc T. Radiation Physicist, Dept. of Radiology, The Johns Hopkins Hospital, Baltimore, Md: Personal communication.

15. Curry TS, Dowdey JE, Murry RC. Christensen's physics of diagnostic radiology. 4th Edition. Philadelphia, Pa: Lea & Febiger, 1990; 372-391.

16. Jones DJ, Wall BF. Organ doses from medical x-ray examinations calculated using Monte Carlo techniques. NRPB-R186 (HMSO, London), National Radiological Protection Board, 1985.

17. Zinreich SJ, Kennedy DW, Kumar A, et al. MR imaging of normal nasal cycle: comparison with sinus pathology. JCAT 1988; 12(6):1014-1019.

18. Kennedy D, Zinreich S, Kumar A, et al. Physiologic mucosal changes within the nose and ethmoid sinus: imaging of the nasal cycle by MRI. Laryngoscope 1988; 98(9):928-933.

19. Zinreich S, Kennedy D, Malat J, et al. Fungal sinusitis: diagnosis with CT and MR imaging. Radiology 1988; 169(2):439-444.

20. Som P, Curtin H. Chronic inflammatory sinonasal diseases including fungal infections: the role of imaging. Radiol Clin North Am 1993; 31(1):33-44.

21. Som P. Imaging of paranasal sinus fungal disease. Otolaryngol Clin North Am 1993; 26(6):983-994.

22. Som P, Dillon W, Curtin H, et al. Hypointense paranasal sinus foci: differential diagnosis with MR imaging and relation to CT findings. Radiology 1990; 176:777-781.

23. Weber A. Inflammatory diseases of the paranasal sinuses and mucoceles. Otolaryngol Clin North Am 1988; 21(3):421-437.

24. Shankar L, Evans K, Hawke M, et al. An atlas of imaging of the paranasal sinuses. Imago Publishing Ltd, 1994; 41-72.

25. Stammberger H. Functional Sinus Surgery. Philadelphia, Pa: B C Decker Inc, 1991; 273-282.

26. Kennedy DW, Zinreich SJ. The functional endoscopic approach to inflammatory sinus disease: current perspectives and technique modifications. Am J Rhinol 1988; 2(3):89-93.

27. Harnsberger R. Imaging for the sinus and nose. In: Head and neck imaging handbook. St. Louis, Mo: Mosby–Year Book, 1990; 387-419.

28. Hosemann W. Dissection of the lateral nasal wall in eight steps. In: Wigand ME, ed. Endoscopic surgery of the paranasal sinuses and anterior skull base. New York, NY: Thieme Medical Publishers Inc, 1990; 36-41.

29. Yousem D. Imaging of sinonasal inflammatory disease. Radiology 1993; 188(2):303-314.

30. Buus D, Tse D, Farris B. Ophthalmic complications of sinus surgery. Ophthalmology 1990; 97:612-619.

31. Hudgins P. Complications of endoscopic sinus surgery: the role of the radiologist in prevention. Radiol Clin North Am 1993; 31(1):21-31.

32. Hudgins P, Browning D, Gallups J. Endoscopic paranasal sinus surgery: radiographic evaluation of severe complications. AJNR 1992; 13:1161-1167.

33. Maniglia A. Fatal and major complications secondary to nasal and sinus surgery. Laryngoscope 1989; 99:276-283.

34. Maniglia A. Fatal and other major complications of endoscopic sinus

surgery. Laryngoscope 1991; 101:349-354.

35. Laine F, Smoker W. The ostiomeatal unit and endoscopic surgery: anatomy, variations, and imaging findings in inflammatory diseases. AJR 1992; 159(4):849-857.

36. Benson ML, Oliverio PJ, Zinreich SJ. Techniques of imaging of the nose and paranasal sinuses. In: Advances in otolaryngology-head and neck surgery. Volume 10. St. Louis, Mo: Mosby–Year Book, 1996. (In press.)

37. Mafee M. Preoperative imaging anatomy of the nasal-ethmoid complex for functional endoscopic sinus surgery. Radiol Clin North Am 1993; 31(1):1-20.

38. Bolger W, Butzin C, Parsons D. Paranasal sinus bony anatomic variations and mucosal abnormalities: CT analysis for endoscopic sinus surgery. Laryngoscope 1991; 101(1/1):56-64.

39. Yousem D, Kennedy D, Rosenberg S. Ostiomeatal complex risk factors for sinusitis: CT evaluation. J Otolaryngol 1991; 20(6):419-424.

40. Laine FJ, Kuta AJ. Imaging the sphenoid bone and basiocciput: pathologic considerations. Semin Ultra CT MRI 1993; 14(3):160-177.

41. Dessi P, Moulin G, Triglia JM, et al. Difference in height of the right and left ethmoidal roofs: a possible risk factor for ethmoidal surgery: prospective study of 150 CT scans. Laryngol Otol 1994; 108:261-262.

42. Johnson DW, Hopkins RJ, Hanafee WN, et al. The unprotected parasphenoidal carotid artery studied by high-resolution computed tomography. Radiology 1985; 155:137-141.

43. Kennedy DW, Zinreich SJ, Hassab MH. The internal carotid artery as it related to endonasal sphenoethmoidectomy. AJR 1990; 4(1):7-12.

44. Delano M, Fun FY, Zinreich SJ. Optic nerve relationship to the posterior paranasal sinuses: a CT anatomic study. AJNR. (In press.)

45. Evans F, Sydnor J, Moore W, et al. Sinusitis of the maxillary antrum. N Engl J Med 1975; 293(15):735-739.

46. Gullane P, Conley J. Carcinoma of the maxillary sinus: a correlation of the clinical course with orbital involvement, pterygoid erosion or pterygopalatine invasion and cervical metastases. J Otolaryngol 1983; 12:141-145.

47. Babbel R, Harnsberger H, Sonkens J, et al. Recurring patterns of inflammatory sinonasal disease demonstrated on screening sinus CT. AJNR 1992; 13(3):903-912.

48. Scuderi A, Babbel R, Harnsberger H, et al. The sporadic pattern of inflammatory sinonasal disease including postsurgical changes. Semin Ultrasound CT MR 1991; 12(6):575-591.

49. Stammberger H, Wolf G. Headaches and sinus disease: the endoscopic approach. Ann Otol Rhinol Laryngol Suppl 1988; 134:3-23.

50. Lidov M, Som P. Inflammatory disease involving a concha bullosa (enlarged pneumatized middle nasal turbinate): MR and CT appearance. AJNR 1990; 11(5):999-1001.

51. Moloney J, Badham N, McRae A. The acute orbit, preseptal, periorbital cellulitis, subperiosteal abscess, and orbital cellulitis due to sinusitis. J Laryngol Otol 1987; 12:1-18.

52. Centeno R, Bentson J, Mancuso A. CT scanning in rhinocerebral mucormycosis and aspergillosis. Radiology 1981; 140(2):383-389.

53. Osguthorpe J, Hochman M. Inflammatory sinus diseases affecting the orbit. Otolaryngol Clin North Am 1993; 26(4):657-671.

54. Walters E, Waller P, Hiles D, et al. Acute orbital cellulitis. Arch Ophthalmol 1976; 94:785-788.

55. Weber A, Mikulis D. Inflammatory disorders of the paraorbital sinuses and their complications. Radiol Clin North Am 1987; 25(3):615-631.

56. Patt B, Manning S. Blindness resulting from orbital complications of sinusitis. Otlaryngol Head Neck Surg 1991; 104(6):789-795.

57. Vinning EM, Kennedy DW. Surgical management in adults: chronic sinusitis. Immunology and Allergy Clinics of North America 1994; 14(1):97- 112.

58. Panje WR, Anand VK. Endoscopic sinus surgery indications, diagnosis, and technique. In: Anand VK, Panje WR, eds. Practical endoscopic sinus surgery. New York, NY: McGraw-Hill Inc, 1993; 68-86.

59. Neuhaus R. Orbital complications secondary to endoscopic sinus surgery. Ophthalmology 1990; 97:1512-1518.

60. Stankiewicz J. Complications of endoscopic intranasal ethmoidectomy. Laryngoscope 1987; 97:1270-1273.

61. Stankiewicz J. Complications in endoscopic intranasal ethmoidectomy: an update. Laryngoscope 1989; 99:668- 670.

62. Mettler FA, Guiberteau MJ. Essentials of nuclear medicine imaging. Ed 3. Philadelphia, Pa: W B Saunders Co, 1991; 73-74.

63. Kennedy D, Shaman P, Hen W, et al. Complications of ethmoidectomy: a survey of fellows of Otolaryngology-Head & Neck Surgery. Otolaryngology-Head & Neck Surgery. (In press.)

64. Zinreich S, Tebo S, Long D, Brem H, et al. Frameless stereotaxic integration of CT imaging data: accuracy and initial applications. Radiology 1993; 188(3):735-742.

4

Sinonasal Cavities: Inflammatory Diseases, Tumors, Fractures, and Postoperative Findings

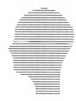

PETER M. SOM
MARGARET BRANDWEIN

126

SECTION ONE
NONNEOPLASTIC DISORDERS

INFLAMMATORY CONDITIONS
Acute Viral and Bacterial Rhinosinusitis

The common cold is the most frequent infectious malady of the upper respiratory tract and is one of the major causes of missed working days. The clinical manifestation of this viral infection is primarily a watery, profuse nasal discharge that usually persists less than a week. The evoked inflammatory changes are completely reversible. The most commonly implicated viruses are rhinoviruses, parainfluenza and influenza viruses, adenoviruses, and respiratory syncytial virus.[1] The typical cold remains primarily a viral rhinitis with little significant sinusitis. However, if a mucopurulent discharge develops, a secondary bacterial infection has occurred. In cases of noncomplicated viral infections, imaging of the sinonasal cavities usually shows that they are normal or shows minimal sinus mucosal thickening, but the mucosa in the nasal fossae is thickened and usually there is swelling of the turbinates. If this swollen mucosa causes obstruction of a sinus ostium, the oxygen tension within the sinus decreases and the normal bacterial flora becomes altered. This results in an acute bacterial sinusitis. Direct sinus puncture or open surgical biopsy yields the most accurate bacterial cultures for a sinusitis because these procedures prevent contamination by nasal flora.[2] The most commonly implicated pathogens from such studies are *Streptococcus pneumoniae* (pneumococcus), *Haemophilus influenzae*, and beta hemolytic streptococcus. Rarely, *Staphylococcus aureus* and *Pseudomonas* infections occur.[3] Pathogenic anaerobes are rare in acute sinusitis. However, in cases of chronic sinusitis with persistently low intrasinus oxygen tensions, anaerobes predominate. These anaerobes include peptostreptococci, *Bacteroides sp. lanchnicus*, and fusobacteria.[4,5] In the case of the maxillary sinus, it is estimated that 10% to 20% of the infections are secondary to

dental infection or are the result of a complication of a tooth extraction.[6]

If the sinus ostial obstruction is transient, the bacterial sinusitis often resolves within 4 to 7 days with conservative treatment. The bacterial sinusitis may be the cause of pain that is usually localized over the affected sinus. By comparison, headache is estimated to occur in only 3% of patients with sinusitis; in these cases, it usually is either a frontal headache secondary to a frontal sinusitis or a suboccipital headache secondary to posterior ethmoid or sphenoid sinusitis.[7] A generalized headache can occur, but it is unusual and is rarely due to secondary intracranial infection.

Because acute bacterial sinusitis results from sinus ostial obstruction, it is in effect a sinus-by-sinus event rather than a generalized process. Thus it is more common to find contiguous unilateral sinusitis than it is to encounter a pansinusitis. Even when both antra are affected, one is usually more severely afflicted. Thus in general, asymmetric sinusitis is a hallmark of bacterial disease. By comparison, pansinusitis is usually found in patients with an allergic sinusitis, possibly because the allergic process is usually a systemic rather than a local event.

Chronic sinusitis results from either persistent acute inflammation or repeated episodes of acute or subacute sinusitis. It is estimated that up to one third of patients with acute sinusitis develop chronic sinusitis. Chronic disease can result in an atrophic, sclerosing, or hypertrophic polypoid mucosa. These varied mucosal changes most often coexist with one another and with areas of acute inflammation of either an infectious or allergic etiology. Because chronically inflamed and scarred mucosa loses some of its ciliary function, it becomes less resistent to future infection. Thus a vicious cycle of infection and reinfection is often present in patients with chronic sinusitis. The bony sinus walls around a chronically infected sinus usually become thickened and sclerotic with reactive new bone formation. This bony change is found with all chronic inflammation regardless of etiology and presumably is a response to periosteal involvement by inflammation.

Allergic sinus disease is associated with nasal polyposis, and there is a tendency toward symmetric involvement. Nasal polyps are uncommon in patients with routine bacterial sinusitis. In addition, most allergic polyps are multiple whereas most inflammatory nonallergic polyps are solitary.

Nearly 10% of the general population has allergic rhinitis and sinusitis. The most common form is seasonal pollinosis, and the prevalent form in North America is ragweed allergy. Spores, molds, and mites are also important antigens.[8] Allergic reactions are manifestations of type I immunologic disorders, which reflect an IgE reagin-antibody reaction with a resulting release of mediators that produce symptoms of sneezing, nasal obstruction, and watery rhinorrhea. Profuse secretions associated with nasal obstruction can result in some retained secretions and eventual infection.[8] Thus the coexistence of bacterial and allergic sinusitis is not uncommon. The resulting hypertrophic, thickened, and redundant allergic sinus mucosa is often referred to as hypertrophic polypoid mucosa, which is less capable than normal mucosa of resisting subsequent infections. Rarely, in the maxillary sinus, hypertrophic mucosa can become so redundant that it prolapses into the nasal fossa, simulating an antrochoanal polyp.[9]

In the recent decade there has been great interest in the prevalence and type of paranasal sinus inflammatory disease in HIV-positive patients.[10] Minimal sinus inflammatory disease as seen on imaging may be clinically disasterous for these patients. Any degree of mucosal disease must be reported so that appropriate and early treatment can be initiated. HIV specifically infects T helper-lymphocytes. One of the many ripple effects of the loss of T helper-cells is dysfunction of the B lymphocytes, which results in unusually severe bacterial infections. The B cells are unable to repond normally to antigenic stimulation, possibly relating to the loss of lymphokine-induced stimulation. In addition to the bacteria associated with sinusitis in normal patients, bacterial sinusitis in patients with AIDS has been caused by *Pseudomonas aeruginosa* and *Legionella pneumophila*, which are considered opportunistic bacterial pathogens rarely causing sinusitis in normal hosts.[11,12]

In the pediatric patient, sinus opacification and mucosal thickening have a questionable correlation with the presence of active infection. This is particularly true in children less than 4 years of age (especially children less than 2 years of age) in whom tears, retained normal secretions, and normal redundant mucosa may account for these imaging findings.[13-16] Thus in all such pediatric patients, paranasal sinus imaging findings should be very carefully evaluated in light of the clinical setting before a diagnosis of active infection is made.

Persistent sinusitis in a pediatric patient may indicate the presence of cystic fibrosis (mucoviscidosis). In these patients, persistent nasal obstruction and sinusitis often lead to hypoplasia of the frontal sinuses, presumably secondary to insufficient aeration. Additional conditions to consider in children with repeated episodes of sinusitis include immune deficiency syndromes, HIV infection, allergic sinusitis, unusual allergies such as aspirin intolerance, and immobile cilia syndrome. In ruling out the latter syndrome, it may be useful to recommend that the clinician submit a brush biopsy from the lateral nasal wall for electron microscopy. Brush biopsies submitted in gluteraldehyde are superior to routine forceps biopsies for visualizing the ultrastructure of ciliated cells. Lastly, children under the age of 10 years rarely develop allergic nasal polyps. Thus the presentation of a nasal polyp in the first few years of life raises the suspicion of an encephalocele, and the appearance of nasal polyposis suggests the diagnosis of cystic fibrosis.[17,18]

In all patients, regardless of age, the radiologist should very cautiously apply the adjectives acute or chronic to the diagnosis of sinusitis, when such a diagnosis is based only on the findings of a single examination. This approach can be fraught with error. For example, on a single imaging study the presence of sinus mucosal thickening may represent any of the following different clinical situations: either the mucosal disease is in a patient who had normal sinuses several days earlier, and thus it represents acute disease; the mucosal thickening is in a sinus that several days earlier was completely opacified, and thus it represents either resolving acute or subacute disease; or lastly the mucosal thickening is unchanged on serial examinations, and thus it represents allergic inflammation or scarred, noninfected mucosa. Unless clinical correlation to and comparison with recent examinations can be made, the radiologist should report only mucosal thickening. Even if chronic reactive thickened bone is identified around a sinus cavity, there may not be any active disease present in the sinus, and any thickened soft tissue may represent fibrotic, scarred mucosa. The radiologist may confidently diagnose acute sinusitis only when an air-fluid level is seen in a patient with clinical signs and symptoms of acute bacterial sinusitis.

Imaging of Abnormal Sinus Mucosa

It must be remembered that although imaging can be highly suggestive of inflammatory disease, it is not possible to identify a specific pathogen or, even in the vast majority of cases, the cause of the inflammation based on the imaging. Thus the pathologist and microbiologist are necessary to establish a definitive diagnosis.

The normal sinus mucosa is very thin compared with the thick bony sinus walls and the adjacent normal volume of sinus air. Normal sinus mucosa is rarely identified on plain films, CT scans, or MR images. On all of these studies, in a normal sinus the air appears to abut directly against the bony sinus walls. Thus it is a relatively simple task to evaluate whether or not the sinus mucosa is normal; no soft-tissue density separating the sinus air and bony wall is consistent with normal mucosa. The one exception to this statement occurs on enhanced MR images, where normal mucosa occasionally will be identified. However, on a study of sinus mucosal thickening seen on brain MR imaging, it was found that mucosal thickening up to 3 mm may be present in clinically normal patients. In addition, clinically silent focal areas of ethmoid mucosal thickening were found in 66% of

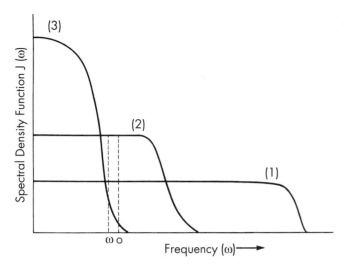

FIG. 4-1 Diagram of a spectral distribution curve for physiologic solutions. The number of molecules at a specific frequency J(ω) is graphed against the range of frequencies (ω). Curve *(1)* is for water and illustrates that a wide range of frequencies are present, but there is not a preponderance of molecules at any one frequency. Curve *(2)* shows what happens as macromolecular proteins are added to the water system. The molecules are present at a more limited number of frequencies. The higher frequencies drop out because the large, slowly tumbling molecules affect the system. Curve *(3)* illustrates that when a large number of macromolecular proteins are added to the systems, most of the molecules have a very limited range of slower frequencies. ωo, Lamor frequency.

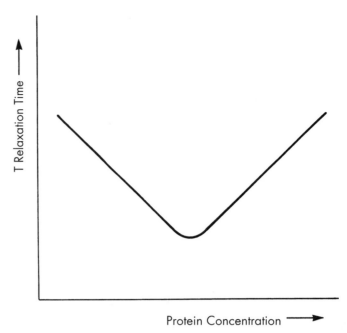

FIG. 4-2 Graph of T1 relaxation time versus macromolecular protein concentration. As protein is added to a water system the T1 relaxation slows until the net frequency of the lattice is that of the Lamor frequency. At that protein concentration the T1 relaxation time is the most efficient (shortest). As still more protein is added the net frequency of the system slows below that of the Lamor frequency, and the T1 relaxation time again becomes less efficient.

ically normal patients. In addition, clinically silent focal areas of ethmoid mucosal thickening were found in 66% of patients.[19] Another series of 263 patients found clinically silent areas of mucosal thickening in nearly 25% of the cases.[20] Thus even minimal degrees of sinus mucosal thickening may not be clinically relevant. The overall evaluation of the sinus mucosa is more easily and thoroughly performed on CT and MRI than it is on plain films.

Magnetic Resonance of Protein Solutions

To understand both the benefits of and problems created by the MRI signal intensities of acute and chronic sinonasal inflammatory disease, a brief, simplified review of T1 and T2 relaxation times in macromolecular protein solutions is warranted. The term *lattice* simply refers to the overall magnetic environment of the system being studied. A proton spin system can be excited by the addition of energy, and the most efficient way to transfer that energy to the protons is to choose that the exciting pulse be at the Larmor frequency. Once excited, the spin system tends to rid itself of the excess energy and return to an equilibrium state. This excess energy is absorbed by the lattice, and a measure of the time it takes for this process to occur is referred to as the spin-lattice or T1 relaxation time.

The most efficient absorption of the excess energy from the excited protons to the lattice occurs when the net molecular rotation of the lattice is at the Larmor frequency. Thus if a system does not have many molecules rotating at the Larmor frequency, the energy absorption is inefficient and

the spin-lattice relaxation time is long. Conversely, if the system has most of its molecules rotating at the Larmor frequency, the T1 relaxation time is efficient and short. A study of the number of molecules in a system that are rotating at various frequencies yields a spectral distribution function that can be graphed as the number of molecules at a specific rotational frequency versus the range of frequencies (Fig. 4-1).

Analysis of pure water shows that these small molecules have a wide range of net rotational frequencies, but there is not a preponderance of molecules at any one frequency, including the Larmor frequency. Thus pure water has a long T1 relaxation time. As large physiologic macromolecular proteins with relatively slow tumbling frequencies are added to pure water, for a variety of reasons the net rotational motion of the system slows. This effect continues as more macromolecular protein is added, until a protein concentration is reached at which there is a maximum number of molecules with a net rotational frequency at the Larmor frequency. At this concentration the T1 relaxation time is the shortest for the system. As more macromolecular protein is added, the net rotational frequency of the system continues to slow and falls below the Larmor frequency. Consequently, for these more concentrated protein solutions the T1 relaxation time is long. Thus for such physiologic solutions, as one proceeds from low macromolecular protein concentrations to high concentrations, the T1 relaxation time goes from long to short to long (Fig. 4-2). This is reflected as the T1-weighted (T1W) signal intensity goes from low to high to low.

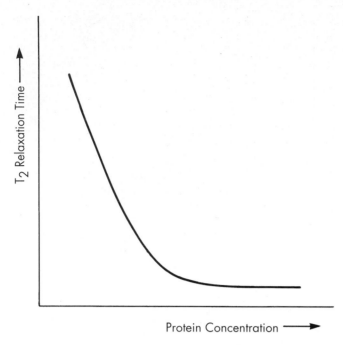

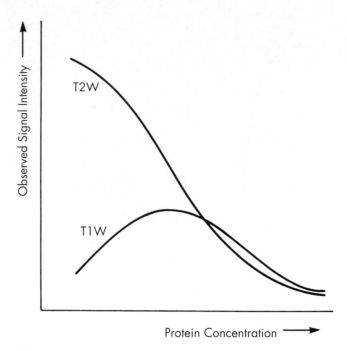

FIG. 4-3 Graph of T2 relaxation time versus macromolecular protein concentration. The more protein added to the system, the lower (faster) is the T2 relaxation time. This relationship holds until the system becomes a solid. As a solid the T2 relaxation time is the fastest it can be, and the T2 relaxation time is a plateau.

FIG. 4-4 Graph of laboratory observed T1W and T2W signal intensities versus macromolecular protein concentrations. These curves reflect the relaxation times shown in Figs. 4-2 and 4-3.

With reference to the T2 relaxation time, initially, after the spin system has been excited, all of the protons can be considered as precessing at the same frequency. However, variations in the local magnetic environment of each proton cause the speed of precession to change by varying amounts, and the result of these magnetic inhomogeneities is that the protons start to precess at a wider and wider range of frequencies. This interaction is referred to as spin-spin relaxation or dipole-dipole dephasing, and the T2 relaxation time is a measure of this process. For pure water, all the molecules are the same, and they are moving so rapidly that they have little effect on the local magnetic fields of particular protons. Hence in pure water the protons precess in phase for a long time and the T2 relaxation time is long. As macromolecular solute is added, the net frequencies slow so that there is more time for spin-spin interactions. In addition, more molecular nonhomogeneity is introduced into the system. Thus as the protein concentration increases, the T2 relaxation time decreases. However, in viscous solutions and solids the T2 effects reach a maximum and the T2 relaxation time plateaus at its shortest time (Fig. 4-3). In fact the T2 relaxation falls from the milliseconds range for physiologic protein solutions to the microseconds range for solids. Such rapid dephasing does not allow any magnetic signal to be detected on MR imaging, and a signal void is observed. Lastly, when the T2 relaxation times are ultrashort in the microseconds range, this effect dominates any observed T1 relaxation and signal voids are also observed on T1 weighted MR imaging. This phenomenon is often referred to as the T2 effect on T1 relaxation time. With this simpli-

fied background, one can approach the MR signal intensities of sinonasal secretions (Fig. 4-4).

Normal sinonasal secretions form a complex solution that is in equilibrium with the interstitial fluids.[9] By weight, about 95% of these secretions is water and 5% is solids; virtually all of these solids are macromolecular proteins, predominantly (60%) mucous glycoproteins. Thus normal sinonasal secretions are predominantly water, and on MR imaging they have long T1 and T2 relaxation times. These are observed as low T1W and high T2W signal intensities.

When normal sinonasal secretions become chronically obstructed, a number of predictable changes occur that alter the protein concentration, the amount of free water (that fraction of the water molecules that magnetically are independent of the effects of the macromolecular proteins), and the viscosity. These changes in the secretions occur as a result of alterations in the composition and function of the obstructed sinus mucosa, which increases the number of goblet cells that are responsible for the production of the mucous glycoproteins. There is also decreased clearance of the mucous glycoproteins. With time the sinus mucosa also reabsorbs the free water in the secretions. As a result of these changes the concentration of these proteins increases in the secretions, and they progressively change from a primarily watery serous composition to a thick mucous collection, and finally into a dessicated, stonelike mucous plug. Accentuating these effects is the intrinsic viscosity of sinonasal secretions, which increases clinically into a sludgelike consistency when the protein content is above about 35%.

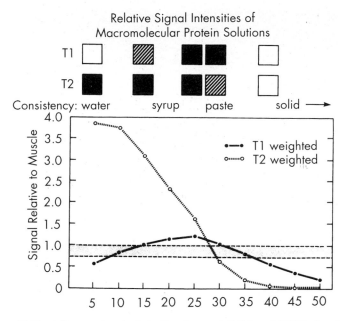

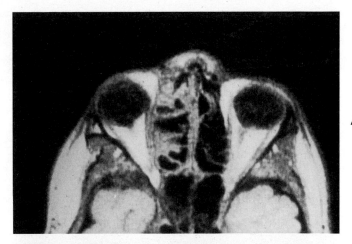

A

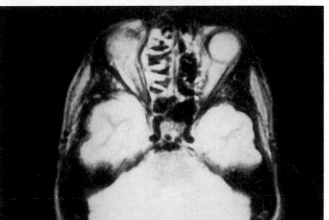

B

FIG. 4-5 Graph of clinically observed T1W and T2W signal intensities versus macromolecular protein concentration. The horizontal zone of gray represents the intermediate range of signal intensity compared with brain. The relationship of the relative physical consistency of the solutions to the signal intensities is shown at the top of the graph. These curves parallel those in Fig. 4-4.

These changes are predictable, but their course of evolution cannot be predicted. In some patients, such changes occur more rapidly in one sinus than in another, but in other patients, all of the chronically obstructed secretions appear to undergo these changes at nearly the same rate. The clinical significance of these changes is not clear. However, what is known is that if one notes the T1W and T2W signal intensities of such secretions, the protein concentration can be very accurately determined. In fact, graphs of observed T1W and T2W signal intensities reflect the signal intensities predicted in the prior discussion of the T1 and T2 relaxation times (Fig. 4-5).

As the protein content rises from 5% to about 25%, both the T1 and T2 relaxation times shorten as predicted. However, this T2 shortening is not seen on the MR images because the T2W signal intensity overall is so high that subtle gradations in the corresponding whiteness are not appreciated. The rise of the T1W signal intensity is more easily observed on the scans.

At about 25% to 30% protein content, significant crosslinking occurs between protein molecules. This phenomenon is noted clinically as an increase in the consistency of the secretions. These changes also slow the macromolecular motion, which in turn allows dipole-dipole dephasing to become a more significant factor. As a result the T2 relaxation time and signal intensity plummet. The T1W signal intensity falls back to a low value between the protein content range of 25% to 40%. Above 35% to 40% protein content, virtually all of the free water has been eliminated from the secretions and direct macromolecular protein-protein

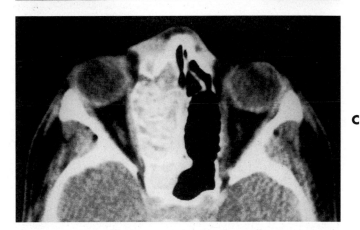

C

FIG. 4-6 Axial T1W (**A**), T2W (**B**), and CT scans (**C**) show apparant scattered areas of aeration in the right ethmoid sinuses and right sphenoid sinus (**A** and **B**). However, these sinuses are completely opacified with desiccated secretions (**C**). Also note that within each sinus (**C**) the dense secretions are separated from the sinus wall by a thin zone of mucoid-density material. Chronic sinusitis.

binding occurs. This results in a sudden increase in the consistency of the secretions. These semisolid and solid protein mixtures have ultrashort T2 relaxation times, and these are noted first as low T2W signal intensities and then as signal voids on both T1W and T2W MR images.

Once the secretions have become chronically thickened

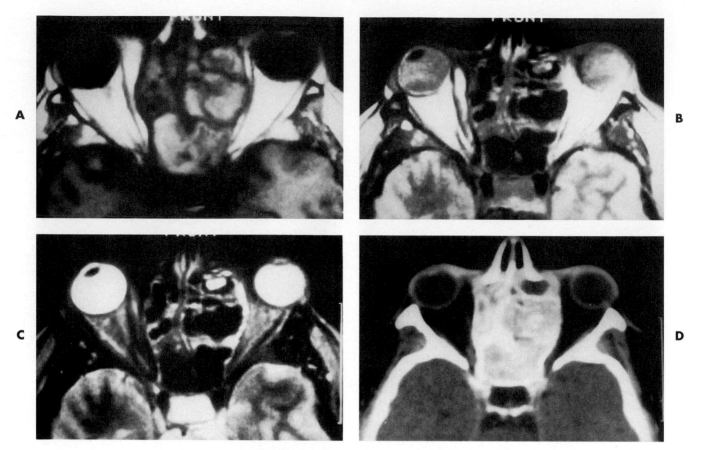

FIG. 4-7 Axial T1W (**A**), proton density (**B**), T2W (**C**) MR scans and CT scan (**D**) show that the expanded ethmoid and sphenoid sinuses are opacified (**A**). However, if a proton density and T2W series were the only MR scans taken, the dried secretions easily seen on CT (**D**) could be mistaken for aerated sinuses in (**B** and **C**). Chronic sinusitis.

and concentrated as previously described, the MRI signal intensities vary according to the protein concentration and thus are quite variable. However, when the secretions become so concentrated that they have signal voids on both T1W and T2W MR scans, distinction from an aerated sinus may be impossible on MRI (Figs. 4-6, 4-7). Although the cause of a signal void with air is due to a paucity of protons whereas the signal void observed with the desiccated secretions is secondary to its ultrashort relaxation times, radiographically the "blackness" is the same. Thus the radiologist can easily underestimate the presence of such chronic secretions and the severity of the sinus disease if MRI is the only imaging examination used. But on CT, such dried secretions are dense, reflecting their high protein concentration and air is black so that distinction is easily made between an aerated sinus and a chronically obstructed sinus (Figs. 4-6, 4-7). Because of this fact and the more accurate and easier CT diagnosis of any chronic bone changes, it is suggested that CT, not MRI, be the first modality with which to image a patient with chronic inflammatory disease.[21-23]

If MR contrast is used, it must be remembered that normal sinus mucosa can enhance, and the relevance of any such enhancing mucosa must always be questioned in light of the patient's complaints. Inflamed sinus mucosa also enhances but entrapped secretions do not (Fig. 4-8). However, as discussed previously, it may be impossible to differentiate an aerated sinus with some mucosal thickening from a totally obstructed sinus containing desiccated secretions.

Sinus and Nasal Mucosal Thickening and Adjacent Bone Changes

There are a number of pathologic conditions that can cause the sinus mucosa to become sufficiently thick to be identified on imaging. These conditions include infection, noninfected inflammation (e.g., allergy, chemical irritation), fibrosis, tumor, or a combination thereof. On plain films the earliest sign of thickened mucosa is often a hazy or vaguely "clouded" appearance of the involved sinus. In these cases, a thickened mucosal margin per se may not be identified. If one can be certain that this appearance is not the result of technical or extrinsic factors (the entire film looks hazy, there is overlying swelling of the soft tissues of the cheek, etc.), then this sinus is abnormal. Commonly this appearance results from the combination of retained secretions and minimal mucosal thickening (Fig. 4-9). Once the mucosa is thick enough to be distinctly identifiable as such on plain films, it usually appears as a uniform soft-tissue density zone that separates the sinus air from the bone (Fig. 4-10).

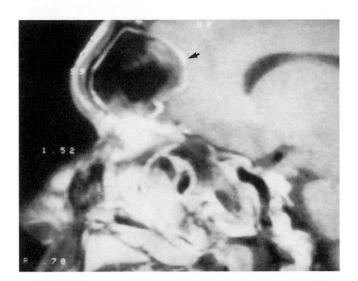

FIG. 4-8 Sagittal T1W contrast MR shows the enhancing mucosa of a frontal sinus mucocele *(arrow)*, surrounding the entrapped secretions, most of which are desiccated and have a signal void intensity.

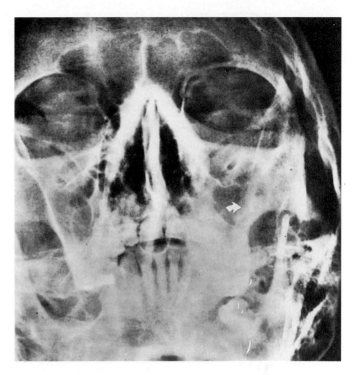

FIG. 4-9 Waters view shows "clouded" right maxillary sinus. Distinct mucosal thickening is not identified. The left antrum is also "hazy," but there is a definite area of mucosa thickening seen along the lateral sinus wall *(arrow)*. Sinusitis.

On plain films this type of change is usually easily identified in the frontal sinuses and along the lower lateral walls of the maxillary sinuses. However, care should be taken not to over interpret haziness that is often seen in the antral zygomatic recesses. These areas of the antra have less air and thicker surrounding bone than the main sinus cavity and almost always appear slightly clouded when compared with the main body of the sinus.

Hypoplasia of the maxillary sinus may cause this sinus to appear diseased on plain film studies. Although in most cases, the greater downward angulation of the lateral aspect of the orbital floor (antral roof), and the larger ipsilateral orbit (and often the larger superior orbital fissure) allow antral hypoplasia to be diagnosed on plain films. Precise evaluation of the mucosa within a hypoplastic sinus may be impossible without CT or MRI. In addition, sectional imaging in the axial plane allows pathology in the cheek to be separated from that in the antral walls or in the sinus mucosa.[24,25]

The unique anatomy of the ethmoid complex can also lead to underdiagnosis of pathology on plain films because there are numerous individual ethmoid sinus cavities, which are small and closely packed together. The increased density associated with mucosal thickening in an isolated group of ethmoidal cells may be almost completely nullified by air-containing surrounding cells and the adjacent sphenoid sinus.

The sensitivity of the plain film examination of the ethmoid sinuses may be increased by paying close attention to the appearance of the intrasinus septa. Poorly visualized septa may belie the presence of mucosal thickening or fluid (Fig. 4-11). However, definitive diagnosis of minimal or focal ethmoid cell disease requires sectional imaging. The lack of visualization of these ethmoid septa with no obvious soft-tissue mass may also result from pneumosinus dilatans, mucocele, or previous ethmoidectomy.

In the sphenoid sinuses, minimal mucosal thickening is usually not identifiable on plain films because these sinuses are partially obscured by many overlapping bone and soft-tissue structures. Air-fluid levels can be identified on films taken in the erect position, but CT or MRI is required in most cases to identify mucosal disease.

Sinus mucosal disease may vary from only a 1- to 2-mm thick mucosa to a hypertrophic polypoid thickening that fills the entire sinus cavity. However, a "thick" mucosa radiographically may be caused by one or all of the following three factors: (1) actual mucosal thickening, (2) a submucosal edematous component, and (3) surface secretions. There seems to be no correlation with the degree of submucosal edema present and the clinical outcome of the patient. Some patients have the sinus cavity filled with redundant mucosa and only a small amount of secretions, and other patients have a sinus cavity primarily filled with retained secretions and only minimal mucosa thickening (i.e., mucocele). The clinical significance between these different responses to inflammation is unclear (Figs. 4-12, 4-13).

When active infection has been present for several days, the associated increased mucosal vascularity presumably results in an increased mobilization of calcium in the adjacent sinus wall. Plain films reveal a "washing out" of the thin mucoperiosteal white line. This is most evident in the frontal sinus and the maxillary sinus along the medial antral wall. In the antrum, it is least likely to involve the posterior or infratemporal walls.[26]

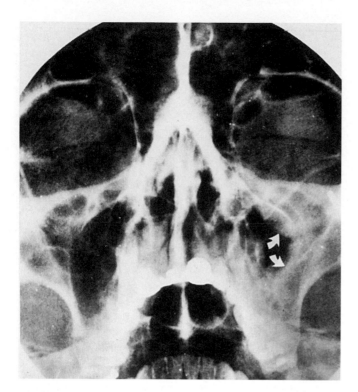

FIG. 4-10   Waters view shows mucosal thickening *(arrows)* in the left antrum. As the mucosa becomes progressively thickened, it heaps up into polypoid masses. Sinusitis.

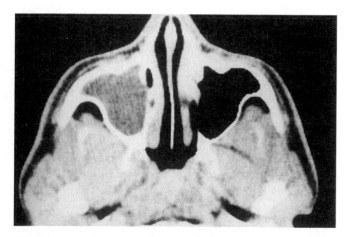

FIG. 4-12   Axial CT scan shows a fluid-filled right maxillary sinus. Because the sinus cavity is not larger than normal, this should not be called a mucocele. Obstructed sinus.

Conversely, when inflammation has been present for many months or years, thickened, dense reactive bone develops in the sinus wall, especially in the frontal bone (Fig. 4-14). In the maxillary sinus the thickened, sclerotic bone may decrease sinus size, a finding confirmed on CT scans (Fig. 4-15).

In the sphenoid sinus, chronic infection may result in a thickened, sclerotic bony reaction around the involved sinus and along the sphenoid sinus septum (Fig. 4-16). Patients with sphenoid sinusitis may report suboccipital pain or

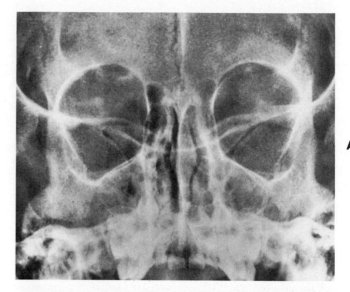

A

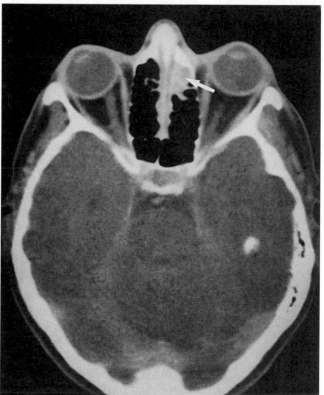

B

FIG. 4-11   **A,** Waters view shows opacification of the left hypoplastic frontal sinus and ethmoid sinuses (compare with normal right side). The maxillary sinuses are also almost totally opacified. Sinusitis. **B,** Axial CT scan on different patient with normal plain films. There is localized inflammatory disease in the left anterior ethmoid cells *(arrow).* The middle and posterior left ethmoid sinuses and the left sphenoid sinus are normal and well aerated. Because this air negates the soft-tissue density of the localized disease, the frontal plain films may appear normal.

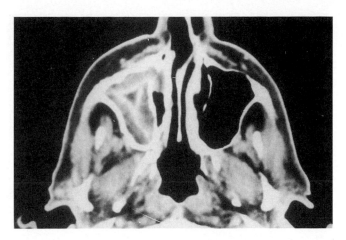

FIG. 4-13 Axial CT scan shows an obstructed right maxillary sinus. Centrally within the sinus there is a triangular area of mucoid density that is entrapped sinus secretions. About this area is a region of thin, uniform enhancement that is the inflammed sinus mucosa. Between this mucosa and the bony sinus wall is a zone of submucosal edema. Acute sinusitis.

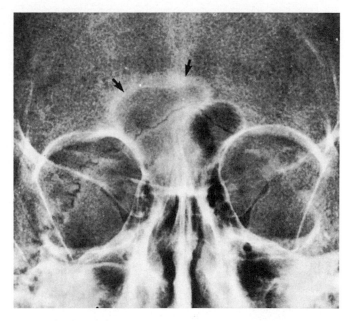

FIG. 4-14 Caldwell view shows a zone of reactive sclerosis around the right frontal sinus *(arrows).* The sinus clouding could be due to acute or chronic infection or fibrosis. Minimal clouding is also present in the right posterior ethmoid sinuses. Chronic sinusitis.

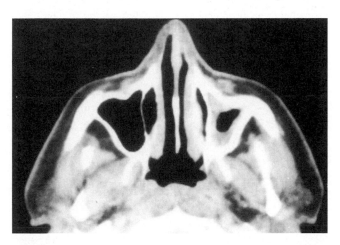

FIG. 4-15 Axial CT scan shows thickening and sclerosis of the walls of the left maxillary sinus. There is also some mucosal thickening in the left antrum that may be active disease, noninfected edematous mucosa, or scarred mucosa. This type of bone reaction indicates that there has been chronic inflammation in this sinus. Chronic sinusitis.

headaches. Rarely, cavernous sinus thrombophlebitis and thrombosis can develop as a complication of sphenoid sinusitis. Eventually, signs and symptoms of meningismus and meningitis can occur. In any such patient, a scan performed to evaluate the brain should always include the skull base and paranasal sinuses.

Osteomyelitis of the bones of the face and sinonasal cavities is an unusual event, but occasional focal sites of osteomyelitis occur. The involved bone has a mottled, irregular appearance on both plain films and CT (Fig. 4-17). There may be sequestra, and the adjacent bone is often thickened and sclerotic. One should search for mottled areas with sequestra as a possible cause of chronic pain.

More commonly, osteomyelitis may be posttraumatic or

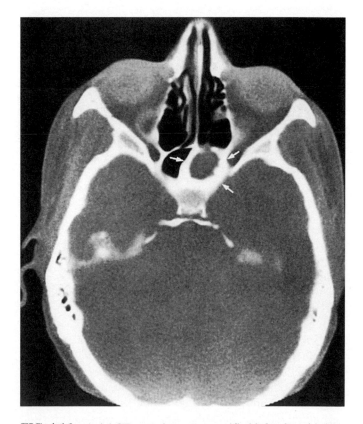

FIG. 4-16 Axial CT scan shows an opacified left sphenoid sinus with reactive, sclerotic thickening of the sphenoid intersinus septum and the walls of the left sphenoid sinus *(arrows).* Chronic sinusitis.

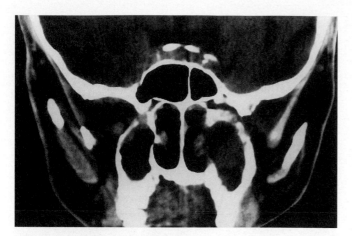

FIG. 4-17 Coronal CT scan shows mucosal thickening in the left maxillary sinus associated with thickened, sclerotic sinus walls. In addition there are areas of rarefaction and early sequestrum formation along the upper antral wall. Incidently noted is minimal mucosal disease in the right maxillary sinus. Chronic sinusitis with osteomyelitis.

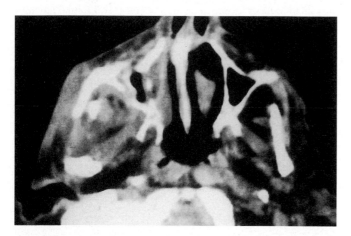

FIG. 4-19 Axial CT scan shows fragmentation of the bony walls of the right maxillary sinus. The bone is slightly thickened and sclerotic. Mucosal thickening is also present in the sinus. Radiation osteitis and sinusitis.

iatrogenic. This is most often following the osteoplastic flap procedure for frontal sinus surgery; a poorly vascularized bone flap over a chronically infected sinus may cause osteomyelitis of the flap. This is a recognized complication of this procedure.

A related condition is postirradiation osteitis, which is rarely seen today in the facial bones because of megavoltage equipment and improved radiation treatment planning. Radiation osteitis is probably most commonly encountered in the mandible, usually in patients irradiated for carcinomas of the tongue and floor of the mouth. In patients irradiated for antral carcinomas, the first manifestation of sinus osteomyelitis may be the development of swelling and inflammation over the zygoma and maxilla, which may initially suggest tumor recurrence. Eventually a bone

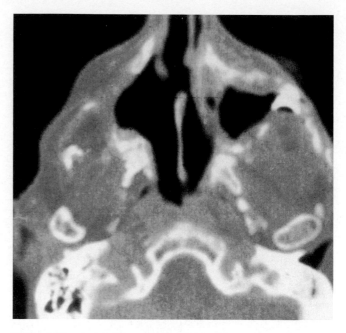

FIG. 4-18 Axial CT scan shows extensive sclerosis and fragmentation of the facial bones. Some of the osseous structures have been extruded as sequestra. Radiation osteitis.

sequestrum is extruded, and symptoms temporarily improve. Multiple sequestra may be extruded. The diagnosis of radiation osteitis may be clinically established after the identification of the sequestra. It is not uncommon for the osteitis to become manifest up to 1 or 2 decades after irradiation. On CT the involved facial bones appear shattered, fragmented, and sclerotic (Figs. 4-18, 4-19). Superficial sequestra should be identified and localized.

When evaluating mucosal thickening on postcontrast CT scans, if the thickened mucosa does not enhance, it is probably not actively infected and usually is fibrotic. Active infection usually has a thin zone of mucosal enhancement with submucosal edema (Fig. 4-13). If these changes are seen in a sinus opacified with sinus secretions, the sinus often has the appearance of roughly concentric rings; for example, an outer bony dense ring, a low mucoid attenuation (10 to 18 HUs) submucosal ring, a thin infected mucosal enhancing ring, and a central zone of entrapped mucoid secretions (Fig. 4-13). Although most minimal to moderate mucosal thickening gives a fairly uniformly thick soft-tissue zone on sectional imaging, thicker, more redundant mucosa can appear almost nodular or "wavelike." In these instances, all of the sinus walls tend to be uniformly involved, unlike the focal nodularity often seen with tumors.

In all cases, the sinuses should be viewed at wide window settings so that disease that opacifies a sinus is not obscured and falsely interpreted as a hypoplastic or aplastic sinus (Fig. 4-20).

On MRI the thickened, inflamed mucosa typically has a low signal intensity on T1W images an intermediate intensity signal on PD images, and a high intensity signal on the T2W images (Figs. 4-6, 4-7, 4-21, 4-22). These changes

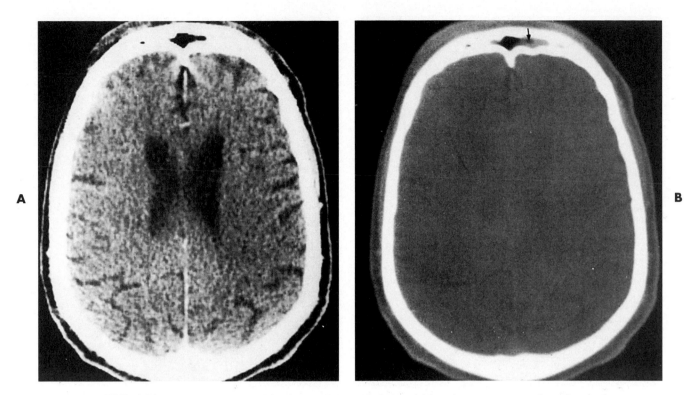

FIG. 4-20 **A,** Axial CT scan viewed at "soft-tissue" window setting shows an apparently well-aerated frontal sinus. **B,** Axial CT scan, same image as **A,** viewed at "bone" window setting shows inflammatory mucosal thickening in the left frontal sinus *(arrow).*

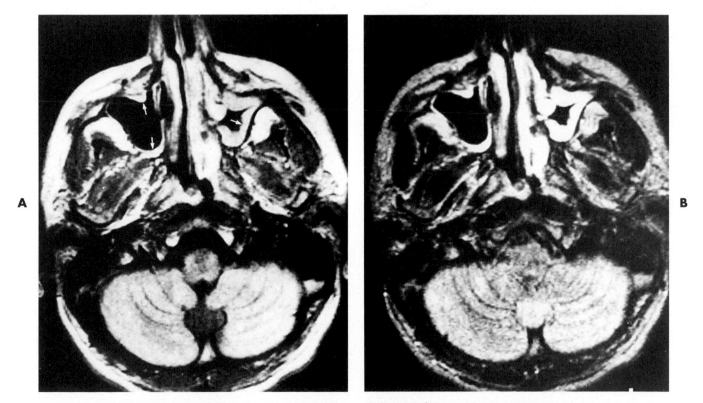

FIG. 4-21 Axial proton density **(A)** and T2W MRI **(B)** scans show mucosal thickening in both maxillary sinuses *(arrows).* The changes are more pronounced on the left side. In **A** the mucosa has an intermediate signal intensity, whereas in **B** it has a high signal intensity. Sinusitis.

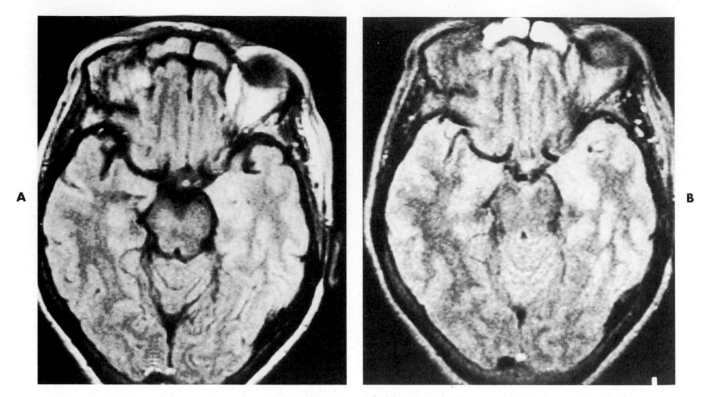

FIG. 4-22   Axial proton density **(A)** and T2W MRI **(B)** scans show opacification of both frontal sinuses with sinusitis and obstructed secretions that have intermediate **(A)** and high **(B)** signal intensities.

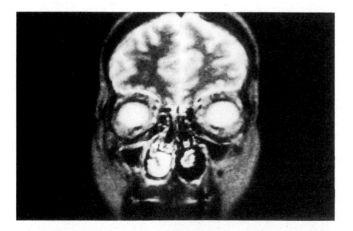

FIG. 4-23   Coronal T2W MR scan shows swelling of the right inferior and middle turbinates and a shrucken appearance to the left-sided turbinates. Normal nasal cycle.

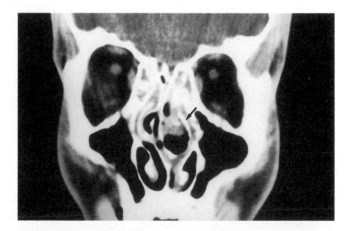

FIG. 4-24   Coronal CT scan shows soft-tisuue mucosal thickening in both ethmoid sinuses and in both nasal fossae. The left middle turbinate *(arrow)* is enlarged (concha bullosa), there is mucosal thickening within the turbinate, and the surrounding air is obliterated. Ethmoid and concha bullosa sinusitis.

reflect the high water content and specific protein concentration of the inflamed tissues. The intensely long T2W signal is helpful in differentiating inflamed tissues from almost all sinonasal tumors that have intermediate T2W signal intensity. By comparison, fibrosis usually gives a low to intermediate signal intensity on all imaging sequences. This is useful in differentiating it from inflammation on the T2W images. However, because both tumor and vascularized scar tissues may give low to intermediate intensity signals on

T2W images, they cannot at present be confidently differentiated by MRI.

Swelling of one nasal turbinate, especially in the absence of concurrent paranasal sinus disease, most probably reflects the normal nasal cycle. Usually a physiologically enlarged turbinate has a thin column of air separating it from the nasal septum and the lateral nasal wall. If this air space is not present, the turbinate probably is pathologically enlarged. Clinical correlation can help resolve any issue.[27]

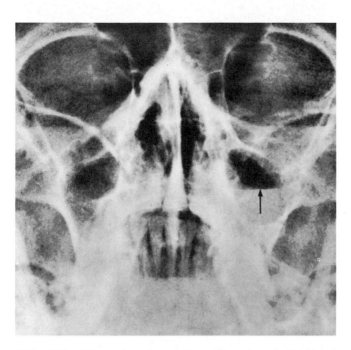

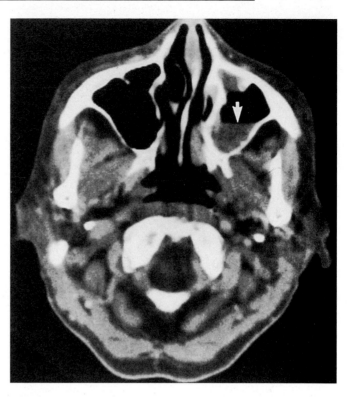

FIG. 4-25 Waters view shows left maxillary sinus air-fluid level *(arrow)* with minimal mucosal thickening. The remaining sinuses are normal. Acute bacterial sinusitis.

FIG. 4-26 Axial CT scan shows left maxillary sinus air-fluid level *(arrow)* of a mucoid density. Minimal mucosal thickening is also present in the anterior left antrum. The right maxillary sinus is normal. Acute bacterial sinusitis.

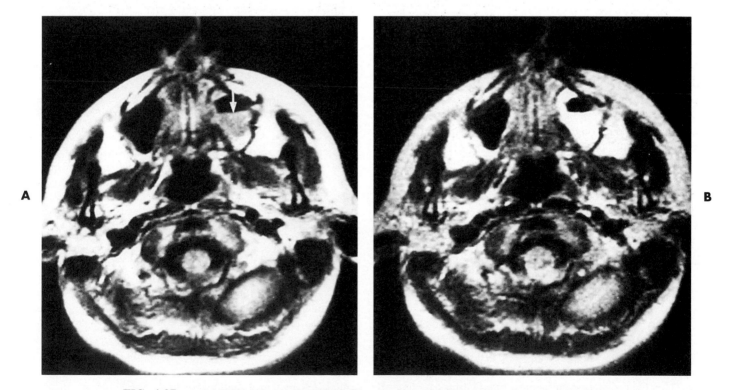

FIG. 4-27 Axial T1W **(A)** and T2W MRI **(B)** scans show a left maxillary sinus air-fluid level *(arrow)*. The fluid has low to intermediate signal intensity in **A** and high signal intensity in **B**. Also seen on **B** is some mucosal thickening in the anterior left antrum and the posterior right antrum. Acute bacterial sinusitis.

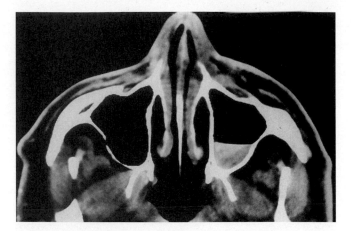

FIG. 4-28 Axial CT scan shows an air-fluid level in the left maxillary sinus. The fluid is quite dense and is acute blood in this patient who received blunt trauma.

On postcontrast CT scans, whether the turbinate is physiologically or pathologically enlarged it will enhance; on MR scans it will give low signal intensity on T1W images, and high signal intensity on T2W images (Figs. 4-23, 4-24). Nasal turbinate swelling may also represent an allergy to contrast material on postcontrast CT scans. This is particularly easy to diagnose if on an initial noncontrast scan, the turbinates appeared normal.[28]

A few patients have been described as having atelectasis of the maxillary sinus with enophthalmos and midface depression. It was hypothesized that this was secondary to osteomeatal complex obstruction creating a negative sinus pressure. However, this concept is still controversial.

Air-Fluid Levels

Most air-fluid levels are visualized in the maxillary sinuses and result from acute bacterial sinusitis. Bacterial sinusitis clearly is the most common cause of a paranasal sinus air-fluid level, even though it occurs in less than half of the patients with this affliction (Figs. 4-25 to 4-27). The next most common cause is postsinus lavage for the treatment of acute bacterial sinusitis. Warm saline is flushed into the sinus (almost exclusively the maxillary sinus) to wash out debris and promote drainage. This saline takes at least 2 to 4 days to empty from the sinus. Thus if a follow-up film is taken within 4 days of such a lavage, the radiologist can not determine if the fluid within the sinus is retained saline or reaccumulated inflammatory secretions. To avoid this problem, follow-up studies should not be obtained until at least 5 to 7 days after an antral lavage.

A mucosal tear or rent can occur with physical trauma regardless of whether sinus wall fracture occurred. An air-fluid level, consisting of secretions and blood, usually indicates a mucosal tear in light of an appropriate trauma history. However, coincidental acute sinusitis in a patient with trauma may confuse the radiologist. This confusion may be settled by MRI. On CT scans the intrasinus blood is denser than mucosal edema and inflammatory secretions (Fig. 4-

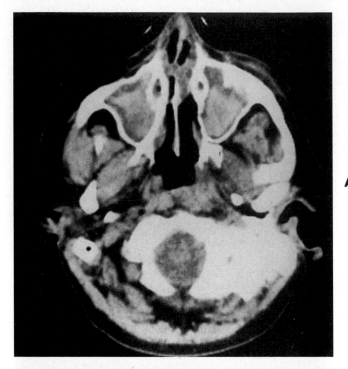

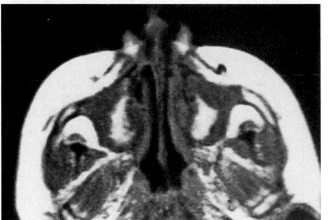

FIG. 4-29 **A,** Axial CT. There are central areas of increased attenuation in both maxillary sinuses that are separated from the sinus walls by a thin zone of low attenuation (mucoid) material. This picture is consistent with desiccated sinus secretions, mycetoma, and hemorrhage. **B,** T1W MRI. The central areas of the antra have high T1W signal intensity with surrounding low signal intensity material, establishing the diagnosis of hemorrhage with inflammation.

28); on MRI T1W images, intrasinus blood (after 24 to 48 hours) has a high signal intensity (Fig. 4-29). By comparison, acute inflammatory related tissues give only a low signal intensity on T1W images. Thus sectional imaging can resolve questionable cases of sinus hemorrhage.[29-31]

In patients with severe trauma, and especially in those with loss of consciousness, treatment usually involves placement of a nasotracheal tube, a nasogastric tube, or both and bed rest in a supine position. These factors interfere with normal sinus drainage, and within 24 hours air-fluid levels can be seen in any or all of the paranasal sinuses.[14] After several days the sinuses may become completely filled

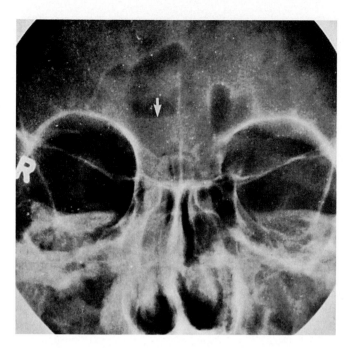

FIG. 4-30 Caldwell view shows soft-tissue clouding of both frontal sinuses and the right ethmoid sinuses. There is also a right frontal sinus air-fluid level *(arrow)*. Acute bacterial sinusitis.

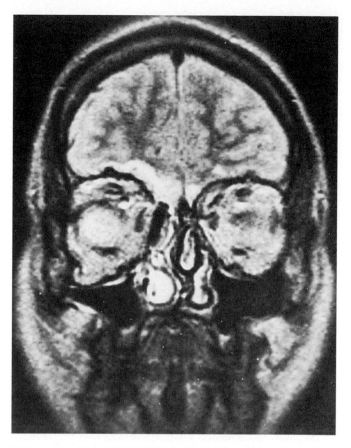

FIG. 4-31 Coronal T2W MRI shows an area of high signal intensity above the right orbit and in the base of the midline anterior cranial fossa. Cerebritis secondary to frontal sinusitis.

with secretions, and films will reveal an apparent pansinusitis. These sinus opacifications usually clear within a few days after the nasal tubes are removed and the patient has started to vary head position.

Barotrauma is a disorder that affects aviators, parachutists, divers, and caisson workers. It most often is associated with an upper respiratory tract infection (34%) accompanied by swelling of the mucosa around the sinus ostium; this anatomic substrate prevents rapid pressure equilibration across this ostium. Mucosal and submucosal hemorrhage occurs, usually associated with pain over the involved sinus. Epistaxis is the second most common symptom. The frontal sinus is involved in 68% of cases, the ethmoid sinus in 16%, and the maxillary sinus in 8%. On plain film studies, mucosal thickening can be detected in the frontal sinuses (24%), the ethmoid sinuses (15% to 19%), and in the antrum (74% to 80%); however, an air-fluid level (present in 12% of cases) appears to be seen only in the maxillary sinus.[32]

Hemorrhage can also result from bleeding disorders such as von Willebrand's disease, in which bleeding tends to occur at mucosal surfaces. Hemophilia, on the other hand, tends to involve internal bleeding and is not associated with a sinus air-fluid level. Coagulation disorders and acute leukemia may also produce air-fluid level. Rarely, chemically induced sinusitis can produce an air-fluid levels. Chromates and other industrial pollutants have been implicated in such cases. Despite the rhinitis and rhinorrhea associated with allergy, few air-fluid levels are seen in allergic patients.

The significance of an air-fluid level varies, depending on the paranasal sinus involved. In the frontal sinuses an air-fluid level usually means acute bacterial sinusitis (Fig. 4-30). Because of the rich venous emissary network that exists between the frontal sinus mucosa and the dural spaces of the adjacent anterior cranial fossa, intracranial complication of frontal sinusitis can occur readily, often within 48 to 72 hours (Figs. 4-31, 4-32).[33] The clinician should be alerted immediately if there is a frontal sinus air-fluid level because these patients require prompt, vigorous treatment, often including intravenous antibiotics. Failure of clinical resolution within another 48 to 72 hours after the onset of treatment usually mandates trephination.

An ethmoid sinus air-fluid level is rare and usually is not associated with either trauma or acute infection. However, if an ethmoid mucocele ruptures and partially drains into the nasal fossa, an air-fluid level may result in what is invariably a mucopyocele. This unusual occurrence is the most common cause of an ethmoid air-fluid level (Fig. 4-33).

In the sphenoid sinus an air-fluid level may indicate the presence of acute sinusitis or nasal cavity obstruction. An air-fluid level in a sick or unconscious patient who has been supine for several days only may indicate poor drainage of this sinus because its ostium is on the anterior sinus wall. In a trauma patient a sphenoid sinus air-fluid level may also signify the presence of either hemorrhage or cerebrospinal

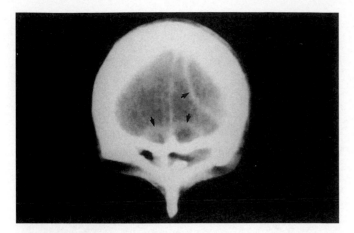

FIG. 4-32 Coronal CT scan shows an osteoma obstructing the left frontal sinus and three epidural abscesses *(arrows)* that occurred within 48 hours of the initial frontal sinus symptoms.

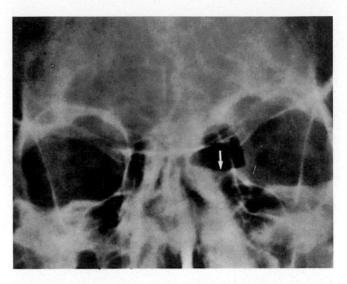

FIG. 4-33 Caldwell view shows clouding of the left frontal sinus. The left ethmoid complex is widened, and there is an ethmoid air-fluid level *(arrow)*. Ruptured left ethmoid mucopyocele.

fluid (CSF) from a skull base fracture. Most often these fractures involve the floor of the anterior cranial fossa or the mastoid portion of the temporal bone, not the sphenoid sinus walls. In the case of anterior skull base fractures, because the dura is firmly attached to the bone, a fracture here is likely to cause a rent in the dura itself, causing CSF rhinorrhea.[34] With the patient supine, CSF escapes through the rent and drains back into the sphenoethmoidal recess; and into the sphenoid sinus. In the case of a temporal bone fracture with an intact tympanic membrane, the CSF drains into the hypotympanum of the middle ear, then escapes via the eustachian tube into the upper nasopharynx and nasal fossa, and then into the sphenoid sinus. Thus CSF rhinorrhea or a sphenoid sinus air-fluid level may reflect a temporal bone fracture.

Cysts and Polyps

The most frequent complications of inflammatory sinusitis are polyps and cysts. The mucous retention cyst is the most common; it is found incidentally on routine plain film examinations in about 10% to 35% of patients.[7] Mucous retention cysts result from the obstruction of submucosal mucinous glands. The cyst wall is the duct epithelium and capsule of the gland itself.[35,36] Although by strict pathologic criteria this qualifies a retention cyst to be called a "mucocele," the radiographic and clinical findings between mucous retention cysts and mucoceles are sufficiently different to merit distinction. Mucous retention cysts can occur in any paranasal sinus along any wall, most commonly in the maxillary sinus.

Serous retention cysts result from the accumulation of serous fluid in the submucosal layer of the sinus mucosal lining. In distinction from the mucous retention cyst, the wall of a serous retention cyst is the mucosa of the sinus. These cysts tend to occur in the base of the maxillary sinuses.

Polyps result from an expansion of fluids in the lamina propria of the Schneiderian mucosa. Polyps may be the result of allergy, atopy, infection, or vasomotor impairment.[37] Paranasal sinus and nasal polyps have the identical

histology. Allergic polyps tend to have a significant population of eosinophils, more than what is usually seen in inflammatory polyps. Also, allergic polyps may be associated with allergic mucin, a sea of eosinophils in mucin and Charocot-Leydin crystals, which are the result of eosinophil degranulation. Radiographically, as mentioned, allergic sinusitis tends to cause diffuse symmetrical disease rather than localized disease. Inflammatory and allergic polyps rarely bleed and are not damaged by manipulation or compression. Fibrosis and neovascularization of polyps (especially nasal polyps) can result in a lesion that pathologically mimics an angiofibroma. However, anatomic location (nasal vs. nasopharynx) and the angiographic and sectional imaging appearance (inflammatory and allergic polyps are poorly vascularized and do not extend into the pterygopalatine fossa) distinguish these lesions from angiofibromas.[38]

The intrasinus polyp and the retention cyst cannot be differentiated clearly on either plain films or sectional imaging. However, this is of little consequence because both are common benign entities.

On plain films, CT, and MR scans, polyps and retention cysts are homogeneous soft-tissue masses with smooth, outwardly convex borders (Figs. 4-34 to 4-45). Multiple or single lesions may be present, and most are small and clearly do not fill the entire sinus cavity. If a cyst occurs in the antral roof of a patient with a history of recent trauma, the plain film examination may simulate a blow-out fracture (Fig. 4-36). However, coronal imaging will demonstrate an intact orbital floor with the cyst or polyp in the antral mucosa. On the Waters view a prominent infraorbital canal (with its attendant soft-tissue contents) can mimic a cyst in the roof of the antrum. Similarly the nasal alae can simulate a medial wall antral cyst, and unerupted teeth, the lips, or a mustache can simulate a cyst on the floor of the maxillary sinus. The coronoid process of the mandible can simulate a cyst on the

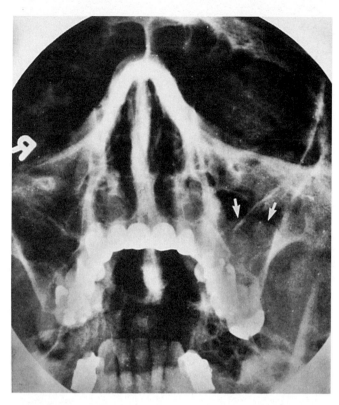

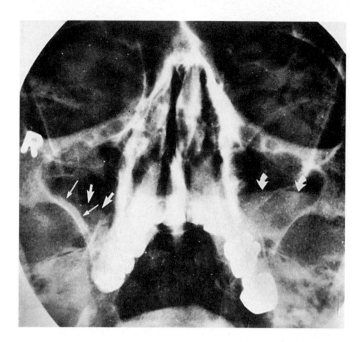

FIG. 4-35 Waters view shows a large "flat" retention cyst *(curved arrows)* in the left antrum. This can simulate an air-fluid level if careful attention is not paid to its slightly convex upper surface. There is minimal mucosal thickening in the right antrum *(thin arrows)*, and another small retention cyst is present in the lower right maxillary sinus *(arrows)*.

FIG. 4-34 Waters view shows a solitary left antral retention cyst or polyp *(arrows)*. This cyst typically has a smooth, outwardly convex contour. The remaining antrum and the other sinuses are normal.

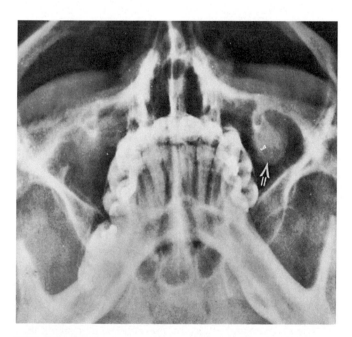

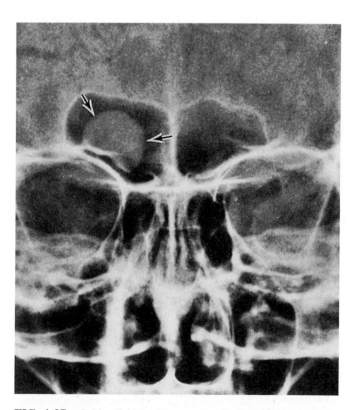

FIG. 4-36 Waters view shows a retention cyst *(arrow)* in the roof of the left antrum.

FIG. 4-37 Caldwell view shows a retention cyst *(arrows)* in the right frontal sinus. Note that this sinus is otherwise normal.

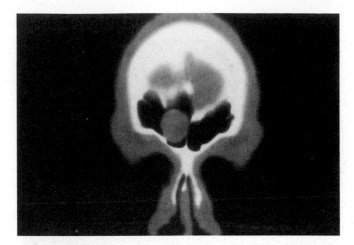

FIG. 4-38   Coronal CT scan shows a solitary retention cyst or polyp in the right frontal sinus. Note the the lesion does not obstruct the sinus.

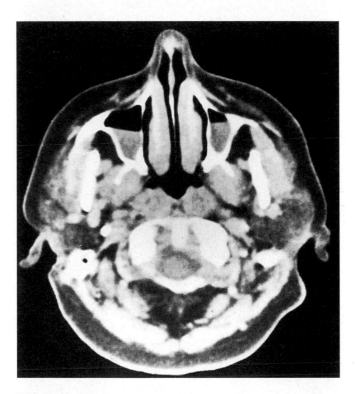

FIG. 4-40   Axial CT scan shows a solitary retention cyst in each maxillary sinus. These cysts may simulate air-fluid levels if their upper slightly convex contour and their nonparallel relationship to the plane of the floor are not noted.

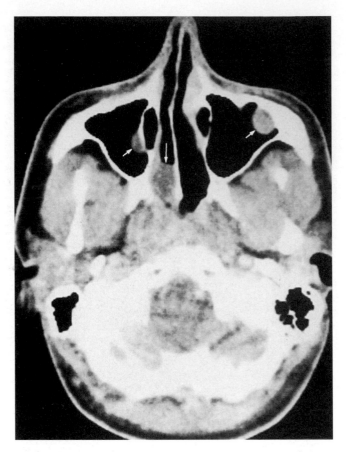

FIG. 4-39   Axial CT scan shows a retention cyst or polyp in the left and right maxillary sinuses *(small arrows)*. There also is a small polyp *(arrow)* in the posterior right nasal fossa.

posterior floor of the antrum on a lateral plain film taken with the patient's mouth closed.

When a cyst becomes moderately large (i.e., about half of the volume of the antrum), it behaves like a water-filled thin balloon in that its upper surface flattens out, somewhat resembling an air-fluid level (Figs. 4-40, 4-42). However, careful evaluation will reveal a slightly convex upper border, and on sectional imaging the convex polypoid appear-

ance is even better seen along the upper and lower portions of the lesion. A true air-fluid level is a fluid level throughout the entire involved sinus. Additionally the planar surface of the fluid will directly reflect gravity in every head position. On MRI these cysts or polyps usually have characteristics similar to those of mucosal inflammation, again reflecting the high water and low specific-protein content. Thus they tend to have low to intermediate signal intensity on T1W images and high signal intensity on T2W images. If the protein content of the cyst fluid increases because of infection or the passage of time, the T1W signal intensity becomes high, reflecting the shortening of the T1 relaxation time (Figs. 4-42 to 4-45).

Retention cysts and polyps are usually asymptomatic and are incidental radiographic findings. However, if they become large enough to fill the sinus cavity, they may obstruct sinus drainage and become symptomatic. Rarely these lesions can remodel the sinus walls to cause some expansion of the sinus cavity. But in most cases on sectional imaging, some small pockets of remaining sinus air can be identified, overlying a part of the convex margin of the lesion (Fig. 4-41). This distinguishes such a cyst from a mucocele, although when a cyst is this large, the distinction is of more intellectual interest than clinical significance.

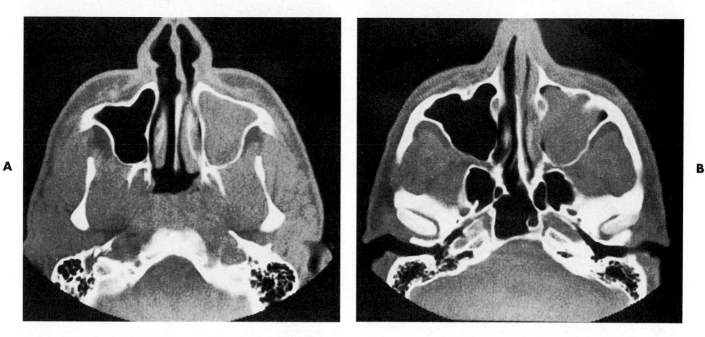

FIG. 4-41   Axial CT scans in the midsinus (**A**) and in the upper portion of the left maxillary sinus (**B**). In **A** the sinus appears to be opacified. However, in **B,** air can be seen outlining the upper surface of a large retention cyst or polyp.

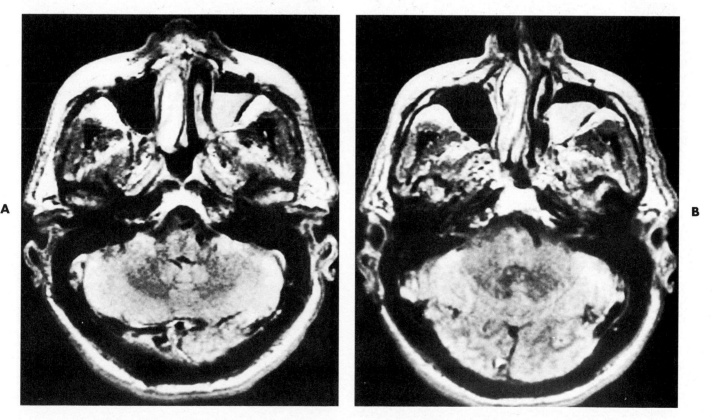

FIG. 4-42   Axial proton density MRI scans low in the antrum (**A**) and higher in the antrum (**B**) show a retention cyst in the left antrum. If the contour of the upper surface is not clearly noted on all scans, this cyst could be mistaken for an air-fluid level.

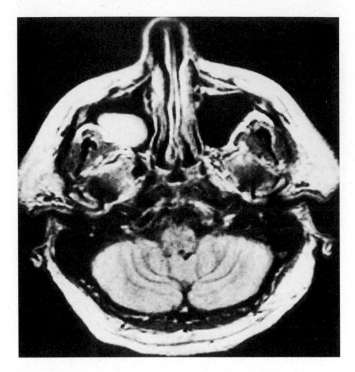

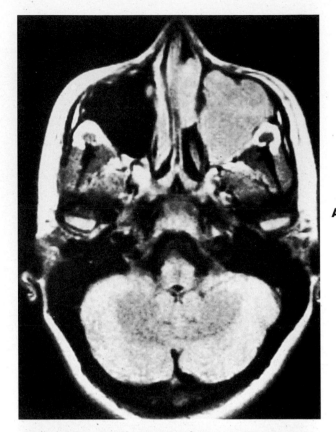

A

FIG. 4-43 Axial proton density MRI scan shows a solitary retention cyst or polyp with an intermediate signal intensity, filling about half of the right antrum.

On occasion an antral polyp may expand and prolapse through the sinus ostium, presenting as a nasal polyp. These are referred to as antrochoanal polyps, which represent 4% to 6% of all nasal polyps. Most are unilateral, solitary lesions, but bilateral antral inflammatory disease is found in as many as 30% to 40% of cases. Almost 8% of these patients have additional nasal polyps, and 15% to 40% of patients have a history of allergy.[39-41] These latter statistics have prompted the suggestion that there is an etiologic relationship to allergy, but this theory has not been borne out. Most antrochoanal polyps occur in teenagers and young adults. If such a polyp is surgically snared in the nasal fossa like a routine nasal polyp without regard to its antral stalk, 20% to 30% of the cases will recur, usually within 2 years.[41] The proper treatment is via a Caldwell-Luc or endoscopic intraantral approach.

Small, antrochoanal polyps radiographically appear as soft-tissue masses that completely fill one maxillary sinus. The infundibular region widens with slight extrusion of the antral mass into the lateral wall of the nasal fossa. At this stage, it can be confused with hypertrophic polypoid antral mucosa that may also extend through the sinus ostium. As the polyp continues to grow, it fills the ipsilateral nasal fossa and extends back into the nasopharynx (Figs. 4-46 to 4-49). Rarely, it may grow sufficiently to hang down into the oropharynx. Although the medial antral wall may be destroyed eventually, the remaining antral walls are rarely remodeled. This can be a difficult diagnosis on plain films, but it is rarely misdiagnosed on sectional imaging.

Sphenochoanal polyps have also been described. They

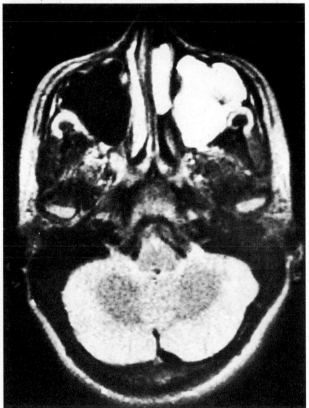

B

FIG. 4-44 Axial proton density image (A) and T2W MRI (B) scans show multiple polyps or cysts, filling the left maxillary sinus. These lesions have the typical intermediate (A) and high (B), signal intensities usually found with cysts and polyps.

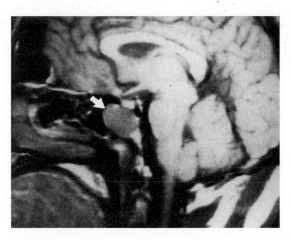

FIG. 4-45   Sagittal T1W MR scan shows a solitary nonobstructing retention cyst or polyp *(arrow)* in the sphenoid sinus.

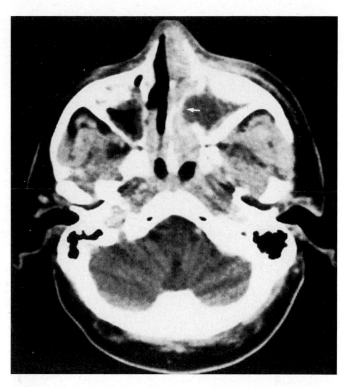

FIG. 4-46   Axial postcontrast CT scan shows a low attenuation (mucoid secretion) mass in the left maxillary sinus that is bulging into the left nasal fossa *(arrow)*. There are inflammatory mucosal changes seen in both nasal fossae and in the right antrum. Left antrochoanal polyp.

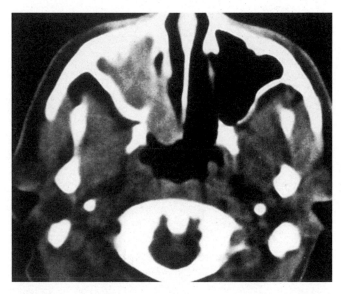

FIG. 4-47   Axial CT scan shows a right antral soft-tissue mass that has prolapsed into the posterior right nasal fossa. Antrochoanal polyp.

are rare, and their etiology appears to be similar to that of the antrochoanal polyp.[42]

Nasal polyps are most often associated with allergy, and when found in this clinical setting, they are usually numerous rather than solitary. Histologically there are a number of secondary changes that can occur with these polyps—infarction, surface ulceration, mucoid liquification, stromal cell atypia, and metaplasia of the surface epithelium. Carcinoma arising from surface metaplasia is very rare and is almost always associated with an external carcinogenic promoter, either smoking or some occupationally related promoter. Atypia of stromal cells may be misinterpreted as a malignancy because of its microscopic resemblance to rhabdomyosarcoma or myxoid sarcoma.[37,39]

Polyps are the most common expansile lesions in the nasal cavity. Although they usually are small and cause lit-

tle deformity, if left unattended in the presence of progression, they can become highly deforming. Eventually they may remodel, disrupt, and destroy the central facial region. They can destroy the medial antral walls, cause hypertelorism, and break through intracranially either via the roof of the nasal cavity and ethmoid complex or via the sphenoid sinus. This degree of marked destruction may be found among the medically underserved patients with intractable allergic polyps and patients with a high level of denial. Destruction secondary to polyposis is an indolent process, causing little if any pain. Although surgery is the treatment of choice for large polyps, in allergic patients, desensitization has in some cases shown dramatic results in reducing the number and size of these polyps.[41]

Etiologically, polyps have been associated with vasomotor rhinitis, infectious rhinosinusitis, diabetes mellitus, cystic fibrosis, aspirin intolerance, and nickel exposure in addition to allergy.[41] In vasomotor rhinitis an instability of the autonomic nervous system has been implicated as the underlying problem. Nasal congestion, watery discharge, and eventually nasal polyps can be responses to emotional stress, endocrine imbalance, atmospheric pressure changes, irritants, and as a reaction to medications.[42] Infectious rhinosinusitis is caused by a variety of agents that produce an acute and chronic inflammation with secondary polyp formation. These patients commonly have a secretory IgA deficiency.[43] There is evidence to suggest a relationship between

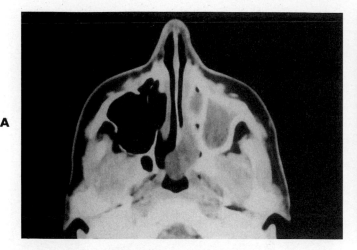

A

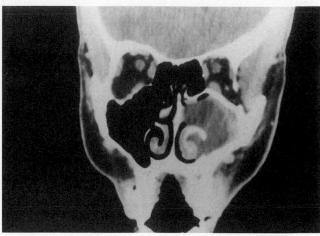

B

FIG. 4-48   Axial CT scan **(A)** shows a mucoid-density mass filling the left antrum and the left nasal fossa and nasopharynx. Coronal CT scan **(B)** shows the polyp widening the left infundibulum and extending into the nasal cavity. Antrochoanal polyp.

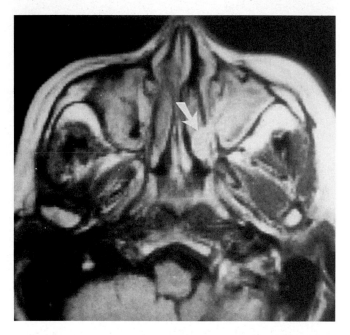

FIG. 4-49   Axial proton density MRI scan shows inflammatory changes in both maxillary sinuses. On the left side a polypoid mass *(arrow)* is seen, extending into the nasal fossa. Antrochoanal polyp.

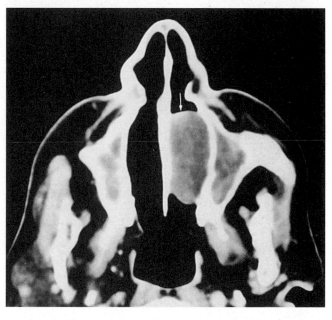

FIG. 4-50   Axial CT scan shows a solitary mucoid attenuation left nasal mass *(arrow)*. There is also inflammatory disease in both antra. Nasal polyp and sinusitis.

nasal polyps and diabetes mellitus. Fluctuating glucose levels in concert with other factors (allergy, infection) may promote polyposis.[44] Between 10% and 20% of children with cystic fibrosis have nasal polyps. In general, nasal polyps are uncommon in children; 29% of such cases are associated with cystic fibrosis. Thus the presence of chronic sinusitis and nasal polyps in a child should prompt an investigation to rule out cystic fibrosis.[45,46] Aspirin intolerance may be a systemic disease rather than a simple allergic response. It is classically characterized by intolerance to aspirin, nasal polyps, and bronchial asthma. About 20% of patients with nasal polyps have asthma, and conversely, about 30% of

asthmatic patients have polyps.[45-47] Nickel workers who have worked 10 years or more in the nickel-refining process have a 4% incidence of nasal polyps and an increased risk for developing carcinomas in the lung, nasal fossa, and larynx.[48]

Radiographically the polyps are often seen on plain films only as a vague increased soft-tissue density within the nasal fossa. On sectional imaging they usually can be identified as discrete single or multiple broad-based, soft-tissue masses (Figs. 4-50 to 4-53). On CT the majority of the polyps tend to have a mucoid attenuation (10 to 18 HUs) with mucosal enhancement occasionally seen at the polyp's surface. However, those polyps that have had sufficient time to develop

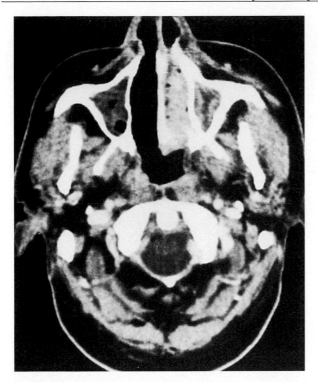

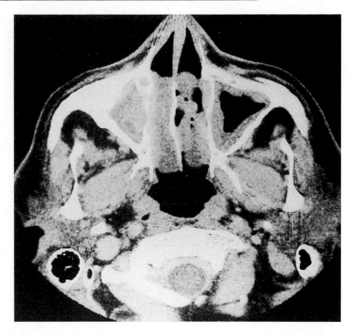

FIG. 4-52 Axial CT scan shows multiple bilateral nasal polyps with inflammatory mucosal thickening in the left antrum and opacification of the right antrum. Polyposis and sinusitis.

FIG. 4-51 Axial postcontrast CT scan shows an enhancing left nasal fossa mass. There is active inflammation (mucosal enhancement) in the left antrum and mucoid secretions in the right antrum. Nasal polyp and sinusitis.

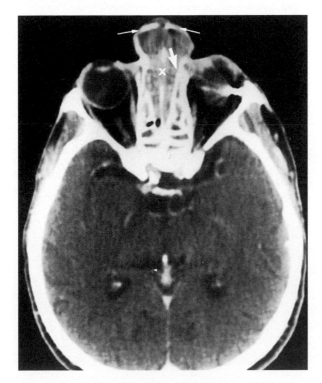

FIG. 4-53 Axial postcontrast CT scan shows bilateral nasal masses that have displaced the nasal bones anterolaterally *(small arrows)* and eroded part of the nasal septum *(x)*. The upper nasal fossae are also widened, and the medial aspect of the ethmoid sinuses has been displaced laterally *(arrow)*. Polyposis and sinusitis.

stromal collagen and fibrous tissue tend to have a higher overall attenuation (20 to 35 HUs). On MRI, typically the dominant feature is the high water and low protein content that gives the polyps a low to intermediate signal intensity on T1W images and high signal intensity on T2W images (Fig. 4-54). However, when multiple polyps are present (often intermixed with mucoceles), the entrapped secretions can have variable T1W and T2W signal intensities. It is the variable imaging appearance that distinguishes such polypoid masses from tumors, which tend to have more homogeneous signal intensities. (Figs. 4-50 to 4-58).[21,49,50]

On CT, when there are multiple polyps crowded within the nasal vault, they can form an overall conglomerate mass that may be difficult if not impossible to distinguish from a tumor. This is especially true of bulky lesions such as inverting papillomas and lymphomas that tend to remodel the surrounding bone. However, there are two appearances of sinonasal polyps that, if present, allow their diagnosis to be established firmly on CT studies. The first of these is the ethmoid polypoid mucocele in which there is either unilateral or bilateral involvement of the ethmoid labyrinth, which is characterized by widening of the ethmoid complex with little if any destruction of the delicate ethmoid septa.[51,52] The individual ethmoid cells are filled with polypoid mucosa and entrapped mucoid secretions. Often the CT appearance of each sinus cavity is that of a central high attenuation region (desiccated secretions) separated from the bony sinus wall by a thin zone of lower mucoid attenuation. By comparison a solid mass (either a single polyp or a tumor) will destroy these septa, and in this latter circumstance it is impossible to distinguish a benign lesion from a low-grade malignant process. The preservation of ethmoidal septa as

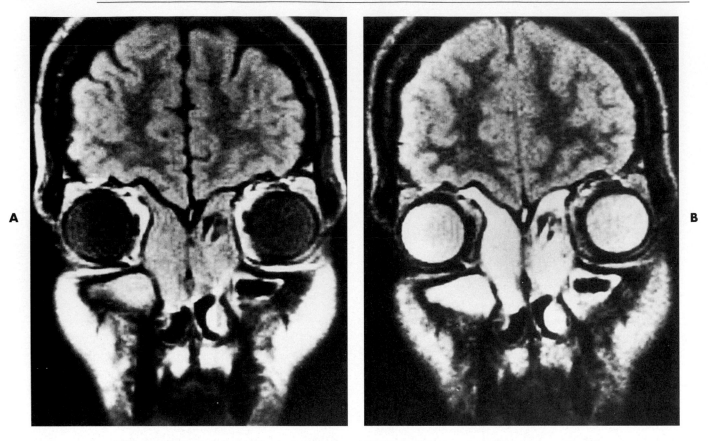

FIG. 4-54   Coronal proton density image (**A**) and T2W MRI (**B**) scans show bilateral nasoethmoid expansile masses causing hypertelorism. These masses have the same signal intensities as the mucosal thickening in the left antrum and the material in the right antrum, namely an intermediate signal intensity in **A** and a high signal intensity in **B**. Polyposis and sinusitis.

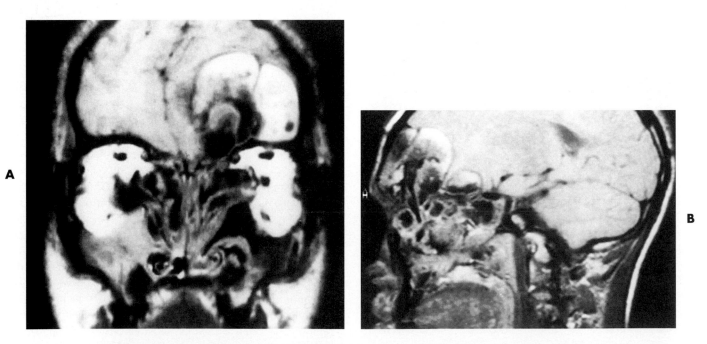

FIG. 4-55   Coronal (**A**) and sagittal (**B**) T1W MRI scans show multiple sinonasal polypoid masses that have broken into the medial aspect of each orbit, as well as intracranially. These are areas of high, intermediate, and low signal intensity throughout the lesion. There are also areas of signal void. Polyposis.

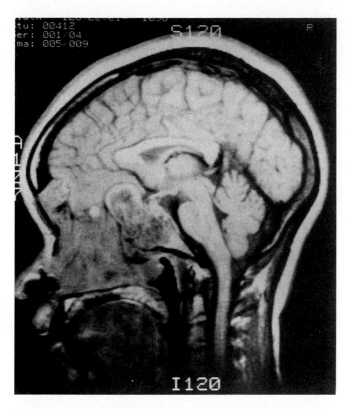

FIG. 4-56 Sagittal T1W MR scan shows a nonhomogeneous signal intensity polypoid mass in the sphenoid sinus, breaking intracranially. Increased soft tissues are also present in the nasal fossae. Polyposis.

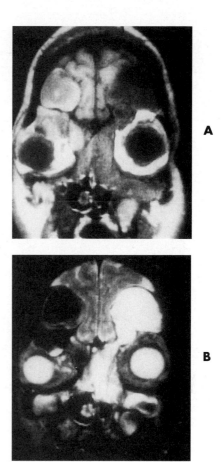

FIG. 4-57 Coronal T1W (**A**) and T2W (**B**) MR scans show bilateral polypoid masses that have broken intracranially and into the left orbit from the frontal sinuses and down into the right orbit from the right supraorbital ethmoid sinuses. The signal intensities indicate that the left-sided lesions are more watery, and the right-sided lesions contain thicker, inspissated secretions. Polyposis.

seen in polypoid mucoceles unequivocally signifies the presence of benign disease (Figs. 4-59 to 4-61). The second circumstance of a unique CT appearance of benign disease is the presence of either a unilateral or bilateral expansile sinonasal mass with cascading, looping, or curvilinear soft-tissue polypoid lesions of fairly high attenuation in a background matrix of mucoid attenuation (10 to 18 HUs) secretions. For the most part the polypoid masses are separated from the adjacent bones by a thin zone of mucoid material. This finding allows the distinction of polyps from tumors on CT, the latter directly abut the bone and either remodel or destroy it (Figs. 4-62 to 4-64). This unique CT appearance is seen in about 20% of patients with nasal polypoid masses.

On MR the signal intensity is determined by the degree of desiccation of the secretions entrapped within the sinuses and between the polyps. The resulting variable appearance of signal intensity is diagnostic of inflammatory disease. The primary diagnostic problem arises when semi-solid or completely desiccated secretions are present. These dried secretions give signal voids on T2W images and, depending on the degree of dessication, either low signal intensity or signal voids on T1W studies. Possible confusion with an aerated sinus can occur unless a CT study is available for comparison (Figs. 4-6, 4-7, 4-65).

The CT appearance of a high attenuation central region separated from the sinus wall by a thin zone of mucoid

attenuation material can be seen in three distinct cases: chronic inspissated secretions, a mycetoma (usually from aspergillosis), and intrasinus hemorrhage (Figs. 4-29, 4-66 to 4-68).[53] Although a specific diagnosis may not always be possible on CT, this appearance reliably indicates that the soft-tissue mass is not a tumor.[37] On MRI a central intrasinus region of signal void or low T1W and T2W signal intensity can represent either desiccated secretions in chronic sinusitis, a mycetoma in a patient with sinus fungal disease, a sinolith, or an intrasinus tooth (antrum) (Figs. 4-6, 4-7, 4-66 to 4-73).

The mycetomas are semisolid and have paramagnetic ions, both of which contribute to their having low signal intensity or signal voids on all imaging sequences. Any inflammatory reaction around the mycetoma will have the typical MRI characteristics of infections or polyps.[54] An intrasinus hemorrhage initially has a low signal intensity on all imaging sequences; but when the blood is oxidized to methemoglobin (by 24 to 48 hours after the trauma), it has a high signal intensity on T1W images and an intermediate signal intensity on T2W images (Fig. 4-29). Thus by using

A

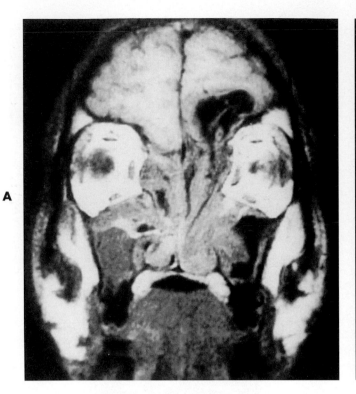

B

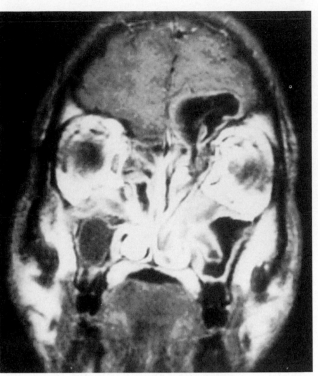

FIG. 4-58   Coronal T1W MRI scans without contrast (**A**) and with contrast (**B**). There are polypoid masses in the nasal cavity and the maxillary and ethmoid sinuses, which have broken intracranially. There are areas of high, intermediate, and low signal intensity. In **B** the mucosal surfaces of the polyps enhance. Polyposis.

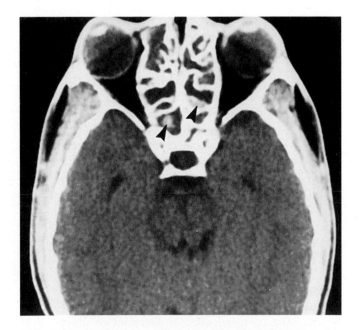

FIG. 4-59   Axial CT scan shows opacification of ethmoid sinuses with widening of the anterior and middle ethmoid complex. The lamina papyracea remain intact. Several discrete polyps (*arrowheads*) are seen within the mucoid secretions filling the ethmoid cells. The delicate intercellular septa are intact. Polypoid mucocele.

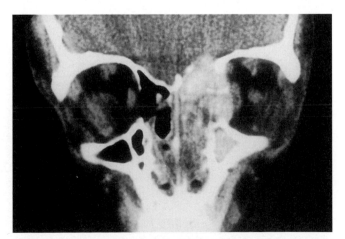

FIG. 4-60   Coronal CT scan shows a left nasal fossa, ethmoid and maxillary sinus mass that has expanded into the left orbit and the left anterior cranial fossa. Although this was at first thought to be a tumor, the CT appearance suggested polyposis. Polyposis.

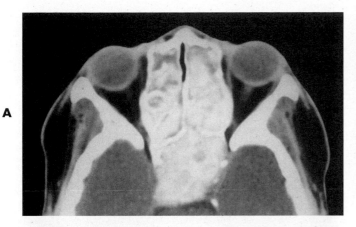

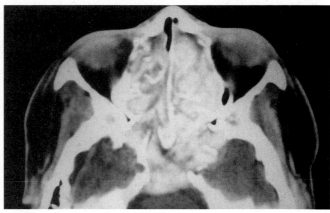

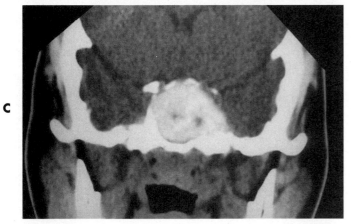

FIG. 4-61 Axial CT scans through the midorbit **(A),** the skull base **(B),** and a coronal CT scan **(C)** through the sphenoid sinus show expansion and remodeling of the ethmoid cells by multiple polyps. The walls of the sphenoid sinuses and the central skull base appear eroded but were only deossified from the chronic pressure. Polyposis.

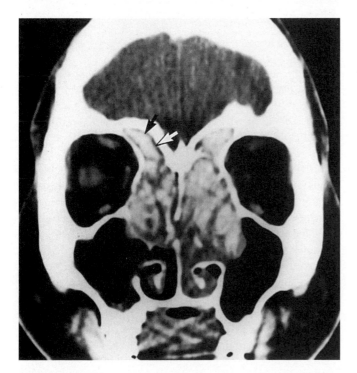

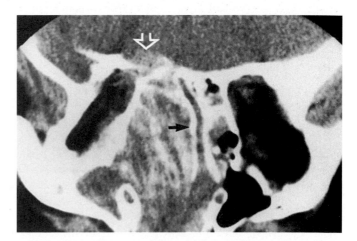

FIG. 4-62 Coronal CT scan shows multiple soft-tissue masses in the ethmoid sinuses and nasal fossa bilaterally. The polypoid masses are separated from the bone by a thin zone of mucoid attenuation material *(arrows)*. The polyps are also imbedded within a matrix of this mucoid material. Polyposis.

FIG. 4-63 Coronal CT scan shows an expansile right nasoethmoid mass that has displaced the nasal septum to the left *(arrow)*. The mass has also focally broken into the floor of the anterior cranial fossa *(open arrow)*. Within the mass are discrete polypoid densities embedded within a mucoid matrix. Polyposis.

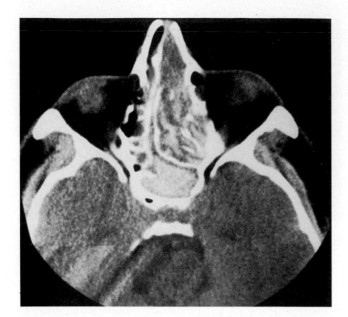

FIG. 4-64 Axial CT scan shows a soft-tissue mass (polyp) in the sphenoid sinus that is for the most part separated from the bone by a zone of mucoid attenuation. There is an expansile left nasoethmoid process that has discrete polypoid soft-tissue masses seen within a mucoid matrix. Polyposis.

MRI, intrasinus hemorrhage can be distinguished in almost all cases from these other lesions (Fig. 4-74).[30,31]

Mucoceles

Mucoceles are the most common expansile lesions to develop in any paranasal sinus. Pathologically they are defined as being composed of a mucous-secreting respiratory epithelium that surrounds mucoid secretions. Histopathologically, mucoceles and mucous retention cysts are identical.[51] It is the clinical and radiographic features that allow for the distinction. Classically a retention cyst is a spherical mucoid-filled cyst that develops when a mucous gland of the sinus mucosa becomes obstructed. The epithelium of the duct and gland capsule are the cyst wall. These cysts are common, usually incidental findings identified in at least 10% of people. Although they can occur in any sinus, they are most common in the antrum. There usually is some remaining sinus air, and rarely the sinus cavity is expanded or the bony sinus walls are remodeled.

By comparison, a mucocele develops from the obstruction of a sinus ostium or a compartment of a septated sinus. The wall of the lesion is the sinus mucosa. The sinus is completely filled, leaving no remaining sinus-cavity air, and the sinus cavity is expanded as the bony walls are remodeled. Mucoceles occur primarily in the frontal sinuses (60% to 65% of cases), but they also are found in the ethmoid sinuses (20% to 25% of cases), maxillary sinuses (10% of cases), and the sphenoid sinuses (1% to 2% of cases).[55-58] When a sinus becomes obstructed and completely filled with secretions, at least three possible outcomes can occur: (1) the sinus ostium will open as the inflammation resolves,

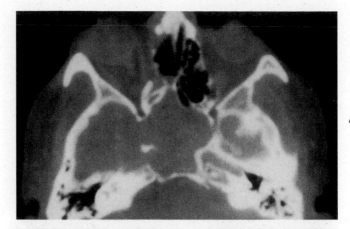

A

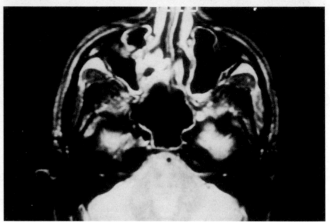

B

FIG. 4-65 Axial CT scan (**A**) of the sphenoid sinus shows the sinus to be opacified, and there is an apparant area of erosion of the skull base along the right side of the sinus. Axial T2W postcontrast MR scan (**B**) shows enhancement of the sinus mucosa and no erosion of the adjacent skull base. The dried sinus secretions have a signal void and could easily be overlooked if only MR was available.

(2) the secretion will become desiccated, or (3) a mucocele develops, which enlarges the involved sinus. Thus the radiologic definition of a mucocele is reserved for the sinus that is airless, filled with mucoid secretions, and has an enlarged sinus cavity. This sinus cavity expansion is the result of pressure necrosis from expanding entrapped secretions, slow erosion of the inner-sinus bony wall, and new bone production from the outer periostium. This remodeling leads to slow sinus expansion. At some point the sinus cavity may become so large that periostial repair can no longer keep the sinus wall ossified. This causes areas of deossification, which appear radiographically as eroded bone. A rare retention cyst may become so large that it completely fills the antrum and widens the infundibular region, making distinction from an early mucocele impossible. This is of no clinical significance because the surgical treatment of both is identical.

The classical mucocele is a noninfected lesion that presents with signs and symptoms that result from the mass itself, for example, proptosis, bossing of the forehead, a mass in the superomedial orbit, nasal obstruction (unilateral or bilateral), and a change in voice quality (nasal sound).

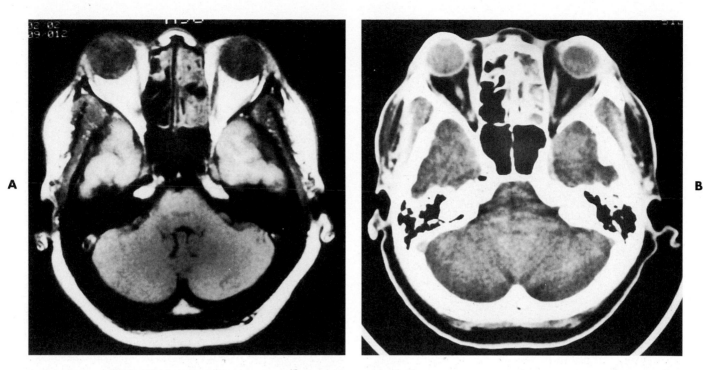

FIG. 4-66 Axial T1W MR scan (**A**) shows disease in the left ethmoid complex with apparant aeration of some midethmoid cells. Axial CT scan (**B**) shows total opacification of the left ethmoid sinuses. The mid-ethmoid cells contain soft-tissue density material. Aspergillosis with ethmoid aspergilloma.

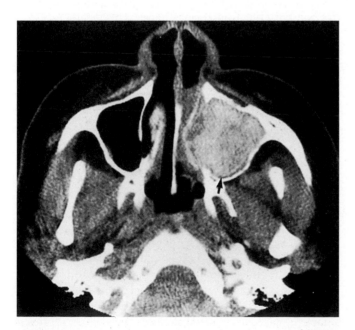

FIG. 4-67 Axial CT scan shows soft-tissue mass in the left antrum, which is separated from the sinus wall by a thin zone of mucoid attenuation material *(arrow)*. There is some remodeling of the medial antral wall. Aspergilloma.

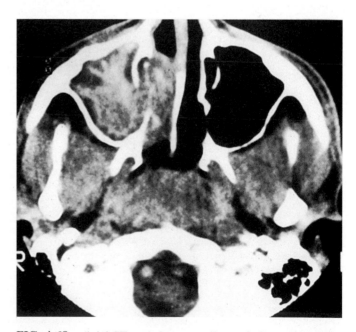

FIG. 4-68 Axial CT scan shows a stellate soft-tissue mass in the right antrum and nasal fossa. The mass is separated from the bone by a thin zone of mucoid attenuation material. There is focal destruction of the medial antral wall. Aspergilloma.

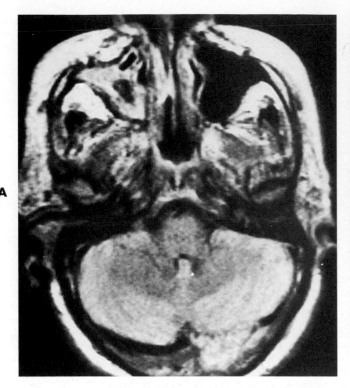
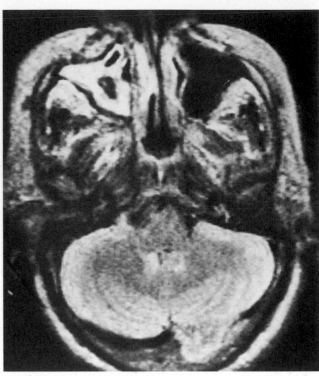

FIG. 4-69 Axial proton density image (**A**) and T2W MR (**B**) scans show inflammatory-type mucosal thickening (**A** is intermediate and **B** is high signal intensity) in the right maxillary sinus. In the center of the sinus is an ovoid mass with low signal intensity. This is a mycetoma (aspergilloma) with surrounding inflammation. Aspergillosis.

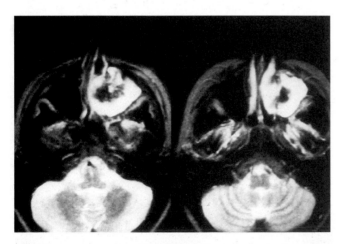

FIG. 4-70 Axial T2W MR scans show inflammatory fluid in the left maxillary sinus with a central region of low signal intensity and signal void. Aspergillosis with an aspergilloma.

Pain is rare and when noted indicates the presence of an infected mucocele or a pyocele (mucopyocele).

Plain Films

On plain films a frontal sinus mucocele first appears as a slightly clouded sinus with a smooth, ovoid, or rounded contour rather than the normal scalloped margin. The normal thin mucoperiosteal white line becomes poorly seen, and if chronic sinusitis was present before the development of the

mucocele, a zone of dense reactive bone may surround the sinus. As the mucocele erodes the sinus contour in the vertical plate of the frontal bone, it also slowly erodes the anterior and posterior frontal sinus tables. This results in a loss of bone density on frontal plain films that more than compensates for the soft-tissue density of the mucoid secretions. Thus a frontal sinus mucocele tends to maintain a radiodensity that is equal to or slightly less than the normal density of the adjacent frontal sinus bone. If an expansile frontal sinus mass that is denser than the adjacent frontal bone is seen, the imager should consider a fibroosseous lesion rather than a mucocele. Radiolucent frontal sinus mucoceles are seen only when one becomes so large as to erode most of the sinus tables (Figs. 4-75 to 4-79). In a hypoplastic frontal sinus there is usually only a single, smooth, centrally concave sinus border that could simulate the appearance of a mucocele. The normally scalloped margins of larger sinuses are not present for assessment of possible erosion. However, whether the sinus is small or large the normal frontal sinus should never violate the orbital contour. Any downward and outward displacement of the superomedial orbital rim (and a similar displacement of the eye) should be considered presumptive evidence of a frontal sinus mucocele until proved otherwise. Similarly the base of the frontal intersinus septum is normally in the midline, and any displacement of this portion of the septum to one side should suggest the presence of a frontal sinus mucocele (Fig. 4-76).

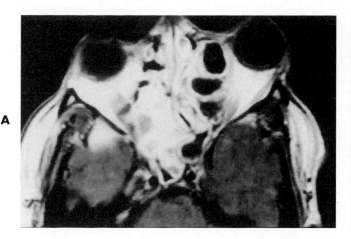
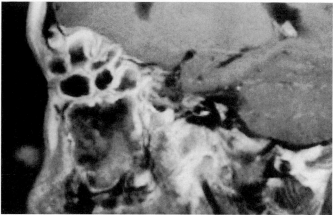

FIG. 4-71 Axial (**A**) and sagittal (**B**) postcontrast T1W MR scans show widening of the ethmoid complex by a polypoid mass that has also broken into the floor of the anterior cranial fossa. Enhancing mucosa is seen surrounding areas of signal void. The maxillary sinuses are also involved by the process. None of the sinuses were aerated on CT. Aspergillosis with an aspergilloma.

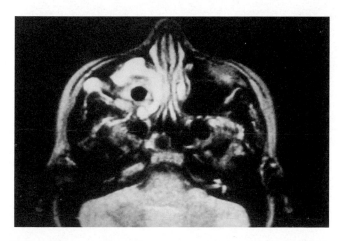

FIG. 4-72 Axial T2W MR scan shows a slightly expanded right maxillary sinus, filled for the most part with high signal intensity material. Within the sinus is an area of signal void. This was a tooth in this dentigerous cyst.

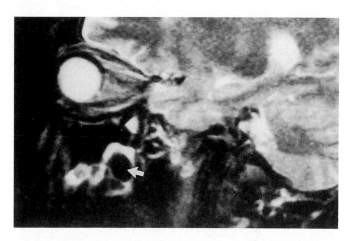

FIG. 4-73 Sagittal T2W MR scan shows an area of signal void (*arrow*), elevating the inflamed maxillary sinus mucosa. Undescended molar tooth.

The midline segments of the anterior and posterior frontal sinus tables are seen on lateral plain films. Significant erosion of these tables off the midline can occur and remain undetected on plain films. Because the absence of an intact posterior frontal sinus wall is of importance to the surgeon, preoperative sectional imaging of a suspected frontal sinus mucocele should always be performed. At times, large, clinically silent intracranial extension of a mucocele can be fortuitously discovered.

Mucoceles can extend posteriorly into the horizontal plate (orbital roof) of the frontal bone, as well as up into the vertical plate. Once in the orbital roof, a mucocele can extend both cranially into the floor of the anterior cranial fossa and caudally. If this extension is not appreciated at the time of surgery, which is usually performed extracranially for the more obvious vertical plate disease, complications from an orbital roof mucocele may require a second opera-

tion and an intracranial approach. In the event that frontal sinus surgery was performed without preoperative sectional imaging and if retrospective review of the plain films suggests that horizontal recess disease is present, a postoperative scan is strongly recommended to resolve this issue and provide an important baseline study with which any further examinations can be compared.

Ethmoid mucoceles usually arise in the anterior rather than the posterior ethmoid cells.[59] This presumably reflects the fact that the anterior ethmoid ostia are the smallest of any in the paranasal sinuses.[60] The viscosity of mucus also plays an etiologic role, and this may explain why ethmoid mucoceles are most common in patients with cystic fibrosis (mucoviscidosis).[61] The typical ethmoid mucocele is an expansile lesion that thins and remodels the lamina papyracea, bowing it into the orbit. As a result the eye is laterally displaced. Although such a mass is obvious clinically,

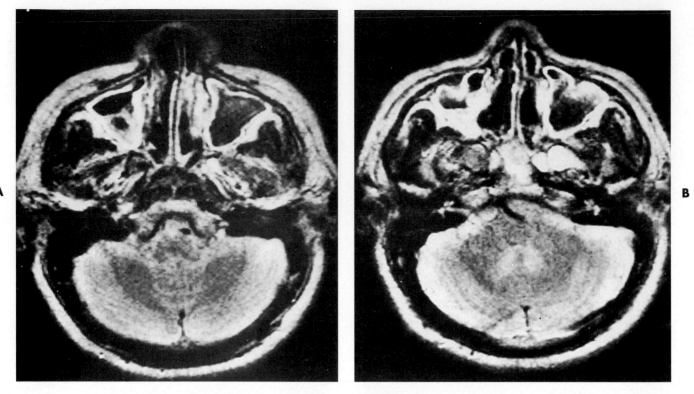

FIG. 4-74 Axial proton density **(A)** and T2W MRI **(B)** show material with a low signal intensity on both images, filling the left antrum (fresh blood). Both maxillary sinuses are lined by a thin mucosal layer of high signal intensity on both images. There is also an air-fluid level in the right antrum, which has mixed signal intensity in **A** and high signal intensity in **B** (sinus secretions and fresh blood).

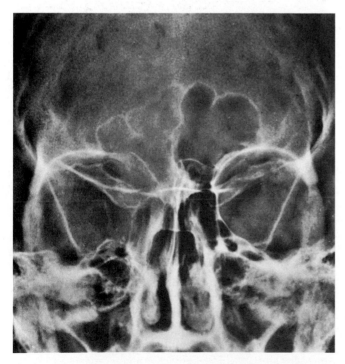

FIG. 4-75 Caldwell view shows clouding of the right frontal sinus and right ethmoid sinuses. There is thinning or erosion of the right superomedial orbital rim. Sinusitis and right frontal sinus mucocele.

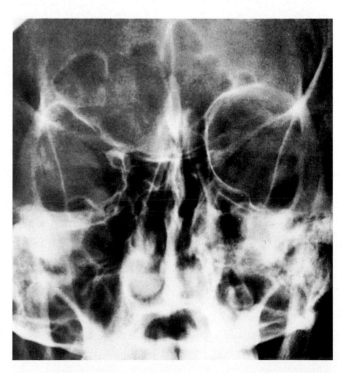

FIG. 4-76 Caldwell view shows slight haziness in the right frontal sinus and flattening of the right superomedial orbital rim. The frontal intersinus septum is also displaced to the left side. Right frontal sinus mucocele.

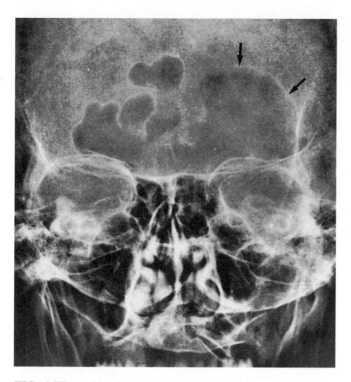

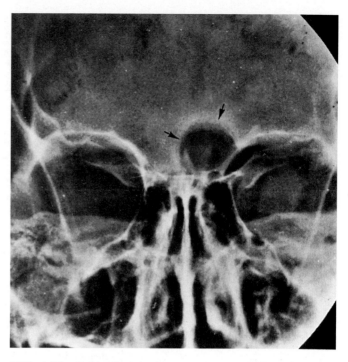

FIG. 4-77 Caldwell view shows a loss of the normal sinus scalloping *(arrows)* and portions of the normal white mucoperiostial line in the left frontal sinus. Left frontal sinus mucocele.

FIG. 4-78 Caldwell view shows a left hypoplastic frontal sinus that has lost the normal thin white line, has a vague zone of surrounding sclerosis *(arrows)*, and is smoothly concave. There is also erosion of the left superomedial orbital rim. Frontal sinus mucocele.

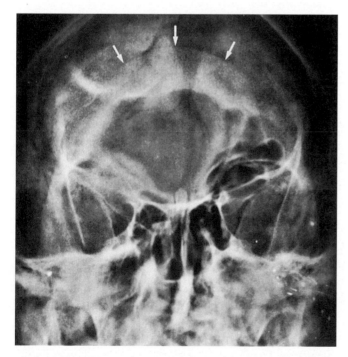

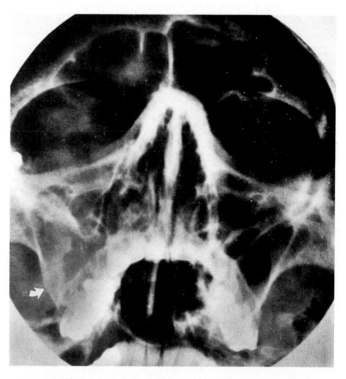

FIG. 4-79 Caldwell view shows a smoothly contoured, enlarged frontal sinus. There is a surrounding zone of sclerosis, and only the lateral most portion of the left frontal sinus appears normal. There is erosion of the right superior and superomedial orbital rim, and a mound of soft tissue is seen above the mass *(arrows)*. Frontal sinus mucocele elevating the forehead and causing right proptosis.

FIG. 4-80 Waters view shows opacified right maxillary sinus with thinning of the lower lateral sinus wall *(arrow)* and some expansion of the sinus cavity. Maxillary sinus mucocele.

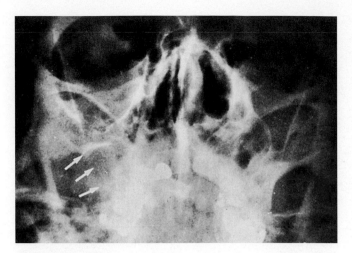

FIG. 4-81 Waters view shows an opacified right maxillary sinus with erosion of the lower lateral sinus wall *(arrows)*. This looks like a carcinoma but was actually an antral mucocele.

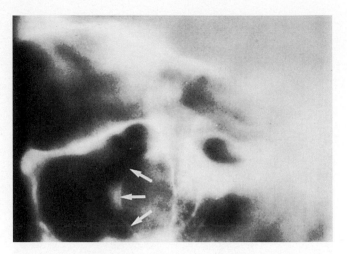

FIG. 4-82 Lateral view multidirectional tomogram shows an expanded compartment *(arrows)* in the posterior portion of the maxillary sinus. Mucocele of a sinus compartment.

it may be very difficult to diagnose on plain films. This is because the obliquely oriented lamina papyracea is seen poorly on frontal films and also because the ethmoid cells surrounding the mucocele may be normal; their air density can partially nullify the soft-tissue density of the mucocele. If an air-fluid level is seen in the ethmoid complex, it may indicate rupture of an ethmoid mucocele with partial drainage into the nasal cavity and adjacent ethmoids. In these cases a mucopyocele is usually present at the time of discovery (Fig. 4-33).[62] Ethmoid mucoceles also can arise in supraorbital ethmoid cells. These are best demonstrated on Caldwell films or coronal images. The obstructing process that leads to the development of these mucoceles is usually an infection or a polyp in the lower portion of the supraorbital cell. These mucoceles typically erode through the orbital roof and displace the globe inferiorly. The entire ethmoid complex, either unilaterally or bilaterally, can be involved by polypoid mucoceles. Characteristically, sectional imaging reveals the preservation of most of the ethmoid septa in an opacified, expanded ethmoid complex. The plain film findings may be only diffuse opacification of the ethmoid complex.

The typical antral mucocele totally opacifies the maxillary sinus and expands the sinus cavity (Fig. 4-80). Unchecked antral mucoceles may eventually overtake the outer maxillary periostium's ability to produce new bone, and frank bone destruction may result. In this circumstance, plain film distinction from tumors may be difficult (Fig. 4-81). If the orbital floor is elevated, the patient may experience diplopia. Rarely, if the mucocele spontaneously collapses after thinning the orbital floor, the globe may descend, causing enophthalmos and diplopia. In an antrum that has been compartmentalized by a septum a mucocele can develop within only one of these sinus sections. This may have significant clinical implications if this mucocele is in a posterior compartment; this region usually eludes the

surgeon when the sinus is surgically explored. In such cases the radiologist may be the only physician to detect this "hidden" mucocele and to direct the surgeon to it (Fig. 4-82).[63]

Sphenoid sinus mucoceles are the least common of the paranasal sinus mucoceles; however, because of their proximity to the optic nerves, they have the highest complication rate after surgical correction. Most sphenoid mucoceles expand anterolaterally into the posterior ethmoids and the orbital apex. Less commonly, expansion may occur upward into the sella turcica and cavernous sinuses or downward into the nasopharynx and posterior nares. Intracranial extension in rare cases can even result in areas of brain necrosis.[64,65] Rarely they may extend into the sphenoid sinus recesses in the greater wings and the pterygoid processes.[66] If sufficiently large, sphenoid sinus mucoceles may cause optic canal and orbital apex syndromes. The critical role of the radiologist is to accurately localize the relationship of the optic nerve to the mass, thereby guiding the surgeon during decompression. Blindness is the most serious major postoperative complication. Radiographic assessment of a sphenoid mucocele requires sectional imaging.

Multiple mucoceles have been reported in several patient's sinuses after facial fractures and in patients with severe allergies. The allergic patient with aspirin intolerance seems to be particularly prone to developing multiple mucoceles.[67]

Sectional Imaging

On CT scans a mucocele appears as an expanded, airless sinus cavity that is filled with fairly homogeneous mucoid attenuation (10 to 18 HUs) secretions.[68] In a few cases the mucocele secretions may be particularly viscid and proteinaceous, and the attenuation may be in the 20 to 45 HU range, similar to muscle attenuation. The sinus walls are remodeled and may be of almost normal thickness, thinned, or partially eroded. In these latter cases the sinus mucosa and the sinus wall periostium are all that contain the mucous secretions

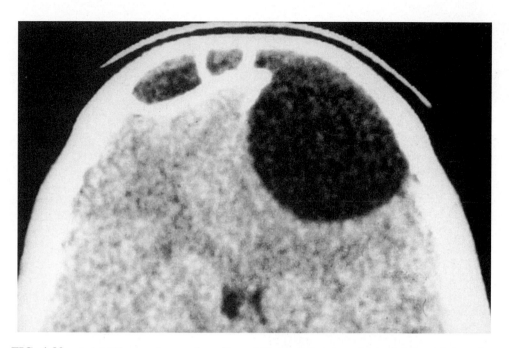

FIG. 4-83   Axial CT scan shows a large "mucoid" attenuation mass in the left frontal sinus that has extended intracranially. A smaller mucocele that extended down into the orbit is present on the right side. Mucoceles.

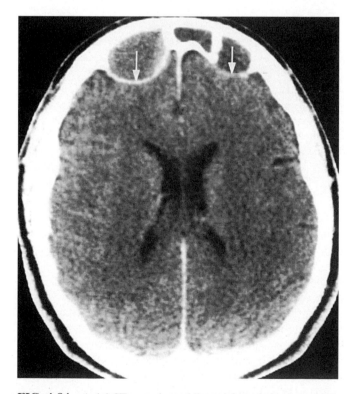

FIG. 4-84   Axial CT scan shows bilateral frontal sinus expansile masses. Each mass has thinned and remodeled the posterior sinus wall *(arrows)* and extended intracranially. The posterior sinus wall appeared intact on the plain film studies. Bilateral frontal sinus mucoceles.

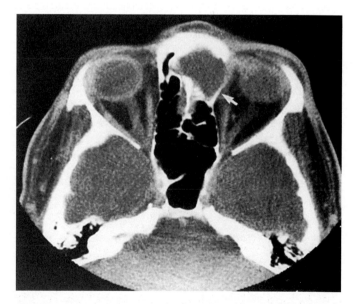

FIG. 4-85   Axial CT scan shows an expansile left frontal sinus mass that is bulging into the upper left orbit. There is primarily bone remodeling *(arrow)* rather than bone destruction. Mucocele.

(Figs. 4-83 to 4-90). If a mucopyocele is present, the inflamed sinus mucosa is seen as a thin line of enhancement just inside the bony sinus walls and establishes the diagnosis of an infected mucocele (Fig. 4-91).[48]

In the patient who has had a prior Caldwell-Luc procedure a fibrous septum may develop between the lateral margin of the anterior sinus wall bony surgical defect and the posterior sinus wall. This septum often is initiated by the development

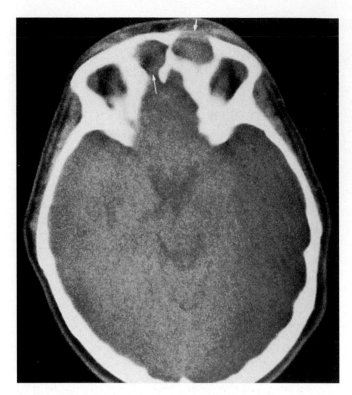

FIG. 4-86   Axial CT scan shows an expansile mass in both the left and right frontal sinuses. The left mass has broken through the anterior sinus wall *(small arrow)* and the right-sided mass has broken through the posterior sinus wall *(arrow)*. Bilateral frontal sinus mucoceles.

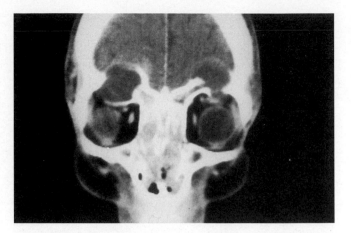

FIG. 4-87   Coronal CT scan shows soft tissue–density material in both ethmoid sinuses and nasal fossae. In addition there are "mucoid" density expanded areas in the roof of each orbit, breaking both intracranially and intraorbitally. Bilateral supraorbital ethmoid mucoceles.

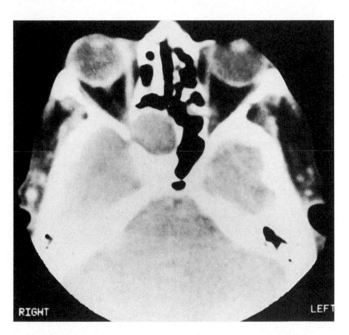

FIG. 4-89   Axial CT scan shows an expansile right sphenoid sinus mass that encroaches on the orbital apex. Sphenoid mucocele.

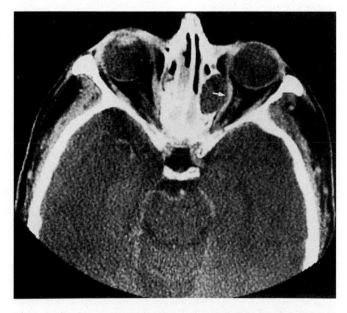

FIG. 4-88   Axial CT scan shows an expansile left ethmoid sinus mass that has extended into the orbit and displaced the medial rectus muscle *(arrow)*. Ethmoid sinus mucocele.

of synechia that progressively form a solid fibrous wall. This septum obstructs the sinus drainage from the lateral portion of the sinus, but the sinus cavity medial to the septum drains normally. Thus the classical findings in such a patient are an expansile mass in the lateral maxillary sinus. When large enough, it may extend into the body of the zygoma and present in the cheek as a soft-tissue mass or it may extend into the lateral, inferior orbit (Figs. 4-92, 4-93).

On MRI the signal intensities are dominated initially by the high water content of the mucous secretions (about 95% water). Thus there usually is a low signal intensity on T1W images, an intermediate signal intensity on PD images, and

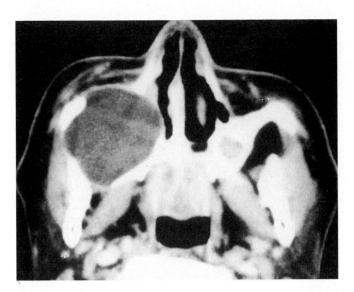

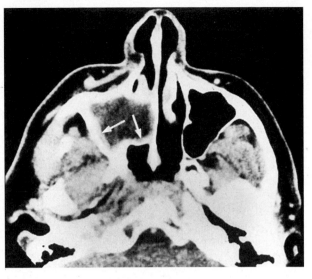

FIG. 4-90 Axial CT scan shows a large expansile mucoid attenuation right antral mass. Portions of the antral wall are thinned. Antral mucocele.

FIG. 4-91 Axial postcontrast CT scan shows an expansile right antral mucoid attenuation mass that has a thin enhancing rim *(arrows)*. Antral mucopyocele.

a high signal intensity on T2W images. However, as discussed previously, with time the secretions become more concentrated and viscous and, depending upon these factors, the signal intensities vary. The relaxation time shortening can be used to approximate the viscosity of the secretions. A long T1 relaxation time (low signal intensity) signifies watery secretions, an intermediate T1 relaxation time (intermediate signal intensity) indicates thick secretions, and a short T1 relaxation time (low signal intensity) indicates desiccated secretions. The T2W signal intensity remains high in most of these lesions. However, when the secretions become progressively more viscid, first the T2W signal intensity and then the T1W signal intensity become low, evenually becoming signal voids.[21] Thus mucoceles can have the following progressive MRI signal intensities: low T1, high T2; intermediate T1, high T2; high T1, high T2; intermediate to high T1, low T2; low T1, low T2; and finally T1 and T2 signal voids (Figs. 4-94 to 4-101).[21] If a mucopyocele is present, the infection appears to cause increased viscosity with a resulting shortening of the relaxation times.

Fungal Diseases

The imaging characteristics of mycotic sinusitis vary from being nonspecific to being highly suggestive of the diagnosis.[69,70] In the early stages of infection a nonspecific mucosal inflammation may be present either in the nasal fossa or paranasal sinus(es) (Figs. 4-71, 4-102). Most often either the maxillary sinus or ethmoid sinuses are involved. Occasionally the sphenoid sinuses are affected, and rarely the frontal sinuses are the only involved sinuses.[71] Air-fluid levels are very uncommon, and when present they suggest a bacterial infection. The surrounding bone in mycotic sinusitis may be thickened and sclerotic, eroded, or remodeled. Most often it

is the combination of these bone changes that suggests either an unusual infection or fungal disease.[72] The associated soft-tissue disease is often found both in the nasal fossa and the paranasal sinuses. In antral mycotic sinusitis the nasal disease may act as a bridge to extension of infection into the cheek. Because the more common forms of antral bacterial sinusitis rarely extend into the soft tissues of the cheek and face, this finding should suggest an aggressive infection or fungal disease.[73] Intrasinus concretions within a mycetoma can be seen occasionally on plain films and CT (Fig. 4-102).[74,75] As previously discussed, when mycetomas are present, its signal void with the surrounding sinus inflammation mimics the MR appearance of chronic infection with desiccated secretions (Figs. 4-55 to 4-58, 4-69 to 4-71).

A variety of fungal diseases involve the sinonasal cavities. These include aspergillosis, mucormycosis, candidiasis, histoplasmosis, cryptococcosis, coccidioidomycosis, myospherulosis, North American blastomycosis, and rhinosporidiosis.[76] There are four clinicopathologic classifications of mycotic sinonasal disease: (1) acute invasive, fulminant disease, (2) chronic invasive infection, (3) noninvasive mycotic colonization ("fungus ball"), and (4) allergic mycotic sinusitis. These four types of infections can be seen with any fungus but are most commonly a result of *Aspergillus* infection. Not infrequently the pathologic diagnosis of mycotic disease requires heightened clinicopathologic suspicion. From a pathologic viewpoint, hyphae may be sparse in allergic mycotic sinusitis, found only beneath the mucosal surface or only within the mucin, or they may be confined to vessels in early invasive sinusitis. Thick sinonasal mucus of unusual color (green, brown, or black) should raise suspicions of mycotic infection. Hyphal fragments may be impossible to classify without culture confirma-

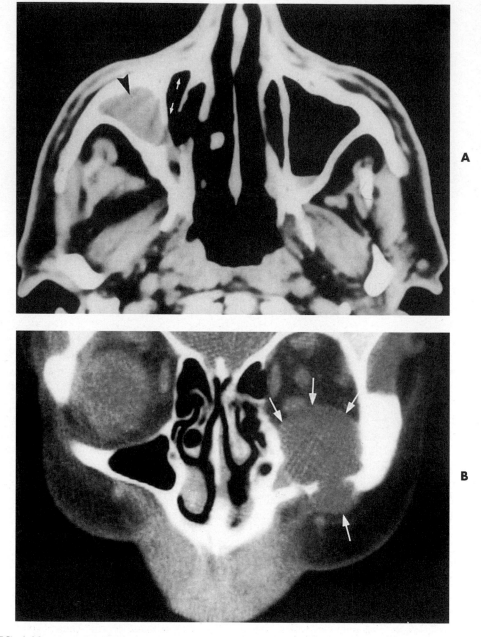

FIG. 4-92   A, Axial CT scan on a patient after a right Caldwell-Luc procedure. There is an expansile mass *(arrowhead)* in the lateral portion of the sinus. The medial portion of the sinus *(small arrows)* is aerated. Postoperative mucocele. **B,** Coronal CT scan on a patient after a left Caldwell-Luc procedure. There is an expansile mass that has broken into the left orbit and the cheek *(arrows).* Postoperative mucocele.

tion. On the other hand, pathologic correlation is necessary to distinguish clinical infection from laboratory contamination.

Fungal Hyphal Diseases

Aspergillosis infection is caused by the fungus *Aspergillus*, a member of the Ascomycetes class. It is an ubiquitous organism frequently found in soil, decaying food, fruits, and plants. The spores are also common contaminants of the respiratory tract and the external auditory canal. *A. fumigatus* is the major pathogen. Of culture-confirmed cases of mycotic sinusitis 87% contained some *Aspergillus* species as sole pathogen or copathogen.[77] *A. flavus* and *A. niger* can also cause human infections.

Acute fulminant *Aspergillus* sinusitis occurs in the immunosuppressed, especially granulopenic patients with hematologic malignancies. Initial complaints are those of acute sinusitis such as nasal discharge, sinus pain, and periorbital swelling. Examination of the nasal cavity and palate

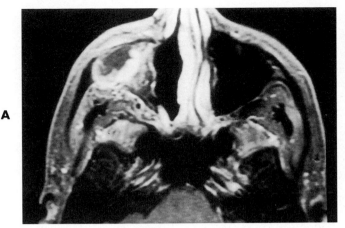
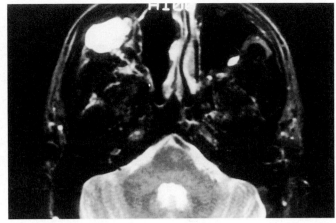

FIG. 4-93   Axial T1W (**A**) and T2W (**B**) MR scans show the patient status post a right partial maxillectomy. There is a nonhomogeneous collection in the zygomatic region of the remaining sinus cavity. The medial portion of this cavity remains well aerated. Postoperative antral mucocele.

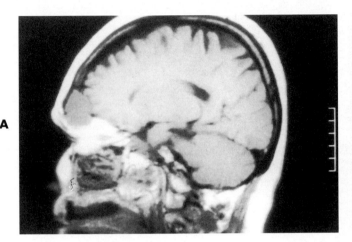
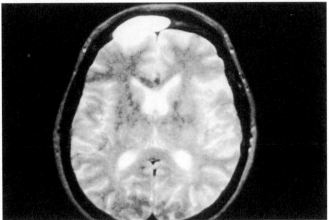

FIG. 4-94   Sagittal T1W (**A**) and axial T2W (**B**) MR scans show an expanded, airless frontal sinus, filled with material that has a low T1W and a high T2W signal intensity. The posterior sinus wall appears to be eroded but was just deossified by the chronic pressure. Frontal sinus mucocele.

reveals pale ischemic tissue that may progress to gray and blackened gangrenous tissue. The ability of *Aspergillus* to invade vessels is aided by its production of elastase and proteases. As the infection spreads through vascular and neuronal routes, orbital nerve invasion occurs, progressing to blindness. Treatment involves surgical debridement and antifungal agents. The tissue at debridement is typically bloodless due to hyphal thrombosis. The prognosis for these patients is usually grave.

Chronic invasive sinusitis can be seen in normal hosts in highly endemic areas such as Sudan or Saudia Arabia. Asymptomatic nasal colonization has been demonstrated. The Middle Eastern cases are quite distinctive in that they occur in immunologically normal patients, probably because of prolonged exposure to large inocula of spores. In the United States, chronic invasive sinusitis is most commonly seen in mildly immunosuppressed patients such as

diabetics. Most patients respond to surgical debridement and antifungal therapy.[78-80]

Mycetoma is the benign fungal colonization of a cavity or space. In the sinonasal tract a mycetoma may occur with changes in local microenvironment such as after surgery or radiotherapy. Anecdotally, sinus aspergillomas have been related to smoking marijuana. Patients with mycetomas may complain of chronic sinusitis, or they may be entirely asymptomatic. Therapy is conservative curettage, but benign recolonization may occur.

Patients with allergic mycotic sinusitis have a history of allergic sinusitis, polyposis, and possibly allergic asthma. Serum eosinophilia, elevated IgE, cutaneous sensitivity to fungal antigens, and the presence of fungal-specific serum precipitins support the diagnosis of allergic mycotic sinusitis. Conservative curettage and systemic steroid therapy are recommended.[81] Histopathologically, hyphae are sparse and

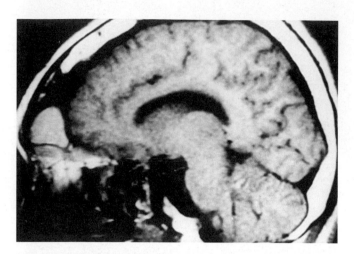

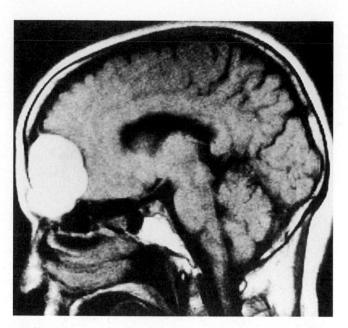

FIG. 4-95   Sagittal T1W MRI scan shows an expansile frontal sinus mass with an intermediate signal intensity. This mass had a high T2W signal intensity. Frontal sinus mucocele.

FIG. 4-96   Sagittal T1W MRI scan shows an expansile frontal sinus mass with high signal intensity. There was also high T2W signal intensity. Frontal mucocele.

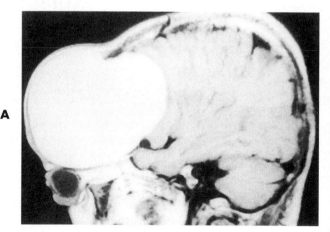

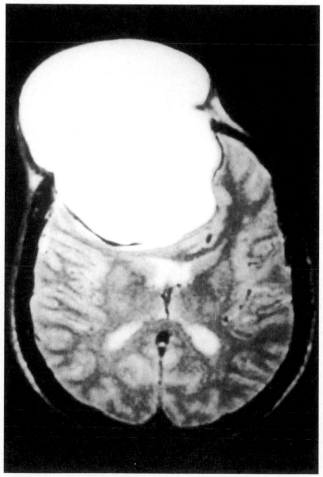

FIG. 4-97   Sagittal T1W (**A**) and axial T2W (**B**) MR scans show a huge expansile frontal sinus mass. There was no hemorrhage within this mucocele; the high signal intensity was due to the macromolecular protein concentration. (Courtesy Dr. Ilka Gerrero.)

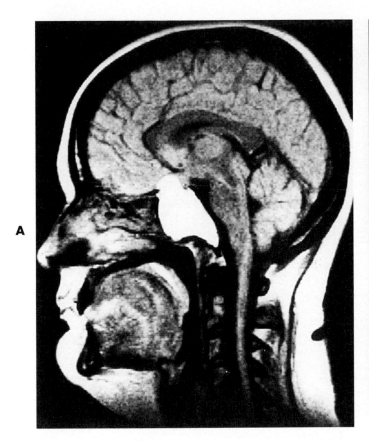
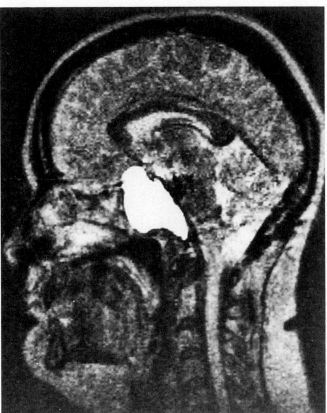

FIG. 4-98   Sagittal T1W (**A**) and T2W MR (**B**) scans show an expansile sphenoid sinus mass that has high signal intensity on both sequences. Sphenoid mucocele.

noninvasive; they may be seen only after special stains are examined. Culture confirmation is necessary because the hyphal fragments do not allow for definitive identification. Because of the environmental prevalence of *Aspergillus*, it is the assumed cause of most allergic fungal sinusitis cases. However, the dematiaceous fungi may also cause allergic sinusitis.

Rhinocerebral mucormycosis (also phycomycosis or zygomycosis) is a disease caused by several genera of the fungi of the class Zygomycetes (formerly Phycomycetes) and the family Mucoraceae. The genera in order of decreasing frequency are *Rhizopus, Mucor,* and *Absidia*. The members of the class Zygomycetes can be found in decaying fruit (especially those with a high sugar content), vegetables, soil, old bread, and manure. This fungus has been isolated sporadically in some studies of indoor environments. Various spices, herbal teas, and birdseed harbor *Rhizopus* and *Absidia*. Iatrogenic subcutaneous wound infections by *Rhizopus* can be caused by ElastoplastR bandages.

The Zygomycetes have a propensity for infecting uncontrolled diabetic patients. Besides affecting diabetics, sinonasal mucormycosis also occurs in patients with hematologic malignancies (e.g., acute leukemia); chronic renal failure and acidosis; malnutrition; cancer; cirrhosis; and prolonged antibiotic, steroid, or cytotoxic drug therapy. *Rhizopus* grows favorably in an acidic, high-glucose environment, which

relates to its elaboration of ketone reductase. The acidosis, in addition to being a favorable growth environment, also further impairs polymorphonuclear leukocyte function.

Sinus murcormycosis occurs predominantly as an invasive rhinocerebral infection. The clinical course may be acute, invasive, and fulminant, just as in aspergillosis. The organism tends to spread rapidly from the nasal fossa to the paranasal sinuses. It invades blood vessels, causing endothelial damage that initiates thrombosis, ischemic and hemorrhagic infarction, and finally purulent inflammation. From these sinuses, eventually there is invasion of the orbits and cavernous sinuses via the ophthalmic vessels. Invasion of the base of the brain is an end-stage event. The entire progression of the disease can occur in only a few days.

However, diabetic patients may develop a more chronic invasive sinusitis, amenable to debridement and antifungal therapy. Mucormycosis is a rare infection in AIDS patients, whose neutrophil function is largely intact.[82] Clinically, black crusting, necrotic tissue is seen over the turbinates, septum, and palate. In immunosuppressed patients, focal ischemic areas may be found instead of the more typical black crusts. In the cases occurring in nondiabetic patients, pulmonary and disseminated infections are more common. Among survivors there is a high incidence of blindness, cranial nerve palsies, and hemiparesis. The best available ther-

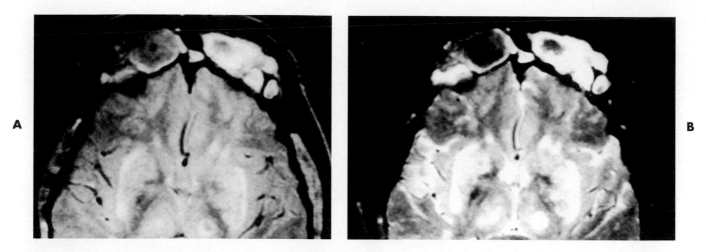

FIG. 4-99   Axial T1W (**A**) and T2W MR (**B**) scans show bilateral expansile frontal sinus masses. On the right side the mass has low to intermediate T1W and low T2W signal intensities. On the left side the mass has high signal intensity on both T1W and T2W scans. Frontal sinus mucoceles.

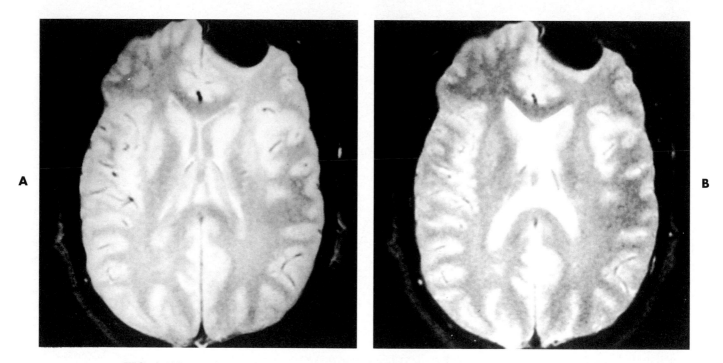

FIG. 4-100   Axial proton density (**A**) and T2W MRI (**B**) scans show an expansile mass in the left frontal sinus that has signal void on both scans. This was a frontal sinus mucocele with dried, desiccated secretions.

apy is adequate surgical debridement and systemic intravenous therapy with amphotericin B.[76]

Murcormycoses has been occassionally documented in nondiabetic, nonimmunosuppressed patients. A preexisting foreign body, marijuana use, or previous surgery or radiotherapy may be predisposing factors in these unusal cases.[83,84]

Fungi from the order Entomophthorales, which are also Zygomycetes, may cause granulomatous rhinoentomophthoromycosis in normal hosts from tropical climates. Cases have been reported in U.S. inhabitants with no history of travel. Entomorphthora species have been isolated from

algae, ferns, insects, and reptiles (*B. ranarum* and *B. haptosporus*). Entomophthorales infection begins as a submucosal nasal mass that slowly expands, causing enormous erosion, destruction, and deformity of the nasal and labial soft tissues. The rhinocerous-like midface expansion is similar to that seen in advanced cases of rhinoscleroma.

Petrillidium boydii (formerly called *Allescheria boydii*) is the current nomenclature for this fungus of the Ascomycetes family. It is a ubiquitous organism in nature most commonly found in rural areas, and it is isolated from soil, poultry, cattle manure, and polluted waters. *P. boydii* sinusitis, which

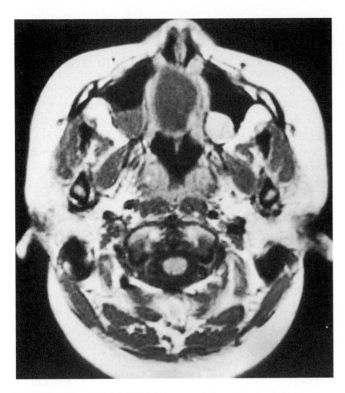

FIG. 4-101 Axial T1W MR scan shows an expansile process that arose in a pneumatized middle turbinate (concha bullosa). This mucocele has a low T1W signal intensity and also had a high T2W signal intensity. Also present is a small retention cyst in the posterior recess of each antrum. On the right side the cyst has low T1W signal intensity, and on the left side the cyst has an intermediate signal intensity.

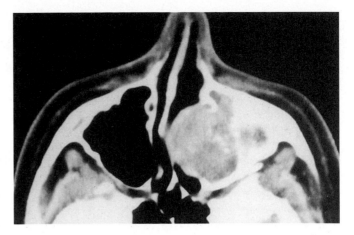

FIG. 4-102 Axial CT scan shows a soft-tissue mass in the left antrum that has thickened the posterior bony wall and thinned or destroyed the medial wall. Within the mass are several discrete calcifications. Aspergillosis.

may be fulminant and lethal, has been reported in immunocompromised patients. It has also been described in normal patients and may resolve with adequate therapy. As in aspergillosis this disease may be either saprophytic or invasive. *P. boydii* has been reported to involve the maxillary, ethmoid, and sphenoid sinuses. The present treatment of choice is miconazole with surgical debridement if necessary.[85,86]

Fungal Yeast Forms

The yeasts of the genus *Candida* are part of the normal mucocutaneous flora. However, under certain circumstances they may produce either a minor or a life-threatening disease. Minor infections may result as overgrowths in patients on antibiotic therapy. The more severe *Candida* infections occur almost exclusively in patients with compromised immune systems. Today, candidiasis represents the most common and most lethal of the opportunistic fungal infections among immunocompromised patients.[76] Most infections are caused by *Candida albicans*, but *C. tropicalis*, *C. stellatoidea*, and *C. krusei* may also cause disease. When the paranasal sinuses are affected, it is usually in otherwise healthy patients who have been on broad-spectrum antibiotics. The maxillary sinuses are almost exclusively

involved, and orbital and intracranial complications are rare. Infections can also occur after maxillary trauma. The treatment of choice for the sinus disease is antral lavage with topical nystatin.[87]

Histoplasma capsulatum is present worldwide. In the United States it is endemic in the Midwest, Central, and Southeast regions. Exposure to *H. capsulatum* occurs through exposure to aerosolized bird or bat droppings and contaminated soil or fertilizers. As with most inhaled mycotic pathogens the most common manifestation of histoplasmosis is as a subclinical pulmonary infection, usually a function of a small exposure source and the state of patient immunity. Patients may develop acute pneumonia after massive inhalation. Chronic cavitating and fibrosing pulmonary infection, sclerosing mediastinitis, and disseminated infection with involvement of bone marrow and adrenals (resulting in Addison's disease) are more serious sequelae of histoplasmosis. Before the AIDS epidemic, disseminated histoplasmosis was rarely seen, and when it was seen, it was usually in elderly patients or those immunosuppressed by chemotherapy or hematologic malignancy. Disseminated histoplasmosis and extrapulmonary histoplasmosis in the face of HIV seropositivity has been included as criteria for AIDS. Disseminated histoplasmosis presents with fever, septicemia, pneumonia, hepatic or renal failure, CNS infection, or skin lesions. It is thought to be due to reinfection from an endemic focus or less frequently reactivation of latent disease. Head and neck manifestations of disseminated disease in AIDS patients include cervical adenopathy, pharyngitis, tonsillitis, and ulcerating oral lesions. Non-AIDs patients may also develop histoplasmosis of the oral cavity and larynx. However, rarely there can be involvement of the nasal mucous membranes, resulting in edema and nasal obstruction. Even more rarely, pansinusitis can occur. The current treatment of choice is amphotericin B.[76,88,89]

Cryptococcus neoformans is a ubiquitous yeast of worldwide distribution. It is associated with pigeon excreta and pigeon nesting sites, and human infection results from inhalation of aerosolized droppings.[76] It may cause asymptomatic, localized pulmonary granulomata; cryptococcal pneumonia or disseminated disease can develop in the immunosuppressed. The meningeal infection seen in the AIDS population is thought to follow respiratory infection. The frontal and maxillary sinuses were documented sources of infection in an AIDS patient with crytococcal meningitis. Sinonasal disease is uncommon and identical to that of histoplasmosis. The treatment is the same as for histoplasmosis.[90,91]

Coccidioidomycosis is a disease caused by the dimorphic fungus *Coccidioides immitis*. The pathogenesis and clinical manifestation of the disease are almost identical to that of histoplasmosis. *C. immitis* is endemic in the southern United States and in northern Mexico, as well as a few sites in Central America and South America. It has been estimated that 20% of cases reported yearly are diagnosed outside the endemic areas, thus widening the relevancy of this organism. *Cocciodioides* is extremely infectious. Illness ranges from subclinical infections to disseminated and often lethal infections, depending on patient immune status, infectious dose, nationality, and other factors such as pregnancy. Most of the head and neck disease affects the laryngotracheal axis with or without concurrent pulmonary disease. Sinonasal involvement is rare.[92,93]

Myospherulosis is not a fungal disease but rather an iatrogenic condition that is caused by the interaction of red blood cells with petrolatum, lanolin, or traumatized human adipose tissue.[76] Large sporangium-like sacs filled with spherules are produced that can be mistaken for a fungi. The disease was first recognized as skin lesions in East Africans; however, in the United States the disease has involved the nose, paranasal sinuses, and middle ear. In these patients there was always prior surgery (i.e., Caldwell-Luc procedure), and the surgical defect was packed with gauze impregnated with petrolatum. The importance of this disease is to recognize it as an innocuous iatrogenic process so that it is not confused with a true fungal disease and given unwarranted therapy.

Infectious-Destructive Sinonasal Diseases, or Granulomatous Diseases

This group includes bacterial, mycobacterial, fungal, protozoan, autoimmune, and lymphoma-related diseases.

Actinomyces and Nocardia

Actinomycosis is a commensural organism of human and bovine hosts; unlike most true fungi they have not been identified as environmental saprophobes. The human pathogen, *Actinomyces israelii* (and less often *A. eriksonii*) is normally present around teeth, especially carious teeth, and in tonsilar crypts. It is classified as a filamentous bacteria rather than a fungus because (1) it reproduces by fission

rather than sporulation (as do perfect fungi) or filamentous budding (as do imperfect fungi), and (2) muramic acid is present in its cell walls and mitochondria are absent, both of which are features of bacteria.

Actinomyces is thought to have limited potential as a pathogen in the normal host. Antecedent trauma or other precursors are necessary predisposing factors for invasive infection. There are three forms: cervicofacial, thoracic, and abdominal; the cervicofacial is the most common form of infection. Soft-tissue abscesses and draining cervical fistulae develop as a result of secondary *Actinomyces* infection of periapical abscesses. Actinomycosis can also present in the neck without the chartacteristic sinuses. These sinuses can occasionally have long tracts, communicating with the soft tissues of the back and chest. Aspiration of oral actinomycosis from carious teeth may lead to pulmonary abscess formation and pneumonia. Rarely, *Actinomyces* may be the cause of sinonasal, laryngeal, or pharyngeal disease.

The pale yellow sulfur granules or grains observed clinically are microcolonies of bacilli. On hematoxylin and eosin (H&E) stain, only blue amorphous masses are visible. The slender, filamentous nature of these bacilli is apparent on Brown and Brenn stain or Gomori methenamine silver stain (GMS). The filaments may mimic fungi in their tendency to branch. *Actinomyces* are routinely not acid-fast, although occasionally they may be weakly acid-fast. This point can help distinguish *Actinomyces* on tissue sections from *Nocardia*. The latter filamentous bacteria does not stain well with H&E, but does stain well with a modified Ziehl-Neelson. The distinction between these two filamentous bacteria is important because their sensitivities to antibiotics differ; penicillin is the drug of choice for *Actinomyces*, but *Norcardia* (most human infection is caused by *N. asteroides*) is unresponsive to penicillin and can be treated with sulfa drugs. The diagnosis of actinomycosis is confirmed by an aerobic culture.[76,94-96]

Tuberculosis (TB) is caused by *Mycobacterium tuberculosis* and *M. bovis,* which are strict aerobes and stain acid-fast. The disease has a worldwide distribution. *M. tuberculosis* is spread through aerosolized repiratory droplets from patients with cavitary TB. *M. bovis* and probably *M. tuberculosis* can cause infection via oral ingestion, although mucosal breaks are probably required. A definite resurgence has been reported in the United States as a result of (1) immigrant populations from endemic countries, (2) reactivation of disease in the elderly population, and (3) the AIDS pandemic. More than 25,000 cases were reported in the United States in 1993 (10 cases per 100,000 people), a 14% increase over reported rates in 1985, which were at a nadir since national reporting began in 1953.[97] The common pulmonary disease may be asymptomatic or cause fever, weight loss, and bloody sputum. Head and neck involvement in TB is rare and thought to be the result of direct infection from expectorated sputum and also hematogenous-lymphatic spread. The sinus disease may be nonspecific; however, when bone involvement occurs, the dominant symptom is pain. The treatment is prolonged antituberculous chemotherapy. Nasopharyngeal and sinonasal TB may clinically and histologically mimic Wegener's granulomatosis. This distinction is of grave consequence because administering the steroid and immunosuppressive agents indicated for active Wegener's may result in miliary progression of unrecognized TB. Also nasopharyngeal TB can be accompanied by lymphadenopathy. This may clinically mimic nasopharyngeal carcinoma, especially in the Asian population at risk for this neoplasm.[98]

Syphilis is a worldwide disease that has been rising in incidence since the 1980s.[99] In 1977 the rate per 100,000 in the United States was 10.4. The rate per 100,000 population has been between 40 to 60 from 1988 to 1992, and more than 110,000 cases were reported in the United States in 1992. Changing patterns in sexual promiscuity and prostitution have lead to the disease resurgence. Syphilis is caused by *Treponema pallidum*, which is usually transmitted through sexual relations, although it can be transmitted through blood transfusions also. By contrast, *T. pertenue* is transmitted through nonvenereal, direct contact.

Syphilis may be divided clinically into three distinct phases: primary, secondary, and tertiary. The first two stages may escape clinical notice. Primary acquired syphilis develops within 1 week to 3 months following exposure. A charcteristic chancre develops at the site of infection. Chancres can also develop after orogenital contact. Oral sites include the lips, palate, gingiva, tongue, and tonsil. Chancre has also been reported in the nose.[76,100] Secondary syphilis occurs weeks to months after the primary chancre and is the result of systemic infection. There is a macular-papular rash that coalesces into warm, moist areas to form hyperplastic lesions: condyloma lata or flat condylomata. Head and neck manifestations of secondary syphilis include condyloma lata, which may occur in the larynx, ears, and nasolabial folds. Tertiary syphilis is a late manifestation seen years to decades after primary infection. Erosive gummas may develop and are ulcerated with indurated margins. The gumma represents a destructive usually painless granulomatous process, which most likely represents a hypersensitivity reaction to *T. pallidum*, as well as the progression of the secondary stage of the disease to the tertiary phase. It tends to develop in intramembranous bones such as the scalp, face, nose, nasal septum, and paranasal sinuses.[76,100,101] Without awareness of patient serology, the radiologist should be aware that this disease can mimic Wegener's granulomatosis or sinonasal fungal disease. Mandibular resorption has been reported and may lead to spontaneous fracture. The treatment of choice remains penicillin.

Congenital syphilis may develop if transplacental infection occurs after the fourth fetal month (when immune competence develops) and within 2 years since the acquired maternal infection.[66] The primary manifestations are in the mucocutaneous tissues and bones; in the head and neck the stigmata include frontal bossing (of Parrot), small maxilla, high palatal arch, Hutchinson's triad (Hutchinson incisors), interstitial keratitis, eighth nerve deafness, saddle nose, and

mulberry molars.[67] The spirochete causes a periostitis that interferes with bone development.[102]

The differential diagnosis of syphilis includes yaws *(framboesia tropica),* a nonvenereally transmitted infection by *T. pertenue,* which occurs in children and young adults primarily in nongenital, unclothed areas. It is endemic in Central and West Africa and Southeast Asia. Uncommonly the late stages of the disease produce granulomas in the mucous membranes of the sinonasal cavities. These granulomas produce severe ulcerations of the nasal region (gangosa) and proliferative exostoses along the medial wall of the maxillary sinus (goundou). The treatment is penicillin. Histologically the spirochetes of *T. pertenue* tend to be more epidermotropic than those of *T. pallidum,* which can be present mainly at the dermal-epidermal junction and dermis. However, clinical history is probably most helpful in distinguishing between syphilis and yaws.

Rhinoscleroma, which is caused by *Klebsiella rhinoscleromatis,* a gram-negative bacterium, is an infection that is endemic at tropical latitudes (Central America, Chile, and Central Africa) at subtropical latitudes (India, Indonesia, Egypt, Algeria, and Morroco) in temperate latitudes (Eastern and Central Europe), and the Russian republics. *K. rhinoscleromatis* is an organism of low infectivity and not a normal commensual organism. Human to human transmission is assumed to be the only mode of contact, and the infection results only after prolonged exposure.

Rhinoscleroma affects the nasal cavity and sinuses; however, it can involve the entire upper repiratory tract, so much so that the general name scleroma had been advocated. The natural course of this infection evolves through three stages. The early stage is the atrophic catarrhal stage; the involved mucosa is reddened and atrophic, with foul purulent discharge and crusting. The clinical differential diagnosis in this early stage includes infection with *K. ozaenae.* The granulomatous stage may appear, months to years later, as waxy, ulcerating inflammatory masses that distend and deform the mucosal surfaces. The inflammatory masses extend through the external nares in severe cases and may distort the soft tissues of the midface resulting in a rhinoceros-like appearance. The clinical differential diagnosis includes leprosy and syphilis. The final sclerotic stage is characterized by fibrosis along with the inflammation, culminating in stenosis.[103]

Rhinosclerosis has been reported in AIDS patients, but the mucocutaneous infections do not appear to differ from cases occurring in the usual hosts.[76,104] The treatment of choice is surgical excision to open the airway and long-term antibiotic therapy, usually with tetracycline.[76]

North American blastomycosis is caused by *Blastomyces dermatitidis,* and the disease is endemic in the Ohio and Mississippi River basins. The disease is not confined to North America and has been detected in South America and Africa. A noted increase of blastomycosis has been seen among avid bird watchers. Based on point source–case studies, it appears that close proximity between the individual's face and soil (e.g. picking up objects off the ground to examine them) makes one more vulnerable to infection.

Blastomyces may cause disease either through inhalation or through traumatic inoculation into skin. Clinically, blastomycosis may present as the acute onset of pneumonia with fever, productive cough, and myalgias. Patients with insidious infection have symptoms such as weight loss, malaise, anorexia, and a chronic cough that may clinically mimic tuberculosis. Most of the head and neck lesions involve the skin, but involvement of the larynx and nasal cavity has been reported. The laryngeal disease may appear clinically identical to carcinoma. Oral lesions may have associated draining sinuses, mimicking actinomycosis. The primary treatment of choice is amphotericin B.[76,105]

South American blastomycosis (paracoccidioidomycosis) is caused by the dimorphic fungus *Blastomyces brasiliensis*. The disease is endemic to South America, especially Brazil, Columbia, Venezuela, Uruguay, and Argentina. As with coccidioidomycosis, a wide range of disease can be seen from subclinical to clinical disease in immunologically normal patients, patients who are immunosuppressed, and patients with AIDS. Aspiration with subsequent hematogenous dissemination is thought to be the mode of transmission because pulmonary involvement is common. It may produce painful, destructive granulomas of the alveolar process, gingiva, nasal cavity, and rarely the paranasal sinuses.[5,106,107] The primary treatment is with amphotericin B, which cures more than 90% of the cases.[108]

Leprosy is caused by the pleomorphic acid-fast bacterium *Mycobacterium leprae*. The disease occurs in almost all tropical and warm temperate regions, including Latin America, South and Southeast Asia, Saharan Africa, the Mediterranean basin, and Northern Europe. In the United States, endemic states include Florida, Louisiana, Texas, California, and Hawaii. Leprosy affects more than 11 million people worldwide; the rate of indigenous cases in the United States has remained stable (10 to 29 cases per year) over the last two decades. However, the rate of imported cases reported in the United States has dramatically increased (up to 300 cases per year) since the late 1970's. This increase in imported cases did not lead to increased transmission among the U.S. population.

Leprosy is a disease of low infectivity transmmitted through prolonged exposure either through nasal secretions or through injured skin. Immunologically, leprosy can be graded by the host response as tuberculoid leprosy (characterized by a robust immunologic response with few bacilli and with the possibility for spontaneous cures), borderline leprosy, and lepromatous leprosy (characterized by anergy to lepromin test and abundant bacilli). Clinically there is a widespread, symmetrical facial distribution of lesions, leading to a coarsening of features. The earlobes and nose are especially enlarged and infiltrated. Intranasal and paranasal sinus involvement is common and occurs after cutaneous nasal involvement. The changes in the sinonasal cavities are those of nonspecific chronic sinusitis and rhinitis. Later

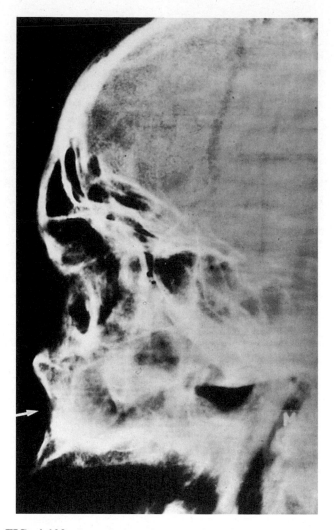

FIG. 4-103 Lateral view shows erosion of the anterior nasal spine *(arrow)*. There is also soft-tissue disease in the maxillary sinuses and nasal fossa. Leprosy.

changes resemble those of a chronic granulomatous disease. A characteristic finding is progressive erosion of the anterior nasal spine. If previous surgery, trauma, and congenital maxillonasal dysplasia are not applicable to the patient, this finding is pathognomonic of leprosy (Fig. 4-103). Retrograde laryngeal involvement usually follows nasal disease. The treatment of choice remains the long-term administration of sulfone derivatives (dapsone).[108]

Rhinosporidiosis is caused by the fungus yeast form *Rhinosporidium seeberi*.[109] The disease has a worldwide distribution but is endemic in places like India, Sri Lanka, Malaysia, Brazil, and Argentina. In the United States, cases have been reported in the rural south and west. Preceeding mucosal trauma (e.g., by digital contamination or dust storms) is considered necessary in establishing infection.[110] Patients with Rhinosporidiosis generally are otherwise healthy. *Rhinosporidium* most commonly infects the conjunctiva and nasal cavity, with resultant friable, lobulated polyps that may cause obstruction of the nasal fossae and

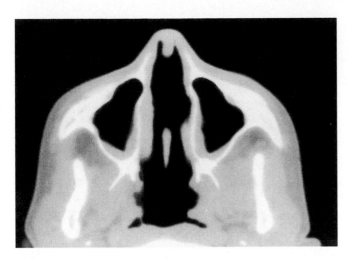

FIG. 4-104 Axial CT scan shows a large erosion of the nasal septum and minimal mucosal thickening in the maxillary sinuses. Cocaine granuloma.

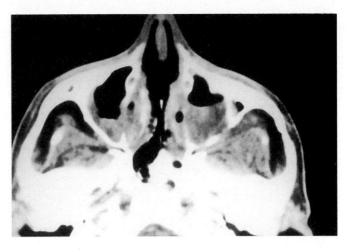

FIG. 4-105 Axial CT scan shows moderated degrees of mucosal disease in both maxillary sinuses and in the nasal fossae. There is a nasal septal erosion and some focal erosion of the bone in the posterior left antrum. Sarcoidosis.

may be confused with neoplasms, especially cylindrical cell papilloma.[76] The nasal polyps are sessile, soft, pinkish, and usually unilateral; and they may diminish aeration in the paranasal sinuses. The treatment of choice is surgical excision or electrocautery.

Glanders, or farcy, is caused by the bacterium *Pseudomonas mallei*. It is contracted by contact with horses, mules, or donkeys. In humans the disease is characterized either by an acute fulminant febrile illness that may lead to death or a chronic indolent granulomatous disease. Farcy refers to the nodular abscesses found in the skin, lymphatics, and subcutaneous tissues.[108] The nasal manifestations of glanders are nasal cellulitis and necrosis that produce septal perforations. The treatment is with sulfonamides.

Leishmaniasis causes mucocutaneous infection (*Leishmania tropica* known as, Oriental sore or "Old World" sore), (*L. mexicana* or *L. brasiliensis* known as, espundia or "New World" sore). The disease is endemic to Central and South America. After initial primary cutaneous sores, metastatic lesions develop in the nose and mouth; these sores are painful, mutilating erosions that can secondarily involve the sinuses.[108,111] Scarring may eventually constrict the nose or mouth, producing gross deformities that interfere with swallowing. The majority of the oronasal diseases are caused by *L. brasiliensis*, and the treatment of this established oronasal disease is with amphotericin B.

Noninfectious Destructive Sinonasal Disease

Wegener's granulomatosis is a necrotizing granulomatous vasculitis that usually affects the upper and lower respiratory tracts and causes a renal glomerulonephritis. A limited form of Wegener's may occur with a more benign course in which only the sinonasal tract is affected. The initial disease may present as a chronic, nonspecific inflammatory process of the nose and sinuses and may remain as such for 1 to 2 years. Usually the nasal septum is first affected. The

process becomes diffuse, and septal ulceration and perforations may result in a "saddle nose" deformity. Secondary bacterial infections complicate the clinical and imaging pictures.

The diagnosis of Wegener's may be difficult to establish early in the disease course or during periods of inactivity. The radiologist can suggest biopsying the paranasal sinuses as opposed to the nasal cavity. Although this site is not as readily accessible as the nasal cavity, it has a greater yield of specific diagnostic features that aid the pathologist. Serum antineutrophil cytoplasmic antibodies (ANCA) are elevated during periods of active disease. In the absence of a specific diagnosis of Wegener's, it behooves the pathologist and the clinician to rule out infectious and malignant causes of destructive sinonasal disease. The disease is probably autoimmune in origin, and the treatment of choice is cyclophosphamide, steroids, and possibly other cytotoxic drugs. Long-term remissions have been achieved; however, it is impossible to predict how long a remission will last.[108,112]

Lethal midline granuloma, which at one time was classified as a granulomatous disease, is now referred to as malignant midline reticulosis or polymorphic reticulosis.[112,113] This disease is discussed in the tumor section.

Sarcoidosis is a systemic, multisystem disease characterized by noncaseating epithelial granulomas[114] An infectious etiology has been sought for these granulomas. Two decades ago, experimental data was presented, suggesting the transmissability of these granulomata, hence fulfilling one of Kock's postulates in an infectious etiology. Patients with sarcoidosis have elevated antibodies to mycobacterium paratuberculosis. However, direct innoculation of sarcoid tissue into a thymic mouse has failed to isolate an infectious agent, so at the present time no known agent has been successfully directly implicated in the etiology of sarcoid.

Sarcoid has a predilection for the Scandinavian countries and for the rural Southeastern United States. It is most com-

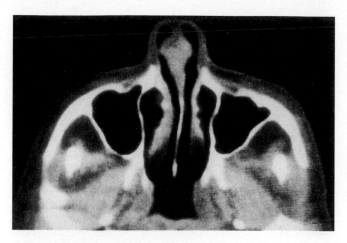

FIG. 4-106   Axial CT scan shows a localized soft-tissue thickening of the anterior nasal septum. Wegener's granulomatosis.

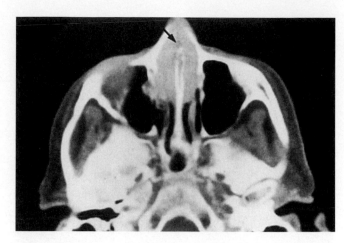

FIG. 4-107   Axial CT scan shows a minimally enhancing bilateral nasal fossa mass that has caused erosion *(arrow)* of the anterior nasal septum. Wegener's granulomatosis.

mon in African-American females with a median age of 25 years. Nasal sarcoid occurs in 3% to 20% of the patients with systemic sarcoidosis. When it occurs, there are multiple small granulomas of the nasal septum and turbinates. There may be nasal discharge, obstruction, and epistaxis. Polypoid degeneration of the nasal fossa mucosa may occur, but the paranasal sinuses are rarely affected. Sarcoid is not generally a destructive disease in the sinonasal tract; however, destruction of the nasal septum and turbinates can occur in unusual cases. Rarely, sharply defined, lytic bone lesions may occur in the calvarium and facial skeleton. Steroid therapy may suppress the inflammatory reaction and provide symptomatic improvement, but fibrous organization of the granulomas may lead to organ dysfunction.[76,115]

Exposure to beryllium may result in chronic granulomas of the nasal fossa. These granulomas may be indistinguishable from those of tuberculosis, leprosy, and sarcoidosis.[111] Chromate salts have been implicated in causing nonspecific granulomas of the nasal cavity. Involvement of the paranasal sinuses is a late and unusual event. Cocaine abuse has become a major worldwide problem. Cocaine causes a necrotizing vasculitis and subsequent granuloma of the nasal septum, which with prolonged exposure usually results in septal erosion. A nonspecific mucosal inflammation may also occur in the nasal fossa. A mucosal reaction to talc used to "cut" the cocaine can also occur.

As a group the destructive and granulomatous diseases that affect the sinonasal cavities first exhibit nasal cavity involvement that can vary from a nonspecific inflammatory-type reaction with mucosal thickening and nasal secretions to a localized soft-tissue mass. The nasal septum may be focally thickened by a bulky soft-tissue mass or septal erosion may be present. The paranasal sinuses usually are involved only after the nasal fossa, and the maxillary and ethmoid sinuses are most often affected. Uncommonly the sphenoid sinuses are involved, and the frontal sinuses are

almost always spared. When the sinuses are involved, there is usually nonspecific inflammatory mucosal thickening; air-fluid levels are rare. The bones of the nasal vault and affected paranasal sinuses may be thickened and sclerotic, reflecting the chronic nature of the inflammatory reaction. Sinus obliteration by reactive bone may occur.[116,117] Similarly there may be areas of bone erosion, reflecting either an osteomyelitic process or necrosis from a granuloma. If the nasal disease becomes a bulky soft-tissue mass, there may, in addition, be remodeling of the adjacent bones (Figs. 4-104 to 4-107).[104]

Cholesteatomas

In addition to mucoceles, there are several other entities that can enlarge an entire sinus cavity or a localized portion thereof. An epidermoid, or cholesteatoma, is a cystic mass with a stratified squamous epithelial wall and a central cavity filled with keratin. In the frontal bone they probably arise from a congenital rest or as a posttraumatic implant. They may develop either in the diplöe or less frequently in the outer table of the skull. On plain films the net effect of the bone loss secondary to the expansile process and the increased density secondary to the deposition of the keratin material with displacement of air within the sinus results in a lucent-appearing lesion when compared with the adjacent normal frontal bone. The margins are slightly scalloped, and there is a thin, uniform white line that identifies the lesion's contour. These latter two findings help differentiate a cholesteatoma from a mucocele (Fig. 4-108). Such confusion may occur if a cholesteatoma arises within or adjacent to the frontal sinus.[118,119]

Rarely a cholesteatoma may occur within a paranasal sinus, usually the maxillary antrum, as a result of squamous metaplasia of the sinus mucosa, presumably secondary to chronic sinusitis. In the antrum, invasion of buccal epithelium via an oroantral fistula has also been proposed as a pos-

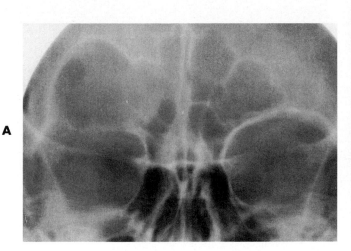

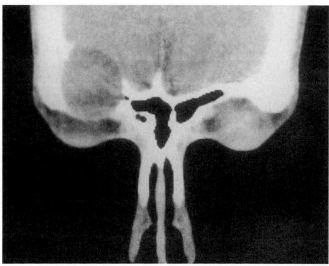

FIG. 4-108 Caldwell view **(A)** shows a smoothly expansile lesion in the lateral right frontal sinus, which is thinning and depressing the right orbital roof. A thin white mucoperiosteal line surrounds the mass. Coronal CT scan **(B)** shows the localized, expansile, homogeneously "mucoid" attenuation mass, which is depressing the right orbital roof. Cholesteatoma.

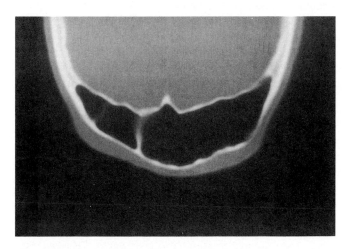

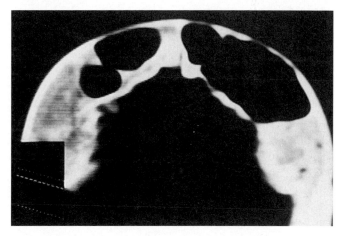

FIG. 4-109 Coronal CT scan shows a very large, normally aerated frontal sinus. Despite its size there was no bossing of the forehead or remodeling of the inner table. Hypersinus.

FIG. 4-110 Axial CT scan shows large frontal sinuses in a patient with a dense cortical calvarium and hyperostosis interna. Despite the size of these sinuses there was no deformity of the forehead. Hypersinuses.

sible etiology.[119] A type of cholesteatoma or pseudo-cholesteatoma may also result in a chronically infected sinus after the active infection subsides. The breakdown products of the purulent exudate may contain cholesterol products and appear as cholesteatomatous debris.[120,121]

On CT a cholesteatoma is an expansile lesion that has soft tissue, mucoidlike attenuation (usually 10 to 25 HUs) and may be indistinguishable from a mucocele (Fig. 4-108). On MRI, depending on the fatty components of the cholesterol, there can be an intermediate to high signal intensity on T1W images and there usually is an intermediate intensity signal on T2W images.[122,123]

Enlarged Aerated Sinuses

A paranasal sinus may be enlarged with normal sinus mucosa and either be normally aerated or hyperaerated. This unusual situation is the result of one of the entities referred to as hypersinus, pneumosinus dilatans, or pneumocele. Part of the confusion arises from a lack of certainty as to how large a sinus may be before it should be called abnormal, and part arises from the lack of a pathologically confirmed etiology for these processes. A study of plain films on 100 normal patients judged a sinus to be abnormally large if its size exceeded that of 99% of the normal population.[124,125] Taking into account magnification factors for films taken

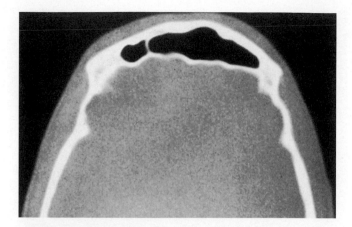

FIG. 4-111   Axial CT scan shows an enlarged left frontal sinus that has not thinned the bone of either the anterior or posterior sinus walls. However, the anterior wall has been bowed forward, causing a bulge in the forehead. Pneumosinus dilatans.

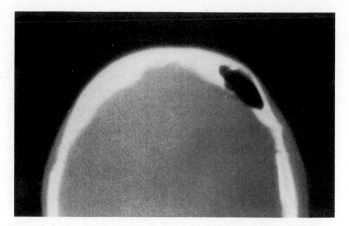

FIG. 4-112   Axial CT scan shows the cranial region of a large left frontal sinus with normal mucosa. A portion of the posterior sinus wall is thinned. Pneumocele.

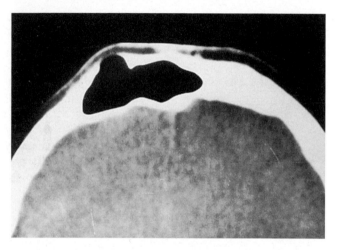

FIG. 4-113   Axial CT scan shows a normal-sized right frontal sinus that has focally thinned the anterior sinus wall to cause a bulge in the forehead. Pneumocele.

on a Franklin head unit (3.4%) and a standard 40 inch focal-distance Caldwell view (10.3%), if a line drawn from the base of the crista galli to a point of maximum distance along the perimeter of the sinus exceeds 74.4 mm (head unit) or 79.3 mm (PA skull film), the sinus is larger than 99% of normal frontal sinuses and may be referred to as a hypersinus. This term refers to a larger than normal sinus that does not expand the normal contours of the bone in which the sinus is located (Figs. 4-109, 4-110).

The term pneumosinus dilatans refers to an aerated sinus that is abnormally expanded (either the entire sinus or a portion of the sinus) and whose walls, although intact and of normal thickness, have been outwardly displaced (remodelled) from their normal boundaries. This causes such problems as frontal bossing, diplopia, or a nasal mass, depending on which sinus is involved and which portion of this sinus is

expanded. Accordingly it is this extension of the sinus beyond the normal bony boundaries that differentiates pneumosinus dilatans from hypersinus. If the entire sinus is not involved, the remaining sinus dimensions are usually normal (Fig. 4-111).[126,127]

Pneumocele refers to an aerated sinus with either focal or generalized sinus cavity enlargement and thinning of the bony sinus walls. It is this latter feature that differentiates pneumosinus dilatans from a pneumocele (Figs. 4-112 to 4-116). This distinction has been developed in the clinical literature where the integrity, or lack of integrity, of the sinus wall was observed. Although a "valve" theory has been suggested as an etiology for the delayed pressure equilibration that apparently occurs in pneumoceles, no such valve has been demonstrated physiologically.

At present there is no clear understanding of the factors that either influence the development of normal sinuses or signal the normal cessation of sinus growth. Consequently the etiology of excessive sinus aeration and growth that produces hypersinus, pneumosinus dilatans, and pneumocele is unclear.[125] The pneumocele's growth can be arrested by creating a surgical window (i.e., antrostomy, ethmoidectomy, sphenoid-sinusotomy) to allow rapid pressure equilibration. The cosmetic deformity that may result from either a pneumosinus dilatans or a pneumocele can be dealt with surgically if necessary by collapsing the sinus.

In the sphenoid sinus the planum sphenoidale may be bowed cranially by an overlying meningioma.[128] This may simulate a pneumosinus dilatans. However, only the roof of the sphenoid sinus is involved and the presence of the intracranial tumor will be demonstrated on CT or MRI. Additionally the bone is usually thickened if related to the presence of an overlying tumor.

An enlarged frontal sinus has also been associated with acromegaly. Although the sinus is large, the sinus mucosa is usually normal (Fig. 4-117).

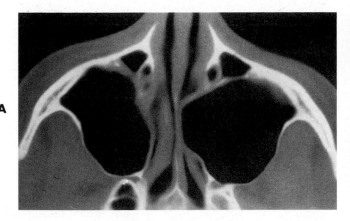
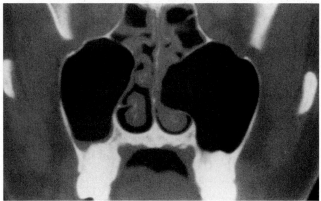

FIG. 4-114   Axial **(A)** and coronal **(B)** CT scans show an aerated, expanded left maxillary sinus. The sinus walls are thinned. Pneumocele.

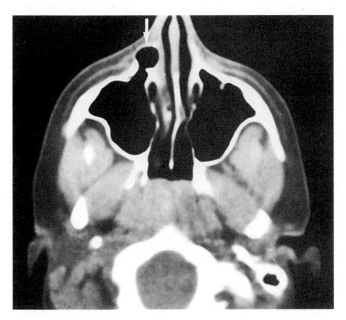

FIG. 4-115   Axial CT scan shows a focal anterior enlargement of the right maxillary sinus *(arrow)* that has thinned the sinus wall and caused a cheek mass. Pneumocele.

Complications of Inflammatory Paranasal Sinus Disease Affecting Adjacent Areas

In the present antibiotic era, most acute paranasal sinus infections are successfully treated. It is only in a few cases that surgical intervention is required to help control an acute infection. However, a delay in initiating proper treatment, organisms resistant to the chosen antibiotics, and incomplete treatment regimens all can allow an initially localized infection to spread to adjacent regions.[129,130]

About 3% of patients with paranasal sinusitis experience some related orbital or preseptal inflammatory disease. These various complications include retention edema of the eyelids, preseptal cellulitis, preseptal abscess, orbital cellulitis, subperiosteal orbital abscess, orbital abscess, and cavernous sinus thrombosis.[129,131] Such orbital complica-

tions are discussed in Chapter 10. In addition, 15% to 20% of the cases of retrobulbar neuritis are secondary to posterior ethmoid and sphenoid sinusitis, and in some of these cases the neuritis can apparently occur without other manifestations of orbital inflammatory disease.[56,132]

The ethmoid sinuses are clearly those most often implicated as the source of infection for orbital complications. The thin lamina papyracea and the anterior and posterior valveless ethmoidal veins allow rapid access of infection into the orbit.[133] When implicated as a source of orbital infection, in descending order of frequency the remaining paranasal sinuses are the sphenoid, frontal, and maxillary.

On rare occasions, mucosal thickening in the nasal fossae and paranasal sinuses is seen in patients with concurrent orbital pseudotumor. These mucosal changes may be noninfectious and consistent with pseudotumor.[29] The association of the orbital and sinonasal disease may suggest this diagnosis; however, more commonly, orbital pseudotumor is either an isolated finding or is associated with routine, unrelated sinonasal inflammatory disease. Maxillary sinus pseudotumor can also occur without associated orbital complications. Unlike its orbital counterpart, which rarely involves the adjacent bone, antral pseudotumor usually presents with areas of bone erosion, sclerosis, and remodeling, often mimicking the imaging appearance of an antral malignancy (Figs. 4-118, 4-119).[134]

Intracranial complications of sinusitis also occur infrequently, and these include meningitis, epidural abscess, subdural abscess, cerebritis, and cerebral abscess (Fig. 4-31).[135] Only 3% of intracranial abscesses originate from sinonasal cavity disease, and only 3% of headaches are reported to result from sinusitis.[129] Intracranial spread of inflammatory disease in the paranasal sinuses most often stems from frontal sinusitis. As has been stated, this is because of the rich emissary network (Beçhet's plexus) that connects the posterior sinus mucosa with the meninges; acting as a source for intracranial inflammatory disease, in decreasing order of frequency for causing intracranial disease the remaining paranasal sinuses are the sphenoid, ethmoid, and maxillary.

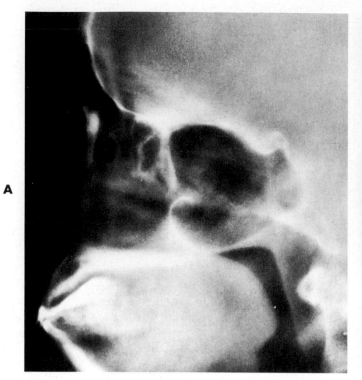

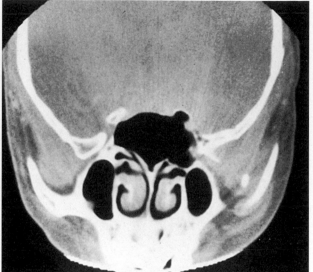

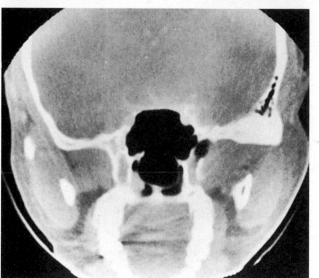

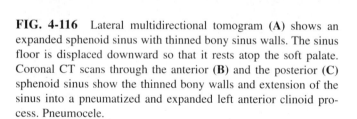

FIG. 4-116 Lateral multidirectional tomogram (**A**) shows an expanded sphenoid sinus with thinned bony sinus walls. The sinus floor is displaced downward so that it rests atop the soft palate. Coronal CT scans through the anterior (**B**) and the posterior (**C**) sphenoid sinus show the thinned bony walls and extension of the sinus into a pneumatized and expanded left anterior clinoid process. Pneumocele.

Osteomyelitis is also a complication of sinusitis and is most often encountered today in patients who have chronic, incompletely treated sinusitis or fungal disease. Less commonly it can occur in patients who were previously irradiated in the facial area. The dominant clinical finding is persistent pain; the radiographic manifestations include focal rarefaction of bone, sequestrum formation, reactive thickening of the bone, bony sclerosis, and ultimately fragmentation of the bone. Over the frontal sinus, a subgaleal abscess can form secondary to sinusitis. This occurs via osteothrombophlebitis and may or may not be associated with frank osteomyelitis. This subgaleal abscess is also called a Pott's puffy tumor.[136]

Whether the complications are intracranial or intraorbital they are more likely to occur in patients with acute sinusitis rather than in cases of chronic inflammatory disease. Only the osseous complications are more common in chronic infections.

Opacified Maxillary Sinuses

When a patient has signs and symptoms of rhinitis and sinusitis, they often seek the advice of an otolaryngologist. Most of these specialists prefer to obtain a plain film examination of the paranasal sinuses to map the disease and provide a graphic means of following its response to treatment; however, increasingly, limited coronal CT studies are being obtained. On these initial films the sinus most severly affected is the maxillary sinus, and frequently the antrum is totally opacified, presumably as a result of polypoid mucosal thickening and retained secretions.[137] The clinician most often treats these patients with decongestants, antihistamines, nasal sprays, and antibiotics. Within 3 to 7 days the presenting symptoms usually have abated, and the assumption is that the opacified sinus has also cleared. However, if follow-up sinus films are obtained on these now asymptomatic patients, the antrum remains opacified in 20% of cases, and in 80% of the people, some resolution of the

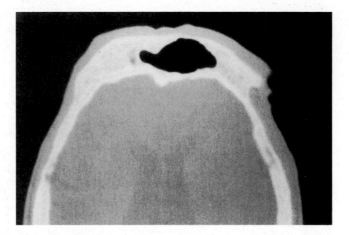

FIG. 4-117   Axial CT scan shows an expanded left frontal sinus in a patient with a thick, cortical-type calvarium. The sinus mucosa is normal. Acromegaly.

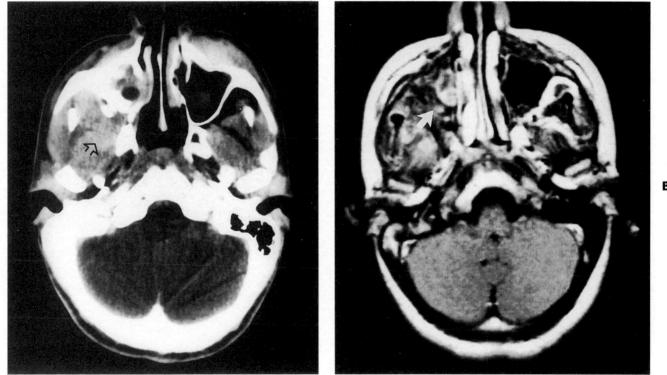

FIG. 4-118   Axial CT scan (**A**) shows an infiltrating lesion in the right infratemporal fossa *(open arrow)*, thickening of the right antral bony walls, and soft-tissue disease in this sinus. Axial T1W MR scan (**B**) shows the soft-tissue disease; however, the thickened, sclerotic bone is almost unde-tected *(arrow)*. Antral pseudotumor.

sinusitis is noted by the radiographic observation of the presence of sinus aeration.[138]

The primary reason the antrum remains opacified, despite the resolution of the patient's symptoms, is that there is an underlying process in the sinus that causes periodic obstruction of the sinus ostium. This in turn causes the bacterial sinusitis that produces the patient's symptoms. If the underlying problem is not resolved, the patient will continue to have repeated episodes of antral sinusitis. This cycle will only be broken if the underlying disease in the antrum is identified and cured. To identify the 20% of patients who have such an underlying problem, a follow-up plain film Waters view should be obtained 1 to 3 weeks after the initiation of therapy. If the sinus remains opacified, either a CT

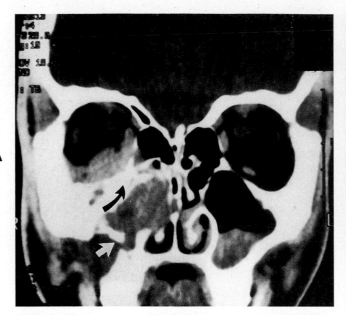
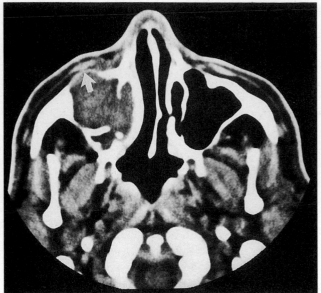
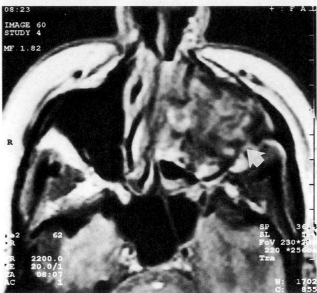

FIG. 4-119   Coronal (**A**) and axial (**B**) CT scans show a soft-tissue mass in the right maxillary sinus. There are areas of bone thickening and sclerosis *(black arrow),* sequestration *(arrow* **A**), and bone remodeling *(arrow* **B**). Axial T1W MR scan (**C**) on a different patient shows a nonhomogeneous soft-tissue mass in the left antrum, focally eroding the posterior wall *(arrow)* to extend into the infratemporal fossa. Antral pseudotumors.

scan or an MRI scan of the sinonasal cavities should be obtained to diagnose the clinically "occult" underlying sinus pathology. The lesions to consider as causes of intermittent obstruction include nasal polyps, an antrochoanal polyp, one or more large retention cysts or polyps, a mucocele, or a tumor. Each of these lesions, other than tumors, is discussed in detail in this chapter.

FOREIGN BODIES

A great variety of foreign bodies have been reported in the sinonasal cavities. Some are made of plastic materials (e.g., beads) or other nonradiopaque materials (e.g., gauze) that cannot be visualized on plain films, and others are radio-

dense (i.e., metallic) and can be localized easily on routine radiographic examinations (Fig. 4-120). If a foreign body is present for a sufficiently long time, it may act as a nidus and become encrusted with mineral salts. As such these calcified masses are referred to either as rhinoliths or sinoliths depending on whether they are respectively located in the nasal fossa or a paranasal sinus (Figs. 4-121 to 4-123).[139,140] If on CT a solitary calification is seen within a sinus cavity, invariably it is the result of infection. Similarly, nearly one half of the times that multiple discrete intrasinus calcifications are present the cause is infection (Fig. 4-102).[141] Far less commonly, intrasinus ossification can occur (Fig. 4-124). The implications of this occurrence are the same as for the calcifications.

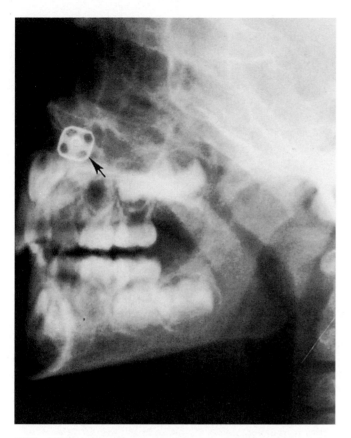

FIG. 4-120 Lateral view shows a nasal metallic snap foreign body *(arrow)*.

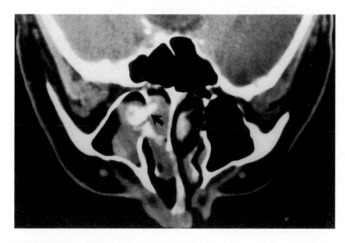

FIG. 4-122 Coronal CT scan shows inflammatory mucosal thickening in the right antrum and nasal fossa. A rhinolith (or sinolith) also is present at the level of the sinus ostium *(arrow)*. Sinusitis and rhinolith.

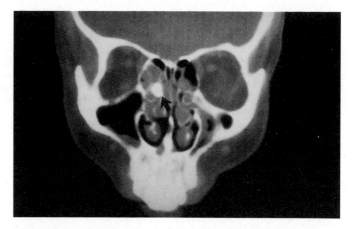

FIG. 4-121 Coronal CT scan shows mucosal thickening in the ethmoid and maxillary sinuses and in the upper nasal fossae. In addition a rhinolith *(arrow)* is present on the right side. Sinusitis and rhinolith.

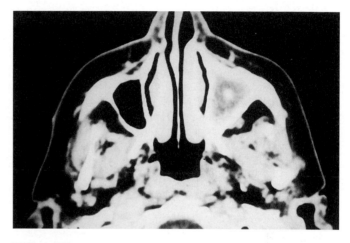

FIG. 4-123 Axial CT scan shows opacification of the left maxillary sinus. Within the center of this sinus is a solitary calcification. Sinusitis and sinolith.

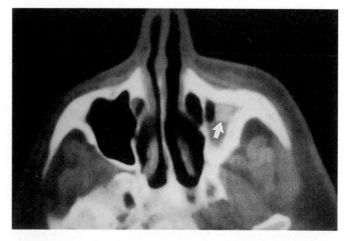

FIG. 4-124 Axial CT scan shows some mucosal thickening in the left antrum and an ossification *(arrow)* in the sinus. Sinusitis and sinolith.

ANOSMIA

The two most common causes of anosmia are idiopathic and sinonasal inflammatory disease. Usually, imaging shows either essentially normal sinonasal cavities or sinonasal inflammatory mucosal thickening that obliterates the nasal olfactory recess(es). However, anosmia can also be caused by sinonasal tumors and a variety of intracranial diseases. Among these, Kallman's syndrome has recently received attention in the literature.[142-144] This syndrome consists of a primary eunuchoidism, secondary to hypogonatropic hypogonadism, and associated congenital anosmia, usually with abscence of the olfactory bulbs and tracts. Coronal MRI best shows the absence of these olfactory structures and allows differentiation of this syndrome from the other more common causes of anosmia.

References

1. Potsic WP, Wetmore RF. Pediatric rhinology. In: Goldman JL, ed. The principles and practice of rhinology. New York, NY: John Wiley & Sons Inc, 1987; 801-845.
2. Carpenter JL, Artenstein MS. Use of diagnostic microbiologic facilities in the diagnosis of head and neck infections. Otolaryngol Clin North Am 1976; 9:611-629.
3. Fried MP, Relly JH, Strome M. Pseudomonas rhinosinusitis. Laryngoscope 1984; 94:192-196.
4. Evans FO, Sydnor JB, Moore WEC et al. Sinusitis of the maxillary antrum. N Engl J Med 1976; 293:735-739.
5. Frederick J, Braude AI. Anaerobic infection of the paranasal sinuses. N Engl J Med 1974; 290:135-137.
6. Van Alyea OE. Nasal sinuses: anatomic and clinical considerations. Baltimore, Md: Williams & Wilkins, 1942.
7. Batsakis JG. Tumors of the head and neck: clinical and pathological considerations. 2nd Edition. Baltimore, Md: Williams & Wilkins, 1979.
8. Stahl RH. Allergic disorders of the nose and paranasal sinuses. Otolaryngol Clin North Am 1974; 7:703-718.
9. Nino-Murcia M, Rao VM, Mikaelian DO et al. Acute sinusitis mimicking antrochoanal polyp. AJNR 1986; 7:513-516.
10. Chong WK, Hall-Craggs MA, Wilkinson ID et al. Prevalence of paranasal sinus disease in HIV infection and AIDS on cranial MR imaging. Clin Radiol 1993; 47:166-169.
11. O'Donnell JG, Sorbello AF, Condoluci DV et al. Sinusitis due to Pseudomonas aeruginosa in patients with HIV Infection. Clin Infect Dis 1993; 16:404-406.
12. Schlanger G, Lutwick, Kurzman M et al. Sinusitis caused by legionella pneumophilia in a patient with AIDS. Am J Med 1984; 77:957-960.
13. Towbin R, Bunbar JS. The paranasal sinuses in childhood. Radiographics 1982; 2:253-279.

14. Odita JC, Akamaguna AI, Ogisi FO et al. Pneumatization of the maxillary sinus in normal and symptomatic children. Pediatr Radiol 1986; 16:365-367.
15. Glasier CM, Ascher DP, Williams KD. Incidental paranasal sinus abnormalities on CT of children: clinical correlation. AJNR 1986; 7:861-864.
16. Glasier CM, Mallory GB Jr, Steele RW. Significance of opacification of the maxillary and ethmoid sinuses in infants. J Pediatrics 1989; 114:45-50.
17. Shugar JMA. Embryology of the nose and paranasal sinuses and resultant deformities. In: Goldman JL, ed. The principles and practice of rhinology. New York, NY: John Wiley & Sons Inc, 1987; 113-131.
18. Johnson JT. Infections. In: Cummings CW, Fredrickson JM, Harker LA et al, eds. Otolaryngology head and neck surgery. Vol. 1. St. Louis, Mo: CV Mosby Co, 1986; 887-900.
19. Rak KM, Newell JDII, Yakes WK et al. Paranasal sinus on MR images of the brain: significance of mucosal thickening. AJR 1991; 156:381-384.
20. Moser FG, Panush D, Rubin JS et al. Incidental paranasal sinus abnormalities on MRI of the brain. Clin Radiol 1991; 43:252-254.
21. Som PM, Dillon WP, Fullerton GD et al. Chronically obstructed sinonasal secretions: observations on T1 and T2 shortening. Radiology 1989; 172:515-520.
22. Dillon WP, Som PM, Fullerton GD Hypointense MR signal in chronically inspissated sinonasal secretions. Radiology 1990; 174:73-78.
23. Som PM, Dillon WP, Curtin HD et al. Hypointense paranasal sinus foci: differential diagnosis with MR imaging and relation to CT findings. Radiology 1990; 176:777-781.
24. Bassoiouny A, Newlands WJ, Ali H et al. Maxillary sinus hypoplasia and superior orbital fissure asymmetry. Laryngoscope 1982; 92:441-448.

25. Modic MT, Weinstein MA, Berlin AJ et al. Maxillary sinus hypoplasia visualized with computed tomography. Radiology 1980; 135:383-385.
26. Silver AJ, Baredes S, Bello JA et al. The opacified maxillary sinus: CT findings in chronic sinusitis and malignant tumor. Radiology 1987; 163:205-210.
27. Kennedy DW, Zinreich SJ, Kumar AJ et al. Physiologic mucosal changes within the nose and ethmoid sinus: imaging of the nasal cycle by MRI. Laryngoscope 1988; 98:928-933.
28. Brock JG, Schabel SI, Curry N. CT diagnosis of contrast reaction. J Comput Tomogr 1981; 5:63-64.
29. Eshaghian J, Anderson RL. Sinus involvement in inflammatory orbital pseudotumor. Arch Ophthalmol 1981; 99:627-630.
30. Som PM, Shugar JMA, Troy KM et al. The use of MR and CT in the management of a patient with intrasinus hemorrhage. Arch Otolaryngol 1988; 114:200-202.
31. Zimmerman RA, Bilaniuk LT, Hackney DB et al. Paranasal sinus hemorrhage: evaluation with MR imaging. Radiology 1987; 162:499-503.
32. Fagan P, McKenzie B, Edmonds C. Sinus barotrauma in divers. Ann Otol Rhinol Laryngol 1976; 85:61-64.
33. Remmier D, Boles R. Intracranial complications of frontal sinusitis. Laryngoscope 1980; 90:1814-1824.
34. Tamakawa Y, Hanafee WN. Cerebrospinal fluid rhinorrhea: significance of an air-fluid level in the sphenoid sinus. Radiology 1980; 135:101-103.
35. Fascenelli FW. Maxillary sinus abnormalities: radiographic evidence in an asymptomatic population. Arch Otol Laryngol 1969; 90:190-193.
36. Zizmor J, Noyek AM. Inflammatory diseases of the paranasal sinuses. Otolaryngol Clin North Am 1973; 6:459-485.
37. Som PM, Sacher M, Lawson W et al. CT appearance distinguishing benign

nasal polyps from malignancies. J Comput Assist Tomogr 1987; 11:129-133.

38. Som PM, Cohen BA, Sacher M et al. The angiomatous polyp and the angiofibroma: two different lesions. Radiology 1982; 144:329-334.

39. Batsakis JG. The pathology of head and neck tumors: nasal cavity and paranasal sinuses. Part 5. Head Neck Surg 1980; 2:410-419.

40. Smith CJ, Echevarria R, McLelland CA: Pseudosarcomatous changes in antrochoanal polyps. Arch Otolaryngol 1974; 99:228-230.

41. Barnes L, Verbin RS, Gnepp DR. Diseases of the nose, paranasal sinuses and nasopharynx. In: Barnes L, ed. Surgical pathology of the head and neck. Vol 1. New York, NY: Marcel Dekker Inc, 1985; 403-451.

42. Weissman JL, Tabor EK, Curtin HD. Sphenochoanal polyps: evaluation with CT and MR imaging. Radiology 1991; 178:145-148.

43. Ballenger JJ. Diseases of the nose, throat and ear. 12th Edition. Philadelphia, Pa: Lea & Febiger, 1977; 105-114, 155-167.

44. Smith MP. Dysfunction of carbohydrate metabolism as an element in the set of factors resulting in the polysaccharide nose and nasal polyps (the polysaccharide nose). Laryngoscope 1971; 81:636-644.

45. Schramm VL, Jr, Effron MZ. Nasal polyps in children. Laryngoscope 1980; 90:1488-1495.

46. Jaffe BF, Strome M, Khaw KT et al. Nasal polypectomy and sinus surgery for cystic fibrosis: a 10 year review. Otolaryngol Clin North Am 1977; 10:81-90.

47. Moloney JR: Nasal polyps, nasal polypectomy, asthma and aspirin sensitivity: their association in 445 cases of nasal polyps. J Laryngol Otol 1977; 91:837-846.

48. Torjussen W. Rhinoscopical findings in nickel workers, with special emphasis on the influence of nickel exposure and smoking habits. Acta Otolaryngol (Stockh)1979; 88:279-288.

49. Som PM, Curtin HD. Chronic inflammatory sinonasal diseases including fungal infections: role of imaging. Radiol Clin North Am 1993; 31:33-44.

50. Som PM, Dillon WP, Sze G et al. Benign and malignant sinonasal lesions with intracranial extension: differentiation with MR imaging. Radiology 1989; 172:763-766.

51. Som PM, Shugar JMA. The CT classification of ethmoid mucoceles. J Comput Assist Tomogr 1980; 4:199-203.

52. Jacobs M, Som PM. The ethmoidal "polypoid mucocele." J Comput Assist Tomogr 1982; 6:721-724.

53. Naul LG, Hise JH, Ruff T. CT of inspissated mucous in chronic sinusitis. AJNR 1987; 8:574-575.

54. Zinreich SJ, Kennedy DW, Malat J et al. Fungal sinusitis: diagnosis with CT and MR imaging. Radiology 1988; 169:439-444.

55. De Juan EE, Green WR, Iliff NT. Allergic periorbital mycopyocele in children. Am J Ophthalmol 1983; 96:299-303.

56. Finn DG, Hudson NR, Baylin G. Unilateral polyposis and mucoceles in children. Laryngoscope 1981; 91:1444-1449.

57. Zizmor J, Noyek AM. Cysts, benign tumors and malignant tumors of the paranasal sinuses. Otolaryngol Clin North Am 1973; 6:487-508.

58. Rogers JH, Fredrickson JM, Noyek AM. Management of cysts, benign tumors and bony dysplasia of the maxillary sinus. Otolaryngol Clin North Am 1976; 9:233-247.

59. Lloyd DM, Bartram CI, Stanley P. Ethmoid mucoceles. Br J Radiol 1974; 47:646-651.

60. Ritter FN. The paranasal sinuses: anatomy and surgical technique. St. Louis, Mo: The CV Mosby Co, 1973.

61. Canalis RF, Zajtchuck JT, Jenkins HA. Ethmoid mucoceles. Arch Otolaryngol 1978; 104:286-291.

62. Zizmor J, Noyek AM, Chapnik JS. Mucocele of the paranasal sinuses. Can J Otolaryngol 1974; 3 (suppl).

63. Som P, Sacher M, Lanzieri CF et al. The hidden antral compartment. Radiology 1984; 152:463-464.

64. Close LG, O'Connor WE. Sphenoethmoidal mucoceles with intracranial extension. Otolaryngol Head Neck Surg 1983; 91:350-357.

65. Osborn AG, Johnson L, Roberts TS. Sphenoidal mucoceles with intracranial extension. J Comput Assist Tomogr 1979; 3:335-338.

66. Chui MC, Briant TDR, Gray T et al. Computed tomography of sphenoid sinus mucocele. J Otolaryngol 1983; 12:263-269.

67. Price HI, Batnitzky S, Karlin CA et al. Multiple paranasal sinus mucoceles. J Comput Assist Tomogr 1981; 5:122-125.

68. Perugini S, Pasquini U, Menichelli F et

al. Mucoceles in the paranasal sinus involving the orbit: CT signs in 43 cases. Neuroradiology 1982; 23:133-139.

69. Demaerel P, Brown P, Kendall BE et al. Case report: allergic aspergillosis of the sphenoid sinus: pitfall on MRI. Brit J Radiol 1993; 66:260-263.

70. Chang T, Teng MMH, Wang SF et al. Aspergillosis of the paranasdal sinuses. Neuroradiol 1992; 34:520-523.

71. Romett JL, Newman RK. Aspergillosis of the nose and paranasal sinuses. Laryngoscope 1982; 92:764-766.

72. Centeno RS, Bentson JR, Mancuso AA. CT scanning in rhinocerebral mucormycosis and aspergillosis. Radiology 1981; 140:383-389.

73. Shugar JMA, Som PM, Robbins A et al. Maxillary sinusitis as a cause of cheek swelling. Arch Otolaryngol 1982; 108:507-508.

74. Kopp W, Fotter R, Steiner H et al. Aspergillosis of the paranasal sinuses. Radiology 1985; 156:715-716.

75. Stammberger J, Jakse A, Beaufort F. Aspergillosis of the paranasal sinuses: x-ray diagnosis, histopathology and clinical aspects. Ann Otol Rhinol Laryngol 1984; 93:251-256.

76. Myerowitz RL, Guggenheimer J, Barnes L. Infectious diseases of the head and neck. In: Barnes L, ed. Surgical pathology of the head and neck. Vol 2. New York, NY: Marcel Dekker Inc, 1985; 1771-1822.

77. Waxman JE, Spector JG, Sale SR et al. Allergic aspergillus sinusitis: concepts in diagnosis and treatment of a new clinical entity. Laryngoscope 1987; 97:261-266.

78. Daghistani KJ, Jamal TS, Zaher S et al. Allergic aspergillus sinusitis with proptosis. J Laryngol Otol 1992; 106:799-803.

79. Milroy CM, Blanshard JD, Lucas S et al. Aspergillosis of the nose and paranasal sinuses. J Clin Pathol 1989; 42:123-127.

80. Kameswaran M, Al-Waddei A, Khurana P et al. Rhinocerebral aspergillosis. J Laryngol Otol 1992; 106:981-985.

81. Blitzer A, Lawson W. Fungal infections of the nose and paranasal sinuses. Part I. Otolaryngol Clin No Am 1993; 26:1007-1035.

82. Blatt SP, Lucey DR, DeHoff D et al. Rhinocerebral zygomycosis in a patient with AIDS. J Infect Dis 1991; 164:215-216.

83. Tyson JC, Gittelman PD, Jacobs JB et

al. Recurrent mucormycosis of the paranasal sinuses in an immunologically competant host. Otolaryngol Head Neck Surg 1992; 107:115-119.

84. Pafrey N. Improved diagnosis and prognosis of mucormycosis: a clinocopathologic study of 33 cases. Medicine 1986; 65:113-123.

85. Mader JT, Ream RS, Heath PW. *Petriellidium boydii (Allescheria boydii)* sphenoidal sinusitis. JAMA 1978; 239:2368-2369.

86. Travis LB, Roberts GD, Wilson WR. Clinical significance of pseudallescheria boydii: a review of 10 years experience. Mayo Clin Proc 1985; 60:531-537.

87. Chapnick JS, Bach MC. Bacterial and fungal infections of the maxillary sinus. Otolaryngol Clin North Am 1976; 9:43-54.

88. Wheat LJ, Conolly-Stringfield PA, Baker RL et al. Disseminated histoplasmosis in AIDS: clinical findings, diagnosis and treatment, and review of the literature. Med 1990; 69:361-374.

89. Oda D, McDougal L, Fitsche T et al. Oral histoplasmosis as a presenting disease in AIDS. Oral Surg Oral Med Oral Pathol 1990; 70:631-636.

90. Browning DG, Schwartz DA, Jurado RL. Cryptococcosis of the larynx in a patient with AIDS: an unusual cause of fungal laryngitis. South Med J 1992; 85:762-764.

91. Lynch DP, Naftolin LZ. Oral Cryptococcus neoformans infection in AIDS. Oral Surg Oral Med Oral Pathol 1987; 64:449-453.

92. Boyle JO, Coulthard SW, Mandel RM. Laryngeal involvement in disseminated coccioidomycosis. Arch Otolaryngol Head Neck Surg 1991; 117:433-438.

93. Fish DG, Ampel NM, Galgiani JN et al. Coccidiodomycosis during HIV infection: a review of 77 patients. Med 1990; 69:384-390.

94. Richtsmeier WJ, Johns ME. Actinomycosis of the head and neck. In: Batsakis J, Savory J, eds. Critical review in clinical laboratory sciences. Vol 11. CRC Press Inc, 1979.

95. Bhatia PL, Obafunwa JO. Rare infections of the nose and paranasal sinuses. Trop Geograph Med 1990; 42:289-293.

96. Kingdom TT, Tami TA. Actinomycosis of the nasal septum in a patient infected with HIV. Otolaryngol Head Neck Surg 1994; 71:675-677.

97. MacGregor RR. A year's experience with tuberculosis in a private urban teaching hospital in the post-sanatorium era. Am J Med 1975; 58:221-228.

98. Bath AP, O'Flynn P, Gibbin KP. Nasopharyngeal tuberculosis. J Laryngol Otol 1992; 106:1079-1080.

99. Centers for Disease Control. Annual summary 1980. Morbidity-Mortality Weekly Report 1981; 19:3.

100. McNulty JS, Fassett RL. Syphilis: an otolaryngologic perspective. Laryngoscope 1981; 91:889-905.

101. Olansky S. Syphilis rediscovered. In: Disease-a-month. Chicago, Ill: Year Book Medical Publishers, 1967; 1-30.

102. Larsen S. Syphilis. Clin Lab Med 1989; 9:545-557.

103. Andraca R, Edson RS, Kern EB. Rhinoscleroma: a growing concern in the US? Mayo Clin Proc 1993; 68:1151-1157.

104. Becker TS, Shum TK, Waller TS et al. Radiological aspects of rhinoscleroma. Radiology 1981; 141:433-438.

105. Reder PA, Neel HB. Blastomycosis in otolaryngology: review of a large series. Laryngoscope 1993; 103:53-58.

106. Lazow SK, Seldin RD, Solomon MP. South American blastomycosis of the maxilla: report of a case. J Oral Maxillofac Surg 1990; 48:68-71.

107. Sposto MR, Scully C, Almeida OP et al. Ora; paracoccidioidomycosis. A study of 36 South American patients. Oral Surg Oral Med Oral Pathol 1993; 75:461-465.

108. Beeson PB, McDermott W: Textbook of medicine. 14th Edition. Philadelphia, Pa: WB Saunders Co, 1975; 164-539.

109. Lasser A, Smith HW. Rhinosporidiosis. Arch Otolaryngol 1974; 102:308.

110. Thianprait M, Thagerngpol K. Rhinosporidiosis. Curr Top Med Mycol 1989; 3:64-85.

111. Harrison TR: Harrison's principles of internal medicine. 9th Edition. New York, NY: McGraw-Hill Inc, 1980.

112. Fauci AS, Wolff SM. Wegener's granulomatosis and related diseases. Disease of the Month 1977; 23:1.

113. Harrison DFN. Midline destructive granuloma: fact or fiction? Laryngoscope 1987; 97:1049-1053.

114. Gordon WW, Cohn AW, Greenberg SD et al. Nasal sarcoidosis. Arch Otolaryngol 1976; 102:11-14.

115. Mailland AAJ, Geopfert H. Nasal and paranasal sarcoidosis. Arch Otolaryngol 1978; 104:197-201.

116. Green WH. Mucormycosis infection of the craniofacial structure. AJR 1967; 101:802-806.

117. Paling MR, Roberts RL, Fauci AS. Paranasal sinus obliteration in Wegener granulomatosis. Radiology 1982; 144:539-543.

118. Zizmor J, Noyek A. Radiology of the nose and paranasal sinuses. In: Paparella MM, Shumrick DA. Otolaryngology. Vol 1. Philadelphia, Pa: WB Saunders Co, 1973; 1043-1095.

119. Taveras JM, Wood EH. Diagnostic neuroradiology. Baltimore, Md: Williams & Wilkins, 1964; 141-142.

120. Dodd GD, Jing BS. Radiology of the nose, paranasal sinuses and nasopharynx. Baltimore, Md: Williams & Wilkins, 1977; 131-133.

121. Verbin RS, Barnes L. Cysts and cyst-like lesions of the oral cavity, jaws and neck. In: Barnes L, ed. Surgical pathology of the head and neck. Vol 2. New York, NY: Marcel Dekker Inc, 1985; 1278-1281.

122. Koenig H, Lenz M, Sauter R. Temporal bone region: high resolution MR imaging using surface coils. Radiology 1986; 159:191-194.

123. Latack JT, Kartush JM, Kemink JL et al. Epidermoidomas of the cerebellopontine angle and temporal bone: CT and MR aspects. Radiology 1985; 157:361-366.

124. Urken ML, Som PM, Lawson W et al. The abnormally large frontal sinus I: a practical method for its determination based upon an analysis of 100 normal patients. Laryngoscope 1987; 97:602-605.

125. Urken ML, Som PM, Lawson W et al. Abnormally large frontal sinuses II: nomenclature, pathology and symptoms. Laryngoscope 1987; 97:606-611.

126. Dross PE, Lally JF, Bonier B. Pneumosinus dilatans and arachnoid cyst: a unique association. AJNR 1992; 13:209-211.

127. Benedikt RA, Brown DC, Roth MK et al. Spontaneous drainage of an ethmoid mucocele: a possible cause of pneumosinus dilatans. AJNR 1991; 12:729-731.

128. Lombardi G. Radiology in neuro-ophthalmology. Baltimore, Md: Williams & Wilkins, 1967.

129. Kutnick SL, Kerth JD. Acute sinusitis and otitis: their complications and surgical treatment. Otolaryngol Clin North Am 1976; 9:689-701.

130. Carter BL, Bankoff MS, Fisk JD.

Computed tomographic detection of sinusitis responsible for intracranial and extracranial infections. Radiology 1983; 147:739-742.

131. Zimmerman RA, Bilaniuk LT. CT of orbital infection and its cerebral complications. Am J Roentgenol 1980; 134:45-50.

132. Rothstein J, Maisel RH, Berlinger NT et al. Relationship of optic neuritis to disease of the paranasal sinus. Laryngoscope 1984; 94:1501-1508.

133. Bilaniuk LT, Zimmerman RA. Computer assisted tomography: sinus lesions with orbital involvement. Head Neck Surg 1980; 2:293-301.

134. Som PM, Brandwein MS, Maldjian C et al. Inflammatory pseudotumor of the maxillary sinus: CT and MR findings in six cases. American Journal of Roentgenology 1994;

163:689-692.

135. Kaufman DM, Litman N, Miller MH. Sinusitis: induced subdural empyema. Neurology 1983; 33:123-132.

136. Williams HL. Infections and granulomas of the nasal airways and paranasal sinuses. In: Paparella MM, Shumrick DA. Otolaryngology. Vol 3. Head and neck. Philadelphia, Pa: WB Saunders Co, 1973; 27-32.

137. Kay NJ, Setia RN, Stone J. Relevance of conventional radiography in indicating maxillary antral lavage. Ann Otol Rhinol Laryngol 1984; 93:37-38.

138. Eichel BS. The medical and surgical approach in management of the unilateral opacified antrum. Laryngoscope 1977; 87:737-750.

139. Price HI, Batnitzky S, Karlin LA et al. Giant nasal rhinolith. AJNR 1981; 2:371-373.

140. RSNA case of the day: case IV, rhinolith. Radiology 1983; 146:251-252.

141. Som PM, Lidov M. The significance of sinonasal radiodensities: ossification, calcification, or residual bone? American Journal of Neuroradiology 1994; 15:917-922.

142. Yousem DM, Turner WJD, Snyder PJ et al. Kallmann's syndrome: MR evaluation of olfactory system. AJNR 1993; 14:839-843.

143. Li C, Yousem DM, Doty RL et al. Neuroimaging in patients with olfactory dysfunction. AJR 1994; 162:411-418.

144. Knon JR, Ragland RL, Brown RS et al. Kallmann syndrome: MR findings. AJNR 1993; 14:845-851.m

Section Two
TUMORS AND TUMORLIKE CONDITIONS

Carcinomas of the nasal cavity and paranasal sinuses are rare, comprising only 0.2% to 0.8% of all malignancies and about 3% of all tumors that arise in the head and neck.[1,2] The SEER (surveillance, epidemiology, and end results) program of the National Institute of Health tabulated more than 50,000 upper aerodigestive tract malignancies from 1973 to 1987, the majority of which were carcinomas. Only 3.6% of these malignancies occurred in the sinonasal tract.[3] Despite their statistically small incidence, sinonasal tumors are a clinically significant group of tumors because of their poor prognosis. The grave outlook for these patients stems from the advanced stage of the tumor at the time of diagnosis and the reluctance of surgeons to pursue aggressive treatment for fear of creating either an undesirable cosmetic deformity, a prolonged morbidity, or gross dysfunction. Furthermore the complex, compact anatomy of the region often limits the extent of surgical resection and may lead to unwanted complications of radiation therapy caused by the difficulties of placing adequate treatment fields.[4,5] Although chemotherapy is starting to play a bigger role in the treatment of patients with sinonasal tumors, the primary treatment modality remains surgery. Because sinonasal tumors often coexist with chronic inflammatory disease, the tumor can clinically be overshadowed by the infection, often adding to a delay in tumor diagnosis. Pain is commonly associated with infection and is not routinely associated with these tumors. However, pain may signify perineural tumor invasion, especially with adenoid cystic carcinoma. When tumor pain is present, it usually signifies relatively advanced tumor growth. Pain in the teeth or gums may indicate the presence of an antral tumor, whereas a headache may signify skull base and intracranial invasion. Inexplicably, pain is not often associated with the bone destruction that accompanies these tumors. Complaints of patients with sinonasal tumors include diplopia, decreasing vision, proptosis, nasal stuffiness, anosmia, nasal-quality voice, epistaxis, and a facial mass. Patients with antral and ethmoidal cancers have an average delay of 6 months between the onset of symptoms and the establishment of a final diagnosis.[4] Most often these tumors are not diagnosed until they are at a high stage and there is invasion of locoregional structures. Antral tumors may cause trismus, epiphora, orbital pain and displacement, or trigeminal or sphenopalatine ganglion-related deficits secondary to dorsal tumor spread. Ethmoid tumors cause nasal stuffiness, orbital complaints, and headache from intracranial spread. Frontal sinus tumors deform the face, spread intracranially, or extend into the orbits. Sphenoid sinus tumors extend into the nasopharynx, intracranially (especially to the cavernous sinuses), the orbit, and the orbital apex.

As imaging technology has improved, superior tumor mapping and staging have provided more accurate information that permits more realistic treatment planning with regard to cure versus palliation.[6] Surgical techniques have also improved, and with detailed tumor mapping, better tumor extirpation can be attained with less morbidity and deformity. More accurate placement of radiation fields can also be attained. To provide the tumor mapping necessary to make a decision about operability and curability, the radiologist must be aware of the critical areas of potential tumor extension that will alter a surgical or treatment approach. These areas include any tumor extension into the floor of the anterior and middle cranial fossae, the pterygopalatine fossae, the orbits, and the palate.[7] In addition, because of the proximity of the various paranasal sinuses to one another and their free communication via the nasal fossae, tumors may spread with ease from one sinus to another. Thus the radiologist must detail the precise sinus involvement, remembering that tumor mapping may alter not only the surgical approach but the radiation treatment plan as well. New color 3-D reconstructions allow the colorized tumor to be visualized within the framework of the facial bones and skull base. Although this is primarily a communication tool with the clinicians, newer treatment-planning computers are able to take advantage of the 3-D data.

Nodal metastasis from sinonasal carcinomas is one of the gravest prognostic signs. Although the primary lymph nodes draining the paranasal sinuses and nasal vault are the retropharyngeal nodes, these nodes or their lymphatic channels are frequently obliterated in adults by repeated childhood infections. Because of this, in adults the secondary nodes, the upper internal jugular and submandibular groups, are the ones most often involved by tumor. Metastasis to these nodes occurs in about 15% of patients and usually signifies tumor extension to the skin, alveolar buccal sulcus, or pterygoid musculature, areas well demonstrated by sectional imaging techniques.[5] The radiologist should be thorough and precise in reporting tumor extension in these sites. With sinonasal carcinomas, distant metastases were present in 34% of autopsied patients. The presence of cervical nodal disease correlated best with such distant metastases.[8]

Precise tumor mapping is necessary to make accurate decisions about irradiation fields or planned surgery. This requires the radiologist to distinguish tumor from adjacent inflammatory disease. Inherent differential CT attenuation values may allow some distinction between a cellular tumor and the lower attenuation of watery secretions. However, if the secretions are desiccated or there is primarily inflamed mucosa, the attenuation values may be similar. A more accurate differentiation may be achieved on contrast CT. But even in these cases, similar tumor and inflammatory attenuation values often raise serious doubts as to where the actual tumor margin is located. It is here that T2W MRI has great application. Because inflammatory infiltrates have high water content, they have high T2W signal intensities on MRI. By comparison, virtually all of the sinonasal tumors are highly cellular and at most have an intermediate intensity signal on T2W studies (Fig. 4-125).[9,10] High T2W signal intensities can be present with benign or low-grade minor salivary gland tumors, some schwannomas, rare hemangiomatous lesions, and polypoid tumors such as inverted papillomas. A diagnosis of one of these tumors should alert the radiologist that distinction between tumor and inflammation based solely on T2W signal intensity may not be accurate.

When tumors are small, they may often elude detection by both the clinician and the radiologist. Unfortunately, it is at this early stage that tumors may be the most curable.[5] However, based on imaging criteria, unless bone involve-

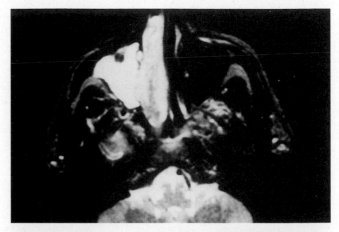

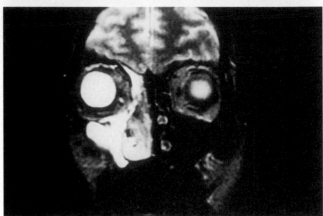

FIG. 4-125   Axial (**A**) and coronal (**B**) T2W MR scans show a polypoid, nonhomogeneous right nasal fossa mass that has intermediate signal intensity. The right maxillary sinus, the right lateral ethmoid sinuses, and the lower nasal fossa have high signal intensity material that represents obstructed secretions. The tumor does not extend directly to the orbital margin. Such a high degree of tumor mapping was not possible on CT, where the secretions and tumor had similar attenuations. Inverted papilloma and obstructed secretions.

ment is detected it may not be possible to confirm a malignant diagnosis. When the tumor becomes large enough to affect the adjacent bone, the pattern of bony involvement may suggest a particular pathologic differential diagnosis. This concept that the radiographic pattern of bone destruction can be related to various tumors is not new. However, it was not until the CT era that the radiologist could achieve highly detailed bone resolution in multiple planes, allowing distinction between aggressive bone destruction and bone remodeling.[11-13]

If the bone is aggressively eroded or destroyed so that only small fragments remain of the sinus wall or nasal vault, the most likely tumor is a squamous cell carcinoma (Figs. 4-126 to 4-128). Far less common tumors such as some sarcomas and lymphomas and metastases from lung and breast tumors can also aggressively destroy bone. Most sinonasal sarcomas, mucoceles, polyps, inverted papillomas, and rarer lesions such as minor salivary gland tumors, schwannomas,

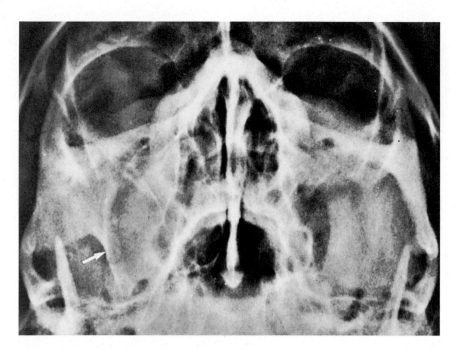

FIG. 4-126 Waters view shows that the lateral wall of the left maxillary sinus is totally destroyed. The right lateral antral wall *(arrow)* is intact. This is an example of aggressive bone destruction. Left antral squamous cell carcinoma.

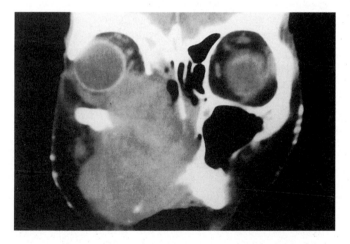

FIG. 4-127 Coronal CT scan shows a highly destructive mass in the right maxillary sinus. The orbital floor is eroded, and the orbit is invaded. The medial and lateral sinus walls are also destroyed, and the tumor has invaded the ethmoid sinuses, the nasal fossa, and the cheek. The bone is not remodeled. Antral squamous cell carcinoma.

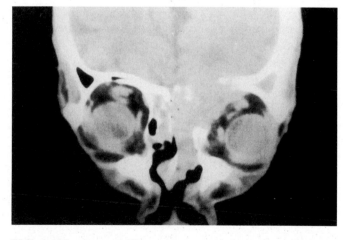

FIG. 4-128 Coronal CT scan shows a highly destructive mass in the left ethmoid sinuses, breaking into the left orbit, the nasal fossa, and the anterior cranial fossa. The involved bone is destroyed rather than remodeled. Ethmoid squamous cell carcinoma.

extramedullary plasmacytomas, most lymphomas, esthesioneuroblastomas, and hemangiopericytomas tend to remodel bone rather than aggressively destroy it (Figs. 4-129 to 4-130). Most tumors with bony involvement have either an aggressively destructive appearance or a remodeling pattern. The radiologist can use this pattern of bone involvement to occasionally question some histologic diagnoses. For example, if a patient has a unilateral polypoid nasal mass, a biopsy read as "large cell lymphoma," and a

predominantly aggressive pattern of bone destruction on imaging, the radiologist should question the diagnosis and request that the surgeon obtain a second biopsy specimen for electron microscopy and immunohistochemistry. The diagnosis in reality may be an anaplastic carcinoma or melanoma, two tumors that are included in the pathologic differential diagnosis of large cell lymphoma. Immunohistochemistry and electron microscopy are very helpful in establishing an accurate pathologic diagnosis. The former

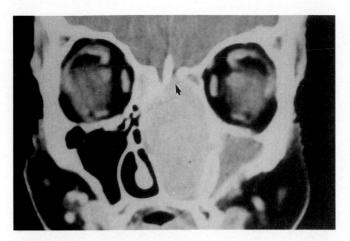

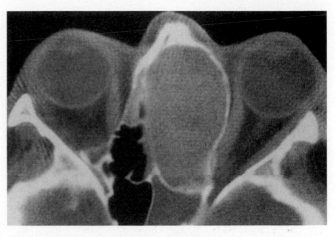

FIG. 4-129 Coronal CT scan shows an expansile left nasal fossa mass that has obstructed the left maxillary sinus, which is filled with lower attenuation secretions. Most of the bone around the tumor is intact and remodeled about the lesion. There is a focal area of bone erosion in the cribriform plate *(arrow)*. Olfactory neuroblastoma.

FIG. 4-130 Axial CT scan shows and expansile nasal fossae and left ethmoid sinus mass, around which the facial bones are remodeled. This is not the appearance expected of a typical squamous cell carcinoma. Schwannoma.

method may be performed on unstained slides from the original biopsy (if it is adequate); the latter method is best performed on tissue specifically minced and fixed in cold gluteraldehyde solutions. Other lesions to be considered in the differential diagnosis include embryonal rhabdomyosarcoma, extramedullary plasmacytoma, esthesioneuroblastoma, and Ewing's sarcoma. Many institutions routinely perform electron microscopic and immunohistochemical testing on all round cell, undifferentiated tumors.

Tumor biology and prognosis are multifaceted issues. Host immune surveillance may limit tumor growth for a variable period of time, sometimes for many years. The successive activation of tumoral oncogenes can correlate with tumor progression or the acquisition of aggressive features. In addition to tumor biology, the critical anatomic location of the neoplasm has prognostic significance. For instance, a lesion confined to the antrum generally has a better prognosis than one located in the pterygopalatine fossa or central skull base. Certain tumors though are highly aggressive regardless of location or even benign appearance on imaging. For example, a nasal fossa melanoma usually has a benign polypoid imaging appearance, yet the 5-year survival prognosis is abysmal. The pathologic diagnosis may be more important in predicting prognosis than predicting the manner by which the tumor destroys or remodels bone. The lethal propensity of certain tumors is, unfortunately, poorly understood. On the other hand, the overall pattern of bone involvement can be used by the imager to suggest a specific differential diagnosis.

In addition to noting the pattern of bone involvement, any alteration of bone density also should be described because sclerotic bone reactions are uncommon with sinonasal tumors. Most often, dense bone in the facial skeleton reflects the presence of chronic inflammation and is usually found with chronic bacterial sinusitis. However, if cou-

pled with areas of focal bone erosion or remodeling, these bone changes should suggest a more aggressive infection such as fungal disease or a granulomatous disease. Although uncommon, frank osteomyelitis in the sinonasal cavities can occur and usually appears as foci of bone rarefaction and sclerosis, often with sequestra. Radiation osteitis also can produce sclerotic bone; however, extensive bony fragmentation is common. Sinonasal bony sclerosis secondary to a tumor is rare. It has been seen with anaplastic carcinomas, nasopharyngeal carcinomas, and osteosarcomas. The dense expanded bone of fibrous dysplasia and ossifying fibroma is usually characteristic. The facial bone changes of Paget's disease may be indistinguishable from those of osteoblastic metastatic prostate cancer. Osteoblastic metastases from breast carcinoma can occur; however, such lesions are usually a mixed blastic and lytic process. Dense osteoblastic bone may also be found as a reaction to meningiomas.

Tumoral calcifications are uncommon in the sinonasal cavities. Discrete solitary or multiple, calcifications usually signify a chronic inflammatory process, either bacterial or fungal. They have also been reported with osteoblastomas, osteochondromas, chondromas, chondrosarcomas, and esthesioneuroblastomas. Diffuse calcifications within a lesion with well-defined margins invariably signifies a benign fibroosseous disease. Alternately, diffuse calcifications in a lesion with poorly defined or invasive margins augers a sarcoma.[14] One problem for the radiologist is that a suspected calcification may actually represent ossification or residual bone. CT cannot distinguish between these possibilities.

Although there is a constant attempt on the part of a radiologist to correlate the imaging appearance with a specific pathologic diagnosis, in only rare instances is this truely possible. This statement reflects the similarity in the CT and MR appearances of different tumors that in most cases prohibits a confident pathologic diagnosis from being made.

Thus the primary contribution of the radiologist is to accurately map the tumor, to be aware of the critical anatomic sites that will influence the treatment planning, and finally to suggest a possible diagnosis that may allow treatment planning to proceed until a final pathologic diagnosis is made.

PAPILLOMAS

The mucosa of the nasal fossae and paranasal sinuses is of ectodermal origin. During maturation the mucosa differentiates into ciliated columnar epithelium and into the mucous Bowman's glands. This unique mucosa may give rise to three distinct histomorphologic papillomas: fungiform, inverted, and cylindric cell. Collectively they are often called Schneiderian papillomas.[1,2] These papillomas are not the result of allergy, chronic infection, smoking, or other noxious environmental agents because the papillomas are almost invariably unilateral in location. It has been suggested that their rarity in children mitigates against a viral etiology.[15-17] However, many sensitive and specific viral studies confirm the association of fungiform and inverted papillomas with human papilloma virus.[18,19] Schneiderian papillomas are uncommon, representing only 0.4% to 4.7% of all sinonasal tumors, which is 25 to 50 times less common than the pedestrian polyp.[2]

Fungiform papillomas (septal, squamous, or exophytic) comprise 50% of Schneiderian papillomas. They usually occur in males between the ages of 20 to 50 years and 95% arise on the nasal septum. They are solitary (75%), unilateral (96%), have a warty or verrucous appearance, and are quite unlikely to undergo malignant transformation.[2,15,20] Histologically, fungiform papillomas have stratified keratinized squamous mucosa on fibrovascular stalks.

Inverted papillomas (endophytic papillomas) comprise 47% of Schneiderian papillomas and most commonly occur in males between the ages of 40 to 70 years. Characteristically, they arise from the lateral nasal wall near the middle turbinate and extend into the sinuses. This secondary extension involves the maxillary and ethmoidal sinuses, but extension into the sphenoid and frontal sinuses has been documented.[2,15] Rarely an isolated inverted papilloma may arise within a sinus without any nasal involvement.[2,15] Inverted papillomas arise from the medial septal wall only rarely and fewer than 4% occur bilaterally. The most common presenting symptoms are nasal obstruction, epistaxis, and anosmia. Secondary sinusitis and tumor extension into the sinuses and orbits can cause pain, purulent nasal discharge, proptosis, diplopia, and a nasal vocal quality.

Microscopically, hyperplastic squamous epithelium can be seen replacing seromucinous ducts and glands, resulting in an endophytic growth pattern. The surrounding mucosa usually reveals squamous metaplasia and hyperplasia-incipient inverted papilloma-like changes. For this reason, mere polypectomy results in high recurrence rates that vary from 27% to 73%.[2] The lateral rhinotomy with en bloc resection of the lateral nasal wall and mucosa is the preferred procedure for all but the smallest localized lesions. Using a more extensive surgical approach has dropped recurrence rates to 0% to 14%, with most relapses occurring within 2 years of surgery.[2,15]

Carcinoma-exinverted papilloma has been reported in 3% to 24% (average 13%) of cases. Carcinoma may be concurrent with an inverted papilloma or develop subsequent to treated inverted papilloma. Most reported malignancies are of squamous cell carcinomas, but verrucous carcinoma, mucoepidermoid carcinoma, spindle cell, clear cell, and adenocarcinomas may occur.[2]

Cylindric cell papillomas represent only 3% of the Schneiderian papillomas. They have many similarities to inverted papillomas, including an affinity for the lateral nasal wall, age of onset, and predominance in males. Microscopically, one sees stratified, tall (cylindrical) oncocytic cells with numerous small intraepithelial cysts, which are filled with mucin and neutrophils. The cysts occasionally cause confusion with rhinosporidiosis; but slightly less than superficial perusal at high power can resolve this confusion.[2]

The imaging findings for all of these papillomas can vary from a small nasal polypoid mass to an expansile nasal mass that has remodeled the nasal vault and extended into the sinuses, causing secondary obstructive sinusitis.[21] The MR findings are nonspecific for this tumor.[22,23] Although calcifications have been reported within the inverted papillomas, these radiodensities are in reality residual bone fragments.[14,24] The nasal septum usually remains intact but may be bowed to the opposite nasal vault wall (Figs. 4-125, 4-131 to 4-133).

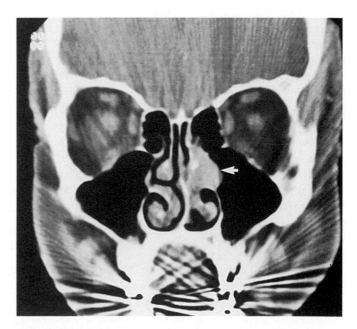

FIG. 4-131   Coronal CT scan shows a small polypoid mass in the left nasal fossa *(arrow)*. There is no associated bone destruction. Inverted papilloma.

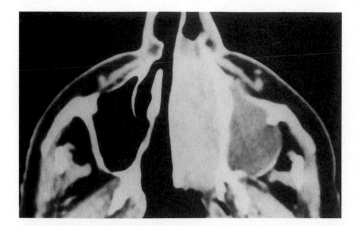

FIG. 4-132 Axial CT shows a large expansile, enhancing mass in the left nasal fossa, which has obstructed the left maxillary sinus, causing a mucocele to form as noted by the modeled left antral wall. The nasal vault bones are intact. Inverted papilloma.

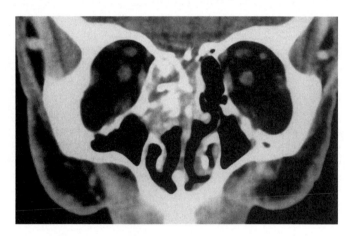

FIG. 4-133 Coronal CT scan shows a soft-tissue mass in the right ethmoid sinuses and adjacent upper nasal fossae. There are apparent calcifications within the tumor; however, at pathology these were all residual pieces of bone. Also note that the adjacent right lamina papyracea remains intact. Inverted papilloma.

ANGIOFIBROMAS

The nasopharyngeal angiofibroma (juvenile angiofibroma) is an uncommon, highly vascular, nonencapsulated, polypoid mass that is histologically benign but locally aggressive. It represents 0.05% of all head and neck neoplasms and almost exclusively occurs in males.[2] However, a few cases have been documented in females, and it has been suggested that when such a diagnosis is made, the patient should have sex chromosome studies to confirm that she is not a he or a mosaic.[25] The typical patient is a male between 10 and 18 years of age, although it may occasionally present in older patients.[2] The presenting symptoms include nasal obstruction, epistaxis, facial deformity, proptosis, nasal voice, sinusitis, nasal discharge, serous otitis media, headache, and anosmia.[2] Almost all angiofibromas originate from the posterior choanal tissue near the pterygopalatine fossa and

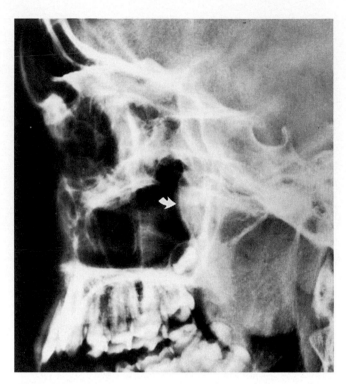

FIG. 4-134 Lateral view shows large nasopharyngeal mass that has displaced the posterior antral wall anteriorly *(arrow)*. The mass also extends into the sphenoid sinuses. Angiofibroma.

sphenopalatine foramen and fill the entire nasopharynx. Its growth is not symmetric, and one side is always the primary site of involvement. Extension into the pterygopalatine fossa occurs in 89% of the cases and results in widening of this fossa with resultant anterior bowing of the posterior ipsilateral antral wall.[26] Although other slowly growing lesions may also similarly widen the pterygopalatine fossa, (e.g., lymphomas, lymphoepitheliomas, schwannomas, and fibrous histiocytomas), 99% of the time the antral bowing is caused by nasopharyngeal angiofibromas.[27] The sphenoid sinus is involved by extension through the roof of the nasopharynx in 61% of cases. Angiofibromas also spread into the maxillary and ethmoid sinuses, 43% and 35% repectively.[25] Intracranial extension occurs in 5% to 20% of cases and primarily involves the middle cranial fossa.[2] Most often this extension progresses from the pterygopalatine fossa into the orbit (through the inferior orbital fissure) and then intracranially through the superior orbital fissure. Direct intracranial extension from the sphenoid or ethmoid sinuses is uncommon. Biopsy should not be attempted in an outpatient or office facility because of tumor vascularity. Sectional imaging and angiography are sufficient to establish the diagnosis.[28] Histologically, one sees thick-walled vessels embedded in densely collagenized fibrous stroma. The differential diagnosis includes a fibrosed antrochoanal or nasal polyp.

Plain-film findings of angiofibromas include a soft-tissue nasopharyngeal mass, widening of the pterygopalatine fossa

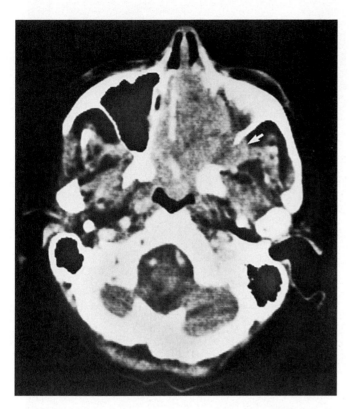

FIG. 4-135 Axial postcontrast CT scan shows a left nasopharyngeal and nasal fossa enhancing mass that has widened the left pterygopalatine fossa and extended into the left infratemporal fossa *(arrow)*. Angiofibroma.

with anterior bowing of the posterior antral wall, and opacification of the sphenoidal sinus (Fig. 4-134). A polypoid nasal mass may cloud the ipsilateral ethmoid and maxillary sinuses. If the superior orbital fissure is widened, intracranial extension will be present.

Contrast CT shows an enhancing mass with the anatomic distribution described above (Figs. 4-134 to 4-137). Intraorbital or intracranial extension is much better visualized on CT than on plain films. On contrast CT the imaging must be done while contrast material is flowing freely. If scanning is delayed, the rich vascular tumor network washes out the contrast medium. Dynamic scanning also identifies the highly vascular nature of these tumors.[29] MRI reveals a mass of intermediate signal intensity on T1W and T2W sequences, with multiple-flow voids that represent the major tumor vessels (Figs. 4-137, 4-138). The primary task of the imager is to map the lesion for the surgeon and in particular to document any intracranial spread. Skull base tumor extension is generally resectable by current surgical techniques.

Angiography demonstrates that the major feeding vessels are the internal maxillary artery and ascending pharyngeal artery on the dominant side (Fig. 4-139). Cross-circulation from contralateral branches of the external carotid artery and occasional feeding branches from the internal carotid arteries are found. The latter is usually associated with intracranial tumor extension. Subselective angiography is usually necessary to identify all of the feeding vessels. Preoperative embolization of the external carotid artery nutrient branches greatly reduces the blood loss at surgery.[2]

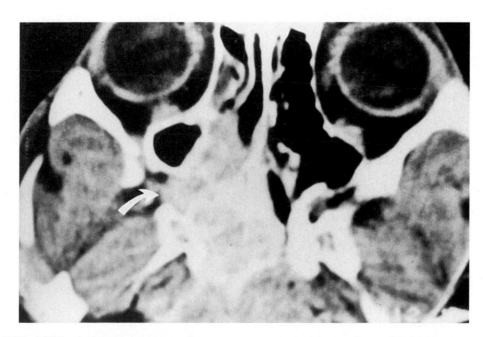

FIG. 4-136 Axial postcontrast CT scan shows an enhancing nasopharyngeal mass that has widened the right pterygopalatine fossa *(arrow)* and extended into the sphenoid sinus. Anteriorly there is minimal extension into the right nasal fossa. Angiofibroma.

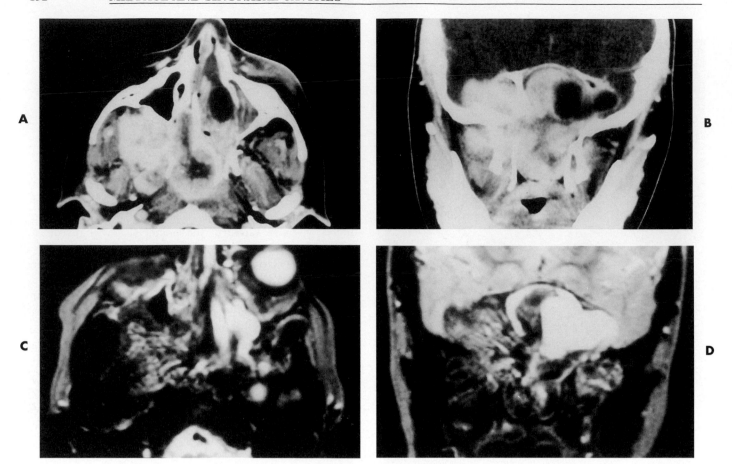

FIG. 4-137   Axial (**A**) and coronal (**B**) CT scans show a large enhancing mass that fills the nasopharynx and nasal fossae, bows the posterior wall of the right maxillary sinus forward, and extends into the right infratemporal fossa. The tumor has also destroyed the floor of the sphenoid sinus and the right middle cranial fossa. There is a nonenhancing region in the vicinity of the left sphenoid sinus. Axial (**C**) T2W and coronal (**D**) proton density MR scans show that the mass is filled with signal voids, reflecting its highly vascular nature. The left sphenoid sinus is filled with fluid. Large angiofibroma with a left sphenoid sinus mucocele. The skull base floor was not destroyed but deossified from the chronic pressure of the tumor. Both cavernous sinuses were intact but elevated by the mass.

The treatment of choice is surgery. Unresectable intracranial disease, if present, can be irradiated. Control rates of 78% using a dose of 30 to 35 Gy have been reported, and an additional 15% of the cases can be controlled by a second course of radiotherapy.[30] Although the radiation affects tumor vascularity, the fibrous tumor component remains unchanged.[2] Experts disagree over the effect of estrogen therapy on angiofibromas. Although some cases of decreased tumor size and vascularity have been reported after estrogen therapy, this response is not achieved in most patients.[2] Similarly the role of chemotherapy remains unclear.

ANGIOMATOUS POLYPS

The angiomatous polyp is a fibrosed and vascularized nasal polyp, presumably the response to minor trauma.[31] The significance of this lesion is that histologically it can be confused with a nasopharyngeal angiofibroma.[26] Several points differentiate these two lesions.

1. The angiomatous polyp is located primarily in the nasal fossa and not in the nasopharynx.
2. The polyp does not extend into the pterygopalatine fossa and only rarely protrudes into the sphenoid sinuses. In these cases the tumor enters the sinus through the anterior wall and not the sinus floor, as with angiofibromas.
3. These polyps do not extend intracranially.
4. On angiography the polyps have only a few demonstrable feeding vessels compared with the rich vascular supply of the angiofibroma.
5. On CT the angiomatous polyp does not enhance as well as the angiofibroma.
6. Vascular flow voids are not seen on MRI.
7. These polyps are easily "shelled out" surgically as is a routine nasal polyp, whereas the nasopharyngeal angiofibroma is difficult to remove from its primary attachment site.
8. Angiography and embolization are not necessary in

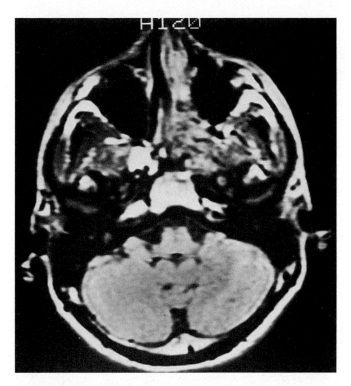

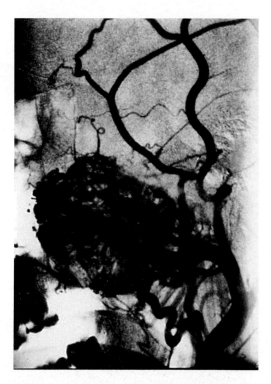

FIG. 4-138 Axial T1W MR through the skull base shows a nasopharyngeal and nasal fossa mass that extends through the left pterygopalatine fossa into the infratemporal fossa. The mass has low to intermediate signal intensity and multiple areas of signal (flow) void. Angiofibroma.

FIG. 4-139 Lateral subtraction angiogram shows the typical, highly vascular tumor appearance of an angiofibroma.

patients with angiomatous polyps (Fig. 4-140). Thus because the pathologist may confuse these lesions if a biopsy is attempted, the radiologist may be the first physician to identify the tumor and thereby render further diagnostic procedures unnecessary.

SQUAMOUS CELL CARCINOMAS

When the distribution of sinonasal carcinomas is analyzed, 25% to 58% of the tumors arise in the antrum; however, the maxillary sinus is secondarily involved by extension in at least 80% of all patients. The nasal cavity is the site of origin in 25% to 35% of cases, the ethmoid complex in 10% of cases, and only only 1% of tumors arise in the sphenoid and frontal sinuses.[1,2] The incidence of squamous cell carcinoma of the nose has an epidemiologic relationship with nickel exposure. Workers exposed to nickel have a 40 to 250 times greater chance of developing this cancer.[32] Workers involved in the production of wood furniture, chromium, mustard gas, isopropyl alcohol, and radium are also at risk for developing carcinomas of the nasal cavity and paranasal sinuses. The latency period from onset of occupational exposure to tumor discovery may be up to three decades. Some 15% to 20% of the patients have a history of chronic sinusitis and polyposis; however, it is doubtful whether a cause-and-effect relationship exists.[2] Coexistant inverted and cylindric cell papillomas, previous radiation, and

immunosuppression (i.e., lack of immune surveillance) may increase the risk of sinonasal carcinoma development.[2,33]

Nasal cavity carcinomas have a predisposition for males between 55 and 65 years of age. Most are low-grade tumors arising on the nasal septum near the mucocutaneous junction. The middle turbinate is also a common site.[33,34] Patient prognosis relates to tumor stage rather than exact site within the nasal cavity.

The treatment may be surgery, radiation, or both. Local recurrences are found in 20% to 50% of the cases, and about 80% of these develop within the first year. Only 15% develop nodal metastases and only 10% have distant metastases. The overall 5-year survival rate is 62%. Metachronous or synchronous tumors are seen in 15% of patients with sinonasal carcinomas; 40% of the secondary tumors occur in the head and neck, and 60% occur below the clavicles in the lungs, gastrointestinal tract, and breasts.[2]

Squamous carcinoma of the maxillary sinus has been the most extensively studied of the sinonasal malignacies. The specific site of origin of antral carcinomas is thought to have prognostic significance and is important in planning therapy and in comparing the treatment results of various medical centers. Initially the antrum was divided into an infrastructure and a suprastructure; however, this classification was soon modified into an infrastructure, mesostructure, and suprastructure, with the lines of division being drawn on a coronal view of the sinuses through the antral floor and the

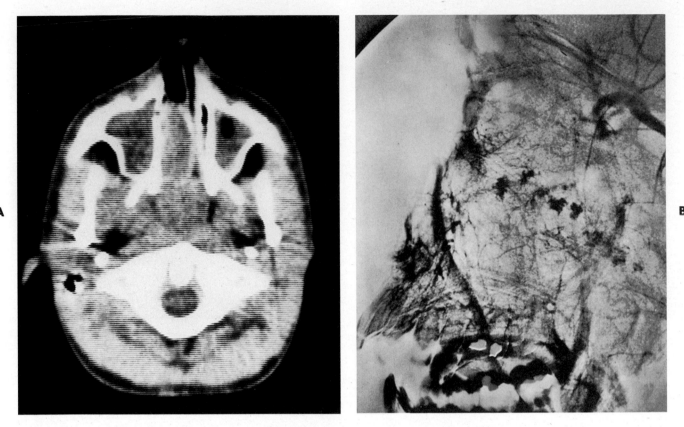

FIG. 4-140   A, Axial CT scan shows a right nasopharyngeal and nasal fossa mass that displaces the nasal septum to the left. The mass does not extend into the pterygopalatine fossa or the sphenoid sinus. A biopsy was read as an angiofibroma. **B,** A lateral subtraction angiogram shows only focal areas of increased vascularity without the typical vascular appearance of an angiofibroma. Angiomatous polyp.

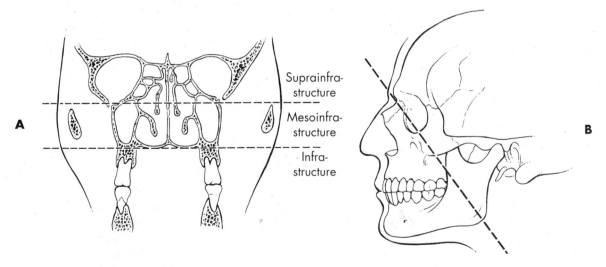

FIG. 4-141   A, Diagram of coronal view of the sinonasal cavities. The lines divide the maxillary sinuses into suprainfrastructure, mesoinfrastructure, and infrastructure portions. Tumors limited to and below the mesoinfrastructure usually can be resected by a partial or total maxillectomy without an orbital exenteration. **B,** Diagram of lateral view of skull with Ohngren's line drawn. Tumors anterior to this line tend to have a better prognosis.

antral roof (Fig. 4-141).[35] Using this system, tumors limited to the mesostructure and infrastructure require a partial or total maxillectomy, whereas tumors that involve the suprastructure require a total maxillectomy and orbital exenteration. Ohngren divided the antrum into posterosuperior and anteroinferior segments by drawing a line on a lateral view of the face from the medial canthus to the angle of the mandible (Fig. 4-141). He suggested that tumors limited to the anteroinferior segment had a better prognosis.[35] It was not until the early 1960s that the TNM system was first applied to antral cancers, and in 1976 The American Joint Committee on Cancer developed a TNM system based on Ohngren's line.[35] Harrison has criticized this TNM classification because it does not correspond to the clinical experience with these tumors.[36] He suggested that a T-1 tumor is limited to the antral mucosa without bone erosion and without regard to Ohngren's line because clinically it is often impossible to evaluate a tumor with regard to this line. A T-2 tumor has bone erosion but no extension beyond the bone, and a T-3 tumor has extension to the orbit, ethmoid complex, or facial skin. Finally a T-4 tumor extends to the nasopharynx, sphenoidal sinus, cribriform plate, or pterygopalatine fossa.

Antral carcinomas are almost twice as common in men as in women, and nearly 95% occur in patients over age 40 years.[2,37] The radioactive contrast medium Thorotrast is clearly established as an etiologic factor for antral carcinoma. Occupational exposures are also important promoters, as with nasal cavity carcinoma. Chronic sinusitis, polyposis, acute trauma, and chronic draining oroantral fistulas are less established as causative factors.[2]

When the tumors are small, they often are misdiagnosed as chronic sinusitis, nasal polyposis, lacrimal duct obstruction, tic douloureux, or cranial arteritis. By the time of diagnosis, between 40% and 60% of patients have facial asymmetry, a tumor bulge in the oral cavity, and tumor extension in the nasal cavity. At least one of these findings is present in almost 90% of cases.[38] The treatment of choice appears to be surgery combined with radiation. Despite controversy in the literature, it appears that survival rates are about the same for either preoperative or postoperative radiation. Postoperative radiation is associated with fewer complications.[2] The 5-year survival rate varies from 20% to almost 40%, with mean figures ranging from 25% to 30%.[39] The main cause of failure is local recurrence, and 75% of these occur within 5 months of initial treatment. Orbital exenteration is only performed if tumor involvement of the orbital periosteum is documented during surgery by frozen section evaluation. Curative surgery generally is not attempted if there is central skull base destruction, tumor in the pterygopalatine fossa, tumor extension into the nasopharynx, regional or generalized metastases, advanced patient age, poor general patient health, or the patient refuses to accept treatment.[2,40]

Although more than 100 cases of primary frontal sinus carcinoma have been reported, it is still a rare entity. The presenting symptoms are similar to those of acute frontal sinusitis; patients have pain and swelling over the frontal sinus. However, in patients with frontal sinus carcinoma the frontal bone erodes rapidly and few patients survive more than 2 years.[5]

Primary sphenoid sinus carcinoma is rare. It is often difficult to distinguish primary sphenoid carcinoma from secondary extension from a posterior ethmoid or nasal fossa carcinoma. As with frontal sinus carcinomas, few of these patients survive longer than 1 or 2 years.

Poorly differentiated or the anaplastic form of carcinoma can be confused histologically with rhabdomyosarcoma, melanoma, large cell lymphoma, esthesioneuroblastoma, and poorly differentiated extramedullary plasmacytoma.[41] As mentioned, immunohistochemistry and electron microscopy are helpful in confirming the diagnosis.

On plain films, all patients with paranasal sinus carcinoma have a soft-tissue mass in the sinus cavity, and 70% to 90% have evidence of bone destruction.[37,42] The primary reason to perform sectional imaging on these patients is to better visualize the extent of spread beyond the sinus cavity. On contrast CT, carcinomas enhance little if at all. On MRI these tumors have an intermediate T1W signal intensity and a slightly higher T2W signal intensity. Sinus carcinomas are fairly homogeneous; however, larger tumors may have areas of necrosis and hemorrhage (Figs. 4-126 to 4-128, 4-142 to 4-157). On contrast MR, most of these tumors enhance only minimally. The characteristic imaging feature of these carcinomas is their strong tendency to aggressively destroy bone regardless of tumor differentiation. Bone remodeling is uncommon. Usually the area of bone destruction is substantial compared with the size of the soft-tissue tumor mass.

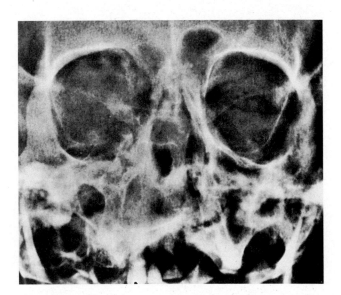

FIG. 4-142   Caldwell view shows clouding of the right ethmoid and maxillary sinuses with destruction of the right lamina papyracea and a portion of the floor of the right orbit. Squamous cell carcinoma.

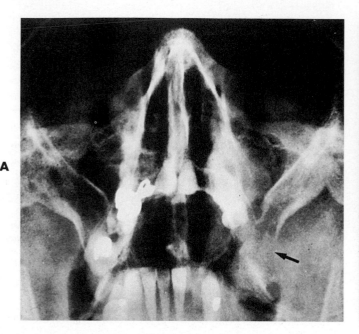

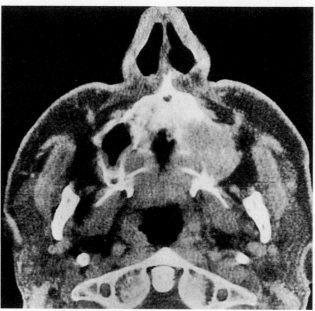

FIG. 4-143   A, Waters view shows destruction of the lower lateral wall of the left maxillary sinus *(arrow)*. **B,** Axial CT scan shows an aggressively destructive lesion of the lower antrum and palate. Squamous cell carcinoma.

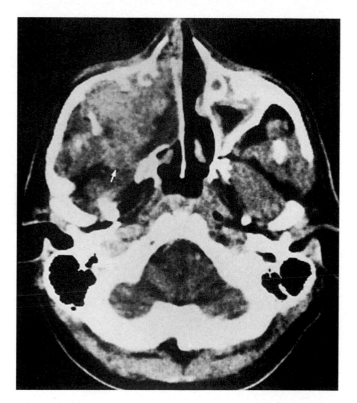

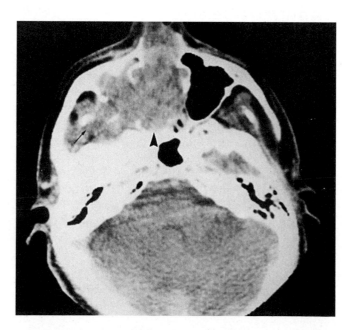

FIG. 4-144   Axial postcontrast CT scan shows a fairly homogeneous mass in the right antrum that has destroyed the medial and lateral walls of the sinus and extended into the infratemporal fossa *(arrow)*. Squamous cell carcinoma.

FIG. 4-145   Axial CT scan shows a destructive lesion of the nasal cavity and right antrum that has extended into the infratemporal fossa *(arrow)*, and the pterygopalatine fossa and eroded the skull base *(arrowhead)*. Squamous cell carcinoma.

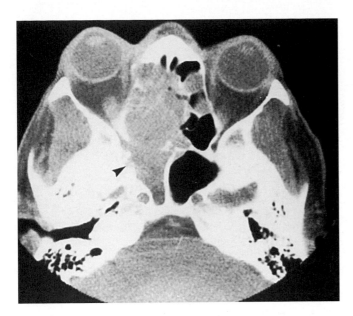

FIG. 4-146 Axial CT scan shows a destructive lesion of the right ethmoid sinus that has extended into the nasal fossa and the sphenoid sinus. There is focal erosion of the skull base *(arrowhead)*. Squamous cell carcinoma.

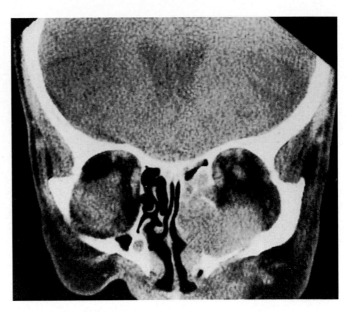

FIG. 4-147 Coronal CT scan shows a destructive lesion of the left ethmoid sinus that has extended into the orbit. Squamous cell carcinoma.

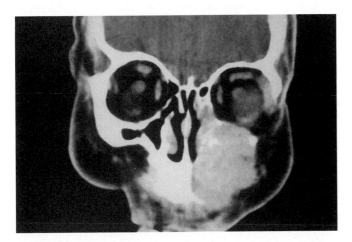

FIG. 4-148 Coronal CT scan shows a soft-tissue mass in the left maxilla, destroying the walls of the sinus and extending into the lower orbit, the cheek, and the nasal fossa. The left hard palate is also destroyed. This small degree of orbital invasion may escape clinical detection but is extremely important to note in the report of this study. In most cases this indicates that an orbital exenteration will have to be performed. Squamous cell carcinoma

ADENOCARCINOMAS

Approximately 10% of all sinonasal tumors are of glandular origin.[2] Sinonasal adenocarcinomas are either minor salivary gland tumors (e.g., adenoid cystic carcinomas, mucoepidermoid carcinomas, acinic cell carcinomas, and benign and malignant pleomorphic adenomas) or tumors known as intestinal-type adenocarcinomas. The minor salivary gland

tumors can arise anywhere within the sinonasal cavities. Most commonly they develop in the palate and then extend into the nasal fossae and paranasal sinuses. Tumors of the minor salivary glands, in order of decreasing frequency, include adenoid cystic carcinoma, adenocarcinoma, pleomorphic adenoma, mucoepidermoid carcinoma, adenocarcinoma not otherwise specified (NOS), acinic cell carcinoma, carcinoma ex-pleomorphic adenoma, and oncocytoma.[43]

Adenoid cystic carcinomas (cylindromas) account for about 35% of minor salivary gland tumors.[44] Of the primary sinonasal lesions, 47% arise in the maxillary sinuses, 32% involve the nasal fossae, 7% reside in the ethmoidal sinuses, 3% occur in the sphenoidal sinuses, and 2% are found in the frontal sinuses.[2] Adenoid cystic carcinomas usually arise in Caucasians between 30 and 60 years of age, although these neoplasms have been reported in an age range of 4 days to 86 years. Symptoms last an average of 5 years and relate to the mass effect and neural involvement of the tumor. A dull pain signals perineural tumor invasion, which is characteristic of this tumor. "Skip lesions" within nerves are known to occur; thus "clean" surgical margins have little prognostic significance. The local postsurgical recurrence rate is 62% within 1 year and 67% to 93% within 5 years.[2] Adenoid cystic carcinomas may recur 10 to 20 years after their initial treatment. As a result, 5-year survival data may give an erroneous indication of the absolute survival rate.[45] Some authorities have stated that no matter how long these patients have a disease-free interval, these patients will eventually die of adenoid cystic carcinoma. A solid or basaloid pattern is associated with poorer outcome. A temporal progression may be observed in patients, progressing from

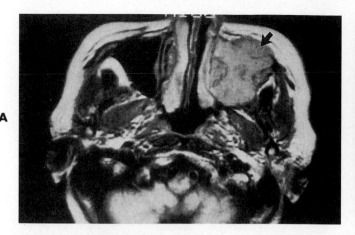

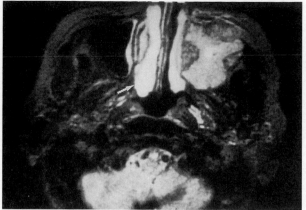

FIG. 4-149   Axial T1W (**A**) and T2W (**B**) MR scans show a destructive lesion *(arrow)* in the left maxillary sinus that extends into the left infratemporal fossa and left cheek. The tumor has an intermediate signal intensity on both images, but appears to brighten on the T2W scans. This is typical of most cellular tumors. Note that the tumor does not have as high a signal intensity as the turbinates *(white arrow)* or the inflamed mucosa along the medial wall of the right antrum. Squamous cell carcinoma.

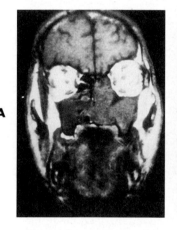

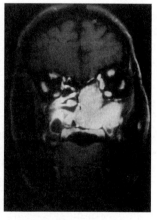

FIG. 4-150   Coronal T1W MR scans without contrast (**A**) and with contrast (**B**) show a mass (**A**) of intermediate signal intensity that has destroyed some of the left antral walls and fills the left nasal fossa. Lower signal intensity material (secretions) fills the right antrum and nasal fossa. This appearance accurately reflected the findings at surgery. The tumor enhances, the inflamed mucosa enhances, and some normal right ethmoid mucosa enhances (**B**). This presents a falsely large impression of the tumor size. Squamous cell carcinoma.

well differentiated (tubular pattern), to moderately differentiated (cribriform pattern), to poorly differentiated.[46] Antral tumors have the worst prognosis; 46% of patients are alive at 5 years, but only 15% are disease free.[2] About half of the sinonasal tumors have distant metastases, primarily to the lungs, brain, cervical lymph nodes, and bone.[2] Wide surgical excision is the treatment of choice. Adenoid cystic carcinomas are radiosensitive, but they are not curable with radiation therapy alone. Despite the fact that overall patient survival may not be affected by radiation treatment, better local tumor control may be achieved if postoperative radiation is given.

Mucoepidermoid carcinomas rank third in frequency among sinonasal malignancies of the minor salivary glands, behind adenoid cystic carcinomas and adenocarcinomas NOS. Most of these tumors involve the antrum and nasal cavity. Almost all minor salivary gland mucoepidermoid carcinomas are of the high-grade or intermediate-grade variety.[43] The biologic activity of these high-grade and intermediate-grade lesions resembles that of the adenocarcinomas.

Benign mixed tumors of the sinonasal cavities are rare; most lesions occur within the nasal fossa. Usually they arise from the nasal septum, although one fifth of the cases originate from the lateral nasal wall. The nasal septal location is curious because the septal submucosa is sparsely populated with minor salivary glands compared with the remainder of the sinonasal tract. A series of 41 cases of nasal cavity pleomorphic adenomas from Japan revealed that 90% of the cases originated from the septum and 10% (4 cases) arose in the lateral nasal wall.[47] The second most common site of origin is the maxillary sinus. Overall, pleomorphic adenomas are statistically the third most common minor salivary gland neoplasms. Intranasal and paranasal pleomorphic tumors are more cellular than their major salivary gland counterparts, and often the minor salivary gland lesions consist almost entirely of epithelial cells with little or no mesenchymal stroma.[45] Wide surgical excision usually prevents recurrences; however, recurrence of the tumor may be delayed well beyond the traditional 5-year period.[3] Malignant change in a sinonasal pleomorphic adenoma is rare. Benign metastasizing pleomorphic adenoma, or metastasizing pleomorphic adenoma, is an infrequent tumor that metastasizes, despite benign histology, usually to the lungs and soft tissues. A benign metastasizing nasal septal pleomorphic adenoma reportedly spread to an ipsilateral submandibular node.[48,49]

Typically, pleomorphic adenomas remodel bone. On CT the less cellular tumors may appear nonhomogeneous

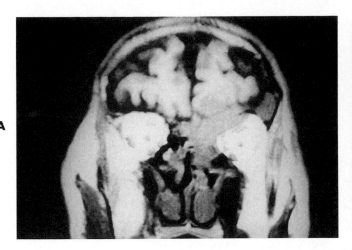
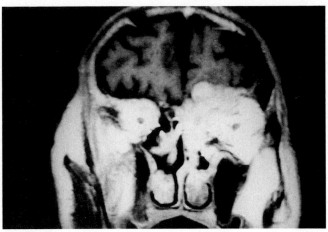

A

B

FIG. 4-151 Coronal T1W MR scans without contrast (**A**) and with contrast (**B**) show a destructive mass in the left ethmoid and nasal fossa. On these non-fat-suppressed scans, the orbital invasion is better seen in **A**; however, the intracranial extention is better seen in **B**. Squamous cell carcinoma.

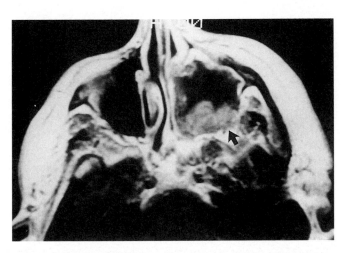

FIG. 4-152 Axial T1W contrast MR scan shows a destructive lesion in the left antrum. The tumor has extended into the infratemporal fossa *(arrow)*. Obstructed (lower signal intensity) secretions fill the sinus. Squamous cell carcinoma.

because of mesenchymal stroma, cystic degeneration, necrosis, or serous and mucous collections.[43] The highly cellular tumor tends to have a homogeneous appearance. On MRI these tumors tend to have an intermediate signal intensity on T1W images. The T2W signal intensity depends on the cellularity of the neoplasm; highly cellular types usually have an intermediate signal on T2W images, and the stromal or less cellular variety have a high T2W signal intensity (Figs. 4-158 to 4-167).[50]

The diagnosis "intestinal-type adenocarcinoma" of the sinonasal cavities was so named because of this tumor's histologic resemblance to colonic adenocarcinoma. These tumors occur primarily in males (75% to 90% of cases) between 55 and 60 years of age. The tumors are especially common in workers in the hardwood and shoe industries and in people who use certain carcinogenic snuffs, particu-

larly Bantus.[51,52] Workers exposed to wood dust have an almost 900 times greater relative risk of developing adenocarcinoma, and a 20 times greater relative risk of developing squamous carcinoma.[53,54] Intestinal-type adenocarcinoma (ITAC) can be classified as low-grade and high-grade tumors. The papillary variant is invariably associated with a low-grade cytology (grade I) and has a distinctly favorable prognosis. The high-grade colonic or signet cell types especially resemble colonic and gastric carcinomas. In these cases it is wise to rule out metastases from these gastrointestinal sites. Such an event is rare; only 6% of all metastases to the sinonasal cavities are from primary gastrointestinal tract tumors (the most common tumors that metastasize to the head and neck are tumors of the kidney, lung, breast, testis, and gastrointestinal tract).[2,55] Patients with sporadic ITAC tend to have shorter survival times than those patients with occupational exposure–related tumors. The reason for this is related to the initial tumor stage at the time of discovery. Sporadic tumors, not associated with inhaled promoters, are more likely to occur in the maxillary sinus. By contrast, occupational exposure–associated ITAC are more likely to occur in the nasal cavity and ethmoids. The maxillary sinus tumors do not become symptomatic until they are of an advanced stage, unlike the nasal cavity and ethmoid tumors, which may become symptomatic before they invade local structures.[53,54]

MALIGNANT MELANOMAS

Sinonasal melanomas arise from melanocytes that have migrated during embryologic development from the neural crest to the mucosa of the nose and sinuses.[2] These tumors represent less than 3.6% of sinonasal neoplasms. Less than 2.5% of all malignant melanomas occur in the sinonasal cavities. These melanomas are two or three times more common in the nose than in the sinuses and most frequently arise

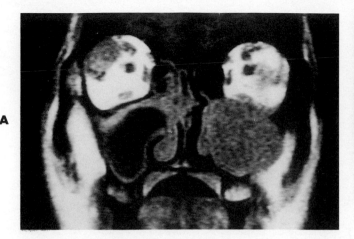
A

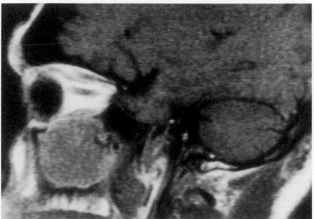
B

FIG. 4-153   Coronal T1W (**A**) and sagittal (**B**) MR scans show an intermediate signal intensity mass destroying the walls of the left maxillary sinus. There is minimal invasion of the orbital floor that was clinically silent. Incidental inflammatory mucosal thickening is present in the right antrum.

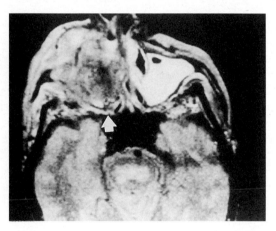

FIG. 4-154   Axial proton density MR scan shows a large, destructive tumor in the right antrum. The zygoma and the soft tissues of the cheek are invaded. However, the fat *(arrow)* in the pterygopalatine fossa remains intact. The lack of invasion of the central skull base greatly improves this patient's chance of cure. Incidently noted are obstructed secretions in the left antrum. Squamous cell carcinoma.

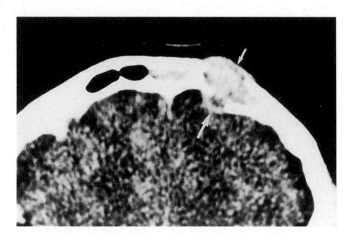

FIG. 4-155   Axial CT scan shows an enhancing left frontal sinus mass that has eroded the anterior *(arrow)* and posterior *(large arrow)* sinus tables. Frontal sinus squamous cell carcinoma.

from the nasal septum.[56,57] Occasionally they develop around the inferior and middle turbinates. The antrum is the site of origin in 80% of paranasal sinus cases. Rare cases develop in the ethmoid sinuses. The frontal and sphenoid sinuses are virtually never involved as primary sites.[2,56,57] Sinonasal melanomas generally develop in patients 50 to 70 years of age. The most common complaints are nasal obstruction and epistaxis, with pain occurring as an initial complaint in only 7% to 16% of patients.[56,57] Between 10% and 30% of these melanomas are amelanotic lesions. Satellite tumor nodules are common. Wide local surgical excision with or without postoperative radiation is the treatment of choice. Up to 40% of patients with sinonasal melanomas present with positive neck nodes.[58,59] Up to 65% of patients with melanoma have a local recurrence or metastases within the first year after surgery. Metastases tend to affect the lungs, lymph nodes, brain, adrenal glands, liver, and skin. Treatment of recurrences yields surprisingly good results.[2] The median survival time is 18 to 34 months.[58,59] Occasional cases may be mysteriously dormant for up to a decade before there is an explosive recurrence. Nasal melanomas have a better prognosis than those tumors originating in the paranasal sinuses; the average survival time of these patients is only 2 to 3 years, and the 10-year survival rate is 0.5%.[56-61] The differential diagnosis of melanoma includes anaplastic carcinoma, lymphoma, embryonal rhabdomyosarcoma, esthesioneuroblastoma, and extramedullary plasmacytoma.[41]

Melanomas tend to remodel bone, although elements of frank bone erosion also may be present. Because of their rich vascular network, melanomas enhance well on postcon-

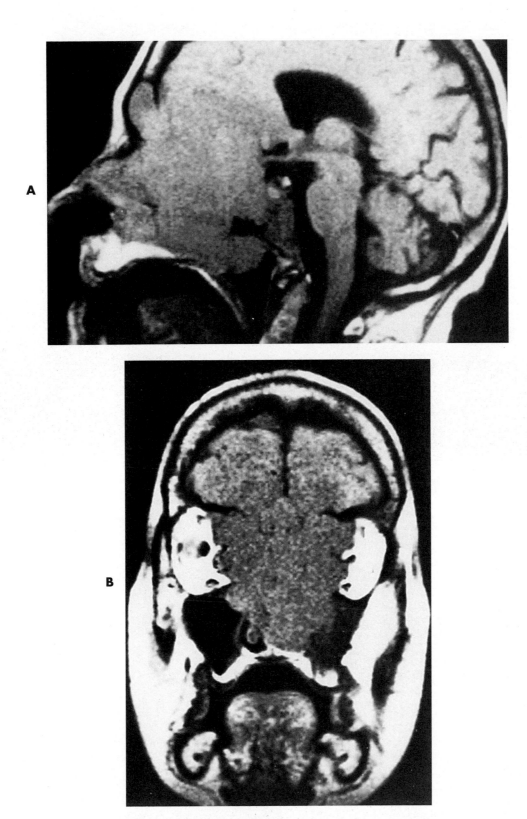

FIG. 4-156   Sagittal (**A**) and coronal (**B**) T1W MRI scans show a large homogeneous destructive lesion of the nasal fossa with a low to intermediate signal intensity. The tumor has eroded the central floor of the anterior cranial fossa and extended into the brain, both orbits, both ethmoids, and both antra. Squamous cell carcinoma.

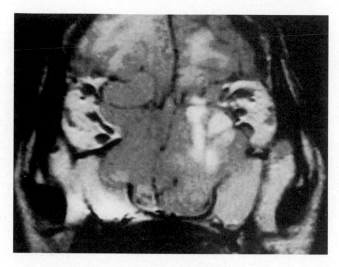

FIG. 4-157   Coronal proton density MRI shows a destructive lesion of the nasal cavity and both maxillary and ethmoid sinuses. The tumor invades both orbits and the anterior cranial fossa. The lesion has a homogeneous intermediate signal intensity except for several well-defined areas of high signal intensity (hemorrhage). Squamous cell carcinoma.

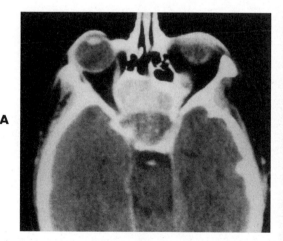

A

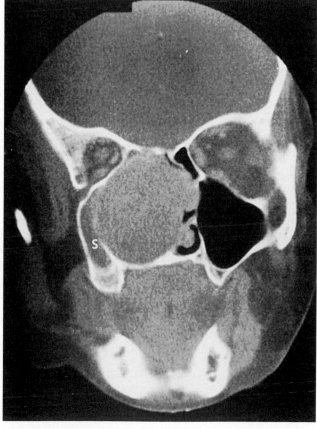

B

FIG. 4-158   Axial CT scan (**A**) shows an enhancing, expansile mass in the posterior ethmoid sinuses. The sphenoid sinuses are obstructed with lower attenuation secretions. There is also some bone remodeling present in the lamina papyracea. Mucoepidermoid carcinoma and a sphenoid mucocele. Coronal CT (**B**) shows an expansile right nasal fossa and ethmoid sinus mass. The lesion has remodeled most of the surrounding bone, and it has obstructed what remains of the right maxillary sinus (*S*). Low-grade mucopidermoid carcinoma.

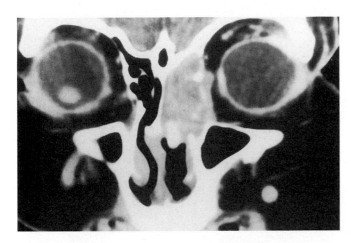

FIG. 4-159   Coronal CT scan shows a mass in the left ethmoid sinuses. Although there is some destruction of the lamina papyracea with minimal invasion of the orbit, there is also an element of widening or remodeling of the ethmoid complex. Mucoepidermoid carcinoma.

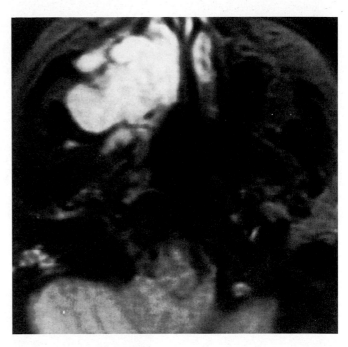

FIG. 4-160   Axial T2W MR scan shows an expansile right maxillary sinus mass that extends into the infratemporal fossa. The tumor has a high signal intensity. Low-grade mucoepidermoid carcinoma.

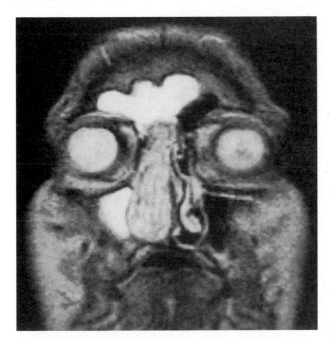

FIG. 4-161   Coronal T2W MR scan shows an expansile right nasoethmoid mass that extends into the base of the right frontal sinus. The lesion obstructs the right frontal and right maxillary sinuses. Adenocarcinoma.

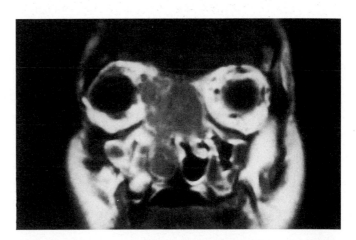

FIG. 4-162   Coronal T1W contrast MR scan shows a nodular, destructive lesion in the nasal fossae and both ethmoid sinuses. The tumor has invaded the right orbit and skull base. Inflammatory disease is present both antra. Adenocarcinoma.

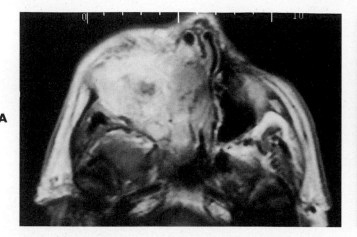
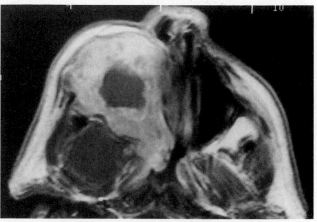

FIG. 4-163   Axial T1W MR scans (**A** and **B**) show a large destructive tumor in the right maxillary sinus that has invaded the overlying skin, the nasal fossa, the infratemporal fossa, and the central skull base. There is an area of residual secretions (**B**) within the sinus. This appearance is similar to that of a squamous cell carcinoma. Adenoidcystic carcinoma.

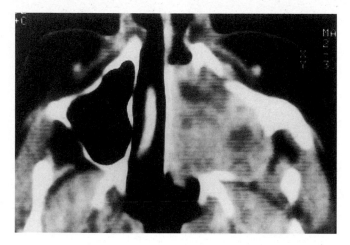

FIG. 4-164   Axial CT scan shows a partially expansile, partially destructive, nonhomogeneous tumor in the left maxillary sinus. The lesion has extended into the nasal fossa and abuts the nasal septum. Adenoidcystic carcinoma.

trast CT and MR scans, and their MRI appearance is usually that of a homogeneous mass of intermediate signal intensity on all imaging sequences. However, some melanomas have high T1W signal intensities primarily because of the presence of hemorrhage (and to a lesser degree because of paramagnetic melanin) (Figs. 4-168, 4-169).

NEUROGENIC NEOPLASMS

One of the difficulties in discussing neurogenic neoplasms (peripheral nerve sheath tumors) is the confusing terminology that has arisen in the literature; many names represent the same lesion. Controversy also has arisen regarding whether nerve sheath tumors arise from Schwann cells or neuroectodermal perineural cells.[62] Today most investigators use the term Schwann cell to describe both of these

cells. It is accepted that a schwannoma, neurinoma, neurilemoma, and perineural fibroblastoma all refer to the same tumor.[1] Peripheral nerve sheath tumors are actually common in the head and neck. Up to 40% of these tumors occur in head and neck sites. Only 4% of these tumors occur in the sinonasal cavities.[63-65]

A schwannoma is a benign, encapsulated, slowly growing nerve sheath tumor that occurs in patients 30 to 60 years of age. It is two to four times more common in women. The most common site of schwannoma is the vagus nerve in the neck, and the eighth cranial nerve. Only about 65 cases of schwannomas have been reported in the sinonasal cavities, and most of these occur in the nasal fossa, maxillary sinuses, and ethmoidal sinuses.[1,62] The most common complaint is a painless mass. Schwannomas rarely if ever undergo malignant change. At surgery the nerve of origin may occasion-

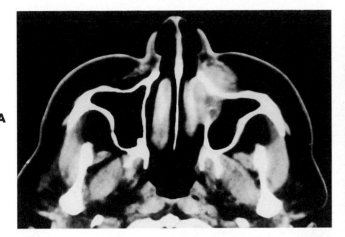

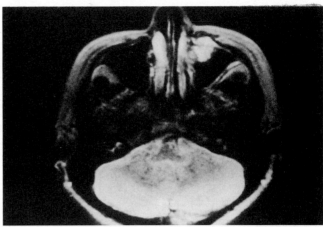

FIG. 4-165   Axial CT (**A**) and T2W MR (**B**) scans show a soft-tissue mass in the anteromedial left orbit and adjacent left cheek. There is some destruction of the medial antral bony wall. Note that the tumor has a high signal intensity in **B**. Adenoidcystic carcinoma.

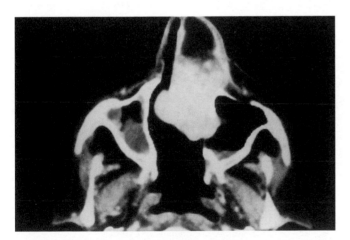

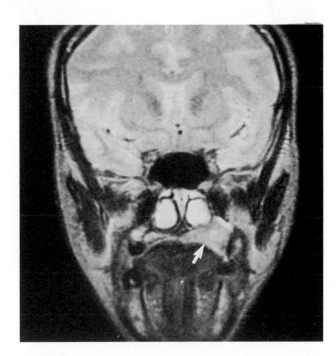

FIG. 4-166   Axial CT scan shows a nodular, bulky mass arising in the nasal septum and laterally displacing the left nose and medial antral wall. Pleomorphic adenoma.

FIG. 4-167   Coronal proton density MR scan shows an expansile and destructive mass in the left palate and lower left antrum *(arrow)*. This mass also had intermediate signal intensity on T2W MRI. High-grade mucoepidermoid carcinoma.

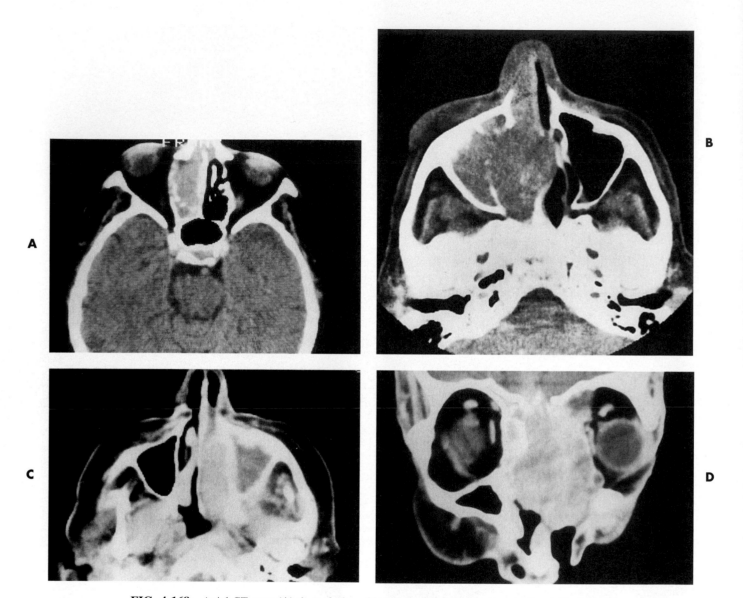

FIG. 4-168   Axial CT scan (**A**) through the orbits shows an expansile mass in the right ethmoid sinuses that is bulging into the right orbit. Most of the lamina papyracea is intact. Malignant melanoma. Axial CT scan (**B**) shows a primarily expansile right nasal fossa mass that obstructs the right antrum. Malignant melanoma. Axial CT scan (**C**) shows an enhancing, expansile polypoid mass in the left nasal fossa. The left antrum is obstructed. There is virtually no bone destruction associated with this benign-appearing lesion. Malignant melanoma. Coronal CT scan (**D**) shows an expansile and destructive enhancing mass in the nasal fossae, ethmoid sinuses, and left maxillary sinus. The tumor has invaded the left orbit and the floor of the anterior cranial fossa. Malignant melanoma.

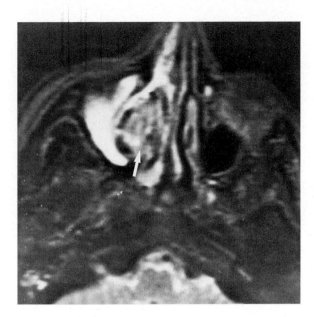

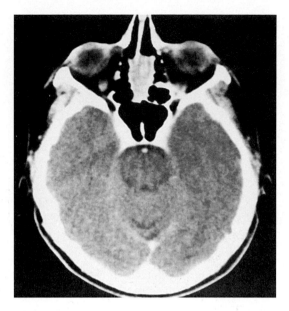

FIG. 4-169   Axial T2W MR scan shows an expansile right nasal fossa mass *(arrow)* that obstructs the right antrum. The tumor has a low to intermediate signal intensity, and the obstructed secretions have a high signal intensity. Malignant melanoma.

FIG. 4-170   Axial CT scan shows an expansile, slightly nonhomogeneous, upper nasal cavity mass. Schwannoma.

ally be stretched over the tumor. In these cases the surgeon may be able to extirpate the lesion while preserving the nerve. By contrast the nerve is an integral part of neurofibromas and must be sacrificed to excise the lesion.[62]

Histologically, schwannomas have two major components: the Antoni A areas, characterized by a compact arrangement of elongated spindled cells, or the Antoni B areas, characterized by a loose myxoid stroma with few spindled cells. This variation is reflected in their CT appearance, which ranges from a variably enhancing homogeneous ovoid mass to a primarily cystic lesion. On postcontrast CT, about one third of the cases enhance more than muscle, one third have attenuation values similar to that of muscle, and one third are primarily cystic.[66] The enhancement on CT and MRI occurs presumably because of extravascular extravasation of the contrast into a poorly vascularized tumor matrix. The MRI characteristics of schwannomas are those of an intermediate signal intensity on T1W images. The T2W signal intensity varies according to whether the lesion is highly cellular (intermediate intensity) or cystic and stromal (nonhomogeneously high intensity). All schwannomas are bone-remodeling lesions, and any site of aggressive bone destruction should raise the possibility of a malignancy rather than a schwannoma (Figs. 4-170 to 4-174).

The neurofibroma is a benign, fairly well-circumscribed, but nonencapsulated nerve sheath tumor. Although it may occur as a solitary lesion, the finding of such a lesion, especially in a young patient, may herald the onset of other tumors with neurofibromatosis (von Recklinghausen's disease). Neurofibromatosis is a hamartomatous disorder that is transmitted as an autosomal dominant trait with variable penetrance. It includes the presence of cafe au lait spots,

multiple neurofibromas, and characteristic bone lesions.[67] Multiple neurofibromas are more likely to be associated with neurofibromatosis.[66] Approximately 8% (5% to 15%) of these tumors may have malignant degeneration.[68,69] The clinical appearance of a plexiform neurofibroma is considered pathognomonic of neurofibromatosis even in the absence of other signs. This tumor usually remains within the confines of the perineurium and resembles a "giant nerve," "bag of worms," or a "string of beads."[62]

Neurofibromas can have a variable CT appearance, depending in part on the degree of cystic degeneration and fatty replacement present within the lesion. On postcontrast CT these tumors may have a variably enhancing homogeneous appearance, contain multiple cystic areas, or have a predominantly fatty attenuation. The degree of fatty replacement within some neurofibromas is far more extensive than that ever seen in schwannomas and may at times cause the radiologist to suggest the diagnosis of a lipoma. Neurofibromas remodel bone and do not cause aggressive bone destruction. If bone has been destroyed, the possibility of a malignant degeneration should be considered. On MR they usually are nonhomogeneous tumors with an overall intermediate T1W signal intensity, and a higher T2W signal intensity. The plexiform lesions in particular often have a fairly high T2W signal intesity.

A traumatic neuroma is not a true neoplasm but a reparative lesion that occurs after disruption of a peripheral nerve. If the proximal portion of the nerve cannot reestablish contact with the distal portion, the proliferating Schwann cells and axons grow haphazardly and form a traumatic neuroma. Excision with approximation of the nerve endings is the treatment of choice.[62]

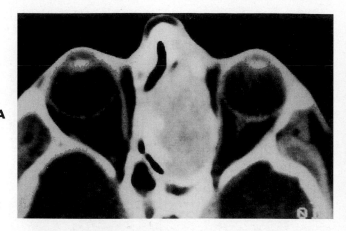
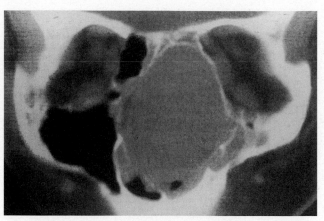

FIG. 4-171   Axial CT scan (**A**) shows an expansile homogeneous mass in the left ethmoid sinuses that has remodeled the surrounding bone. Schwannoma. Coronal CT scan (**B**) shows a large expansile mass in the left nasal fossa and ethmoid sinuses. The left antrum and right ethmoid sinuses are obstructed by the mass. The surrounding bone is remodeled rather than destroyed. Schwannoma.

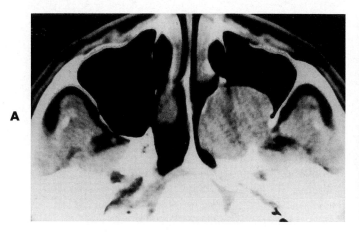
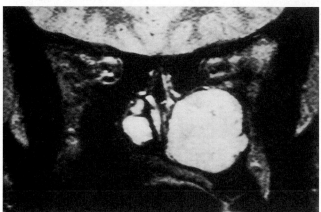

FIG. 4-172   Axial CT (**A**) and coronal T2W MR (**B**) scans show a large, ovoid mass in the left pterygopalatine fossa and posterior antrum. There is primarily bone remodeling about the mass. Schwannoma of V_2.

A malignant peripheral nerve sheath tumor (MPNST) is a neuroectodermal sarcoma that is the malignant counterpart of a neurofibroma.[65] This term replaces the term malignant schwannoma. Although they can occur as isolated lesions, 25% to 50% are associated with neurofibromatosis. They occur primarily in patients 28 to 34 years of age. Only 9% to 14% of MPNSTs are found in the head and neck. The cranial nerves, large cervical nerves, sympathetic chain, and inferior alveolar nerve are the most commonly involved nerves. Symptoms include an enlarging mass, occasional pain, paresthesia, muscle weakness, and atrophy.[62] Because Schwann cells can produce collagen and have a spindle shape, some MPNSTs are confused histologically with fibrosarcomas. However, electron microscopy reveals a redundant basement membrane and cellular processes in MPNSTs and no basement membrane in the fibrosarcoma.[62] MPNSTs associated with neurofibromatosis behave more aggressively than isolated lesions. The 5-year survival rates are 15% to 30% with neurofibromatosis and 27% to 75% without it. Tumors that exceed 7 cm in size, have more than 6 mitoses per 10 high-power fields, and are located near the central body axis have a poorer prognosis. Local recurrences and hematogenous pulmonary metastases are common, whereas lymph node metastases are rare.[70] Their imaging characteristics may be similar to squamous cell carcinoma (Figs. 4-174, 4-175).

Granular cell tumors (myoblastomas) are uncommon lesions that appear primarily in the skin of the nose, eyelids, forehead, scalp, and neck. They also may develop in the lips, floor of the mouth, palate, pharynx, larynx, and trachea. Most occur in patients 35 to 40 years old. These tumors have a female predominance except for the laryngeal granular cell tumors. Treatment is excision; interestingly, many incompletely excised lesions do not recur. Most granular cell tumors reach a size of 1 to 5 cm and are composed of polyhedral cells with eosinophilic granular cytoplasm and

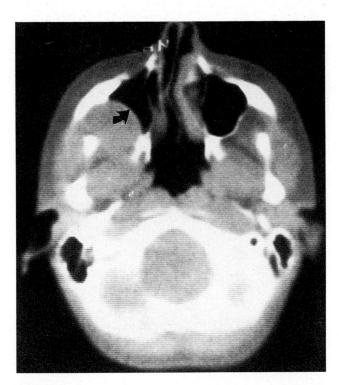

FIG. 4-173 Axial CT scan shows an expansile mass of the right infratemporal fossa, which bows the posterior antral wall anteriorly *(arrow)*. Schwannoma of infratemporal fossa.

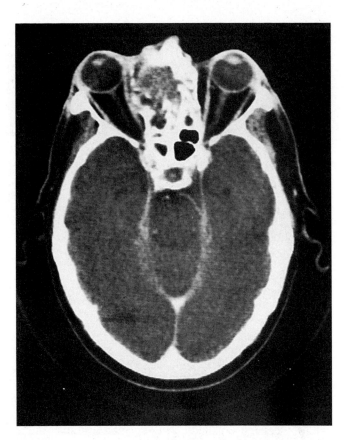

FIG. 4-174 Axial CT scan shows an expansile right anterior ethmoid mass that erodes the lamina papyracea and bulges into the right orbit. Malignant schwannoma.

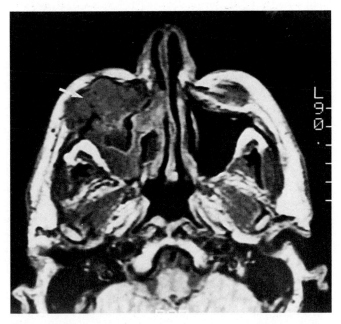

FIG. 4-175 Axial T1W MR scan reveals a destructive lesion originating in the roof of the right antrum *(arrow)*. The mass has a low signal intensity and had an intermediate T2W signal intensity. Malignant schwannoma of V_2.

round to oval nuclei. Intraneural tumor foci can be seen, but this is not a sign of malignancy. No mitoses and necrosis are seen.[62] Ultrastructurally the granules of a granular cell tumor are actually autophagolysosomes, containing myelin-like structures. This confirms the Schwannian lineage. Rarely, malignant granular cell tumors may be encountered. Malignant granular cell tumors are either large yet histologically benign and metastatic, or they are histologically malignant and metastatic.[71]

TUMORS OF NEURONAL ORIGIN

Although these tumors rarely arise in the sinonasal cavities, they have been reported in the head and neck. They most commonly arise in the cervical sympathetic chain as a neck mass or in the orbit, eyelids, tongue, pharynx, and larynx. Secondarily from these sites, the sinonasal cavities may be involved. Sometimes painful, lesions of the sympathetic nervous system may be associated with Horner's syndrome and vagal dysfunction.[62]

The neural plate's central portion invaginates during early embryogenesis to form the neural tube from which the brain, spine, and peripheral nerves develop. The lateral portions of the neural plates are not incorporated into the neural tube and instead form the left and right neural crests from

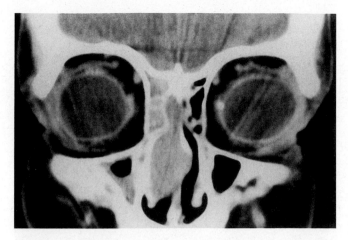

FIG. 4-176 Coronal CT scan shows an expansile right nasal fossa mass obstructing the right ethmoid and maxillary sinuses. The lesion is limited to the sinonasal cavities. Olfactory neuroblastoma.

which the sympathetic and parasympathetic systems develop. The neural crest cells from which the sympathetic system develops are called sympathogonia. They normally differentiate into neuroblasts, which then mature into ganglion cells. A neuroblastoma is a malignancy derived from these neural crest cells. If the tumor partially differentiates into mature ganglion cells, it is called a ganglioneuroblastoma. A tumor composed entirely of mature neural elements is called a ganglioneuroma. The more immature neuroblastoma is the least differentiated tumor of the nervous system lesions. The ganglioneuroblastoma has less malignant potential than a neuroblastoma, and the ganglioneuroma is benign.[62]

Olfactory Neuroblastomas

Olfactory neuroblastoma (ONB) (esthesioneuroblastoma) is an uncommon tumor of neural crest origin that arises from the olfactory mucosa in the superior nasal fossa. The incidence peaks once in the 11- to 20-year age group (16.8% of all tumors) and again in the 50- to 60-year age group (22.8% of all tumors); however, the age of these patients ranges from 3 to 88 years.[62,72] This polypoid tumor may be of variable consistency and may bleed profusely on biopsy. Olfactory neuroblastomas are almost always unilateral and only in highly neglected cases do they appear as a bilateral nasal fossae mass. ONB can be histologically classified as ONB with pseudorosettes (20% of cases), ONB with true rosettes (40% of cases), and ONB with sheets of cells without rosettes (40% of cases). It is this last variety that is most often confused with anaplastic carcinoma, large cell lymphoma, melanoma, extramedullary plasmacytoma, and embryonal rhabdomyosarcoma.[41] However, electron microscopy and immunohistochemical testing can differentiate these lesions. The staging system of Kadish, Goodman, and Wine refers to patients with disease confined to the nasal cavity as stage A, those with disease in the nasal cavity and one or more paranasal sinuses as stage B, and those with disease extending beyond the nasal cavity and

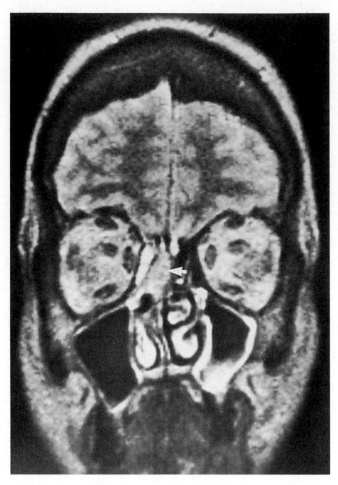

FIG. 4-177 Coronal T2W MR scan shows a small right nasoethmoid mass *(arrow)* of intermediate signal intensity with inflammatory changes in the lateral right ethmoids and both maxillary sinuses (high signal intensity). The tumor extends through the cribriform plate. Olfactory neuroblastoma.

paranasal sinuses as stage C.[73] Using this system, 30% of patients are classified as stage A, 42% as stage B, and 28% as stage C. The respective 5-year survival rates are 75%, 68%, and 41.2%.[72,73] Craniofacial resection performed on all patients may cure more than 90% of cases. This approach takes into account the microscopic presence of intracranial tumor that can occur with an intact and normal-appearing cribriform plate.[74] This is in contrast to performing an extended lateral rhinotomy for stage A and stage B patients, which has a recurrence rate of nearly 50%. The 5-year survival rate for all patients is 69%.[75] When survival is stratified for tumor grade, the 5-year survival for low-grade and high-grade tumors is repectively 80% and 40%.[75] Adjuvant chemotherapy is recommended for patients with high-grade tumors or postive surgical resection margins. Others recommend adjuvant radiotherapy for all patients because combined surgery and irradiation resulted in a 92% disease-free status.[76] Locoregional and distant metastasis occurs in up to 38% of patients.[77] Late recurrences or metastatic disease can occur up to 2 decades after initial presentation. Negative

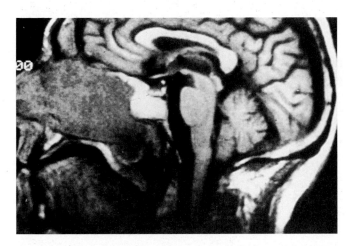

FIG. 4-178 Sagittal T1W MR scan shows a large low to intermediate signal intensity nasoethmoid mass that erodes the floor of the anterior cranial fossa and obstructs the sphenoid sinus (high signal intensity). Olfactory neuroblastoma.

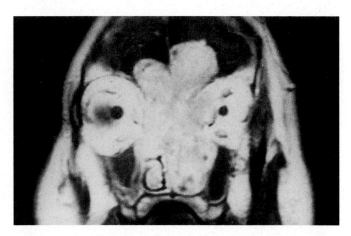

FIG. 4-179 Coronal T1W contrast MR scan shows a large enhancing mass that fills both nasal cavities and the ethmoid sinuses. The tumor extends into the left orbit and breaks intracranially. Both maxillary sinuses contain obstructed secretions. Olfactory neuroblastoma.

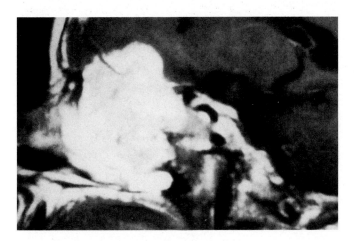

FIG. 4-180 Sagittal T1W contrast MR scan shows a large sinonasal mass that obstructs the frontal and sphenoid sinuses and extends into the anterior cranial fossa. Contrast best shows the extent of intracranial disease and the presence of dural involvement. Olfactory neuroblastoma.

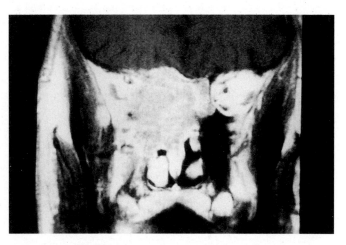

FIG. 4-181 Coronal T1W contrast MR scan shows a right nasoethmoid mass that invades the right orbit and elevates the dura in the floor of the anterior cranial fossa. The tumor extends into the left ethmoid and right maxillary sinus. Aspects of this tumor appear more aggressive than the usual olfactory neuroblastoma and should raise the possible diagnosis of a carcinoma. Olfactory neuroblastoma.

prognostic factors include female sex, age over 50 years at presentation, tumor recurrence, metastasis, high tumor grade, and Kadish stage C at presentation.[76]

The role of imaging in these patients is to map the tumor so as to precisely anticipate surgical boundaries. On CT, olfactory neuroblastomas usually are homogeneous, enhancing masses that primarily remodel bone. They commonly extend into the ipsilateral ethmoid and maxillary sinuses and only rarely involve the sphenoid sinuses. When large, they can extend to involve both sides of the nasal cavity and the paranasal sinuses. Calcifications can occur within the tumor mass.[78] On MRI these tumors have an intermediate signal intensity on all imaging sequences, with the T2W signal intensity being higher.[79] They also enhance with contrast (Figs. 4-129, 4-176 to 4-183). In some of the larger tumors that have intracranial extension, peripheral tumor cysts can occur at the margins of the intracranial mass. These cysts have their broadest base on the tumor, and when seen, they highly suggest the imaging diagnosis of this tumor.[80]

Melanotic Neuroectodermal Tumors of Infancy

The rare melanotic neuroectodermal tumor occurs 92% of the time in patients less than 1 year of age. It is a rapidly growing soft-tissue mass that may invade bone. However, despite this aggressive appearance, it is essentially benign,

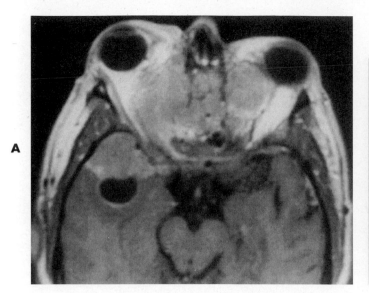

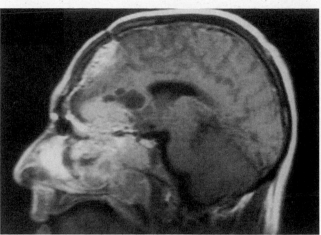

FIG. 4-182   Axial (**A**) and sagittal (**B**) T1W contrast MR scans on a patient who previously had a craniofacial resection for an olfactory neuroblastoma. There is a large enhancing recurrence extending into the orbits and the anterior cranial fossa. Note the small cysts at the intracranial margin of the tumor. In **A** the cyst is broad based against the tumor. Such cysts are highly suggestive of the diagnosis. Olfactory neuroblastoma.

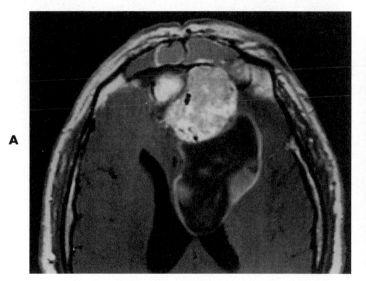

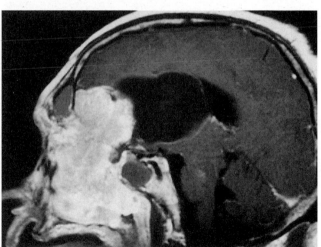

FIG. 4-183   Axial (**A**) and sagittal (**B**) T1W MR scans show a large enhancing sinonasal mass that obstructs the frontal and sphenoid sinuses and extends intracranially. There is a large cyst at the intracranial margin of the tumor (compare with Fig. 4-182). Olfactory neuroblastoma.

requiring local excision with curettage as treatment. Recurrences develop in only 15% of patients, and only two or three malignant cases have been reported with metastases to lymph nodes, liver, bones, adrenal glands, and soft tissues.[62,81] The anterior maxilla is the most common site, accounting for 71% of all cases.

TUMORS OF THE PARAGANGLIOMA NERVOUS SYSTEM

Paraganglioma of the nasal cavity is extraordinarily rare. Secondary involvement of the sphenoid and ethmoid sinuses from a large glomus jugulare is more likely to occur (Fig. 4-184).[82,83] These lesions are discussed in Chapter 18.

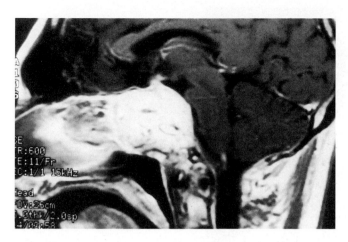

FIG. 4-184 Sagittal T1W contrast MR scan shows an enhancing mass in the sphenoid sinuses. The tumor has invaded the clivus. Vascular flow voids are present within the tumor. Paraganglioma arising in the sphenoid sinus.

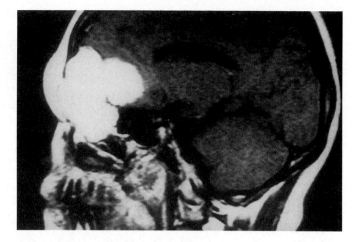

FIG. 4-185 Sagittal T1W MR scan shows an enhancing anterior cranial fossa mass that extends caudally into the sinonasal cavities. The epicenter of this tumor is above the level of the cribriform plate, suggesting the intracranial origin of the lesion. Meningioma.

MENINGIOMAS

Meningiomas are benign, slowly growing tumors that arise from clusters of meningocytes at the tips of the arachnoid villi, usually in relationship to the major dural sinuses. They comprise 13% to 18% of all primary intracranial tumors and are two to four times more common in females; rate of incidence peaks near 45 years of age.[62] These tumors can extend or arise outside of the neuroaxis; however, this is uncommon. Of all the meningiomas that occur outside of the neuroaxis, about one third are direct extensions from an intracranial or intraspinous lesion.[84,85] Primary extracranial meningiomas are quite rare, comprising less than 1% of cases.[86] Most of these extraneuroaxis meningiomas occur in the head and neck and have been reported in the bones of the skull, orbit, nose, paranasal sinuses, oral cavity, middle ear, skin of the scalp, and cervical soft tissues.[62] Very rarely an extracranial meningioma might represent a metastasis from an intracranial meningioma.[87]

The imaging characteristics of these sinonasal lesions show an enhancing mass that remodels bone. Most lesions lie in the nasal vault, and adjacent sclerotic, reactive bone may be a dominant feature. This bone reaction can mimic the imaging appearance of fibrous dysplasia. If the tumor has spread from the intracranial cavity, remodeling of the skull base with tumor extension into the sinonasal cavities is best seen on coronal images. On MRI these tumors have signal intensities similar to that of the brain on all imaging sequences. They enhance and vascular flow voids have only rarely been observed (Figs. 4-185, 4-186).

CHORDOMAS

Chordomas are slow-growing tumors that arise from embryonic notochord remnants. They probably represent about 1% of all malignant bone tumors.[88] The vast majority occur in the skull base (clivus) and in the sacrococ-

cygeal region. Rarely, chordomas have been reported in the maxilla and mandible.[89] In these cases the tumor presumably arises in notochordal remnants that separated from the main notochord during the extreme mesodermal movements of the face that take place in early embryogenesis. These ectopic rests can be located in the paranasal sinuses.[89,90]

On contrast CT the classic chordoma is a minimally enhancing, destructive lesion that has areas of dystrophic calcification and residual bone fragments. The only reported case in the maxillary sinus mimicked a mucocele (Fig. 4-187).[89] On MRI, chordomas are extremely variable in their appearance, and they can have anywhere from a low to high signal intensity on any sequence (Figs. 4-188 to 4-190).[91]

LYMPHOMAS

The term lethal midline granuloma is a clinical, inexact term, indicating a destructive sinonasal process and implying a lack of definitive pathologic diagnosis. Malignant midline reticulosis or polymorphic reticulosis (PR) indicates a necrotic infiltrate of inflammatory cells mixed with an atypical lymphoid infiltrate. In reality, PR is a prelymphomatous state, which generally occurs in a population younger than those patients with sinonasal lymphoma (the mean age for patients with sinonasal lymphoma may be up to 66 years). Subsequent biopsies of PR indicate a progression to a diffuse, high-grade lymphoma.

About 47% of non-Hodgkin's lymphomas occur in the head and neck; 90% of these are cervical nodal lymphomas. Ten percent of non-Hodgkin's lymphomas occur in head and neck extranodal sites, usually in the thyroid and tonsils (71%).[91] Hashimoto's thyroiditis is a common precursor to thyroid lymphoma. Up to 17% of all lymphomas and 44% of all head and neck extranodal lymphomas occur in the sinonasal cavities.[92] There is an equal sex distribution. Lym-

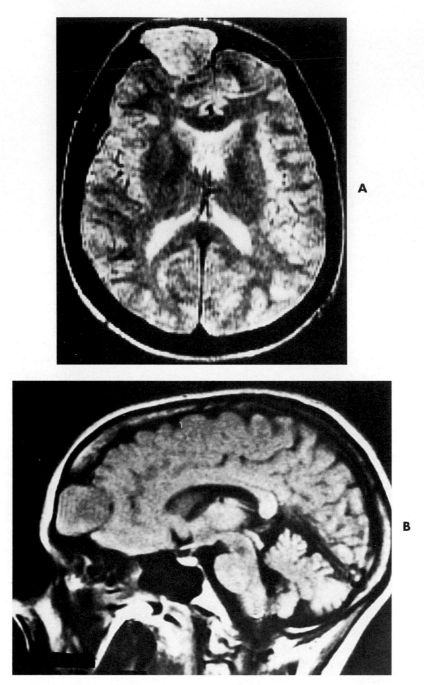

FIG. 4-186   Axial T2W (**A**) and sagittal T1W (**B**) images show an expansile mass in the right frontal sinus that extends intracranially. The mass has low to intermediate, slightly nonhomogeneous signal intensity in **B** and high signal intensity in **A**. Frontal sinus meningioma.

phomas are the only soft-tissue malignancies that are radiocurable.[93] Therefore a confirmed diagnosis of lymphoma spares the patient any further invasive therapy and directs the patient to the oncologist and radiotherapist.

The working formulation, elaborated in 1982, standardizes nomenclature and grades lymphomas based on pattern (follicular versus diffuse) and cell type (small cleaved, large, mixed, small noncleaved).[94] The majority of sinonasal lymphomas are immunotyped as T-cell lymphomas. High-grade

morphology, angiotropism, and necrosis are characteristic features of these lymphomas. Many series of these T-cell sinonasal lymphomas have been reported in Oriental populations and in patients from Peru.[95] These lymphomas have invariably been found to harbor the Epstein-Barr virus (EBV). "Asian population–EBV positive–T-cell lymphoma" is not an absolute rule. European and American patients may also develop sinonasal EBV positive T-cell lymphomas, although the B-cell phenotype is still more com-

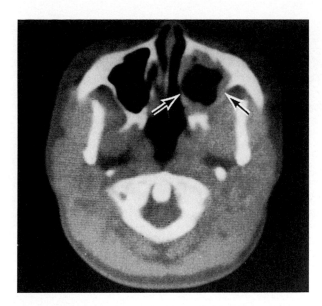

FIG. 4-187 Axial CT scan performed after surgical drainage of a presumed mucocele shows thinning or destruction of the medial and posterior antral walls *(arrows)* with fairly uniform soft tissues lining the antrum. Chordoma of antrum.

mon in these populations. In the Asian population, only a minority of nasal–nasopharyngeal B-cell lymphomas, and no tonsillar–base of tongue B-cell lymphomas, were associated with EBV infection. These latter facts strengthen the role of EBV as a specific cofactor for T-cell sinonasal lymphomas. Patients with sinonasal T-cell lymphomas also had elevated serum EBV viral capsid antigen.[96-99]

Sinonasal lymphomas can occur with or without associated cervical or systemic nodal disease.[100,101] Evidence suggests that the presence of adenopathy with extranodal lymphoma may reduce the 5-year survival rate by 50%.[1] After treatment, overall the 5-year survival rates are 50% to 70%. Chemotherapy is emerging as the initial treatment modality for extranodal sinonasal lymphoma; radiation is being used in cases of incomplete tumor response.

On CT and MRI, lymphomas in the sinonasal cavities tend to be bulky soft-tissue masses that enhance to a moderate degree. These tumors also tend to remodel bone, although occasionally they erode bone.[102-105] Most often the disease is located in the nasal fossae and maxillary sinuses. Less often, lymphoma is found in the ethmoid sinuses, and only rarely is it found in the sphenoid and frontal sinuses. On MRI it tends to have an intermediate intensity signal on all imaging sequences (Figs. 4-191 to 4-195).

Burkitt's lymphoma, a form of non-Hodgkin's lymphoma, has distinct epidemiologic, clinical, and pathologic features. It occurs predominantly in children and is endemic in Central Africa, where it is the most common childhood malignancy and is strongly associated with (EBV). Nonendemic Burkitt's lymphoma is rare, occurs primarily in North America, and is not associated with EBV. Although this disease can involve head and neck structures such as the jaws, orbits, meninges, extradural spaces, nasopharynx, and lymph nodes, it does not primarily involve the sinonasal cavities.[106]

Leukemia is a malignant proliferation of lymphatic or hematopoetic cells and their precursors in the blood or bone marrow. The leukemias are classified as either myeloid or lymphocytic, acute and chronic forms.[106] Rarely do primary leukemic infiltrates penetrate the sinonasal cavities. Instead, most patients with leukemia have involvement of the nose and paranasal cavities secondary to life-threatening infections and hemorrhage.

GRANULOCYTIC SARCOMAS

Granulocytic sarcoma, or chloroma, is a rare, localized, malignant tumor composed of immature myeloid elements. *Chloroma* describes the green hue seen when these tumors are sectioned. The color, caused by the cytoplasmic enzyme myeloperoxidase, fades after exposure to air. Granulocytic sarcoma occurs in only 3% of patients with acute and chronic myeloid leukemia. The mean patient age is 48 years, and most (85%) present with solitary lesions. In the head and neck, osseous lesions have been reported in the skull, face, orbit, and paranasal sinuses, whereas extramedullary tumors have been reported in the nasal cavity, paranasal sinuses, nasopharynx, tonsil, mouth, lacrimal gland, salivary glands, and thyroid gland.[106] An associated myeloproliferative disease is found in 48% of patients, and acute myeloid leukemia occurs in 22% of the cases. However, 30% of patients with granulocytic sarcoma have no hematologic disease at the time of initial diagnosis. The onset of granulocytic sarcoma may be a harbinger for the development of acute blast crisis within a few months of the diagnosis. The prognosis of patients with acute myeloid leukemia is not altered by the development of a chloroma; however, in patients with chronic myeloid leukemia and other myeloproliferative disorders the granulocytic sarcoma is an ominous sign because it is associated with the acute or blastic phase of the disease.[106] On CT, chloromas are enhancing, homogeneous masses.[107] On MRI, they have intermediate to high signal intensities on all imaging sequences.

PLASMA CELL DYSCRASIAS

Multiple myeloma is the most common member of a group of diseases known collectively as plasma cell dyscrasias. These diseases, including Waldenstrom's macroglobulinemia, heavy chain disease, and primary amyloidosis, all have a malignant proliferation of plasma cells or lymphocytoid plasma cells and the presence of monoclonal immunoglobulin or immunoglobulin fragments in the patient's urine. The proliferation of neoplastic cells is associated with bone destruction and involves the bone marrow of the axial skeleton. However, the soft tissues can also be involved. Multiple myeloma usually affects patients over the age of 40 (mean age is 63) and has a roughly equal sex distribution. The most frequent complaints are bone pain (63%), weakness (23%), and weight loss (15%). An extraosseous plasmacytoma is

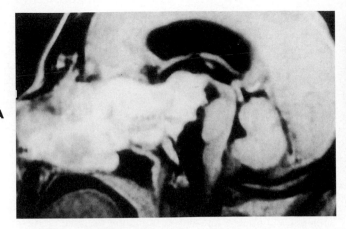
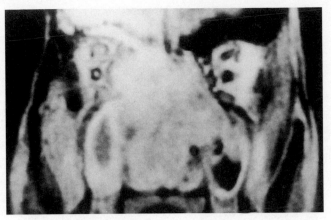

FIG. 4-188   Sagittal (**A**) and coronal (**B**) T1W contrast MR scans show a large enhancing mass that replaces almost the entire clivus and extends forward to fill the sinonasal cavities. There is also a large dorsal extension of this tumor. This is an unusally large chordoma with uncharacteristic exuberant ventral and dorsal growth.

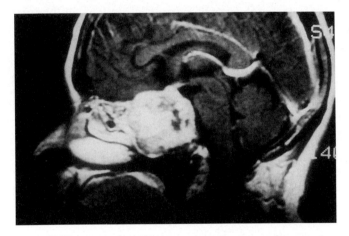
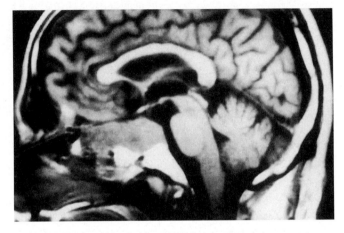

FIG. 4-189   Sagittal T1W contrast MR scan shows a bulky, non-homogeneously enhancing mass in the clivus and sphenoid sinus. This is a more characteristic MR appearance of a chordoma than shown in Fig. 4-188.

FIG. 4-190   Sagittal T1W MR scan shows an intermediate signal intensity mass in the upper clivus and the sphenoid and ethmoid sinuses. There is little intracranial extension. Chordoma.

the initial manifestation of multiple myeloma in only 5% of patients.[106] In the head and neck, soft-tissue masses occur primarily in the nose, paranasal sinuses, nasopharynx, and tonsils. Patients may have oronasal bleeding as a primary manifestation of hyperviscosity. Skeletal lytic lesions are found in 85% of patients, and a combination of lytic bone lesions, osteoporosis, and pathologic fractures is found in 63% of patients at disease onset.[105] An extraosseous tumor at the initial appearance of muliple myeloma is rare, but it is found in two thirds of patients at autopsy. Paraosseous tumor extension through destroyed cortical bone occurs in 50% of patients at autopsy. In 10% to 12% of patients with multiple myeloma, amyloidosis is present. Infection and renal failure are the primary causes of death. With the use of alkylating agents, steroids, and local irradiation, the median survival time is 20 months; 66% of patients are alive after 1 year, 32% after 3 years, and 18% after 5 years.[107] The imag-

ing characteristics appear to be similar to those of lymphomas (Fig. 4-196).

EXTRAMEDULLARY PLASMACYTOMAS

Extramedullary plasmacytoma is a rare soft-tissue malignancy composed of plasma cells. Eighty percent of these tumors occur in the head and neck, mainly in the upper respiratory tract and oral cavity. They represent 3% to 4% of all sinonasal cavity tumors.[108,109] About 20% of the head and neck extramedullary plasmacytomas are initially associated with multiple myeloma, and of these tumors, 95% occur in patients over the age of 40 years (mean is 59 years).[106] The tumors are four times more likely to occur in males than in females, and 90% of the patients are white.[106] The most common presenting symptoms are a soft-tissue mass (80%), airway obstruction (35%), epistaxis (35%), local pain

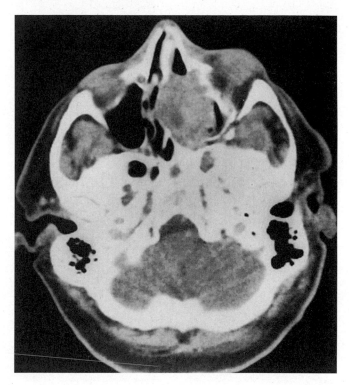

FIG. 4-191   Axial CT scan shows an expansile left nasal fossa mass that extends into the left maxillary and ethmoid sinuses and back to the skull base. Large cell lymphoma.

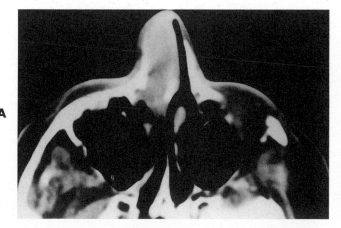
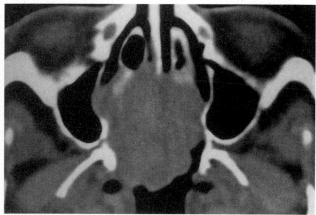

FIG. 4-192   Axial CT scan (**A**) shows a soft-tissue mass in the right nose and anterior nasal cavity. There is widening of the involved right side, and there is no bone erosion. Large cell lymphoma. Axial CT scan (**B**) shows a bulky, lobulated posterior nasal fossa mass, centered on the nasal septum. There is minimal thinning of the medial right antral wall. The dominant finding is expansion of the nasal vault. Large cell lymphoma.

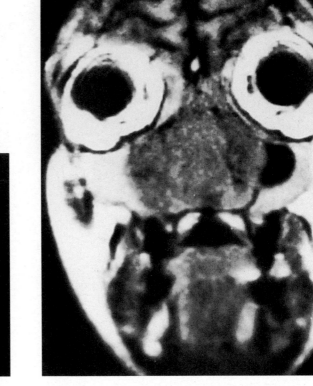

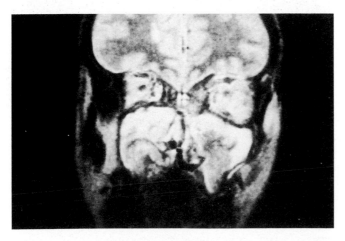

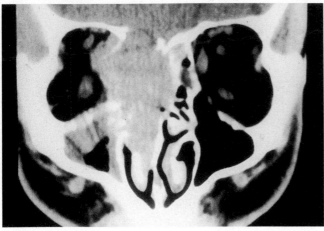

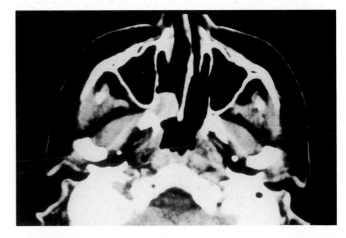

FIG. 4-193   Coronal CT scan shows a bulky soft-tissue mass in the right ethmoid and nasal cavity. The tumor has invaded the right orbit and the floor of the anterior cranial fossa. There is also obstruction of the right antrum. This is a more aggressive appearance of a large cell lymphoma and based on the imaging could be a carcinoma.

FIG. 4-194   Coronal T1W MR scan shows an expansile bilateral nasal cavity mass that extends into the ethmoid and maxillary sinuses. The mass has a low to intermediate signal intensity and had a slightly higher T2W signal intensity. Large cell lymphoma.

FIG. 4-195   Coronal T2W MR scan shows both maxillary sinuses to be opacified. The lower portion of each sinus has intermediate signal intensity tumor, and the remaining upper portion of each sinus has high signal intensity secretions. Large cell lymphoma.

FIG. 4-196   Axial CT scan shows a small polypoid mass along the right posterior lateral nasal wall. There is no associated bone erosion. Extraosseous plasmacytoma.

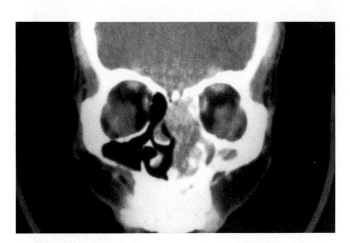

FIG. 4-197 Coronal CT scan shows a soft-tissue mass filling the left nasal cavity and the left ethmoid sinuses and obstructing the left antrum. There is focal erosion of the cribriform plate region, otherwise the marginal bone about the mass is intact. Extramedullary plasmacytoma.

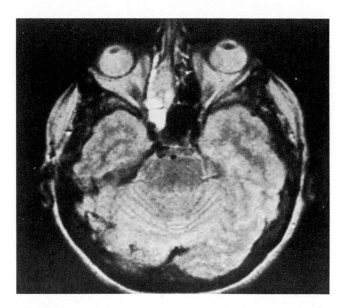

FIG. 4-198 Axial proton density MRI shows a right ethmoid and nasal mass, which has a low to intermediate signal intensity. Surrounding the mass are chronically obstructed secretions with high signal intensity. Extramedullary plasmacytoma.

(20%), proptosis (15%), and nasal discharge (10%). The mean duration of symptoms is 4 1/2 months. Of the head and neck lesions, 28% occur in the nasal cavity and 22% occur in the paranasal sinuses.[106]

The differential diagnosis includes anaplastic carcinomas, esthesioneuroblastomas, melanomas, large cell lymphomas, and embryonal rhabdomyosarcomas, as well as benign lesions such as plasma cell granulomas and pseudolymphomas.[106] Radiation therapy and surgery are the treatments of choice; alkylating agents and steroids help patients with painful bone lesions and patients with systemic disease. Eventually, 35% to 50% of patients with primary extramedullary plasmacytomas develop disseminated disease and regional lymph node disease. Local bone destruction and persistent primary tumors after radiation are not necessarily poor prognostic indicators. Between 31% and 75% of patients are alive after 5 years; however, the median length of survival after the onset of myeloma is less than 2 years.[106]

On CT, extramedullary plasmacytomas of the sinonasal cavities are homogeneous, enhancing, polypoid masses that remodel surrounding bone.[110] On MRI they have an intermediate signal intensity on all imaging sequences, they enhance, and because they are highly vascular, they may have vascular flow voids (Figs. 4-197, 4-198).

MESODERMAL TUMORS AND TUMORLIKE LESIONS

The true incidence of soft-tissue tumors, especially the ratio of benign to malignant tumors, is nearly impossible to determine because many benign tumors such as lipomas and

hemangiomas never undergo biopsy.[111] Sarcomas represent less than 1% of the total cancers reported in the United States. In children under age 16, these tumors represent 7% to 11% of all malignancies.[112] Of all sarcomas, 10% to 15% occur in the head and neck.[113]

HISTOCYTOSIS X

Hystiocytosis X comprises three diseases: eosinophilic granuloma, Letterer-Siwe disease, and Hand-Schüller-Christian disease. Although these diseases have manifestations in the skull and temporal bones, sinonasal disease is virtually unreported.[106]

RHABDOMYOSARCOMAS

Rhabdomyosarcoma is a malignant tumor of skeletal muscle. It accounts for 84% percent of all soft-tissue sarcomas and 35% to 45% of those that occur in the head and neck. It is primarily a pediatric disease, 43% of patients are under 5 years old, and 78% are under 12 years old. About 7% of cases occur in the second decade of life, and 2% to 4% of cases occur in each subsequent decade. Rhabdomyosarcoma is the seventh most common malignancy in children, following leukemia, central nervous system tumors, lymphoma, neuroblastoma, Wilms' tumor, and osteogenic sarcoma.[114] Of the fatal cases, 43.2% originate in the head and neck region, 28.6% in the genitourinary tract, 16% in the trunk, and 12.2% in the extremities.[112]

Embryonal rhabdomyosarcoma occurs primarily in the first decade of life, although 25% of the cases are in persons over the age of 20 years. Of embryonal tumors, 79%

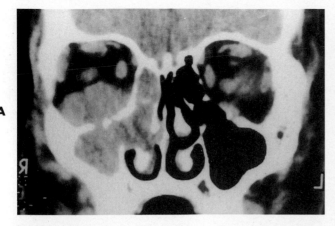

FIG. 4-199 Coronal CT scan (**A**) shows a soft-tissue mass in the right antrum. The medial sinus wall and portions of the antral roof are destroyed, and the tumor extends into the orbit, right ethmoid sinuses, and right nasal cavity. Despite these local areas of destruction, there are large areas where there is intact bone adjacent to the tumor. Rhabdomyosarcoma. Axial T1W MR scan (**B**) shows a homogeneous mass in the left infratemporal fossa extending into the left antrum and the skull base. The mass has an intermediate signal intensity. Rhabdomyosarcoma.

arise in the head and neck or genitourinary tract; with modern chemotherapy and radiation therapy, 5-year survival rates have risen from 8% to 21% to 65%.[115] Between 10% and 38% of these cases metastasize to regional lymph nodes. Embryonal rhabdomyosarcoma can be histologically confused with anaplastic carcinoma, esthesioneuroblastoma, melanoma, large cell lymphoma, and extramedullary plasmacytoma.[41]

Alveolar rhabdomyosarcomas occur primarily in 15- to 25-year-olds. These tumors arise in the extremities in 54% of cases, the trunk in 28%, and the head and neck in 18%.[112] The median survival time is only 8.75 months, and the 5-year survival rate is only 2%.[116] Alveolar rhabdomyosarcomas have a great propensity for lymph node metastases; 33% of cases have regional node involvement at initial tumor presentation and 75% to 85% involve regional or distant nodes during the course of the disease.[112]

The pleomorphic rhabdomyosarcoma occurs primarily between ages 40 and 60; only 6% of the tumors are found in patients under age 15. Most of these tumors develop in the extremities, and only 7% develop in the head and neck. The 5-year survival rate is 25% to 35%. Most metastases result from hematogenous spread and only 9% involve regional lymph nodes.[112]

In the head and neck the most common sites for all rhabdomyosarcomas are the orbit (36%), nasopharynx (15.4%), middle ear and mastoid (13.8%), sinonasal cavities (8.1%), face (4.5%), neck (4.1%), and larynx (4.1%). In the nasal cavity and paranasal sinuses, the most common presenting findings are nasal obstruction, rhinorrhea, epistaxis, sinusitis, local pain, otalgia, headache, toothache, proptosis, decreased visual acuity, and cranial nerve defects.[112] About

42% of patients have cervical lymph node metastases, and 58% have distant metastases. After treatment, distant metastases may be a greater threat to survival than local recurrence.[117-119]

On imaging, rhabdomyosarcomas usually have elements of both bone remodeling and bone destruction. On contrast CT these tumors enhance little to moderately and are generally homogeneous in appearance. On MRI they are also remarkably homogeneous and have intermediate signal intensities on all imaging sequences (Fig. 4-199).

FIBROSARCOMAS

Fibrosarcomas account for 12% to 19% of all soft-tissue sarcomas and are found predominantly in the lower extremities and trunk; only 15% occur in the head and neck. Most head and neck tumors involve the sinonasal cavities (18.3%), larynx (14.8%), neck (6.1%), and face (4.9%), and they usually arise in patients between 20 and 60 years of age.[112] Fibrosarcomas can be well differentiated with well-developed collagen production and few mitoses (grade I) [fibromatosis or desmoid tumor] or they may be poorly differentiated with little collagen production and frequent mitoses (grades II to III).

A desmoid tumor (fibromatosis, grade I fibrosarcoma) is a unique entity, requiring special recognition. The tumors are histologically very bland and well differentiated with no tendency to metastasize. An isolated biopsy of a desmoid might look like nothing more than scar tissue. The diagnosis is firmly established on biopsy, when the pathologist can identify the bland fibroblasts incidiously infiltrating host tissue. Examination during surgery shows that this white-tan

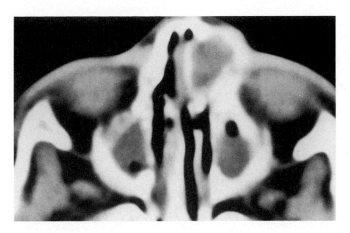

FIG. 4-200 Axial CT scan shows a soft-tissue mass in the left lacrimal duct region, bulging into the left nasal fossa. The bone is remodeled around the lesion. Incidently noted are inflammatory secretions in both maxillary sinuses. Fibromatosis.

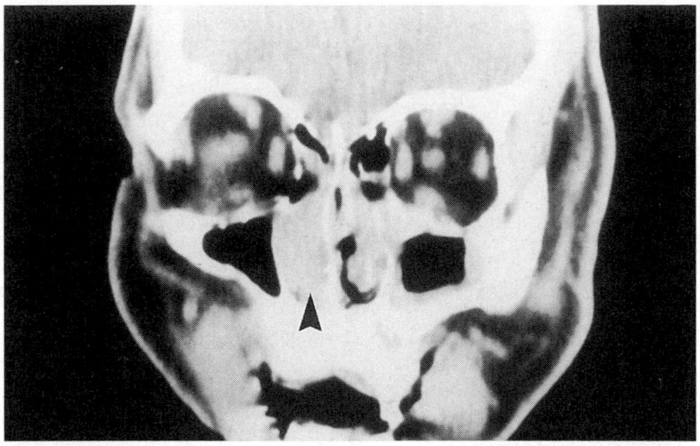

FIG. 4-201 Axial CT scan shows an expansile polypoid mass in the right nasal fossa *(arrowhead)*. There is no bone erosion, and the nasal septum is intact. Inflammatory disease is present in the left antrum and nasal cavity. Fibrous histiocytoma.

scarlike tumor in most cases sends out innumerable tentacles, making complete extirpation virtually impossible. Positive resection margins are the rule.

Fibromatosis occurs most commonly between the fourth and sixth decades of life. Although grade II and grade III fibrosarcomas may be seen occasionally in the pediatric population, fibromatosis (desmoid tumor, grade I fibrosarcoma) is more likely to occur in the pediatric population. In the head and neck, fibromatosis may occur in the sternocleidomastoid muscle and, less likely, in the sinonasal tract. Recurrences after resection are common and in some series are as high as 90%.[120,121] Progression to higher grade fibrosarcoma may occur in occasional unfortunate cases, usually after radiotherapy.

For grade II and grade III fibrosarcomas, local recurrences develop within 18 months of initial treatment and metastases occur within 2 years of local recurrences.[112] The prognosis depends on the adequacy of the surgical resection, the number of mitoses, the size and location of the lesion, male sex, and the presence of pain or cranial nerve symptoms. Of these parameters the resection margins are probably the most important. Complete surgical excision with ample margins is the treatment of choice. Only 1% to 11% of patients develop positive regional lymph nodes; however, the 5-year survival rates are only 33% to 69%.[112] In addition the younger the patient is when the tumor appears, the better is the prognosis.[112] Although the local recurrence rate of pediatric fibrosarcoma is similar to that for adults (17% to 47%), younger patients only have metastases in up to 14% of cases, and they have a higher 5-year survival rate of 85%.

Less than 20% of all fibrosarcomas originate in the skeleton where they account for 3% to 5% of all primary malignant bone tumors. Of these tumors, 15% occur in the head and neck, usually involving the jaw or maxilla. Bony fibrosarcomas tend to spread more aggressively than their soft-tissue counterparts. Most of these tumors arise in males

between 35 to 40 years of age. Those occurring in the older population (30%) are usually the secondary type, arising in previously irradiated or diseased bone such as bone with fibrous dysplasia, Paget's disease, giant cell tumors, bone infarcts, and osteomyelitis. Most are grade II or grade III lesions, and the 5-year survival rate for all of these lesions varies from 27% to 40%. The higher the grade and the larger the tumor, the worse the prognosis. Metastases occur to the lungs and other bones; only 3% spread to regional lymph nodes.[93]

On CT, fibrosarcomas have a generally homogeneous, nonenhancing appearance. They also tend to remodel bone (Fig. 4-200). On MRI they have low to intermediate signal intensities on all imaging sequences.

MALIGNANT FIBROUS HISTIOCYTOMAS

Fibrous histiocytic tumors are neoplasms comprised of an admixture of histiocytes and fibroblasts. Malignant fibrous histiocytoma (MFH) are sarcomas of soft tissue and bone. The vast majority occur in the extremities, retroperitoneum, and abdomen. Only about 3% occur in the head and neck, and most of these occur in the skin, orbit, or sinonasal cavities.[112] Head and neck malignant fibrous histiocytomas have a male predominance and occur at a median age of 46 years. Local recurrences develop in 27% of cases, and 75% of these reccur within 2 years of diagnosis. Cervical nodal metastases occur in 12% and distant metastases in 42% of cases. The 2-year survival rate for all MFH is 60%. An accurate survival rate just for head and neck tumors cannot be obtained because most of the reported tumors in this area have only recently appeared in the literature.[112]

MFH can be histologically classified as myxoid, angiomatoid, inflammatory, and giant cell type. The differential diagnosis of MFH includes pleomorphic rhabdomyosarcomas, pleomorphic liposarcomas, and anaplastic carcinomas. Electron microscopy and histochemical testing

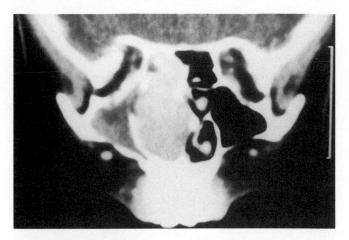

FIG. 4-202 Coronal CT scan shows an enhancing right nasal fossa mass that extends into the right ethmoid sinuses. The right antrum is obstructed. There is primarily bone remodeling about the mass. Hemangiopericytoma.

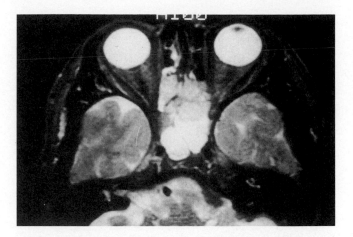

FIG. 4-203 Axial T2W MR scan shows an intermediate signal intensity mass in the posterior ethmoid sinuses and anterior sphenoid sinuses. The remaining obstructed sphenoid sinuses are filled with high signal intensity secretions. Hemangiopericytoma.

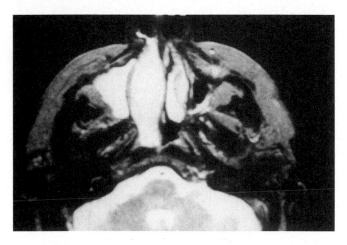

FIG. 4-204 Axial T2W MR scan shows a high signal intensity expansile mass in the right nasal cavity. The right antrum is filled with higher signal intensity obstructed secretions. Minimal inflammatory mucosal thickening is present in the left antrum. Hemangiopericytoma.

may be necessary for a definitive diagnosis. The current treatment of choice is wide surgical excision; the role of radiation therapy remains difficult to assess.[112]

On contrast CT these tumors usually enhance moderately or not at all. Either aggressive bone destruction or bone remodeling can occur, making the CT characteristics nonspecific (Fig. 4-201).[122] On MRI, fibrous histiocytomas usually have intermediate signal intensities on all imaging sequences.

LIPOSARCOMAS

Liposarcomas comprise 15% to 18% of all malignant soft-tissue sarcomas. Before the recognition of MFH, pleomorphic liposarcomas were most frequently diagnosed as soft-tissue sarcomas. Currently it is the second most commonly diagnosed sarcoma. Most occur in men, at an average age of 43 years. Only about 3% of liposarcomas occur in the head

and neck. Of these, only isolated cases have been reported in the sinonasal cavities.[112] Histologically, liposarcomas can be classified as either well differentiated, myxoid, round cell, pleomorphic, or mixed. The 5-year survival rate for liposarcomas is as follows: well-differentiated tumors, 85% to 100%; myxoid, 71% to 95%; round cell, 12.5% to 55%; pleomorphic, 0% to 45%; and mixed, 31% to 33%. The overall incidence of metastases is 25% to 45%, and it is most likely to occur with the round cell or pleomorphic types. The treatment of choice is wide surgical excision. The role of postoperative radiation remains controversial.

Based on the general experience with liposarcomas elsewhere in the body, on CT these lesions have an overall low (fatty) attenuation value (-65 to -110 HUs) and there are irregular areas of soft-tissue density seen within the lesion. The tumor margins may infiltrate adjacent soft tissues. MRI shows a nonhomogeneously high T1W signal intensity and an intermediate T2W signal intensity.[123]

LEIOMYOSARCOMAS

Leiomyosarcomas represent only 5% to 6% of all soft-tissue sarcomas and occur primarily in the uterus, gastrointestinal tract, and retroperitoneum. Only 3% to 10% of these tumors arise in the head and neck; of these, 19% arise in the sinonasal cavities.[112]

Leiomyosarcomas are distinguished from their benign counterparts, leiomyomas, by the presence of more than 10 mitoses per high-power field, atypia, and necrosis. The malignant cells of the epithelioid variant appear less spindled and more cuboidal. This variant is more likely to arise in the stomach or the mesentery but has been found in head and neck sites.[124] In the nose and paranasal sinuses these tumors have an equal sex distribution and an average age incidence of 50 years.[125] The sinonasal symptoms are nonspecific, patients complain of nasal obstruction, bleeding, and pain. Treatment involves radical extirpation. Little

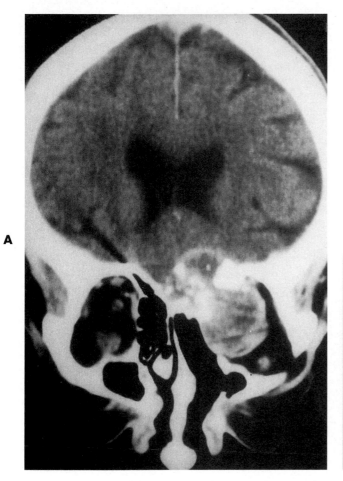

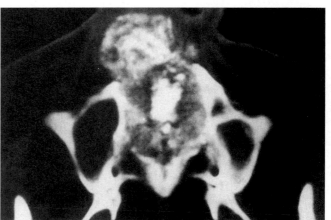

FIG. 4-205 Coronal CT scan (**A**) shows a destructive mass in the left ethmoid sinuses. The tumor has broken into the left orbit and the anterior cranial fossa. Gross, discrete calcifications are also present within the mass. Chondrosarcoma. Axial CT scan (**B**) shows a bulky mass arising in the hard palate and extending ventrally into the nose. There are innumerable calcifications spread throughout the tumor. Chondrosarcoma.

response has been found with either radiation therapy or chemotherapy.[124] About 75% of patients have a local recurrence and 35% develop metastases. At least 50% of these patients die of the disease, usually within 2 years of diagnosis.[125] Prognosis appears to depend most on initial tumor stage. Leiomyosarcomas are bulky lesions that remodel bone and enhance little; they may have multiple areas of necrotic and cystic liquefaction within.[126]

HEMANGIOPERICYTOMAS

Hemangiopericytomas (HPCs) are uncommon vascular lesions that arise primarily in the lower extremities, retroperitoneum, and pelvis. However, 15% occur in the head and neck, and of these, 55% arise in the nasal cavity.[127] HPCs are tumors thought to be derived from the contractive cells that surround the outer aspect of small vessels, Zimmerman's pericytes. The lower extremities and the retroperitoneum-

pelvis are the most common sites for HPCs. The head and neck is the third most common site; tumors occur in the neck, perioral soft tissues, and lastly the sinonasal tract. Sinonasal hemangiopericytomas (SNHPCs) present as gray to tan, spongy, vascular, polypoid masses. Nasal obstruction and epistaxis are common presenting symptoms.[128] Other presenting complaints include watery rhinorrhea, serous otitis media, proptosis, infraorbital anesthesia, and facial pain. SNHPCs generally involve the nasal cavity along with one or more sinuses. A review of the literature revealed an overall recurrence rate of 19% (22 of 115 cases). The majority of recurrences (19 of 22) were single (16%) and most (14 of 19) occurred within the first 5 years after resection. However, first recurrences after the first 10 years have occurred. Multiple recurrences were a rarer finding, seen in only 4 of 115 cases. Overall, three patients (2.6%) developed metastases (usually locoregional sites and local lymph nodes). Four patients (3.5%) ultimately died of disease (usually from a lack of local control). This confirms the general low-grade malignant potential of this neoplasm. It appears that no single feature of SNHPC can predict patient course for this basically low-grade neoplasm. The prognosis of SNHPC most likely strongly depends on tumor stage at initial presentation and completeness of primary resection. Features such as mitotic rate, necrosis, and nuclear pleomorphism are probably significant for high-stage or incompletely resected tumors. The role of chemotherapy is still evolving, but initial reports show promise.[112,128,129]

Microscopically, fusiform or spindle cells can be seen, forming short fasicles and bundles, which become more dense around vessels. The abundant vessels have typical cuffs of perivascular hyalinization. Staghorn vessels may actually be rare. Nuclear pleomorphism is not normally present in SNHPCs.[128]

On CT, hemangiopericytomas are expansile, bone-remodeling lesions with a variably enhancing, fairly homogeneous appearance (Figs. 4-202 to 4-204). On MRI they enhance and have low to intermediate T1W signal intensity and a higher T2W signal intensity.

ANGIOSARCOMAS OF SOFT TISSUE

Angiosarcomas account for only 2% to 3% of all soft-tissue sarcomas. The term angiosarcoma describes malignant tumors that arise from endothelial cells of blood or lymphatic vessels. The hemangioendothelioma or hemangioendothelial sarcoma connote a related vascular sarcoma of somewhat better differentiation. Angiosarcomas have been reported in virtually every site of the body, but most arise in the skin, liver, and breast. Sinonasal tumors are uncommon. They present with epistaxis, nasal obstruction, headaches, and proptosis.[130] The average age of onset is 42 years, and the male to female ratio is 3:2. From the limited number of reported cases, the 5-year survival rate is 60%. Inexplicably, sinonasal tumors appear to have a better prognosis than skin and soft-tissue lesions. Axial skeletal and soft-tissue angiosarcomas have a 30% rate of metastases to regional lymph nodes and 20% metastases to distant sites within 2 to 3 years of initial treatment.[112] There are too few cases of sinonasal angiosarcomas to compare the rates of metastases. Surgery with or without radiation therapy is the treatment of choice, and therapy must take into account that angiosarcomas often extend several centimeters beyond their apparent limits. Sinonasal angiosarcomas are extremely rare.[131,132] They have been reported in patients as young as 8 years old. Presenting symptoms relate to mass effect and include epistaxis. On CT and MRI these tumors are aggressive, bone destroying lesions that enhance well.

ANGIOSARCOMAS OF BONE

Most angiosarcomas arise de novo, although they have been reported at sites of chronic osteomyelitis. They represent less than 1% of all primary malignant tumors of bone and can occur as solitary lesions (77%) or as multifocal tumors, involving several bones (23%). Most multifocal tumors occur in the bones of the extremities, pelvis, and spine. The solitary tumors are twice as common in males, and 60% of patients are between 20 and 49 years of age.[112] Head and neck tumors make up 15% of solitary intraosseous angiosarcomas. Most head and neck tumors arise in the mandible and skull. The symptoms vary with the specific bone involved; however, most patients complain of dull local pain and swelling of the affected region. Complete surgical excision is the treatment of choice; radiotherapy is reserved for inaccessible lesions, incompletely excised tumors, or palliative treatment. Grade I lesions recur locally but do not metastasize, as do grade II and III lesions. For patients with solitary lesions the 5-year survival statistics are 20%, and for patients with multifocal lesions the rate is 36%, reflecting the predominance of grade I tumors in these latter patients. Most metastases are to the lungs and are rarely to other viscera, regional lymph nodes, and bones.[112]

MESENCHYMAL CHONDROSARCOMAS

The mesenchymal chondrosarcoma is a rare neoplasm of bone (60% to 70% of cases) or soft tissues (30% to 40% of cases). The mandible is one of the preferred osseous sites, and the craniospinal meninges and orbital soft tissues are the most common extraskeletal sites. These tumors also have been reported in the ethmoid sinuses. More than half of the patients are between 10 and 30 years of age, and radical excision appears to offer the best chance of cure. Few patients have responded to radiation therapy. Survival is highly variable; most patients die within months, whereas others survive for many years. The 5-year survival figures do not always correspond with clinical cures. Hematogenous metastases are preceded by one or more local recurrences. The osseous and extraosseous lesions do not differ significantly in their clinical behavior.[112]

CHONDROMAS AND CHONDROSARCOMAS

Chondrogenic tumors of the sinonasal cavities are rare and most often malignant. This is in contrast to chondrosarcomas of the larynx, which are usually low grade. The average patient is 44 years old, and males predominate by a 3:2 ratio. About 60% of the tumors arise in the anterior alveolar region of the maxilla, and patients usually consult their physician with complaints of nasal obstruction, epistaxis, chronic nasal discharge, loose teeth, poorly fitting dentures, an expansile painless mass, proptosis, or headache.[88] Most tumors are either grade I or II chondrosarcomas; grade III lesions are uncommon. The incidence for metastases for grades I, II, and III are 0%, 10%, and 71%, respectively.[133] Early, wide excision is the only modality that results in a cure because these lesions are not radiosensitive and chemotherapy results have been unrewarding. The 5-year

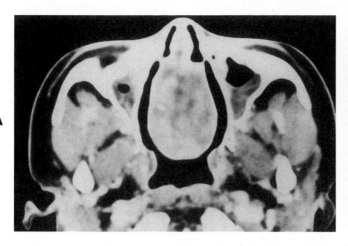
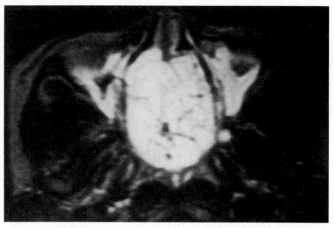

FIG. 4-206   Axial CT (**A**) and axial T2W MR (**B**) scans show a bulky mass arising from the nasal septum. Scattered calcifications are present within the mass. The lesion had an intermediate T1W signal intensity. Unrelated inflammatory changes are present in the maxillary sinuses. Chondrosarcoma.

survival rate is 40% to 60%, and at least 60% of patients have a local recurrence within 5 years. However, some recurrences have been reported 10 to 20 years after initial treatment. Overall, only 7% of sinonasal chondrosarcomas develop metastases, which predominantly go to the lungs and bones. Uncontrolled local disease is the most common cause of death.[88]

True chondromas, that is, fully benign cartilagenous tumors, of the sinonasal cavities have been reported in the nose, ethmoid, sinuses, maxilla, sphenoid sinuses, and nasopharynx. They are equally divided between males and females, and about 60% occur in patients less than 50 years of age. Because 20% of head and neck chondrosarcomas may be misdiagnosed initially as chondromas due to sampling errors, wide surgical excision is the treatment of choice.[133,134]

On CT, calcifications within the tumor matrix are not always seen. These lesions tend to be expansile, remodel bone, and have an attenuation less than muscle but greater than fat.[135,136] They do not provoke sclerotic bone at their margins. On MRI they usually have low T1W and high T2W signal intensity, and they can enhance (Figs. 4-205 to 4-207).

MALIGNANT MESENCHYMOMAS

Malignant mesenchymomas are rare tumors composed of two or more sarcomatous elements that ordinarily are not found together. As diagnostic criteria have become more refined, the frequency of malignant mesenchymoma has declined from a peak incidence in the 1950s and 1960s. Most tumors that were previously diagnosed as malignant mesenchymomas are probably currently classified as malignant fibrous histiocytomas. Collectively the death rate is 60% in adults and 43% in children.[68] Two cases of malignant mesenchymoma studied with CT scans appeared as

aggressive lesions that were indistinguishable from squamous cell carcinomas.

HEMANGIOMAS

Hemangiomas of the nasal cavity occur on the septum (65%), then the lateral wall (18%) and vestibule (16%). Most arise in the anterior septum near Kisselbach's plexus, and most are of the capillary type. Lesions arising on the lateral wall usually are of the cavernous type. Epistaxis and nasal obstruction are the most common patient complaints. Simple excision is generally curative for these lesions, which rarely exceed 2 cm in their greatest dimension. Hemangiomas are diagnosed when small because they cause dramatically severe epistaxis. Rarely, intranasal hemangiomas may develop in the second trimester of pregnancy. Most of these lesions spontaneously regress within 4 to 8 weeks after delivery.[112] Hemangiomas of the paranasal sinuses are very rare; two have been described in the maxillary sinuses and two in the sphenoid sinuses. In the nasal cavity they also tend to develop in the inferior and middle turbinates. On CT they enhance. The sphenoid sinus cases showed destruction of the skull base.[112] Hemangiomas have an intermediate signal intensity on all MR imaging sequences; they enhance, and vascular flow voids occasionally may be present (Fig. 4-208).[137,138]

SOLITARY HEMANGIOMAS OF BONE

The solitary hemangioma lesion accounts for only 0.7% of all primary bone tumors. In the head and neck the most common sites are the skull (53%), mandible (10.7%), nasal bones (9%), and cervical vertebrae (6%). Although many patients have a history of local trauma, a cause-and-effect relationship remains doubtful. The lesions most often occur

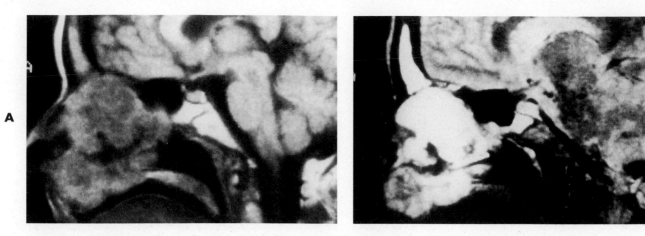

FIG. 4-207 Sagittal T1W (**A**) and T2W (**B**) MR scans show a slightly nonhomogeneous nasal septal mass that has a low to intermediate signal intensity in **A** and a high signal intensity in **B**. The frontal sinuses are obstructed by the tumor. Chondrosarcoma.

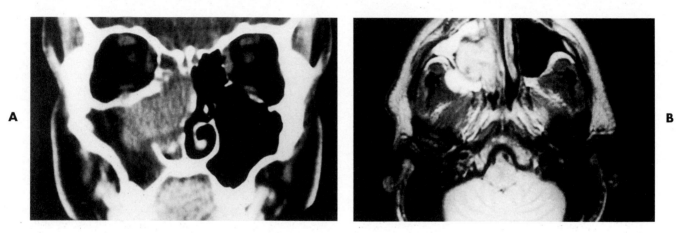

FIG. 4-208 Coronal CT scan (**A**) shows a mass in the right nasal cavity and the right maxillary and ethmoid sinuses. Obstructed secretions are present in both the right antrum and ethmoid sinuses. Most of the bone around the margin of the tumor is intact. Axial proton density MR scan (**B**) shows the tumor to have a high signal intensity, but not as high as the signal intensity of the obstructed secretions in the right antrum. The chronic antral obstruction has lead to the development of a mucocele, which bulges into the right infratemporal fossa. Hemangioma.

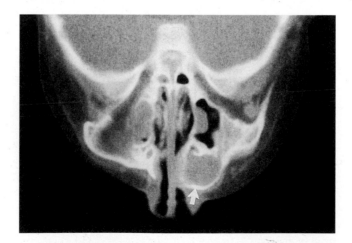

FIG. 4-209 Coronal CT scan shows an expansile mass in the left anterior maxilla (*arrow*). The surrounding bone is intact. Myxoma.

in females by a 2:1 ratio; the average age of onset is 31 years. Most commonly, patients experience a firm, non-painful swelling that is associated with a pulsating sensation. Actual bruits are rarely heard. When hemangiomas involve the facial bones and mandible, angiograms have revealed that the blood supply is from the facial artery or the internal maxillary artery. The inadvertent surgical violation of an intraosseous hemangioma can be associated with exceptionally rapid blood loss, often as much as 3500 ml. Even so, surgery is the primary treatment of choice. Embolization may greatly reduce operative blood loss, provided that the operation is performed shortly after embolization, before a collateral circulation can develop.[88]

Radiographically these lesions have a "soap bubble" or "honeycomb" appearance and enhance on postcontrast CT scans. On MRI they have low to intermediate T1W and high T2W signal intensity. They also enhance.

LYMPHANGIOMAS

Lymphangiomas virtually are unreported in the sinonasal cavities and are located primarily on the neck, face, floor of the mouth, and tongue.[112]

RHABDOMYOMAS

Rhabdomyomas are rare benign tumors with skeletal muscle differentiation. Clinically and pathologically they may be divided into adult and fetal forms. Adult rhabdomyomas are most commonly encountered in the heart and are associated with tuberosclerosis. Extracardiac adult rhabdomyomas are rare but have a tendency to affect head and neck sites such as the oral cavity and the larynx. In a series of 27 cases collected by Kapidia, et al the sinonasal tract was not affected in any case, but two cases did involve the nasopharynx. Although these tumors are benign, they may be multinodular. Of the cases, 42% recurred. The fetal form occurs at a median age of 4 years. The most common site in a series of 24 cases was the facial soft tissues. No cases affected the sinonasal tract, but the nasopharynx was involved in three cases. Only one of these recurred. The histologic distinction between fetal rhabdomyoma and adult rhabdomyoma is obviously of crucial significance. Fetal rhabdomyomas grow in a circumscribed, noninfiltrating pattern and lack the necrosis and nuclear pleomorphism seen in adult rhabdomyomas.[118,119]

LEIOMYOMAS

Leiomyomas are benign smooth-muscle tumors, only eight of which have been reported in the nose and paranasal sinuses. Knifelike pain has been reported with this lesion, and it is believed that the pain is due to spasmodic contraction of the tumor with resultant ischemia. Of the head and neck tumors, 71% are conventional leiomyomas, 27% are angiomyomas, 1.2% are epithelioid leiomyomas, and 0.8% are mesectodermal leiomyomas.[112,139]

LIPOMA AND LIPOMA-LIKE LESIONS

These lesions, which include the ordinary lipoma, myxoid lipoma, angiolipoma, pleomorphic lipoma, spindle-cell lipoma, myelolipoma, hibernoma, and lipoblastomatosis, are of various reported frequencies; however, they have not been reported to arise within the sinonasal cavities.

MYXOMAS

A myxoma is a mesenchymal neoplasm comprised of undifferentiated stellate cells in a myxoid stroma. Only about 130 cases have been documented, and their occurrence in descending order of frequency is in the heart, subcutaneous tissues, bone, genitourinary tract, and skin. Head and neck myxomas are usually intraosseous; those of the jaws represent 40% to 50% of all head and neck myxomas and are followed in frequency by palatal tumors. On CT they are cystic-appearing lesions that do not enhance (Fig. 4-209).[140]

FASCIITIS

These lesions also represent a wide variety of pathologic entities that include nodular fasciitis, proliferative fasciitis, focal myositis, myositis ossificans, and myositis ossificans circumscripta or progressiva. None of these entities have been described in the sinonasal cavities.[112]

FIBROOSSEOUS LESIONS

Of all the nonepithelial tumors that involve the sinonasal cavities, 25% are osseous or fibroosseous lesions.

Osteomas

Osteoma is a benign proliferation of bone that occurs almost exclusively in the skull and facial bones. Of patients with osteomas, 20% to 30% have a history of prior trauma, but this is not thought to be causative.[88] Head and neck osteomas occur mainly in the frontal sinuses, followed in descending order by the ethmoid, maxillary, and sphenoid sinuses. The high prevalence of osteomas in the frontal and ethmoid sinuses may relate to the fact that this region is the junction of membranous and enchondral development of the frontal and ethmoid bones.

Several histologic types of osteomas exist. The compact, or "ivory," type of osteoma is composed of dense, hard, mature bone, with only small amounts of fibrous tissue. The cancellous, or "mature," type of osteoma has sparse intertrabecular spaces that may be empty or filled with fat, fibrous tissue, or hematopoietic elements.[88] Fibrous osteomas contain abundant mature lamellar bone but have greater amounts of intertrabecular fibrous tissue. As a result, on plain films, bone density varies from a very dense, sclerotic lesion for the ivory-type osteoma to a progressively less dense and less ossified lesion for the fibrous osteoma. In

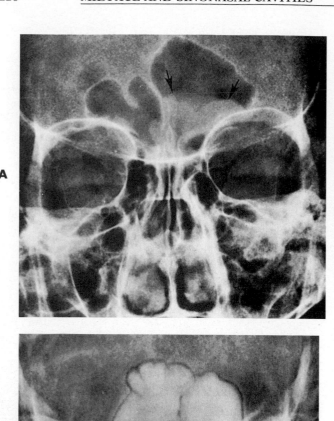

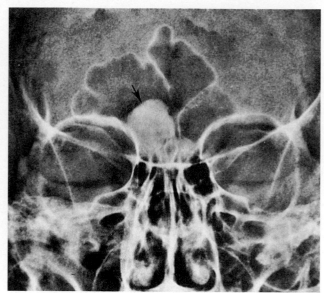

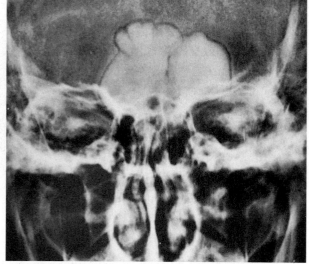

FIG. 4-210   **A,** Caldwell view shows a polypoid mass *(arrows)* that is slightly denser than the adjacent frontal bone. Fibrous "soft" osteoma. **B,** Caldwell view shows an ivory osteoma *(arrow)* in right frontal sinus. The sinus is not obstructed. **C,** PA view shows bilateral frontal osteomas. Note how the osteomas have conformed to the sinus contour.

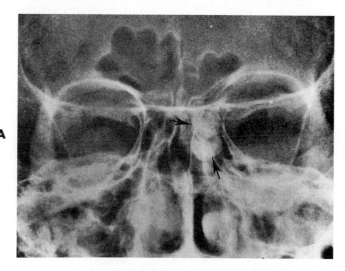

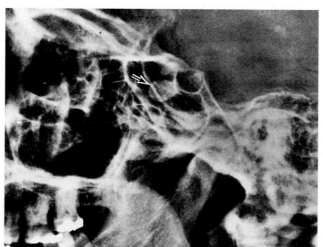

FIG. 4-211   **A,** Caldwell view shows an osteoma in left ethmoid sinuses *(arrows).* **B,** Lateral view shows an osteoma *(arrow)* in sphenoid sinuses.

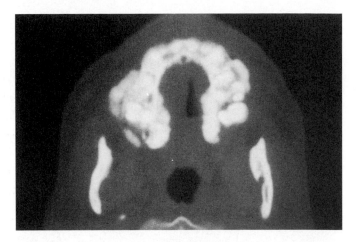

FIG. 4-213 Axial CT scan shows multiple exostoses (osteomas) of the maxillary alveolus. This is a benign condition that only occurs in the jaw. Maxillary exostosis.

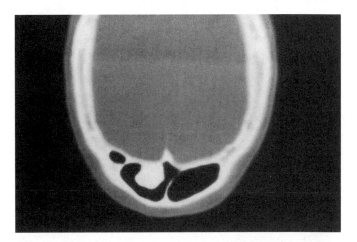

FIG. 4-214 Coronal CT scan shows a nonobstructing osteoma arising from the posterior frontal sinus wall. Osteoma.

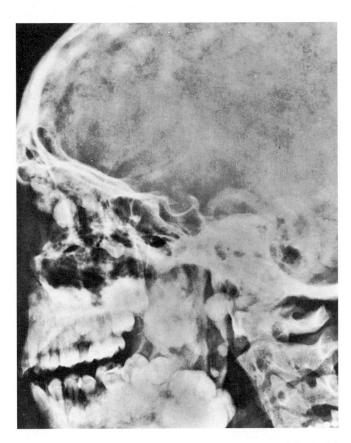

FIG. 4-212 Lateral view shows multiple osteomas of the facial bones, mandible, and calvarium. Gardner's syndrome.

fact, some fibrous osteomas may be confused on plain films with a retention cyst or polyp (Figs. 4-210, 4-211).

Osteomas usually are small and incidental findings on plain films. However, they can obstruct the frontal sinus in 17% of cases, and this results in the need for immediate surgery.[141] Almost all osteomas remain confined to the sinuses, often conforming to the contour of the sinus. However, osteomas are the most common benign paranasal sinus tumors associated with spontaneous cerebrospinal fluid rhinorrhea.[142] When multiple osteomas are seen, primarily in the skull and mandible, the diagnosis of Gardner's syndrome should be considered. The osteomas in this syndrome can arise during the teenage years and be diagnosed before the appearance of intestinal polyps, which often do not arise until the third decade of life (Fig. 4-212). Multiple osteomas can also occur as maxillary exostoses. This benign condition usually presents clinically as a painless bulging of the alveolus, possibly causing ill-fitting dentures (Fig. 4-213).

On CT, osteomas arise from one of the sinus walls or the intersinus septum. The differences between the compact, cancellous, and fibrous types of osteomas correlate with the degree of bone-matrix density seen within the lesion. On MRI these lesions give a nonhomogeneous, low to intermediate signal intensity on all imaging sequences. Based purely on MRI findings their osseous nature may go undetected (Figs. 4-214, 4-215).

Osteochondromas

Osteochondromas represent 40% to 50% of benign osseous lesions and 10% to 15% of all osseous tumors. It is not clear whether they represent a true neoplasm or a developmental abnormality. They can arise from any bone that develops from enchondral ossification. Because most of the craniofacial bones develop by intramembranous ossification, osteochondromas in the sinonasal cavities are rare. Of the approximately 77 cases reported in this region, most arose in the mandible. They have been reported in the sphenoid bone,

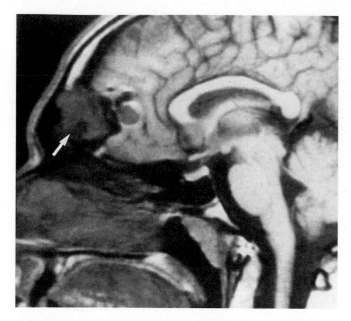

FIG. 4-215   Sagittal T1W MR scan shows a low signal intensity mass in the frontal sinuses that has extended into the anterior cranial fossa, causing pneumocephalus. Osteoma.

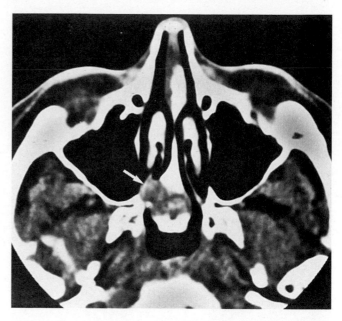

FIG. 4-216   Axial CT scan shows an expansile, partially calcified mass in the posterior nasal septum *(arrow)*. Osteochondroma.

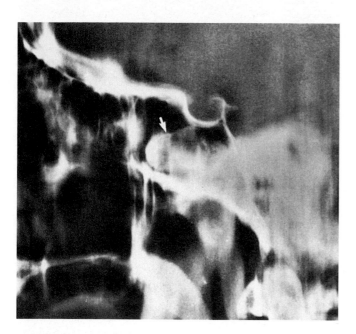

FIG. 4-217   Lateral multidirectional tomogram shows a partially ossified pedunculated mass in the sphenoid sinus *(arrow)*. Osteochondroma.

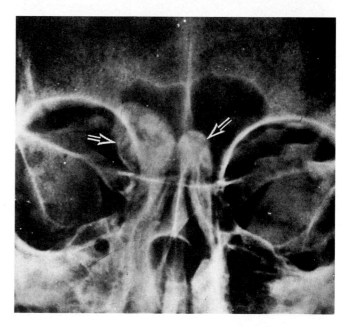

FIG. 4-218   Caldwell view shows bone density masses *(arrows)* in the ethmoid sinuses, which project into the anterior cranial fossa. There is also disease in the ethmoid sinuses. Osteoblastoma.

maxillary tuberosity, zygomatic arch, and nasal septum.[88] Most osteochondromas stop growing with maturation of the remaining skeleton. However, it is not unusual to find a lesion that either stops growing before or continues to grow after skeletal maturation. Surgery is the treatment of choice, and only 1% to 2% of lesions recur. Similarly, only 1% to 2% of solitary osteochondromas undergo malignant change, usually into chondrosarcomas.[88] Radiographically these tumors tend

to have a pedunculated, mushroom shape. The cartilaginous cap is often not visible and when seen may be focally calcified. On MRI they have a nonhomogeneous low to intermediate signal intensity on all imaging sequences (Figs. 4-216, 4-217).

Osteoid Osteomas

These lesions represent 11% of benign bone neoplasms. They occur twice as commonly in males, and 80% of the

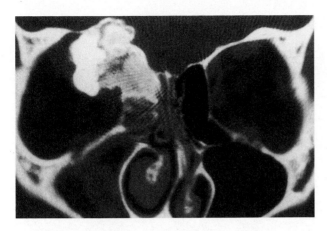

FIG. 4-219 Coronal CT scan shows a bony-density lesion in the right frontal and ethmoid bones. The bone is expanded, and the cortices are intact. Part of the lesion has a "ground glass" appearance; however, the remaining portion of the mass has a large, very dense bone production. Benign osteoblastoma.

patients are between 5 and 25 years of age. Only 26 cases have been reported in the head and neck, most of which were in the mandible and cervical vertebrae. Osteoid osteomas have been reported in the frontal, ethmoid, and maxillary bones. Patients describe a dull pain that usually worsens at night, is intensified by activity, and is relieved by rest. On plain films and CT the classic lesion is a dense cortical ovoid mass with a 1 to 2 mm, low-density nidus. However, the nidus also may be dense and difficult to identify.[88] Histologically the nidus is recognized as a tangled array of new osteoid bony trabecula surrounded by reactive bone. Surgery is the treatment of choice.

Osteoblastomas

Osteoblastomas represent only 3% of all benign bone tumors and possess histologic features that are virtually identical to osteoid osteoma. Those lesions greater than 2 cm in diameter usually are diagnosed as osteoblastomas. Most osteoblastomas occur in the vertebrae (30% to 40%); however, at least 15 cases have been reported in the maxilla, ethmoid, and sphenoethmoid regions.[88] In contrast to osteoid osteomas, the pain of osteoblastomas usually is more severe, is not nocturnal, and is not relieved by aspirin. Osteoblastomas are divided into the classic benign type and the aggressive type. Conservative surgery, consisting of local excision or curettage, cures 80% to 90% of the cases of benign osteoblastoma. The aggressive type recurs locally but unlike osteogenic sarcoma it does not metastasize.[88] The pathologic distinction between aggressive osteoblastoma and a well-differentiated osteogenic sarcoma may at times be difficult.

Radiographically these tumors have a variable appearance; some lesions have large discrete areas of organized bone density and others have a mixed osseous and fibrous appearance. The latter is more nodular and more coarsely organized than most ossifying fibromas and some fibrous

dysplasias. The lesions tend to be expansile and remodel the adjacent bone (Figs. 4-218, 4-219).[142-144]

Osteogenic Sarcomas

Osteosarcomas (OS) comprise 2% of all primarily malignant bone neoplasms. They are the second most common malignant tumor of the skeleton after multiple myeloma. OS is twice as common as chondrosarcoma, three times more common than Ewing's sarcoma, and four to six times more common than an osseous fibrosarcoma. It can arise as a primary lesion or be related to prior irradiation, exposure to Thorotrast, or a variety of benign conditions that include Paget's disease, fibrous dysplasia, giant cell tumor, osteoblastoma, bone infarct, and chronic osteomyelitis.[88,145] OSs represent between 0.5% and 1% of all sinonasal tumors. Head and neck lesions account for 5% to 9% of OSs, and the mandible and maxilla are the most common locations. In the maxilla the most common sites are the alveolar ridge, the anterior midline, and the sinus. Pain occurs in half of the cases, and 25% of patients have dental symptoms.

Head and neck OSs occur primarily in males in their third or fourth decades of life, in contrast to axial skeletal OSs, which occur usually during the second decade. Before current aggressive chemotherapeutic regimes, mandibular and maxillary OSs were thought to have a better prognosis than axial skeletal OSs, which tend to metastasize early, especially to the lungs. This no longer holds true because the general prognosis of axial skelatal OS has improved. The prognosis of mandibular-maxillary OS depends on tumor stage and grade at presentation. The 5-year survival figures for tumors of the craniofacial bones range from 23% to 59%. Of the head and neck tumors, 11% are grade I, 41% are grade II, 41% are grade III, and 7% are grade IV. This compares with 85% of the extrafacial tumors being grade III or grade IV. Of the osteosarcomas, about 53% are osteoblastic, 24% are chondroblastic, 24% are fibroblastic, and 2% to 11% are telangiectatic.[88]

The radiographic appearance depends on the degree of osteoblastic tumor present. As a result these tumors vary from a purely lytic, aggressively destructive mass to an osteoblastic tumor within the facial bones. Classically the rapid tumor growth can cause a "sunburst" periosteal bone reaction. Variable-sized areas of dense calcification or bone can be seen within some tumors (Fig. 4-220).

On CT these lesions appear as soft-tissue, aggressively destructive masses. In about 25% of cases, regions of amorphous and irregular calcification occur both in the central and peripheral regions of the tumor. New tumor bone is present in only 25% of cases; however, purely blastic lesions can be seen, especially in the posterior maxillary alveolus (Fig. 4-221).[145] On MRI these tumors usually have a nonhomogeneous appearance of low to intermediate signal intensity on all imaging sequences. However, densely ossified regions of the tumor will have lower signal intensities, and the "nonossified" regions usually have higher signal intensities on all sequences (Fig. 4-222).

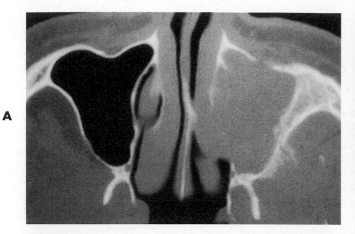

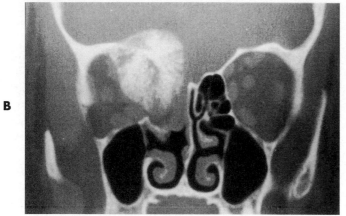

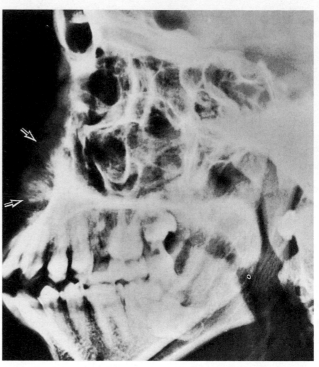

FIG. 4-220   Axial CT scan **(A)** shows a poorly defined thickening of the posterior wall of the left maxillary sinus. Aggressive periosteal bone production is present and is best seen along the infratemporal fossa margin of the sinus. Osteogenic sarcoma. Coronal CT scan **(B)** on a patient who previously had a craniofacial resection shows a recurrent bony tumor with aggressive periosteal production. Osteogenic sarcoma. Lateral view **(C)** shows an aggressive tumor of the maxilla that has caused a "sunburst" periosteal reaction. Osteogenic sarcoma.

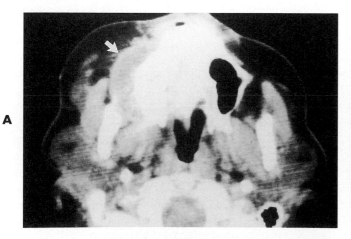

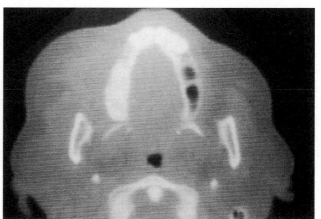

FIG. 4-221   Axial CT scans viewed at "soft tissue" **(A)** and "bone" **(B)** window settings show a nonossified mass along the outer margin of the right maxillary alveolus *(arrow)*. The alveolus in this area is minimally enlarged and dense. Osteogenic sarcoma.

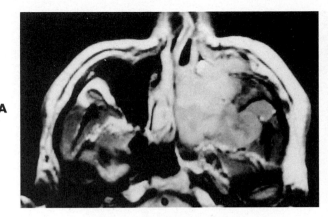

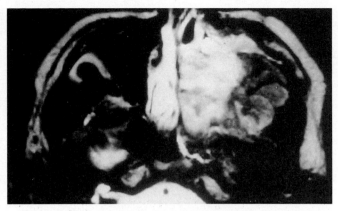

FIG. 4-222 Axial proton density (**A**) and T2W (**B**) MR scans show a large mass in the left maxillary sinus that has destroyed the medial sinus wall and portions of the anterior and posterior sinus walls, infiltrating into the infratemporal fossa. There are two components of the lesion. The anteromedial region has higher signal intensity in both **A** and **B** and is the nonossified portion of the tumor. The posterolateral region of the tumor was partially ossified on CT. Osteogenic sarcoma.

Paget's Disease

Paget's disease is a bone disorder of unknown etiology. Increased osteoclastic and osteoblastic activity results in the disorderly production of highly characteristic abnormal bone.[105] The disease usually occurs in patients over the age of 50 years, and it primarily involves the vertebrae (76%), calvaria (65%), pelvis (43%), femur (35%), and tibia (3%). Its incidence increases with age; between 3% and 3.7% of people older than 40 years of age are affected.[146] In 80% of patients the degree of skeletal involvement is limited and found fortuitously on radiographic studies or at autopsy. The facial bones are rarely involved; however, whenever the maxilla and mandible are affected, the calvarium is also involved.[147] The reduced size of the cranial cavity secondary to bony ingrowth of the calvaria and skull base can lead to altered patient mentality, dementia, and other neurologic abnormalities. Basilar invagination is associated with cranial nerve deficits. Encroachment into the orbits, neurovascular canals, and sinonasal cavities has lead to proptosis, visual loss, neurologic deficits, facial deformity, and nasal congestion. Despite the thickness of the bone, it is extremely vascular and fragile and may be prone to fracture.

The initial radiographic and CT appearance of Paget's disease of the calvarium often reveals a lytic phase that produces osteoporosis circumscripta, usually involving the frontal region to the greatest degree. A "mixed" phase may follow. This phase shows foci of sclerotic, woven bone within areas of lower density, which represent sites of fibrous myeloid production. The remaining bone often gives a moderately diffuse radiopacity. The calvaria are thickened; usually the greatest degree of thickening is anterior. One side of the skull tends to be more affected than the other. Inner table irregularity is usually greater than that of the outer surface. The sclerotic form of Paget's usually affects the facial bones. This form results in a thickened, dense bone with slightly irregular cortical surfaces (Figs. 4-223, 4-

224).[147] On MRI the dense foci of bone give rounded foci of signal void on all imaging sequences. The marrow tissues give high T1W and fairly high T2W signal intensity. This reflects the fat and blood protein in these regions. The background matrix gives an intermediate signal intensity on all imaging sequences. The facial area demonstrates a mixed, low to intermediate signal intensity on all imaging sequences.[147] The lesion usually enhances nonhomogeneously.

Sarcomas may develop in 5% to 10% of patients who have multifocal Paget's disease and in less than 2% of patients with limited bone involvement. The prognosis of Paget's sarcoma is grave; most patients die within 2 years. The development of multiple tumors is frequent; autopsy studies suggest a multicentric rather than a metastatic origin for these tumors. Most Paget's sarcomas are osteogenic sarcomas (50% to 60%) or fibrosarcomas (20% to 25%). In the facial area, benign giant cell tumors can also occur. On plain films and CT, giant cell tumors usually appear as sharply localized, nonosseous masses. Because the bone seen in Paget's disease, as well as the sarcomas, tends to give intermediate signals on all imaging sequences, it is more difficult to diagnose and map these malignancies or tumors on MRI than on CT (Fig. 4-224).[147]

Fibrous Dysplasia

Fibrous dysplasia is an idiopathic skeletal disorder in which medullary bone is replaced and distorted by poorly organized, structurally unsound, fibroosseous tissue that is composed of woven-type bone with few osteoclasts. The disease can occur in a monostotic form, a polyostotic form, and as part of Albright's syndrome. The monostotic type accounts for 75% to 80% of all cases and most often involves the ribs and femurs. Of monostotic fibrous dysplasia cases, 20% to 25% occur in the head and neck; the maxilla and mandible are the most common sites.[148]

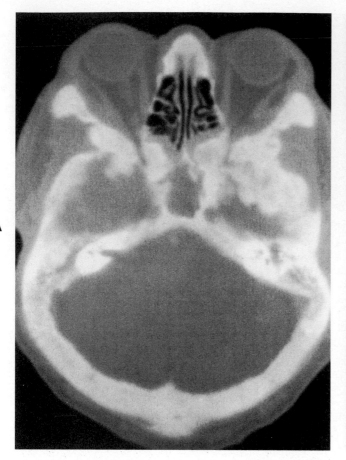

A

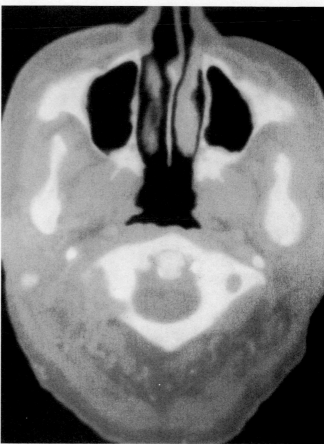

B

FIG. 4-223   Axial CT scans through the orbits **(A)** and the maxillary sinuses **(B)** show the bones of the skull base, upper cervical vertebra, and face to be thicker and more dense than normal. There is a slightly irregular contour to the bones. Paget's disease.

Polyostotic disease accounts for 20% to 25% of all cases. Usually there is unifocal bony involvement, except in severe cases where bilateral disease can occur. Of these patients, 40% to 60% have involvement of the skull and facial bones.[146,148] Albright's syndrome consists of polyostotic fibrous dysplasia, cutaneous pigmentation, and sexual precocity. It occurs almost exclusively in females. The ratio of monostotic fibrous dysplasia to Albright's syndrome is 40:1. The skin pigmentations have irregular margins (coast of Maine) as opposed to the smoother bordered pigmentations (coast of California) of neurofibromatosis. For all types of fibrous dysplasia, most patients are under 30 years of age when the disease is discovered.[146] Bone expansion can encroach on the paranasal sinuses, nasal fossae, orbits, and neurovascular canals. When there is extensive involvement of the facial bones, the resulting distortion of the face has been referred to as the "lion face," or leontiasis ossea. It was not appreciated until recently that fibrous dysplasia is a cause of mucoceles, especially of the frontal and sphenoid sinuses.

Bone affected with fibrous dysplasia undergoes malignant transformation in about 0.5% of cases. This occurs more often with the polyostotic form. About 50% of the sar-comas that complicate the monostatic disease occur in the skull and facial bones, whereas 62% of the sarcomas associated with polyostotic disease occur in the femur.[149] Malignant transformation can be hastened by irradiation. The average interval from the diagnosis of fibrous dysplasia to the appearance of the sarcoma is 13½ years. Of the sarcomas, 65% are osteogenic sarcomas, 18% are fibrosarcomas, 10% are chondrosarcomas, and 7% are giant cell sarcomas.[146] It is generally accepted that the appearance of new fibrous dysplasia lesions decrease or cease after skeletal growth has ended. Radiographically these lesions become more sclerotic with time. However, some lesions continue to grow after skeletal maturation and after they become sclerotic. Serial biopsies in fibrous dysplasia do not reveal maturation of woven bone into lamellar bone.[146] Surgery is used only to correct deformities, relieve pain, correct functional problems, or resect sarcomatous disease. Fibrous dysplasia recurs in 20% to 30% of cases, usually within 2 to 3 years of initial therapy.[146]

The radiologic appearance varies, according to the degree of fibrous tissue present. Thus the bone texture can range from a nonhomogeneous mixture of bone and fibrous

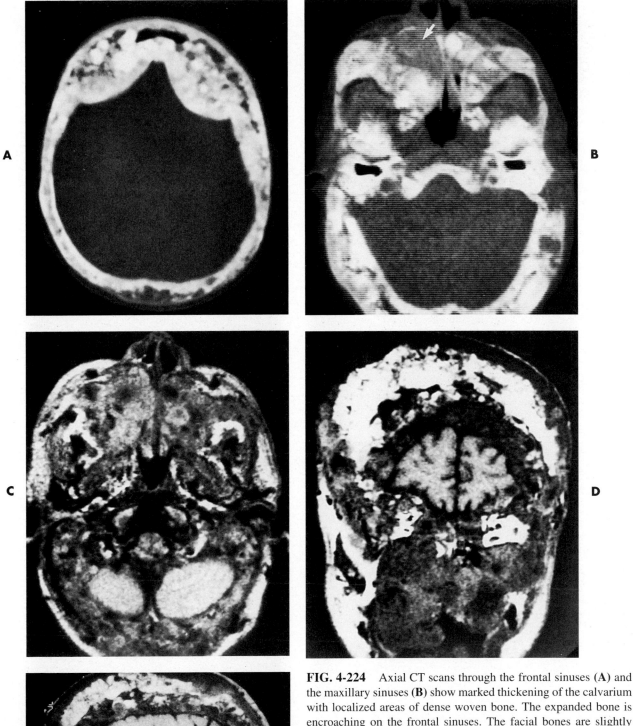

FIG. 4-224 Axial CT scans through the frontal sinuses (**A**) and the maxillary sinuses (**B**) show marked thickening of the calvarium with localized areas of dense woven bone. The expanded bone is encroaching on the frontal sinuses. The facial bones are slightly thickened and dense, and the expanded bones have obliterated the maxillary sinuses and most of the nasal fossa. A localized area of nonossified tissue is seen in the right maxilla *(arrow)*, which was an osteogenic sarcoma. Axial proton density (**C**) coronal (**D**) and sagittal (**E**) T1W MR scans show diffusely thickened bone in the facial region and the calvarium. The areas of high signal intensity in the calvarium on **D** and **E** correspond to marrow. The thickened calvarium has reduced the size of the intracranial compartment. The majority of the abnormal bone has a nonhomogeneous low to intermediate signal intensity. Paget's disease with osteogenic sarcoma in the right maxilla.

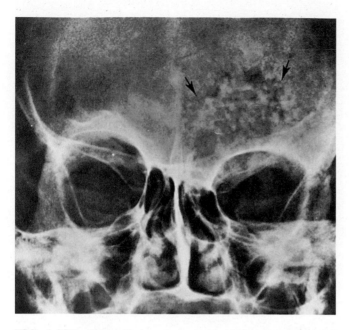

FIG. 4-225 Caldwell view shows a mixed "lytic" and "blastic" expansile lesion in the left frontal bone *(arrows)* that has depressed the superior orbital margin. Fibrous dysplasia.

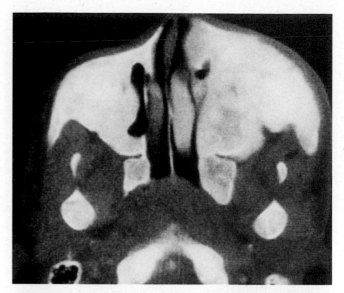

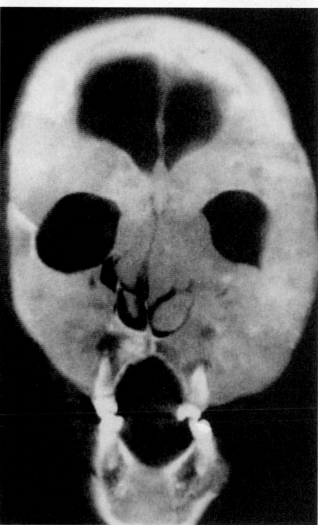

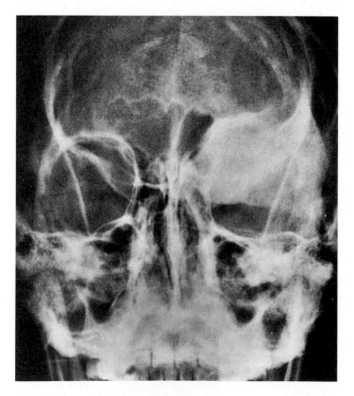

FIG. 4-226 Caldwell view shows a very dense expansile lesion of the left frontal and zygomatic bones that has encroached on the left orbit. Fibrous dysplasia.

FIG. 4-227 Axial **(A)** and coronal **(B)** CT scans show a ground glass density expansile bony process that has encroached on the orbits and obliterated the ethmoid and maxillary sinuses. Fibrous dysplasia (Leontiasis ossea).

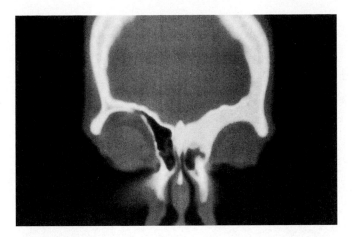

FIG. 4-228 Coronal CT scan shows that the left frontal and ethmoid bones are expanded. The cortices are intact. The widening occurs in the medullary space, which has a "ground glass" appearance. Fibrous dysplasia.

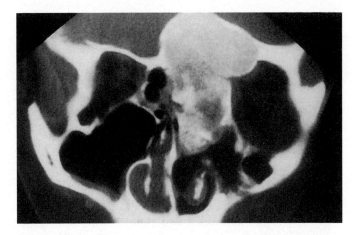

FIG. 4-229 Coronal CT scan shows expanded ground glass bone in the left frontal and ethmoid bones. The cortices are intact. Fibrous dysplasia.

tissues to a predominantly fine bony (ground-glass) appearance. The disease expands the diploic or medullary space and widens the bone. A thin, intact rim of cortical bone is often seen over the margins of the involved bone. MRI usually shows a low to intermediate intensity signal on all imaging sequences, and often the cortical bone, overlying the medullary disease, can be identified as a zone of low signal intensity. There usually is intense enhancement with contrast. If areas of high T2W signal intensity are present within the obstructed or involved sinus, the presence of a mucocele should be considered (Figs. 4-225 to 4-235).[150,151]

Ossifying Fibromas

Ossifying fibroma is a densely cellular, well-circumscribed fibrous tumor that ossifies, starting at the periphery. The ossification is made of immature woven bone that matures into lamellar bone. On CT the lesion is expansile and usually has larger nonossified areas of fibrous tissue density than does fibrous dysplasia.[146] The internal organization of the lesion shows discrete zones of either osseous or fibrous tissue. However, in some cases the CT appearance is indistinguishable from fibrous dysplasia, and the pathologist also may have difficulty differentiating these lesions. Compared with fibrous dysplasia, ossifying fibroma has a greater tendency to behave aggressively (grow faster and recur more quickly after surgery) and to expand internally toward the orbits, nasal fossae, and sinus cavities rather than to deform the outer surface bones (Figs. 4-236 to 4-238).

The differential diagnosis of ossifying fibroma is with fibrous dysplasia and also fibrous osteoma. Fibrous dysplasia is usually not radiographically well circumscribed or discrete, as is an ossifying fibroma. Biopsy or resection reveals that the bony trabeculae of fibrous dysplasia are abnormally shaped and are composed of immature woven bone. The bone of a fibrous osteoma is mature, dense, and abundant, with intramedullary fibrosis.

Cherubism

Cherubism is an autosomal dominant disease with variable expressivity often referred to as congenital fibrous dysplasia. This term is a misnomer though because histopathologically this lesion is a giant cell tumor. Some of the cases may arise as a result of a spontaneous mutation, which results in a nonsex-linked dominant gene.[146] Usually a 50% to 75% penetrance exists in females and 100% in males. The disease appears between the ages of 6 months to 7 years and is characterized by bilateral fullness of the jaws. The eyes appear to look upward as the lower sclera are exposed. The disease often develops rapidly until age 7 years and then gradually regresses. First the mandible is involved, which is followed by the maxilla in about two thirds of the cases. Most of the radiographic changes occur in the mandible, where expansile cystic masses are seen in the angles and ramus. As the disease progresses to the maxilla, the sinus opacifies and the orbital floor may be bulged upward. This latter finding is one of the causes of the upward-looking eye of cherubism.[146]

GIANT CELL TUMORS

True giant cell tumors (osteoclastomas) make up 4% to 5% of all primary bone neoplasms. They are usually benign, but occasionally cases recur aggressively and metastasize. More than 75% are located in the epiphyseal region of long bones, with half of the cases occurring about the knee.

True giant cell tumors (GCT) of the head and neck are extraordinarily rare. This diagnosis must actually be scrutinized when not associated with Paget's disease. The differential diagnosis of a GCT of the head and neck includes giant cell reparative granuloma, "brown tumor" of hyperparathyroidism, or more rarely a giant cell-rich osteogenic sarcoma. The distinctions between these entities may be impossible to make on a biopsy without radiographic and clinical correlation.

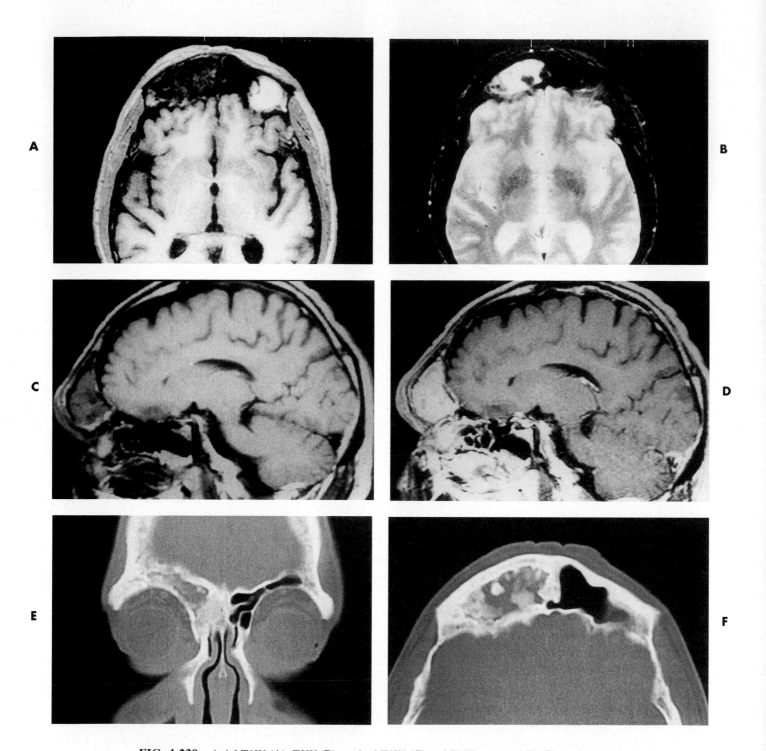

FIG. 4-230   Axial T1W (**A**), T2W (**B**), sagittal T1W (**C**) and T1W contrast MR (**D**), and coronal (**E**) and axial (**F**) CT scans show a nonhomogeneous right frontal sinus mass that has low signal intensity in **A,** high signal intensity in **B,** and diffusely enhances in **C.** The CT scans show the bone to be expanded, with intact cortices, and a medullary space filled with ossified and nonossified regions. Fibrous dysplasia.

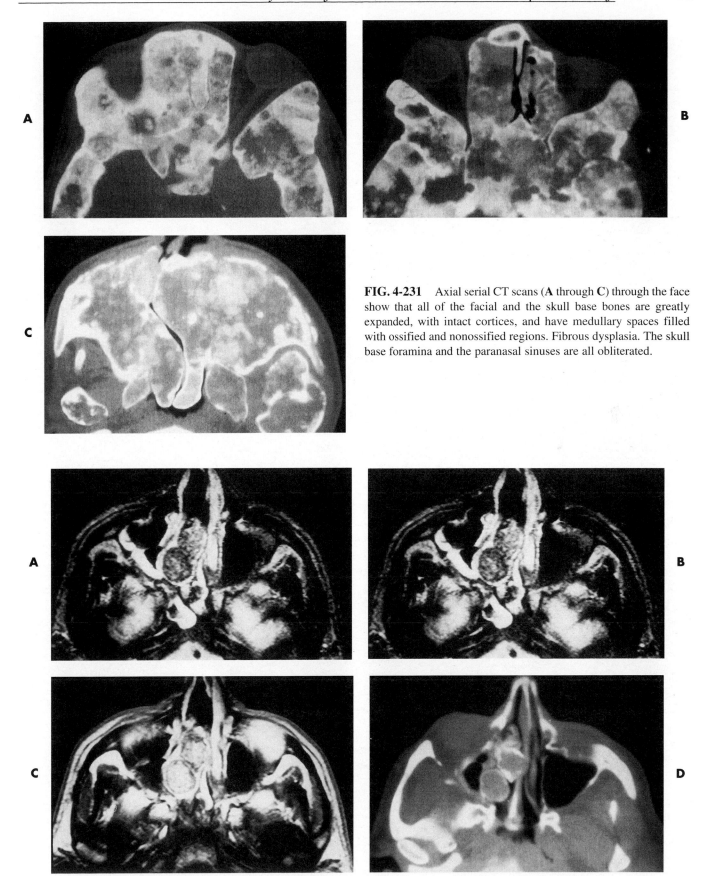

FIG. 4-231 Axial serial CT scans (**A** through **C**) through the face show that all of the facial and the skull base bones are greatly expanded, with intact cortices, and have medullary spaces filled with ossified and nonossified regions. Fibrous dysplasia. The skull base foramina and the paranasal sinuses are all obliterated.

FIG. 4-232 Axial T1W (**A**), T2W (**B**), T1W contrast MR (**C**) and axial CT (**D**) scans show a polypoid right posterior nasal cavity mass that has low T1W and intermediate T2W signal intensity and diffusely enhances (**C**). The CT scan shows the lesion to have an intact bony cortex and nonossified central regions. Fibrous dysplasia.

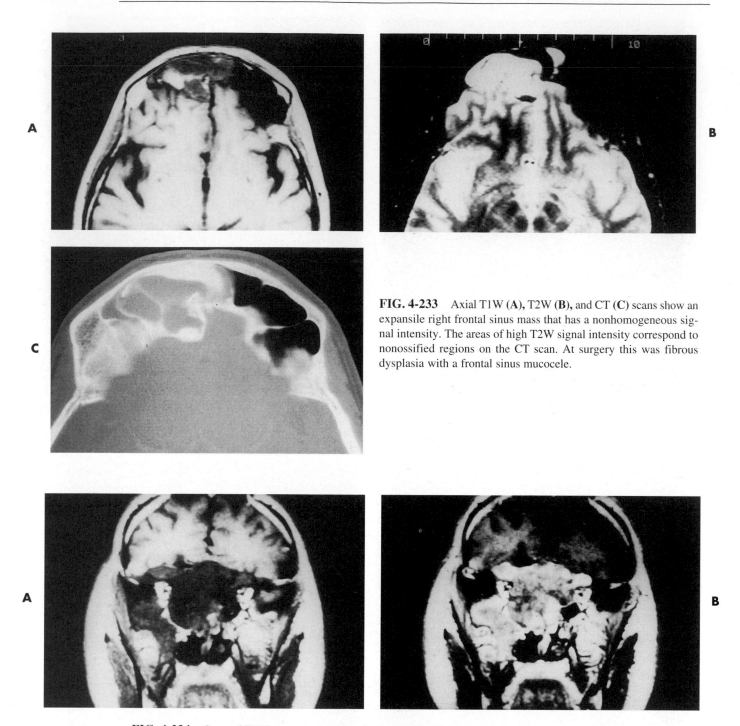

FIG. 4-233 Axial T1W (**A**), T2W (**B**), and CT (**C**) scans show an expansile right frontal sinus mass that has a nonhomogeneous signal intensity. The areas of high T2W signal intensity correspond to nonossified regions on the CT scan. At surgery this was fibrous dysplasia with a frontal sinus mucocele.

FIG. 4-234 Coronal T1W noncontrast (**A**) and postcontrast (**B**) MR scans show an expansile mass involving the sphenoid, ethmoid, and frontal bones. The mass has a low signal intensity and diffusely (and nonhomogeneously) enhances. Fibrous dysplasia.

Approximately 10% to 15% of GCTs show clinical or histologic evidence of malignancy. These malignant lesions can be primary or can arise secondarily as a malignant transformation in a benign tumor. Almost all of the secondary type have been irradiated previously. The recommended treatment of choice is complete surgical excision or curettage. Because most tumors are not radiosensitive and this treatment may induce malignant transforma-

tion, radiation therapy should be reserved only for surgically inaccessible tumors. Based on all GCTs occurring in the body, 30% to 50% recur with curettage and most local failures recur within 2 years of initial therapy.[112]

On CT the tumors enhance moderately and they tend to destroy and remodel bone.[152,153] On MR they usually have fairly low signal intensity on all sequences, and they enhance.

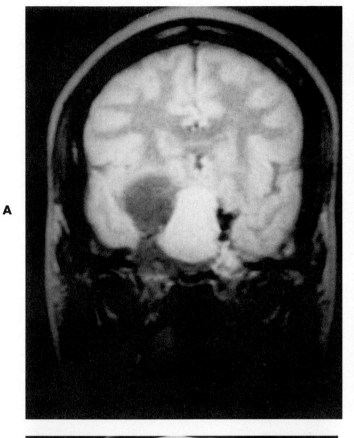

A

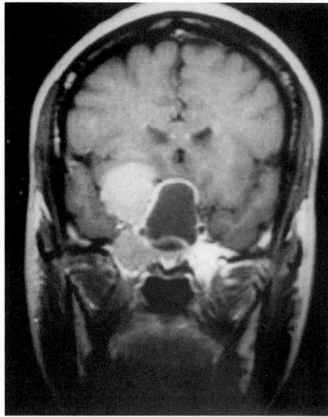

B

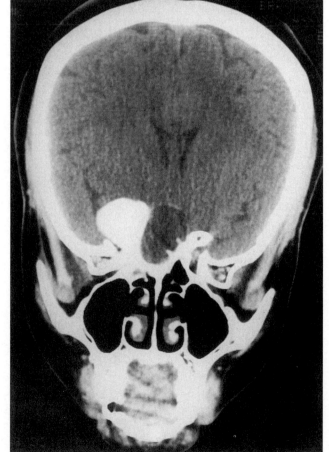

C

FIG. 4-235 Coronal proton density (**A**), T1W contrast MR (**B**), and CT scans (**C**) show a low signal intensity mass in the right sphenoid bone and a high signal intensity process in an expanded left sphenoid sinus (**A**). The right-sided mass diffusely enhances, but only the mucosa enhances surrounding the secretions in the left sphenoid sinus (**B**). The CT shows the right-sided mass to be densely ossified (**C**). Fibrous dysplasia causing a left sphenoid sinus mucocele.

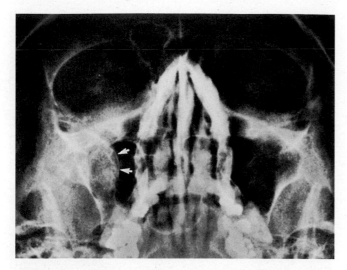

FIG. 4-236 Waters view shows an expansile bony mass in the lateral wall of the right maxillary sinus. The mass has displaced the lateral sinus wall toward the midline *(arrow)*. Ossifying fibroma.

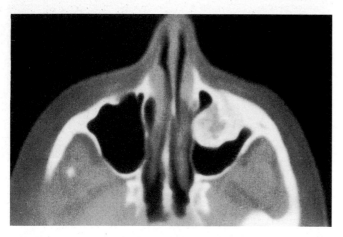

FIG. 4-237 Axial CT shows an osseous mass extending into the left antrum from the anterior sinus wall. The central region of the lesion is only partially ossified. Ossifying fibroma.

GIANT CELL REPARATIVE GRANULOMAS

Giant cell reparative granuloma (GCRG) may be either peripheral or central and occurs in the mandible or the maxillary alveolus. The peripheral (soft tissue) type is four times more common than the central type and involves the gingiva and alveolar mucosa. Underlying bone is rarely involved in peripheral lesions. The tumor usually develops in women over 20 years of age and is related to a prior tooth extraction or an ill-fitting denture. Central GCRG can have extensive bone destruction and most often manifests in patients 10 to 20 years of age. Typically it has a multiloculated plain film appearance (Fig. 4-239).[112,152-155] The central GCRG is unrelated to trauma.

Pathologically, GCRG characteristically has a hemorrhagic fibroblastic type of background with innumerable osteoclastic giant cells. This background is helpful in distinguishing GCRG from a GCT. The latter lacks the diffuse

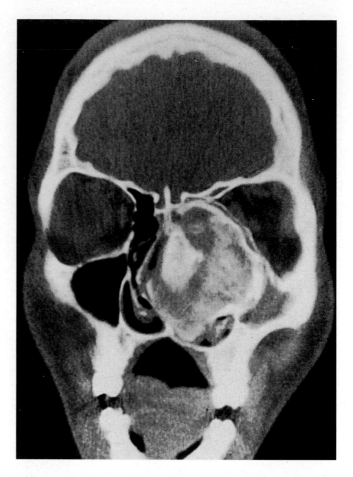

FIG. 4-238 Coronal CT scan shows an expansile left nasal fossa mass that has encroached upon the left ethmoid sinuses, the maxillary sinus, and the orbit. The surrounding bone is intact and the central portion of the lesion has both ossified and nonossified segments. Ossifying fibroma.

hemorrhage, hemosiderin, and fibroblasts, and the background cells are identical to the nuclei of the osteoclastic giant cells. The giant cells of a GCT are diffusely and evenly dispersed throughout the tumor. In distinction the brown tumor of hyperparathyroidism has uneven clumps of osteoclasts, has perivascular hemorrhage, and has hemosiderin deposition. It is useful to know the serum calcium and parathyroid hormone levels when dealing with any giant cell lesion. In hyperparathyoidism the calcium will be elevated, unless the patient is already severely calcium depleted. Serum parathyroid homone (PTH) is of course elevated with a brown tumor of hyperparathyroidism and is normal with other GCTs. PTH is also normal in tumor-induced osteomalacia, which radiologically can mimic severe hyperparathyroidism.

On CT these lesions enhance, are bulky, and can aggressively erode the maxillary sinus walls or have an expansile, remodeling appearance (Fig. 4-240). On MRI they have low to intermediate signal intensity on both T1W and T2W images. Their MR appearance may mimic that of squamous cell carcinoma.[156]

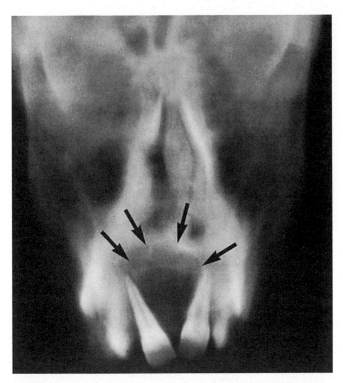

FIG. 4-239 Coronal multidirectional tomogram shows an expansile lesion in the maxillary alveolus and hard palate *(arrows)*. Central type giant cell granuloma.

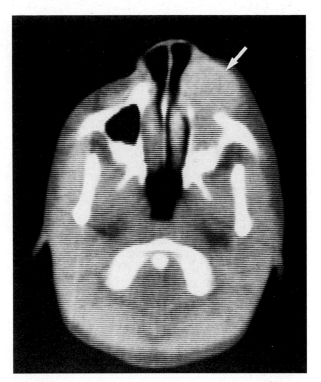

FIG. 4-240 Axial CT shows a bulky lesion of the left antrum, which has destroyed the anterior maxillary wall and extended into the cheek *(arrow)*. Giant cell granuloma.

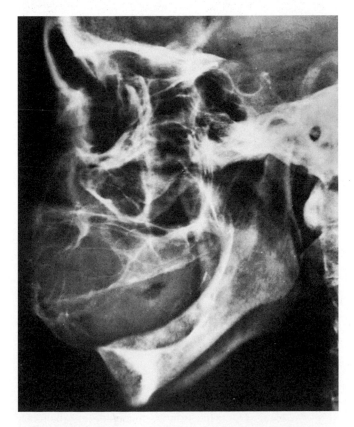

FIG. 4-241 Lateral view shows an expansile, loculated, and destructive lesion of the maxilla. Aneurysmal bone cyst.

ANEURYSMAL BONE CYSTS

An aneurysmal bone cyst is neither an aneurysm nor a true cyst, but it does occur in bone. Rather, it is a benign, nonneoplastic osseous lesion characterized by the presence of numerous blood-filled, usually nonendothelialized cavities. This lesion occurs mainly in females over the age of 20 years and represents only 1% to 2% of all primary bone tumors. Between 3% and 12% of aneurysmal bone cysts occur in the head and neck, and they have been reported in the maxilla, orbit, ethmoid, and frontal bones.[63] They can be slowly or rapidly enlarging masses, and nonthrobbing pain is usually present. Surgical excision or curettage are the treatments of choice; in the jaws this treatment approach has resulted in a 26% recurrence rate. Recent use of cryosurgery and curettage has produced better results, with a recurrence rate of only 8%.[88] Radiographically this lesion may be unilocular or demonstrate a multilocular "soap bubble" or "honeycomb" radiolucency (Fig. 4-241). The peripheral bone margins demonstrate bone remodeling and destruction. On MR the classical findings are those of multiple cysts with fluid-fluid levels (Figs. 4-242, 4-243).

THALASSEMIA

Thalassemia can reduce either the alpha chains of globulin (alpha-thalassemia) or the beta chains (beta thalassemia).

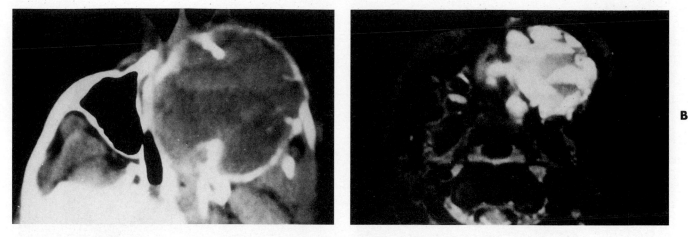

FIG. 4-242 Axial CT scan (**A**) and axial T2W MR (**B**) show an expansile mass in the left maxillary sinus. The surrounding bone is remodeled and not eroded. On MR, multiple cystic components with fluid-fluid levels are seen within the lesion. Aneurysmal bone cyst. (Courtesy of Drs. Revel and Vanel.)

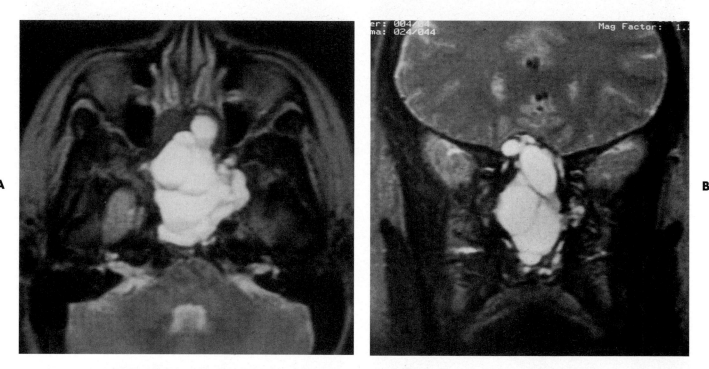

FIG. 4-243 Axial (**A**) and coronal (**B**) T2W MR scans show a mass in the sphenoid bone and sphenoid sinus. This lesion is comprised of multiple cystic areas each with a fluid-fluid level. Aneurysmal bone cyst.

The beta form has major osseous abnormalities caused by marrow space expansion. Beta thalassemia is an autosomal recessive disorder that occurs primarily in patients of Mediterranean origin. Patients who have thalassemia major are homozygous for the trait and have the most severe form of the disease, resulting from active marrow hyperplasia. Patients with thalassemia intermedia are also homozygous but have a milder form of the disease. Patients with the mildest form, thalassemia minor, are heterozygous for the trait and are usually asymptomatic.

The classic radiographic changes of thalassemia in the skull include a thickened calvarium and a "hair-on-end" appearance. In the facial area, sinus pneumatization is delayed and the maxilla is expanded secondary to marrow expansion, which can result in both malocclusion and a cosmetic deformity. On CT, soft-tissue density material (marrow) is seen filling and expanding the maxillae, and this process may extend into the central skull base and mandible (Fig. 4-244).[157] Often the frontal, sphenoid, and maxillary sinuses are poorly developed.

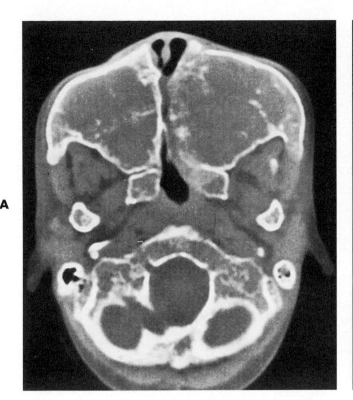

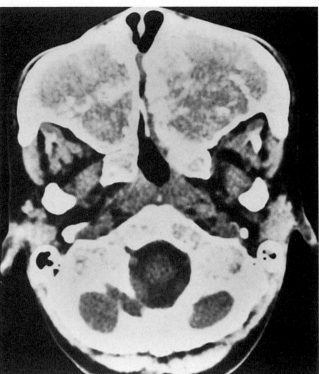

FIG. 4-244   Axial CT at wide **(A)** and narrow **(B)** window settings show markedly expanded maxilla with no development of the maxillary sinuses. The surrounding cortical bone is intact. The central portions of each maxilla are filled with expanded marrow. Thalessemia.

EWING'S SARCOMA

Ewing's sarcoma is a highly malignant, small, round cell tumor that accounts for 5% to 10% of all primary osseous malignancies. About 60% of cases occur in the lower extremities and pelvis. At the time of diagnosis, almost 90% of patients are between 5 and 30 years of age. Only 1% to 4% of all Ewing's sarcomas occur in the head and neck. Most commonly the mandible is involved, followed in frequency by the maxilla, calvarium, and cervical vertebrae.[88] Patients typically have pain and localized swelling; radiographically a destructive lesion shows periosteal "onion skinning" or a "sunburst" appearance. Ewing's sarcoma (ES) is related to primitive neuroectodermal tumor (PNET). The distinction between ES and PNET is based only on immunophenotypic and ultrastructural findings. PNET has some evidence of neuroendocrine differentiation such as neurosecretory granules and cellular processes by electron microscopy (EM), and evidence of expression of two or more neuroendocrine markers. (This neuroendocrine differentiation is quantatively a fraction of that seen, for instance, in an olfactory neuroblastoma.) ES on the other hand reveals no evidence of any kind of differentiation. The present treatment of choice for ES and PNET is local excision with radiation therapy for the incompletely excised lesions. Micrometastases, which are present in 15% to 30% of patients, are treated with chemotherapy. The 5-year survival

rates have risen from less than 10% in the prechemotherapy era to the current 60% to 79%. Ewing's sarcoma recurs locally in 13% to 20% of patients (65% at postmortem), usually coinciding with the completion of chemotherapy. The tumors metastasize to the lungs (86%), skeleton (69%), pleural cavity (46%), lymph nodes (46%), dura and meninges (27%), and central nervous system (12%).[88] Because of its rarity in the facial area, Ewing's sarcoma of the sinonasal cavities probably should be considered a metastasis from an infraclavicular primary tumor until proven otherwise. The significance in the distinction between ES and PNET is that PNET is somewhat more chemosensitive than ES and is associated with a longer mean survival after multimodality therapy. PNET occurs most commonly as a soft tumor of the lower truck or lower extremities. Association with a major nerve trunk has been seen in one third of the cases. PNET does occur in the head and neck, usually in the sinonasal cavities. Survivors of retinoblastoma are at risk for a host of secondary neoplasms; sinonasal PNET has been reported in these survivors (Fig. 4-245).[158-161]

KAPOSI'S SARCOMA

Before the aquired immunodeficiency syndrome (AIDS) epidemic, Kaposi's sarcoma (KS) was rarely encountered in the head and neck. The classic form of KS is an indolent

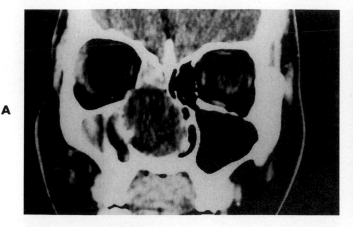

A

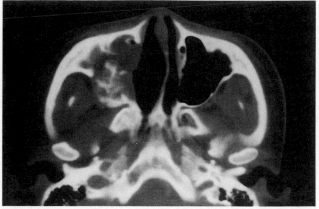

B

FIG. 4-245   Coronal CT scan **(A)** shows a mucoid attenuation mass expanding the right nasal fossa. There is some bony thickening present along the adjacent right nasal vault wall. Axial CT scan **(B)** taken after biopsy of the mass, shows irregular tumoral bone within the right antrum, bulging into the infratemporal fossa. Primitive neuroectodermal tumor.

tumor that occurs most commonly as soft, red nodules on the lower limbs and less commonly on the upper limbs. Lesions may be multicentric and coalescent, but they rarely exceed 2 cm. Patients with classic KS usually have long survivals and die of something other than KS. From the literature and the files of the Armed Forces Institute of Pathology (AFIP), Gnepp, Chandler, and Hyams compiled a total of 83 cases of classic KS, which affected the head and neck.[162] Of all classic KS cases, 8% affected cutaneous sites on the head and neck, and only 2% affected the mucosal surfaces. Mucosal sites included the conjunctiva, palate, tongue, gingiva, and tonsil; skin sites included the eyelids, nose, ears, and face. By comparison, AIDS KS cases commonly affected skin of the head and neck (32%) and upper airway mucosal surfaces (19%). Common sites for AIDS KS cases in the head and neck include the palate, gingiva, buccal mucosa, tongue, larynx, trachea, and sinuses.[163-166] Patients with classic KS are usually over the age of 50 at the time of tumor diagnosis, although 3% to 4% of the cases of the classic form are diagnosed in patients less than 15 years old. Patients with AIDS diagnosed with head and neck KS tend to be decades younger than the classic cases (mean age 38 years), though of course there is overlap in both age groups.[162,167]

ODONTOGENIC CYSTS

Odontogenic cysts arise from the various components of the dental apparatus. As a group they are uncommon, and only those that grow sufficiently large to extend into the maxillary sinuses and palate are discussed here. Odontogenic cysts can be classified as follicular cysts, periodontal cysts, odontogenic keratocysts, and calcifying odontogenic cysts.

Follicular Cysts

These cysts can be subclassified as primordial or dentigerous. The primordial cyst represents 5% of follicular cysts

and 1.75% to 6.9% of all odontogenic cysts. This cyst develops as a result of degeneration of the enamel organ. Because this cyst occurs before any calcified dental structures have been formed and before the tooth germ has erupted, the cyst is located in the jaw at a site normally occupied by an adult tooth. Only if a primordial cyst arises from a supernumerary tooth germ will the patient have a normal complement of teeth.[117,168] The cyst usually is an incidental finding on radiographs, since almost all are asymptomatic unless secondarily infected. The lesions are unilocular and well circumscribed. They are differentiated from residual cysts by the patient's history (with this latter cyst) of a prior tooth extraction in the area of the missing tooth. Treatment involves thorough curettage.

The dentigerous cyst represents 95% of follicular cysts and nearly 34% of all odontogenic cysts. Most of these cysts occur during the second and third decades of life. The cyst arises in an unerupted tooth, after the crown of the tooth has developed. Radiographically it is a cyst into which the crown of the tooth projects. As the cyst grows, it pulls the unerupted tooth with it. When small, dentigerous cysts are unilocular. When large, they may be multilocular, the tooth within the cyst may be displaced from its normally expected location, and there may be resorption of the roots of neighboring teeth.[168] Only the permanent teeth are affected. The most common locations are the mandibular third molar, the maxillary canine, and third molar teeth.

Radiographically the dentigerous cyst must be distinguished from a normal dental follicle. If a dental follicle measures 2 cm or greater in width, it is highly likely that the unerupted tooth will become a dentigerous cyst. Similarly a pericoronal space of 2.5 mm or more in width signals an 80% chance that the unerupted tooth will become a dentigerous cyst.[114] If the cyst breaks through into the maxillary sinus, it may grow rapidly, remodeling the antral walls. Often the inferior maxillary sinus cortex is elevated over portions of

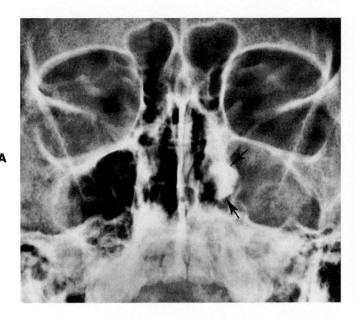

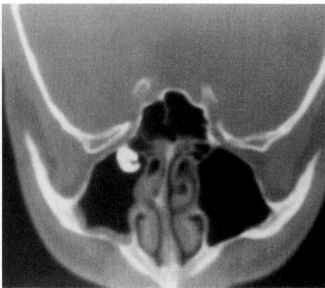

FIG. 4-246   Caldwell view (**A**) shows an expansile process in the left maxillary sinus with a tooth in the medial antral wall *(arrows)*. Dentigerous cyst. Coronal CT scan (**B**) shows an undescended free tooth in the right maxillary sinus. Minimal mucosal thickening is also present in the lower sinus. This should not be confused with a dentigerous cyst.

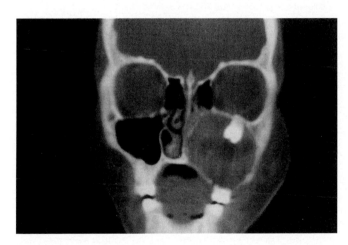

FIG. 4-247   Coronal CT scan shows an expansile mass in the left antrum. A molar tooth is present in the cranial wall of the lesion. Dentigerous cyst.

the cyst. In the axial view this can be detected by noting what appears to be two bony walls in the posterior sinus. In these instances the most posterior bone is the true sinus wall, and the more anterior bone is the elevated sinus floor. If multiple dentigerous cysts are present, the patient should be examined for the basal cell nevus syndrome.

An ameloblastoma may arise within the wall of the dentigerous cyst. This mural or cystic ameloblastoma is often diagnosed only by the pathologist; the radiographic findings in such cases are those of a simple dentigerous cyst.[168,169] There is a familial predisposition toward this tran-

formation. The prognosis of a cystic ameloblastoma arising in a dentigerous cyst is excellent. These lesions are usually cured by currettage. On MRI the cyst fluid has intermediate signal intensity on T1W images and high T2W signal intensity; the displaced tooth gives a signal void on all imaging sequences. In this regard the MRI appearance may be similar to that of an antral aspergilloma (Figs. 4-72, 4-73, 4-246 to 4-249).

Periodontal Cysts (Periapical Cysts or Radicular Cysts)

The periodontal, apical periodontal, periapical, radicular, or dental cyst is the most common cyst of the jaws. It arises in erupted, infected teeth and usually is the sequela of a preexisting periapical granuloma. The cyst most commonly involves the maxillary teeth, and if it breaks through into the maxillary sinus, it can grow rapidly, remodeling the antral walls and elevating portions of the inferior sinus cortex (Fig. 4-250).[168,169]

The residual periodontal cyst generally results from a retained periapical cyst after the involved tooth has been extracted. The residual cyst also occurs most often in the maxilla and is differentiated from a primordial cyst by the history of a tooth extraction. Treatment of these cysts consists of simple enucleation.[168]

The lateral periodontal cyst is a noninflammatory developmental cyst that arises lateral to the tooth root. This cyst probably arises from proliferation of rests of the dental lamina. This cyst occurs most often in adults in the premolar and cuspid area. Radiographically there is an incidental multiloculated cyst along the lateral tooth root.

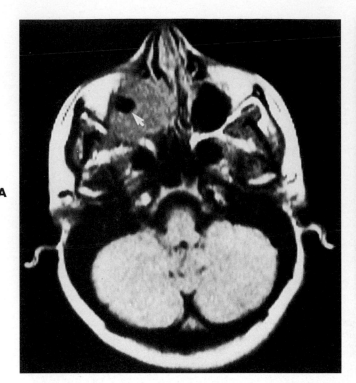
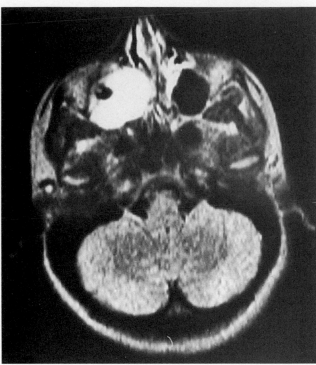

FIG. 4-248   Axial proton density (**A**) and T2W MR (**B**) scans show an expansile mass in the right maxillary sinus. The mass has a low to intermediate signal intensity in **A** and a high signal intensity in **B**. Within the mass is an area *(arrow)* of signal void (tooth) on all images. Dentigerous cyst.

Odontogenic Keratocysts

Most odontogenic keratocysts are of the parakeratotic type. These aggressively growing lesions tend to recur (12% to 62.5%) after removal. These cysts are associated with Marfan's syndrome and the basal cell nevus syndrome, and they may have a neoplastic potential.[113] The parakeratotic odontogenic keratocyst represents 3.3% to 16.5% of all jaw cysts, and most occur in patients in their second and third decades of life. The mandible is affected two to four times more often than the maxilla, and most lesions occur in the posterior aspect of the jaws. The lesion is asymptomatic in half of the patients; the other half of patients frequently complain of pain. The symptoms last an average of 22 months. In the maxilla, parakeratotic odontogenic keratocysts can cause nasal obstruction and extend into the maxillary sinus.[168] These cysts may be destructive and invade the adjacent bone or have a thin reactive sclerotic bony rim, and they can have smooth or scalloped margins. The recurrence rate does not correlate with standard treatments (marsupialization or enucleation). However, no recurrences have been reported of cysts removed in one piece. In 13% of cases the keratocyst is of the orthokeratotic type. These cysts are less aggressive, recur infrequently, and virtually all are unilocular.[168]

Calcifying Odontogenic Cysts

This cyst has a variety of names, including keratinizing

ameloblastoma, keratinizing and calcifying ameloblastoma, and melanotic ameloblastic odontoma.[168] The calcifying odontogenic cyst is an uncommon lesion, affecting the maxilla and mandible equally. About 78% are intraosseous and 22% are confined to the soft tissues. They are either unilocular or multilocular radiolucent cysts that frequently contain radiopaque material, ranging from small flecks to large masses. The lesion can be well circumscribed or poorly demarcated, and it radiographically resembles a calcifying epithelial odontogenic tumor, an odontoma, an ossifying fibroma, and fibrous dysplasia.[113] The lining of a calcifying odontogenic cyst consists of ameloblastic epithelium and "ghost cells," which undergo dystrophic calcification. Treatment can be by curettage, enucleation, or conservative surgical excision; unlike the keratocyst, recurrences are unlikely.

FISSURAL CYSTS

In general, fissural cysts are believed to be derived from entrapped epithelium in the fusion lines of the frontonasal and maxillary processes during facial development. As a group, fissural cysts are uncommon. They are lined by stratified squamous epithelium, respiratory epithelium, or a combination of the two. The capsule is composed of fibrous connective tissue. Because of their histologic similarities, fissural cysts are distinguished from one another by anatomic location.[168] Fissural cysts are classified as midline

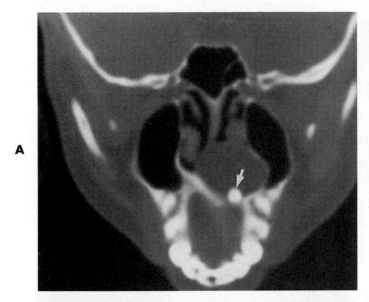

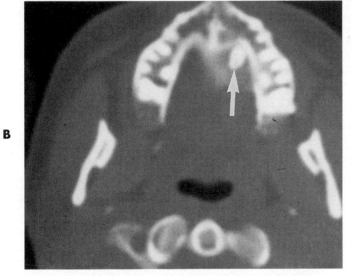

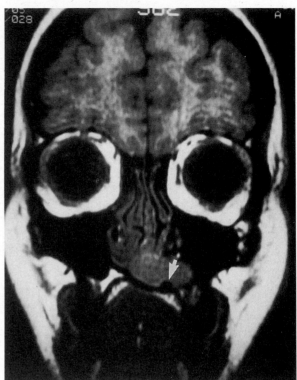

FIG. 4-249 Coronal CT **(A),** axial CT **(B),** and coronal T1W MR **(C)** scans show a cystic mass in the anterior hard palate (premaxilla). Within the cyst is a partially formed tooth *(arrow).* Dentigerous cyst of mesiodent tooth.

or lateral cysts (Fig. 4-251). Those occurring along the midline fusion line of the maxillary processes (nasopalatine cysts [incisive canal cysts, cysts of the palatine papilla] and median palatal cysts) do not extend into the paranasal sinuses. Radiographically they appear as well-delineated cystic lesions within the hard palate (Fig. 4-252). Of the lateral cysts (nasolabial or nasoalveolar cysts and globulomaxillary cysts), only the latter involve the maxillary sinuses. The nasoalveolar cyst is entirely a soft-tissue lesion and thus is not strictly a true fissural cyst (Fig. 4-253). It appears as a small cystic mass in the upper lip and lateral aspect of the nose. The globulomaxillary cyst is found between the maxillary lateral incisor and canine teeth and is believed to be either a true fissural cyst or possibly of odontogenic origin. These cysts represent less than 3% of all cysts of the jaws and 20% of the maxillary fissural cysts. Most occur in patients under 30 years of age, and the lesions are usually painless unless secondary infection develops.[168,169]

Radiographically the globulomaxillary cyst appears as an inverted pear-shaped or ovoid cyst in the maxillary alveolus (Fig. 4-254). The cyst often pushes apart the roots of the lateral incisor and canine teeth and, when large, can distort the lower anterior aspect of the maxillary sinus.

ODONTOGENIC TUMORS

Odontogenic tumors such as odontogenic cysts arise from the dental apparatus; unlike the cysts these tumors also mimic various stages of odontogenesis. A whole host of tumors of various histologic types exists; this section describes only the ameloblastoma, cementoma, odontoma, and fibromyxoma because these are the most common odontogenic tumors to involve the paranasal sinuses.

Ameloblastomas

Ameloblastoma is a slowly growing solid and cystic tumor,

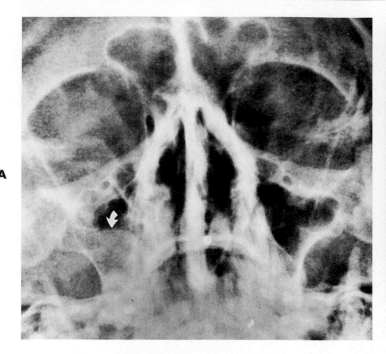

A

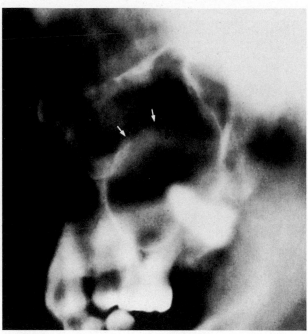

B

FIG. 4-250   **A,** Waters view shows a mass in the lower right antrum that has elevated the inferior mucoperiosteal white line *(arrow)*. This indicates that the mass arose in the alveolus below the sinus. **B,** A lateral multidirectional tomogram shows a cystic mass extending from a partially unerupted tooth and extending into the maxillary sinus. Radicular cyst.

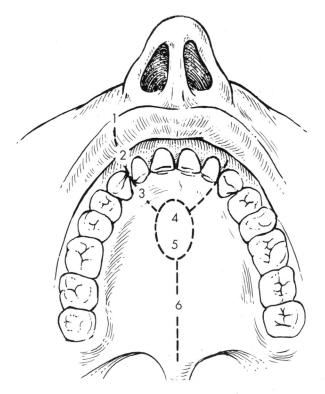

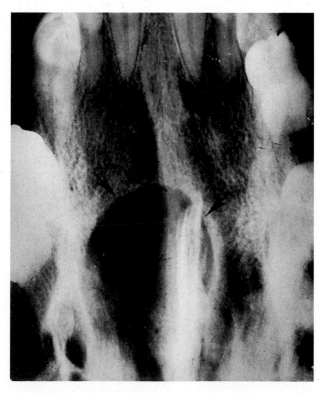

FIG. 4-251   Diagram of distribution of fissural cyst. *1,* Nasolabial cyst; *2,* nasoalveolar cyst; *3,* globulomaxillary cyst; *4,* nasopalatine cyst; *5,* cyst of palatine papilla; and *6,* median palatal cyst.

FIG. 4-252   Intraoral occlusal film shows a well-demarcated cyst *(arrows)* of the palate. Fissural cyst.

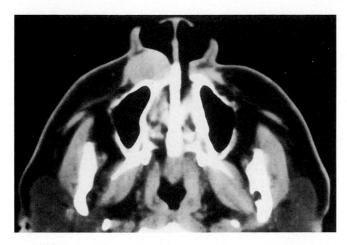

FIG. 4-253 Axial CT scan shows a soft-tissue density ovoid mass in the soft tissues of the right face, deep to the lateral margin of the nose. The adjacent maxillary bone is uninvolved. Nasoalveolar cyst.

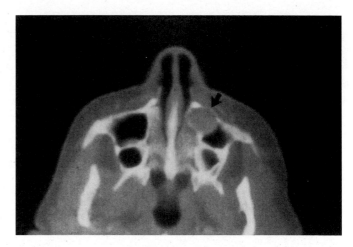

FIG. 4-254 Axial CT scan shows an expansile soft-tissue mass *(arrow)* in the left anterior maxilla. The caudal aspect of the lesion extended down into the alveolus, separating the canine and lateral incisor teeth. This cyst has a thin rim of bone around its margin. Globullomaxillary cyst.

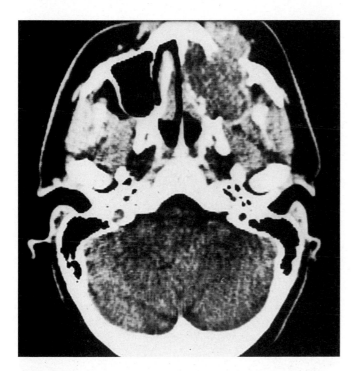

FIG. 4-255 Axial CT scan shows a partially expansile and partially destructive mass in the lower left maxillary sinus. Ameloblastoma.

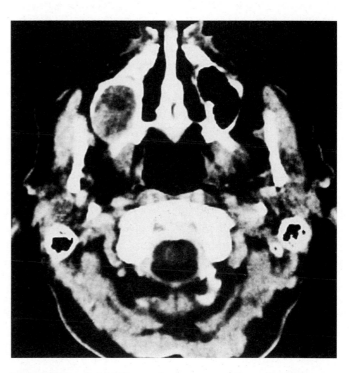

FIG. 4-256 Axial CT scan shows an expansile nonhomogeneous mass in the right maxillary alveolus and lower antrum. Ameloblastoma.

arising from the odontogenic apparatus. No differentiation into actual tooth (hard) structures occurs, hence the previous term for this lesion, adamantinoma (adamantine-unyielding, hard), has been abandoned. Although the ameloblastoma is the most common tumor that arises from the epithelial components of the embryonic tooth, this tumor comprises only 1% of all jaw cysts and tumors. Most occur in patients in the third and fourth decades of life, and 90% of the maxillary lesions involve the premolar-molar area. Few if any early

clinical symptoms appear. As the tumor enlarges a painless swelling forms, and in the maxilla large lesions have caused nasal obstruction. Other signs and symptoms include pain, bleeding, unhealed extraction sites, trismus, and neural involvement.[170,171] Ameloblastomas develop in 17% of dentigerous cysts; however, the percentage drops notably in patients older than 30 years of age. This decrease suggests that the potential for ameloblastoma formation is lost as the cyst's odontogenic epithelium undergoes squamous meta-

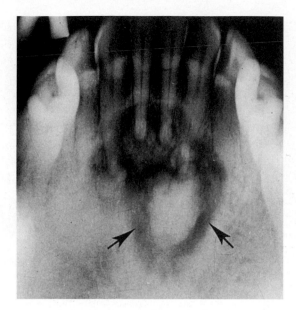

FIG. 4-257 Intraoral occlusal film shows a calcified palatal mass with a surrounding lucent zone *(arrows).* Note the small radiopaque densities, surrounding the tooth roots (hypercementosis). Cementoma.

plasia with age.[171] Primordial and residual cysts rarely develop into ameloblastomas.

Radiographically the ameloblastoma appears as a multiloculated, lytic lesion with no mineralized components. If the tumor extends into the antrum, the sinus is clouded and the sinus walls are remodeled and destroyed. On CT these tumors tend to have a nonenhancing, nonhomogeneous appearance, and on MRI they have nonhomogeneous mixed signal intensities. On T1W images these tumors demonstrate intermediate signal intensity, whereas on T2W studies ameloblastomas have variable intermediate and high signal intensities (Figs. 4-255, 4-256).

Histologic variants of ameloblastoma include the follicular, plexiform, acanthomatous, and granular cell. By and large there are no prognostic distinctions that can be made based on the histologic variants. Although histologically benign, slow-growing, and nonmetastasizing, these tumors tend to recur and can even cause death secondary to skull base invasion with extension to the brain. In rare instances, two malignant variants may be found: the malignant ameloblastoma and the ameloblastic carcinoma.

The malignant ameloblastoma histologically resembles benign ameloblastoma, but it metastasizes. These metastases are also histologically benign and occur after a long history of multiple unsuccessful attempts at surgical cure or after radiation therapy. Most metastases go to the lungs, pleura, and regional lymph nodes.[171] The ameloblastic carcinoma is an obviously histologic malignancy, and the metastases are less well differentiated than the primary tumor. Complete surgical resection is the treatment of choice for all ameloblastomas. Chemotherapy appears to be relatively ineffective against both the primary lesion and the metastases, and most lesions are not radiosensitive.[171]

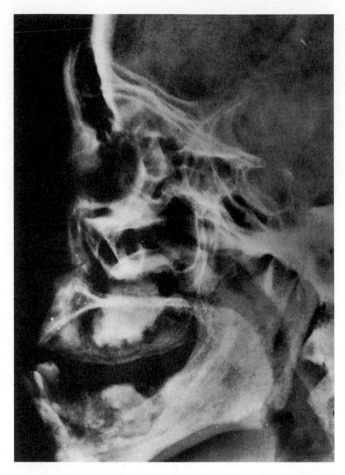

FIG. 4-258 Lateral view shows a calcified mass with a surrounding lucent zone in the maxillary alveolus and in the mandible. Cementoma.

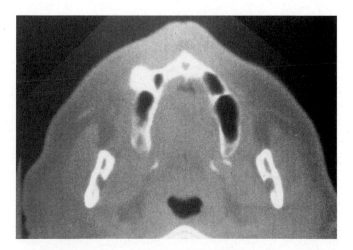

FIG. 4-259 Axial CT scan shows a dense osseous mass arising in the right maxillary alveolus. The lesion is localized to one area, and the remaining alveolus is normal. Cementoma.

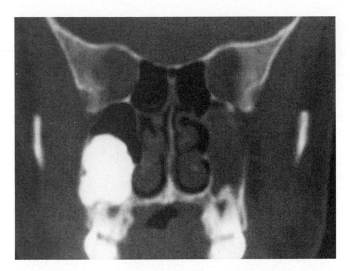

FIG. 4-260   Coronal CT scan shows a very dense mass arising from the right maxillary alveolus and extending into the right antrum. Complex odontoma.

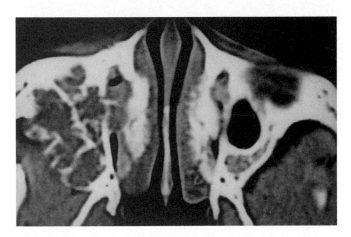

FIG. 4-262   Axial CT scan shows a partially destructive and partially expansile mass in the right maxillary sinus. The lesion contains lacelike areas of calcification. Fibromyxoma.

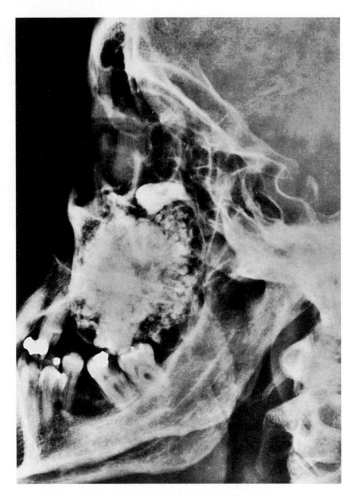

FIG. 4-261   Lateral view shows a large expansile mass in the left maxillary alveolus and antrum. There are innumerable discrete, toothlike densities (denticles). Compound odontoma.

Cementomas

These tumors arise from the mesodermal periodontal ligament. This ligament surrounds and attaches the roots of the teeth to the adjacent alveolar bone. Its cells can form cementum, bone, and fibrous tissue. The four distinct tumor types include the cementifying fibroma, benign cementoblastoma, periapical cemental dysplasia, and gigantiform cementoma.

The cementifying fibroma (cemento-ossifying fibroma) is initially an asymptomatic lesion that is found on routine dental radiographs. When large, these lesions can produce a firm, painless swelling and facial asymmetry. Most lesions occur in the mandibular-premolar-molar region; however, the maxilla can be affected. Because cementifying fibromas contain varying amounts of calcified material, their radiographic appearance varies from a radiolucent process to a radiopaque lesion.[171] In all cases the lesion is well demar-

cated from the adjacent bone, and in most instances it is unilocular and ovoid. This tumor is related to ossifying fibroma and may have areas of ossification, in which case it is referred to as a cemento-ossifying fibroma. The presence of distinct margins differentiates this lesion from fibrous dysplasia, which is histologically similar but has indistinct borders. Conservative excision is the treatment of choice and recurrences are rare (Figs. 4-257 to 4-259). These lesions have been reported in the maxillary sinuses and in the ethmoid sinuses. Whether this latter occurrence results from differentiation of primitive mesenchymal cells or an ectopic periodontal ligament is an unresolved point; however, this lesion is included in the differential diagnosis of fibrous dysplasia and meningioma.

The benign cementoblastoma (true cementoma) is an uncommon cementum-producing lesion that is fused to the root(s) of a tooth. Most of the teeth affected are in the premolar-molar region of the jaws, and the lesion may disrupt the tooth innervation by surrounding the root apex. As a result, many of the involved teeth are not viable.[171]

Radiographically these lesions appear as well-defined radiopaque mass(es) that are continuous with the root apices

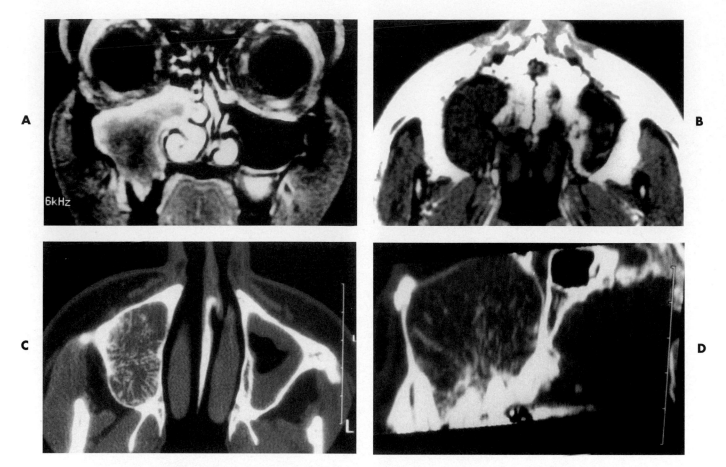

FIG. 4-263   Coronal T1W contrast MR (**A**), axial T1W noncontrast MR (**B**), axial CT (**C**), and reformatted sagittal CT (**D**) scans show an expansile low signal intensity mass, filling the right maxillary sinus. Minimal nonhomogeneity is seen in **B**. Entrapped high signal intensity secretions are present around the lesion. The CT scans show that within the lower portion of the mass there are thin, lacelike calcifications. Odontogenic fibromyxoma.

of affected teeth. A zone of lucency, or a "halo," surrounds each lesion. The radiographic differential diagnosis is primarily with the condition known as hypercementosis. In this process, excessive amounts of cementum accumulate along the surface of the involved tooth root(s). Hypercementosis is associated with Paget's disease, periapical inflammation, and elongation of a tooth as a result of the loss of its antagonistic opposing tooth.[171]

Periapical cemental dysplasia (cementoma, periapical fibrous dysplasia) is more a reactive lesion than a true neoplasm. It is the most frequently encountered cementoid lesion and occurs almost exclusively in females. Initially the lesion appears radiolucent, similar to a periapical cyst or granuloma, but then it calcifies. The involved tooth is always vital to testing, and the radiopaque mass is separated from the tooth root by a narrow radiolucent zone, rather than being on the root surface as in hypercementosis. Periapical cemental dysplasia is a benign self-limiting process and surgical excision is not necessary.

The gigantiform cementoma (familial multiple cementoma) is a rare tumor that may be neoplastic or dysplastic. It is characterized by nodular, irregularly shaped radiopacities in several portions of one or both jaws. Asymptomatic expansion of the cortical plates is frequent, with concomitant, simple bone cysts. The term florid osseous dysplasia has been proposed as a better name for this entity, which is self-limiting, affects only the alveolar process, and seems to be independent of teeth. Paget's disease can be ruled out on the basis of a normal serum alkaline phosphatase level in patients with gigantiform cementoma. Treatment depends on the clinical course. The most common complication is the development of low-grade osteomyelitis in the edentulous areas.

Odontomas

Odontomas contain epithelial and mesenchymal components of the dental apparatus that have complete differentiation, resulting in the presence of enamel, dentin, cementum, and pulp. The complex odontoma has a haphazard arrangement of the elements. In compound odontomas the elements have a normal relationship to one another.[171] Complex and compound lesions occur equally, and 95% are detected in the second decade of life. Most lesions are asymptomatic, and 75% occur in the maxilla. Radiographically the complex

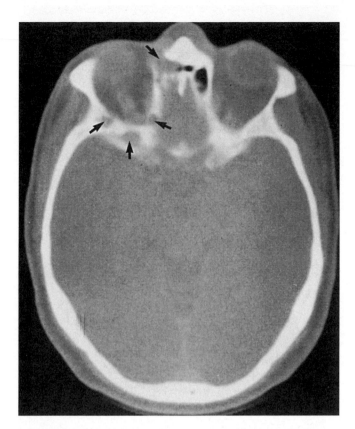

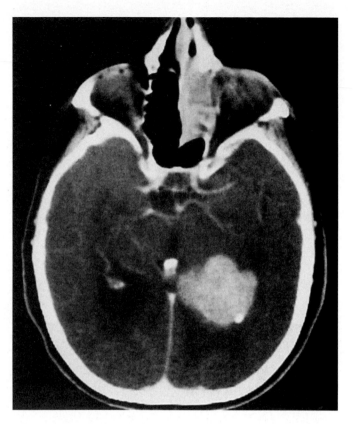

FIG. 4-264   Axial CT scan shows multiple discrete areas of lytic bone destruction *(arrows)*. Metastatic lung carcinoma.

FIG. 4-265   Axial contrast CT scan shows an enhancing mass in the left ethmoid sinuses and nasal cavity and a second mass in the occipital horn. Metastatic melanoma.

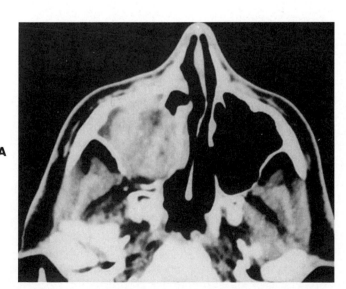

A

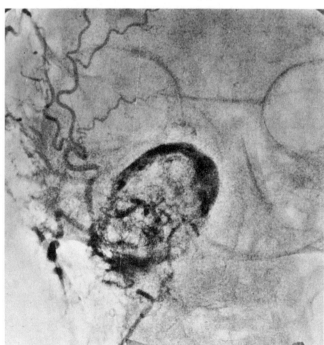

B

FIG. 4-266   Axial contrast CT (**A**) and coronal subtraction angiogram (**B**) scans show an expansile enhancing and vascular mass in the right maxillary sinus. Metastatic hyperhephroma.

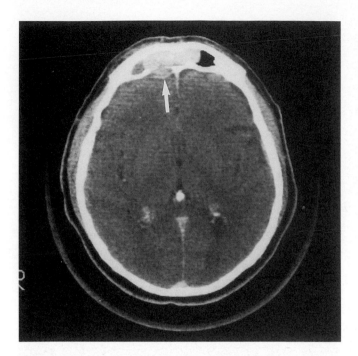

FIG. 4-267   Axial contrast CT scan shows an enhancing frontal sinus mass that eroded the posterior sinus table *(arrow)*. Metastatic hypernephroma.

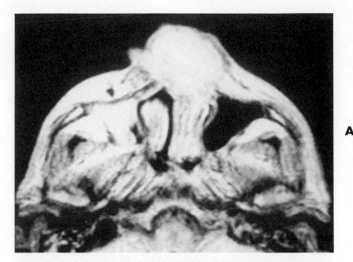

A

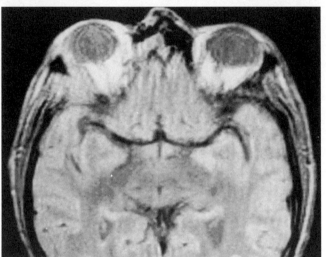

B

FIG. 4-268   Axial proton density MRI through the level of the lower nasal fossa (**A**) and the orbits (**B**) show two distinct masses: one in the nose and one in the right lateral orbital wall. Both masses are homogeneous and of an intermediate to high signal intensity. Metastatic lung carcinoma.

odontoma appears as an amorphous radiopacity. The compound odontoma has anywhere from 3 to 2000 miniature teeth (or denticles), with only single roots or no roots. All odontomas are surrounded by a thin, radiolucent halo that represents the fibrous capsule. Treatment involves complete surgical excision; recurrences are rare (Figs. 4-260, 4-261).

Fibromyxomas

The term fibromyxoma applies to several lesions, which as a group are fibrous variants of a myxoma. These tumors include the nonossifying fibroma, the desmoplastic fibroma, and the odontogenic fibroma.[172] Possibly the odontogenic myxoma also should be included in this group. Fibromyxomas tend to occur during the second and third decades of life. When they appear in the maxilla and paranasal sinuses, these tumors can be locally aggressive and have a high recurrence rate.

Radiographically, fibromyxomas are primarily expansile when they involve the sinuses, although focal areas of aggressive bone destruction may be present. These lesions usually have flecks or thin strands of calcification dispersed within the tumor substance. Complete surgical excision is the treatment of choice (Figs. 4-262, 4-263).

METASTASES TO THE SINONASAL CAVITIES

Metastasis from primary tumors below the clavicles to the sinonasal cavities is infrequent. Only about 100 have been reported. The most common primary tumor with signs and symptoms referable to the sinonasal cavities is the renal cell carcinoma. Tumors found in the sinonasal cavities precede the diagnosis of the primary tumor in 8% of patients.[173] Next in frequency are tumors of the lung and breast; these are followed considerably less frequently by tumors of the testis, prostate, and gastrointestinal tract.[2,174] The average age of patients with metastases from renal cell tumors to the sinonasal cavities is near the end of the sixth decade of life, similar to that of patients with breast carcinoma metastases. Bronchogenic and gastrointestinal tract metastases generally appear in the fifth decade of life. Symptoms of metastases

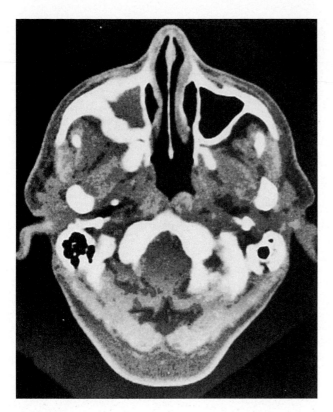

FIG. 4-269 Axial CT scan shows thickened, sclerotic bone in the right maxilla, zygoma, and lateral pterygoid plate. The right antrum is obstructed. Metastatic prostate carcinoma.

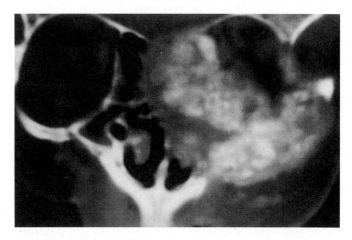

FIG. 4-270 Coronal CT scan shows diffuse, irregular tumoral calcification in the left face, invading the ethmoid, anterior cranial fossa floor, nasal fossa, orbit, maxillary sinus, and cheek. Metastatic sarcoma with calcium deposition.

are nonspecific, except for the renal cell lesions, which commonly cause epistaxis.[175] The presence of metastases in the sinonasal cavities does not appear to alter the prognosis in patients with generalized carcinomatosis. However, if a sinonasal metastasis is the only one from a primary renal cell carcinoma, the surgical removal of the metastasis and the primary tumor may result in a good survival time.[176] Squamous and basal cell carcinomas of facial and scalp skin may metastasize to the central skull base, usually along neurogenic pathways. These metastases can occur despite clean specimen margins of the resected primary skin tumor. In these cases, the most accurate prognostic finding is perineural tumor invasion in the primary lesion.[177-179] Skin melanomas in rare instances metastasize to the sinonasal cavities. Along with the metastases from renal cell carcinomas, these lesions are the most vascular metastases and often manifest with epistaxis.

On CT, metastases from lung, breast, distal genitourinary tract, and gastrointestinal tract tumors are aggressive, bone-destroying, soft-tissue masses that enhance minimally if at all. The metastases are usually indistinguishable from a primary sinonasal squamous cell carcinoma. By comparison, metastases from primary renal cell carcinomas and melanomas are enhancing masses that may remodel the sinonasal walls, as well as destroy them. Prostate carcinoma is one of the few primary tumors that may give a purely blastic metastasis to the facial bones and skull. Although a soft-tissue mass may occur, often only a sclerotic, slightly thickened bone with an abnormal, irregular trabecular pattern is seen. On CT this pure bone disease can be overlooked unless wide windows are used to evaluate the bone.

The most important radiographic indication of metastasis is the presence of more than one lesion, particularly because sinonasal tumors usually do not erode multiple areas of bone. Rather, contiguous sites of bone erosion spread from an area of initial involvement. Thus two areas of bone erosion with intervening normal bone suggests metastatic disease (Figs. 4-264 to 4-270).

References

1. Batsakis JG. Tumors of the head and neck: clinical and pathological considerations. 2nd Edition. Baltimore, Md: Williams & Wilkins, 1979; 177-187.

2. Barnes L, Verbin RS, Gnepp DR. Diseases of the nose, paranasal sinuses, and nasopharynx. In: Barnes L, ed. Surgical pathology of the head and neck. Vol 1. New York, NY: Marcel Dekker Inc, 1985; 403-451.

3. Muir C, Weiland L. Upper aerodigestive tract cancers. Cancer (Suppl) 1995; 75:147-153.

4. Harrison DFN. The management of malignant tumors of the nasal sinuses. Otolaryngol Clin North Am 1971; 4:159-177.

5. Harrison DFN. Problems in surgical management of neoplasms arising in the paranasal sinus. J Laryngol 1976; 90:69-74.

6. Jeans WD, Gilani S, Bullimore J. The effect of CT scanning on staging of tumours of the paranasal sinuses. Clin Radiol 1982; 33:173-179.

7. Curtin HD, Williams R, Johnson J. CT of perineural tumor extension: pterygopalatine fossa. AJNR 1984; 5:731-737.

8. Nishijima W, Takooda S, Tokita N et al. Analysis of distant metastases in squamous cell carcinoma of the head and neck and lesions above the clavicle at autopsy. Arch Otolaryngol Head Neck Surg 1993; 119:65-68.

9. Lloyd GAS, Lund VJ, Phelps, PD et al. Magnetic resonance imaging in the evaluation of nose and paranasal sinus disease. Br J Radiol 1987; 60:957-968.

10. Som PM, Shapiro MD, Biller HF et al. Sinonasal tumors and inflammatory tissues: differentiation with MR. Radiology 1988; 167:803-808.

11. Dubois PJ, Schultz JC, Perrin RL et al. Tomography in expansile lesions of the nasal and paranasal sinuses. Radiology 1977; 125:149-158.

12. Som PM, Shugar JMA. When to question the diagnosis of anaplastic carcinoma. Mt Sinai J Med 1981; 48:230-235.

13. Som PM, Shugar JMA. The significance of bone expansion associated with the diagnosis of malignant tumors of the paranasal sinuses. Radiology 1980; 136:97-100.

14. Som PM, Lidov M. The significance of sinonasal radiodensities. ossification, calcification, or residual bone? American Journal of Neuroradiology 1994; 15:917-922.

15. Hyams VJ. Papillomas of the nasal cavity and paranasal sinuses: a clinicopathologic study of 315 cases. Ann Otol Rhinol Laryngol 1971; 80:192-206.

16. Lasser A, Rothfeld PR, Shapiro RS. Epithelial papilloma and squamous cell carcinoma of the nasal cavity and paranasal sinuses: a clinicopathologic study. Cancer 1976; 38:2503-2510.

17. Vrabec DP. The inverted schneiderian papilloma: a clinical and pathological study. Laryngoscope 1975; 85:186-220.

18. Brandwein M, Steinberg B, Thung S et al. HPV 6/11 and 16/18 in Schneiderian inverted papillomas. Cancer 1989; 63:1708-1713.

19. McLachlin CM, Kandel RA, Colgan TJ et al. Prevalence of HPV in sinonasal papillomas. A study using PCR and in-situ hybridization. Modern Pathology 1992; 5:406-409.

20. Norris HJ. Papillary lesions of the nasal cavity and paranasal sinuses. I. Exophytic (squamous) papillomas: a study of 28 cases. Laryngoscope 1962; 72:1784-1797.

21. Momose KJ, Weber AL, Goodman M et al. Radiological aspects of inverted papilloma. Radiology 1980; 134:73-79.

22. Yousem DM, Fellows DW, Kennedy DW et al. Inverted papilloma: evaluation with MR imaging. Radiology 1992; 185:501-505.

23. Woodruff WW, Vrabec DP. Inverted papilloma of the nasal vault and paranasal sinuses: spectrum of CT fingings. AJR 1994; 162:419-423.

24. Lund VJ, Lloyd GAS. Radiological changes associated with inverted papillomas of the nose and paranasal sinuses. Br J Radiol 1984; 57:455-461.

25. Apostol JV, Frazell EL. Juvenile nasopharyngeal angiofibroma, Cancer 1965; 18:869-878.

26. Som PM, Cohen BA, Sacher M et al. The angiomatous polyp and the angiofibroma: two different lesions. Radiology 1982; 144:329-334.

27. Som PM, Shugar JMA, Cohen BA et al. The nonspecificity of the antral bowing sign in maxillary sinus pathology. JCAT 1981; 5:350-352.

28. Bryan RN, Sessions RB, Horowitz BL. Radiographic management of juvenile angiofibromas. AJNR 1981; 2:157-166.

29. Som PM, Lanzieri CF, Sacher M et al. Extracranial tumor vascularity: determination by dynamic CT scanning. II. The unit approach. Radiology 1985; 154:407-412.

30. Fitzpatrick PJ, Briant DR, Berman JM. The nasopharyngeal angiofibroma. Arch Otolaryngol 1980; 106:234-236.

31. Batasakis JG. Tumors of the head and neck: clinical and pathological considerations. 2nd Edition. Baltimore, Md: Williams & Wilkins, 1979; 139-143.

32. Barton RT. Nickel carcinogenesis of the respiratory tract. J Otolaryngol 1977; 6:412-422.

33. Penzin KH, Lefkowitch JH, Hui RM. Bilateral nasal squamous carcinoma arising in papillomatosis: report of a case developing after chemotherapy for leukemia. Cancer 1981; 48:2375-2382.

34. Weimert TA, Batsakis JG, Rice DH. Carcinoma of the nasal septum. J Laryngol Otol 1978; 92:209-213.

35. Baredes S, Cho HT, Som ML. Total maxillectomy. In: Blitzer A, Lawson W, Friedman WH, eds. Surgery of the paranasal sinuses. Philadelphia, Pa: WB Saunders Co, 1985; 204-216.

36. Harrison DFN. Critical look at the classification of maxillary sinus carcinoma. Ann Otol 1978; 87:3-9.

37. Chaudhry AP, Gorlin RJ, Mosser DG. Carcinoma of the antrum: a clinical and histopathologic study. Oral Surg Oral Med Oral Pathol 1960; 13:269-281.

38. Larsson LG, Martensson G. Maxillary antral cancers. JAMA 1972; 219:342-345.

39. St Pierre S, Baker SR: Squamous cell carcinoma of the maxillary sinus: analysis of 66 cases, Head Neck Surg 1983; 5:508-513.

40. Som ML. Surgical management of carcinomas of the maxilla. Arch Otolaryngol 1974; 99:270-273.

41. Ogura JH, Schenck NL. Unusual nasal tumors: problems in diagnosis and treatment. Otolaryngol Clin North Am 1973; 6:813-837.

42. Conley J. Concepts in head and neck surgery. Stuttgart, Germany: Georg Thieme Verlag, 1970.

43. Klintenberg C, Olofsson J, Hellquist H

et al. Adenocarcinoma of the ethmoid sinuses: a review of 38 cases with special reference to wood dust exposure. Cancer 1984; 54:482-488.

44. Spiro RH, Koss LG, Hajdu SI et al. Tumors of minor salivary origin: a clinicopathologic study of 492 cases. Cancer 1973; 31:117-129.

45. Conley J, Dingman DL. Adenoid cystic carcinoma in the head and neck (cylindroma). Arch Otolaryngol 1974; 100:81-90.

46. Yamamoto Y, Saka T, Makimoto K et al. Histological changes during progression of adenoid cystic carcinoma. J Laryngol Otol 1992; 106:1016-1020.

47. Suzuki K, Moribe K, Baba S. A rare case of pleomorphic adenoma of nasal cavity in Japan. Nippon Jibiinkoka Gakkai Kaiho 1990; 93:740-745.

48. Freeman SB, Kennedy KS, Parker GS et al. Metastasizing pleomorphic adenoma of the nasal septum. Arch Otolaryngol Head Neck Surg 1990; 116;1331-1333.

49. Compagno J, Wong RT. Intranasal mixed tumors (pleomorphic adenomas): a clinicopathologic study of 40 cases. Am J Clin Pathol 1977; 68:213-218.

50. Sigal R, Monnet O, de Baere T et al. Adenoid cystic carcinoma of the head and neck: evaluation with MR imaging and clinical-pathologic correlation in 27 patients. Radiology 1992; 184:95-101.

51. Acheson ED, Gowdell RH, Jolles B. Nasal cancer in the Northamptonshire boot and shoe industry. Br Med J 1970; 1:385-393.

52. Hadfield EH. A study of adenocarcinoma of the paranasal sinuses in woodworkers in the furniture industry. Ann R Coll Surg Engl 1970; 46:301-319.

53. Franquemont DW, Fechner RE, Mills SE. Histologic classification of sinonasal intestinal-type adenocarcinoma. Am J Surg Pathol 1991; 15:368-375.

54. Barnes L. Intestinal-type adenocarcinoma of nasal cavity and paranasal sinuses. Am J Surg Pathol 1986; 10:192-202.

55. Batasakis JG. Tumors of the head and neck: clinical and pathologic considerations. 2nd Edition. Baltimore, Md: Williams & Wilkins, 1979; 76-99.

56. Freedman HM, DeSanto LW, Devine KD et al. Malignant melanoma of the nasal cavity and paranasal sinuses. Arch Otolaryngol 1973; 97:322-325.

57. Batsakis JG, Sciubba J. Pathology. In: Blitzer A, Lawson W, Friedman WH, eds. Surgery of the paranasal sinuses. Philadelphia, Pa: WB Saunders Co, 1985, 74-113.

58. Welkosky HJ, Sorger K, Knuth AM et al. Malignant melanoma of the mucus sinuses of the upper aerodigestive tract. Clinical, histological and immunohistochemical characteristics. Laryngorhinootologie 1991; 70:302-306.

59. Franquemont DW, Mills SE. Sinonasal malignant melanoma: a clinicopathologic and immunohistochemical study of 14 cases. Am J Clin Pathol 1991; 96:689-697.

60. Holdcraft JH, Gallagher JC. Malignant melanomas of the nasal and paranasal sinus mucosa. Ann Otol Rhinol Laryngol 1969; 78:1-20.

61. Gallagher JC. Upper respiratory melanoma pathology and growth rate. Ann Otol 1970; 79:551-556.

62. Barnes L. Verbin RS, Gne DR. Diseases of the nose, paranasal sinuses, and nasopharynx. In: Barnes L, ed. Surgical pathology of the head and neck. Vol 1. New York, NY: Marcel Dekker Inc, 1956; 659-724.

63. Hillstrom RP, Zarbo RJ, Jacobs JR. Nerve sheath tumors of the paranasal sinuses: electron microscopy and histopathologic diagnosis. Otolaryngol Head Neck Surg 1990; 102:257-263.

64. Donnelly MJ, Saler MH, Blayney AW. Benign nasal schwannoma. J Laryngol Otol 1992; 106:1011-1015.

65. Hellquist HB, Lundgren J. Neurogenic sarcoma of the sinonasal tract. J Laryngol Otol 1991; 105:186-190.

66. Som PM, Biller HF, Lawson W et al. An approach to parapharyngeal space masses: an updated protocol based upon 104 cases. Radiology 1984; 153:149-156.

67. Hunt JC, Pugh DG. Skeletal lesions in neurofibromatosis. Radiology 1961; 76:1-19.

68. Oberman HA, Sullenger G. Neurogenous tumors of the head and neck. Cancer 1967; 20:1992-2001.

69. D'Agostino AN, Soule EH, Miller RH. Sarcomas of the peripheral nerves and somatic soft tissues associated with multiple neurofibromatosis (von Recklinghausen's disease). Cancer 1963; 16:1015-1027.

70. Guccion JG, Enzinger FM. Malignant schwannoma associated with von Recklinghausen's neurofibromatosis. Virchows Arch 1979; 383:43-57.

71. Cadotte M. Malignant granular cell myoblastoma. Cancer 1974; 33:1417-1422.

72. Elkon D, Hightower SI, Lim ML et al. Esthesioneuroblastoma. Cancer 1979; 44:1087-1094.

73. Kadish S, Goodman M, Wine CC. Olfactory neuroblastoma: a clinical analysis of 17 cases. Cancer 1976; 37:1571-1576.

74. Som PM, Lawson W, Biller HF et al. Ethmoid sinus disease: CT evaluation in 400 cases. III. Craniofacial resection. Radiology 1986; 159:605-609.

75. Morita A, Ebersold MJ, Olsen KD et al. Esthesioneuroblastoma: prognosis and management. Neurosurgery 1993; 32:706-715.

76. Dulgurov P, Calcaterra T. Esthesioneuroblastoma: the UCLA experience 1970-1990. Laryngoscope 1992; 102:843-849.

77. Mack EE, Prados MD, Wilson CB. Late manifestations of esthesioneuroblastoma in the central nervous system: report of two cases. Neurosurgery 1992; 30:93-97.

78. Regenbogen VS, Zinreich SJ, Kim KS et al. Hyperostotic esthesioneuroblastoma: CT and MR findings. JCAT 1988; 12:52-56.

79. Derdeyn CP, Moran CJ, Wippold FJ II et al. MRI of estesioneuroblastoma. JCAT 1994; 18:16-21.

80. Som PM, Lidov M, Brandwein M et al. Sinonasal esthesioneuroblastoma with intracranial extension: marginal tumor cysts as a diagnostic MR finding. Am J of Neuroradiology 1994; 15:1259-1262.

81. Stowens D, Lin TH. Melanotic progonoma of the brain. Hum Pathol 1974; 5:105-113.

82. Alarcos A, Matesanz A, Alarcos E et al. A glomus tumor of the nasal fossa and ethmoid sinus. Acta Otorrinolaringol Esp 1992; 34:291-295.

83. Straehler HJ. Paraganglioma of the nasal cavity. Laryngol Rhinol Otol 1985; 64:399-402.

84. Farr HW, Gray GT Jr., Vrana M et al. Extracranial meningioma. J Surg Oncol 1973; 5:411-420.

85. Lopez DA, Silvers DN, Helwig EB.

Cutaneous meningioma: a clinicopathologic study. Cancer 1974; 34:728-744.

86. Taxy JB. Meningioma of the paranasal sinuses: a report of two cases. Am J Surg Pathol 1990; 14:82-86.

87. Som PM, Sacher M, Strenger SW et al. "Benign" metastasizing meningioma. AJNR 1987; 8:127-130.

88. Barnes L. Verbin RS, Gnepp DR. Diseases of the nose, paranasal sinuses, and nasopharynx. In: Barnes L, ed. Surgical pathology of the head and neck. Vol. 1. New York, NY: Marcel Dekker Inc, 1985; 912-1044.

89. Shugar JMA, Som PM, Krespi YP ct al. Primary chordoma of the maxillary sinus. Laryngoscope 1980; 90:1825-1830.

90. Wright D. Nasopharyngeal and cervical chordoma: some aspects of their development and treatment. J Laryngol 1967; 81:1337-1355.

91. Yuh WTC, Flickinger FW, Barloon TJ et al. MR imaging of unusual chordomas. JCAT 1988; 12:30-35; and McGurk M, Goepel JR, Hancock BW. Extralnodal lymphoma of the head and neck: a review of 49 consecutive cases. Clin Radiol 1985; 36:455-458.

92. Fellbaum C, Hansmann ML, Lennert K, Malignant lymphomas of the nasal and paranasal sinuses. Virch Arch A Pathol Anat Histopathol 1989; 414:399-405.

93. Bortnick E. Neoplasms of the nasal cavity. Otolaryngol Clin North Am 1973; 6:801-812.

94. Non-hodgkin's lymphoma pathologic classification project. Cancer 1982; 49:2112-2135.

95. Arber DA, Weiss LM, Albujar PF et al. Nasal lymphoma in Peru: high incidence of T-cell immunophenotype and Epstein-Barr virus infection. Am J Surg Pathol 1993; 17:392-399.

96. Ye YL, Zhou M, Lu XY et al. Nasopharyngeal and nasal malignant lymphoma: a clinicopathological study of 54 cases. Histopathology 1992; 20:511-516.

97. Ho FC, Choy D, Loke SL et al. Polymorphic reticulosis and conventional lymphomas of the nose and upper aerodigestive tract: a clinicopathologic study of 70 cases, and immunophenotypic studies of 16 cases. Hum Pathol 1990; 21:1041-1050.

98. Furukawa M, Sakshita H, Kimaur Y et al. Association of Epstein-Barr virus with polymorphic reticulosis. Eur Arch Otorhinolaryngol 1990; 247:261-263.

99. Ratech H, Burke JS, Blayney DW et al. A clinicopathologic study of malignant lymphomas of the nose, paranasal sinuses, and hard palate, including cases of lethal midline granuloma. Cancer 1989; 64:2525-2531.

100. Lee Y-Y, Van Tassel P, Nauert C et al. Lymphomas of the head and neck: CT findings at initial presentation. AJNR 1987; 8:665-671.

101. Wilder WH, Harner SG, Banks PM. Lymphoma of the nose and paranasal sinuses. Arch Otolaryngol 1983; 109:310-312.

102. Harnsberger HR, Bragg DG, Osborn AG et al. Non-Hodgkin's lymphoma of the head and neck: CT evaluation of nodal and extranodal sites. AJNR 1983; 8:673-679.

103. Kondo M, Hashimoto T, Shiga H et al. Computed tomography of sinonasal non-Hodgkin's lymphoma. JCAT 1984; 8:216-219.

104. Duncavage JA, Campbell BH, Hanson GH et al. Diagnosis of malignant lymphomas of the nasal cavity, paranasal sinuses and nasopharynx. Laryngoscope 1983; 93:1276-1280.

105. Marsot-Dupuch K, Raveau V, Aoun N et al. Lethal midline granuloma: impact of imaging studies on the investigation and management of destructive mid facial disease in 13 patients. Neuroradiology 1992; 34:155-161.

106. Barnes L, Verbin RS, Gnepp DR. Diseases of the nose, paranasal sinuses, and nasopharynx. In: Barnes L, ed. Surgical pathology of the head and neck. Vol. 1. New York, NY: Marcel Dekker Inc, 1985; 1045-1209.

107. Pomeranz SJ, Hawkins HH, Towbin R et al. Granulocytic sarcoma (chloroma): CT manifestations. Radiology 1985; 155:167-170.

108. Castro EB, Lewis JS, Strong EW. Plasmacytoma of paranasal sinuses and nasal cavity. Arch Otolaryngol 1973; 97:326-329.

109. Fu Y-S, Perzin KH. Nonepithelial tumors of the nasal cavity, paranasal sinuses and nasopharynx: a clinicopathologic study—IX plasmacytomas. Cancer 1978; 42:2399-2406.

110. Kondo M, Hashimoto S, Inuyama Y et al. Extramedullary plasmacytoma of the sinonasal cavities: CT evaluation. JCAT 1986; 10:841-844.

111. Enziger FM, Weiss SW. Soft tissue tumors. 2nd Edition. St Louis, Mo: The CV Mosby Co, 1988.

112. Barnes L, Verbin RS, Gnepp DR. Diseases of the nose, paranasal sinuses, and nasopharynx. In: Barnes L, ed. Surgical pathology of the head and neck. Vol 1. New York, NY: Marcel Dekker Inc, 1985; 725-880.

113. Rosenberg SA et al. Sarcomas of the soft tissue and bone. In: De Vita VT, Hellman S, Rosenberg SA, eds. Cancer: principles and practice of oncology. Philadelphia, Pa: JB Lippincott Co, 1982; 1036-1093.

114. Young JL Jr, Miller RW. Incidence of malignant tumors in US children. J Pediatr 1975; 86:254-258.

115. Hajdu SI. Soft tissue sarcomas: classification and natural history. Cancer 1981; 31:271-280.

116. Enzinger FM, Shiraki M. Alveolar rhabdomyosarcoma: an analysis of 110 cases. Cancer 1969; 24:18-31.

117. Makishima K, Iwasaki H, Horie A. Alveolar rhabdomyosarcoma of the ethmoid sinus. Laryngoscope 1975; 85:400-410.

118. Kapidia S, Meis JM, Frisman D et al. Adult rhabdomyoma (RM) of the head and neck: a clinicopathologic and immunophenotypic study. Human Pathol 1993; 24:608-617.

119. Kapidia S, Meis JM, Frisman D et al. Fetal rhabdomyoma (FRM) of the head and neck: a clinicopathologic and immunophenotypic study. Human Pathol 1993; 24:754-765.

120. Enzinger F, Weiss S. Soft tissue tumors. 3rd Edition, St Louis, Mo: Mosby-Year Book, 1995; Chapter 10.

121. Heffner DK, Gnepp DR. Sinonasal fibrosarcomas, malignant schwannomas, and "Triton" tumors: a clinicopathologic study of 67 cases. Cancer 1992; 70:1089-1101.

122. Merrick RE, Rhone DP, Chilis TJ. Malignant fibrous histiocytoma of the maxillary sinus. Arch Otolaryngol 1980; 106:365-367.

123. Dooms GC, Hricak H, Sollitto RA et al. Lipomatous tumors and tumors with fatty component: MR imaging potential and comparison of MR and CT results. Radiology 1985; 157:479-483.

124. Kuruvilla A, Wenig BM, Humphrey DM et al. Leiomyosarcoma of the sinonasal tract: a clinicopathologic study of nine cases. Arch Otolaryngol Head Neck Surg 1990; 116:1278-1286.

125. Dropkin LR, Tang CK, Williams JR. Leiomyosarcoma of the nasal cavity and paranasal sinuses. Ann Otol Rhinol Laryngol 1976; 85:399-403.

126. McLeod AJ, Zornoza J, Shirkhoda A. Leiomyosarcoma: computed tomographic findings. Radiology 1984; 152:133-136.

127. Enzinger FM, Smith BH. Hemangiopericytoma: an analysis of 106 cases. Hum Pathol 1976; 7:61-82.

128. El-Naggar AK, Batsakis JG, Garcia GM et al. Sinonasal hemangiopericytomas: clinicoopathologic and DNA content study. Arch Otolaryngol Head Neck Surg 1992; 118:134-137.

129. Kauffman SL, Stout AP. Hemangiopericytoma in children. Cancer 1960; 13:695-710.

130. Kimura Y, Tanaka S, Furuka M. Angiosarcoma of the nasal cavity. J Laryngol Otol 1992; 106:368-369.

131. Kurien M, Nair S, Thomas S. Angiosarcoma of the nasal cavity and maxillary antrum. J Laryngol Otol 1989; 103:874-876.

132. Solomons NB, Stearns MP. Haemangiosarcoma of the maxillary antrum. J Laryngol Otol 1990; 104:831-834.

133. Evans HL, Ayala AG, Romsdahl MM. Prognostic factors in chondrosarcoma of bone: a clinicopathologic analysis with emphasis on histologic grading. Cancer 1977; 40:818-831.

134. Chaudhry AP, Robinovitch MR, Mitchell DF et al. Chondrogenic tumors of the jaws. Am J Surg 1961; 102:403-411.

135. McCoy JM, McConnel FMS. Chondrosarcoma of the nasal septum. Arch Otolaryngol 1981; 107:125-127.

136. Gay I, Elidan J, Kopolovic J. Chondrosarcoma of the skull base. Ann Otol Rhinol Laryngol 1981; 90:53-55.

137. Dillon WP, Som PM, Rosenau W. Hemangioma of the nasal vault: MR and CT features. Radiology 1991; 180:761-765.

138. Ghosh LM, Samanta A, Nandy T et al. Haemangioma of the maxilla. J Laryngol Otol 1988; 102:725-726.

139. Harcourt JP, Gallimore AP. Leiomyoma of the paranasal sinuses. J Laryngol Otol 1993; 107:740-741.

140. Shugar JMA, Som PM, Meyers RJ et al. Intramuscular head and neck myxoma: report of a case and review of the literature. Laryngoscope 1987; 97:105-107.

141. Fu Y-S, Perzin KH. Nonepthelial tumors of the nasal cavity, paranasal sinuses and nasopharynx: a clinicopathologic study. Cancer 1974; 33:1289-1305.

142. Osguthorpe JD, Hungerford GD. Benign osteoblastoma of the maxillary sinus. Head Neck Surg 1983; 6:605-609.

143. Som PM, Bellot O, Blitzer A et al. Osteoblastoma of the ethmoid sinus: the fourth reported case. Arch Otolaryngol 1979; 105:623-625.

144. Coscina WF, Lee BCP. Concurrent osteoblastoma and aneurysmal bone cyst of the ethmoid sinus: case report. CT J Comput Tomogr 1985; 9:347-350.

145. Oot RF, Parizel PM, Weber AL. Computed tomography of osteogenic sarcoma of nasal cavity and paranasal sinuses. JCAT 1986; 10:409-414.

146. Barnes L. Verbin RS, Gnepp DR. Diseases of the nose, paranasol sinuses, and nasopharynx. In: Barnes L, ed. Surgical pathology of the head and neck. Vol. 1. New York, NY: Marcel Dekker Inc, 1985; 883-1044.

147. Som PM, Hermann G, Sacher M et al. Paget disease of the calvaria and facial bones with an osteosarcoma of the maxilla: CT and MR findings. JCAT 1987; 11:887-890.

148. Dehner LP. Fibro-osseous lesions of bone. In: Ackerman LU, Spjut HJ, Abell MR, eds. Bones and joints. International Academy of Pathology, Monograph No. 17. Baltimore, Md: Williams & Wilkins, 1976; 209-235.

149. Schwartz DT, Alpert M. The malignant transformation of fibrous dysplasia. Am J Med Sci 1964; 274:1-20.

150. Som PM, Lidov M. The benign fibro-osseous lesion: its association with paranasal sinus mucoceles and its MR characteristics. Journal of Computer Assisted Tomography 1992; 16:871-876.

151. Sterling KM, Stollman A, Sacher M et al. Ossifying fibroma of sphenoid bone with coexistent mucocele: CT and MRI. Journal of Computer Assisted Tomography 1993; 17:492-494.

152. Som PM, Lawson W, Cohen BA. Giant cell lesions of the facial bones. Radiology 1983; 147:129-134.

153. Rhea JT, Weber AL. Giant cell granuloma of the sinuses. Radiology 1983; 147:135-137.

154. Friedman WH, Pervez N, Schwartz AE. Brown tumor of the maxilla in secondary hyperparathyroidism. Arch Otolaryngol 1974; 100:157-159.

155. Smith GA, Ward PH. Giant cell lesions of the facial skeleton. Arch Otolaryngol 1978; 104:186-190.

156. Som PM, Brandwein MS, Maldjian C et al. Inflammatory pseudotumor of the maxillary sinus: CT and MR findings in six cases. American Journal of Roentgenology 1994; 163:689-692.

157. Smithson LV, Lipper MH, Hall JA Jr. Paranasal sinus involvement in thalassemia major: CT demonstration. AJNR 1987; 8:564-565.

158. Saw D, Chan JKC, Jagirdar J et al. Sinonasal small cell neoplasm developing after radiation therapy for retinoblastoma: an immunohistologic, ultrastructural and cytogenetic study. Human Pathol 1992; 23:896-899.

159. Klein EA, Anzil AP, Mezzacappa P et al. Sinonasal primitive neuroectodermal tumor arising in a long-term survivor of heritable unilateral retinoblastoma. Cancer 1992; 70:423-431.

160. Chowdry K, Manoukian JJ, Rochon L et al. Extracranial primitive neuroectodermal tumor of the head and neck. Arch Otolaryngol Head Neck Surg 1990; 116: 475-478.

161. Schmidt D, Herrmann C, Jurgens H et al. Malignant peripheral neuroectodermal tumor and its necessary distinction from Ewing s sarcoma. A report from Kiel Pediatric Tumor Registry. Cancer 1991; 68:2251-2259.

162. Gnepp DR, Chandler W, Hyams V. Primary Kaposi's sarcoma of the head and neck. Ann Inter Med 1984; 100:107-114.

163. Lothe F, Murray JF. Kaposi's sarcoma: autopsy findings in the African. Acta Unio Internat Contra Cancrum 1962; 18:429-452.

164. Greenberg JE, Fischl MA, Berger JR. Upper airway obstruction secondary to AIDS-related Kaposi's sarcoma. Chest 1985; 88:638-640.

165. Levy FE, Tansek KM. AIDS-associated Kaposi's sarcoma of the larynx. J Ear Nose Throat 1990; 69:177-183.

166. Fliss DM, Parikh J, Freeman JL. AIDS-related Kaposi's sarcoma of the sphenoid sinus. J Otolaryngol 1992; 21:235-237.

167. Barnes L, Verbin RS, Gnepp DR. Diseases of the nose, paranasal sinuses, and nasopharynx. In: Barnes L, ed. Surgical pathology of the head and neck. Vol. 1. New York, NY: Marcel Dekker Inc, 1985; 1834-1836.

168. Barnes L, Verbin RS, Gnepp DR. Diseases of the nose, paranasal sinuses, and nasopharynx. In: Barnes L, ed. Surgical pathology of the head and neck. Vol. l. New York, NY: Marcel Dekker Inc, 1985; 1233-1329.

169. Stafne EC, Gibilisco JA: Oral roentgenographic diagnosis. 4th Edition. Philadelphia, WB Saunders Co, 1975; 147-168.

170. Botsakis JG. Tumors of the head and neck: clinical and pathological consideration. 2nd Edition. Baltimore, Md: Williams & Wilkins. 1979; 531-560.

171. Mehlisch DR, Dahlin DC, Masson JK. Ameloblastoma: a clinicopathologic report. J Oral Surg 1972; 30:9-22.

172. Barnes L, Verbin RS, Gnepp DR. Diseases of the nose, paranasal sinuses, and nasopharynx. In: Barnes L, ed. Surgical pathology of the head and neck. Vol. 1. New York, NY: Marcel Dekker Inc, 1985; 1331-1409.

173. Barnes L, Verbin RS, Gnepp DR. Diseases of the nose, paranasal sinuses and nasopharynx. In: Barnes L, ed. Surgical pathology of the head and neck. Vol. 1. New York, NY: Marcel Dekker Inc, 1985: 410.

174. Som PM, Norton KI, Shugar JMA et al. Metastatic hypernephroma to the head and neck. AJNR 1987; 8:1103-1106.

175. Batsakis JG. Tumors of the head and neck: clinical and pathological considerations. 2nd Edition. Baltimore, Md: Williams & Wilkins. 1979; 240-251.

176. Bernstein JM, Montgomery WW, Balogh K. Metastatic tumors to the maxilla, nose and paranasal sinus. Laryngoscope 1966; 76:621-650.

177. Cottel WI. Perineural invasion by squamous cell carcinoma. J Dermatol Surg Oncol 1982; 8:589-600.

178. Goepfert H, Dichtel WJ, Medina JE et al. Perineural invasion in squamous cell skin carcinoma of the head and neck. Am J Surg 1984; 148:542-547.

179. Hanke CW, Wolf RL, Hochman SA et al. Chemosurgical reports: perineural spread of basal cell carcinoma. J Dermatol Surg Oncol 1983; 9:742-747.

Section Three
FRACTURES

The paranasal sinuses develop within and are protected by the facial bones. These bones also serve as attachments for the facial muscles, support the maxillary dentition, and surround the orbits, nasal fossae, and mouth. The facial skeleton is a somewhat honeycombed structure of varying thicknesses and form that develops strength along stress zones by forming buttressed arches. In general the most superficial portion of the facial skeleton is physically the strongest and serves the additional function of protecting the more delicate central part of the face.[1,2] The honeycombed construction of the middle third of the facial skeleton evolved to resist the vertical masticatory forces, and in this regard it provides excellent stability. However, external, axial impact forces directed toward the midface can disrupt this central structure, and the fracture of even one buttress can weaken the entire lattice, causing it to collapse. Fortunately, such collapse is often prevented by the strong craniocaudal facial buttresses and the support of the skull base.[3]

Facial Buttresses

The facial skeleton can be analyzed in terms of the supporting buttresses that comprise its structure. There are two main sagittal buttresses on each side of the face. A medial buttress extends from the anterior maxillary alveolus up the lateral wall of the pyriform aperture and into the medial orbital wall. This nasomaxillary buttress is thus formed by the lower maxilla, the frontal process of the maxilla, the lacrimal bone, and the nasal process of the frontal bone. A lateral buttress, the zygomaticomaxillary buttress, is formed on each side by the lateral wall of the maxilla, the body of the zygoma, and the orbital process of the frontal bone in the lateral orbital wall.[2] A third buttress has been suggested, the pterygomaxillary buttress, which extends from the posterior maxillary alveolus (tuberosity) cranially along the pterygoid plates to the skull base. These buttresses have evolved as mechanical adaptations of the skull to masticatory forces, and the greatest occlusal forces are absorbed by the zygomaticomaxillary buttress as evidenced by the thick cortical bone present in the lateral maxillary-zygomatic region when compared with the more fragile medial maxillary wall. In addition to the sagittal buttresses already described, some authors believe that there is also a median buttress formed by the nasal septum. Overall these craniocaudal buttresses are curved, and analysis suggests that they need reinforcement by axial struts. Thus these sagittal buttresses are interconnected by three axial (horizontal) struts that are formed by the floor of the anterior cranial fossa, the orbital floor and zygomatic arches, and the maxillary alveolus and hard palate. In addition the skull base, which is oriented at approximately a 45° angle to the occlusal plane of the maxilla, acts as an additional axial buttress. Together these buttresses or struts form an interconnecting facial support system. The facial skeleton can also be conceptualized as being formed by two coronal buttresses: an anterior plane formed by the frontal bone (glabellar region), the orbital rims, the anterior maxilla, and the alveolus; and a posterior plane formed by the posterior wall of the maxilla and pterygoid processes.[3,4]

Such analyses, first studied experimentally by Le Fort, have led to an understanding of the three major lines of weakness in the midfacial skeleton and help explain why certain fractures follow an overall predictable course.[5] The efforts of Le Fort are recognized today by the Le Fort types I, II, and III fractures. The forces he used experimentally are similar to the low-velocity impact forces that occur today in fist fights and sporting events. However, at present there are also high-velocity impact injuries such as those that occur in high-speed vehicular accidents and with violence involving blunt devices or gunshot wounds. Depite the much greater order of magnitude of these imact forces, the same fracture lines are still encountered, albeit in various combinations other than those Le Fort observed.[3]

Clinical Diagnosis and Treatment

The actual diagnosis of facial fractures usually is accomplished by a combination of clinical and imaging examinations. The clinician is primarily concerned with the detection of malocclusion, abnormal mobility, and crepitation as signs of fracture. Often, deformity of the facial skeleton is initially concealed by overlying edema, hemorrhage, and soft-tissue injury. Any evidence of a palpable step-off at the orbital rim, diplopia, hypertelorism, midfacial elongation, cerebrospinal fluid (CSF) rhinorrhea, or flattening of the cheek further helps the clinician identify the type of fracture present. However, only after radiographic studies can the fractures be completely identified and characterized. It is now recognized that the information gained from CT is of greater net value than that gained from a combination of routine radiographs and clinical examination, and thus imaging is essential for proper treatment planning.[3,6] In many instances, clinicians wait several days after the trauma before reducing the fracture(s). This delay allows some of the soft-tissue injury to subside and may be necessary if the patient has other life-threatening injuries that require immediate attention (before the less critical facial fractures are addressed). However, if possible, a delay of more than 7 days is to be avoided because after this time fibrous fixation of the fracture occurs and fracture reduction becomes more difficult, often requiring refracturing to attain normal positioning.

The basic principles of treating midfacial fractures are (1) reduction of the fractures and (2) fixation of the fractured bones to one another and to the skull. Absolute immobilization of the fractures is the main prerequisite for rapid and undisturbed healing because the main interferences with fracture healing are local mechanical factors. In the early phase of fracture healing, mobility can disturb the normal course of bone regeneration and lead to faulty differentiation of the callus.[3,7,8] Of primary clinical concern is the

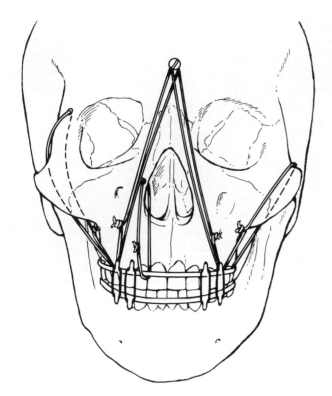

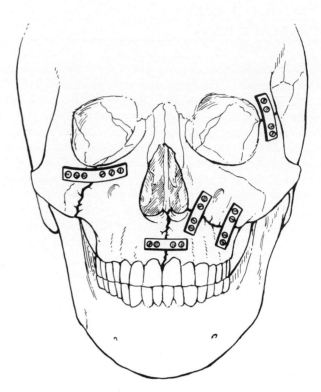

FIG. 4-271   Frontal diagram of the different types of intraosseous wiring. The maxillary and mandibular teeth are fitted with arch bars, which are held together with rubber bands. With the patient in good occlusion, fixation can be achieved by frontomalar suspension, glabella (screw) suspension, pyriform aperture suspension, or circumzyomatic suspension.

FIG. 4-272   Frontal diagram of the use of microplates or miniplates as they are used in the fixation of midfacial fractures at typical fracture sites.

restoration of occlusion and facial form, because these provide a means of restoring the essential masticatory function. Midfacial restoration is accomplished by means of arch bars applied to the maxillary and mandibular teeth and then after manipulation is held in good occlusion by fixing the arch bars together with small rubber bands. Such fixation of the midface must be maintained until bony union and consolidation are achieved. If internal wire fixation is used, immobilization usually takes 6 to 8 weeks (Fig. 4-271). Intermaxillary fixation alone requires 3 to 4 weeks to prevent further occlusal malalignment.[7] Today most internal fixation is accomplished by the use of microplates or miniplates and screws (Fig. 4-272).[7,9] If this technique is used, intermaxillary fixation is accomplished without a waiting interval. In addition the growing use of microplate fixation has almost made obsolete the complex internal fixation schemes accomplished with wire sutures and wire suspensions (suspension wires extended from the maxillary arch bars to the zygomatic processes of the frontal bones, or to the zygomatic arches from a glabella screw, or to the margins of the pyriform aperture) and external fixation using a halo frame with fixation bars.

Infections of the fracture line are among the most serious complications of facial fractures. Any fracture must be considered potentially infected if it traverses the alveolus, the walls of the nasal skeleton or the paranasal sinuses, or com-

municates with a soft-tissue wound. Such fractures are called compound fractures. Appropriate antibiotic therapy reduces the chances of infection in compound fractures.[3,8] With good treatment the risk of infection of a maxillary or midfacial fracture is only about 2%, and the risk of osteomyelitis is 0.5%. However, a treatment delay of 2 to 3 weeks raises the incidence of osteomyelitis to 1.3%.[8] Similarly, posttraumatic sinusitis occurs in 7.25% to 9% of all the patients with midfacial fractures, and proper maintenance of sinus drainage must be a therapeutic consideration.[7]

IMAGING

CT is the modality of choice for the most complete evaluation of the facial skeleton, facial soft tissues, and brain and dural spaces, which so often have associated damage in the severe accidents that cause facial trauma.[10] Axial and coronal CT scans currently provide the clinician most diagnostic information.[11] A single-plane CT study (i.e., axial or coronal) does not provide as much information as an orthogonal two-plane examination; specialized sagittal or oblique plane studies, although helpful in specific cases, are considered optional.[8] If direct coronal CT cannot be obtained because of the patient's clinical status, coronal CT reconstructions from the axial study are acceptable albeit less desirable alternatives. Helical CT provides a means of obtaining bet-

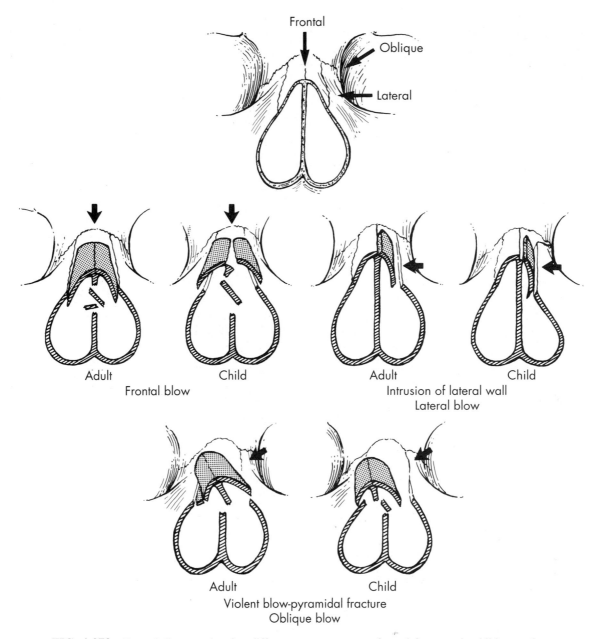

FIG. 4-273 Frontal diagram showing different common types of nasal fractures in children and adults that result from frontal, lateral, and oblique blows.

ter quality 2D reconstructions in any plane and provides excellent 3D reconstructions. Although some detail is lost as part of the smoothing algorithm, the 3D images serve as an excellent communication tool with the surgeons.[12] It allows clinicians to visualize the fracture segments and their relationship to one another better than on a series of 2D scans in any one plane. With the newer 3D software the fracture segments can be manipulated on screen so that the clinician can evaluate a particular treatment approach or the results of a treatment plan. The latter is especially true when evaluating a planned repair of a midfacial congenital defect. In addition, 3D models can now be constructed from the CT data, allowing hands-on preoperative planning in complex cases.[12]

MRI can be helpful in differentiating blood from inflammatory reactions and edema fluid. This is especially true if the imaging is performed at least 48 hours after the injury, when intrasinus blood has a high methemoglobin content. In this state, blood has a high T1W signal intensity, and edema and infection have intermediate to low T1W signal intensities.[13] However, such a distinction is rarely of clinical importance, and because MRI does not visualize the bone directly, small yet unstable nondisplaced facial fractures may not be seen. As a result, CT scanning is the modality of choice in facial trauma patients.[14]

The skull base also must be carefully examined because fractures of the anterior cranial fossa are found in 7.1% of central midfacial fractures, 14.7% of centrolateral midfacial fractures, and 1.1% of lateral midfacial fractures.[7] The midfacial area is formed by the paired maxillae, palatal bones, inferior turbinates, lacrimal bones, nasal bones, zygomas,

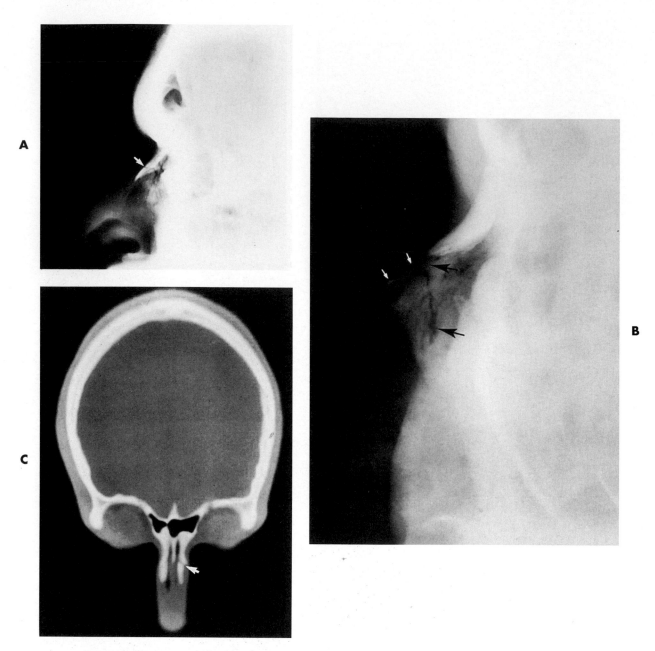

FIG. 4-274   Lateral view. **A,** Nondisplaced fracture *(arrow)* is seen extending from the midline nasal bones laterally. **B,** Lateral view shows communicated nasal bone fractures *(small arrows)* with extension into the frontal processes of the maxilla *(arrows).* **C,** Coronal CT scan shows an isolated minimally depressed left nasal fracture *(arrow).*

solitary vomer and ethmoid bones. Central midfacial fractures include all forms of fractures that occur between the root of the nose and the alveolar processes of the maxillae, without involvement of the zygomas. These fractures include the alveolar process fracture of the maxilla with detachment of teeth, the transverse fracture just above the floor of the nasal cavity with separation of the palate and alveolus (Le Fort I, or Guérin's, fracture), the median or paramedian sagittal fracture of the hard palate, the pyramidal fracture with separation of the midface either with the nasal bones (Le Fort II and Wassmund II) or without the nasal bones (Wassmund I), and fractures of the nasal bones and nasoethmoidal region.[7]

NASAL FRACTURES

Nasal injuries are the most common fractures of the facial skeleton; about 50% of facial fractures are isolated fractures of the nasal pyramid.[9,14] Nasal fractures can occur as isolated fractures or with other facial injuries. A distinction should be made between fractures of the cartilaginous nasal structures and those of the nasal bones because they represent different types of injuries.[3] The extent of disruption of the nasal structure relates to the direction and degree of the force causing the injury (Fig. 4-273). The lateral imact injury is more common than the frontal injury; 66% of nasal fractures result from a lateral force, but only 13% were

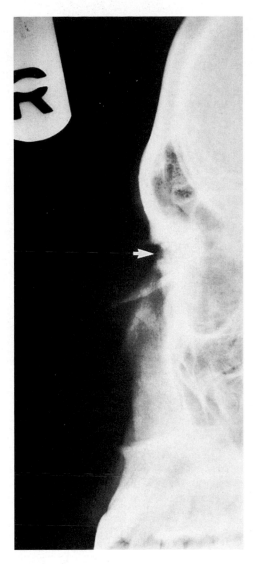

FIG. 4-275 Lateral view shows a nasal fracture through the frontonasal suture *(arrow)* with posterior displacement of the nasal bones.

result from a frontal impact.[15] A classification system divides the frontal injuries into 3 types. In plane 1 injuries the injury does not extend dorsal to a plane that extends from the caudal tip of the nasal bones to the anterior nasal spine. The majority of the impact is absorbed by the lower nasal cartilages and the nasal tip. Separation and avulsion of the upper lateral nasal cartilages occurs, and occasionally there is posterior dislocation of the septal and alar cartilages. In plane 2 injuries the external nose, the nasal septum, and the anterior nasal spine are involved. There is splaying or flattening of the nasal bones, septal cartilage tears, and overriding may occur. In plane 3 injuries the orbital and possibly the intracranial structures are also involved. There typically is comminution of the nasal bones and fractures of the frontal process of the maxilla, the lacrimal bones, and the ethmoid labyrinth. Nasal septal injuries are severe, and upward extension may involve the cribriform plate and orbital roof.[15] With lateral (oblique) impacts, plane 1 injuries result from the weakest force and involve only the

ipsilateral nasal bone. Typically the lower nasal bone, the frontal process of the maxilla, and possibly the pyriform aperture margin are medially displaced. Lateral plane 2 injuries result from a greater force than plane 1 injuries. The fracture results in medial displacement of the ipsilateral nasal bone and lateral displacement of the contralateral nasal bone and nasal septum. Lateral plane 3 injuries are still more severe, with comminution of the nasal bones and involvement of the nasal septum, the frontal process of the maxilla, and the lacrimal bone.[15]

In summary the majority of nasal bone fractures involve the thinner, distal third of the nasal bones, and the nasoethmoid margin remains intact.[3,9] A lateral blow to the nose usually causes a simple cartilage depression or fracture of only the ipsilateral nasal bone (Fig. 4-274). However, an anteriorly placed nasal blow usually fractures both nasal bones at their lower ends, and because the force is absorbed by the nasal septum, the septum is also displaced and fractured. With a greater force, the entire nasal pyramid, including the frontal processes of the maxillae, may become detached (Fig. 4-275).[9] When the nasal bones and septum are displaced posteriorly, a saddle nose deformity and splaying of the nose result.[3] In more severe fractures, traumatic hypertelorism and telecanthus may occur and hemorrhage caused by rupture of the anterior or posterior ethmoidal arteries may be severe.

In adults the internasal suture is solidly ossified so that the nasal bones function as a unit between the frontal processes of the maxilla. However, in children the internasal suture is not yet ossified, and the nasal bones are essentially hinged on each other while resting on the frontal processes of the maxillae. As a result the frontal processes usually are not fractured in childhood nasal injuries.[3] In fact, it has been noted that in children there is a less prominent nasal projection (nasal bone length is almost equal to width); there is increased elasticity and stability of the midface due to the presence of developing bone, the relative lack of sinus pneumatization, and the state of mixed dentition; there is an increased shielding of the facial skeletal structure due to the disproportionate amount of soft tissue relative to bone; and the small weight and size of the child decreases inertial impact forces.[15]

If the nose is struck from the side and near its base, the lateral cartilaginous walls may be displaced and this type of injury is not identified radiographically. Further, edema and hemorrhage usually fill in the resulting surface depression and obscure clinical detection of the deformity. If these injuries and simple nasal fractures initially go undetected, especially if they are in conjunction with more serious injuries, the inadequately treated nasal trauma may result in cosmetic deformity and functional impairment.[3]

If the nasal trauma results in buckling of the nasal septal cartilage, the fractured cartilage fragments may overlap one another, thereby separating the perichondrium from the cartilage. This event allows a hematoma to develop in the space between the perichondrium and the cartilage, and this hematoma interferes with the cartilage's overlying muco-

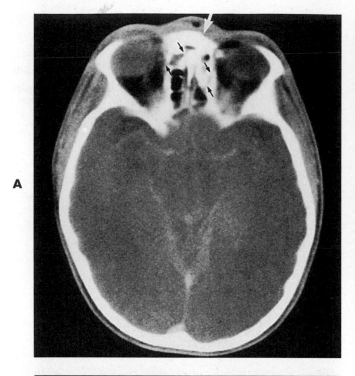

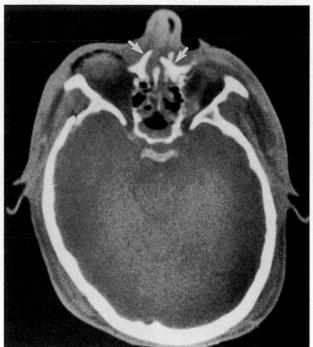

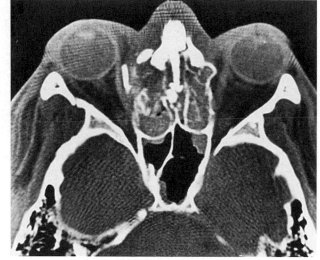

FIG. 4-276 **A,** Axial CT scan shows a nasoorbital fracture with posterior displacement of the nasion *(arrow)* and fractures through the fovea ethmoidalis *(small arrows).* **B,** Axial CT scan shows a nasoorbital fracture with posterior and medial displacement of the nasal bones and frontal processes of the maxilla *(arrows).* There are also fractures of the ethmoids with some hypertelorism. **C,** Axial CT scan shows a nasoorbital fracture with posterior displacement of the nasal bones and fractures and hypertelorism of the ethmoids.

periostial vascular supply. Eventual cartilage necrosis occurs. If a septal hematoma is not initially identified and treated, it becomes an organized hematoma, which leads to an unyielding thickening of the septum and impaired breathing.

If a septal hematoma becomes infected after mucosal injury, a septal abscess will develop. This event may lead to the onset of fever, pain, septal swelling, and eventual cartilage necrosis, which results in a loss of nasal support and a saddle nose deformity.[3] To avoid this complication, it is essential to have careful clinical examination of the nasal septum and early evacuation of a septal hematoma. If imaging studies of the nose and nasal fossae are also performed, the radiologist should always direct attention to the nasal septum to identify any localized septal swelling or deviation.[3]

One study demonstrated that, based on clinical examination, 25% of patients required surgical reduction of a nasal fracture or dislocation despite a negative plain film examination.[16] In addition there is a poor correlation (6.6% to 10%) between the plain film demonstration of a fracture and the need for surgical reduction.[15] In more severe injuries a higher detection rate and better clinical correlation are achieved with the use of CT.

NASOORBITAL FRACTURES

The nasoorbital fracture most often results from a blow over the bridge of the nose. The force displaces the nasal pyramid posteriorly, fracturing the nasal bones, frontal processes of the maxillae, lacrimal bones, ethmoid sinuses, walls of the

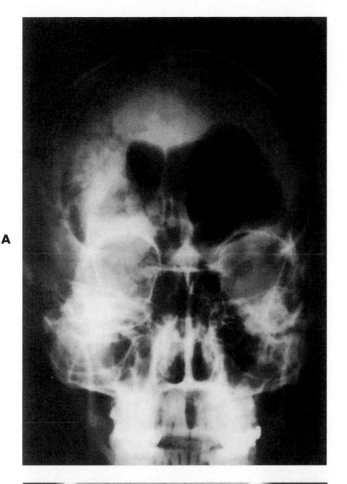

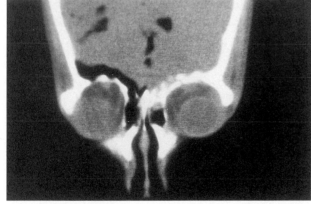

FIG. 4-277   **A,** Caldwell view shows massive intracranial air in a patient who had a nasoorbital fracture. **B,** Coronal CT scan shows intracranial air in a patient with a nasoorbital fracture.

frontal sinuses, cribriform plate, and nasal septum. The ethmoid lamina usually fractures on itself in an accordion fashion, and this is best visualized on CT in the axial plane. Posttraumatic hypertelorism and telecanthus may result, as well as associated damage to the lacrimal apparatus and the medial canthal tendon (Fig. 4-276). Careful attention also should be given to any fractures involving the bones near the optic canal because a surgical attempt at repositioning the displaced facial bones might displace such an optic canal fracture and cause blindness.

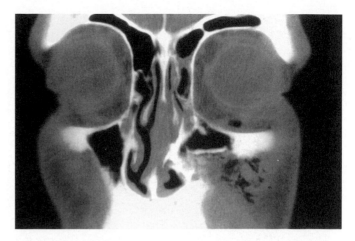

FIG. 4-278   Coronal CT scan shows a maxillary fracture involving the anterior lower antral wall. The fracture segments are prolapsed into the antrum and nasal cavity. There is also orbital and subcutaneous emphysema.

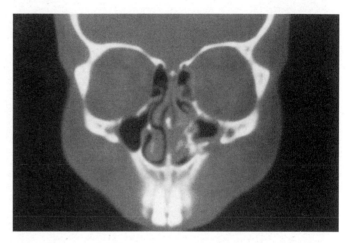

FIG. 4-279   Coronal CT scan shows comminuted maxillary fractures involving the left anteromedial maxilla.

In the floor of the anterior cranial fossa the dura is thin and firmly adherent to the bone. Thus the skull base and dura in the anterior cranial fossa function as a unit, and a fracture through this region invariably tears the dura. Dural tears provide a pathway for CSF rhinorrhea and the development of an intracranial pneumocele or infection (Fig. 4-277).[3] In one series, motor vehicle accidents accounted for nearly 70% of these cases and 63% of the patients had associated severe nonfacial injuries. In addition, 51% of the cases had central nervous system injury; 42% of the patients had CSF leakage.[17] Telecanthus is present in 12% of the cases.[18]

MAXILLARY FRACTURES

Alveolar fractures are the most common isolated maxillary fractures. An upward blow to the mandible can thrust the mandible into the maxilla and push the maxillary teeth upward and outward. This movement in turn fractures the

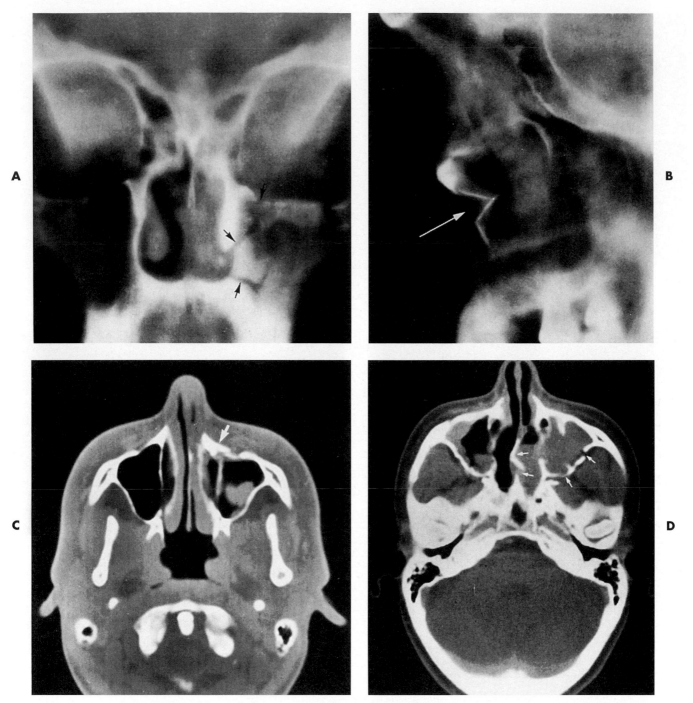

FIG. 4-280   **A,** Coronal multidirectional tomogram shows comminuted fractures of the left anterior and medial maxilla *(arrows)*. **B,** Lateral multidirectional tomogram shows an isolated fracture of the anterior maxillary sinus wall *(arrow)*. This type of fracture usually results from a blow from a narrow object. **C,** Axial CT scan shows an isolated fracture of the anteromedial left maxilla *(arrow)*. Hemorrhage is present in the left antrium. **D,** Axial CT scan shows fractures of the left maxillary sinus posterolateral and medial walls and a fracture of the nasal septum *(arrows)*.

alveolus. Because of the strong soft-tissue support over the alveolus, these isolated fractures rarely are displaced. The involved teeth often are displaced or devitalized, and such alveolar fractures in children may damage the tooth germs.[7] Partial fractures of the maxilla can result from a blow deliv-

ered by a narrow object directly over the anterior maxillary wall. The fractures involve the anterior and lateral antral walls and extend toward the pyriform aperture and down into the maxillary alveolus (Figs. 4-278 to 4-280). Sagittal fractures of the palate result from either an axial or an

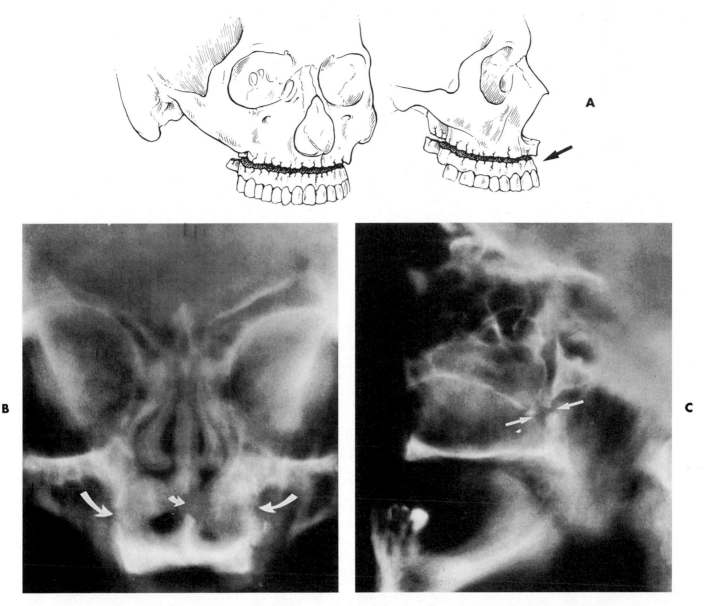

FIG. 4-281   **A,** Diagram of a Le Fort I fracture, which results in a "floating" palate. **B,** Coronal multidirectional tomogram shows a Le Fort I fracture *(arrows)*. **C,** Lateral multidirectional tomogram shows the Le Fort I fracture and its extension through the pterygoid plates *(arrows)*.

oblique blow to the chin or a direct blow to the upper jaw. The fracture passes through the weakest portion of the palatine process of the maxilla, which is sagittally oriented just off of the midline. The midline itself is reinforced by the vomer, whereas the lateral hard palate is supported by the alveolus. In more violent trauma a sagittal midline fracture can occur; comminuted palatal fractures are associated with other central or centrolateral facial fractures.[7]

LE FORT I FRACTURES

The Le Fort I fracture (Guérin's fracture) results from a blow delivered over the upper lip region and is characterized

by detachment (from the caudal portions of the maxillary sinuses) of the upper jaw with the tooth-bearing segments (at a level just above the floor of the nasal cavity). The fracture extends through the lower nasal septum, the lower walls of the maxillary sinuses, and the lower pterygoid plates. Thus the fracture segment includes the entire palate, maxillary alveolus and teeth, and portions of the pterygoid plates. This "floating palate" is displaced posteriorly, resulting in malocclusion and hemorrhaging into the antra (Fig. 4-281).[7]

LE FORT II FRACTURES

A strong, broad blow over the central facial region causes a

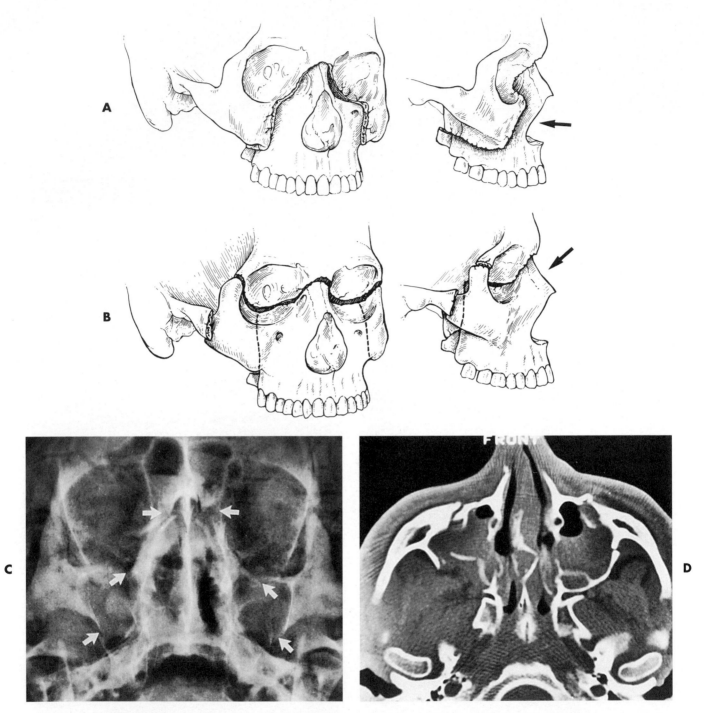

FIG. 4-282   **A,** Diagram of a Le Fort II fracture. The midfacial fracture segment is pyramidal in shape, and these fractures are often called pyramidal fractures. **B,** Diagram of Wassmund I fracture. This is the same type of fracture as Le Fort II, except that the nasal bones are spared. **C,** Waters view shows a Le Fort II fracture *(arrows)* that creates a pyramidal-shaped fracture segment. **D,** Axial CT scan shows a Le Fort II fracture. On more caudal scans the pterygoid plates were fractured, and on more cranial scans the ethmoid sinuses and orbital floors were fractured.

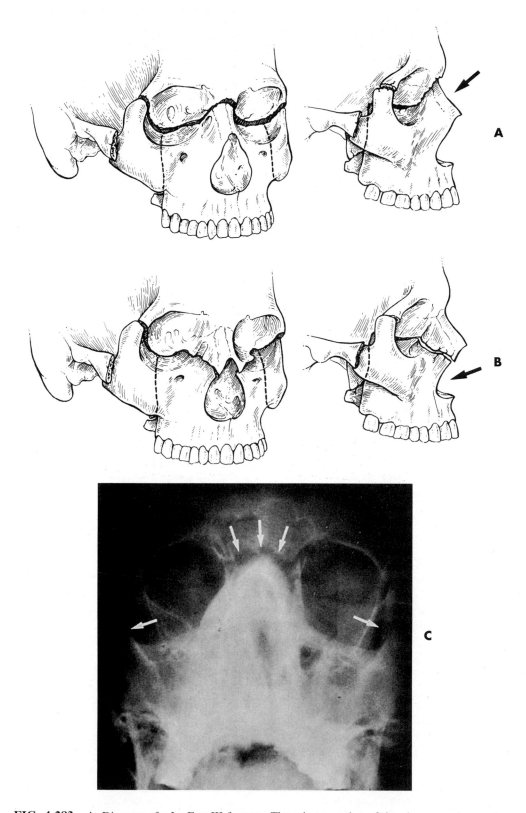

FIG. 4-283 **A,** Diagram of a Le Fort III fracture. There is separation of the viscerocranium and the facial bones. The dotted fracture lines extend down the posterior maxillary sinus walls. **B,** Diagram of Wassmund III fracture. This is a similar fracture to the Le Fort III, except the nasal bones are not involved. The dotted fracture lines extend down the posterior maxillary sinus walls. **C,** Waters view shows a Le Fort III fracture *(arrows)*. Hemorrhage is present in both antra.

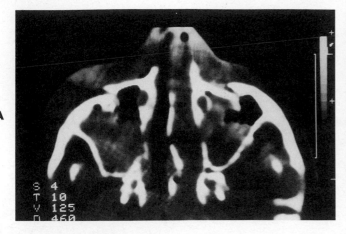
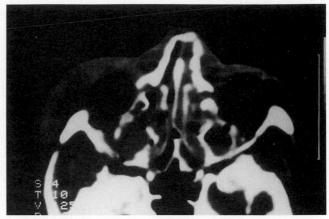

FIG. 4-284   Axial CT scans show a Le Fort III fracture. The more caudal aspects of the fracture (**A**) are similar to a Le Fort II fracture. However, the more cranial fractures (**B**) separate the facial bones from the cranium.

pyramidal fracture, one of the most severe midfacial fractures. The high, central midface fracture (Le Fort II) is characterized by a fracture line that extends through the root of the nose, then runs bilaterally to involve the lacrimal bones and medial orbital walls. On each side the fracture line then turns anteriorly along the floor of the orbit near the infraorbital canal and extends down the zygomaticomaxillary suture and the anterior wall of the maxilla; posteriorly the fracture goes down across the infratemporal surface of the maxilla and finally extends through the lower pterygoid plates. This creates a pyramid-shaped central facial fracture segment. The deep central midface (Wassmund I) fracture spares the nasal bones and extends from the lateral edges of the pyriform aperture back across to the lacrimal bones and into the medial orbital walls. From this point the fracture is the same as the Le Fort II (Fig. 4-282).[7] In the Le Fort II and Wassmund I fractures the zygomatic bones remain attached to the cranium. The pyramidal-shaped fracture segment (the central midface) is posteriorly displaced, resulting in a "dishface" deformity, malocclusion, and hemorrhage. Anesthesia or paresthesia of one or both of the infraorbital nerves occurs in 78.9% of the cases.[9]

LE FORT III FRACTURES

Centrolateral midfacial fractures are characterized by separation of the entire facial skeleton from the skull base. Such a craniofacial dysjunction usually has a fracture line, extending through the root of the nose, then bilaterally across the lacrimal bones and medial orbital walls, and then posterolaterally across the floor of the orbits to the inferior orbital fissure. At this point, one portion of the fracture line extends laterally and upward across the lateral orbital walls to end near the zygomaticofrontal sutures. A second fracture line extends from the orbital floor down across the back of the maxillae to the lower portion of the pterygoid plates. The zygomatic arches also are fractured, thereby completing the

separation of the viscerocranium. Such a fracture is called a Le Fort III or Wassmund IV fracture (Figs. 4-283, 4-284). The same fracture without inclusion of the nasal bones is called a Wassmund III fracture (Fig. 4-283), and the fracture line extends from each side of the pyriform aperture up to the lacrimal bones. The fracture then continues as a Le Fort III fracture. Thus the distinguishing feature between the Le Fort III fracture and the Le Fort II fracture is the inclusion in the Le Fort III fractured segment of the zygomas and lateral orbital walls. These patients have a dishface deformity, CSF rhinorrhea, hemorrhage, damage to the lacrimal apparatus, and malocclusion. The infraorbital nerves are involved in 69.3% of cases.[9]

Lateral midfacial fractures include the zygomatic fractures (trimalar, or tripod), zygomatic arch fractures, zygomaticomaxillary fractures, zygomaticomandibular fractures, and fractures of the floor of the orbit (blow-out fractures).[19]

TRIMALAR (ZYGOMATIC) FRACTURES

Zygomatic fractures are the second most common facial fractures after nasal bone trauma. The fracture lines in a zygomatic fracture extend along the lateral orbital wall (zygomaticofrontal suture and the zygomaticosphenoid suture) from the inferior orbital fissure to the orbital floor near the infraorbital canal, then down the anterior maxilla near the zygomaticomaxillary suture, and up the posterior maxillary wall back to the inferior orbital fissure. There is also a fracture through the weakest part of the zygomatic arch, which is about 1.5 cm dorsal to the zygomaticotemporal suture. The infraorbital nerve is impaired in 94.2% of the cases.[9] These fractures are usually referred to as trimalar fractures because there are the following three fractures: (1) through the lateral orbital wall, (2) separating the zygoma and maxilla, and (3) through the zygomatic arch. The term quadramalar fracture has rarely been used and refers to the fractures extending through four suture lines (zygomati-

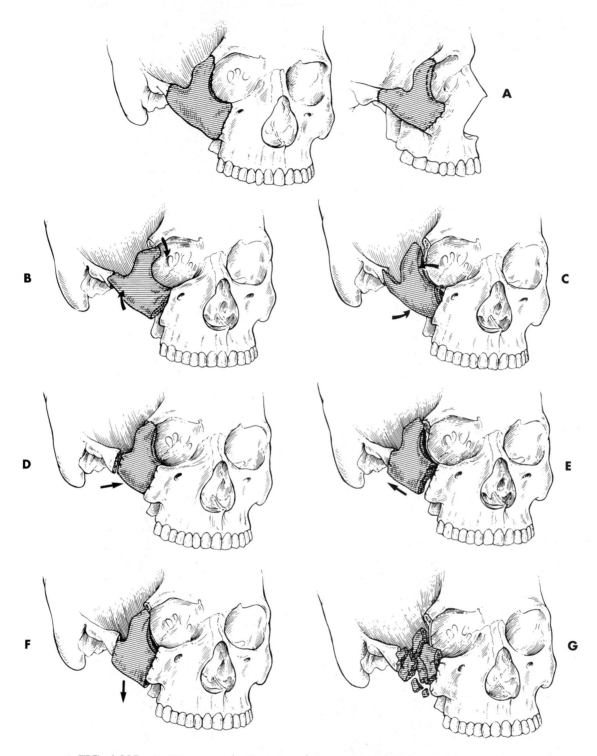

FIG. 4-285 **A,** Diagram of nondisplaced trimalar zygomatic fracture. **B,** Diagram of zygomatic fracture with clockwise (medial) rotation around a horizontal axis (anterior to posterior) through the zygoma. **C,** Diagram of zygomatic fracture with counterclockwise (lateral) rotation around a horizontal axis (anterior to posterior) through the zygoma. **D,** Diagram of zygomatic fracture with pure medial displacement. **E,** Diagram of zygomatic fracture with pure posterior displacement. **F,** Diagram of zygomatic fracture with pure inferior displacement. **G,** Diagram of zygomatic comminuted (complex) fracture.

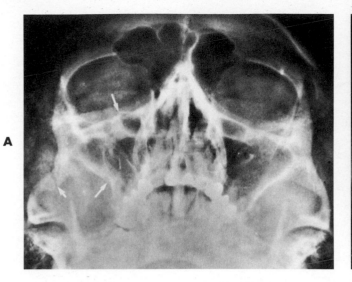

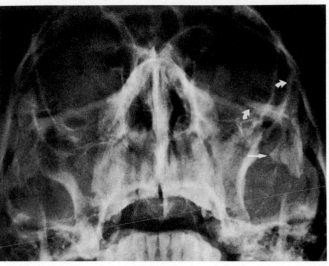

FIG. 4-286 **A** Waters view shows a nondisplaced right zygomatic fracture. The fractures through the maxilla and the zygomatic arch are seen *(arrows)*. However, the zygomaticofrontal fracture is not visualized because there was only a slight diastasis at this point. **B,** Waters view shows a left zygomatic fracture that is laterally displaced *(arrow)* and slightly clockwise (laterally) rotated *(curved arrows)*.

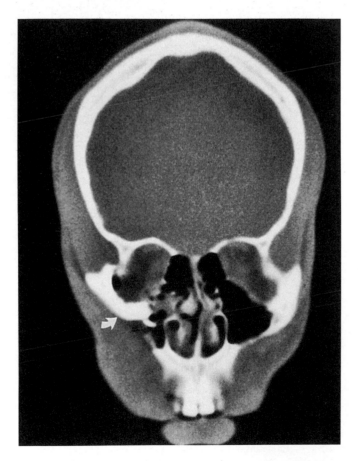

FIG. 4-287 Coronal CT scan shows a right zygomatic fracture, which is superiorly displaced and considerably counterclockwise (laterally) rotated *(arrow)*. There is also subcutaneous emphysema.

cofrontal, zygomaticosphenoid, zygomaticotemporal, and zygomaticomaxillary). In one study, as many as one third of all patients who suffer comminuted malar fractures had an ocular disorder, but only 16.7% of patients with a "blow-out" fracture had ocular problems. Decreased visual acuity was the primary problem accompanying the majority of significant eye injuries.[20]

Several classifications of lateral midface fractures have been proposed.[19,21,22] Each considers the displacement of the zygoma as it relates to the clinical severity of the fracture and how malar position may be used to plan the treatment. Zygomatic fractures account for 49% to 53% of the midface fractures, and in one study 69% of midfacial fractures involved the zygomatic complex either alone or in combination with other midface fractures.[7,21] The reports vary considerably as to the frequency of the different malar fracture positions. One of the more complete classifications, including the fracture type, frequency, and postreduction stability, is shown in Table 4-1.[21] Before the use of miniplates and microplates, use of this type of classification allowed the clinician to better predict the postoperative stability of the fracture and thus influence the degree of fixation needed (Figs. 4-285 to 4-290). When the malar emminence is rotated in more than one axis or displaced in more than one direction, the primary rotation and displacement is usually used to classify the fracture. However, these complex cases point out the limitation of any of these classification systems. In the present era, when the use of miniplates and microplates is common, there is less reliance on a classification system to determine treatment type. But some sur-

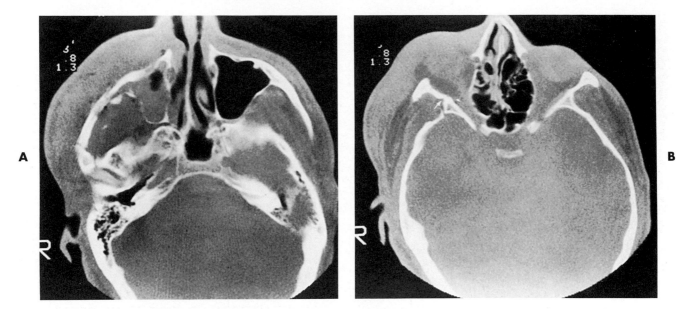

FIG. 4-288 **A,** Axial CT scan shows a right zygomatic fracture with posterior displacement and clockwise (medial) rotation of the zygoma. **B,** Axial CT scan, more cranial than **A,** shows the zygomatico-frontosphenoid fracture *(arrow)*.

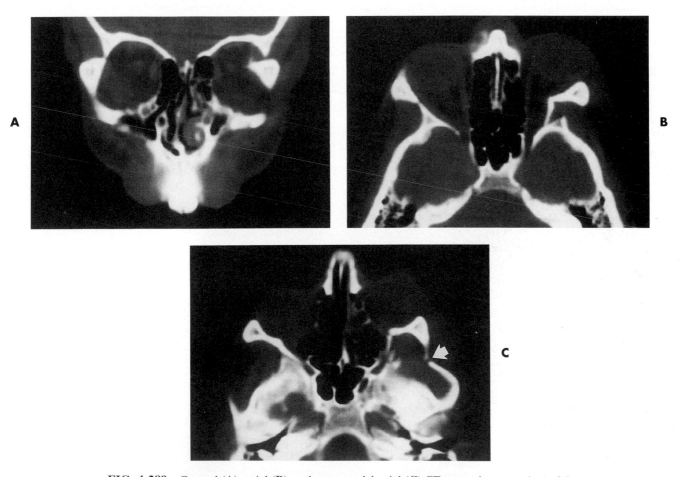

FIG. 4-289 Coronal **(A),** axial **(B),** and more caudal axial **(C)** CT scans show a variant of the classical trimalar fracture. The lateral orbital wall is dorsally displaced and rotated counterclockwise. The zygomatic arch is also fractured (arrow in C). Rather than the more common fracture which extends through the zygomaticomaxillary suture region, this fracture extends through the lateral zygoma or lower lateral orbital wall.

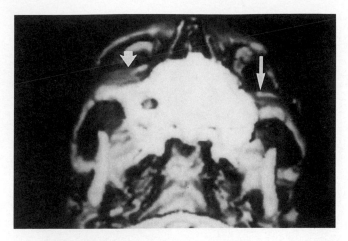

FIG. 4-290   Three dimensional reconstruction on a patient with a left trimalar fracture. The zygoma is posteriorly displaced *(long arrow)* compared with the normal right side *(short arrow).* The white area in the center of the picture is the hard palate seen en-face. Most of the mandible was removed from the computerized picture.

TABLE 4-1
Type, Frequency, and Postreduction Stability
of Zygomatic Fractures

Fracture Type	Frequency (%)	Postreduction Stability (%)
Nondisplaced	11	100
Isolated arch	16	93
Rotation around vertical axis	12	
Medial	3.5	57
Lateral	8.5	88
Rotation around horizintal axis	6	
Medial	1	0
Lateral	5	50
Displacement without rotation	31	
Medial	11.5	39
Lateral	1	0
Posterior	12	92
Inferior	6.5	0
Isolated rim	9.5	47
Complex	14.5	0

geons still utilize a classification system to predict postoperative stability because these surgeons do not believe that all zygomatic fractures need fixation after reduction. It is generally believed that the primary cause of movement of a reduced but nonfixed malar fracture is the masseter muscle's pulling force on the zygoma.[23]

Zygomaticomaxillary fractures differ from trimalar fractures in that the former fractures include a maxillary segment. In distinction to the trimalar fracture line, zygomaticomaxillary fractures involve the orbital floor, extend down the anterior maxilla near the infraorbital foramen, run to the premolar region, and then extend across the palate to the maxillary tuberosity and lower pterygoid plates.

Zygomaticomandibular fractures differ from zygomatic fractures only by the additional fracture of the mandibular condyle, coronoid process, or both.[19]

When there are isolated fractures of the zygomatic arch, there usually are at least three discrete fracture lines, creating two fracture segments. These pieces are displaced medially and downward, reflecting the direction of the impact force. The fracture pieces may impinge on the temporalis muscle or coronoid process of the mandible and interfere with movement of the lower jaw (Figs. 4-291, 4-292). Trismus is reported in 45% of zygomatic arch fractures and in about 33% of all zygomatic fractures.[23]

Fractures of the orbital floor may occur as either simple or comminuted fractures in conjunction with midfacial fractures, with atypical periorbital fractures (orbital roof), or as isolated blow-out fractures.

BLOW-OUT AND BLOW-IN FRACTURES

The term orbital blow-out fracture describes the injury that results from a blow to the orbit by an object that is too large to enter the orbit (fist, baseball, etc.). The force of the blow is absorbed by the orbital rim and is transmitted to the thin-

ner orbital floor, which shatters, usually in the middle third near the infraorbital canal. As the eye is pushed back into the conical orbital apex, it increases infraorbital pressure and this "blows out" the fractured floor into the maxillary sinus. Usually the orbital rim is not fractured (pure blow-out fracture) and the globe remains undamaged. Less commonly the inferior orbital rim also is fractured; this is referred to as an impure blow-out fracture. Blow-out fractures represent only 3% to 5% of all midface fractures (Figs. 4-293 to 4-297).[19,24] Herniation of orbital fat, inferior rectus muscle, and inferior oblique muscle can occur with occasional muscle entrapment in the fracture line, resulting in diplopia on upward gaze. However, diplopia is the most frequent complaint in all patients with blow-out fractures and may occur solely because of periorbital edema and hemorrhage, which exert pressure on the globe. This type of diplopia resolves in several days, whereas entrapment diplopia remains. If the cause of diplopia is in doubt, a traction test can be performed on the inferior muscles. Rarely a depression fracture of the orbital roof or superior orbital rim can impinge on the upper globe, prohibiting upward gaze and clinically mimicking an inferior muscle entrapment (Fig. 4-298). Imaging studies clarify this situation.[25] In these latter cases, communication with the base of the anterior cranial fossa can lead to CSF leakage into the orbit or herniation of meninges or brain through the fracture line. Rarely the orbital floor fracture segments can herniate upward into the orbit, impinging on the inferior orbital muscles or the globe. This unusual occurrence has been called a blow-in fracture, and on imaging it must be clearly identified so that the clinician can reposition this fractured bone.[9,26,27]

Fractures of the medial orbital wall can occur either as isolated fractures or in conjunction with orbital floor fractures. Such medial wall fractures may be present in as many as 50% of orbital floor fractures. Often the ethmoid fracture is poorly visualized on plain films, with only some clouding

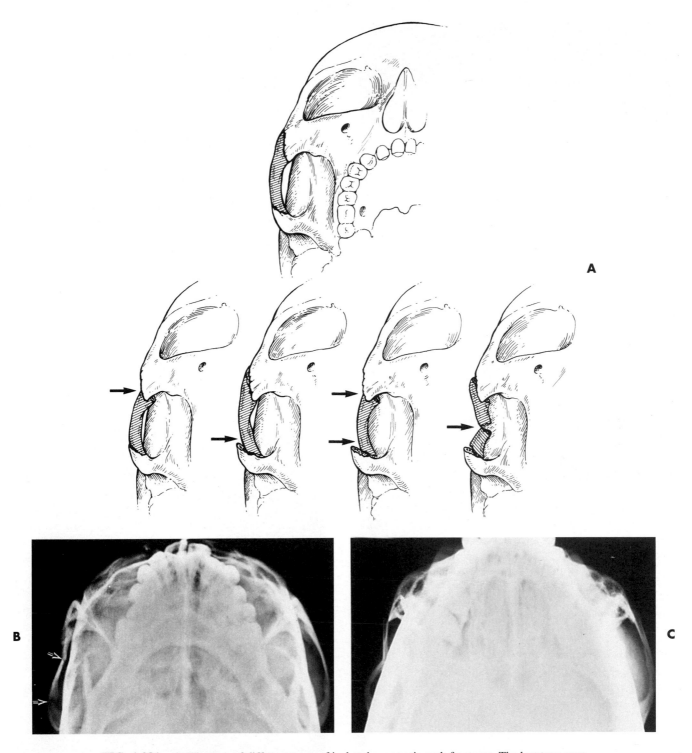

FIG. 4-291   A, Diagram of different types of isolated zygomatic arch fractures. The last type may impinge medially on the coronoid process of the mandible. **B,** Underpenetrated base view shows slightly depressed right zygomatic arch fractures *(arrows).* **C,** Underpenetrated base view shows markedly depressed right zygomatic arch fractures.

of the ethmoid cells being evident. Even on CT scans, if there is no bone displacement, the actual fractures may not be identified. However, on CT, fat that has herniated into the fractured ethmoid complex is well visualized (Figs. 4-299 to 4-302). Herniated fat can also be identified on MRI, although the small fracture segments may not be identified. Muscle

entrapment in these fractures is rare.[28] The only imaging differential diagnosis is with a congenital dehiscence of the lamina papyracea. In this case, although on CT and MRI portions of the lamina papyracea are not visualized and orbital fat lies in the ethmoid complex, the margins of the defect are smooth and usually there is no history of trauma.

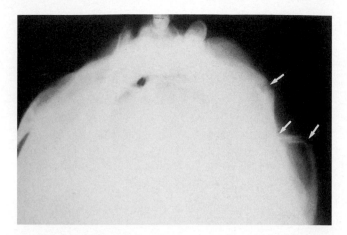

FIG. 4-292   Underpenetrated base view shows three fractures of the left zygoma. The bone segments are very medially displaced, locking mandiblar motion.

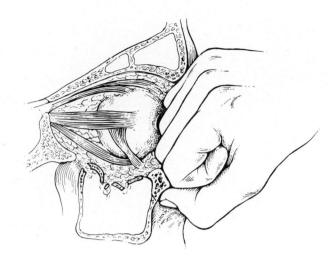

FIG. 4-293   Diagram of blow-out fracture. The impacting object is larger than the orbital rim diameter. The blow fractures the orbital floor and pushes the eye back. The eye then displaces the fractured floor into the antrum.

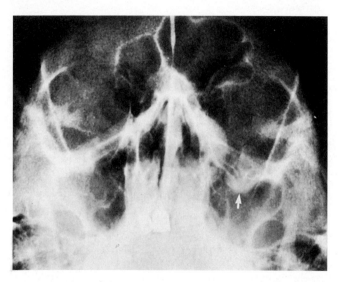

FIG. 4-294   Waters view shows polypoid soft-tissue mass in the roof of the left antrum *(arrow)*. Blow-out fracture.

Medial wall fractures can also be inferred by the presence of orbital emphysema. Such orbital air most commonly comes from an ethmoid sinus fracture and only rarely results from an isolated maxillary fracture (Figs. 4-297, 4-299, 4-300, 4-303). The infrequent occurrence of orbital emphysema with orbital floor blow-out fractures is attributed to the rapid sealing of the fracture by edema, hemorrhage, and periorbital herniation of orbital fat and muscle. Orbital emphysema develops after an ethmoid fracture when nose blowing by the patient increases intranasal pressure, which in turn raises the intrasinus pressure and forces air into the orbit. In most patients, refraining from nose blowing allows the fracture line to seal and the orbital air to resorb.[9,19] Rarely, air can enter the orbit from a complex fracture, involving the frontal or sphenoid sinuses. However, these cases are associated with severe facial trauma, and the source of the air becomes evident on imaging studies.

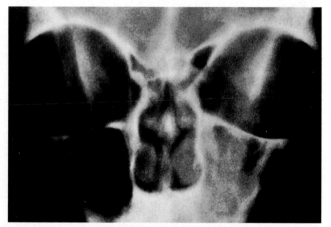

A

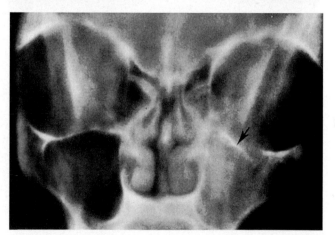

B

FIG. 4-295   Coronal multidirectional tomograms show **(A)** an intact orbital rim anteriorly and **(B)** a trapdoor-type orbital floor fracture *(arrow)* posteriorly behind the rim. Pure blow-out fracture.

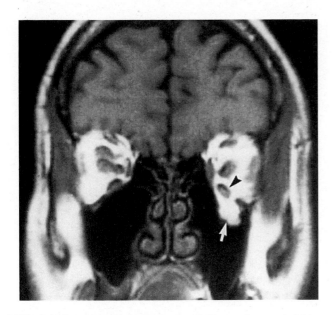

FIG. 4-296 Coronal proton density MRI scan shows a left blow-out fracture. Fat has herniated into the left antrum *(arrow)*, and there is minimal depression of the inferior rectus muscle *(arrowhead)*.

The two clinical indications for immediate surgery on an orbital blow-out fracture are definite muscle entrapment and acute enophthalmos. In the most dramatic case the globe is almost completely displaced into the maxillary sinus, and there is one report of complete globe herniation into a fractured ethmoid sinus.[29,30] However, milder and more common degrees of acute enophthalmos may take several days to clinically confirm because of the presence of periorbital edema and hemorrhage.[24] The development of chronic enophthalmos is also to be avoided because it leads to cosmetic deformity and in some cases diplopia. Chronic enophthalmos develops when too much orbital fat has herniated from the orbit. Although initially the increased orbital volume clinically goes unnoticed because of compensatory intraorbital edema, the subsequent loss of edema and scarring and lipogranulation of the herniated tissues eventually cause sufficient volume loss that the globe recedes. The patients who are at greatest risk are those who have sizable herniations of fat into one sinus (maxillary or ethmoid) or moderate herniations into both medial wall and orbital floor fractures. The imager must draw the clinician's attention to

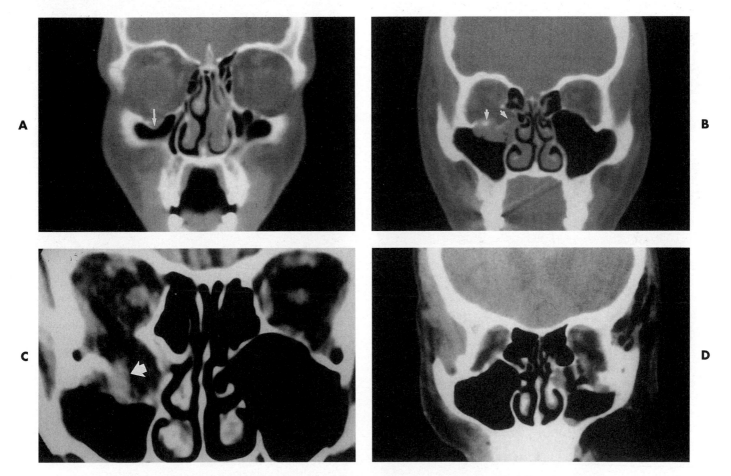

FIG. 4-297 Coronal CT scans. **A,** A small blow-out fracture of the right orbital floor *(arrow)*. **B,** A comminuted right orbital floor fracture that also involves the lower medial orbital wall *(arrows)*. **C,** A large right orbital floor blowout fracture. The inferior rectus muscle *(arrow)* is depressed into the fracture. This muscle was entrapped on the lateral fracture margin. **D,** A blow-out fracture in the floor and medial wall of the left orbit. Orbital emphysema is also present.

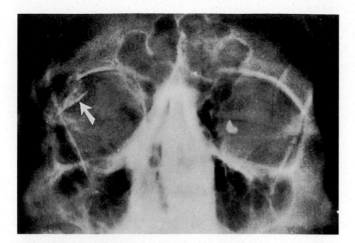

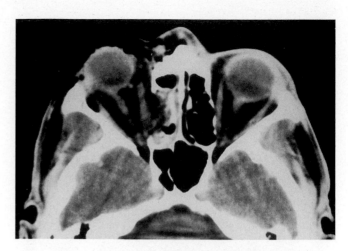

FIG. 4-298   Waters view shows a depressed orbital roof fracture *(arrow)* that impinged on the globe and clinically mimicked a blow-out fracture of the orbital floor with entrapment. A foreign body is also seen in the left eye.

FIG. 4-299   Axial CT scan shows a medial wall blow-out fracture of the right orbit. There is herniation of the orbital contents into the right ethmoid. There is also orbital emphysema.

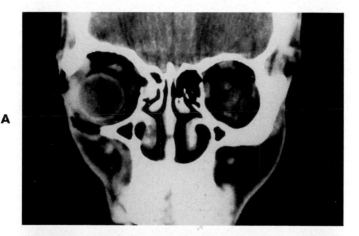

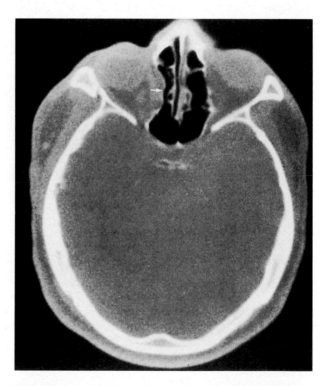

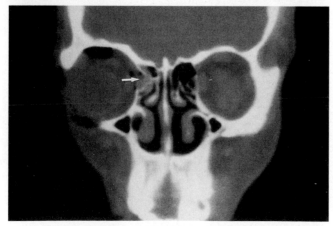

FIG. 4-300   Coronal CT scans at soft tissue (**A**) and bone (**B**) settings show a medial wall right blow-out fracture *(arrow)*. There is also orbital emphysema. Notice how difficult it is to detect the findings in **A**.

FIG. 4-301   Axial CT scan shows an old right medial wall blow-out fracture *(arrow)*, or possibly a congenital dehiscence of the lamina papyracea.

any such cases that may have the potential to develop chronic enophthalmos, even in the absence of acute enophthalmos or muscle entrapment.[24] Alloplasts are often used to reconstruct the orbital wall. The products most often used include Teflon, Silastic, and Marlex mesh, all of which have the benefit of not being absorbed.[17] However, these alloplasts have the disadvantages of extrusion and infection. They can be identified on CT, which is a useful modality to detect early displacement of the graft.

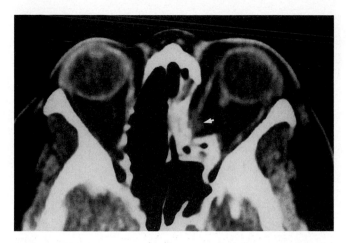

FIG. 4-302   Axial CT scan shows a left medial wall blow-out fracture. The medial rectus muscle is entrapped in the fracture *(arrow)*.

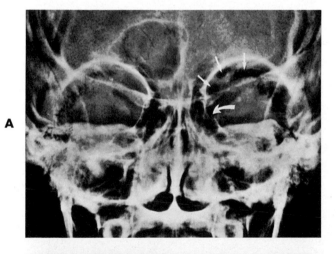

A

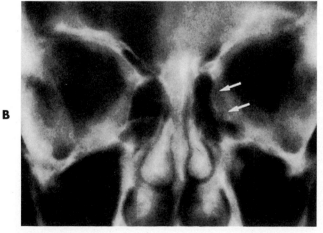

B

FIG. 4-303   Caldwell view **(A)** and coronal multidirectional tomogram **(B)** show orbital emphysema *(three arrows)* and a defect in the left lamina papyracea *(curved arrow)*. The tomogram better shows the medial wall depressed fracture *(two arrows)*.

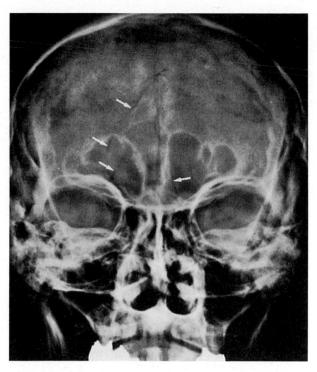

FIG. 4-304   Caldwell view shows a comminuted fracture of the frontal bone *(arrows)* that extends into the frontal sinus.

On plain films, soft-tissue swelling over the inferior orbital rim, antral opacification with or without an air-fluid level, and subcutaneous emphysema in the cheek are often the only indirect signs of a blow-out fracture. An actual depressed or displaced orbital floor bone fragment may not be seen. Occasionally a soft-tissue polypoid density can be visualized in the antral roof. This may represent the site of the blow-out fracture filled with orbital contents and hemorrhage, or it may represent an unrelated antral cyst or polyp. Only on coronal CT or MRI can the actual fracture and herniated tissue be clearly seen. A completely displaced piece of bone, a trapdoor fracture, or hinged fracture can then be identified, as can the typical "teardrop" herniation of orbital contents. On CT the orbital fat may be of a higher attenuation than expected because of hemorrhage; in rare cases an antral air-blood level may be present.[13] On MRI the high T1W signal intensity of the orbital fat and any hemorrhage can be well seen; however, a small bone fracture segment may not be identified.

FRONTAL SINUS FRACTURES

Frontal sinus fractures are either the result of direct trauma or an extension of a calvarial fracture into the sinus. Of all fractures involving the frontal sinuses, 67% are limited to the anterior table, 28% involve both the anterior and posterior sinus walls, and only 5% are limited to the posterior sinus table.[31] Most commonly a linear fracture occurs in the anterior sinus wall.[32] This tears the mucosa and produces hemorrhage, edema, and sinus opacification. The fracture line may extend downward, often involving the superome-

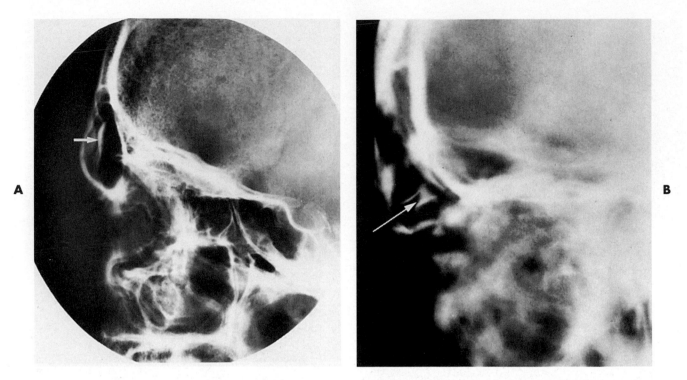

FIG. 4-305   **A,** Lateral view shows a depressed anterior frontal sinus wall fracture *(arrow)*. **B,** Lateral view shows a depressed fracture *(arrow)* of the anterior wall and floor of the frontal sinus.

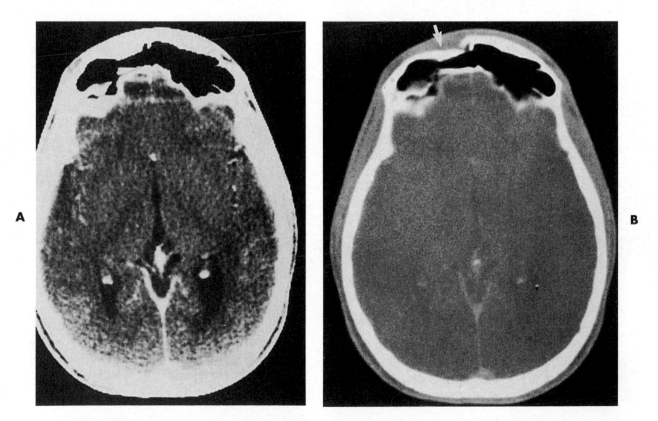

FIG. 4-306   Axial CT scans at narrow window settings **(A)** and wide window settings **(B)** show that the fracture of the anterior wall of the right frontal sinus *(arrow)* can be missed on soft-tissue settings because hemorrhage and edema fill in the forehead defect.

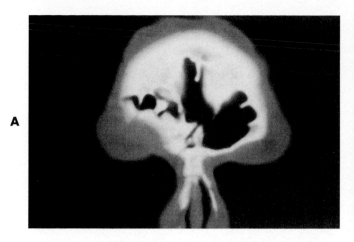

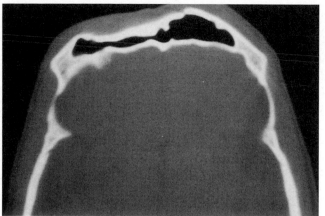

FIG. 4-307   Coronal (**A**) and axial (**B**) CT scans show a depressed fracture of the right anterior frontal sinus table that also involves the right orbital roof.

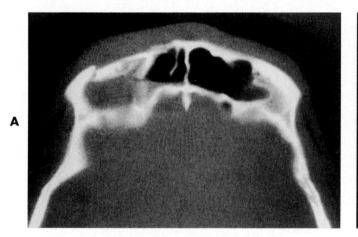

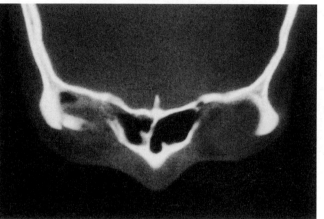

FIG. 4-308   Axial (**A**) and coronal (**B**) CT scans show a fracture involving the right orbital roof and the lower anterior frontal sinus table.

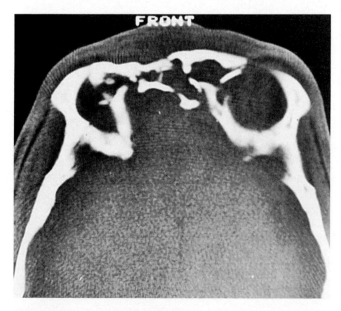

FIG. 4-309   Axial CT scan shows a comminuted midfacial fracture that involves the frontal bone and frontal sinuses.

dial orbital rim (Figs. 4-304 to 4-309). Comminuted fractures of the anterior wall also occur and frequently reflect the size and shape of the object causing the fracture. On plain film Caldwell and Waters views, only a vague density may appear in the frontal sinus. However, on a lateral view, bone fragments may be identified. Axial CT most clearly confirms the presence of such depressed fractures, which often are clinically unobserved because the forehead soft-tissue depression is filled by edema and hemorrhage.[33] Complex fractures of both the anterior and posterior frontal sinus tables usually are associated with other midfacial fractures. Isolated fractures of the posterior sinus wall are rare. They occur either as an extension of a skull base fracture or as an extension of a calvarial fracture.[34,35] Any fracture involving the posterior frontal sinus wall opens communication with the dural spaces. CSF leakage into the sinus and intracranial infection or pneumocele can develop. Rarely, orbital emphysema or CSF leakage can result from frontal sinus fractures. In one study of CT scans on patients with suspected intracranial posttraumatic injuries, 90% of the patients had a frontal sinus fracture identified on the initial CT. Complex fractures involving the anterior and posterior walls accounted for 65% of the cases, and isolated anterior wall (24%) or posterior wall (11%) fractures were less common.[33] This study reflects the severity of the trauma that led to both the fractures and the intracranial damage. In fact, it has been determined that it takes two to three times the force to fracture the frontal sinus than it does to fracture the zygoma, maxilla, or mandible.[36]

In general, nondisplaced frontal sinus fractures are treated conservatively. Uncomplicated anterior table fractures with cosmetic deformity are treated by fragment reduction and stabilization, usually with microplates or miniplates. Nasofrontal duct obstruction is usually managed by sinus obliteration. Finally, comminuted, displaced anterior and posterior table fractures, especially those associated with persistent CSF leakage, are often treated by frontal sinus cranialization.[35]

SPHENOID SINUS FRACTURES

Fractures of the sphenoid sinus seldom occur, but when they do, they are associated with severe cranial trauma and basilar skull fractures. Rarely, milder trauma to the midfacial region may extend back into the sphenoid sinus. Sinus opacification or a sphenoid sinus air-fluid level may indicate the presence of CSF, hemorrhage, or simply poor sinus drainage. If the fracture injures the adjacent internal carotid arteries or cavernous sinuses, these events may be life threatening.

PEDIATRIC FACIAL FRACTURES

When compared with the adult skeleton, the pediatric facial bones behave differently with regard to fracture patterns, healing, and treatment. The inherent elasticity of the facial

bones in the young patient is advantageous in trauma because the bone yields more easily and does not fracture as readily as it does in an adult.[3] When a fracture does occur, the thick, elastic periosteum usually prevents bone displacement and a green-stick fracture results. Fractures heal faster in children than in adults, so the period of immobilization is shorter. However, if treatment is delayed, the fragments may become fixed, making fracture reduction more difficult. Malocclusions in the primary dentition that are not completely corrected may be spontaneously compensated for by the secondary dentition or may be treated by orthodontic therapy.[3] Although children have many advantages in terms of healing, they are at a disadvantage with regard to dentition. In 30% to 50% of pediatric facial fractures the tooth germs lie in the fracture. These teeth fall out during healing or have delayed development and deformities that do not manifest clinically until the permanent teeth erupt. Facial fractures also can damage the bony growth centers and result in osseous hypoplasia, functional abnormalities, and cosmetic deformities. Some clinicians believe that the child's parents should be informed of these potential problems at the time of the initial injury.

Children generally have too few teeth for fixation splints. Treatment plans must be modified from those used in adult patients. No wire ligatures can be placed in children under 2 years old. After this age, it may be possible to fix interdental wires and arch bars, if the primary teeth have not been damaged by caries or their crowns have an adequately retentive form. However, with the appearance of interdental spaces caused by eruption of the secondary teeth, the possibility of fixing dental splints becomes less likely. Similarly, erupted permanent teeth can only accept such ligatures after their greatest convexity has passed the gingival margin. This period lasts from about the fifth to eighth years of life.[3]

References

1. Smith HW, Yanagisawa E. Paranasal sinus trauma. In: Blitzer A, Lawson W, Friedman WH, eds. Surgery of the paranasal sinuses. Philadelphia, Pa: WB Saunders Co, 1985; 299-315.

2. Mancuso AA, Hanafee WN. Computed tomography and magnetic resonance imaging of the head and neck. 2nd Edition. Baltimore, Md: Williams & Wilkins, 1985; 42-60.

3. Stanley RB Jr. Maxillofacial Trauma. In: Cummings CW, Fredrickson JM, Harker LA et al. Otolaryngology-head and neck surgery. 2nd Edition. St. Louis, Mo: Mosby-Year Book, 1993; 374-402.

4. Gentry LR, Manor WF, Turski PA et al. High-resolution CT analysis of facial struts in trauma. I. Normal anatomy. AJR 1983; 140:523-532.

5. Le Fort R. Etude experimentale sur les fractures de la machoire superieure. Rev Chir 1901; 23:208, 360, 479.

6. Manson PN. Dimentional analysis of the facial skeleton. In: Manson PN ed. Cranio-maxillofacial trauma: problems in plastic and reconstructive surgery. Philadelphia, Pa: JB Lippincott, 1991.

7. Schwenzer N, Kruger E. Midface fracture. In: Kruger E, Schilli W, Worthington P, eds. Oral and maxillofacial traumatology. Vol 2. Chicago, Ill: Quintessence Publishing Co Inc, 1986; 107-136.

8. Kreipke DL, Moss JJ, Franco JM et al. Computed tomography and thin-section tomography in facial trauma. AJNR 1984; 5:185-189.

9. Rowe NL, Williams JL, eds. Maxillo

facial injuries. Vol 1. Edinburgh, Scottland: Churchill Livingstone Inc, 1985; 363-558.

10. Brant-Zawadzki MN, Minagi H, Federle MP et al. High-resolution CT with image reformation in maxillofacial pathology. AJR 1982; 138:477-483.

11. Zilkha A. Computed tomography in facial trauma. Radiology 1982; 144:545-548.

12. Solar P, Ulm C, Lill W et al. Precision of three-dimensional CT assisted model production in the maxillofacial area. Eur Radiol 1992; 2:473-477.

13. Zimmerman RA, Bilaniuk LT, Hackney DB et al. Paranasal sinus hemorrhage: evaluation with MR imaging, Radiology 1987; 162:499-503.

14. Manson PN, Markowitz B, Mirvis S, et al. Toward CT-based facial fracture treatment. Plast Reconstr Surg 1990; 85:202-212.

15. Arden RL, Mathog RH: Nasal fractures. In: Cummings CW, Fredrickson JM, Harker LA et al, eds. Otolaryn-gology-head and neck surgery. 2nd Edition. St. Louis, Mo: Mosby-Year Book, 1993; 737-753.

16. Clayton MI, Lesser THJ. The role of radiography in the management of nasal fractures. J Laryngol Otol 1986; 100:797-801.

17. Lew D, Sinn DP. Diagnosis and treatment of midface fractures. In: Foneseca RJ, Walker RV, eds. Oral and maxillofacial trauma. Vol 1. Philadelphia, Pa: WB Saunders Co, 1991; 515-542.

18. Stranc MF. Primary Treatment of nasoethmoid injuries with increased intercanthal distance. Br J Plast Surg 1970; 23:8-25.

19. Fugii N, Yamashiro M. Classification of malar complex fractures using computed tomography. J Oral Maxillofacial Surgery 1983; 41:562-567.

20. al-Qurainy IA, Stassen LF, Dutton GN et al. The characteristics of midfacial fractures and the association with ocular injury: a prospective study. British Journal of Oral & Maxillofacial Surgery 1991; 29:291-301.

21. Yanagisawa E. Symposium on maxillofacial trauma. III. Pitfalls in the management of zygomatic fractures. Laryngoscope 1973; 83:527-546.

22. Knight JS, North JF, Chir B. The classification of malar fractures: an analysis of displacement as a guide to treatment. Br J Plast Surg 1961; 13:325-339.

23. Ellis E. Fractures of the zygomatic complex and arch. In: Foneseca RJ, Walker RV, eds. Oral and maxillofacial trauma. Vol 1. Philadelphia, Pa: WB Saunders Company, 1991; 435-514.

24. Smith B, Grove A, Guibor P. Fractures of the orbit. In: Jones IS, Jakobiec FA, eds. Diseases of the orbit. Hagerstown, Md: Harper & Row, Publishers Inc, 1979; 571-580.

25. McClury FL Swanson PJ. An orbital roof fracture causing diplopia. Arch Otolaryngol 1976; 102:497-498.

26. Gruss JS, Hurwitz JJ. Isolated blow-in fracture of the lateral orbit causing globe rupture. Ophthalmic Plastic & Reconstructive Surgery 1990; 6:221-224.

27. Walker J, Davidorf FH, Kelly DR et al. Laceration of the globe due to a blow-out fracture. Archives of Ophthalmolgy 1990; 108:1522-1523.

28. Coker NJ, Brooks BS, Gammel TE. Computed tomography of orbital medial wall fractures. Head Neck Surg 1983; 5:383-389.

29. Berkowitz RA, Putterman AN, Patel DB. Prolapse of the globe into the maxillary sinus after orbital fracture Am J Ophthalmol 1981; 91:253-257.

30. Raghav B, Vashisht S, Keshav BR et al. The missing eyeball—CT evaluation (a case report). Indian J Ophthalmol 1991; 39:188-189.

31. Shockley WW, Stucker FJ JR., Gage-White L et al. Frontal sinus fractures: some problems and some solutions. Laryngoscope 1988; 98:18-22.

32. Valvassori GE, Hord GE. Traumatic sinus disease. Semin Roentgenol 1968; 3:160-171.

33. Olson EM, Wright DL, Hoffman HT et al. Frontal sinus fractures: evaluation of CT scans in 132 patients. American Journal of Neuroradiology 1992; 13:897-902.

34. Bergeron RT, Rumbaugh CL. Skull trauma. In: Newton TH, Potts DG, eds, Radiology of the skull and brain. St Louis, Mo: The CV Mosby Co, 1971; 763-818.

35. Rohrich RJ, Hollier LH. Management of frontal sinus fractures: changing concepts. Clinics in Plastic Surgery 1992; 19:219-232.

36. Nahum AM. The biomechanics of maxillofacial trauma. Clin Plast Surg 1975; 2:59-64.

Section Four
POSTOPERATIVE SINONASAL CAVITIES RADIOGRAPHIC EVALUATIONS

To properly evaluate the postoperative patient, the radiologist must be knowledgeable about a number of facts, some of which are often obscure at the time of radiologic examination or film interpretation. Ideally the radiologist should know what operation was performed, when the surgery was done, and the disease that prompted the surgery. Familiarity with the various surgical procedures enables the radiologist to determine which bone, if any, can be expected to be removed, what soft-tissue defects may be created, and what soft tissue or foreign material is usually placed to repair the surgical defect. This knowledge is essential for proper film interpretation and should help prevent the erroneous diagnosis of a surgical defect as a site of bone erosion or a muscle-fascia graft as a tumor recurrence.

The interval between the surgery and the time of imaging helps the radiologist determine the type of soft-tissue reaction present. For recent surgery the primary healing reaction is an active inflammation with edema and possible hemorrhage. However, if the surgery was performed months to years ago, the primary expected healing reaction is a mature granulation tissue or vascularized scar with varying degrees of fibrosis. In addition the reactive bony sclerosis that may occur after those procedures that denude mucosa from bone require time to develop and produce bone thickening that may reduce sinus cavity size. Finally, knowledge of the disease process that initially prompted the surgery allows the radiologist to anticipate the types of imaging changes to be expected. Thus if the initial disease was chronic infection, one may commonly expect recurrent sinus mucosal thickening, reactive bone sclerosis and thickening, and possible nasal polyposis. If the initial disease was a granulomatous process, one may expect sinus mucosal thickening, nasal mucosal changes, septal erosions, and bone erosions intermixed with areas of reactive bony changes. If the initial disease was a tumor, the concern will be characterizing any nodular or localized soft-tissue disease, differentiating recurrent tumor from infection, and observing the presence of progressive bone erosion or soft-tissue extension to areas not normally involved by the surgery.

The best and most efficacious way to interpret a postoperative imaging study is to compare it with a prior examination. During the first postoperative years, this is best accomplished by comparing a follow-up study with a baseline scan. This baseline scan is thus very important for the imaging monitoring of a patient after surgery because this scan provides an anatomic reference with which all future examinations can be compared. If this baseline study is obtained too close to the time of surgery, although there is little chance for recurrence of the disease that prompted surgery, the imaging findings are dominated by the postoperative soft tissue changes of hemorrhage and edema and thus give a false impression of what the eventual stable postoperative appearance will be. The best compromise appears to be a postoperative waiting period of 6 to 8 weeks. This time allows most of the hemorrhage and edema to resolve, whereas few if any tumors (or chronic inflammatory diseases) will recur within this period.[1-3] Although the baseline study is less important in patients with inflammatory disease, it still provides a reference standard against which future imaging studies can be compared. On subsequent follow-up CT or MR scans, any progressive soft-tissue resolution can be interpreted as a further reduction of any postoperative changes or a resolution of inflammatory disease. However, the appearance of any new soft tissue changes, or sites of bone erosion, must be considered recurrent disease until proven otherwise. Patients who have been operated on for inflammatory disease usually do not need periodic follow-up scans and are only imaged if symptoms reappear. By comparison, those patients who have been operated on for tumors should have scheduled, periodic follow-up scans, if early tumor recurrences are to be diagnosed. The time interval between these examinations usually is 4 to 6 months for the first 3 postoperative years, and then 6- to 12-month intervals for the next 2 to 3 years.[1,2]

Plain films do not allow detailed evaluation of the postoperative patient because of the overall survey nature of these films and the unique anatomy of the paranasal sinuses, where focal soft-tissue disease is best assessed by its relationship to the adjacent bone (which may now be resected) and sinus cavity air (which may be obscured by fibrosis or disease). Thus CT and MRI are the examinations of choice in monitoring the course of postoperative patients. CT allows the detailed evaluation of bone and a fairly accurate assessement of the soft tissues, provided both axial and coronal views are available. The use of contrast is desirable because it provides some distinction between inflammatory tissue,

tumor, and scar. However, such differentiation is not always easily accomplished. MRI offers the possibility of further differentiating recurrent tumors from sites of active infection. However, even when using contrast, vascularized scar and tumors can not be easily distinguished with MRI, and early bone erosions may go undetected.[4] Conversely, early tumor invasion into marrow-containing bone is usually detected earlier on MRI than on CT. Ultimately the examination of choice depends on the surgical procedure and the disease. Is bone erosion is an important diagnostic consideration? Is the major diagnostic problem differentiating tumor from active infection or scar? Is the diagnostic challenge simply mapping the presence of inflammatory mucosal disease?

Following recurrent inflammatory disease with imaging is best done on CT. The appearance of mucosal thickening is easily identified, and interval changes can be assessed by comparison with a previous CT study. However, the radiologist is presented with more serious diagnostic problems when following a patient with tumor. The distinction between inflammatory disease, scar, and tumor becomes of critical importance.

On noncontrast CT, inflammatory secretions and reactions tend to have a lower attenuation than most sinonasal tumors, whereas on contrast CT, active inflammatory changes tend to enhnace more than most tumors. However, variations in this pattern commonly exist, and vascularized scar tissues cannot be confidently differentiated from either inflammatory tissue or tumor.

On MRI, inflammatory tissues usually have a low to intermediate T1W signal intensity and a high T2W signal intensity. As mentioned earlier in this chapter, about 95% of sinonasal tumors have an intermediate signal intensity on all imaging sequences. Thus in most cases a good distinction can be made between tumor and adjacent inflammation.[5] On contrast MRI the inflammatory tissues intensely enhance, and they tend to line or parallel the sinus cavity wall. Tumors, on the other hand, usually enhance less and have a distinct mass configuration. Unfortunately, the vascularized scar tissue that often develops in the postoperative sinonasal cavities has the identical imaging characteristics as tumor on CT and MRI, with or without contrast. Ultimately the distinction between these tissues is made either by comparing the imaging findings on serial studies or biopsying any suspicious regions.

OPERATIVE PROCEDURES
Nasal Surgery

Although surgery on the nose is primarily cosmetic, post-traumatic airway reconstruction accounts for many procedures. Surgery confined to the nasal or septal cartilages rarely leaves an imaging identification. Only those operations that remodel the nasal bone have any noticeable imaging manifestations. During rhinoplasty, the saw, chisel, and file remove bone and may leave some slight irregularity of the midline nasal bones; this may give a slightly nodular,

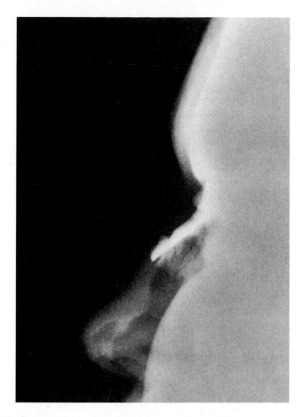

FIG. 4-310 Lateral view shows a patient who has had a prior rhinoplasty. The irregularity of the nasal bone contour is postsurgical in etiology.

somewhat unusual nasal bone profile best seen on lateral plain films of the nose (Fig. 4-310). The nasal bones are also purposely fractured in cases of nasal bone " hump" removal. Once this bony mound has been removed, the resulting broad nasal base is cosmetically too wide. Because of this, the lateral nasal walls are fractured and turned inward, recreating a thin, midline nasal contour. Such iatrogenic fractures may mimic a recent traumatic fracture, and only the patient's history may resolve any confusion. After 6 to 12 months, the sharp edges of all nasal fractures become smooth, and the fracture lines are less sharply identified. Old fractures also can prove confusing when there has been recent nasal trauma.[3,6]

In more severe nasal injuries in which the nasal bones have been crushed, cartilage or rib implants may be used to reconstruct a normal nasal contour. These implants give a unique radiographic appearance that once identified indicates to the imager that reconstructive surgery was performed (Figs. 4-311 to 4-313).

The topic of endoscopic sinonasal surgery was covered in Chapter 3. The following discussion regards those more classical, nonendoscopic operations.

Frontal Sinus Surgery

Statistically, most frontal sinus disease stems from infection and can be classified as acute or chronic. In acute infections, especially if an air-fluid level is found on plain films or imaging, factors such as the time to diagnosis and the imme-

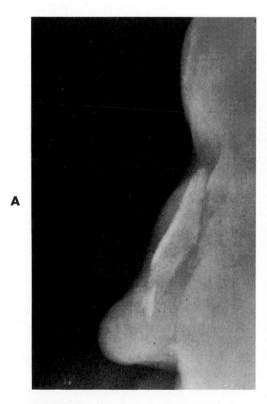
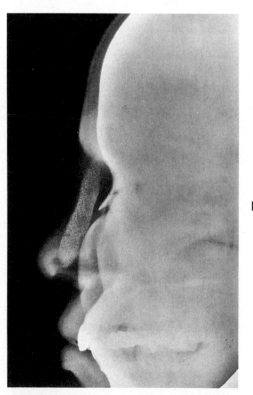

FIG. 4-311 **A,** Lateral view shows a patient with a rib nasal graft replacing badly fractured nasal bones. **B,** Lateral view shows a patient with a partially calcified cartilage nasal graft replacing badly fractured nasal bones.

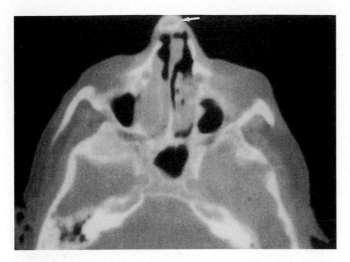

FIG. 4-312 Axial CT scan shows a rib *(arrow)* used in a nasal reconstruction. There is unrelated inflammatory disease in the nasal cavities.

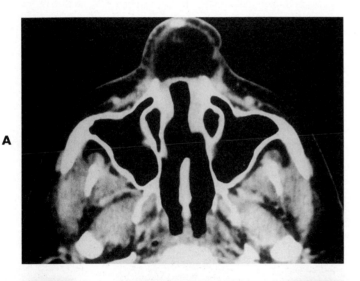

A

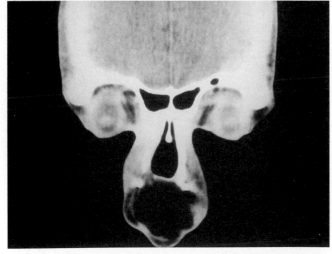

B

FIG. 4-313 Axial **(A)** and coronal **(B)** CT scans show a free flap reconstruction of the nose. The bulk of the graft is fatty.

diate patient response to treatment determine whether or not a trephination (essentially an incision and drainage) procedure should be performed. The operation consists of drilling a small hole 0.5 to 1 cm to the side of the midline, usually near the upper edge of the eyebrow. After the sinus is entered and drained (the sinus mucosa is not stripped), a drainage tube or cannula is placed in the sinus for 8 to 14 days, after which it is removed to prevent a foreign body reaction in the sinus mucosa.[3] Most often the surgeon determines by means of a Caldwell view the sinus size and the presence of any sinus loculations. Care must be taken so that the drill does not enter either the orbit below, the anterior cranial fossa through the posterior sinus wall, or, for a small sinus, outside of the sinus margin. The surgical defect is poorly visualized on coronal and axial CT unless the scans happen to pass directly through the site (Fig. 4-314). If the scan is performed while the drain is in place, the drain can be followed to its exit point from the sinus.

In patients with chronic inflammatory disease, two types of procedures can be performed: those that do not obliterate the sinus cavity and the more commonly performed procedures that obliterate the sinus cavity.

Although not commonly performed today, there are mainly three frontal sinus nonobliterative procedures: the Lynch, Killian, and Riedel approaches.

The Lynch procedure primarily is utilized in the ethmoid sinuses and supraorbital ethmoid cells. However, it also provides good entrance into a small- to moderate-size frontal sinus. The Lynch incision is buried in the creases and concavity of the lateral nose and superomedial orbital margin. The frontal sinus is entered from below and behind the orbital rim, and the region of the nasofrontal duct is exposed by a lateral (external) ethmoidectomy. The diseased frontal sinus and ethmoid mucosa is removed, and a tube is placed in the nasofrontal duct to promote sinus drainage through a reconstructed duct. This tube remains in place for 6 to 8 weeks and then is removed intranasally (Figs. 4-315 to 4-317).[3,6] If the frontal sinus is too large for all of its mucosa to be effectively removed by the standard Lynch procedure, an extended Lynch incision can be used, extending the incision more laterally over the orbit or a larger bony defect can be made in the anterior frontal sinus wall, using either the Killian or Riedel procedures.

In a moderately large frontal sinus the Killian procedure can be used. Via two bony defects this approach creates a larger entrance into the frontal sinus than can be obtained with an extended Lynch procedure. In the Killian approach the first bony defect is created above the orbital rim in the anterior frontal sinus wall, and the second defect is created below and behind the orbital rim in the frontal sinus floor (via a standard Lynch incision). The intact superior orbital rim partially prevents the overlying soft tissues of the forehead from collapsing into the sinus, and when compared with the Reidel procedure, the resulting cosmetic deformity is minimized (Fig. 4-318). However, the soft tissues of the forehead region do partially prolapse into the sinus cavity and

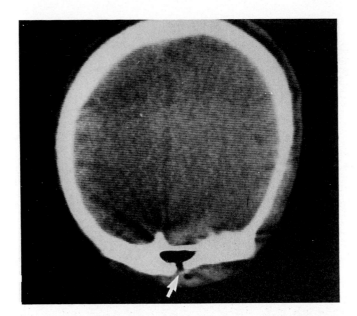

FIG. 4-314 Coronal CT shows a posttrephination frontal sinus. The site of the trephination is seen as a hole in the anterior sinus wall *(arrow)*.

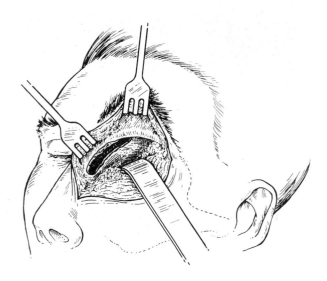

FIG. 4-315 Diagram of a Lynch procedure. The ethmoid sinuses, supraorbital ethmoid cells, and small frontal sinuses can be approached by this procedure. The incision is buried in the creases of the lateral nose and superomedial orbital rim.

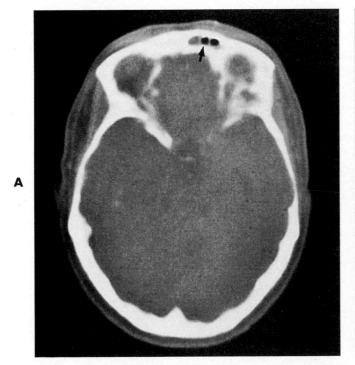

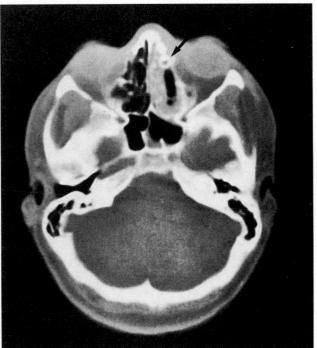

FIG. 4-316 **A,** Axial CT scan shows a tube *(arrow)* in the left frontal sinus. The sinus is partially filled with secretions. **B,** Axial CT scan through the ethmoid sinuses of same patient shows the drainage tube *(arrow)* extending down into the nose. The anterior lamina papyracea has been removed as have most of the ethmoid septa because the patient has had an external ethmoidectomy. The ethmoid cavity and the left sphenoid sinus have inflammatory changes.

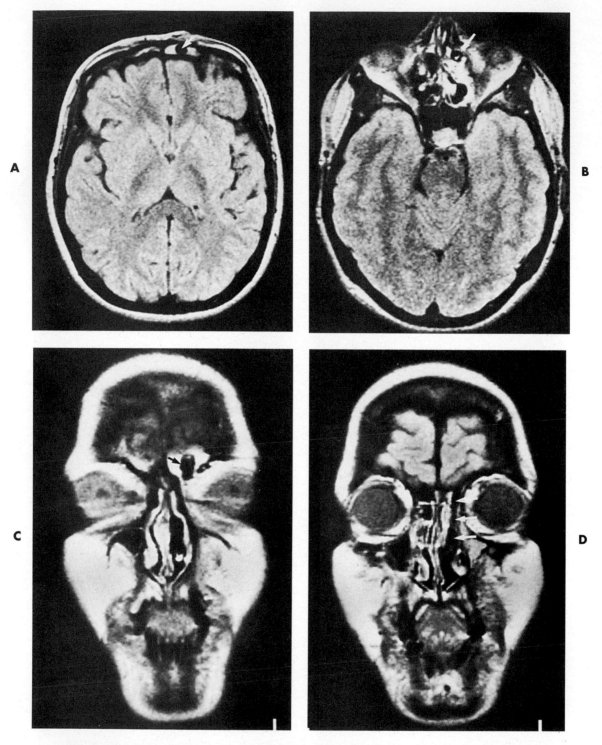

FIG. 4-317 **A,** Axial proton density MR scan shows a drainage tube in the left frontal sinus *(arrow).* Inflammatory secretions are present in the sinus. **B,** Axial proton density MR scan shows the drainage tube in the ethmoid sinuses *(arrow)* and inflammatory changes in the ethmoid sinuses. It is almost impossible to appreciate that an external ethmoidectomy has been performed. **C,** Coronal proton density MR scan shows the frontal sinus tube *(arrow)* and frontal sinus secretions. **D,** Coronal proton density MR scan, posterior to **C,** shows the drainage tube extending through the ethmoid sinuses into the nasal fossa *(arrows).*

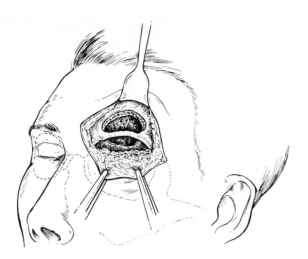

FIG. 4-318 Diagram of a Killian procedure. Because of the forehead deformity, this procedure has for the most part been abandoned.

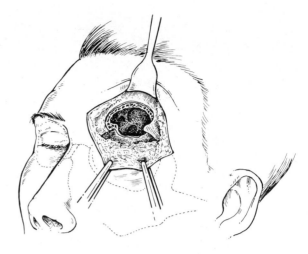

FIG. 4-319 Diagram of a Riedel's procedure. Because this operation causes a large deformity of the forehead, it has been almost entirely abandoned.

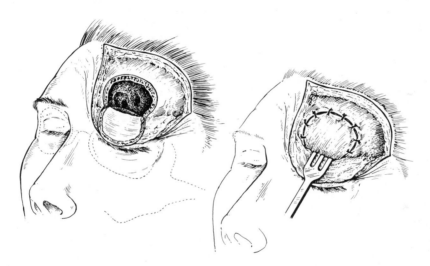

FIG. 4-320 Diagram of an osteoplastic flap procedure. The anterior sinus wall is flipped down with the inferior periosteum left intact. After the sinus mucosa and disease are removed, the sinus is obliterated with fat and then the flap is replaced. This procedure leaves almost no cosmetic deformity.

create a noticeable cosmetic deformity, which is well seen on axial scans. As in the Lynch procedure, the nasofrontal duct is reconstructed through an external ethmoidectomy.

For the reliable removal of diseased sinus mucosa in a large frontal sinus, the Riedel procedure can be used. In this approach the two surgical defects created in the Killian procedure are joined into one large defect, which includes the superior orbital rim (Fig. 4-319). At the completion of the procedure the soft tissues of the forehead are laid on the posterior frontal sinus wall, which has been denuded of its mucosa. This effectively obliterates the upper sinus cavity but creates a cosmetically undesirable soft-tissue defect in the forehead. The nasofrontal duct is reconstructed as in the Lynch procedure.[3,6]

Because of the cosmetic deformities associated with these procedures, particularly the latter two techniques, and because the nasofrontal duct becomes obstructed postoperatively in about 50% of these patients, the cosmetically less-deforming obliterative osteoplastic flap procedure has gained great recent popularity, especially in the moderate to large frontal sinuses in which mucosa cannot be removed by a Lynch approach.

The osteoplastic flap incision is either a curved coronal scalp incision that is hidden in the scalp hair or through an incision that extends between the eyebrows, crossing the intervening skin crease near the root of the nose. Once the periosteum over the frontal bone is exposed, a template made from a Caldwell view is used to trace the frontal sinus

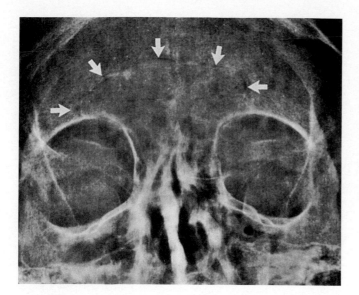

FIG. 4-321   Waters view shows a patient's status post a bilateral osteoplastic flap. The flap margins can barely be identified (arrows).

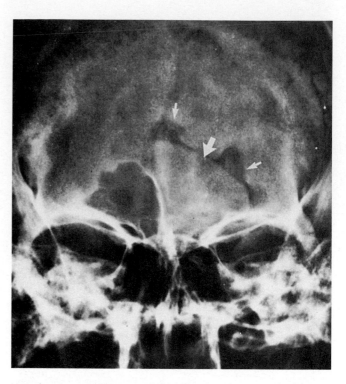

FIG. 4-322   Caldwell view shows a patient's status post a left ostcoplastic flap. The margins of the flap are well seen (arrows). The space between the flap and the sinus margin is a normal postoperative finding, resulting from the bone removal that occurs during surgery.

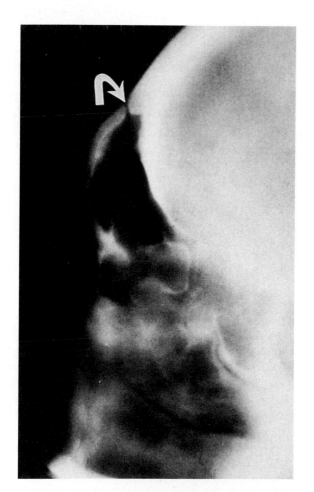

FIG. 4-323   Lateral multidirectional tomogram shows a patient's status post an osteoplastic flap procedure. The surgical margin of the flap (arrow) is seen and may simulate a fracture.

contour on the bone and periosteum. This template should come from a film taken on a dedicated head unit such as the Franklin head unit, which has a magnification factor of only 3.4% (compared with 10.3% on a standard 40-inch posteroanterior Caldwell film).[7] The traced outline of the sinus should be made so that the bone incision lies just inside the sinus contour. The periosteum is incised on all except its inferior margin, and the frontal sinus contour is drilled into the anterior frontal sinus table. The drill line is beveled medially and downward to ensure that the frontal sinus and not the anterior cranial fossa is entered. The inferior margin of this anterior wall is not drilled but is fractured from side to side and turned downward off of the sinus with its overlying periosteum intact. This technique yields a viable bone flap. The sinus mucosa is then drilled out, and the sinus cavity is obliterated with fat or muscle, usually taken from the abdominal wall. The anterior sinus wall is then replaced, the periosteum sutured, and the skin closed, leaving literally no cosmetic deformity (Fig. 4-320). The fat gradually undergoes fibrosis until the fibrosis represents one third to one half the volume of the obliterating material. More extensive fibrosis of the fat does not appear to normally occur. Throughout this process, no volume loss occurs so that the sinus remains obliterated. Infection of the bone flap or the operative margins, with or without associated osteomyelitis, and infection of the obliterating fat are the two most significant complications of the osteoplastic flap procedure. When

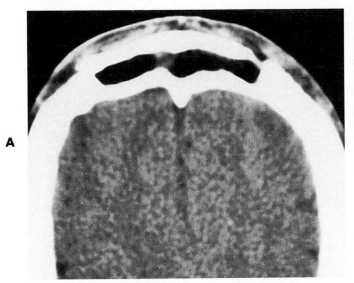
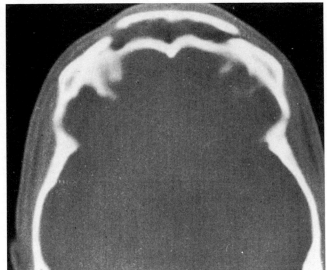

FIG. 4-324   Axial CT scans at narrow (**A**) and wide (**B**) window settings. The sinus is filled with fat, and the flap is sharply seen in good position.

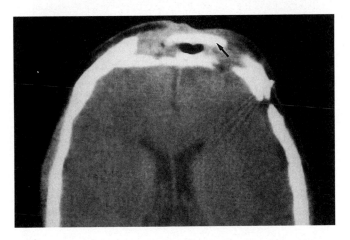

FIG. 4-325   Axial CT scan shows an infected osteoplastic flap. There is swelling of the overlying forehead soft tissues, and the bone flap has been partially eroded *(arrow)*. In addition, just dorsal to the flap there is air, which should not be present in an obliterated sinus. The defect in the left posterior sinus table was related to the surgery.

such infection occurs, it is often necessary to reoperate to remove the infection. This second procedure often results in removal of the anterior sinus wall bone flap with some resulting inward prolapse of the forehead soft tissues. A plastic reconstruction can be performed at a later date, once the infection is cured. If the osteoplastic flap procedure was performed to obliterate a mucocele that thinned or destroyed a portion of the posterior or anterior sinus tables, these defects, as well as the surgically related anterior wall defect, are visualized on subsequent imaging studies.

On plain films the osteoplastic bone flap is identified by a variably thin zone of lower density at its margins. This zone represents the surgically removed portion of the ante-

rior sinus table (Figs. 4-321, 4-322). In a few cases the flap fit may be so good as to make visualization of the surgical margin almost impossible on Caldwell or Waters views. However, a lateral view clearly shows the beveled surgical defect. In fact, if a history of prior surgery is not obtained, this defect may be misinterpreted as an anterior frontal table fracture (Fig. 4-323). If the sinus margin was altered before surgery, it will remain so after surgery. Thus the mucoperiosteal white line may be absent or replaced by a thick zone of sclerosis, and the sinus contour may be remodeled. Although this appearance can be confusing and suggests that whatever caused these changes is still present in the sinus, these sinus alterations merely reflect whatever process originally necessiated the surgery. The fat used to obliterate the sinus usually causes the sinus to have a plain film hazy soft-tissue density, suggesting sinusitis. The surgical bony margins should be sharp and of a normal texture even though the bone flap does not fit precisely against the adjacent frontal bone. An air-fluid level indicates reinfection of the sinus, a serious complication.

On CT the bone flap may go unnoticed if only narrow windows are used. At wide window settings the bone flap should have a normal texture (Fig. 4-324). However, the edges of the flap and the adjacent frontal bone occasionally have a ragged, irregular appearance that reflects the beveling surgical procedure. Without any associated clinical or soft-tissue changes of infection, this irregular bone should not elicit a diagnosis of osteomyelitis. Frank osteomyelitis appears as areas of bone demineralization, erosion, or sequestration accompanied by swelling and cellulitis of the overlying forehead soft tissues. There usually is also evidence of infection in the underlying fat (Figs. 4-325, 4-326). The bone flap should be in a normal alignment with the adjacent frontal bone, that is, the flap should not be either depressed into the sinus or elevated over the adjacent frontal

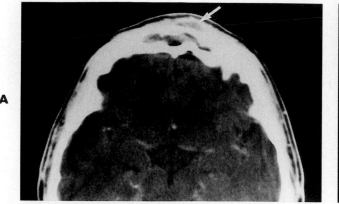
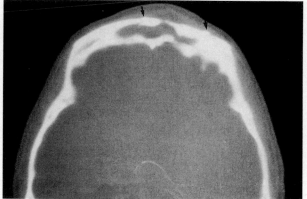

FIG. 4-326 Axial CT scans at soft tissue (**A**) and bone (**B**) window settings show a patient who had a left osteoplastic flap. The small wire sutures stabilizing the flap can barely be seen in **B** *(small arrows)*. There is erosion of the midanterior flap, and an abscess is present in the forehead *(arrow in A)*. The fat used to obliterate the sinus is also dense, reflecting infection.

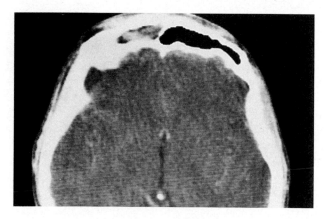

FIG. 4-327 Axial contrast CT scan shows a patient's status post a right osteoplastic flap. The obliterating fat is dense. Early postoperative infection of the fat.

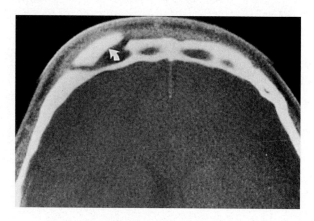

FIG. 4-328 Axial CT scan shows elevation of the top of a right osteoplastic flap *(arrow)*. This usually indicates swelling and infection of the obliterating fat.

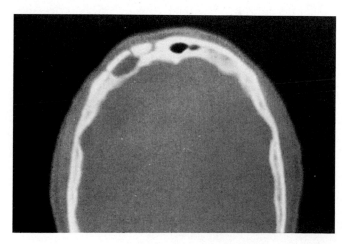

FIG. 4-329 Axial CT scan shows a fracture of the osteoplastic flap on the right side. This occurred at surgery and is a normal postoperative finding.

bone. When the flap is elevated, infection of the underlying obliterating fat must be considered. The obliterated sinus is best examined at both narrow and wide windows. The entire sinus cavity should be airless and filled with fat that has randomly scattered strands of soft-tissue density fibrous tissue. Whenever a focal mass of soft-tissue density is seen within the fat or whenever more than half the fat content is of fibrous density, the imager should raise the possibility of infection of the obliterating material (Figs. 4-326, 4-327). This type of infection is usually associated with elevation of the flap secondary to swelling of the fibrous fatty material (Fig. 4-328). In these cases the intracranial compartment should also be examined for evidence of spread of the infection. Occasionally the osteoplastic flap fractures during surgery; however, as long as the overlying periosteum remains intact, the fracture pieces usually remain viable. In such cases, the imager should verify that the bony pieces have a normal texture, that there are no sites of osteomyelitis, and that the bone fragments are not elevated (Fig. 4-329).

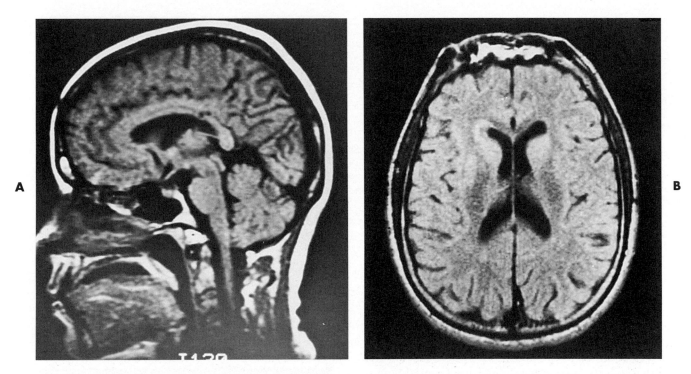

FIG. 4-330   Sagittal T1W (**A**) and axial proton density (**B**) MRI scans show (fat) high signal intensity material within the obliterated sinus. The flap is often hard to identify on MRI scans.

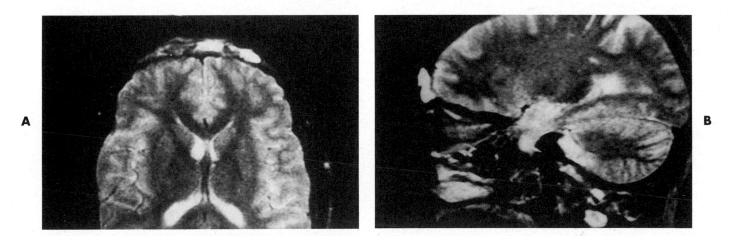

FIG. 4-331   Axial (**A**) and sagittal (**B**) T2W MR scans on a patient who has had an osteoplastic flap. The right side of the obliterated sinus has a normal fat signal intensity. However, the middle and left regions of the sinus have high signal intensity. This usually indicated the presence of infection, but this patient was asymptomatc. Such high T2W signal intensity may be a normal postoperative MRI finding.

In rare instances, after many years, some calcification can occur in the obliterating fat; this in and of itself should only be considered a normal postoperative variant.

On MRI the signal intensities in the normal postosteoplasic flap sinus reflect the obliterating fat. Thus there is a high T1W signal intensity and an intermediate T2W signal intensity (Fig. 4-330). Although infection in the fat will produce a high T2W signal intensity, occasionally areas of such high T2W signal intensity are seen in noninfected sinuses

(Fig. 4-331). The precise cause of this signal is unclear. Infection should be considered if there is high T2W signal intensity in the obliterating fat and swelling and inflammation in the surrounding forehead tissues.

Ethmoid Sinus Surgery

The ethmoid complex can be partially resected via three major approaches: the external, the internal (intranasal), and the transmaxillary (transantral) (Fig. 4-332). These proce-

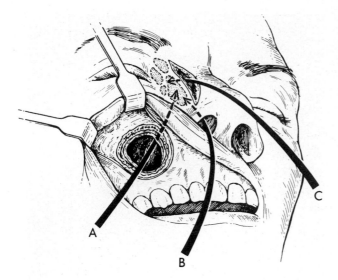

FIG. 4-332 Diagram of the three major surgical approaches to the ethmoid sinuses. **A,** Transmaxillary or transantral. **B,** Internal or intranasal. **C,** External (Lynch).

dures are performed for inflammatory disease, and the aim is to progressively remove the disease from each cell until all of the pathologic material is removed. The primary areas of complication are entrance into the floor of the anterior cranial fossa and damage to the orbital contents.[1,3,7]

The external approach provides the best overall access and visualization of the ethmoid cells. After a Lynch incision, the periorbita is elevated and the surface of the lamina papyracea is viewed to identify prior fractures and any areas of dehiscence or erosion. The anterior and posterior ethmoidal canals are exposed. A line connecting these canals lies just below the floor of the anterior cranial fossa, and if the surgeon stays caudal to this line, intracranial entrance should not occur. The surgical field can be enlarged to the frontal sinus, supraorbital cells, orbit, anterior sphenoid sinus, or base of the skull; the nasofrontal duct is best opened with this approach. In this approach the anterior cells are first entered through the lamina papyracea, and then the posterior cells are progressively opened as needed. Because a Lynch incision must be made, this external approach has a scar hidden in the crease of the medial orbital margin.

The internal ethmoidectomy is an intranasal approach and includes resection of the middle turbinate to provide better access to the ethmoid and sphenoid cells. The ethmoid complex is usually entered via the bulla ethmoidalis; the more posterior cells are then opened, and then the anterior cells are resected. Although in experienced hands, the lamina papyracea is not violated in this procedure; dehiscence of the lamina papyracea or a prior external ethmoidectomy are contributing factors to inadvertant entrance into the orbit. The internal ethmoidectomy approach is used for isolated ethmoid sinus disease, for biopsies in patients who do not have coexistent antral disease, and in patients who do not wish to have an external incision.

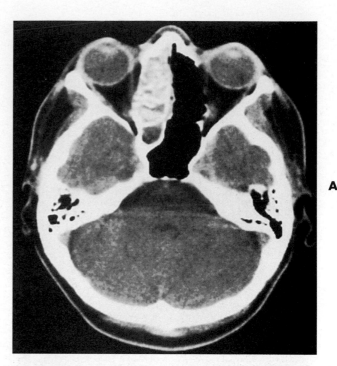

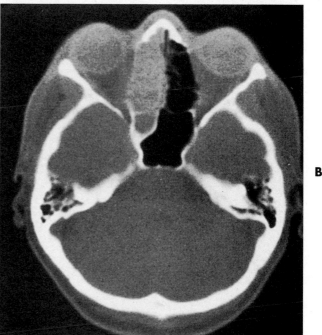

FIG. 4-333 Axial CT scans at **A,** narrow and **B,** wide window settings show inflammatory disease in the right ethmoid and sphenoid sinuses and, in **A,** an apparent prior left sphenoethmoidectomy. However, in **B** the left ethmoid septa and the anterior sphenoid sinus wall are intact, indicating that no surgery was performed.

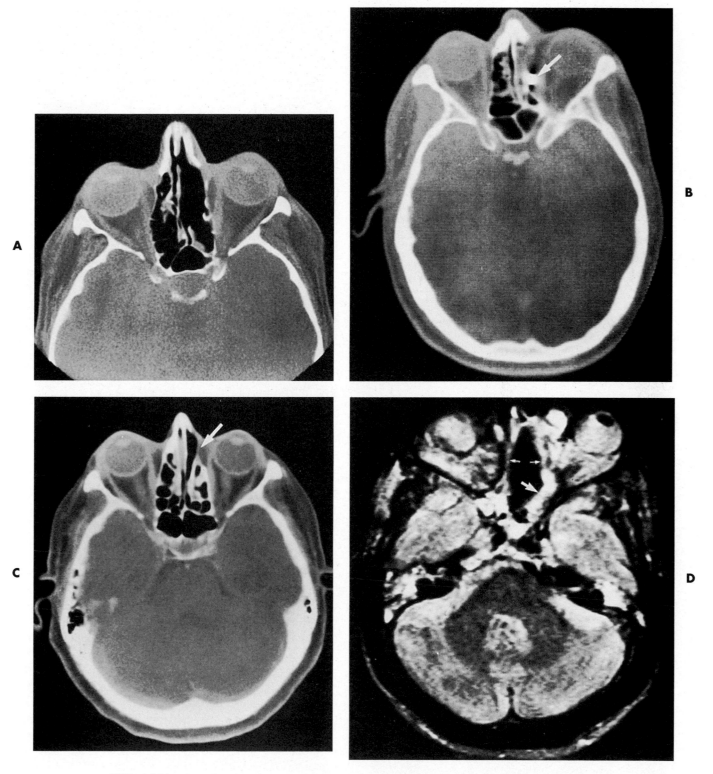

FIG. 4-334   A, Axial CT scan shows the postoperative appearance of a complete left internal ethmoidectomy. **B,** Axial CT scan shows a patient's status post a left external ethmoidectomy. The surgical clip *(arrow)* is used to control bleeding from the ethmoidal vessels. The soft tissue in the anterior ethmoid cavity is fibrosis and granulation tissue. **C,** Axial CT scan shows the postoperative appearance of a left external ethmoidectomy. The anterior lamina papyracea has been surgically removed and is replaced by fibrosis *(arrow)*. **D,** Axial T2W MR scan shows the appearance of prior complete bilateral internal ethmoidectomies. Part of the postoperative cavity is lined with fibrotic tissue *(small arrows),* and other areas have inflammatory tissue with a high T2W signal intensity *(arrow).*

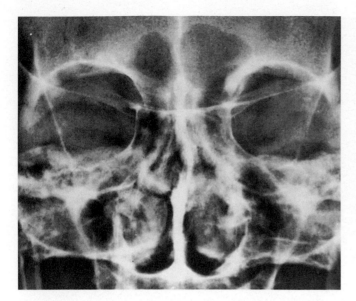

FIG. 4-335 Caldwell view shows clouding of the left ethmoid sinuses. This appearance suggests infection. However, in this patient this was due to fibrosis after an ethmoidectomy.

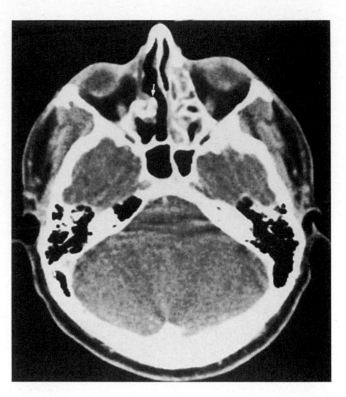

FIG. 4-336 Axial CT scan shows a patient who has had a right ethmoidectomy. There is a focal area of bone production within the postoperative cavity *(arrow)*. This represents reactive bone in response to surgery and has no pathologic significance.

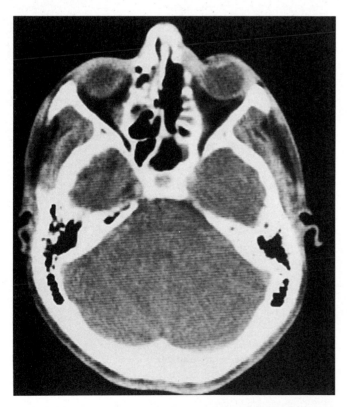

FIG. 4-337 Axial CT scan shows the appearance of a left ethmoidectomy. Several of the posterior and more cranial ethmoid septa are still seen. This is a common finding, and these areas may be sites of residual disease.

The transantral approach is used when the antral cavity has coexistent sinusitis or when the intranasal approach is not possible because of anatomic or technical reasons. The antrum is entered using a Caldwell-Luc approach, and the medial, upper maxillary sinus wall (ethmoidomaxillary plate) is taken down so that the ethmoid cells can be entered. The ethmoid cells are then progressively resected.

In virtually all of these procedures the surgeon is forced to blindly cut through the most inaccessible ethmoid septa, those located at the cranial and posterior margins of the ethmoid complex. Even when the surgeon believes that the resection extended back into the sphenoid sinus, CT scans often show that the most posterior ethmoid cells and the sphenoid sinus remain untouched by the procedure (as often do the most cranial ethmoid cells). This discrepancy points out the difficulty of intraoperatively estimating one's precise anatomic position, and it is because of this limitation that postoperative scans should be obtained if the patient's symptoms persist or recur (Figs. 4-333 to 4-338).[1] Because of the small, boxlike anatomy of the ethmoid cells, postoperative hemorrhaging can fill some unresected cells, and on occasion rather than resorb, the blood becomes fibrosed or even ossified. Such en bloc fibrosis does not often occur after surgery in the other paranasal sinuses but is fairly common in the ethmoid complex. The imaging differentiation of recurrent disease from fibrosis can be difficult. In general, on CT, recurrent inflammation enhances and the

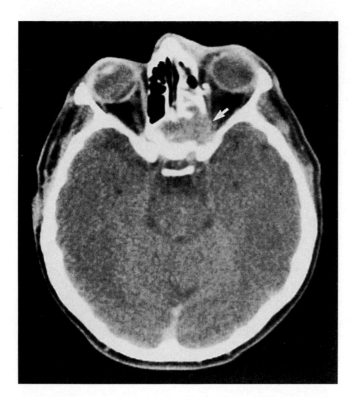

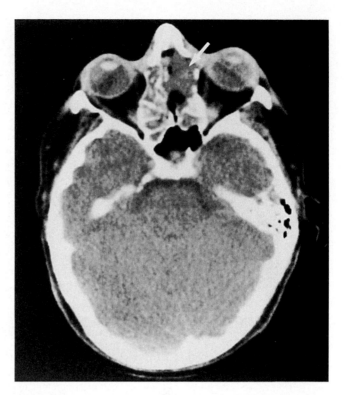

FIG. 4-338 Axial CT scan shows a destructive mass in the left posterior sphenoethmoid region *(arrow)*. This patient had a limited left ethmoidectomy for suspected infectious disease. No preoperative scan was obtained. It was only when postoperative left eye signs developed that a scan was obtained. Infection and carcinoma.

FIG. 4-339 Axial CT scan shows the appearance of a left ethmoidectomy that has an accumulation of mucoid material within the postoperative cavity *(arrow)*. Postoperative mucocele.

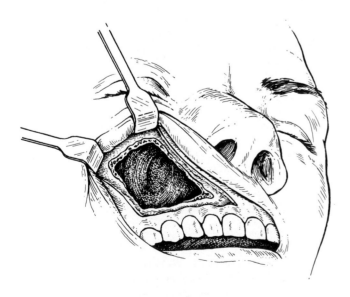

FIG. 4-340 Diagram of Caldwell-Luc approach. The maxillary sinus is entered anteriorly from the canine fossa. The hole in the sinus can be of a variable size.

fibrosis does not. However, the differences in attenuation values frequently are not sufficient to establish a definitive diagnosis. Occasionally a dense fibrous scar develops within the postoperative ethmoid bed. This scar usually has low T1W and T2W signal intensity and thus can be distinguished from active infection on the T2W scans. Rarely the denuded ethmoid bone develops a hyperostotic reaction that produces variable amounts of bone. In some cases a localized osteoma-like bone develops; in other cases the entire postoperative cavity may be obliterated by the bone production (which often mimics the appearance of fibrous dysplasia). This type of bone reaction also occurs in the maxillary sinus and to a lesser degree in the sphenoid sinus. It is rare that this reactive bone develops in the postoperative frontal sinus.

In addition to noting the degree of ethmoid septal removal, the imager should anticipate (1) an absent anterior third to half of the lamina papyracea from an external approach, (2) an absent medial ethmoid wall and probable absent middle turbinate from an internal approach, and (3) a Caldwell-Luc defect in the lower anterior antral wall, absent bone in the upper medial antral wall, and possibly an absent middle turbinate from a transantral approach. Any residual soft tissues in the remaining ethmoid cells should be clearly noted by the imager for future reference.

If a postethmoidectomy cavity becomes obstructed after mucosal reepithelialization, a postoperative mucocele develops (Fig. 4-339). This mucocele usually does not behave

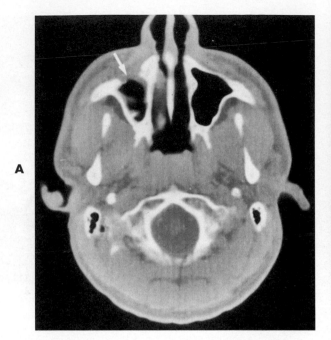

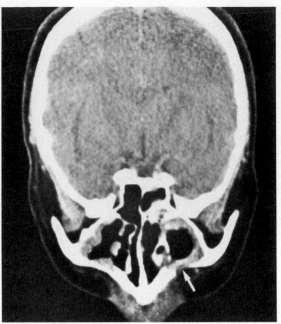

FIG. 4-341 **A,** Axial CT scan shows the anterior sinus wall Caldwell-Luc defect *(arrow).* The soft tissues in the sinus were senechia. **B,** Coronal CT scan shows the Caldwell-Luc defect in the anterior sinus wall *(arrow)* and inflammatory mucosal thickening in both antra.

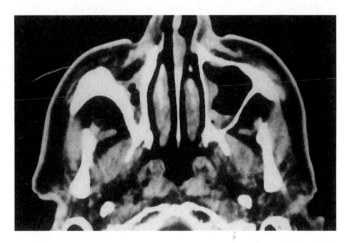

FIG. 4-342 Axial CT scan shows a patient's status post a right Caldwell-Luc procedure. Fat from the cheek has partially prolapsed into the defect, and some inflammatory mucosal thickening is present bilaterally.

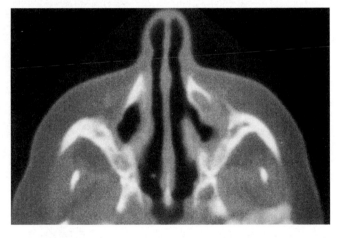

FIG. 4-343 Axial CT scan shows a patient's status post bilateral Caldwell-Luc procedures. The thickening of the posterolateral sinus bony walls is a reaction to the denuding of the sinus mucosa during the procedure.

like a typical ethmoid mucocele, which tends to expand laterally into the orbit. Rather this postoperative mucocele takes the course of least resistance and expands within the enlarged postoperative ethmoid cavity. It is only after the entire ethmoid cavity is filled that the mucocele bulges into the orbit. On imaging, characteristically there is a collection of entrapped secretions within the postoperative ethmoid. However, at times the appearance may be similar to routine inflammation on both CT and MRI.[8]

Maxillary Sinus Surgery

Today the most common diagnostic and therapeutic procedures performed on the antrum and the osteomeatal complex are endoscopic techniques. However, intranasal antrostomy and the Caldwell-Luc operation are still performed. The endoscopic techniques are discussed in Chapter 3.

In an intranasal antrostomy the membranous and bony lateral nasal wall of the inferior meatus is partially resected in an attempt to create better gravity drainage of the sinus.

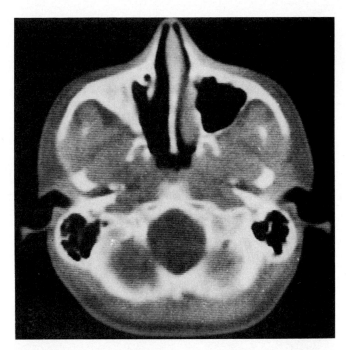

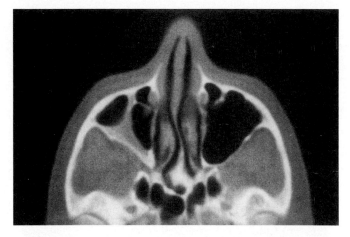

FIG. 4-345 Axial CT scan on a patient's status post a right Caldwell-Luc procedure. On this more cranial scan through the antrum a septum *(arrow)* has formed between the anterior and posterior sinus walls. If this septum completely obstructs the lateral portion of the sinus, a postoperative mucocele will develop.

FIG. 4-344 Axial CT scan shows a post Caldwell-Luc right maxillary sinus in which the remaining antral wall bone has reactively thickened to almost obliterate the sinus cavity.

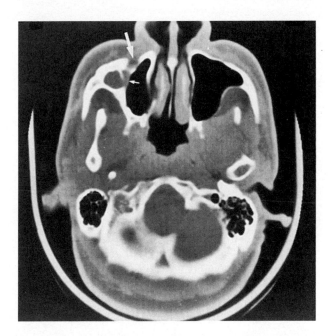

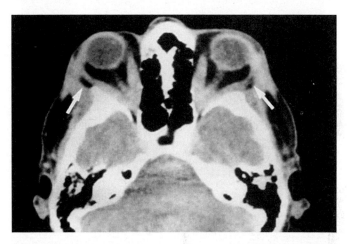

FIG. 4-347 Axial CT scan shows a patient with the changes of thyroid ophthalmopathy. All of the extraocular muscle bellies are enlarged; there is tapering at the tendon insertions, and there is bilateral proptosis. The lateral orbital walls *(arrows)* have been surgically removed. Patient status post bilateral lateral orbitotomies (Kronlein approaches).

FIG. 4-346 Axial CT scan shows the anterior Caldwell-Luc defect in the right maxillary sinus wall *(large arrow)*. There is an expansile mass in the lateral portion of the right antrum *(small arrow)*. Postoperative antral mucocele.

In the Caldwell-Luc procedure, in addition to the intranasal antrostomy the maxillary sinus is entered via the canine fossa region in the lower anterior antral wall. Because this entrance scar is intraoral, there is no facial scarring (Fig. 4-340). Once the sinus is entered, the diseased mucosa is removed. Initially the anterior wall bony defect is

closed by a hematoma that eventually undergoes fibrosis (Figs. 4-341 to 4-344).

However, this hematoma can uncommonly become infected, and in rare instances an oroantral fistula may be created. If this unusual complication occurs, it is usually within the first or second postoperative week. Via the Caldwell-Luc approach the bone of the posterior sinus wall can be removed to provide access for internal maxillary artery ligation or to expose the pterygopalatine fossa, vidian nerve, and pterygopalatine ganglion.[3] In such cases a bony defect in the upper, medial, and posterior antral wall also can be seen on imaging.

In some patients, synechiae develop between the posterior maxillary sinus wall and the lateral margin of the canine

A

B

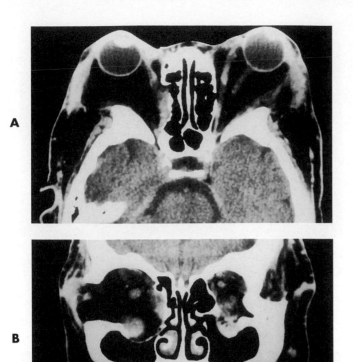

FIG. 4-348 Axial **(A)** and coronal **(B)** CT scans show a patient with bilateral thyroid ophthalmopathy and bilateral Kronlein and orbital floor decompression procedures. A medial right ethmoid decompression was also performed.

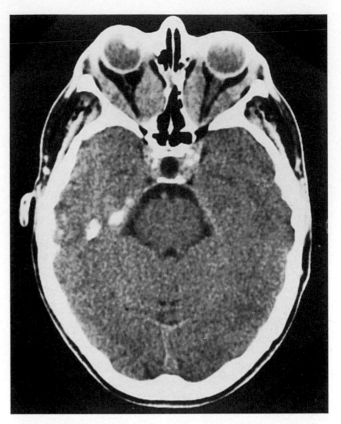

FIG. 4-349 Axial CT scan shows large muscle bellies in the extraocular muscles with tapering at the anterior tendon insertions. The ethmoid complexes have been collapsed for decompression. Thyroid ophthalmopathy.

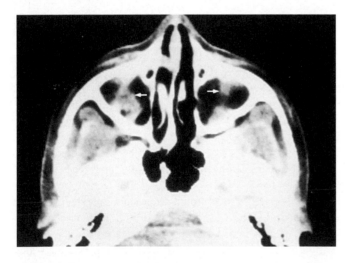

FIG. 4-350 Axial CT scan through the upper maxillary sinuses shows the inferior rectus muscles *(arrows)* and orbital fat in the upper antra. The orbital floors have been surgically removed. Thyroid ophthalmopathy in a patient status post bilateral orbital floor decompressions.

fossa—Caldwell-Luc defect in the anterior sinus wall. Persistent synechiae may form the basis for a membrane that extends across the sinus between the anterior and posterior walls. Once formed, this membrane obstructs the drainage of the lateral portion of the maxillary sinus and leads to the appearance of a postoperative antral mucocele (Figs. 4-92, 4-345, 4-346).

As previously mentioned, once the sinus mucosa has been stripped from the sinus wall a bony reaction may be elicited that results in reactive bone formation, thickening of the sinus wall, and reduction or obliteration of the sinus cavity. Such a reaction is an expected consequence of the procedure and should not necessarily signify to the radiologist that active infection is present (Figs. 4-341 to 4-344).[9]

Optic nerve compression and decreased visual acuity in patients with thyroid ophthalmopathy may be treated by surgical decompression of the orbit. The procedures most commonly employed are a lateral orbitotomy (Krönlein's procedure); an antral (orbital floor) decompression, using a Caldwell-Luc approach; an ethmoid decompression, using an external ethmoidectomy approach; and an orbital roof decompression accomplished via a craniotomy. Of these operations the greatest degree of decompression from a single procedure is obtained from the orbital floor approach.

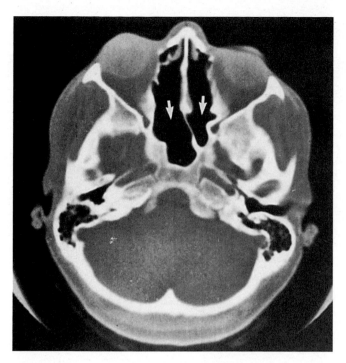

FIG. 4-351   Axial CT scan shows a patient with bilateral eth-moidectomies and sphenoid sinusotomies. The anterior sphenoid sinus walls have been removed *(arrows)*.

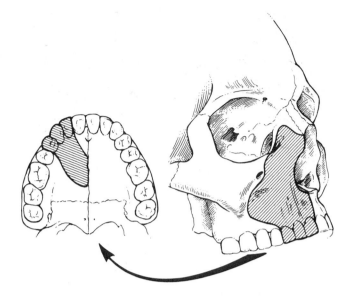

FIG. 4-352   Diagram of a typical medial maxillectomy resection. A portion of the palate is removed if needed to obtain a tumor-free margin. The medial antral wall and inferior turbinate are also included in the resection.

However, this procedure must be performed bilaterally so that the visual axes are not made asymmetric, resulting in diplopia and cosmetic deformity. The lateral and ethmoid decompressions can be combined with antral decompressions to achieve maximal relief of exophthalmos and a decrease in intraorbital pressure. The orbital roof approach provides relatively little decompression, and because it is a more extensive surgical approach, it is reserved for only the most severe cases.

On sectional imaging the absence of the lateral portion of the orbital wall may at first elude detection, the imager's attention being drawn by pronounced proptosis with muscle enlargement. However, careful evaluation of the bony orbital walls will show that a Krönlein procedure was performed (Figs. 4-347, 4-348). The ethmoid decompression has the same appearance as an external ethmoidectomy, and it is the orbital muscle findings of thyroid ophthalmopathy that suggests the diagnosis (Figs. 4-348, 4-349). The antral decompression reveals prolapse of the orbital fat and inferior muscles into the upper maxillary sinuses. Without history, on axial scans this operation may present a confusing picture, often mimicking an unusual antral disease. However, coronal scans reveal that most of the orbital floor bone is missing, a finding that differentiates this postoperative appearance from the rare event of bilateral orbital floor blow-out fractures, where the displaced fracture's segments can be identified (Figs. 4-348, 4-350).

Sphenoid Sinus Surgery

The sphenoid sinuses can be approached through the anterior sinus wall for biopsy, to improve sinus drainage, or to

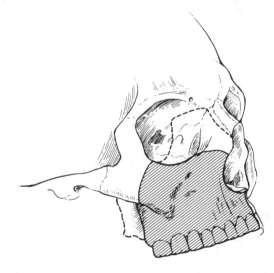

FIG. 4-353   Diagram of a typical total maxillectomy resection. Variable portions of the zygoma and pterygoid plates may be included in the resection. Similarly the orbital floor may be taken in its entirety, and an ethmoid resection *(dotted line)* may also be included to obtain a tumor-free margin.

remove inflammatory tissue. The sphenoid sinusotomy opens the anterior wall of the sinus and creates a wide, open cavity that leads into the nasopharynx (Fig. 4-351). The sinus can be reached by intranasal, transseptal, transmaxillary, or transethmoidal approaches.

In the transnasal approach, portions of the posterior middle turbinate, the superior turbinate, and some of the posterior ethmoid cells are removed to gain exposure. In the transseptal approach, portions of the cartilaginous and bony nasal septum (vomer) are removed. The transmaxillary

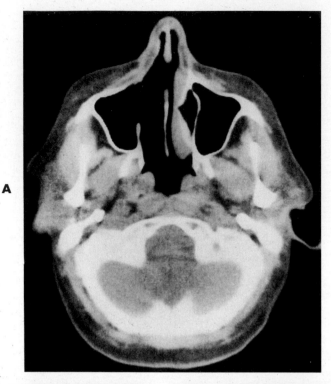

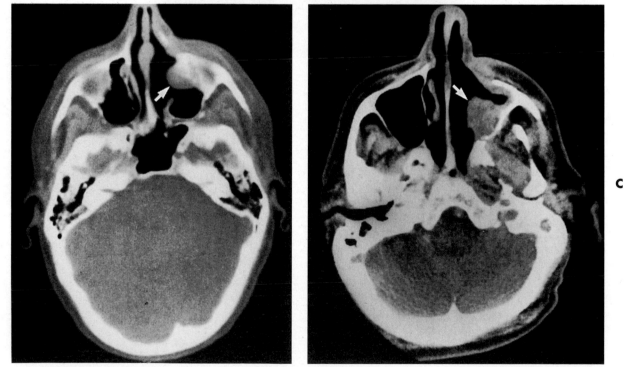

FIG. 4-354 **A,** Axial CT scan shows the normal postpartial right maxillectomy appearance. The soft tissues in and around the antrum should be smooth. **B,** Axial CT scan shows a postpartial left maxillectomy with a nodular mass *(arrow)* in the antrum. Although this could be an inflammatory mass, the suspicion of tumor should be raised until proven otherwise. Tumor Recurrence. **C,** Axial CT scan shows a postpartial left maxillectomy with an irregularly nodular tumor recurrence *(arrow)* in the antrum. The smooth soft tissues lining the anterior left antrum represented scar tissue.

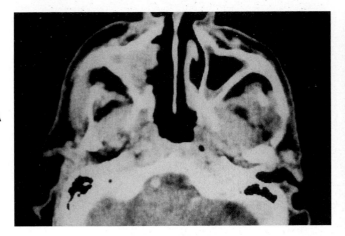
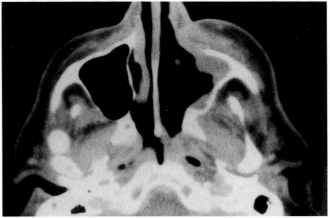

A   B

FIG. 4-355 Axial CT scan (**A**) on a patient's status post a right medial maxillectomy. The soft tissues within the right sinus have a nodular contour and are suggestive of recurrent inverted papilloma. Inflammatory disease is present in the left antrum. Axial CT scan (**B**) on a patient's status post a left medial maxillectomy. There is a nodular fullness in the soft tissues, filling the post operative cavity. This smooth nodule was a retention cyst and not recurrent tumor.

approach is an extension of a Caldwell-Luc procedure in which a transmaxillary ethmoidectomy is extended to include the anterior sphenoid sinus wall. The transethmoidal approach is simply a posterior extension of an external ethmoidectomy procedure. Thus depending on the approach used, in addition to an absence of one or both anterior sphenoid sinus walls, the respective surgical defects just described should be observed on scans.[3,6]

When a sphenoid sinusotomy is performed, care must be taken to avoid trauma to the carotid artery. In 17% of patients the bony wall, separating the sinus and artery, is so thin that it provides little if any protection from trauma. Carotid artery damage may lead to a posttraumatic aneurysm or a carotid-cavernous fistula.[10,11] Similarly, damage can occur to the cavernous sinus and to the vidian nerve in those patients who have this nerve running within the sinus floor.

A transsphenoidal hypophysectomy can be performed as an extension of the sphenoid sinusotomy. Once the sphenoid sinus cavity is surgically exposed, portions of the anterior wall and floor of the sella turcica can be removed and the pituitary fossa entered from below. Muscle, fat, cartilage, or bone may be used to seal the surgical defect. On sectional imaging, in addition to the site of surgical bone removal, sclerotic thickening of the remaining portions of the anterior wall and floor of the sella turcica may be observed. Some postoperative prolapse of sellar contents into the sphenoid sinus can occur, and without benefit of the surgical history, the imaging picture can simulate that of a large pituitary tumor with extension into the sphenoid sinus. In the preoperative evaluation of patients being considered for a transsphenoidal hypophysectomy, the imager must direct special attention to the thickness of the bone forming the anterior wall of the sella turcica. In nearly 99% of patients the sphenoid sinus development extends back to within 1 mm of the anterior wall or under the sellar floor. However,

in the 1% of patients in whom a thick margin of bone remains between the sinus and sella, the transsphenoidal approach is not desirable and instead an intracranial approach is used often.[12]

Surgery for Sinus Malignancy

The type of tumor-curative operation performed on the maxillary sinus varies, depending upon the precise location of the primary neoplasm. For localized nasal tumors that only involve the lower portion of the medial antral wall, a partial maxillectomy (medial maxillectomy) is usually performed. Occasionally, portions of the adjacent hard palate and maxillary alveolus must also be included in the resection (Fig. 4-352). Thus in a partial maxillectomy, the medial antral wall, the inferior turbinate, often the middle turbinate, the lower ethmoid cells, and if appropriate portions of the hard palate and alveolus are absent on the scans. The lateral portion of the antrum and its mucosa remain intact.

For more extensive tumors, a total maxillectomy can be performed (Fig. 4-353). In addition to resection of the maxilla there is some variation as to what is included in the resection. Such surgery may include the body of the zygoma, the ipsilateral hard palate and alveolus, the inferior turbinate, and often the pterygoid plates and portions of the ethmoid sinuses.[1,2,13] Modifications are made to fit the specific tumor location. Thus the orbital floor may be left in place, or it may be included along with an orbital exenteration. The latter is performed when there is gross tumor extension into the orbit. Depending on the specific tumor, any erosion of the orbital bone, even without gross penetration of the orbit, may lead to an orbital exenteration. For squamous cell carcinoma, any involvement of the orbital bone usually results in an orbital exenteration. If the orbit is not exenterated, tumor recurrence is often at the orbital margin. With other tumors such as olfactory neuroblastomas, initial involvement of the orbital wall need not result in an exen-

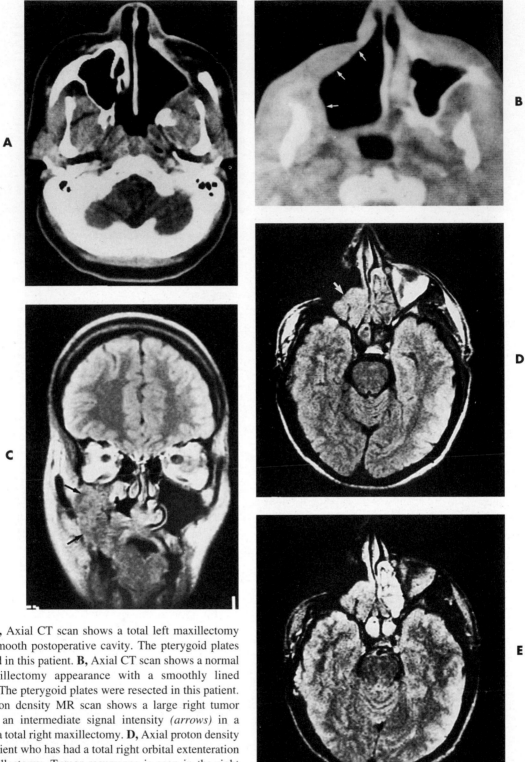

FIG. 4-356   **A,** Axial CT scan shows a total left maxillectomy with a normal smooth postoperative cavity. The pterygoid plates were not resected in this patient. **B,** Axial CT scan shows a normal total right maxillectomy appearance with a smoothly lined *(arrows)* cavity. The pterygoid plates were resected in this patient. **C,** Coronal proton density MR scan shows a large right tumor recurrence with an intermediate signal intensity *(arrows)* in a patient who had a total right maxillectomy. **D,** Axial proton density MRI shows a patient who has had a total right orbital extenteration and a total maxillectomy. Tumor recurrence is seen in the right orbital apex *(arrow).* However, it is impossible to tell if the left ethmoid sinuses and the sphenoid sinuses are also involved. **E,** Axial T2W MRI on same patient shows high signal intensity in the left ethmoid sinuses and both sphenoid sinuses, indicating the presence of entrapped inflammatory secretions and not tumor. The actual tumor is seen as an intermediate signal intensity mass.

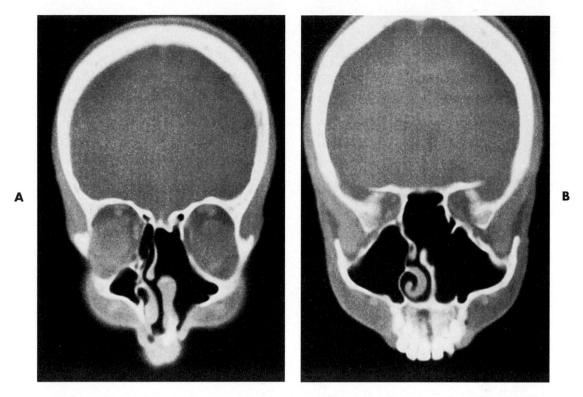

FIG. 4-357   Coronal CT scan through the anterior antrum (**A**) and posterior antrum (**B**) and sphenoid sinus in a patient who has had a left lateral rhinotomy.

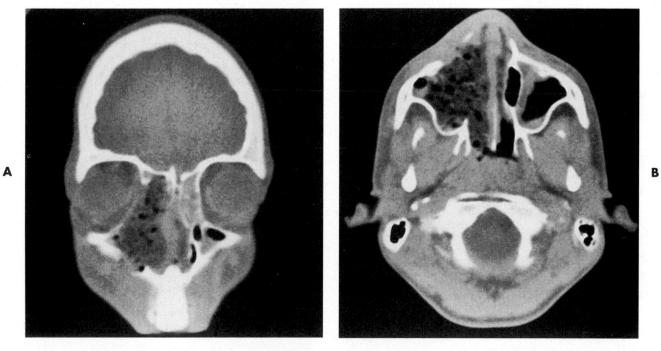

FIG. 4-358   Coronal (**A**) and axial (**B**) CT scans show a patient who has had a right lateral rhinotomy. The postoperative cavity is filled with postoperative packing.

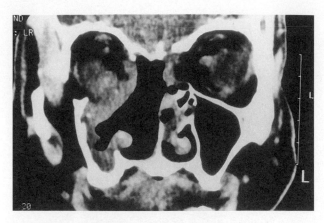

FIG. 4-359 Coronal CT scan on a patient's status post an extended right lateral rhinotomy. The floor of the right orbit has been removed. The thickened soft tissues along the orbital margin could be either scar or recurrent tumor. The best way to evaluate this disease is to compare this scan with a previous study. Biopsy may be necessary. No tumor was present in this case.

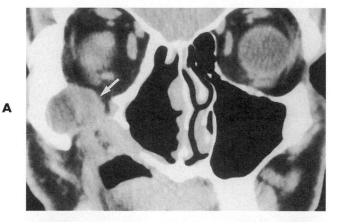

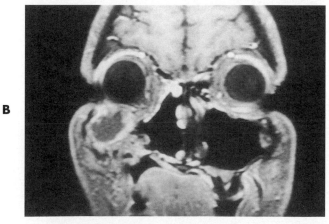

FIG. 4-360 Coronal CT **(A)** and coronal T1W postcontrast fat-suppressed MR **(B)** scans show a patient's status post an extended right lateral rhinotomy. No nodularity is present within the postoperative cavity. However, there is a mass *(arrow)* in the right zygomatic recess of the antrum, which has broken into the floor of the right orbit. The lesion has surrounding mucosal enhancement, but the secretions within it do not enhance. Postoperative mucocele.

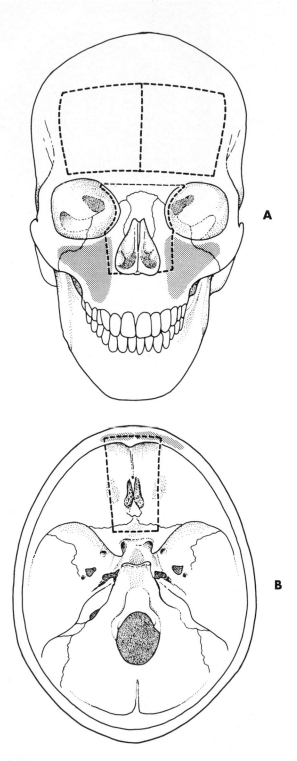

FIG. 4-361 Diagrams of the skull in the frontal view **(A)** and axial view **(B)** as seen from above with the calvarium removed. The osteotomies typically performed in the craniofacial procedure *(dashed lines)* are outlined.

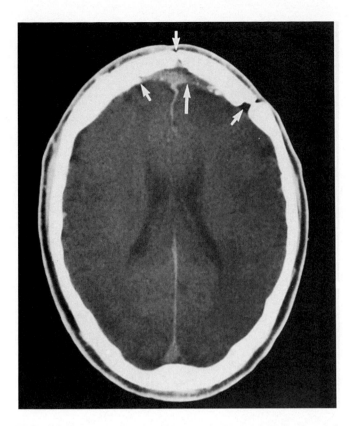

FIG. 4-362   Axial contrast CT scan shows dural thickening and enhancement *(large arrow)* that normally is seen as a postoperative finding in a patient who has had a craniofacial resection. The osteotomy sites in the frontal bones are also seen *(arrows)*.

teration. If there is a good preoperative tumor response to chemotherapy and the tumor no longer lies against the orbit, in most cases, tumor resection without an exenteration may be curative. After the bone resection the postmaxillectomy surgical cavity is lined with a split-thickness skin graft to have an immediate epithelial surface lining the defect. If the orbital floor was removed, various synthetic grafts can be placed to help support the orbital contents. Similarly, prostheses are placed to fill the surgical defects created in the hard palate and alveolus. These foreign substances can cause imaging problems either because they may degrade the image quality or because, in the case of some plastics and musculofascial grafts, on MRI they may simulate normal bone. Eye prostheses also may cause degradation artifacts on scans.

The sinus cavity in a partial maxillectomy patient is lined by normal mucosa. The created sinus cavity after a total maxillectomy is lined by a split-thickness skin graft. In both cases, after the 6- to 8-week postoperative interval, nearly all of the edema and hemorrhage have subsided, and a baseline scan should be performed. This scan maps the patient's new anatomy and establishes the contour and thickness of the postoperative mucosal surfaces. The normal postoperative mucosa is smooth and moderately thin. Any localized

area of soft-tissue nodularity or mucosal-submucosal thickening must be suspected of representing recurrent tumor, until proven otherwise. If such an area develops that was not noted on the baseline scan, the imager should direct the clinician specifically to this site for biopsy (Figs. 4-354 to 4-356). This approach has led to more positive biopsy specimens than obtained with the multiple blind–biopsy technique. The routine postoperative imaging follow-up of patients has also lead to identification of small, early recurrences that were overlooked on routine clinical follow-up.[14]

Extensive Nasoethmoid Surgery

The lateral rhinotomy provides access to the entire nasal cavity and the maxillary, ethmoid, and sphenoid sinuses. Modifications and extensions of this approach can be used to include access to the frontal sinuses. The typical incision extends from just below the medial end of one eyebrow, caudally between the nasal dorsum and medial canthus of the eye, down the nasofacial crease, and along the nasal alar rim. The incision is then extended down the upper lip if necessary.[15] The nose is turned to the side, thereby exposing the pyriform aperture. This procedure gives access to the entire lateral nasal wall and nasal septum. Usually removed at surgery are the medial antral wall, the ethmoid cells, and the inferior and middle turbinates. The anterior sphenoid wall can be resected via this procedure, and the operation can be extended to include the entire nasal septum and contralateral nasal cavity structures, resulting in a total rhinotomy. In general the operation of choice for a unilateral nasal tumor is a medial maxillectomy with a lateral rhinotomy and ethmoidectomy. Despite the extent of the resection, the cosmetic and functional results are excellent. Regarding patient follow-up, as in the postmaxillectomy patients, the same general imaging rules of suspecting tumor at sites of soft-tissue nodularity and mucosal thickening apply (Figs. 4-357, 4-360).

Craniofacial Resection

This large operation is reserved for patients with tumors of the superior nasal cavity, ethmoid sinuses, frontal sinuses, anterior sphenoid sinuses, and orbits. The operation essentially combines a frontal craniotomy with resection of the midportion of the floor of the anterior cranial fossa, with an extended lateral rhinotomy. The surgery is often performed by a skull-base team comprised of a neurosurgeon and an otolaryngologist. Initially, one of several types of frontal or bifrontal craniotomies are performed, the frontal lobes are elevated, and any tumor extension into the brain is resected. The bone and dura are then incised and the typical resection includes the posterior wall of the frontal sinuses, the cribriform plates, both foveae ethmoidalis, and as much of the medial orbital roof as is necessary to obtain a margin around the tumor. The posterior incision runs along the posterior roof of the sphenoidal sinus. An extended lateral rhinotomy that includes the ethmoid sinuses and medial orbital wall, the nasal septum, and if necessary a portion of the medial orbital roof or the medial maxilla is then performed. Once

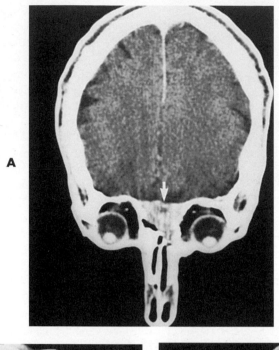

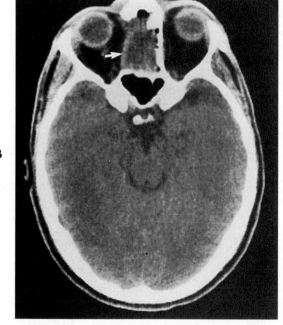

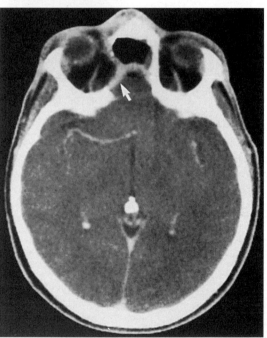

FIG. 4-363 **A,** Coronal contrast CT scan on a patient who has had a craniofacial resection. The fascial and muscle graft and the dural enhancement are seen *(arrow),* filling the surgical defect in the floor of the anterior cranial fossa. The graft hangs down into the postoperative nasoethmoidal cavity. **B,** Axial CT scan shows a soft-tissue mass *(arrow)* in the postoperative upper nasoethmoid cavity. This is the fascial-muscle graft of an osteoplastic flap as it prolapses slightly below the level of the anterior skull base. **C,** Axial contrast CT scan shows dural and granulation tissue enhancement *(arrow)* just below the level of the fascial-muscle graft in a patient who has had a craniofacial resection. The air anteriorly is actually in the upper postoperative nasoethmoid cavity.

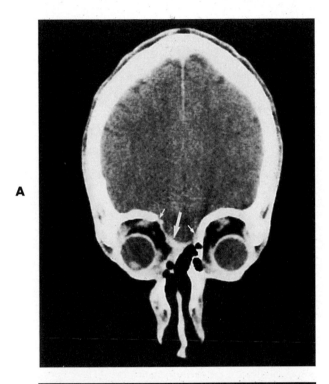

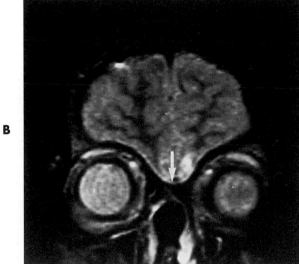

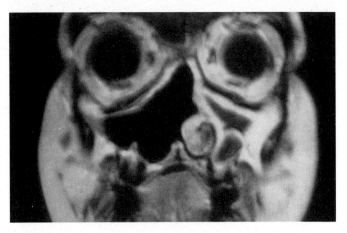

FIG. 4-365   Coronal T1W postcontrast fat-suppressed MR scan shows a patient's status post a craniofacial resection. The mucosa lining the postoperative nasal cavity and the right maxillectomy cavity is smooth and normal. There is a sinusitis with entrapped secretions in the left antrum. The graft in the floor of the anterior cranial fossa enhances minimally. If not careful, one may overlook the extent of the removed bone, especially in the skull base.

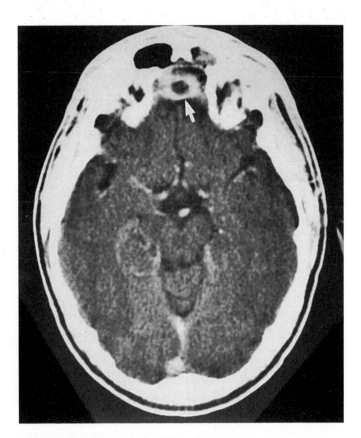

FIG. 4-364   **A,** Coronal contrast CT scan shows fascial-muscle-dural enhancement *(large arrow)* and margins of the bony resection *(small arrows)* in this patient who has had craniofacial resection. **B,** Coronal T2W MRI scan shows same region as in **A.** The fibrosed graft *(arrow)* cannot be clearly delineated from the adjacent intact bone.

FIG. 4-366   Axial contrast CT scan shows a ring-enhancing mass *(arrow)* just cranial to the fascial-muscle graft in a patient who has had a craniofacial resection. Postoperative abscess.

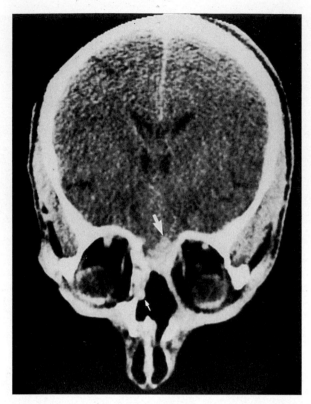

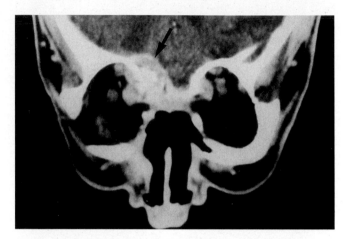

FIG. 4-367   Coronal contrast CT on patient who has had a craniofacial resection. The upper fascial-muscle graft contour is nodular
(arrow). This should raise the suspicion of an early tumor recurrence
(compare with Figs. 4-363, *A* and 4-364, *A*). Recurrent tumor.

FIG. 4-368   Coronal CT scan on a patient's status post a craniofacial resection. There is a soft-tissue mass *(arrow)* along the graft
margin in the floor of the anterior cranial fossa. The mass has also
invaded the right orbit. Recurrent adenocarcinoma.

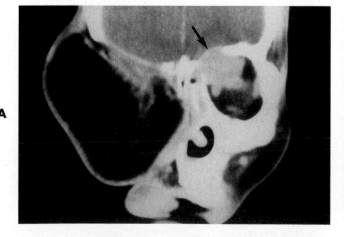

A

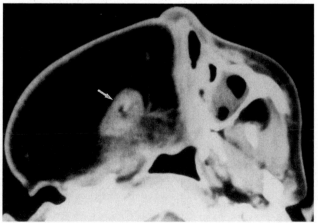

B

FIG. 4-369   Coronal (**A**) and axial (**B**) CT scans on a patient who has had multiple recurrences of
rhabdomyosarcoma, after chemotherapy, irradiation, and numerous operations. Finally a large
myocutaneous graft was used to replace her entire right facial region. The bulk of this graft makes
clinical detection of a recurrence within it extremely difficult. Imaging shows the muscle *(arrow* in
B) within the graft and no evidence of a graft recurrence. However, a recurrence is now present on
the left side *(large arrow* in **A**).

the entire specimen has free margins, the surgeons proceed with an en bloc extirpation. An anterior dural flap and a temporalis free musculofascial graft are used to close and support the cranial floor defect, and the lateral rhinotomy is closed separately (Fig. 4-361).[2,16,17]

Postoperative CT scans contain several areas that may cause diagnostic difficulties. First the anterior dura adjacent to the frontal osteotomy becomes thickened and enhances on contrast studies. This appearance may persist indefinitely and relates to a low-grade reactive process that obliterates the dural spaces (Fig. 4-362). Second the musculofascial flap that supports the central region of the floor of the anterior cranial fossa can bulge slightly downward into the upper postoperative nasoethmoid cavity (Fig. 4-363). This can simulate a tumor mass on axial CT scans and MRI but usually can be identified as representing the graft region on coronal studies. This is especially true during the period before the free flap becomes completely fibrosed, usually between 2 to 8 months after the surgery. Although the CT appearance is not effectively altered once the flap is completely fibrosed, the MRI findings are changed. The initial intermediate T1W and high (inflammatory) T2W signal intensities are gradually replaced by low signal intensities or signal voids on all imaging sequences. This change corresponds to the graft being replaced by scar. The thickness of the fibrosed graft may occasionally be sufficiently similar to

that of the remaining bony floor of the adjacent anterior cranial fossa that on coronal MR images the radiologist may not detect that bone has been removed (Fig. 4-364). Only the altered contour of the bony floor of the anterior cranial fossa (absent crista galli) may signify that the surgery included the bone in this region (Fig. 4-365). Such bone defects are seen easily on coronal CT. Any nodularity along the cranial or nasal margin of the graft or postoperative sinonasal cavity must be suspected of representing tumor. Progressive thickening of the graft or an upward convexity along the cranial margin of the graft are possible signs of tumor recurrence. Unfortuneately, a vascularized scar tissue develops postoperatively that has similar imaging findings to recurrent tumor on both CT and MRI, with or without contrast. Thus, tumor recurrence in these patients is better detected by a change in the mucosal or graft surface contour or thickness.[2] In the more radical surgical cases, it is especially helpful to compare studies with a baseline examination. Any alteration from these initial postoperative CT and MRI appearances should raise the possibility of a postoperative infection or tumor recurrence (Figs. 4-366 to 4-368).

Although technically large graft replacements of the facial area can be performed, the cure rate of such major surgery is often disappointing. Tumor recurrences can occur either deep within the graft or adjacent to the surgical bed (Fig. 4-369).

References

1. Som PM, Lawson W, Biller HF et al. Ethmoid sinus disease: CT evaluation in 400 cases. II. Postoperative findings. Radiology 1986; 159:599-604.
2. Som PM, Lawson W, Biller HF et al. Ethmoid sinus disease: CT evaluation in 400 cases. III. Craniofacial resection. Radiology 1986; 159:605-609.
3. Naumann HH, Buckingham RA. Head and neck surgery: indications, techniques, pitfalls. Vol 1. Face and facial skull. Philadelphia, Pa: WB Saunders Co, 1980; 173-462.
4. Som PM, Urken ML, Biller H et al. Imaging the postoperative neck. Radiology 1993; 187:593-603.
5. Som PM, Shapiro MD, Biller HF et al. Sinonasal tumors and inflammatory tissues: differentiation with MR. Radiology 1988; 167:803-808.
6. Ballantyne JC, Harrison DFN, eds. Operative surgery: nose and throat. London, England: Butterworth Publishers, 1986; 1-177.
7. Urken ML, Som PM, Lawson W et al.

The abnormally large frontal sinus. I. A practical method for its determination based upon an analysis of 100 normal patients. Laryngoscope 1987; 97:602-605.
8. Som PM, Shugar JMA. The CT classification of ethmoid mucoceles. JCAT 1980; 4:199-203.
9. Unger JM, Dennison BF, Duncavage JA et al. The radiological appearance of the post Caldwell-Luc maxillary sinus. Clin Radiol 1986; 37:77-81.
10. Johnson DM, Hopkins RJ, Hanafee WN et al. The unprotected parasphenoidal carotid artery studied by high-resolution computed tomography. Radiology 1985; 155:137-141.
11. Pedersen RA, Troost BT, Schramm VL. Carotid-cavernous sinus fistula after external ethmoid-sphenoid surgery. Arch Otolaryngol 1981; 107:307-309.
12. Yanagisawa E, Smith AW. Normal radiographic anatomy of the paranasal sinuses. Otolaryngol Clin North Am 1973; 6:429-457.

13. Baredes S, Cho HT, Som ML. Total maxillectomy. In: Blitzer A, Lawson W, Friedman WH, eds. Surgery of the paranasal sinuses. Philadelphia, Pa: WB Saunders Co, 1985; 204-216.
14. Som PM, Shugar JMA, Biller HF. The early detection of antral malignancy in the postmaxillectomy patient. Radiology 1982; 143:509-512.
15. Lawson W, Biller HF. Lateral rhinotomy. In: Blitzer A, Lawson W, Friedman WH, eds. Surgery of the paranasal sinuses. Philadelphia, Pa: WB Saunders Co, 1985; 197-203.
16. Lund VJ, Howard DJ, Lloyd GAS. CT evaluation of paranasal sinus tumors for craniofacial resection. Br J Radiol 1983; 56:439-446.
17. Nuss DW, Janecka IP. Surgery of the anterior and middle cranial base. In: Cummings CW, Fredrickson JM, Harker LA et al. Otolaryngology-head and neck surgery. 2nd Edition. Vol 4. St. Louis, Mo: Mosby, 1993; 3300-3337.

PART II

Mandible and Temporomandibular Joints

5

Mandible: Anatomy, Cysts, Tumors, and Nontumorous Lesions

Alfred L. Weber
Steven J. Scrivani

SECTION ONE
NORMAL ANATOMY

The mandible is a tubular structure formed by dense cortical bone that is filled with trabecular bone and bone marrow. The mandible is bilaterally symmetric and has a horseshoe configuration when viewed axially. When viewed from the side, it is L-shaped with a horizontal body and a vertical ascending ramus; posteriorly, where the body and ascending ramus join is the mandibular angle. The body is capped by the alveolar process, which contains the tooth sockets. Cranially the ascending ramus ends posteriorly in the condyle and anteriorly in the coronoid process. The condyle and coronoid process are separated by the mandibular or signoid notch. The condyle is further subdivided into head and neck portions. The lateral pterygoid muscle inserts anteriorly on the neck, and the temporalis muscle inserts anteriorly on the coronoid process. Anteriorly, on each side of the outer body of the mandible near the level of the first premolar tooth, is the mental foramen, which contains the mental nerves and vessels. The portion of the mandible between the mental foramina is referred to as the mandibular symphysis. The midline mental protuberance and the two mental tubercles on either side are all situated along the caudal anterior border of the symphysis.

On the inner surface of the middle third of the ascending ramus is the mandibular foramen, which is the origin of the mandibular canal. The canal contains the inferior alveolar nerves and vessels. The mylohyoid groove, which contains the mylohyoid nerve and vessels, extends obliquely downward and forward from the mandibular foramen.

On the lingual or inner midline cortex are the genial tubercles for the origins of the geniohyoid and genioglossus muscle. On either side of the lower lingual cortex are the digastric fossae for the origins of the anterior bellies of the digastric muscles. Also located along the lingual cortex on either side, at the level of the tooth sockets, is the mylohyoid line for the attachment of the mylohyoid muscles. The angle and ascending ramus of the mandible serve as the main insertion of the muscles of mastication. The masseter muscle inserts on the outer cortex of the coronoid process, ramus, and angle of the mandible; the medial pterygoid inserts on the inner surface of the lower ramus and angle, and the temporalis inserts on the anterior coronoid process and ramus.

The mandible has several weak areas that predispose it to fractures. These areas include the level of the mental foramen, the tooth sockets, crypts of impacted teeth, and the condylar neck. The most common areas for fracture are the body and the condylar process, which account for approximately two thirds of all mandibular fractures.

A detailed discussion of the tooth anatomy and the attachments of the teeth to the mandible is given in Chapter 6. Germain to this discussion, it should be noted that there are two sets of teeth (dentition) that develop during life. The first set consists of 20 deciduous teeth that erupt between the ages of 6 and 36 months. There are two incisor, one canine, and two molar deciduous teeth in each quadrant of the mouth. The permanent dentition develops with additional teeth that have no deciduous predecessors. The permanent teeth erupt between the ages of 6 to 21 years and consist of a central incisor, a lateral incisor, one canine, two premolars, and three molars in each quadrant of the mouth, making a total of 32 adult teeth.[1-6]

References

1. Mustoe TM, Thaller SR. General concepts: overview of anatomy and basics of history and physical examination. In: Thaller SR, Montgomery WW. Guide to dental problems for physicians and surgeons, Baltimore, Md: Williams & Wilkins, 1988.
2. Kerr D, Marsh M, Millard HD. Oral diagnosis. St. Louis, Mo: C.V. Mosby Co, 1974.
3. Montgomery WW. Surgery of the upper respiratory system. Vol 2. 2nd Edition. Philadelphia, Pa: Lea & Febiger, 1989; 1-31.
4. Scott JH, Barrington N, Symons B. Introduction to dental anatomy. 7th Edition. London, England: Churchill Livingstone, Inc, 1974.
5. Sicher H, DuBrul EL. Oral anatomy. St. Louis, Mo: C.V. Mosby Co, 1975.
6. Reed GM, Sheppard VF. Basic structures of the head and neck: a programmed instruction in clinical anatomy for dental professionals. Philadelphia, Pa: WB Saunders, 1976.

SECTION TWO
IMAGING

RADIOLOGIC EXAMINATION

Although CT and MRI provide certain detail that the plain films cannot, the best survey examination of the mandible is still the plain film study.[1-8] Radiologic examination of the mandible can be performed on a head unit or on a horizontal radiography table, and intensifying screens are used to achieve bone detail. The film cassette is placed either on the tabletop or in the film holder of the head unit. The standard radiologic evaluation of the mandible includes the posteroanterior (PA) view, the left and right lateral oblique views, and the lateral view. When indicated, these views can be supplemented by plain films of the temporomandibular joints (TMJ), panoramic radiographs, and intraoral dental views.

Posteroanterior View

The PA view (Fig. 5-1) provides a frontal view of the ascending ramus, angle, and body of the mandible. Because of the superimposition of the cervical spine, the symphysis of the mandible is poorly seen. Depending on the area of interest, this can be partially circumvented by turning the patient's head slightly to the left or right. The PA view is obtained with the patient's forehead and nose on the cassette. The sagittal plane of the head is perpendicular to the plane of the cassette, and the cental ray is perpendicular to the cassette.

Lateral Oblique View

The lateral oblique view (Fig. 5-2) is the most commonly employed and the most useful of the conventional projections. It is obtained by placing a 5 × 7 inch film cassette at the side of the lower jaw. The tube is angled 30° cranially, with the central beam at the angle of the mandible. This view depicts the body of the mandible, alveolus, angle, ascending ramus, sigmoid notch, mandibular condyle, and coronoid process. Portions of the mandibular canal are also well seen.

Lateral View

The lateral view (Fig. 5-3) provides limited information because of the superimposition of both halves of the mandible. The film cassette is placed on the side of the face and jaw. The tube points toward the face from a straight lateral position, and the central beam is focused on the angle of the mandible. This view offers some information regarding any asymmetry of the mandible and the relationship of the skull base and midface to the mandible.

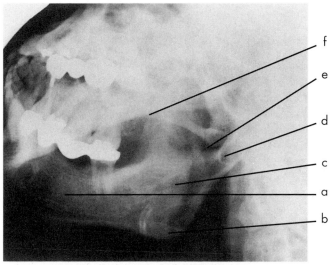

FIG. 5-2 Oblique view of the mandible demonstrates normal anatomy. *a*, Body of mandible; *b*, angle of mandible; *c*, ramus; *d*, mandibular condyle; *e*, sigmoid notch; and *f*, coronoid process.

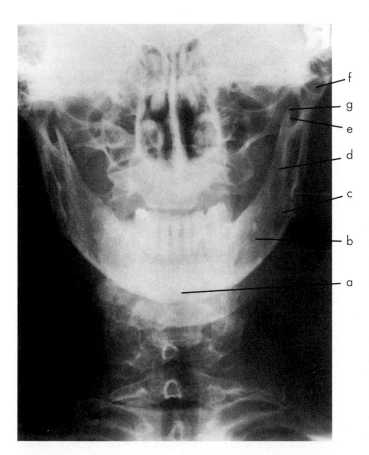

FIG. 5-1 PA view of the mandible demonstrates normal anatomy. *a*, Symphysis of mandible; *b*, body of mandible; *c*, angle of mandible; *d*, ramus; *e*, sigmoid notch; *f*, mandibular condyle; and *g*, coronoid process.

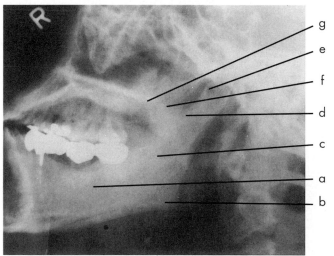

FIG. 5-3 Lateral view of the mandible demonstrates normal anatomy. *a*, Body of mandible; *b*, angle of mandible; *c*, ramus; *d*, neck of mandibular condyle; *e*, mandibular condyle; *f*, sigmoid notch; and *g*, coronoid process.

Panoramic Radiography

The panoramic unit produces a curved planar tomogram of the upper and lower jaws (Fig. 5-4). The image is obtained by a synchronous and reciprocal movement of the x-ray tube and the film cassette around the lower region of the patient's head. This single film provides a survey examination of the mandible, maxilla, lower portions of the nasal fossae, and maxillary antra. The anterior teeth and symphysis are not well seen because of the overlying image of the cervical spine. This study is also regarded as a good survey examination of the TMJs. However, because of distortion, the more lateral the point of interest is from the midline, the less accurate is the study.

INTRAORAL RADIOGRAPHY

Intraoral dental radiography is performed with small dental film packets that contain no screen, high-speed film, and a sheet of lead foil to reduce back scatter. The dental radiography machine consists of a small, lightweight, freely movable tube head with a tube current of 10 to15 mA and a range of 60 to100 kVp. There are three basic intraoral projections: the periapical, the bite wing, and the occlusal. The periapical and bite wing views evaluate the anatomy of the tooth apices and the adjaent bone, and the relationship of the tooth to any pathology constitutes an important diagnostic parameter. The occlusal view depicts the lingual and outer surface of the anterior mandible, can localize stones in the anterior submandibular ducts, and can demonstrate the anterior hard palate.

COMPUTED TOMOGRAPHY

Computed tomography (CT) has become an important diagnostic tool in the assessment of many mandibular lesions, especially malignant tumors both within and adjacent to the mandible.[5-8] The examination is performed as 3 to 5 mm axial contiguous scans in a plane parallel to the inferior mar-

gin of the body of the mandible. The scans should extend from the level of the TMJs to the hyoid bone. Coronal scans should also be obtained from the external auditory canals to the anterior margin of the mandibular symphysis. The scan plane should be oriented perpendicular to the orbitomeatal line (Fig. 5-5). CT shows areas of bone expansion and destruction and is especially useful when evaluating the lingual and outer mandibular cortices. Extraosseous extension of both benign and malignant lesions is also well seen on CT. The use of three dimensional (3D) imaging techniques allow presurgical planning of reconstructive surgery for congenital and acquired deformities of the mandible. This data can be further utilized with computer assisted design-computer assisted manufacturing (CAD-CAM) programs to preoperatively plan and fabricate alloplastic implant materials, and models of the mandible can be made to preoperatively plan the best reconstructive approach.

MAGNETIC RESONANCE IMAGING

Magnetic resonance imaging (MRI) has limited application with most mandibular lesions because they are either osseous in nature or contain calcifications. However, MRI is most useful for evaluating whether or not there is an abnormality of the mandibular marrow, for assessing the presence of tumors in the adjacent soft tissues, and for helping determine whether a mass is cystic or solid. On T1-weighted (T1W) images, fluid-filled cysts usually have a low to intermediate signal intensity and a high T2W signal intensity. Tumors usually have low to intermediate T1W signal intensity, and intermediate T2W signal intensity. Distinction between a cyst and a tumor may be especiallty useful in a young patient who has a hemorrhagic bone cyst, a lesion that usually does not require surgical intervention. Some tumors, including ameloblastomas, can exhibit an aggressive behavior with extraosseous extension. If the tumor is not completely extirpated, recurrence is likely, and MRI nicely visualizes any extraosseous extension before surgery.

The mandible frequently is eroded by carcinomas arising in the gingiva, floor of mouth, and tongue, and this topic is discussed in detail in Chapter 9. MRI is also the modality of choice for evaluating the TMJ, which is discussed in detail in Chapter 7.[9-11]

RADIONUCLIDE SKELETAL SCINTIGRAPHY (BONE SCAN)

Bone scanning often complements other diagnostic procedures when evaluating the bony structures of the maxillofacial skeleton.[12-14] Radionuclide techniques have a greater sensitivity than many other imaging techniques, yet the decreased specificity for abnormal findings in the maxillofacial skeleton is of some concern and poses some limitations. Radiopharmaceuticals are given intravenously in a standard fashion and become localized by absorption to apatite crystals in the bone matrix. The degree of absorption

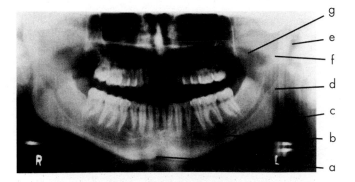

FIG. 5-4 Panorex view of the mandible demonstrates normal anatomy. *a,* Symphysis of mandible; *b,* body of mandible; *c,* angle of mandible; *d,* ramus; *e,* mandibular condyle; *f,* sigmoid notch; and *g,* coronoid process.

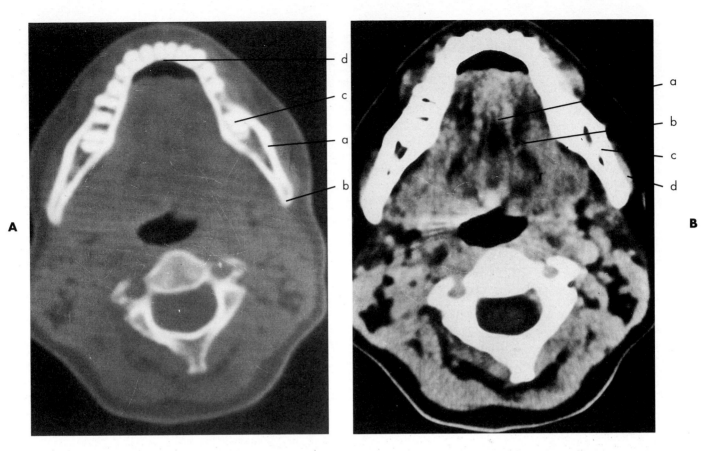

FIG. 5-5 **A,** Axial CT scan through the normal mandible (bone window setting). *a,* Ascending ramus; *b,* angle of mandible; *c,* body of mandible; and *d,* symphysis of mandible. **B,** Axial CT scan of the normal mandible (soft tissue window setting). *a,* Tongue; *b,* floor of mouth; *c,* mandible; and *d,* masseter muscle.

can depend upon the amount of blood flow to the tissue; the osteoblastic cavity; the permeability factors of the vascular membranes of the tissues; and various hormonal, physiologic, and pathophysiologic factors of the tissues being imaged. Planar views are obtained in multiple projections with numerous methods available to magnify and enhance resolution. Single photon emission computed tomography (SPECT) is a particular advance in studying the maxillofacial region because it can provide information in 3D, avoids some of the difficulties of overlapping structures, and has a higher specificity than planar images.

In addition, radionuclide images can be superimposed with other imaging techniques to give more diagnostic information. To gain the full value from the information obtained from radionuclide scintigraphy, there should be careful coordination and cooperation between the radiologist and the clinician. Information regarding the patient's clinical presentation, history, physical examination, and the results of other imaging and appropriate laboratory data are essential to better interpret the scintigraphy and achieve an accurate and meaningful diagnosis.

References

1. Stafne EC, Gibilisco JA. Oral roentgenographic diagnosis. 4th Edition. Philadelphia, Pa: WB Saunders Co, 1975.

2. Weber AL, Easter KM. Cysts and odontogennic tumors of the mandible and maxilla. I. Contemporary Diagnostic Radiology 1982; 5(25):1.

3. Weber AL, Easter KM. Cysts and odontogenic tumors of the mandible and maxilla. II. Contemporary Diagnostic Radiology 1982; 5(26):1.

4. Blaschke DP, Osborn AG. The mandible and teeth. In: Bergeron RT, Osborn AG, Som PM, eds. Head and neck imaging excluding the brain. St. Louis, Mo: Mosby–Year Book, 1984.

5. Weber AL. Radiologic evaluation. In: Thaller SR, Montgomery WW, eds. Guide to dental problems for physicians and surgeons. Baltimore, Md: Williams & Wilkins, 1988.

6. Osborn AG, Hanafee WN, Mancuso AA. Normal and pathologic CT anatomy of the mandible. AJR 1982; 139(3):555-559.

7. Hanafee WN, Mancuso AA. Pictorial essay: normal and pathologic CT anatomy of the mandible. AJR 1982; 139:555-559.

8. Seldin EB. Radiology of the mandible. In: Taveras JM, Ferrucci JT, eds. Radiology: diagnosis, imaging, intervention. Vol 3. Philadelphia, Pa: JB Lippincott Co, 1987.

9. Schellhas KP, Wilkes CH. Temporomandibular joint inflammation: comparison of fast scanning with T1- and T2-weighted imaging techniques. AJR 1989; 153:93-98.

10. Tasaki M, Westesson P-L. Temporomandibular joint: diagnostic accuracy with sagittal and coronal MR images. Radiology 1993; 186:723-729.

11. Westesson P-L, Katzberg RW, Tallents RH, et al. CT and MRI of the tempomandibular joint: comparison with autopsy specimens. AJR 1987; 148:1165-1171.

12. Krasnow AZ, Collier BD, Kneeland JB, et al. Comparison of high resolution MRI and SPECT bone scintigraphy for noninvasive imaging of the temporomandibular joint. J Nucl Med 1987; 28:1268-1274.

13. Cisneros GJ, Kaban LB. Computerized skeletal scintigraphy in assessment of mandibular asymmetry. J Oral Maxillofac Surg 1984; 42:513-520.

14. O'Mara RE. Scintigraphy of the facial skeleton. In: Westesson P-L. Contemporary maxillofacial imaging. Oral and Maxillofacial Surgery Clinics of North America 1992; 51-60.

SECTION THREE
PATHOLOGY

The proper management of pathologic lesions of the mandible is predicated on a number of factors, not the least of which is making an accurate diagnosis. A logical sequence of diagnostic studies should be performed to better guide management. There should be proper clinical evaluation, including whenever possible a tissue diagnosis and precise imaging of the involved area. Imaging in at least two planes is necessary to properly analyze the lesion and adjacent tissues.

CYSTS
Definition and Classification

A cyst is pathologically characterized as an epithelial lined cavity that usually contains fluid or semisolid material.[1] In most cases microscopic examination of the lining tissue, as well as the clinical and radiographic findings, are necessary to achieve a diagnosis.

Cysts frequently occur in the jaw, and they appear radiographically as unilocular or multilocular lucent areas of varying size and definition. Cysts of the mandible can come to clinical attention by destroying bone and weakening the mandible, by causing functional disturbances, or by the effects of secondary cyst infection. Delayed tooth eruption and displacement and resorption of tooth roots are often seen on imaging. A cyst's relationship to a tooth is an important differential diagnostic feature. On the basis of development, cysts have been subdivided into odontogenic and nonodontogenic types.

Odontogenic cysts arise from tooth derivatives.[2] Histologic analysis of the epithelial layers, the presence of cyst calcification, and the clinical findings allow further subdivision. The term residual cyst is frequently applied to any cyst (specifically to a periodontal apical cyst) that remains or develops after surgical removal of a tooth.

Nonodontogenic cysts are developmental in origin. The fissural variety, as the name implies, arise along lines of fusion of the various bones and embryonic processes, and they are classified according to their anatomic location.

Developmental cysts include other cyst types derived from embryologic structures (e.g., dermoid cysts) and cysts arising from other causes (e.g., solitary bone cysts, Stafne cysts, and aneurysmal bone cysts).

Odontogenic Cysts
Dentigerous (Follicular) Cysts

After the radicular, or periodontal cysts, which are discussed in the next section, the dentigerous cyst is the most common odontogenic cyst.[3,4] Most dentigerous cysts become evident during the third and fourth decades of life, and most (75%) are located in the mandible. They have been noted to occur in association with the crown of an unerupted tooth, and in the usual case the tooth crown projects into the lumen of the cystic cavity. However, with continued cyst growth, only a limited portion of the tooth may be attached to the cyst surface (Fig. 5-6). Multiple cysts may occur.

Dentigerous cysts vary greatly in size, ranging from less than 2 cm in diameter to cysts that cause massive expansion of the jaw. They may cause displacement of teeth, but apical resorption of tooth structures is uncommon. Fractures and superimposed infection may develop in the cyst. Dentigerous cysts do not demonstrate an extracystic soft-tissue mass as seen in ameloblastomas, but ameloblastomas, mucoepidermoid tumors, and carcinomas may develop on the wall of the cyst.

A mandibular dentigerous cyst appears as a circumscribed, unilocular area of osteolysis that incorporates the crown of a tooth (Fig. 5-7). The adjacent teeth are displaced, and uncommonly they may be partly eroded. Dentigerous cysts in the maxilla often extend into the antrum, displacing and remodeling the bony sinus wall. Large cysts may project into the nasal cavity or infratemporal fossa and may elevate the floor of the orbit. On MRI the contents of the cyst show a high signal intensity on T2W images and low to intermediate signal intensity on T1W images. The tooth itself is an area of signal void.

Periodontal (Radicular) Cysts

Periodontal cysts can be further classified as periapical (radicular) or lateral cysts.[5] Radicular cysts are by far the most common odontogenic cyst. They may form at any time during life, although the peak incidence is in patients between 30 and 50 years of age; there is no sex predilection. This cyst is most often associated with carious teeth, and it may originate from a persistent periapical granuloma. Most of these cysts are discovered incidentally on radiography,

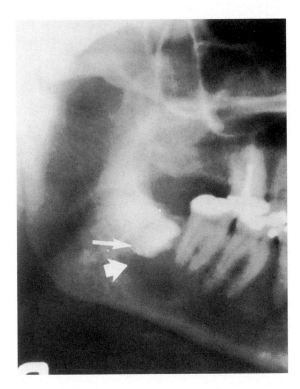

FIG. 5-6 Dentigerous cyst. Panorex view of the mandible shows a sharply marginated, oval-shaped cyst in the body of the right mandible *(short arrow)*. The crown of the impacted third molar tooth is incorporated into the posterior portion of the cyst *(long arrow)*.

but expansion of the cyst may cause a clinically noticeable displacement of teeth, and swelling and pain may occur when the cyst enlarges or becomes secondarily infected.

Radiographically a radicular cyst is a well-circumscribed radiolucency arising from the apex of the tooth and bounded by a thin rim of cortical bone (Fig. 5-8); large lesions may expand the cortical plates. A radicular cyst can displace tooth structures and may cause slight root resorption. If the cyst occurs in the maxilla, extension into the maxillary sinus may be observed (Fig. 5-9). Radiographically, radicular cysts cannot be differentiated from periapical granulomas, which usually are less than 1.6 cm in diameter.

Odontogenic Keratocysts

Odontogenic keratocysts account for 3% to 11% of all jaw cysts, and they occur twice as often in the mandible as the maxilla.[6,8] These cysts are found in patients of all ages, but the peak incidence is in patients in the second and third decades of life. This cyst has been classified as a separate type of bone cyst because of its aggressive biologic behavior and histologic structure. Histologically the cysts are lined by a stratified, keratinizing, squamous epithelium. The epithelium is characteristically thin, six to eight cell layers, and the keratinization is usually parakeratinizing. The interface between the epithelium and the connective tissue is flat, without rete ridge formation. The basal layer is prominent, with palisading cells containing darkly staining and enlarged nuclei. Daughter cysts or microcysts are often observed microscopically. The recurrence rate has been variously reported as being between 20% and 60%. This high recurrence rate is thought to be the result of their specific abnormal biology, and many varied hypotheses have been reported in an attempt to solve this problem.

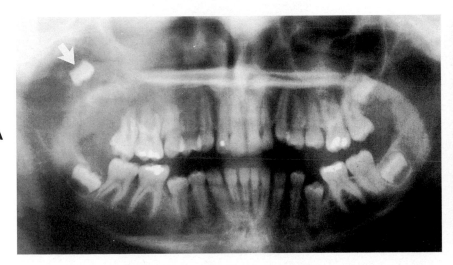
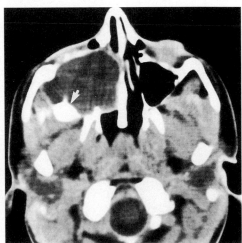

A

B

FIG. 5-7 Dentigerous cyst. **A,** Panorex view of the mandible and maxilla shows a displaced tooth in the upper lateral aspect of the right maxilla *(arrow)*. There is a poorly defined expansile lesion in the same region. **B,** Axial CT demonstrates an expansile cystic lesion within the right antral cavity with extension into the right nasal cavity and infratemporal fossa. Note a localized density at the posterior margin of this cyst, representing a tooth that is incorporated into the cyst *(arrow)*.

The diagnosis depends on the cyst's microscopic features and is independent of its location and radiographic appearance. This cyst is a radiolucent lesion that is often multiloculated, has a smooth or scalloped border (Fig. 5-10), is characteristically located in the body and ramus of the mandible, and often occurs in conjunction with an impacted tooth (Fig. 5-11).

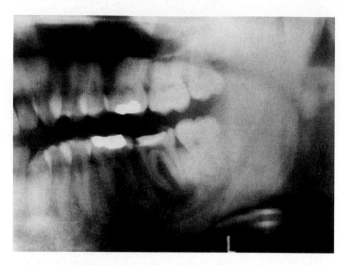

FIG. 5-8   Radicular cyst of left mandibular second molar tooth. Panorex view of the mandible demonstrates a cystic, well-defined lesion around the apices of the lower left mandibular tooth. Note sclerosis around the cyst and adjacent mandibular teeth, which is secondary to chronic osteitis.

Basal Cell Nevus Syndrome

Basal cell nevus syndrome is a genetic disorder, inherited as an autosomal dominant trait with variable penetrance and expressivity.[9,10] The syndrome becomes apparent between 5 and 10 years of age; there is no sex predilection, and many patients with this syndrome have slight mental retardation. The syndrome consists of a number of features that are classically grouped into five categories: cutaneous, skeletal, ophthalmologic, neurologic, and sexual. Among the most common features are multiple cysts of the jaw, multiple basal cell carcinomas, skeletal abnormalities, and ectopic calcifications. At least two of these findings must be present to establish a diagnosis.

The multiple jaw cysts develop early in childhood; they may be either unilocular or multilocular and often prove to be keratocysts varying in size from 1 mm to several centimeters (Fig. 5-12). Many investigators have suggested that the odontogenic keratocysts in basal cell nevus syndrome are histologically and biologically different from the solitary type of odontogenic keratocysts not associated with this syndrome. However, this concept is not universally agreed upon, and many investigators feel that those cysts associated with this syndrome are just larger, multilocular, and tend to have more frequent satellite microcysts that may account for their clinical behavior. The nevoid basal cell carcinomas appear later than the cysts, usually before 30 years of age, and they are found especially on the face, trunk, neck, and arms. The most common skeletal abnormalities are bifid ribs, synostosis of ribs, kyphoscoliosis, vertebral fusion,

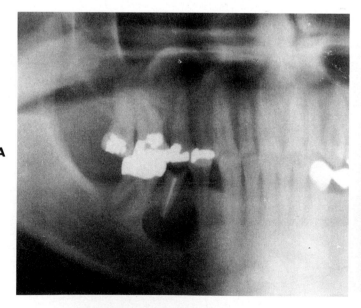
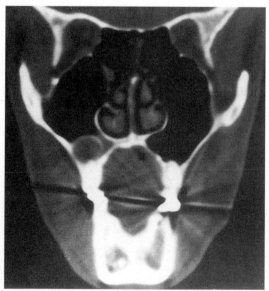

A   B

FIG. 5-9   Radicular cyst. **A,** Panorex view of the mandible and maxilla shows a radicular cyst around the apex of the right second premolar tooth within the mandible and around the apex of the upper right second premolar tooth. The upper radicular cyst bulges into the right antral cavity. **B,** Coronal CT of the paranasal sinuses shows the maxillary radicular cyst projecting into the floor of the right antrum.

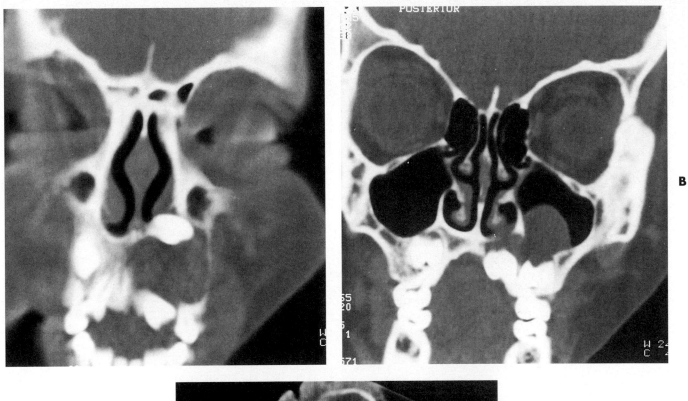

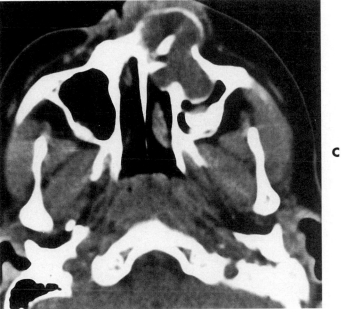

FIG. 5-10   Keratocyst of the left maxilla. **A,** Coronal CT (bone window setting) demonstrates an expansile lesion in the left maxilla causing displacement of teeth superiorly and inferiorly. **B,** Coronal CT demonstrates a cystic lesion extending into the left maxilla. **C,** Axial CT (soft-tissue window setting) demonstrates the expansile cyst in the left maxilla, anterior portion of the left nasal cavity, and adjacent maxillary antrum. Note the low attenuation of the cyst and the tooth remnants at the medial aspect of the cyst.

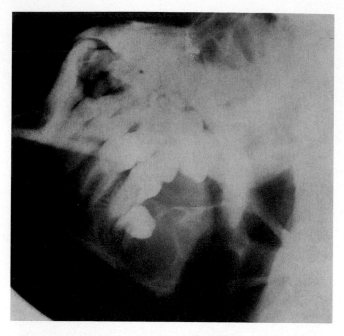

FIG. 5-11   Keratocyst. Oblique view of the mandible shows a multiloculated cyst in the posterior body of the mandible, angle of the mandible, and ramus. The third molar tooth is incorporated into the anterior part of the cyst. There is encroachment upon the posterior aspect of the second molar tooth. Note that there is also expansion with thinning of the anterior wall of the ascending ramus.

mild ocular hypertelorism, prognathism, polydactyly, and frontal and temporoparietal bossing. The ectopic calcifications occur most frequently in the falx cerebri and other areas of the dura.

The surgical management of odontogenic keratocysts demands special attention because of the aggressive biologic behavior of these benign lesions. Surgical treatment over the years has included decompression and marsupialization, enucleation and curettage, and local and en block resection and reconstruction. Various adjuvant methods of treatment have been used to decrease the potential for recurrence or to deal with a recurrence. These include extraction of teeth in continuity with the cyst, excision of overlying mucosa, and treatment of the surrounding bone with peripheral ostectomy, chemical cautery, or cryosurgery. Many of these lesions, especially recurrences, are treated with some combination of these surgical techniques. No matter what management strategy is employed nor what the surgical outcome, these patients must be closely followed for many years.

Nonodontogenic Cysts
Fissural Cysts

A nasopalatine duct cyst (incisive canal cyst) is a nonodontogenic developmental cyst in the incisive canal near the anterior palatine papilla.[11,12] The cysts probably arise from epithelial remnants in the incisive canal. The cysts can occur at any age but are most frequently found in patients in the

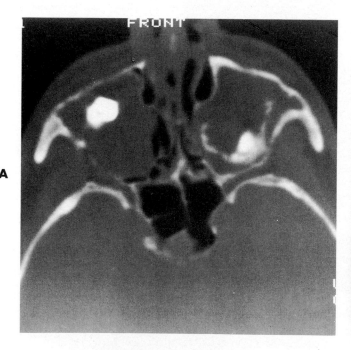

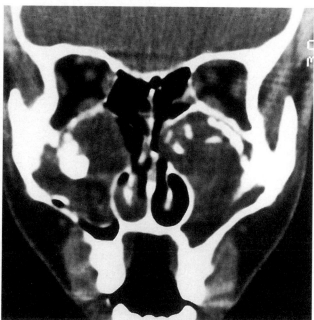

A

B

FIG. 5-12   Bilateral maxillary keratocysts in a patient with the basal cell nevus syndrome. **A,** Axial CT (bone window setting) through the maxillary antra shows slightly expansile lesions in both antral cavities reflected by a cystic bony rim in the left antral cavity and some lateral expansion and thinning of the right antral bone. Note displaced teeth on the left and right within the cystic lesions. **B,** Coronal CT (soft-tissue window setting) demonstrates bilateral cystic lesions in the maxillary antra with part of a thin rim of surrounding bone seen in the left antrum. Note the displaced tooth in the upper part of the right antral cavity and low attenuation of the cyst contents.

fourth and sixth decades of life, with no sex predilection. These cysts are usually asymptomatic, but some patients note swelling in the palate, especially when the cyst is primarily in the incisive papilla. Occasionally, patients notice a discharge of mucoid material and a salty taste through what are thought to be remnants of embryonic ductal structures on the palate.

Many of these cysts are small, found on routine radiographic surveys. It may be difficult on imaging to differentiate between an enlarged incisive fossa and an incisive canal cyst. The incisive canal cyst is always located at or close to the midline and usually is round or ovoid, although it may be heart-shaped (Fig. 5-13). A condensed rim of cortical bone is often seen along the periphery, and the lesion may displace the roots of the central incisors.

A globulomaxillary cyst is a cyst located between the lateral incisor and the canine tooth, at the site that corresponds to a developmental suture between the lateral nasal and maxillary processes.[13,14] Today there is evidence that these fissural cysts are probably of odontogenic origin from epithelial remnants. Such a cyst usually extends toward the crest of the alveolar ridge and may cause the roots of the adjacent teeth to diverge. The cyst usually assumes a pear shape as it increases in size (Fig. 5-14). If a globulomaxillary cyst extends over the apex of the incisor or canine tooth (or both), the vitality of these teeth must be determined to help differentiate a globulomaxillary cyst from a radicular cyst. These cysts are generally treated with simple enucleation, taking care not to damage any nearby vital functional structures. The resulting bony defect usually heals with new

bone over several months, and further reconstructive intervention is rarely needed.

Solitary, Simple, or Hemorrhagic Bone Cysts

Solitary, simple, or hemorrhagic bone cysts are seen more frequently in men than in women, and they usually are found in young people, with 70% occurring in patients in their second decade of life.[15,16] The etiologic factors of this lesion are usually obscure. Yet, whether this cyst results from an injury unassociated with a fracture that causes an intramedullary hematoma that disintegrates and produces the cyst within the bone, aseptic necrosis, or degeneration of an earlier benign tumor the end result appears to be the same. A hemorrhagic bone cyst is a unilocular cavity that can be empty or partly filled with a clear or sanguineous fluid. The cyst lining consists of a loose vascular connective tissue that may have areas of recent or old hemorrhage.

Because these cysts often are asymptomatic, most are discovered incidentally during examination of the teeth. It is believed that some of these solitary bone cysts regress spontaneously. These lesions are most commonly located in the mandibular marrow space that extends posteriorly from the premolar region. Less often they may occur in the incisor area of the mandible. Radiographically these cysts are slightly irregular in shape and size and have poorly defined borders. The outline of the cyst between the roots of the teeth has a scalloped appearance (Fig. 5-15). Larger cysts may extend into the interdental space and the ramus, and the mandible may be slightly expanded. The radiographic features are not sufficiently specific to be diagnostic.

These lesions are usually surgically investigated with a single diagnostic and therapeutic procedure. Using a minimally invasive surgical technique, the surgeon can evaluate the lesion and sample tissue; healing usually takes place with reossification.

Aneurysmal Bone Cysts

These lesions are far more common in children than in adults, in females than in males, and in the mandible than in the maxilla or zygoma.[17-20] They usually present with a

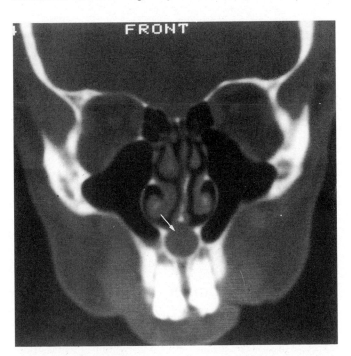

FIG. 5-13 Nasopalatine cyst. Coronal CT (bone window setting) shows a cyst with bony expansion in the nasopalatine duct between the upper central incisor teeth. There is a slight bulge into the adjacent nasal cavity.

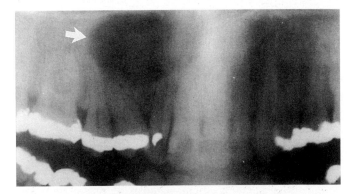

FIG. 5-14 Globulomaxillary cyst. Panorex view shows a cystic structure *(arrow)* in the right maxilla causing divergence of the roots of the lateral incisor and canine tooth.

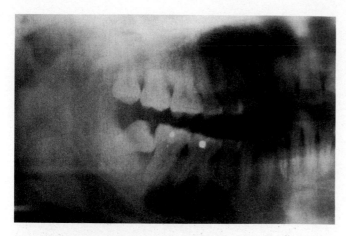

FIG. 5-15 Hemorrhagic bone cyst in the body of the right mandible. Panorex view of the mandible shows a sharply defined, oval-shaped cyst around the apices of the molar and premolar teeth of the right mandible.

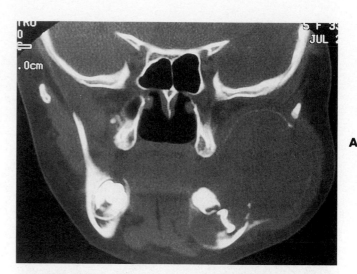

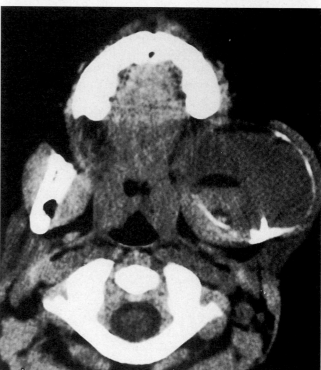

FIG. 5-16 Aneurysmal bone cyst of the left mandible. **A,** Coronal CT through the posterior portion of the mandible shows an expansile lesion in the left mandible. Note the thin bony rim around the cyst and misplacement of teeth in the mandible at the lower aspect of the cyst. **B,** Axial CT through the ascending ramus of the mandible shows a cystic, expansile lesion with several fluid-fluid levels.

rapidly growing swelling that can be markedly disfiguring, and there is usually no pain or paresthesia. There can be spontaneous bleeding from around the teeth or from areas of mucosal trauma. Although there is often a history of prior trauma, these cysts can occur without this history, and they may be associated with a preexistent intraosseous pathologic processes (aneurysmal bone cyst plus). Radiographically these lesions are large, often multiloculated large areas of bone destruction (Fig. 5-16). Histologically they are epithelial-lined, blood-filled cavities with accumulations of immature connective tissue, multinucleated giant cells, areas of osteoid, and inflammatory cells. Numerous approaches have been used to treat these lesions, including interventional radiologic procedures, low-dose radiation therapy, and multiple types of surgical enucleation and resection. More recently these and other types of giant cell lesions have been treated with calcitonin, interferon, and direct intralesional steroid injections.

Static Bone Cavities (Stafne Cysts)

A Stafne cyst appears as an elliptical, ovoid, or round radiolucency usually located in the posterior mandible, often near the angle of the mandible below the mandibular canal (Fig. 5-17). Stafne cysts occur more frequently in men than in women and have been reported in patients from 20 to 70 years of age (most are discovered by 50 years of age). These asymptomatic lesions are usually detected incidentally on routine radiographs of the mandible.[21] The bone defect is open on the lingual surface of the mandible, and submandibular salivary gland tissue has been demonstrated within the bone cavity of some Stafne cysts. Bilateral lesions have been described.

Radiographically the radiolucency has a well-defined border, often showing slight sclerosis at the margin, and varying in size from 1 to 2 cm. Diagnostic evaluation is usually needed to rule out other benign, malignant, or metastatic disease, which can present similarly in this location.

BENIGN ODONTOGENIC TUMORS

Odontogenic tumors result from an abnormal proliferation of the cells and tissues involved in odontogenesis.[22,23] They represent a diverse group of lesions, which are classified according to the origin of the various layers of tooth development. Based on the histologic findings, these tumors have been divided into epithelial, mesodermal, and mixed tissue tumors of odontogenic origin. The radiographic appearance

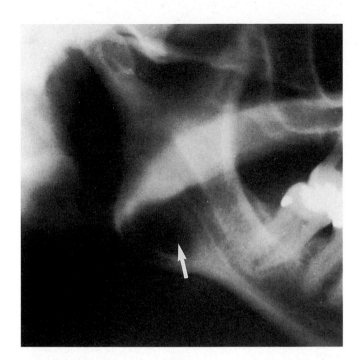

FIG. 5-17 Static bone cavity (Stafne cyst). Oblique view of the mandible shows an oval-shaped cavity in the angle of the mandible *(arrow)* below the mandibular canal.

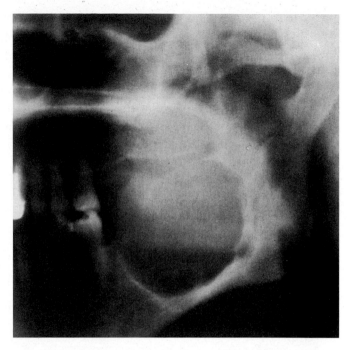

FIG. 5-18 Ameloblastoma. Oblique view of the mandible shows a large cystic lesion in the body and ramus of the mandible with attentuation and loss of bone superiorly. The lesion has broken through the upper part of the mandible.

of odontogenic tumors varies, and many of them cannot be differentiated from the cysts previously described.

Ameloblastomas

An ameloblastoma is a benign epithelial odontogenic tumor thought to arise from ameloblasts.[24-26] It is found with about equal frequency in men and women and has a peak incidence in the third and fourth decades of life, with two thirds of cases occurring before 40 years of age. Ameloblastomas account for approximately 18% of odontogenic tumors; 81% are located in the mandible, and the remaining 19% are found in the maxilla. Half of the mandibular lesions are located in the molar regions. An ameloblastoma is a slow-growing, painless mass that may reach a considerable size, and swelling is the most common presenting symptom.

Radiographically an ameloblastoma is radiolucent and either multilocular or unilocular (Fig. 5-18). The unilocular lesions occur most often in the maxilla. The multilocular form often has been described as having a honeycombed or bubblelike appearance, and the loculi may be oval or spherical and vary in size. Ameloblastomas can vary in size from a small cyst confined to the alveolus to a large cyst that causes extensive destruction of the mandible or maxilla. The tumor has a tendency to break through the cortex of the bone, with subsequent tumor extension into the adjacent soft tissues (Figs. 5-19, 5-20). There can be bony expansion of variable degrees, sometimes with a scalloped marginal sclerosis, and there is no periosteal new bone formation. Loss of the lamina dura, erosion of the tooth apex, and displacement of the teeth are also commonly seen.

The biologic behavior of these lesions has been of great interest and debate. Numerous clinical and histopathologic studies have evaluated the several varieties of ameloblastomas in an attempt to relate the clinical picture, histologic pattern, and biologic behavior, allowing more appropriately guided treatment. However, at this time there does not seem to be any good correlation, and the treatment strategies remain predominantly surgical. A variety of approaches have been advocated based on the individual patient. These include curettage and adjuvant treatment of the surrounding soft tissues, wide local excision, and large en block excisions with immediate or staged reconstruction. With recurrent tumors and delayed reconstructions, CT, MRI, and technetium bone scanning can be helpful in evaluating whether a soft tissue mass is a recurrence or fibrous healing.

Calcifying Epithelial Odontogenic Tumors (Pindborg Tumors)

A calcifying epithelial odontogenic tumor is composed of polyhedral epithelial cells in a fibrous stroma that contains acidophilic homogeneous structures that commonly calcify.[27-29] At first diagnosis the average age of a patient is about 40 years, with an age range of 12 to 78 years. There is no sex predilection. Many of these tumors are located in the premolar-molar area of the mandible, and in half of the cases they are associated with the crown of an impacted tooth.

Radiographically the lesion usually is a mixed radiolucent and radiopaque mass that may be unilocular but more often is multilocular (honeycombed). It has poorly defined, irregular borders that reflect its aggressive behavior, which

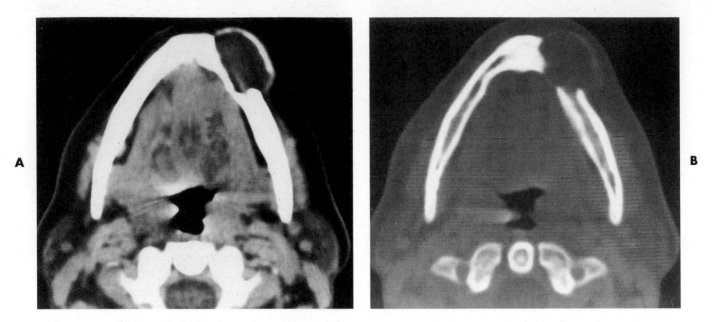

FIG. 5-19 Ameloblastoma. **A,** Axial CT (soft-tissue window setting) shows an expansile lesion in the body of the left mandible and adjacent symphysis with marked lateral expansion. **B,** Axial CT (bone window setting) defines the boundary of this expansile lesion to better advantage. Also, note erosion of the lingual surface of the mandible.

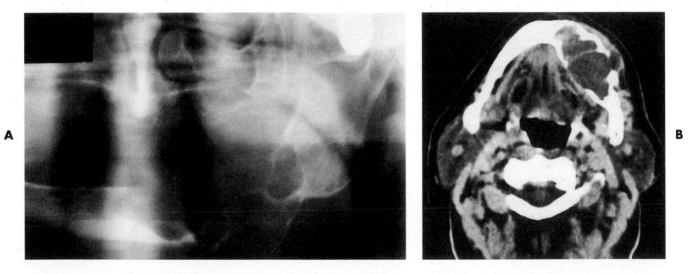

FIG. 5-20 Ameloblastoma. **A,** Panorex view of the mandible shows a multiloculated aggressive lesion in the body and ramus of the mandible with considerable loss of bone. **B,** Axial CT (soft-tissue window setting) shows the expansile lesion in the body and ramus. There is loss of bone medially and laterally. There are low attenuation, slightly septated soft-tissue densities within the lesion. A small component of the tumor has penetrated through the lateral cortex into the adjacent soft tissues.

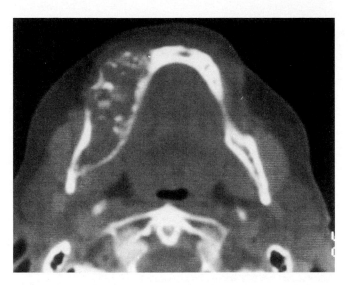

FIG. 5-21 Pindborg tumor. Axial CT (bone window setting) shows marked expansion of the right mandible with loss of bone in the lateral cortex. Multiple calcific densities are noted within the lesion.

is similar to that of the ameloblastoma (Fig. 5-21). Radiopaque densities of varying degrees may be located close to the crown of an impacted tooth. Curettage is the preferred treatment, but recurrence or extensive tumor involvement should be treated by resection.

Odontomas

An odontoma is a benign tumor made up of the various components of teeth (e.g., enamel, dentin, cementum, and pulp). It is also designated as a composite lesion because of the admixture of several types of tissue.[30-33] During its maturation, an odontoma passes through the same stages as a developing tooth, but dentin and enamel are laid down in an abnormal pattern. In the initial stage of development, a radiolucent area develops because of bone resorption by the odontogenic tissues. In the intermediate and late stages, progressive calcification takes place, which is initially characterized by small, speckled calcific densities that eventually form radiopaque masses surrounded by a lucent ring. These tumors may be discovered in any location of the dental arches and are situated between the roots of teeth.

Both forms of odontoma (complex composite and compound composite) are frequently associated with unerupted teeth. It is noteworthy that compound composite odontomas occur most often in the anterior portion of the jaw, whereas complex composite odontomas tend to occur in the posterior jaw. A developing odontoma without calcification or with few calcifications is radiographically difficult to diagnose and usually cannot be differentiated from other similar-appearing lesions.

Complex Composite Odontomas

Complex composite odontomas account for 24% of all odontomas.[31-32] These lesions are composed of dental tissues arranged in a disorderly pattern and bearing no morphologic similarity to normal or rudimentary teeth. Complex composite odontomas most commonly occur in patients aged 10 to 25 years, and males and females are affected equally. The lesion usually is asymptomatic and most frequently is located in the premolar and molar regions in the mandible, although it is sometimes found in the maxilla. Most lesions are small, measuring only a few millimeters, but some may reach a considerable size.

Radiographically these lesions are well-demarcated, radiopaque masses, often with radiating structures. Occasionally the tumor is surrounded by a narrow radiolucent zone, and there usually is a nearby unerupted tooth. The preferred therapeutic treatment is enucleation. Cancellous bone grafting may be appropriate, depending on the size and location of the surgical defect.

Compound Composite Odontomas

Compound composite odontomas consist of dental tissues that have some similarity to a normal tooth, having a more orderly pattern than in complex composite odontomas.[33] The lesion is composed of many toothlike structures, with enamel, dentin, cementum, and pulp arranged as in a normal tooth. The differentiation of teeth varies from case to case, and the number of teeth involved may be surprisingly high.

Most compound composite odontomas (60%) occur in patients in the second and third decades of life, and there is no sex predilection. The tumor frequently is located in the incisor-canine region of the maxilla. It is usually small but may occasionally displace teeth or interfere with their eruption; the lesion is otherwise asymptomatic. Radiographically, several small, rather well-defined, malformed or rudimentary teeth are demonstrated, surrounded by a radiolucent zone that is caused by a fibrous capsule. The teeth contained in a compound composite odontoma are dwarfed and usually distorted with simple roots (Fig. 5-22). Most of these lesions are well encapsulated and easily enucleated, and recurrences are not encountered after enucleation.

Ameloblastic Fibroodontomas

An ameloblastic fibroodontoma is a mixture of ameloblastic tissue and a composite odontoma. It is a rare lesion that can occur at any age but is more prevalent in children, being rare after the age of 13 years. This tumor is more common in the mandible (premolar-molar region) than in the maxilla, and it is always associated with developing teeth. Painless swelling or absence or displacement of teeth are the most common signs leading to its diagnosis.

Radiographically the tumor has a lucent, well-defined margin with a solitary mass or several small radiopaque masses that may resemble miniature teeth (Fig. 5-23). Radiographic differentiation from other odontomas is not possible, and inadequate removal may be followed by a recurrence.

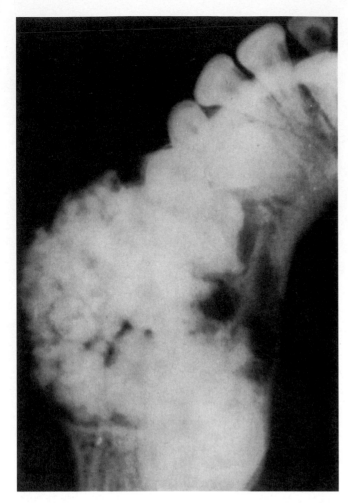

FIG. 5-22 Compound odontoma. Semiaxial view of the mandible shows a calcified lesion arising from the outer cortex of the mandible. The lesion contains multiple malformed teeth. Note the surrounding lucent zone between the expanded cortex and malformed teeth.

Odontogenic Myxomas

An odontogenic myxoma appears to be a true odontogenic tumor, originating from the mesodermal portion of the odontogenic apparatus. This tumor, which is not found in bones outside the jaw, accounts for about 3% to 6% of odontogenic tumors.[34-37] They occur most often in the second and third decades of life, with no sex predilection. The tumor consists of rounded and angular cells lying in an abundant mucoid stroma, and the lesion is painless, locally invasive, and slow growing. If untreated, odontogenic myxomas eventually may cause extensive destruction of bone with marked cortical expansion. The mandible and maxilla are involved with about equal frequency; however, in the mandible the body and ramus are the most commonly affected.

Radiographically, several radiolucent areas of varying size are present, septated by straight or curved bony trabeculae that form triangular-, quadrangular-, or square-shaped compartments (Fig. 5-24). Unilocular cysts have also been described. The radiographic margins of the tumor may be

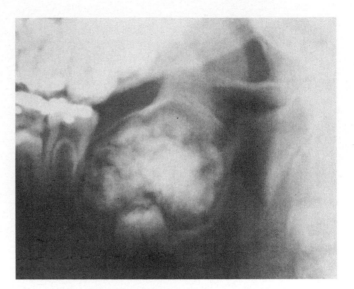

FIG. 5-23 Ameloblastic fibroodontoma. Oblique view of the mandible shows an expansile lesion in the posterior body and ramus of the mandible. Amophous calcific densities are noted within the lesion. There is a radiolucent zone between the calcified mass and the adjacent expanded cortex. Note the impacted third molar tooth, which is incorporated in the inferior part of the lesion.

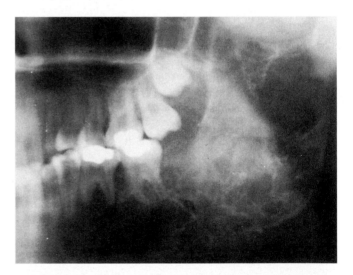

FIG. 5-24 Myxoma of the mandible. Panorex view of the mandible shows multiple small, irregular, lucent areas within the mandible bounded by thickened trabeculae. The lesion more anteriorly demonstrates an ill-defined lucent area beneath the molar teeth. There is extension of this myxoma through the cortex of the mandible, which is best illustrated inferiorly near the angle of the mandible.

well or poorly defined, and the lesion may simulate an ameloblastoma, central giant cell granuloma, or hemangioma. This tumor is benign but very aggressive and rapidly growing. It shows little encapsulation and often extends through bone with a propensity to invade local soft tissues. It may appear to expand in thin layers into and through bone, as well as into the adjacent soft tissues.

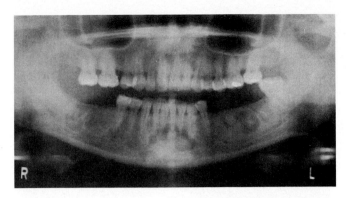

FIG. 5-25 Periapical cemental dysplasia. Panorex view of the mandible shows multiple sclerotic foci within the mandible, especially at the symphysis and body on the left. Some of these sclerotic areas merge imperceptibly with the mandible. Other densities are surrounded by a lucent ring. The radiographic appearance shows the evolution from lucent areas in the early stages, to a mixed stages, and finally sclerotic stage.

Because of its histology and behavior, the treatment of choice has become wide en bloc resection as opposed to simple enucleation. A tumor-free margin must be resected because of the tumor's local invasiveness and its tendency to recur. A recurrence rate of 25% after curettage has been reported.

Cementomas
Periapical Cemental Dysplasias

Periapical cemental dysplasia is a rare lesion that occurs most often in the mandibular region, although in rare cases one may develop in the maxilla.[38-40] It always occurs at the roots of teeth. This lesion is more common in women (average age at diagnosis is 40 years) and among blacks. In almost half of the patients, pain is the initial symptom; other patients may develop a hard swelling that may cause facial asymmetry.

The initial lesion, which is caused by a proliferation of connective tissue from the periodontal membrane, appears as a well-defined radiolucency. However, it subsequently may be transformed into a radiopaque calcified mass. These lesions can be divided radiographically into three stages: (1) a rather well-defined radiolucency at the apex of a tooth (osteolytic stage); (2) a lesion that is partly radiolucent and partly radiopaque with the dense tissue initially central in the lesion (cementoblastic stage); and (3) a lesion that is transformed into a mineralized radiopaque mass surrounded by a narrow radiolucent zone (mature incisive stage) (Fig. 5-25). The involved tooth is normal in color and responds normally to tests of vitality.

Periapical cemental dysplasia does not require treatment unless the lesion becomes infected or other disturbing symptoms occur. The treatment of choice is enucleation, with or without extraction of the involved tooth. No recurrences have been reported.

Cementifying Fibromas

A cementifying fibroma is a slow-growing lesion of mesenchymal origin that is composed of cellular fibroblastic tissue that contains basophilic masses of cementum-like tissues.[41] In some cases varying amounts of bony trabeculae are interspersed within the lesion, reflecting the name cemento-ossifying fibroma. Cementifying fibromas occur most commonly in young and middle-aged adults (most often African-American women), and the mandible is predominantly involved. The tumors usually are 1 to 2 cm in diameter, although larger lesions rarely have been reported.

The radiographic features depend on the tumor's stage of development. In the early stage the lesion appears as a well-circumscribed, well-demarcated, radiolucent lesion with no internal radiopacities. As with an osteoblastoma, the lesion in time becomes surrounded by a well-defined radiolucent zone and contains a varying opacity. These tumors may be treated by enucleation.

Benign Cementoblastomas

Also called a *true cementoma,* a benign cementoblastoma is a rare neoplasm of functional cementoblasts, which is characterized by the formation of a cementum or cementum-like mass connected with a tooth root.[42,43] The lesion occurs most frequently in men under 25 years of age, is solitary, and usually is located in the molar or premolar region, with the mandibular first molar being most frequently involved. Benign cementoblastomas are most often associated with permanent teeth, but primary teeth may also be affected.

Radiographically the tumor is well defined, with central dense radiopaque material being attached to the tooth root and a surrounding radiolucent zone of uniform width, which represents the peripheral unmineralized tissues of the formative cellular layers. These tumors have a tendency to expand the cortical bone of the jaws. The lesion is easily enucleated because it is benign and is surrounded by a capsule.

BENIGN NONODONTOGENIC TUMORS

Benign nonodontogenic tumors are not unique to the jawbone, being found in other parts of the skeleton as well. Their radiographic appearance in the jaw does not differ significantly from their appearance in other bones, if one takes into account any abnormalities the lesions may cause to adjacent tooth structures. The discussion of these lesions is based mainly on their tissue of origin.

Exostoses

Exostoses are localized outgrowths of bone that vary in size and can be either flat, nodular, or pedunculated protuberances on the surface of the mandible or maxilla.[44-46] The cause of these exostoses of the jaw is unknown. Three types of exostoses are identified according to their location: the torus mandibularis, the torus palatinus, and multiple (maxillary) exostoses.

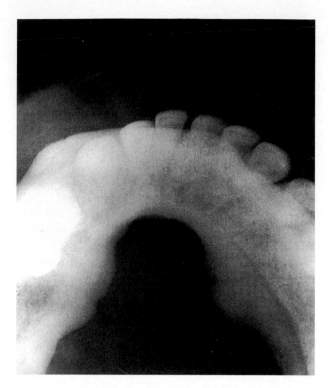

FIG. 5-26 Torus mandibularis. Dental view demonstrates bony exostoses along the lingual surface of the mandible bilaterally.

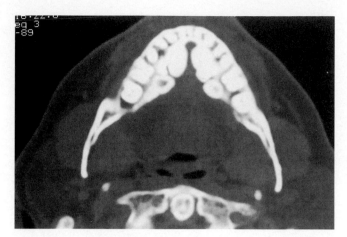

FIG. 5-27 Torus mandibularis. Axial CT (bone window setting) through the mandible demonstrates bilateral bony exostosis of the lingual surface of the mandible.

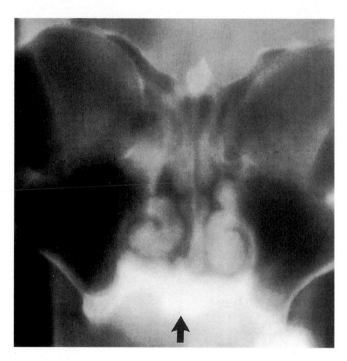

FIG. 5-28 Torus palatinus. Coronal tomographic section shows a bony exostosis of the hard palate *(arrow)* projecting into the upper oral cavity.

Radiographically, exostoses are recognized as areas of increased bony density projecting from the mandible or maxilla. Those exostoses composed of compact bone are of uniform radiopacity, whereas those that contain a marrow space have trabeculations. Some exostoses are difficult to demonstrate radiographically, particulary small ones and those that are superimposed on the teeth. An enostosis is a related lesion that originates from the inner cortex of the jaw as an area of osteosclerosis.

Torus mandibularis is an outgrowth of bone on the lingual surface of the mandible (Figs. 5-26, 5-27). It usually is situated above the mylohyoid line, opposite the bicuspid teeth.[44] The size, shape, and number of exostoses vary. The mandibular tori are usually bilateral, but this condition has been found to be unilateral in 20% of cases. The reported incidence in the United States ranges between 6% and 8%, with no sex predilection.

Torus palatinus is a flat, spindle-shaped, nodular or lobular exostosis that arises in the middle of the hard palate (Fig. 5-28). The cause is unknown, but some theories suggest that it may be a hereditary condition.[44,45] The incidence in the United States varies between 20% and 25%, with women being affected most often. Although the torus palatinus may occur at any age, its peak incidence is before the age of 30 years. Radiographically the torus palatinus is radiopaque with distinct borders and is composed of either dense compact bone or a shell of compact bone with a center of cancellous bone. Often a midline suture can be identified through the lesion. Surgical removal is indicated if the torus interferes with swallowing or if a denture must be constructed for prosthetic tooth replacement.

Multiple exostoses of the jaw arise from the buccal surface of the maxilla primarily, in the molar region.[46] They appear as small, nodular, bony masses.

Osteomas

An osteoma is a benign neoplasm composed of compact or cancellous bone, usually in an endosteal or periosteal location.[47-49] These tumors vary greatly in size and, if large, can cause disfigurement. The average age of patients with osteo-

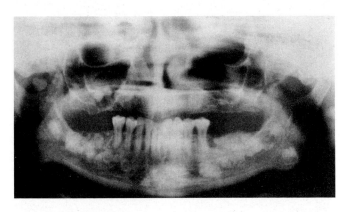

FIG. 5-29 Gardner's syndrome. Panorex view of the mandible and maxilla demonstrates multiple osteomas within the mandible and the alveolar portion of the maxilla. There is some conglomeration of the osteomas, especially in the body of the right mandible.

mas is 50 to 60 years, and twice as many women are affected as men. These lesions occur most often in the paranasal sinuses, especially in the frontal and ethmoid sinuses. The next most common site is the jaw, and the mandible is affected more often than the maxilla.

Osteomas have a characteristic radiographic appearance. They are well-circumscribed, sclerotic bony masses attached by a broad base or pedicle to the surface of the mandible. Root absorption may occur when the osteoma is located in the vicinity of a tooth. The need for surgical removal is determined clinically because they have not been found to become malignant.

Gardner's syndrome, which is inherited as an autosomal dominant trait, consists of multiple osteomas, multiple colonic polyps, epidermoid and sebaceous cysts, desmoid tumors of the skin, and impacted supernumerary and permanent teeth (Fig. 5-29). The multiple osteomas often precede the onset of the colonic polyps, and these polyps almost always eventually become malignant.[50-53] The osteomas have a predilection for the frontal bone, maxilla, and mandible, although they may be observed in any of the bones of the cranium or facial skeleton. The osteomas of the jaw usually appear early in life, most often in the second decade.

Osteochondromas

An osteochondroma is a benign lesion thought to arise from overgrowth of cartilage at a growth site, and these lesions have been reported most frequently in the coronoid and the condylar processes.[54,55] Radiographically they usually appear as radiopaque extraosseous projections. Although it has been suggested that these tumors are very slow growing and may have malignant potential, this is not universally agreed upon. Complete surgical removal is the treatment of choice, and recurrence is rare.

Chondromas

Chondromas are slow-growing lesions that presumably arise from cartilaginous remnants in bone.[56] They produce destruction of normal bone and appear as lytic lesions in the body of the mandible and occasionally in the condyle. Full delineation of condylar lesions often requires CT or MRI. Histologically they are neoplasms of hyaline cartilage that are usually homogeneous in appearance. It may be difficult to distinguish between benign and malignant lesions when unusual mitotic activity is identified. Surgical removal with wide margins is the preferred treatment.

Synovial Chondromatosis

Synovial chondromatosis is a proliferation of synovial tissues with the formation of cartilaginous particles in the synovium that can ossify and migrate into the TMJ space. Symptoms vary widely, but patients often complain of intermittent periarticular swelling, pain, and limitation of motion. Radiographic findings depend on the extent of the proliferative process and include joint effusion, anatomic derangement of the normal joint structures with widening of the joint space, irregularity of the joint articular surfaces, and evidence of calcified or ossified particles within the joint space. Surgical removal of the lesion and synovectomy is the usual treatment, and in most cases the articular disk does not need to be reconstructed. In cases where reconstruction is deemed necessary the most common procedure is a vascularized, pedicled temporalis muscle flap interpositional between the condyle and the articular fossa of the temporal bone.

Giant Cell Lesions

Giant cell lesions of the maxillofacial skeleton make up a continuum of clinically distinct yet histologically very similar pathologic conditions.[57-64] The giant cell granuloma, giant cell tumor, brown tumor of hyperparathyroidism, and cherubism are clinically separate entities that fall into this category. Whether or not the "true" giant cell tumor of long bones exists in the maxillofacial skeleton continues to be a controversy. Most authors now believe that there is an analogy between the two lesions, and that possibly they could represent a spectrum of a similar pathologic process. Several groups have carried out histomorphometric studies to examine the biologic behavior of these lesions to classify them more correctly, with the aim of correlating histologic and clinical behavior. Based on the clinical, radiologic, and histologic findings, the designation of giant cell lesions of the jaws as either aggressive or nonaggressive may be of more help to the clinician than designation of all of these lesions as belonging to one group.

Giant cell granuloma occurs most frequently in the second and third decades of life, and they occur twice as frequently in women as in men. Painless swelling is the most common symptom, but some lesions may be noted as an incidental finding during routine radiographic screening. The mandible is affected in about two thirds of the reported cases, with most tumors being located in the anterior mandible between the second premolar and the second molar, often with extension across the midline. On occasion these lesions may exhibit a more aggressive clinical and radiographic appearance.

Radiographically the lesion most often has a radiolucent, multilocular, honeycombed appearance with tiny bony septae traversing the involved area (Fig. 5-30). When present, the various loculi are irregular in shape and vary in size; however, unilocular tumors without trabeculation do occur. Often there is a rather marked expansion with thinning of the cortical plates, and perforation may occur in large lesions. If the mass is adjacent to teeth, displacement and root resorption are seen. Lesions, especially those in the antral region, produce "ground glass" radiopacities and occasional calcifications (Fig. 5-31). Treatment modalities include enucleation and curettage with local osteotomy, chemical cautery, electrocautery, cryotherapy, and en bloc resection.[63,64] Calcitonin, interferon alfa, and intralesional steroids are newer modalities that have found some success for more aggressive and recurrent lesions.

HISTIOCYTOSIS X (LANGERHAN'S HISTIOCYTOSIS)

Histiocytosis X is a spectrum of disease that has as its primary pathology a proliferation of lipid-laden Langerhan's cells (histiocytes) accompanied by a significant inflammatory response.[65-71] This process can be focal or widely disseminated, acute or chronic, and benign or malignant. The cause of this disease remains unknown, although genetic factors, infectious agents, and immunologic abnormalities have been suggested. Based on the clinical presentation, three variants have been described: Letterer-Siwe disease

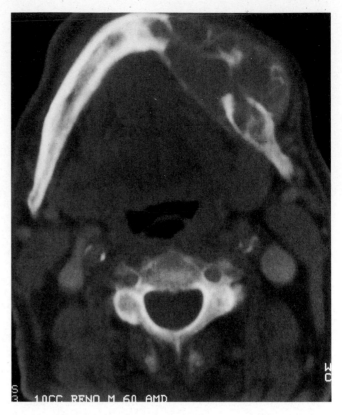

FIG. 5-30   Giant cell granuloma of the left mandible. Axial CT (bone window setting) demonstrates a loculated, expansile lesion involving the ramus, body, and symphysis of the mandible.

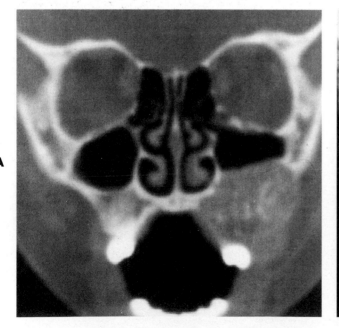
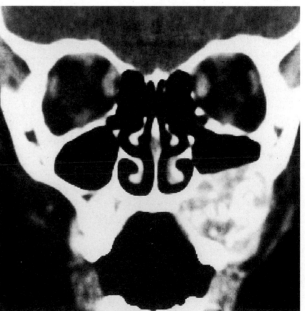

FIG. 5-31   Giant cell granuloma of the left maxilla. **A,** Coronal CT (bone window setting) shows an expansile lesion in the left maxilla bulging into the left lower antrum and adjacent oral cavity. Note calcific densities within the lesion. **B,** Coronal CT (soft-tissue window setting) demonstrates to better advantage the calcific and bony densities within the expansile lesion.

(disseminated acute histiocytosis), Hand-Schüller-Christian disease (disseminated chronic histiocytosis), and Eosinophilic granuloma (localized histiocytosis).

Letterer-Siwe Disease

Letterer-Siwe disease is the acute, widely disseminated form of histiocytosis X.[69] It is generally fatal and usually occurs in infants under 1 year of age. Lesions are usually present in several bones and may appear as multiple small, rounded radiolucencies with well-defined borders. If teeth are present in the affected regions, they are frequently mobile and there is associated gingival bleeding.

Hand-Schüller-Christian Disease

Hand-Schüller-Christian disease is the disseminated chronic skeletal and extraskeletal form of histiocytosis X.[70] It is the intermediate stage between eosinophilic granuloma and Letterer-Siwe disease. It occurs mostly in children (predominantly boys by a ratio of 2:1) from the first to the tenth year of life. The three classic signs of the disease (single or multiple sharply defined calvarial defects, unilateral or bilateral exophthalmos, and diabetes insipidus) are noted in about 10% of patients. Other organs such as the lymph nodes, liver, spleen, lungs, and skin may be involved. The first indication of the disease often appears in the oral structures, either in the form of red spongy gingiva or premature loss of teeth. The typical radiographic appearance is one of irregular, lucent defects in the mandible and maxilla. The affected teeth appear to be "floating in space" as a result of marked destruction of the alveolar bone. The disease is slowly progressive, and the mortality rate may be as high as 60%.

Eosinophilic Granulomas

Eosinophilic granuloma is the mildest and most favorable form of histiocytosis X.[71] There is a predilection for males, and there is a peak frequency in the third decade of life. The average age of patients with eosinophilic granuloma of the jaw is higher than that of patients with lesions in other parts of the body, and frequent sites are the skull and the tooth-bearing areas of the mandible. The lesion may be an incidental radiographic finding and may manifest as local pain, swelling, tenderness, or fever and general malaise. Eosinophilic granuloma of the mandible causes well-demarcated areas of osteolysis that may appear "punched out." Maxillary lesions usually are not as well demarcated as those in the mandible.

The area of bone involvement is characterized by irregular lucent patches having no reactive sclerosis but often showing cortical destruction (Fig. 5-32). These patches may appear as single or multiple areas of rarefaction simulating jaw cysts, periapical granulomas, or periodontal disease (Fig. 5-33). Early radiographic findings include destruction of the alveolar bone crest and interdental septum and loss of the cortical outline of a tooth follicle or the lamina dura. The teeth in the involved regions become loose, float in space, and are exfoliated.

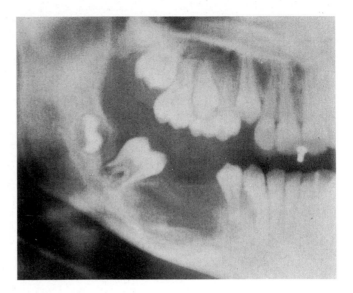

FIG. 5-32 Eosinophilic granuloma in the right mandible. Panorex view of the mandible shows a lucent, irregular area fairly well defined in the body of the mandible between the second molar tooth and the first premolar tooth. There is some loss of the lamina dura of the lower second molar tooth.

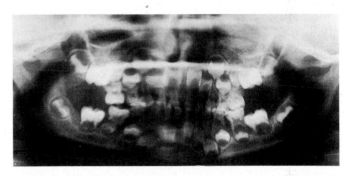

FIG. 5-33 Diffuse eosinophilic granuloma in the mandible. Panorex view of the mandible shows loss of the lamina dura of erupted and partially erupted tooth follicles. This is especially evident at the second lower right molar tooth.

Unifocal lesions may be curetted and packed with cancellous bone. With several recurrences or persistent residual granulomas, low-dose irradiation and cortisone treatment may be beneficial. Cytostatic agents (vinblastine, cyclophosphamide, etoposide) also have been used successfully. Other treatment modalities include immunotherapy (suppressin A, cyclosporin), hormonal therapy, intralesional steroids, and bone marrow transplantation.

FIBROOSSEOUS LESIONS
Fibrous Dysplasia

Fibrous dysplasia is a lesion of unknown cause, diverse histopathology and an uncertain pathogenesis, which is most commonly seen in the first three decades of life.[72-77] It occurs more frequently in the maxilla than in the mandible, where it usually arises in the posterior regions of the bone.

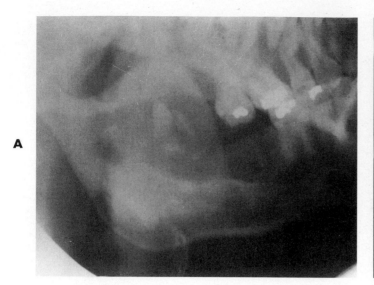
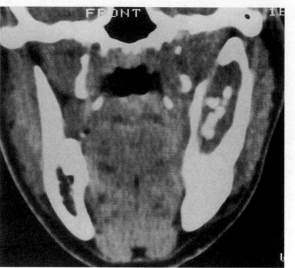

FIG. 5-34 Monostotic fibrous dysplasia in the left mandible. **A,** Oblique view of the left mandible shows a sclerotic expansile lesion in the ramus of the mandible with extension into the coronoid process. There are some calcific densities within the central anterior part of this lesion. **B,** Coronal CT (soft-tissue window setting) shows the expansile nature of the lesion in the ramus. Calcified densities are noted within the lesion.

There are considerable microscopic variations in the different lesions, as evidenced by fibrous tissue alternating with trabeculae of coarse woven bone and less organized lamellar bone. The three forms of fibrous dysplasia are monostotic fibrous dysplasia, polystotic fibrous dysplasia (in which multiple bony lesions, often unilateral, occur) and Albright's syndrome.

Monostotic fibrous dysplasia occurs equally as often in males as females and is encountered frequently in children and young adults, with a mean age of 27 years.[74] The clinical symptoms usually are painless swelling of the involved bone; however, neurovascular compromise may also cause symptoms. Typically there is involvement of the jaw, as noted by bulging of the labial or buccal plates, malalignment and displacement of teeth, protuberance of the maxilla, or enlargement of the maxilla or zygoma with proptosis. There also can be skull base disease.

Polystotic fibrous dysplasia manifests early in life, often with an insidious onset. The disease is characterized by bone deformities, and in some cases there is associated bone pain. In this form of fibrous dysplasia, the skull and face are frequently involved, often with obvious asymmetry secondary to bone expansion. Jaw involvement develops slowly and usually presents with facial deformity, overgrowth of the alveolar bone, and displacement of teeth. There can be marked enlargement of the maxilla, with involvement of the maxillary sinuses, nasal cavities, orbit, and base of skull. Craniofacial fibrous dysplasia is generally not a functionally devastating disease unless the lesion involves the orbit and skull base, where blindness, pituitary dysfunction, and vital neurovascular compromise may occur.

Albright's syndrome is a developmental defect of unknown cause. It is represented by cutaneous pigmenta-

tion, precocious puberty, and multiple skeletal lesions. Young girls are affected most often.

The roentgenographic appearance of fibrous dysplasia can vary considerably, usually depending on the degree of bone present within the lesion. One appearance is that of a unilocular or multilocular, primarily radiolucent lesion, with a well-defined border. Interspersed bony trabeculae are often present within the lucent area, rendering the lesion partially radiopaque (Fig. 5-34). Another appearance is that of a marked, homogeneous increase in bone density associated with bone expansion, which reflects the predominent histologic finding of bony trabeculae with only a few scattered areas of fibrous tissue (Fig. 5-35).

Cystic lesions of appreciable size cause thinning and remodeling of the cortex but rarely perforate the cortex and produce new periosteal bone. Although the lesion may cause resorption of the roots of erupted teeth, this is rare.

The disease is usually self-limiting, often not progressing after the third decade of life. Surgical treatment usually is limited to a cosmetic debulking and recontouring of the bone. However, an accelerated progression of the disease has been noted with early and aggressive surgical manipulation, sometimes mandating additional surgery. Only small lesions can be removed by enucleation. Because there is a low incidence of malignant transformation of fibrous dysplasia, regular and careful follow-up should be maintained.

Ossifying Fibromas (Fibroosteomas)

The ossifying fibroma is an encapsulated, benign neoplasm consisting of fibrous tissue that contains various amounts of irregular bony trabeculae.[78-80] As the lesion matures, the areas of ossification increase in number and coalesce, accounting for the lesion's progressive increased radioden-

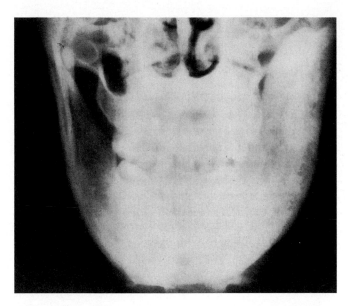

FIG. 5-35 Monostotic fibrous dysplasia. PA view of the mandible shows an expansile sclerotic lesion involving the left ramus of the mandible with extension into the angle and body of the left mandible.

sity. The disorder is found most often in females and may occur at any age, but it is most common in the third and fourth decades of life. The lesion develops predominantly in the mandible and is usually situated at the roots of the teeth or in the periapical region. It generally is asymptomatic, but a progressive increase in size may eventually cause swelling of the jaw.

Radiographically the lesion usually has a distinct boundary, unlike fibrous dysplasia, and in the early stages, it presents as a lucent area. As the lesion matures, bone densities appear, transforming the lesion into a radiopaque mass surrounded by a "halo" of less ossified tissue. One aggressive variety of ossifying fibroma is referred to as *juvenile ossifying fibroma*. This term designates a very actively growing destructive lesion that is histologically identical to the routine ossifying fibroma. This lesion affects individuals younger than 15 years of age and occurs exclusively in the maxilla.

The treatment of ossifying fibroma is usually surgical enucleation, although for some forms of this lesion, especially the juvenile form that is prone to recur, consideration should be given to a broader surgical resection.

Paget's Disease (Osteitis Deformans)

Paget's disease of bone is a chronic disease characterized by abnormal functioning of osteoblasts and osteoclasts resulting in poorly mineralized and deformed bones.[81,82] There is a slightly higher male preponderance, and the incidence increases with age. There are also reports of an occasional familial pattern. Although the exact cause remains unknown, numerous theories have been proposed regarding its development, including a slow virus infection, hormonal abnormalities, a vascular anomaly, an autoimmune-type

connective tissue disorder, and a true neoplasia. Malignant transformation, although not a common occurrence, has been reported in the jaws and is a constant concern.

In the craniofacial skeleton, involvement of the skull, maxilla, and mandible is common. Headache, dizziness, hearing loss, and other cranial nerve abnormalities may result from the skull base involvement. The maxilla is involved more commonly than the mandible. The jaw lesions present as bone enlargement, separation of teeth with generalized widening of the interdental spaces, ill-fitting dentures, and frequently neuralgia-type pain.

Radiographically the jaw lesions have a variable appearance depending on the stage of disease progression. There can be "punched out" radiolucent areas, mixed areas giving a "cotton wool-like" appearance, and more densely sclerotic areas. The jaw lesions frequently show evidence of rarefaction and sclerotic change in the alveolar bone, with loss of the lamina dura surrounding the teeth and hypercementosis of the roots of teeth. Radionuclide scanning can identify the presence of disease based on the presence of areas of biologic activity. Laboratory findings typically include elevations in serum alkaline phosphatase and urinary hydroxyproline. Serum calcium and phosphorus are usually normal.

Clinical management may consist of no more than closely following the patient. When more severe disease exists or when the bone lesions in the craniofacial skeleton cause symptoms, therapeutic intervention is usually indicated. Nonsurgical treatment can include steroids and the use of calcitonins and diphosphonates. Surgical procedures must be carried out with great care because the abnormal bone is often very vascular, and significant bleeding can occur.

VASCULAR LESIONS

Vascular lesions of the head and neck are a perplexing group of problems that over the years have generated significant debate and confusion as to terminology and classification.[81-89] Descriptive, anatomic-pathologic, and embryologic classification schemes have been devised and debated and generally have not offered clinicians significant treatment guidance. The classification developed by Mulliken and Glowaki in 1982 is based on the cellular kinetics of the anomalous vessels and provides a diagnostic and therapeutic approach based on the biologic behavior of the lesion.[86] In this classification, two entities exist: hemangiomas and vascular malformations.

Hemangiomas

Hemangiomas are usually not identified at birth, but they appear soon thereafter. They are present in 12% of all children by 1 year of age. They go through a rapid proliferation phase during the first year of life, and this is followed by a much slower involution phase, which usually reaches partial or complete resolution by 5 to 7 years of age. Hemangiomas are 2 to 2½ times more common in females, and there is no race predilection.

Hemangiomas are found most often in the skull and vertebrae, and although common in the head and neck, they are rarely located in the jaw. They are benign tumors with vessels that have a marked endothelial turnover, and there are increased numbers of mast cells that are thought to play a role in the pathophysiology of these lesions.

Although most hemangiomas can be diagnosed by history and physical findings, some are difficult to fully evaluate clinically and warrant imaging studies. CT and MRI are particulary helpful for deeper lesions and those thought to involve bone. Doppler ultrasound and angiography may also be employed. Angiography of hemangiomas will show a well-circumscribed mass usually with prolonged parenchymal staining and tissue blush.

Treatment is based on correctly identifying the lesion and distinguishing it from a vascular malformation. Kaban and Mulliken pointed out in their review of vascular anomalies of the maxillofacial region that many reported hemangiomas were in fact vascular malformations.[85] Management of maxillofacial hemangiomas often consists of counseling and parental support along with observation. If significant functional problems ensue, treatment approaches consist of steroid therapy, compression therapy, radiotherapy, embolization, and treatment with interferon alfa.[88,89] Surgery is reserved for small lesions and as a secondary procedure to correct a cosmetic deformity.

Vascular Malformations

Vascular malformations are usually present at birth, but they may not be clinically evident until some ensighting event occurs. Their growth parallels normal body growth and is influenced by numerous additional factors. There is no sex predilection. Vascular malformations can be composed solely of capillary, venous, arterial, or lymphatic tissues or can be a combination of these tissues. They are subdivided into high-flow or low-flow lesions based on their clinical and angiographic pattern. In the maxillofacial region they frequently involve bone.

Radiographically the lesion appears as a radiolucent area, often traversed by delicate bony trabeculae forming variously sized small cavities. In large hemangiomas the cortex may be thinned, remodeled, or eroded. If the trabeculae are arranged in a radiating pattern, a sunburst or spoke wheel appearance results. In some cases there may be a single radiolucent lesion with a sclerotic or ill-defined border, which simulates a cyst. Root absorption, loss of the lamina dura, and exfoliation of teeth have also been reported, and over the lesion a bruit may be heard or a thrill palpated. Spontaneous bleeding around the involved teeth is a problem in the jaws.

Management of vascular malformations mandates a thorough knowledge of the pathologic process and the relevant anatomy. Small lesions may be treated with sclerosing agents, radiotherapy, cryotherapy, laser treatment, or conventional surgical techniques. Larger lesions, particularly high-flow and arteriovenous malformations, are best treated with embolization techniques, with or without surgical resection.

NEUROGENIC TUMORS

Benign neurogenic tumors, which include schwannomas (neurilemmommas), neurofibromas, and traumatic neuromas, occasionally are found centrally within the jaw.[90-93] They may occur at any age, and there is little or no sex predilection. Most of these slow-growing lesions arise in the mandible and cause pain or paresthesia.

A schwannoma is usually encapsulated and composed of two distinct histological components: Antoni type A tissue and Antoni type B tissue.[91] A neurofibroma arises from the connective tissue sheath of nerve fibers and has axons traversing the unencapsulated tumor.[92,93] A neurofibroma may occur as a solitary lesion or as multiple lesions associated with neurofibromatosis. Solitary neurofibromas may originate in the oral mucosa or may occur within the jaws.

Radiographically these lesions may present as solitary radiolucencies associated with the inferior alveolar canal or as multilocular radiolucencies that have produced extensive bone damage, with cortical remodeling and even perforation. On occasion the intraosseous tumor may perforate the cortex of the jaw and extend into the overlying soft tissues. A schwannoma, arising from the dental nerve within the inferior alveolar canal, may cause bulbous, elongated enlargement of the canal, and a neurofibroma adjacent to bone may produce a saucer-shaped, erosive defect on the surface of the bone.

Treatment is surgical but depends upon the size and location of the lesion. Smaller lesions can often be removed without significant damage to the nerve or surrounding tissues and without the need for major reconstructive surgery. Larger lesions, especially those with significant bone involvement, usually require a larger surgical exposure with enucleation or en bloc surgical resection, often with additional treatment modalities such as cautery or cyrotherapy of the bone. When these techniques need to be employed, surgical reconstruction is mandatory, often along with a microsurgical nerve repair.

MALIGNANT TUMORS

Malignant tumors can be grouped into three categories: (1) lesions that invade the mandible and maxilla secondarily from adjacent soft-tissue structures of the oral cavity and sinuses, (2) tumors that arise primarily within the mandible and maxilla, and (3) metastatic tumors from distant sites. The radiographic appearance of malignant lesions often allows differentiation from benign tumors and cysts; however, a biopsy is necessary to establish the final diagnosis. For proper treatment planning, it is important to radiographically assess the extent of the malignant tumor before surgery or radiation therapy. CT and MRI have proven valuable in assessing the extent of a tumor outside the mandible and maxilla, as well as assessing disease extension within the bone or metastases to the neck.

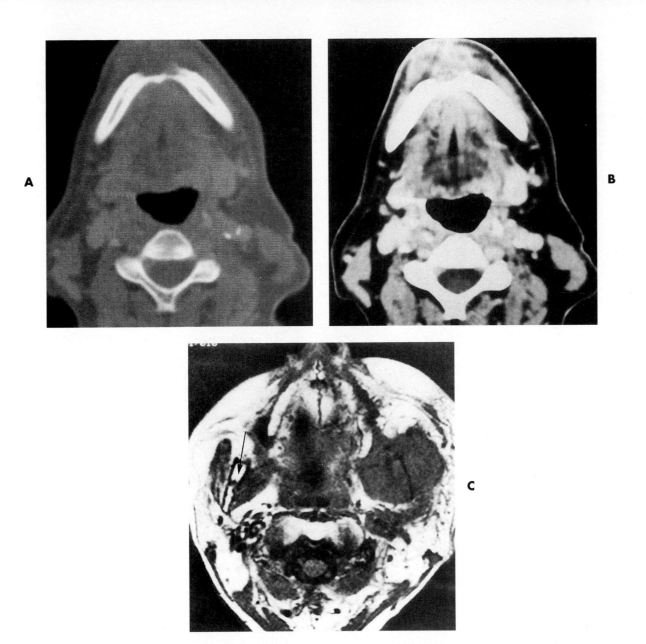

FIG. 5-36 Squamous cell carcinoma of the anterior mouth with secondary invasion of the mandible. **A,** Axial CT of the mandible (bone window setting) shows an erosion in the central and anterior part of the mandibular symphysis. **B,** Axial CT (soft-tissue window setting) demonstrates a lesion in the anterior mouth with extension into the mandible. Again, note the erosion in the anterior cortex and adjacent medullary portion of the mandible. **C,** Another patient. Axial T1W MR scan shows a large squamous cell carcinoma in the left cheek and retromolar trigone, which has infiltrated the ramus of the mandible. The normal high signal intensity of marrow (arrow) is seen on the right side.

Carcinomas

Most carcinomas encountered in the jaw originate in the oral cavity (lip, tongue, buccal mucosa, gingiva, floor of mouth, and palate) and maxillary sinuses, and they secondarily invade the mandible and maxilla.[94-98]

Radiographically the osseous involvement manifests early at the alveolar ridge with a saucer-shaped erosive defect. Initially this defect may be shallow and well defined, but in time an irregular cavity is formed, and there is usually no evidence of bony sclerotic reaction or periosteal reaction. Initially, superficial erosion of the alveolar crest in the tooth-bearing regions may mimic periodontal disease, and pathologic fractures are common complications in advanced cases.

A subgroup of carcinoma is referred to as *central epidermoid carcinoma* of the jaw. This tumor may develop from epithelial components that participated in the development of the teeth or from epithelial cells that have become enclosed within the deeper structures of the jaw during embryonic development. About 90% of these lesions are found in the mandible; they occur more frequently in men than in women, and their peak incidence is in the sixth and seventh decades of life. Although uncommon, this lesion is now recognized as a distinct entity.

Radiographically, carcinoma usually appears as a radiolucency with irregular margins (Fig. 5-36). Permeative disease extension may create a moth-eaten appearance. The

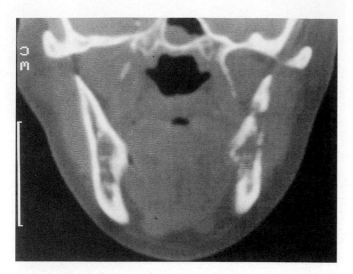

FIG. 5-37 Carcinoma of the breast metastatic to the left mandible. Coronal CT through the mandible (bone window setting) shows a lytic destructive lesion in the ramus of the left mandible. There is no new bone formation.

radiographic findings are nonspecific, and the tumor cannot be differentiated from other malignant lesions.

Carcinomatous transformation of the epithelium in an odontogenic cyst is a rare event, although it has been reported in dentigerous cysts, radicular cysts, residual cysts, and keratocysts. None of the reported cases affected individuals over 40 years of age. Radiographically the lesion appears like a cyst with a circumscribed margin. In the area of malignant degeneration the margin may become ill-defined, irregular, or moth-eaten.

Mucoepidermoid Carcinomas

Mucoepidermoid carcinomas can also affect the jaws.[99,100] Women are affected twice as often as men, and the average age at diagnosis is 46 years. The radiographic changes consist of ill-defined, lytic, or multilocular cystic areas, which are often indistinguishable from squamous cell carcinoma.

CT and MRI are extremely helpful in delineating the extent of disease in the mandible and the surrounding soft tissues, as well as identifying cervical lymph node involvement. An accurate tissue diagnosis is also mandatory to plan appropriate therapy, which usually consists of combined radiation therapy, chemotherapy, and surgery. A pretreatment oral examination and dental evaluation is necessary to diagnose any tooth and gum pathology that needs to be eliminated before initiating radiotherapy or chemotherapy. Also, when surgical resection is planned, appropriate prosthetic reconstruction strategies can be planned before surgery, allowing better functional results and patient satisfaction.

Metastatic Jaw Tumors

Metastatic tumors to the mandible or maxilla may be the first indication of an occult malignancy or the first evidence

of dissemination of a known primary tumor. Patients with metastatic lesions may be asymptomatic or may complain of symptoms similar to those found with other primary malignant tumors. Metastases to the mandible are four times more frequent than to the maxilla, and the most common primary tumors are in the breast, lung, kidney (hypernephroma), thyroid, prostate, and stomach.

In most instances the bone destruction caused by a metastatic lesion is radiographically similar to that of a primary tumor, and the area of destruction within the mandible may be localized, bilateral, or diffuse (Fig. 5-37). On occasion a mixed lesion of lytic and blastic areas may be encountered, usually from a carcinoma of the breast. In rare cases, metastasis from a carcinoma of the prostate may cause diffuse osteoblastic change.

When metastatic disease is suspected, a thorough search for the primary site and other sites of metastatic involvement should be immediately initiated, and a biopsy for definitive tissue diagnosis should be obtained. A team approach with coordination between internist, radiologist, oncologist, surgeon, and other health care providers involved in the care of the cancer patient is the optimal approach to an often difficult problem.[101-106]

Sarcomas
Osteogenic Sarcomas

Osteogenic sarcoma is a malignant tumor of the bone in which neoplastic cells produce a variable amount of osteoid.[107-109] According to the predominant tissue observed microscopically, these lesions are classified as osteoblastic, chondroblastic, or fibroblastic. About 6.5% of osteogenic sarcomas arise in the jaw.

Primary osteogenic sarcoma usually affects children and young adults, with a peak incidence in the second decade. However, osteogenic sarcomas of the mandible and maxilla have their peak incidence a decade later. The mandible is affected more often than the maxilla, and there is no sex predominance. The main symptoms are swelling and pain, but paresthesias, loose teeth, and bleeding have been reported.

Radiographically, osteogenic sarcoma can cause lytic bone destruction with indefinite margins (osteolytic type) (Fig. 5-38), an area of sclerosis (osteoblastic type) (Figs. 5-39, 5-40), or a mixed pattern. The osteoblastic type is the most common in the jaw. Some osteosarcomas show a sunburst effect caused by radiating mineralized tumor spicules. Cortical breakthrough, with tumor outside the jaw, is a common finding in advanced cases. Because a symmetrically widened periodontal membrane may be the earliest radiographic finding of osteogenic sarcoma of the jaw, this tumor must be differentiated from other diseases such as sclerodoma or acrosclerosis that also cause widening of the periodontal membrane.

Osteosarcomas can be easily assessed by CT because this modality identifies lesions that contain calcium, osteoid, or both. However, the extent of tumor spread within the marrow space or outside of the jaw may be seen better with MRI.

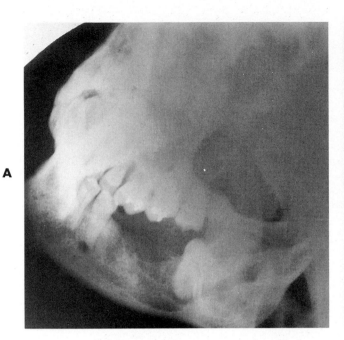

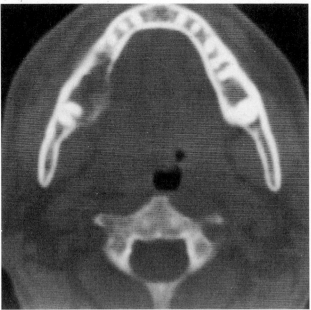

A **B**

FIG. 5-38   Osteogenic sarcoma of the mandible. **A,** Oblique view of the mandible shows an ill-defined lucent area in the body of the right mandible. There is loss of the lamina dura of the remaining third molar tooth. There is also invasion of the mandibular canal. **B,** Axial CT (bone window setting) shows ill-defined destruction with expansion of the body of the right mandible.

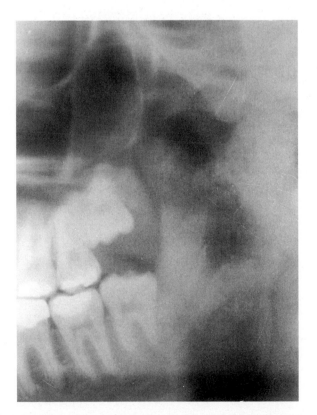

FIG. 5-39   Osteogenic sarcoma of the left mandible. Panorex view of the mandible shows a sclerotic lesion in the ascending ramus of the mandible and coronoid process. The boundaries of the mandible are poorly defined posteriorly. There is extension of this sclerotic tumor into the upper left mandibular canal.

Patients with mandibular osteosarcomas have a better prognosis than those with maxillary tumors; however, patients with mandibular or maxillary osteosarcomas are prone to develop either a recurrence or distant metastases, especially to lungs. Treatment is surgical excision usually followed by radiation therapy and possibly chemotherapy.

Fibrosarcomas

Fibrosarcoma of the jaw is a rare lesion that occurs predominantly in the mandible.[110,111] Onset can occur at any age but is most common before the age of 50 years, with a peak incidence between 20 and 40 years of age. Among these tumors, peripheral and central fibrosarcomas have been differentiated. The rare central form most frequently develops in the mandibular canal and causes central bone destruction, with gradual expansion leading to cortical erosion in larger lesions. The more prevalent peripheral type originates from the periostium or the periodontal membrane, frequently in the body and angle of the mandible. Radiographically, erosive changes are encountered at the alveolar ridge or at the inferior border of the mandible, and the depth of the defect varies depending on the stage of tumor development. Usually an extramandibular soft tissue mass of variable size is palpated.

Ewing's Sarcoma

Ewing's sarcoma occurs predominantly in children and young adults between 5 and 25 years of age, and males are affected twice as frequently as females.[112,113] In one series of studies, jaw involvement occurred in 13% of cases, and this

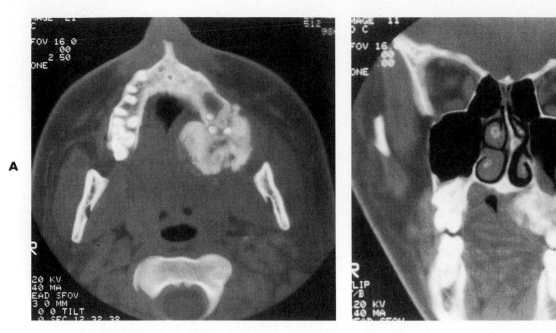

FIG. 5-40 Chondroblastic osteosarcoma of the left maxilla. **A,** Axial CT through the maxilla demonstrates a sclerotic, destructive lesion in the left maxilla with extension into the lower portion of the left antrum. **B,** Coronal CT demonstrates the sclerotic, destructive expansile lesion in the left maxilla and in the lower left maxillary antrum.

lesion occurs 10 times more frequently in the mandible than in the maxilla. Radiographically the lesion has a mottled, irregular, lucent appearance, with sclerosis interspersed in a small percentage of tumors. Perpendicular bony spicules and extensive bone destruction may be found at the cortices. The characteristic onion-peel (onion skin) layering of new subperiosteal bone is often absent in the jaw. This tumor tends to metastasize early, often to multiple bony sites making treatment difficult and the prognosis poor. Treatment is usually by combination of radiotherapy and chemotherapy.

Malignant Lymphomas

Malignant lymphoma is derived from lymphocytes and reticulum (histiocytic) cells that are in different stages of development, and the disease can have either a regional or systemic distribution.[114] Lymphomas in the head and neck occur predominantly in the neck nodes, oral cavity, nasopharynx, and occasionally in the sinuses. However, primary lymphoma of bone may occur in the mandible and maxilla. Such bone lymphomas are predominantly histiocytic (large cell) lymphomas; they occur more frequently in the mandible than in the maxilla, and there is a predominance in males. Radiographically there are no pathognomonic findings. In the mandible, most often there are ill-defined, lytic destructive areas of variable size. Radiation therapy and chemotherapy are the primary treatment modalities.

Multiple Myelomas

Although single lesions may occasionally occur, multiple myeloma is characterized by multiple or diffuse bone

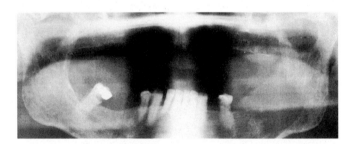

FIG. 5-41 Multiple myeloma of the mandible. Panorex view of the mandible shows a large destructive lesion in the body and ramus of the left mandible with extramandibular extension at the alveolus. There is the suggestion of a pathologic fracture at the anterior aspect of this lytic defect. Also, note multiple punched out lucent areas throughout the mandible, especially in the left ramus consistent with foci of multiple myeloma.

involvement.[115,116] Myeloma occurs most frequently in patients 40 to 70 years of age, with males being affected twice as frequently as females. In patients with multiple myeloma of the jaw, mandibular lesions are far more common, and there is a predilection for the angle, ramus, and molar teeth regions. The typical radiographic appearance is of punched out, regular, circular, or ovoid radiolucencies with no circumferential bone reaction, especially when the skull is involved (Fig. 5-41). The cortex of the mandible may be perforated, but expansion of bone is not demonstrated. If the lesion is extensive, the entire bone may be destroyed and bone destruction frequently is associated with hypercalcemia.

Treatment of multiple myeloma is primarily medical, and chemotherapy is the primary modality, often along with anabolic steroids, fluoride, calcium, and vitamin D. Solitary bone lesions most often are treated with radiation therapy. When surgery of jaw lesions is planned, consideration of the hematologic status of the patient is necessary to avoid untoward complications.

Leukemia

Leukemia may involve the jaw bones, and in one series of patients with acute leukemia, 63% of cases had disease in the jaw.[117-119] An early radiographic finding is loss of the lamina dura with loosening of the teeth. This is often followed by a varying degree of lytic bone destruction. Treatment is primarily medical management, and special attention should be paid to reducing the chance of oral infection and bleeding.

References

1. Weber AL, Easter KM. Cysts and odontogenic tumors of the mandible and maxilla. I. Contemp Diagn Radiol 1982; 5(25):1.

2. Borg G, Persson G, Thilander H. A study of odontogenic cysts with special reference to comparisons between keratinizing and non-keratinizing cysts. Swed Dent J 1974; 67:311-325.

3. Albright CR, Hennig GH. Large dentigerous cyst of the maxilla near the maxilary sinus. J Am Dent Assoc 1971; 83:1112-1115.

4. Mourshed F. A roentgenographic study of dentigerous cysts. Oral Surg 1964; 18:47-54.

5. Stafne EC, Milhon JA. Periodontal cysts. J Oral Surg 1945;102-111.

6. Donoff RB, Guralnick WC, Clayman L. Keratocysts of the jaw. J Oral Surg 1972; 30:800-884.

7. Brannon RB. The odontogenic keratocyst: a clinicopathologic study of 312 cases. I. Clinical features. Oral Surg 1962; 42:54-72.

8. Brennon RB. The odontogenic keratocyst: a clinicopathologic study of 312 cases. II. Histologic features. Oral Surg 1977; 43:233-255.

9. Koutnik AW, Kolodny SC, Hooker SP, et al. Multiple nervoid basal cell epithelioma, cysts, of the jaws, and bifid ribs syndrome: report of a case. J Oral Surg 1975; 33:686-689.

10. Gorlin RJ, Goltz RW. Multiple nevoid basal cell epithelioma, jaw cysts, and bifid ribs. N Eng J Med 1960; 262:908-912.

11. Abrams A, Howell FV, Bullock WK. Nasopalatine cysts. Oral Surg 1963; 16:306-332.

12. Campbell JJ, Baden E, Williams AC. Nasopalatine cyst of unusual size: report of case. J Oral Surg 1973; 31:776-779.

13. Christ TF. The globulomaxillary cyst:

14. Little JW, Jakobsen J. Origin of the globulomaxillary cyst. J Oral Surg 1978; 31:188.

15. Huebner GR, Turlington EG. So-called traumatic (hemorrhagic) bone cysts of the jaw. Oral Surg 1971; 31:254-265.

16. Biewald HF. A variation in the management of hemorrhagic, traumatic or simple bone cyst. J Oral Surg 1987; 25:627.

17. Ellis DJ, Walters PJ. Aneurysmal bone cyst of the mandible. J Oral Surg 1972; 34:26-32.

18. Gruskin SE, Dablin DC. Aneurysmal bone cyst of the mandible. J Oral Surg 1968; 26:523-528.

19. Steidler NE, Cook RM, Reade PC. Aneurysmal bone cysts of the jaws: a case report and review of the literature. Br J Oral Surg 1970; 16:254-261.

20. Reyneke JP. Aneurysmal bone cyst of the maxilla. Oral Surg 1978; 45:441-447.

21. Stafne EC. Bone cavities situated near the angle of the jaw. J Am Dent Assoc 1942; 29:19-69.

22. Regezi JA, Kerr DA, Courtney RM. Odontogenic tumors: analysis of 706 cases. J Oral Surg 1978; 36:771-778.

23. Weber AL, Easter KM. Cysts and odontogenic tumors of the mandible and maxilla. II. Contemporary Diagnostic Radiology 1982; 5(36):1.

24. Small IA, Waldron CA. Ameloblastoma of the jaw. Oral Surg Oral Med Oral Path 1955; 8(3):281-297.

25. Hylton RP, McKean TW, Albright JE. Simple ameloblastoma: report of case. J Oral Surg 1972; 30:59.

26. Mehlisch DR, Dahlin DC, Masson JK. Ameloblastoma: a clinicopathologic report. J Oral Surg 1972; 30:9-22.

27. Franklin CD, Hindle MO. The calcifying epithelial odontogenic tumor: report of four cases: two with long-term follow-up. Br J Oral Surg 1976; 13:230-238.

28. Franklin CD, Pindborg JJ. The calcifiying epithelial odontogenic tumor. Oral Surg 1976; 42:753-465.

29. Pindborg JJ. A calcifying epithelial odontogenic tumor. Cancer 1958; 11:838-843.

30. Tratman EK. Classification of odontomes. Br Dent J 1951; 91:167-173.

31. Curreri RC, Masser JE, Abramson AL. Complex odontoma of the maxillary sinus: report of a case. J Oral Surg 1975; 33:45-48.

32. Caton RB, Marble HB Jr, Topazian RG. Complex odontoma in the maxillary sinus. J Oral Surg 1973; 36(5):658-662.

33. Thompson RD, Hale ML, McLeran JH. Multiple compound composite odontomas of maxilla and mandible: report of case. J Oral Surg 1968; 26:478-480.

34. Gundlach KK, Schulz A. Odontogenic myxoma: clinical concept and morphological studies. J Oral Pathol 1977; 6(6):343-358.

35. Hendler BH, Abaza NA, Quinn P. Odontogenic myxoma, surgical management and an ultrastructural study. Oral Surg 1979; 47:203-217.

36. Davis RB, Baker RD, Alling CC. Odontogenic myxoma: clinical pathologic conference, case 24. I. Oral Surg 1978; 36:534-538.

37. Davis RB, Baker RD, Alling CC. Odontogenic myxoma. clinical pathologic conference, case 24. II. Oral Surg 1978; 36:610.

38. Zegarelli EV, Kutscher AH, Napoli N, et al. The cementoma: a study of 235 patients with 435 cementomas. Oral Surg 1964; 17:219-224.

39. Vegh T. Multiple cementomas (peri-

apical cemental dysplasia). Oral Surg 1976; 42:402-406.

40. Chaudhry AP, Spink JH, Gorlin RJ. Periapical fibrous dysplasia (cementoma). J Oral Surg 1958; 16:483.

41. Hamner JE III, Scofield HH, Cornyn J. Benign fibro-osseous jaw lesions of periodontal membrane origin: an analysis of 249 cases. Cancer 1968; 22:861-878.

42. Cherrick HM, King OH Jr, Lucatorto FM, et al. Benign cemento-blastoma: a clinicopathologic evaluation. Oral Surg 1974; 37:54-63.

43. Eversole LR, Sabes WR, Dauchess VG. Benign cementoblastoma. J Oral Surg 1973; 36:824-830.

44. Suzuki M, Sakai T. A familial study of torus palatinus and torus andibularis. Am J Phys Anthropol 1960; 18:263.

45. King DR, Moore GE. An analysis of torus palatinus in a transatlantic study. J Oral Med 1976; 31:44-46.

46. Bhaskar SN, Cutright DE. Multiple enostosis: report of cases. J Oral Surg 1968; 26:321-326.

47. Weinberg S. Osteoma of the mandibular condyle: report of case. J Oral Surg 1977; 35:929-932.

48. Noren GD, Roche WC. Huge osteoma of the mandible: report of a case. J Oral Surg 1978; 36:375-379.

49. Alling CC, Martinez MG, Ballard JB, et al. Osteoma cutis: clinical pathologic conference, case 5 II. J Oral Surg 1974; 32:195-197.

50. Halse A, Roed-Petersen B, Lund K. Gardner's syndrome. J Oral Surg 1975; 33:673-675.

51. McFarland PH, Scheetz WL, Knisley RE. Gardner's syndrome: report of two families. J Oral Surg 1968; 26:632-638.

52. Neal CG. Multiple osteomas of the mandible associated with polyposis of the colon (Gardner's syndrome). Oral Surg 1969; 28:628-631

53. Witkop CJ. Garner's syndrome and other osteognathodermal disorders with defects in parathyroid functions. J Oral Surg 1968; 26:639-642.

54. Ramon Y, Horowitz I, Oberman M, et al. Osteochondroma of the coronoid process of the mandible. Oral Surg 1977; 43:696-697.

55. Allan JH, Scott H. Osteochondroma of the mandible. Oral Surg 1974; 37:556-565.

56. Chaudry AP, Robinovitch MR, Mitchell DF, et al. Chondrogenic tumors of the jaws. Am J Surg 1961; 102:403-411.

57. Waldron CA, Shafer WG. Central giant cell reparative granuloma of the jaws. Am J Clin Pathol 1966; 45:437-647.

58. Wesley RK, et al. Central giant cell granuloma of the mandible: clinical pathologic conference, case 25 I. Oral Surg 1978; 36:713.

59. Smith GA, Ward PH. Giant-cell lesions of the facial skeleton. Arch Otolaryngol 1978; 104:186-190.

60. Curtis ML, Hatfield CG, Pierce JM. A destructive giant cell lesion of the mandible: report of a case. J Oral Surg 1979; 37:432-436.

61. Chuong R, Kaban LB, Kozakewich H, et al. Central giant cell lesions of the jaws: a clinicopathologic study. J Oral Maxillofac Surg 1986; 44:708-713.

62. Whitaker SB, Waldron CA. Central giant cell lesions of the jaws: a clinical, radiologic, and histopathologic study. Oral Surg Oral Med Oral Pathol 1993; 75:199-208.

63. Pogrel MA. The use of liquid nitrogen cryotherapy in the management of locally aggressive bone lesions. J Oral Maxillofac Surg 1993; 51:269-273.

64. MacIntosh RB. Surgical management of benign nonodontogenic lesions of the jaws. In: Peterson LJ, et al, eds. Principles of oral and maxillo-facial surgery. Vol. 2. 1993; 713-753.

65. Rapidis AD, Langdon JD, Harvey PW, et al. Histiocytosis X. Int J Oral Surg 1978; 7:76-84.

66. Scott J, Finch LD. Histiocytosis X with oral lesions: report of case. J Oral Surg 1972; 30:748-653.

67. Soskolne WA, Lustmann J, Azaz B. Histiocytosis X: report of six cases initially in the jaws. J Oral Surg 1977; 35:30-33.

68. Sigala JL, Silverman S Jr, Brody HA, et al. Dental involvement of histiocytosis. Oral Surg 1972; 33:42-48.

69. Lieberman PH, et al. A reappraisal of eosinophilic granuloma of bone, Hand-Schüller-Christian disease and Letterer-Siwe syndrome. Medicine 1969; 48:375-400.

70. Maw RB, McKean TW. Hand-Schüller-Christian disease: report of case. J Am Dent Assoc 1972; 85:1353-1357.

71. Ragab RR, Rake O. Eosinophilic granuloma with bilateral involvement of both jaws. Int J Oral Surg 1975; 4:73-79.

72. Waldron CA, Giansanti JS. Benign fibro-osseous lesions of the jaws: a clinical-radiologic-histologic review of sixty-five cases. II. Benign fibro-osseous lesions of periodontal ligament origin. Oral Surg 1973; 35:340-350.

73. Cangiano R, Stratigos GE, Williams FA. Clinical and radiographic manifestations of fibro-osseous lesions of the jaws: report of five cases. J Oral Surg 1971; 29:872-881.

74. Hayward JR, Melarkey DW, Megquier J. Monostotic fibrous dysplasia of the maxilla: report of cases. J Oral Surg 1973; 31:625-627.

75. Eversole LR, Sabes WR, Rovin S. Fibrous dysplasia: a nosologic problem in the diagnosis of fibro-osseous lesions of the jaws. J Oral Pathol 1972; 1:189-220.

76. Waldron CA, Giansanti JS. Benign fibro-osseous lesions of the jaws:a clinic-radiologic-histologic review of sixty-five cases. I. Fibrous dysplasia of the jaws. Oral Surg 1973; 35:190-201.

77. Waldron CA, Giansanti JS. Benign fibro-osseous lesions of the jaws: a clinical-radiolog-histologic review of sixty-five cases. II. Benign fibro-osseous lesions of periodontal ligament origin. Oral Surg Oral Med Oral Pathol 1973; 35:340-350.

78. Schlumberger HG. Fibrous dysplasia (ossifying fibroma) of maxilla and mandible. Am J Orthodontics 1946; 32:579-587.

79. Sherman RS, Sternbergh WCA. Roentgen appearance of ossifying fibroma of bone. Radiology 1948; 50:595-609.

80. Waldron CA. Ossifying fibroma of mandible: report of 2 cases. Oral Surg Oral Med Oral Path 1953; 6:467-473.

81. Anderson JT, Dehner LP. Osteolytic form of Paget's disease. J Bone Joint Surg (Am) 1976; 58:994-1000.

82. Gee JK, Zambito RF, Argentieri GW, et al. Paget's disease (osteitis deformans) of the mandible. J Oral Surg 1972; 30:223-227.

83. Lund BA. Hemangioma of the mandible and maxilla. J Oral Surg 1972; 22:234.

84. Macansh JD, Owen MD. Central cavernous hemangioma of the mandible: report of two cases. J Oral Surg 1972; 30:293-296.

85. Kaban LB, Mulliken JB. Vascular anomalies of the maxillofacial region. J Oral Maxillofac Surg 1986; 44:203-213.

86. Mulliken JB, Glowacki J. Hemangiomas and vascular malformations in infants and children: a classification based on endothelial characteristics. Plast Reconstr Surg 1984; 69:412.

87. Boyd JB, Mulliken JB, Kaban LB, et al. Skeletal changes associated with vascular malformations. Plast Reconstr Surg 1984; 74:789-795.

88. Ezekowitz RAB, Mulliken JB, Folkman J. Interferon alfa-2a for life-threatening hemangiomas of infancy. N Engl J Med May 28, 1992.

89. Ricketts RR, Hatly RM, Corden BJ, et al. Interferon alfa-2a for the treatment of complex hemangiomas of infancy and childhood. Ann Surg 1994; 219:605-612.

90. Shklar G, Meyer I. Neurogenic tumors of the mouth and jaws. Oral Surg 1963; 16:1075-1093.

91. Shimura K, Allen EL, Kinoshita Y, et al. Central neurilemmoma of the mandible: report of a case and review of the literature. J Oral Surg 1973; 31:363-367.

92. Prescott GH, White RF. Solitary, central neurofibroma of the mandible: report of case and review of the literature. J Oral Surg 1978; 28:305.

93. Singer CF, Gienger GL, Kulborn TL. Solitary intraosseous neuro-fibroma involving the mandibular canal: report of case. J Oral Surg 1973; 31:127-129.

94. Nolan R, Wood NK. Central squamous cell carcinoma of the mandible: report of a case. J Oral Surg 1976; 34:260-264.

95. Coonar HS. Primary intraosseous carcinoma of maxilla. Br Dent J 1979; 147:47-48.

96. Lapin R, Garfinkel AW, Catania AF, et al. Squamous cell carcinoma arising in a dentigerous cyst. J Oral Surg 1973; 31:354-358.

97. Shear M. Primary intra-alveolar epidermoid carcinoma of the jaw. J Pathol 1969; 97:645-651.

98. Sirsat MV, Sampat MB, Shrikhande SE. Primary intra-alveolar squamous cell carcinoma of the mandible. Oral Surg 1973; 35:366-371.

99. Fredrickson C, Cherrick HM. Central mucoepidermoid carcinoma of the jaws. J Oral Med 1978; 30:80-85.

100. Schultz W, Whitten JB. Mucoepidermoid carcinoma in the mandible: report of case. J Oral Surg 1969; 27:337-340.

101. Adler CI, Sotereanos GC, Valdivieso JG. Metastatic bronchogenic carcinoma of the maxilla: report of case. J Oral Surg 1973; 31:543-546.

102. Al-Ani S. Metastatic tumors to the mouth: report of two cases. J Oral Surg 1973; 31:120-122.

103. Appenzeller J, Weitzner S, Long GW. Hepatocellular carcinoma metastatic to the mandible: report of case and review of literature. J Oral Surg 1971; 29:668-671.

104. Carter DG, Anderson EE, Currie DP. Renal cell carcinoma metastatic to the mandible. J Oral Surg 1977; 35:992-993.

105. Cherrick HM, Demkee D. Metastatic carcinoma of the jaws. J Am Dent Assoc 1973; 87:180-181.

106. Moss M, Shapiro DN. Mandibular metastasis of breast cancer. J Am Dent Assoc 1969; 78:756-757.

107. Garrington GE, Scofield HH, Cornyn J, et al. Osteosarcoma of the jaws: analysis of 56 cases. Cancer 1967; 20:377-391.

108. Caron AS, Hajdu SI, Strong EW. Osteogenic sarcoma of the facial and cranial bones: review of 43 cases. Am J Surg 1971; 122:719-725.

109. Wilcox JW, Dukart RC, Kolodny SC, et al. Osteogenic sarcoma of the mandible. review of the literature and report of case. J Oral Surg 1973; 31:49-52.

110. Taconis WK, van Rijssel TG. Fibrosarcoma of the jaws. Skeletal Radiol 1986; 15:10-13.

111. Wright JA, Kuehn PG. Fibrosarcoma of the mandible. Oral Surg 1973; 36:16-20.

112. Borhgelli RF, Barros RE, Zampieri J. Ewing sarcoma of the mandible: report of case. J Oral Surg 1978; 36:473-475.

113. Carl W, Schaaf NG, Gaeta J, et al. Ewing's sarcoma. J Oral Surg 1971; 31:472-478.

114. Steg RF, Dahlin DC, Gores RJ. Malignant lymphoma of the mandible and maxillary region. Oral Surg Oral Med Oral Path 1959; 12:128.

115. Miller CD, Goltry RR, Shenasky JH. Multiple myeloma involving the jaws and oral soft tissue. Oral Surg 1969; 28:603-609.

116. Tabachnick TT, Levine B. Multiple myeloma involving the jaws and oral soft tissue. J Oral Surg 1976; 34:931-933.

117. Curtis AB. Childhood leukemias: osseous change in jaws on panoramic dental radiographs. J Am Dent Assoc 1971; 88:844-847.

118. Michaud M, Baehner RL, Bixler D, et al. Oral manifestations of acute leukemia in children. J Am Dent Assoc 1977; 95:1145-1150.

119. Sela MN, Pisanti S. Early diagnosis and treatment of patients with leukemia: a dental problem. J Oral Med 1977; 32:46-50.

6

Dental Implants and Multiplanar Imaging of the Jaw

JAMES J. ABRAHAMS

Edentulism is present in almost half of the population that is between 45 and 74 years of age.[1] Traditionally, edentulism has been treated with removable dentures; however, not all patients are candidates for dentures and many have continued difficulty with speech, oral function, and reduced self-esteem. In response to these problems, dentists developed nonremovable bridges that are attached to oral implants, metal posts surgically embedded in the jaw (Fig. 6-1). During the past decade, it has been determined that CT, with a dental reformatting program, is the method of choice for the preoperative assessment of these patients, and as a result of this work, new dialogues and interactions have been created between the radiologist and the dentist and oral surgeon. This in turn has brought new territories and unfamiliar diseases to the radiologist's attention. Radiologists now evaluate the dental aspects of the oral cavity, including implants, periodontal disease, odontogenic tumors, and other lesions of the jaw.[2-8] The goal of this chapter is to present a comprehensive discussion of dental implants, CT reformatting programs, and the anatomy, pathology, and terminology related to this area.

DENTAL IMPLANTS

Dental implants are metal posts that are surgically implanted in the jaw to support a fixed dental prosthesis (Fig. 6-1). In the early development of implants, dentists attempted to imitate the natural anchorage system of the teeth, which are attached to the bony socket by the periodontal ligament. In addition to supporting the teeth this ligament permits slight degrees of tooth motion within the socket. This ligament is visualized on plain radiographs as a thin radiolucent line situated between the lamina dura of the jaw and the tooth. The initial efforts to reproduce this ligament promoted growth of soft tissue between the oral implant and the bone.[9] These implants were often referred to as *pseudoligaments* or *fibrous osseointegrated implants*.[10,11] However, the long-term results of these soft tissue–anchored implants were

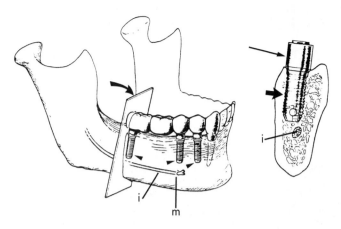

FIG. 6-1 View of the mandible illustrating the plane of orientation of the cross-sectional DentaScan images. The top of the plane *(curved arrow)* would correspond to one of the numbered perpendicular lines on the axial image in Fig. 6-6, *A*. Note how the height and width of the alveolar process and the location of the mandibular canal can be readily determined on the cross sectional image. Three root form implants are seen *(arrowheads)* supporting a four tooth prosthesis. The abutment *(thin arrow)* that is attached to the fixture *(broad arrow)* raises it above the surface of the bone and gingiva and into the oral cavity. Inferior alveolar canal *(i); (m),* mental foramen. (From Langer B, Sullivan D. Osseointegration: its impact on the interrelationship of periodontics and restorative dentistry. Part 1. Int J Periodont Res 1989; 9:86.)

poor, and researchers redirected their efforts toward the possibility of anchoring the implants by direct contact with bone. Early long-term studies with these osseointegrated implants were optimistic, with success rates of 91% in the mandible and 81% in the maxilla.[12] Microscopic sections through bone containing implants demonstrated the ability of osteoblasts to grow and integrate with the titanium posts, resulting in osseointegration.[13] The results of these early studies were corroborated by others, and this paved the road for the osseointegrated implants utilized today.[14]

There are three basic types of implants: root form (Fig. 6-1), blade (Fig. 6-2), and subperiosteal (Fig. 6-3). The osseointegrated, cylinder-shape implants described previously are the root form because they simulate the shape of the root of a tooth. They are the ones most frequently used today and will be the type dealt with in this chapter. The blade implants are rectangular and are similar in shape to a razor blade. From the long side of the rectangle, one or more posts extend into the oral cavity to permit fixation of the prosthesis. The rectangular portion is implanted into the bone via a linear osteotomy, and the posts extend up above the gingiva. Lastly the subperiosteal implants are metallic meshes that are custom built to fit over the alveolar process and under the periosteum. Several metallic posts extend from the mesh into the oral cavity (above the gingiva) to

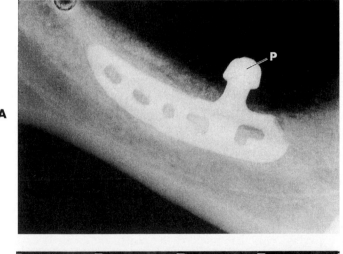

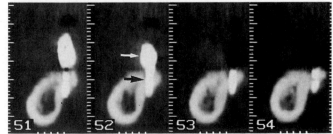

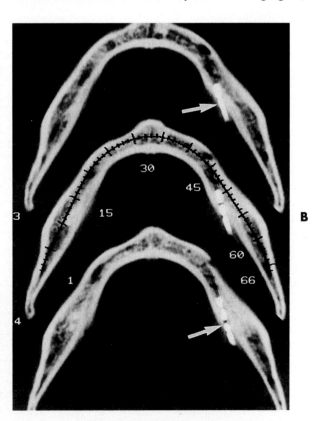

FIG. 6-2 Blade implant in mandible. **A,** Plain film illustrating a single post-blade implant. Note how the blade is inserted in the mandible after a linear osteotomy while the post *(P)* extends above the level of the bone and gingiva. **B,** Axial views demonstrating blade implant in mandible *(arrow).* **C,** Cross-sectional views illustrating the blade within the mandible *(black arrow)* and the post *(white arrow)* extending into the oral cavity above the level of the bone and gingiva.

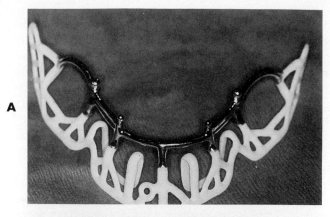

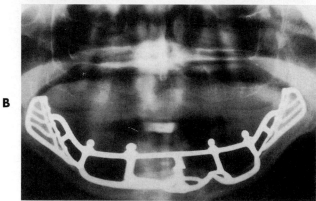

FIG. 6-3 Subperiosteal implant. **A,** Photograph of subperiosteal implant. The white portion will fit under the periosteum and on top of the bone of the alveolar process and the metallic-appearing portion will extend above the gingiva to support the prosthesis. The subperiosteal portion *(white)* is often coated with hydroxyapatite to facilitate bone growth. **B,** Panoramic view demonstrating the subperiosteal implant on a severely atrophic mandible. The prosthesis has not been attached. (Courtesy Dr. Wayne C. Jarvis, Williamsville, NY.)

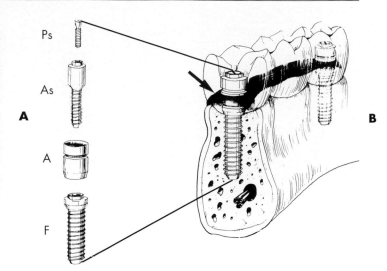

FIG. 6-4 Illustration demonstrating the components of an implant **(A)** and two root form implants supporting a three-tooth prosthesis **(B)**. For illustrative purposes the black portion running through the prosthesis *(arrow)* represents the metal framework within the prosthesis. Prosthesis screw *(Ps)*, abutment screw *(As)*, abutment *(A)*, and fixture *(F)*.

support the prosthesis. To customize these subperiosteal implants, the alveolar process must be surgically exposed so a plaster impression can be obtained to manufacture the implant. After the implant is manufactured, the patient returns for a second surgical procedure that permits placement of the implant. The first surgical procedure can be eliminated if thin-slice axial CT is used to produce a 3D model of the jaw from which the prosthesis can be manufactured.

Osseointegrated root form implants are made up of several components (Fig. 6-4). The fixture is the portion of the implant that is surgically embedded in the osseous tissue of the jaw, and it is made of titanium, a material that promotes osseointegration. The fixtures come in various sizes, typically ranging from 3.25 to 3.75 mm in diameter and 7 to 10 mm in length.[6] The size of the implant chosen is dependent upon the amount of available jaw bone. Dentists prefer the largest possible implant because it increases the surface area and thus provides stronger anchorage and more successful osseointegration. It is also preferable to have 1 to 1.5 mm of bone on either side of the implant and 1 to 2 mm of bone

between the bottom of the implant and the adjacent structures (i.e., maxillary sinus, mandibular canal).[6] Fixtures can be threaded, unthreaded, or even coated with hydroxyapatite.[15]

The next component of the implant is the abutment (Figs. 6-1, 6-4), which is attached to the fixture to increase its height to a level above the gingival surface. This occurs 3 to 6 months after the initial procedure, thus giving the fixture time to heal within the bone. The fixture is surgically exposed, and the abutment is attached with an abutment screw (Fig. 6-4). The top of the abutment screw itself has a small screw hole, which allows the dental prosthesis to be attached by a screw that runs through the prosthesis and into the abutment screw. This screw is designed to be the weakest portion of the implant so that in the event of unforeseen stress it, rather than the fixture, will break. Angled abutments are also available to correct for implants that are inserted at an angle rather than parallel to the residual teeth.

The prosthesis is composed of a strong metal framework (Fig. 6-4) that supports the prosthetic teeth. Because the implants actually support this framework, patients can have a full 14-tooth dental prosthesis supported by only six implants or a three-tooth prosthesis supported by two implants, as shown in Fig. 6-4.

IMPLANT SURGICAL PROCEDURE

Dental implant surgery is a two-stage procedure requiring a 4 to 6 month healing period between stages.[16] The healing period allows time for osseointegration to occur. In the first stage the fixture is installed; in the second stage the fixture is exposed, and the abutment is attached. The procedures are typically performed in the dentist's office, using local anesthetic.

Fixture Placement

The first stage of surgery, fixture installation, is more extensive than the second stage and usually takes about 2 hours, depending on the number of fixtures placed. Anesthesia is obtained by using local infiltration with lidocaine or a nerve block. A linear incision is then made along the buccal or lingual surface of the alveolar ridge, and a soft tissue flap, incorporating the periosteum, is reflected back (Fig. 6-5, *E*). If the exposed bony ridge, has a sharp or pointed surface secondary to buccolingual atrophy, an alveoloplasty may be performed to remove the sharp edge and provide a broad surface to install the fixtures. The anticipated implant site has been radiographically predetermined (Fig. 6-5, *A-D*). Its position is then located on the patient either by measuring from an existing tooth or from another landmark that can be identified both on the films and on the patient or by using a stent with markers (Fig. 6-5, *B*). Refer to the discussion of radiographic and surgical stents.

After the site has been identified on the patient, a series of graduated drill bits produce a hole in the bone. The hole is progressively widened to the appropriate size. A countersink widens the drill hole's entrance to accommodate the fixture head. The hole is then threaded with a titanium tap bur to accommodate the threaded fixture. Both drilling and threading are done at extremely low revolutions per minute (RPM) and with copious irrigation to prevent heating and destruction of osteoblasts because osseointegration can only occur with viable cells. The top of the fixture has a threaded hole (Fig. 6-5, *G*) to accommodate the abutment screw that is inserted during the second stage of the procedure. To prevent soft tissue and bone from growing into the hole while the patient is healing, a cover screw is used (Fig. 6-5, *E*). The implant and cover screw are flush with the surface of the bone. To raise the height of the implant above the gingival surface, an abutment is later attached.

After the fixtures are placed, the tissue flap is sutured closed and the implants are allowed to heal for approximately 4 months in the mandible and 6 months in the maxilla (Fig. 6-5, *F*). This promotes the process of osseointegration, thus forming a strong bond between the bone and the implant. Approximately 1 week after the initial surgery, the skin sutures are removed, and the patient is fitted with an interim prosthesis, which typically is the one used before surgery. Because of the fixture, minor modifications of the old prosthesis may be necessary.

Abutment Connection

The second stage of the procedure tends to be less traumatic for the patient and is typically carried out with only local infiltration of lidocaine. A pointed probe is used to locate the cover screws; after they are located an incision is made to expose and remove them. Alternatively a circular soft-tissue punch can be used to excise the tissue above the cover screw. The abutment is then attached to the fixture using the abutment screw. The top of the abutment screw has a screw hole that permits the prosthesis to be screwed into the fix-

ture (Figs. 6-4, 6-5, *H*). Finally a surgical pack is applied and retained for a short period by a healing cap.

Prosthedontic Procedure

To make the prosthesis, an impression of the jaw with the abutments in place is made, using plaster or hydrocoloid. From this impression a cast of the mandible or maxilla is obtained. From this cast the prosthesis is made, aligning properly with the screw holes and properly aligning the prosthetic teeth with the occlusal plain. After the prosthesis is manufactured, it is fixed to the abutments with screws that typically come out the central fossa of the prosthetic teeth. A white compound is used to cover the screw holes (Fig. 6-5, *I*).

RADIOLOGY FOR ORAL IMPLANTS

To perform the implant procedure, the oral surgeon and dentist need to know the precise height, width, and contour of the alveolar process, as well as its relationship to the maxillary sinus and mandibular canal. Injury to the neurovascular bundle within the mandibular canal results in paresthesia or hypesthesia of the face, whereas perforation into the maxillary sinus increases the likelihood of implant failure and creates the potential for an oroantral fistula and antral infection. The precise dimensions of the alveolar process are important to determine preoperatively because atrophy of the alveolar ridge, which occurs in edentulous patients, may preclude the use of implants.

Before the development of CT dental reformatting programs, attempts were made to obtain this information with panoramic, intraoral, and cephalometric films. However, the panoramic film produced up to 25% distortion, making accurate measurements almost impossible. In addition, the width (thickness) of the alveolar process could not be determined by any of these techniques. Therefore the surgeon had to rely primarily on clinical assessment to determine if the alveolar process was thick enough to accommodate an implant. Unfortunately, it was common to find during surgery that there was insufficient bone for the implants. As a result, radiologists and dentists began to evaluate the efficacy of using CT to assess these patients.[17,18] Axial and coronal images were only marginally helpful because of the streak degradation artifacts created by any dental restorations. However, reformatted images using thin-slice axial CT were found to be extremely useful because the streak artifact could be avoided, the anatomy could be displayed in multiple planes, the width of the alveolar process could be accurately assessed, and accurate reproducible millimeter measurements could be made. Reformatting software programs, which display multiple panoramic and cross-sectional images, soon became available (Figs. 6-6, 6-7).[19-22] The particular program used in this chapter is DentaScan. Although these programs were initially developed to assess implant patients, they have also gained popularity for evaluating all lesions of the jaw (Fig. 6-8).[3,5,7,8]

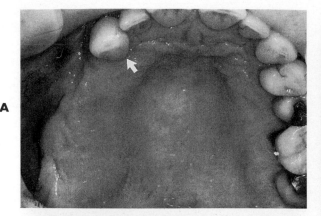

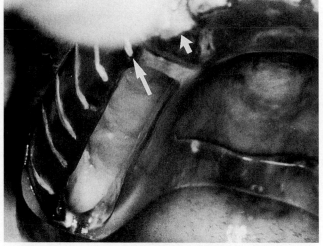

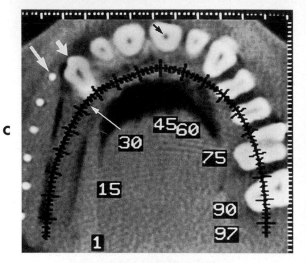

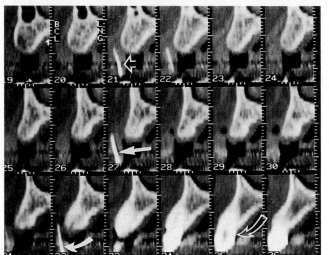

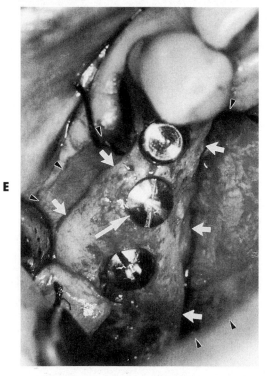

FIG. 6-5 Surgical implant procedure. **A,** This patient, being evaluated for dental implants, is edentulous distal to the right maxillary canine *(arrow)*. **B,** A stent with six vertical markers has been placed over the alveolar ridge and residual teeth. The sixth marker *(long arrow)* is adjacent to the right canine *(short arrow)* and will be demonstrated on the CT images. This marker appears as a dot on the axial image next to perpendicular line 32 (**C**) and as a line on cross-sectional image number 32 (**D**). **C,** Axial view demonstrating the sixth marker *(long thick arrow)* at perpendicular line 32 *(thin arrow)* and adjacent to the right canine *(short white arrow)*. Note the radiolucent pulp in the center of the teeth *(black arrow)*. **D,** Cross-sectional views demonstrating markers 4 *(open arrow)*, 5 *(straight arrow)*, and 6 *(curved arrow)* of the stent. Note that marker number 6 is adjacent to the right canine *(open curved arrow)*. By placing the stent on the patient during surgery, the surgeon knows that the bone under marker 6 is as depicted by cross-sectional image 32. **E,** An incision is made and the gingival and periosteal flap *(arrowheads)* is held back with sutures. This exposes the bone of the alveolar process *(short thick arrows)*. Holes are drilled, and three titanium implants are inserted into the bone. Note that the implants are flush with the bone, and their openings are covered with healing screw caps *(long arrow)*.

(Continued)

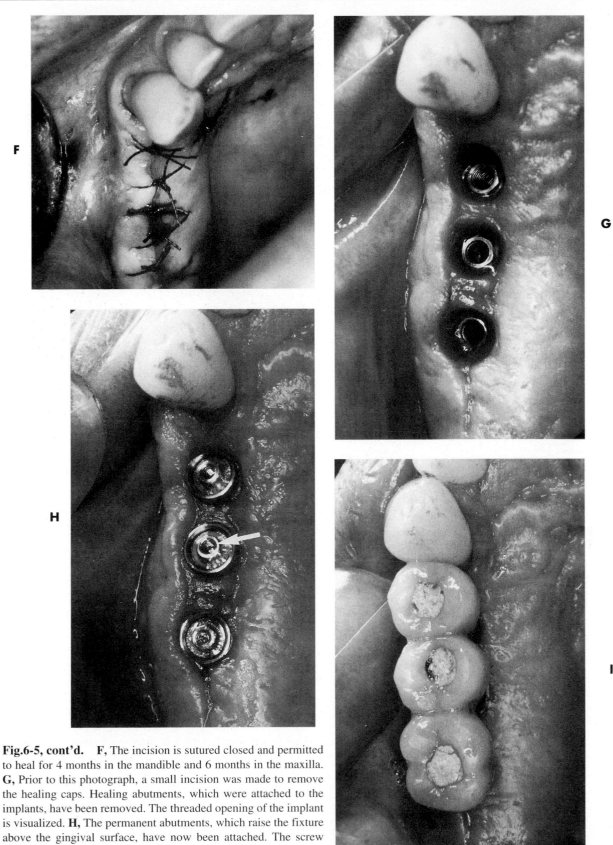

Fig.6-5, cont'd. **F,** The incision is sutured closed and permitted to heal for 4 months in the mandible and 6 months in the maxilla. **G,** Prior to this photograph, a small incision was made to remove the healing caps. Healing abutments, which were attached to the implants, have been removed. The threaded opening of the implant is visualized. **H,** The permanent abutments, which raise the fixture above the gingival surface, have now been attached. The screw hole *(arrow)* in the center of the abutment will accommodate the screw that fixes the prosthesis. **I,** The prosthesis is now attached to the three implants. The screw heads are covered with a white compound. (From Abrahams JJ. The role of diagnostic imaging in dental implantology. Radiol Clinics of North America 1993; 31(1):163-180.)

Dental CT Program
Scan Parameters

The patient is placed supine in the gantry, using a head holder, chin strap, and sponges on either side of the head to prevent motion. The patient is then instructed to remain motionless. A lateral digital scout view is first obtained to define the upper and lower limits of the study and to determine if the scan plane is parallel to the alveolar ridge. Because the DentaScan program does not permit angulation of the gantry, if the scan plane is not correctly positioned, the patient should be repositioned and a repeat lateral digital scout scan should be performed. Once the scan plane is correct, 1-mm contiguous scans are obtained using a bone algorithm, dynamic mode, 15-cm field of view, 512 × 512 matrix, 140 kV and 70 mA. If both the mandible and maxilla are being studied, a separate run should be performed for each because the scan angle of the mandible is slightly different than that of the maxilla.

Running the Dental Program

Programs may vary slightly from manufacturer to manufacturer; however, the following guidelines generally apply. After the axial images are acquired, a curved line along the midportion of the alveolus is superimposed on an axial image of the mandible or maxilla (Figs. 6-6, A, 6-7, A). The axial image chosen should be at the level of the roots of the teeth and should demonstrate the full contour of the mandible or maxilla. The curved line is created on this axial image by depositing the cursor on approximately six different points along the curve of the jaw. The program then automatically connects these points to produce a smooth curve that will be superimposed on the jaw. This curved line defines the plane and location of the reformatted panoramic images (Figs. 6-6, C, 6-7, D). Several images are then reformatted both buccally and lingually to this curve.

The reformatted cross-sectional images (Figs. 6-6, D-F, 6-7, E, F) are defined by multiple numbered lines that the program automatically deposits perpendicular to the curved line (Figs. 6-6, A, 6-7, A). Fig. 6-6, A illustrates the plane and orientation of the cross-sectional images and the distance between the numbered perpendicular lines. The distance between the cross-sectional images can be varied. In general a 2-mm spacing is used. If a stent with radiographic markers is utilized, 1-mm slices may be necessary to visualize the markers. The mandibular canal (neurovascular bundle) is easily visualized on the cross-sectional images, and the width and contour of the jaw can be readily assessed (Fig. 6-6, D-F). Streak artifact, which degrades visualization of bone on direct coronal images, does not degrade the reformatted cross-sectional images because the artifact is projected at the level of the crowns of the teeth and not over the bony alveolus (curved arrow in Fig. 6-6, E).

When the program is completed, three types of images are displayed: axial, cross-sectional, and panoramic. Typically there are approximately 30 to 50 axial images, 40 to 100 cross-sectional images, and 5 panoramic images. It is important to film these images in a consistent fashion to avoid confusing the referring dentist. Life-size (1 to 1 magnification) cross-sectional and panoramic images are preferred. This can usually be accomplished with most programs by filming four images on a 14 × 17 x-ray film. If this does not work, the manufacturer of the program should be consulted. A millimeter scale displayed on the films (mm bottom of Fig. 6-6, D) is used to verify the degree of magnification and to obtain accurate measurements. One can place calipers on the bone image to be measured and transfer this caliper setting to the millimeter scale. Any minification or magnification of the images equally minifies or magnifies the scale and thus does not affect the measurements.

Optimally, filming is done on a laser printer, and usually two original film sets are printed, one for the radiologist and one for the dentist. Most often the axial images are filmed with 12 images per sheet of film, and the cross-sectional and panoramic images are filmed with 4 images per film. Each cross-sectional and panoramic image actually contains multiple images. The images are typically photographed at a width (window) of between 3000 to 4000 and a level (center) of between 300 to 500 (see Figs. 6-6 to 6-10).

Interpretation of Dental CT Program Images and Measurements

An understanding of the anatomy and pathology of the jaw is necessary to appropriately interpret the images displayed by the dental CT programs. It should first be noted that each CT view can be related to the other by a series of scale marks that appear on the films. Marks, which run along the side of the cross-sectional and panoramic images (Figs. 6-6, C, 6-6, D) correspond to the direct axial slices that were used to reformat the images. For example, in Fig. 6-6, 42 axial images were obtained to reformat the images; thus there are 42 scale marks along the side of the reformatted cross-sectional (Fig. 6-6, D) and panoramic images (Fig. 6-6, C). Marks along the bottom of the panoramic images (Fig. 6-6, C) correspond to numbered cross-sectional images. Numbered scale lines correspond to the numbered lines drawn perpendicular to the curve superimposed on the axial image in Fig. 6-6, A. They therefore also correspond to the numbered cross-sectional images in Figs. 6-6, D, E, F. To illustrate how one view can be related to another, note how the right mental foramen (M) in Fig. 6-6, E, which is seen on cross-sectional image 20 (lower right) at the level of the fourteenth scale mark on the side of the image, is also seen in Fig. 6-6, B on axial image 14 at the twentieth perpendicular line. The same process can be applied to the panoramic view.

When the scan is performed as part of the preoperative workup of a dental implant patient, the status of the dentition and the proposed implant sites must be established. It should be stated whether the patient is partially edentulous or completely edentulous. If some teeth remain, their precise location must be noted. In the partially edentulous patient, it is presumed that the implants will be placed in the edentulous segments, and thus measurements are obtained in these

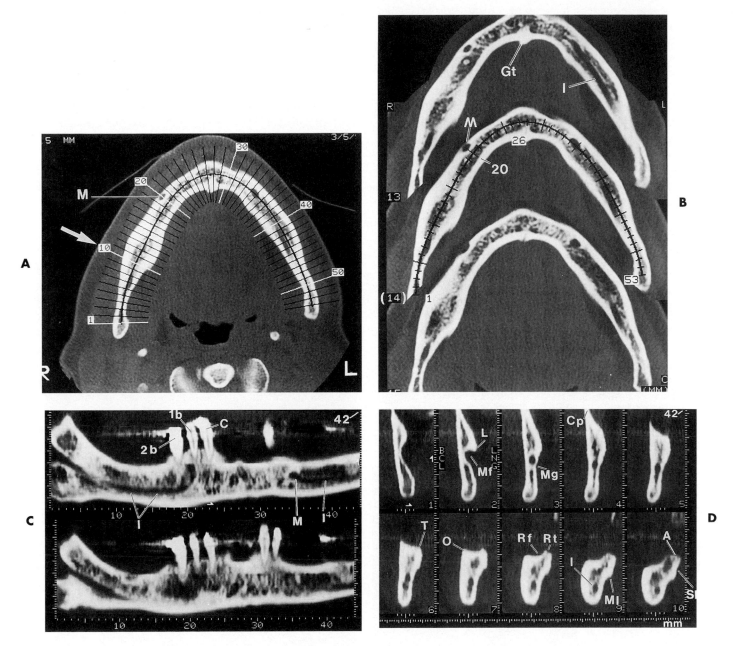

FIG. 6-6   CT (DentaScan) of mandible. The anatomy identified on the mandibular anatomic specimen in Fig. 6-12 is now identified on these CT images. **A,** Axial image of mandible with superimposed curve. The curve defines the plane and location in which the panoramic images in **C** are reformatted. Numbered lines drawn perpendicular to this curve *(arrow)* define the plane and location in which the cross-sectional images viewed in **D** through **F** are reformatted. Mental foramen *(M)*. **B,** Axial images illustrating the inferior alveolar canal *(I)*, the mental foramen *(M)*, and the genial tubercle *(Gt)*. The numbers along the left side of the figure refer to the particular number of the axial image. Note that the mental foramen, which is seen on axial image number 14 at the twentieth perpendicular line, is also seen in **E** on cross-sectional image 20 *(lower right)* at the level of the fourteenth tick mark on the side of the image. The tick marks and numbers allow images to be correlated with one another. **C,** Panoramic views. The numbered tick marks along the bottom of the images correspond to the numbered perpendicular lines displayed on the axial image in **A**. The tick marks along the side of the image correspond to the axial images that were used to reformat these images. Note that there were 42 axial images acquired and thus 42 tick marks along the side of this image. Inferior alveolar canal *(I)*, mental foramen *(M)*, second bicuspid *(2B)*, first bicuspid *(1B)*, and cuspid *(C)*.

Continued

regions. In the edentulous areas, if the cross-sectional images are 2 mm apart, typically measurements are made on every fifth cross-sectional image. If the cross-sectional images are 1 mm apart, measurements are provided for every tenth image. The height and width of the alveolar process are measured as described in the following paragraph.

In the mandible the height in the region distal (posterior) to the mental foramen is measured from the top of the alveolar process to the top to the mandibular canal (Fig. 6-6, *E, arrowheads* in image 17). Methods of locating the mandibular canal, if it is not initially visualized on the cross-sectional images, are discussed later. In the region mesial (anterior) to the mental foramen, the full height of the mandible is obtained because the mandibular canal ends at the mental foramen and thus it is not present mesial to the foramen. Measurements in this area are provided from the top of the alveolar ridge to the bottom of the mandible (Fig. 6-6, *F, arrowheads* in image 30). The width is measured near the top of the alveolar process (Fig. 6-6, *F, arrowheads* in image 30). Occasionally, if the alveolar process comes to a point secondary to atrophy, it may be difficult to obtain a measurement. In this situation the surgeon may choose to remove the top pointed portion of the ridge (alveoloplasty), providing a broad base for an implant. This obviously affects the height of the alveolar ridge, and it is best to let the surgeon estimate how much of the ridge will be removed. Often under these circumstances, one simply states that the ridge is pointed,

and a measurement for the width is not provided.

In the maxilla the height in the distal (posterior) aspect is measured from the top (inferior surface) of the alveolar process to the floor of the maxillary sinus (Fig. 6-7, *E, arrows* in image 7). More mesially (anteriorly) the height is usually not limited by the maxillary sinuses and is measured from the alveolar ridge to the nasal fossa floor (Fig. 6-7, *F, arrows* in image 23). The width is measured in the same manner as that described for the mandible (Fig. 6-7, *F, arrows* in image 22). In the completely edentulous patient, it is more desirable to place the implants centrally because the height of the alveolar process is not limited by the more distal mandibular canal or the maxillary sinuses.

Dictated Report

A complete and comprehensive report should be provided for the referring dentist or oral surgeon. First, the report usually provides a discussion of the density and general health of the jaw. Also described are the presence of such conditions as maxillary sinus disease, periodontal disease, root canal procedures, extraction sockets, retained roots, atrophy, cysts, osteitis condensans, contour irregularities, surgical changes, and anomalies such as torus palatinus or mandibularus. Next the status of the dentition is discussed, and measurements of the alveolar process are provided. Measurements are provided in a tabular fashion, and the mental foramina and incisive foramen are identified for easy inter-

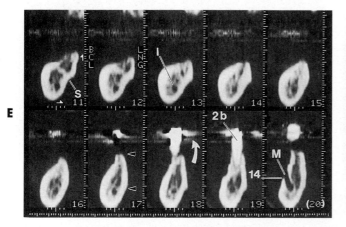   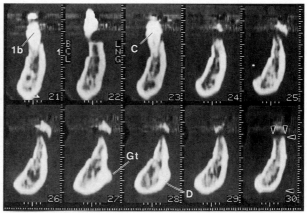

Fig. 6-6, cont'd.   D through **F,** Cross-sectional views. Images 1 through 10 (**D**) are through the posterior right mandible (see perpendicular lines 1 through 10 in **A**). Images 11 through 20 (**E**) are more anterior. Images 21 through 30 (**F**) extend to the midline. The images of the left half of the mandible are not shown. *Arrowheads* in image 17 (**E**) indicate that the height of the mandible distal to the mental foramen is measured from the top of the alveolar process to the top of the mandibular canal, and mesial to the foramen it is measured from the top of the alveolar process to the bottom of the mandible (*arrowheads* in **F,** image 30). Measurement of the width is also demonstrated in image 30 (**F**). *MM* at the bottom of **D** indicates the millimeter scale. Note how streak artifact from dental restoration (*curved arrow* in **E**) does not degrade visualization of the bone. *A* indicates alveolar process; *C,* cuspid; *Cp,* coronoid process; *D,* digastric fossa; *Gt,* genial tubercle; *I,* inferior alveolar canal; *M,* mental foramen; *Mf* mandibular foramen; *Mg,* mylohyoid groove; *Ml* mylohyoid line; *O,* oblique line; *Rf,* retromolar fossa; *Rt,* retromolar triangle; *S,* submandibular fossa; *Sl,* sublingual fossa; *T,* temporal crest; *1B,* first bicuspid; and *2B,* second bicuspid. (From Abrahams JJ. Anatomy of the jaw revisited with a dental CT software program: Pictorial essay. AJNR 1993; 14:979-990.

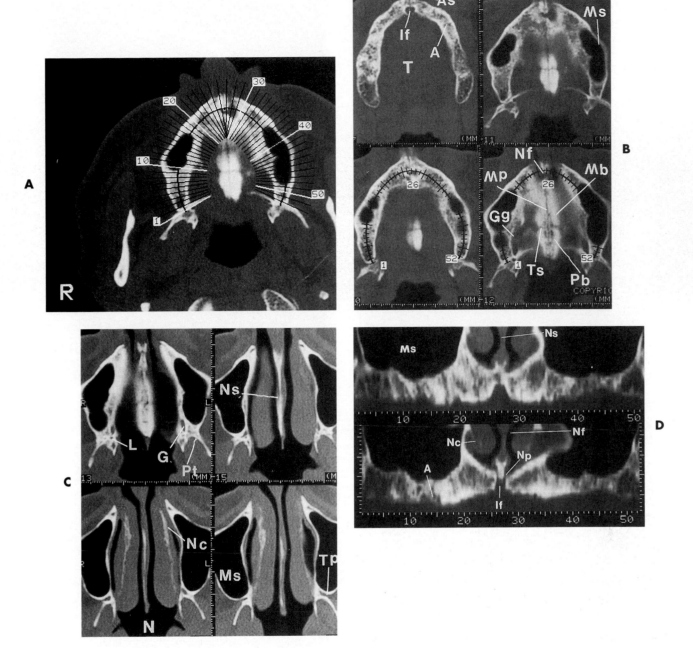

FIG. 6-7   CT (DentaScan) of maxilla. The anatomy identified on the maxillary anatomic specimen in Fig. 6-16 is now identified on these CT images. **A,** Axial image with superimposed curve. The curve defines the plane and location in which the panoramic images seen in **D** are reformatted. Numbered lines drawn perpendicular to this curve define the plane and location in which the cross-sectional images viewed in **E** and **F** are reformatted. **B,**   Axial views through the alveolar ridge and hard palate. *A* indicates alveolar process; *As,* inferior nasal spine; *Gg,* groove for greater palatine nerve; *If,* incisive foramen; *Mb,* maxillary bone—palatine process; *Mp,* median palatine suture; *Ms,* maxillary sinus; *Nf,* nasal fossa; *Pb,* palatine bone—horizontal plate; *Ts,* transverse suture; and *T,* tongue. **C,** Axial views through the maxillary sinuses and the pterygopalatine fossa. *G* indicates greater palatine foramen; *L,* lesser palatine foramen; *Ms,* maxillary sinus; *Nc,* nasal conchi; *Ns,* nasal septum; *Pt,* pterygoid process; and *Tp,* pterygopalatine fossa. **D,** Panoramic views. *A* indicates alveolar process; *If,* incisive foramen; *Ms,* maxillary sinus; *Nc,* nasal concha; *Nf,* nasal fossa; *Np,* nasopalatine canal; and *Ns,* nasal septum.

Continued

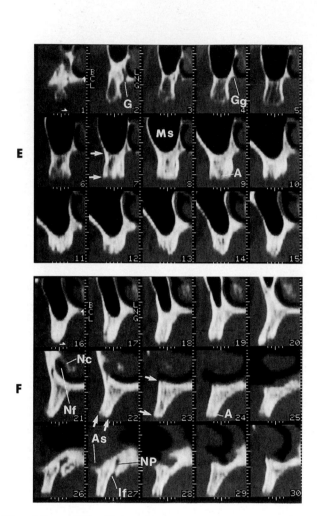

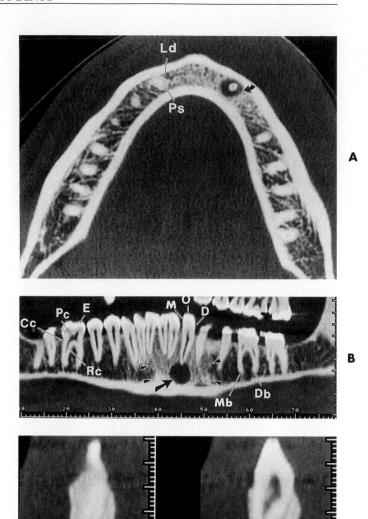

Fig. 6-7, cont'd. E and **F,** Cross-sectional views. Images 1 through 15 (**E**) are through the posterior right maxilla (see perpendicular lines 1 through 15 in **A**); images 16 through 30 (**F**) are more anterior on the right and extend to the midline (see perpendicular lines 16 through 30 in **A**). The *arrows* in image 7 (**E**) indicate how the height of the distal alveolar process is measured from the floor of the maxillary sinus to the top of the alveolar process and the mesial alveolar process (**F** in image 23) is measured from the floor of the nasal fossa to the top of the alveolar process (*arrows* in image 23). The *arrows* in image 22 (**F**) indicate how the width of the alveolar process is measured. *A* indicates alveolar process; *As,* anterior maxillary spine; *G,* greater palatine foramen; *Gg,* groove for greater palatine nerve; *If,* incisive foramen; *Ms,* maxillary sinus; *Nc,* nasal concha; *Nf,* nasal fossa; and *Np,* nasopalatine canal. (From Abrahams JJ. Anatomy of the jaw revisited with a dental CT software program: pictorial essay. AJNR 1993; 14:979-990.)

FIG. 6-8 Mandibular DentaScan demonstrating a radicular cyst surrounding the root apex of the left canine. **A,** Axial view demonstrating the radicular cyst *(black arrow).* The periodontal space *(Ps)* typically not seen on CT can be visualized in this patient between the lamina dura *(Ld)* and the tooth. **B,** Panoramic view illustrating an area of sclerotic osteitis condensans *(arrowheads)* surrounding the radicular cyst *(black arrow).* The cervical constriction *(Cc),* pulp chamber *(Pc),* root canal *(Rc),* and dense enamel *(E)* are nicely demonstrated on the right first molar. The mesial *(M),* occlusal *(O),* and distal *(D)* surfaces of the left canine are demonstrated, as well as the mesiobuccal *(Mb)* and distobuccal *(Db)* roots of the left first molar. The lingual root of the left first molar is not seen in this plane. **C,** Cross-sectional views demonstrating the radicular cyst surrounding the root apex.

pretation and reference. For example, the following measurements were obtained from Figs. 6-6, *E, F*:

Image 17:   Height 14 mm, width 4 mm
Image 20:   Left mental foramen
Image 25:   Height 26 mm, width 4 mm

If a stent with radiopaque markers is utilized, then the markers on the images are numbered with a wax pencil, measurements are obtained on the cross-sectional images where the markers appear, and the image number is provided in the report. In Fig. 6-5, *D*, for example, the measurements at the markers are as follows:

Marker #4 (Image 21):   Height 13 mm, width 6 mm
Marker #5 (Image 27):   Height 12 mm, width 5 mm

The report should end with a brief impression, describing any pertinent pathology and the degree of atrophy and giving a statement that all measurements should be verified before surgery. This statement is included because the surgeon may choose to place the implant at a somewhat different angle than that measured by the radiologist.

Identifying the Mandibular Canal

It is extremely important to identify the mandibular canal on cross-sectional images and to provide measurement from the top of the alveolar ridge to the top of this canal. If the canal is not properly identified, its injury during implant surgery can be quite debilitating for the patient, resulting in permanent paresthesia and hypesthesia of the face. Typically the canal can be readily seen on cross-sectional images. However, there are times when portions of the canal or even the entire canal may be hard to visualize on the cross-sectional images. In this situation the following methods may be helpful in locating the canal.

The first method involves the cortical niche sign, which refers to an indentation along the inner or medullary margin on the lingual cortex of the mandible. This niche is created by the mandibular nerve as it traverses the mandible (Fig. 6-9). However, this niche can be quite subtle, unlike that shown in Fig. 6-9, and it is not identified in all patients. When present, it is a good way to identify the canal. Caution should be taken not to confuse other cortical irregularities with the cortical niche sign. The cortical niche is a continuous defect seen on multiple cross-sectional images. Other cortical irregularities are randomly situated and are not seen consecutively on multiple images. When the canal is identified with the cortical niche sign, its location should be confirmed with the other methods.

The next method, referred to as triangulation, utilizes the scale marks on the films to relate an anatomic structure well seen on one view with its location on another view. With this method the panoramic and axial views can be utilized to identify the canal on the cross-sectional views. For example, in Fig. 6-11, *A*, it is difficult to see the canal on the cross-sectional images, but the canal is readily seen in the panoramic view (Fig. 6-11, *B*). The information from the

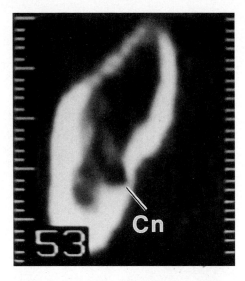

FIG. 6-9   Cortical niche sign. This cross-sectional image of the mandible demonstrates an indentation on the lingual cortex of the mandible called the cortical niche sign *(Cn)*, which is created by the mandibular nerve as it traverses the mandible. This sign, which is often more subtle than this, can be helpful in identifying the location of the mandibular canal. (From Abrahams JJ. CT assessment of dental implant planning. Oral and Maxillofac Surg Clin North Am 1992; 4:1-18.)

panoramic view can be used to triangulate the location of the canal on the cross-sectional image, as shown in Fig. 6-11. To locate the canal on cross-sectional image 14 (Fig. 6-11, *A*), first refer to the fourteenth scale mark along the bottom of the panoramic view (Fig. 6-11, *B*). A vertical line from this point is then drawn up to the bottom of the canal and extended across in a perpendicular direction toward the scale marks on the left side of the panoramic image. Note that this line intersects the twenty-first scale mark along the left side of the image. The level of the canal in cross-sectional image 14 can then be identified by counting up 21 scale marks along the side of the image (Fig. 6-11, *A*). This same process can also be utilized with the axial images.

Finally, if a canal is identified on some cross-sectional images but not on others, the images on which it is identified can be utilized to estimate the position of the canal on the other images. This can be done because the distance from the bottom of the mandible to the bottom of the canal tends to be relatively constant. The only region where the distance is not constant is immediately adjacent to the mandibular foramen and the mental foramen. It is the distance from the top of the canal to the top of the alveolar process that varies secondary to atrophic changes. With this knowledge, one can extrapolate the location of the canal from the images in which it is visualized. For example, in Fig. 6-6, *E*, the distance from the bottom of the canal to the bottom of the mandible in image 11 is 5 mm, and in image 15 it is also 5 mm. Therefore if the canal was not visualized in image 15, its location could be estimated by utilizing the position of the canal that was visible on image 11. Usually

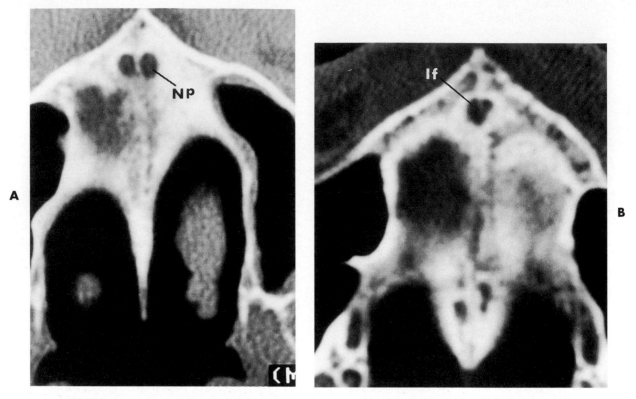

FIG. 6-10   Axial views of the nasopalatine canal and the incisive foramen. **A,** The more superior axial image demonstrates the two nasopalatine canals *(Np)*. **B,** The inferior slice demonstrates their common opening, the incisive foramen *(If)*. (From Abrahams JJ. Anatomy of the jaw revisited with a dental CT software program: pictorial essay. AJNR 1993; 14:979-990.)

the right and left hemimandibles are symmetrical, and the distance from the bottom of the mandible to the bottom of the canal on the right side at a particular point is approximately the same as the distance measured at that same point on the left. Thus if the canal is identified on the cross-sectional images of the right half of the mandible but not on the left side, this information can be used to estimate the position of the canal on the left side. It is recommended that several of these methods be used to confirm the location of the canal, rather than relying on only one method.

Radiographic and Surgical Stents

A *stent* is a clear acrylic device that fits snugly over the residual teeth and alveolar ridge (Fig. 6-5, *B*). It is manufactured by the dentist after an impression of the teeth and ridge has been obtained. Radiopaque markers are attached to the stent to facilitate transfer of information from the DentaScan to the patient. The same radiographic stent is used as a surgical template when the implants are inserted.

The radiographic markers are typically made of guttapercha, a radiopaque material commonly used by dentists as a temporary filling. Other radiopaque material such as pieces of wire may also be used for markers. Ideally the markers are 1 to 2 mm in diameter, vertically oriented, and without a mesial or distal tilt (Fig. 6-5, *B*). The vertical

markers should be attached to the stent in such a way that they extend deep into the buccal vestibule. This aids in their visibility on the cross-sectional images because they overlie the bony alveolus rather than the crowns of the teeth, which may have streak artifacts from restorations. Other types of markers have also been used, including coating a denture with barium.[23] The radiologist can help the dentist place the markers in a manner that yields the greatest information because most dentists are unfamiliar with CT.

Fig. 6-5 illustrates how the stent is used. After the patient is scanned, the markers appear as dots on the axial image (Fig. 6-5, *C*) and as lines on the cross-sectional images (Fig. 6-5, *D*). If the surgeon is interested in putting an implant just distal to the right canine (Fig. 6-5, *A, C, short white arrow*), it is noted that the sixth marker falls in this location (Fig. 6-5, *B, C, long thick arrow*). Next the axial images are examined to see on which cross-sectional image the marker appears. In this case the sixth marker on the stent appears on the axial image at perpendicular line 32 (Fig. 6-5, *C, thin arrow*) and is therefore seen on cross-sectional image 32 in Fig. 6-5, *D*. The surgeon knows that the bone under marker 6 corresponds to cross-sectional image 32.

After the incision is made and the alveolar bone is exposed, this stent can be placed back on the patient and used as a template. This stent is designed with a cut-out over

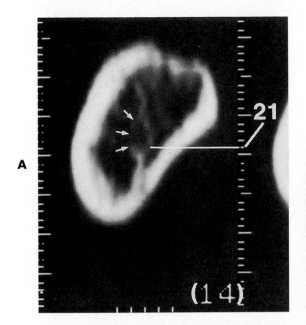

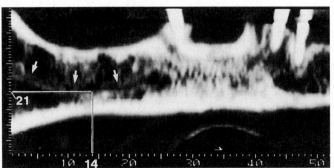

FIG. 6-11   Triangulation. When the inferior alveolar canal is not initially seen on the cross-sectional images as in this case **(A)**, its location can be determined by triangulating from the panoramic **(B)** or axial image as described in the section of text titled Identifying the Mandibular Canal). Inferior alveolar canal is indicated by arrows. (From Abrahams JJ. CT assessment of dental implant planning. Oral and Maxillofac Surg Clin North Am, 1992; 4:1-18.)

the alveolar aspect so that the surgeon can directly mark the area for the implant (Fig. 6-5, *B*). The marker on the cross-sectional image also can be used to help the surgeon estimate the correct facial or palatal angulation of the implant.

Stents and markers are only accurate if the stent fits tightly and if its position in the patient's mouth is the same during scanning and surgery. The dentist should give the patient careful instruction on how to insert the stent properly.

ANATOMY
Dentition and General Consideration

The teeth of the mandible and maxilla are embeded in a horseshoe-shaped bony ridge called the *alveolar process*. Each process divides the oral cavity into two compartments: a more central one adjacent to the tongue called the *oral cavity* proper and a more peripheral one adjacent to the cheeks and lips called the *oral vestibule*. A horseshoe-shaped furrow formed where the mucous membrane of the lip and cheek reflect onto the alveolar process is termed the *fornix vestibuli*. In the midline vertically oriented folds of mucosa, the labial frenula, helps connect the upper and lower lips to the alveolar process. The lingual frer um, or frenulum, is a similar structure in the midline on the under surface of the tongue.

When fully dentured, the jaw contains 32 teeth—16 in the maxilla and 16 in the mandible. The teeth can be referred to by tooth number or by name. They are numbered sequentially starting in the posterior right maxilla with tooth number 1 and continuing to number 16 in the posterior left maxilla. In the mandible they continue with tooth number 17 in the pos-

terior left and end with tooth number 32 in the posterior right. The teeth are named beginning in the midline and moving distally on each side as follows: the central incisor, the lateral incisor, the canine, the first premolar, the second premolar, the first molar, the second molar, and the third molar.

The portion of the tooth exposed in the oral cavity is called the *anatomic crown* (*arrowheads* in Fig. 6-12, *C*) and that portion of the tooth embedded in the bony socket is referred to as the *root* (Fig. 6-8, *B*). Most of the tooth is composed of dentine; however, the outer surface of the crown is covered by the smooth, dense enamel, and the outer surface of the root is covered by dense cementum, a tissue very similar to bone. A constriction where the crown and root meet is referred to as either the *cervical constriction* or the *cementoenamel junction* (*Ce* in Fig. 6-8, *B*). On CT, particularly in young people the dense enamel appears separate from the dentine and looks like a dense band covering the crown of the tooth (*E* in Fig. 6-8, *B*). With age, receding gingiva and bone cause portions of the root to be exposed in the oral cavity. The crown now differs from the original anatomic crown (that portion covered with enamel) and should be referred to as the *functional crown* (*arrows* in Fig. 6-12, *C*). The *arrows* in Fig. 6-12, *C* point to the functional crown, and the *arrowheads* point to the anatomic crown.

The neurovascular bundle of the tooth enters the root apex via the apical foramen and travels through the root canal and into an expanded pulp chamber in the crown. The root canal and pulp chamber are seen on CT as a relatively radiolucent area in the center of the root and crown (Fig. 6-8, *B*). Accessory apical foramina along the side of the root, rather than the apex of the root, may occasionally exist.

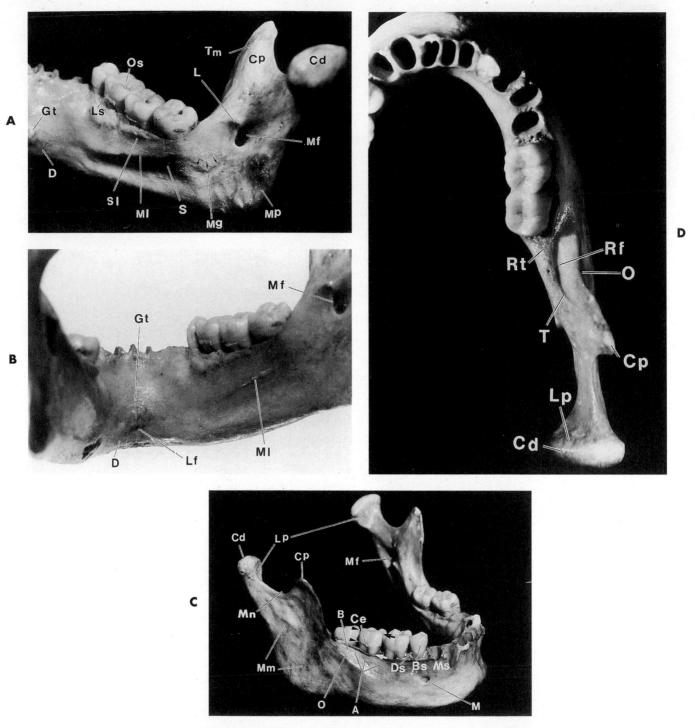

FIG. 6-12   Anatomic specimen demonstrating the lingual (**A** and **B**), buccal (**C**), and superior (**D**) aspects of the mandible. *A* indicates alveolar process; *B,* buccinator muscle insertion; *Bs,* buccal surface; *Cd,* condyle; *Ce,* cemento enamel junction; *Cp,* coronoid process; *D,* digastric fossa; *Ds,* distal surface; *Gt,* genial tubercle; *L,* lingula; *Lf,* lingual foramen; *Lp,* lateral pterygoid muscle insertion; *Ls,* lingual surface; *M,* mental foramen; *Mf,* mandibular foramen; *Mg,* mylohyoid groove; *Ml,* mylohyoid lines; *Mm,* masseter muscle insertion; *Mn,* mandibular notch; *Mp,* medial pterygoid insertion; *Ms,* mesial surface; *O,* oblique line; *Os,* occlusal surface; *Rf,* retromolar fossa; *Rt,* retromolar triangle; *S,* submandibular fossa; *Sl,* sublingual fossa; *T,* temporal crest; *Tm,* temporalis muscle insertion; *arrowheads,* anatomic crown; *black and white arrows,* functional crown; *small black arrows,* mylohyoid groove. (From Abrahams JJ. Anatomy of the jaw revisited with a dental CT software program: pictorial essay. AJNR 1993; 14:979-990.)

Each crown has five free surfaces.[24] The biting surface, or the surface where the upper and lower teeth oppose each other, is referred to as the *occlusal surface* (Figs. 6-8, *B*, 6-12, *A*). The surface facing toward the inside, or toward the oral cavity, is called the *lingual surface* in the mandible and the palatal surface in the maxilla (Fig. 6-12, *A*). The outer surface of the tooth facing toward the lip and cheek is termed the *labial surface* for the incisors and canines and the buccal surface for the premolars and molars (Fig. 6-12, *C*). This surface may more simply be referred to as the *facial surface* for all the teeth. The other tooth surfaces are the contact surfaces where one tooth contacts a neighboring tooth. Of these two surfaces the one closest to the midline is referred to as the *mesial surface,* and the other is referred to as the *distal surface* (Figs. 6-8, *B*, 6-12). The mesial surface in the incisors and canines may also be called the *medial surface,* but in the premolars and molars it is termed the *anterior surface.* Likewise the distal surface in the incisors and canines may be called the *lateral surface,* and in the premolars and molars the *posterior surface.*

Direction also can be described with this terminology. For example, toward the midline would be referred to as *mesial,* or *anterior,* and moving in the direction of the molars would be referred to as *distal,* or *posterior.* When referring to the crown of the tooth, one may move in the occlusal direction (toward the opposing tooth) or in the cervical direction (toward the cervical constriction), and when referring to the root, one may move in the cervical or apical direction. The use of this terminology is nicely exemplified by naming the roots of the teeth. For example, the first molar contains three roots, two buccal and one lingual. Of the two buccal roots, one is termed a *mesiobuccal* and the other is termed the *distobuccal* (Fig. 6-8, *B*). The lingual one is simply called the *lingual root.*

The teeth are held into the bony socket by a highly specialized periodontal ligament that provides the teeth with small degrees of motion or "give" within the socket. On plain films the ligament appears as a radiolucency between the cementum of the root and the lamina dura of the bony socket. The periodontal space normally measures between 0.1 and 0.2 mm and is therefore not typically identified on CT. Fig. 6-8, *A,* however, does show the lamina dura and to a lesser degree the periodontal space. A radiolucency seen on CT between the tooth root and the alveolar bone may represent a pathologic state such as periodontal disease, which is discussed later. In the cervical portion of the tooth, the fibers of the periodontal ligament radiate from the cementum of the root into the gingiva and serve to attach the gingiva to the tooth.

Mandible

The anatomy of the mandible is described first on the anatomic specimen in Fig. 6-12 and on the illustrations of the neurovascular and muscular structures in Figs. 6-13 and 6-14.[18,24-32] This anatomy is then labeled on the cross-sectional, axial, and panoramic CT images in Fig. 6-6.[33]

Anatomic Specimen

Lingual Surface. The mandibular nerve, the third division of the trigeminal nerve (Fig. 6-13, *A*), enters the lingual surface of the mandible through the mandibular foramen (*Mf* in Fig. 6-12, *A*). The foramen is situated in the center of the ramus, 1 to 2 cm posterior to the third molar at the craniocaudal level of the crowns of the teeth. The nerve (and mandibular artery) then travels anteriorly in the inferior alveolar canal (mandibular canal) (Fig. 6-13, *A*). The canal typically hugs the lingual aspect of the mandible until it curves labially to exit the mandible at the mental foramen (*M* in Figs. 6-12, *C*, 6-13, *A*), which on the labial surface of the mandible is between the first and second premolars at the level of the roots. As the neurovascular bundle travels through the mandible, small nutrient canals extend coronally to supply the teeth (Fig. 6-13, *A, arrow*). At the mental foramen the main trunk of the mandibular nerve exits as the mental nerve and supplies sensory fibers to the skin overlying the mandible and lower lip (Fig. 6-13, *A*). A smaller branch, the incisive nerve, continues toward the midline within the mandible in the incisive canal (Fig. 6-15). It is accompanied by the incisive artery. This nerve innervates the canine and lateral incisor teeth, and the artery exits through the lingual foramen, which is located in the midline, inferiorly on the lingual aspect of the mandible (*Lf* in Figs. 6-12, *B*, 6-15, *C*). After exiting the mandible this artery anastomosis with the lingual artery of the tongue (Fig. 6-14, A).

The mylohyoid nerve, a small branch of the mandibular nerve, rather than entering the mandibular foramen with the rest of the nerve, travels anteriorly in the mylohyoid groove on the lingual surface of the mandible (*Mg* in Fig. 6-12, *A*). The mylohyoid nerve supplies the mylohyoid muscle (Fig. 6-14, *A, C, D*), which fans out like a sling to form the functional floor of the oral cavity. This muscle inserts on the mandible along a bony ridge, the mylohyoid line (*Ml* in Fig. 6-12, *A*). This line acts as a landmark, separating the oral cavity from the suprahyoid portion of the neck. Inferior to the mylohyoid muscle is the submandibular fossa (*S* in Fig. 6-12, *A*), a slight concavity in the mandible for the submandibular gland. A small portion of the gland wraps around the posterior aspect of the mylohyoid muscle to enter the sublingual space (Fig. 6-14, *A*). Superior to the mylohyoid line and muscle is the sublingual fossa (*Sl* in Fig. 6-12, *A*), in which is situated the sublingual gland (Fig. 6-14, *A*).

Also above the mylohyoid muscle are the geniohyoid and genioglossus muscles, which insert on a midline bony protuberance called the *genial tubercle* (*Gt* in Figs. 6-12, *B*, 6-15, *C*). It has four bony spines, two superior ones for the right and left genioglossus muscles and two inferior ones for the right and left geniohyoid muscles (Figs. 6-14, *C, D,* 6-15, *C*). Inferior to the mylohyoid muscle and to either side of the genial tubercle are the digastric fossae (*D* in Fig. 6-12, *A, B*), each for the origin of the anterior belly of the digastric muscle (Fig. 6-14, *A*).

The temporalis muscle (Fig. 6-14, *B*) inserts on the coronoid process, the most superoanterior extension of the

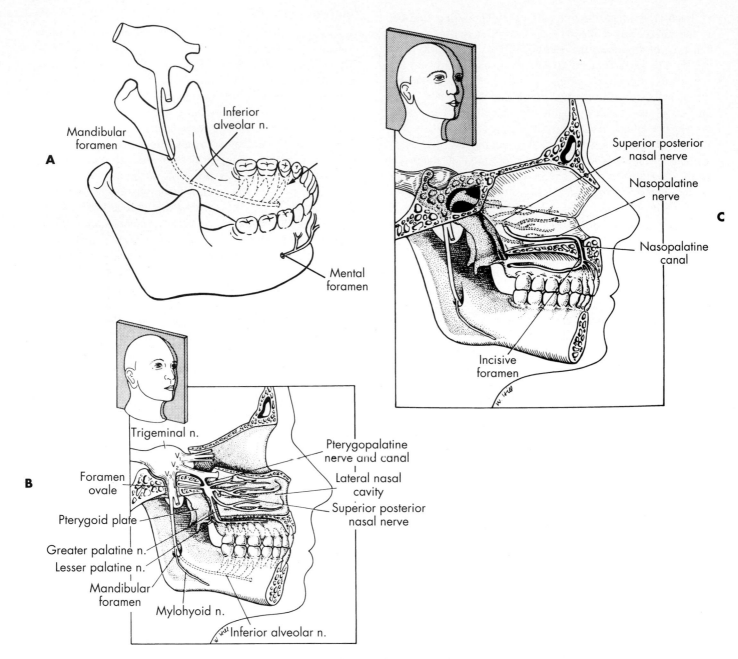

FIG. 6-13 Neurovascular structures. **A,** View of the mandible illustrating the mandibular foramen, the mental foramen, and the nutrient canals, which extend from the inferior alveolar canal toward the teeth. *n* indicates nerve and arrow nutrient canals. **B,** Parasagittal view through the trigeminal nerve and the lateral nasal cavity. Note how the myelohyoid nerve travels on the lingual surface of the mandible rather than entering the mandibular foramen. The greater palatine nerve arises from the pterygopalatine nerve, a branch of V2. **C,** Midsagittal view through the incisive foramen and the nasal septum. Note how the nasopalatine nerve, a branch of the superior-posterior nasal nerve, travels along the nasal septum and through the incisive foramen. (From Abrahams JJ. Anatomy of the jaw revisited with a dental CT software program: pictorial essay. AJNR 1993; 14:979-990.)

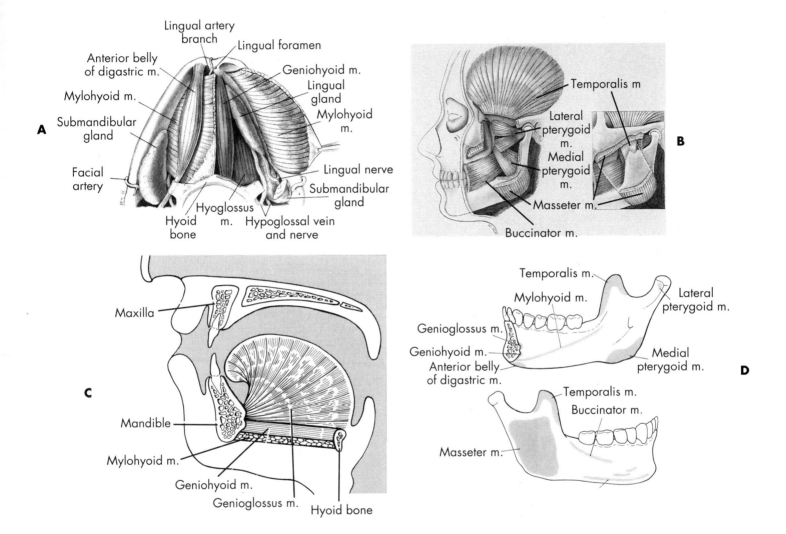

FIG. 6-14   Muscles and insertions. **A,** Mandible viewed from below. *m* indicates muscle. **B,** Lateral view with zygomatic arch and coronoid process removed. **C,** Midline sagittal view through the genial tubercle. **D,** Muscle insertions. Lingual surface (**a**). Buccal surface (**b**). (From Abrahams JJ. Anatomy of the jaw revisited with a dental CT software program: pictorial essay. AJNR 1993; 14:979-990.)

mandibular ramus (*Cp* in Fig. 6-12, *A*, *C*). From here this muscle runs deeps to the zygomatic arch to flare out over the lateral surface of the calvarium. Its function is to elevate the mandible, thus closing the jaw. Between the coronoid process and the more posterior articular condyle is the mandibular notch (*Mn* in Fig. 6-12, *C*). The lateral pterygoid muscle (Fig. 6-14, *B*) inserts on the anterior aspect of the condyle (Figs. 6-14, *D*, *Lp* in 6-12, *C*) and depresses, protrudes, and moves the jaw from side to side. The medial pterygoid (Fig. 6-14, *B*) inserts more inferiorly on the angle of the mandible near the junction of the body and ramus (*Mp* in Figs. 6-12, *A*, 6-14, *D*) and serves to close the mandible along with the temporalis muscle.

Buccal Surface. On the buccal surface a bony ridge, the oblique line (O in Fig. 6-12, *C*), is formed where the coronoid process (*Cp* in Fig. 6-12, *C*) merges with the body of the mandible. The buccinator muscle (Fig. 6-14, *B*), which compresses the cheeks to hold food between the teeth, inserts between the oblique line and the more medially (lingually) situated alveolar process (*B* in Figs. 6-12, *C*, 6-14, *D*). The deep and superficial portions of the masseter muscle (Fig. 6-14, *B*, *D*) insert on the buccal surface of the ramus (*Mm* in Figs. 6-12, *C*, 6-14, *D*), having originated from the inferior and medial aspect of the zygomatic arch. This muscle acts to close the jaw along with the medial pterygoid and temporalis muscles. Portions of the platysma muscle also insert on the buccal aspect of the mandible along a line that runs inferiorly from the region of the molars to the mental protuberance (Fig. 6-14, *D*). Anteriorly, between the first and second premolar teeth, the mental foramen is identified (*M* in Fig. 6-12, *C*).

Superior Surface. The alveolar process, which houses the teeth, forms the most superior portion of the mandibular body. Its curved, or horseshoe, configuration is more acute than that of the body itself. This causes the alveolar process in its posterior (distal) aspect to be medially (lingually) positioned in relation to the mandibular body (Fig. 6-12, *D*). The cross-sectional DentaScan images nicely illustrate how the alveolar process is situated on the lingual aspect of the mandible in image 10 (lower right) of Fig. 6-6, *D*.

Posterior to the teeth the alveolar process tapers to form the retromolar triangle (*Rt* in Fig. 6-12, *D*) that merges with the lingual aspect of the ramus to form the temporal crest (*T* in Fig. 6-12, *D*). Buccal to this the anterior portion of the coronoid process (*Cp* in Fig. 6-12, *D*) merges with the body of the mandible to form the oblique line (*O* in Fig. 6-12, *D*). Between the oblique line and the temporal crest lies the retromolar fossa (*Rf* in Fig. 6-12, *D*). The lateral pterygoid muscle inserts on the anterior lingual aspect of the condyle (*Lp* in Fig. 6-12, *D*).

CT Images

Cross-Sectional View
Lingual Surface. Cross-sectional images 1 through 5 in Fig. 6-6, *D*, are through the distal aspect of the right mandible, near the junction of the ramus and body. The

mandibular foramen *(Mf)*, the lingula *(L)*, and the mylohyoid groove *(Mg)* are clearly seen on these images. More anteriorly (images 9 through 11 in Fig. 6-6, *D*, *E*), the mylohyoid line *(Ml)*, the submandibular fossa *(S)*, and the sublingual fossa *(Sl)* are identified. In the region of the mid-line (images 27 and 28 in Fig. 6-6, *F*), the genial tuber-cle *(Gt)* and the digastric fossa *(D)* can be seen. The superior *(Gt-g)* and inferior *(Gt-h)* processes of the genial tubercle, where the genioglossus and geniohyoid muscles insert, are better visualized in Fig. 6-15, *C*. This figure also demonstrates the lingual foramen *(Lf)* just below the genial tubercle.

Buccal Surface. The oblique line *(O)* that is formed where the coronoid process *(Cp)* merges with the body of the mandible, is seen in the posterior images (images 4 through 7 in Fig. 6-6, *D*). More anteriorly (image 20 in Fig. 6-6, *E*), the mental foramen *(M)* can be seen in cross-section. The course of the neurovascular bundle can be clearly traced on the cross-sectional images as it enters the manibular foramen on the lingual surface, travels through the inferior alveolar canal *(I)*, and finally exits the mental foramen on the buccal surface.

Superior Surface. On the buccal aspect of the superior surface, the coronoid process *(Cp)* is again visualized on the more distal images in Fig. 6-6, *D*. On more anterior images, the coronoid process merges with the mandible to form the oblique line *(O)* seen in image 7 of Fig. 6-6, *D*. On the lingual aspect of the superior surface, the temporal crest *(T)* is visualized on the more distal images (image 6 in Fig. 6-6, *D*). More anteriorly the temporal crest becomes the retromolar triangle *(Rt* in image 8, Fig. 6-6, *D*), and finally the alveolar process (*A* in image 10, Fig. 6-6, *D*). The molars, which are normally seen in the alveolar process at this point, are absent in this edentulous patient. In the posterior mandible the alveolar process (*A* in image 10, Fig. 6-6, *D*) assumes a more lingual position in relation to the body of the mandible. This can be appreciated by comparing the position of the alveolar process in relation to the mandible in image 10 (Fig. 6-6, *D*) and image 17 (Fig. 6-6, *E*). The retromolar fossa *(Rf* in Fig. 6-6, *D*) is identified between the oblique line and the temporal crest.

Internal Anatomy. Internally the inferior alveolar canal *(I)* is seen from its origin at the mandibular foramen to its termination at the mental foramen *(M)*. From the region of the mental foramen a smaller canal, the canal for the incisive artery *(Ia)*, can be seen extending toward the midline (Fig. 6-15, *A*, *B*). On the cross-sectional images the canal distal to the mental foramen is the inferior alveolar canal and the canal mesial to the mental foramen is the canal for the incisive artery (Fig. 6-15, *A*, *B*). In the midline the canal for the incisive artery exits the lingual foramen *(Lf* in Fig. 6-15, *C)* to anastomose with the lingual artery.

Axial View. On the axial view the genial tubercle *(Gt)*, mental foramen *(M)*, and inferior alveolar canal *(I)* are identified in Fig. 6-6, *A*, *B*.

Panoramic View. On the panoramic view the course of the inferior alveolar canal *(I* in Figs. 6-6, *C*, 6-15, *A)* can be traced to its exit point, the mental foramen *(M)*. The canal for the incisive artery *(Ia)* is visualized extending from the mental foramen toward the midline in Fig. 6-15, *A*. Also in Fig. 6-15, *A*, nutrient canals *(N)* can be seen extending cephalad from the inferior alveolar canal *(I)* toward the teeth.

Maxilla

The anatomy of the maxilla is described first on the anatomic specimen in Fig. 6-16 and then on the illustrations of the neurovascular structures in Fig. 6-13.[18,25-32] This anatomy is then identified on the axial, panoramic, and cross-sectional CT images in Fig. 6-7 and 6-10.[3]

Anatomic Specimen

The hard palate is composed of several bones delineated by sutures. The transverse suture (coronally oriented Ts in Fig. 6-16, *A*) separates the horizontal plate of the palatine bone (Pb in Fig. 6-16, *A*) from the palatine process of the maxillary bone (Mb in Fig. 6-16, *A*). The median palatine suture (Mp in Fig. 6-16, *A*), which runs in an AP (sagittal) direction, divides the palate into right and left halves. The pterygoid process of the sphenoid bone (Pt in Fig. 6-16, *A*) is just posterior to the alveolar process. In younger patients a coronally oriented suture also separates the premaxilla from the maxilla. This suture extends from the incisive foramen (If in Fig. 6-16, *A*) to the lateral incisor-cuspid region (arrow in Fig. 6-16, *A*).

As in the mandible the teeth are housed in the alveolar process (A in Fig. 6-16, *A*), a horseshoe-shaped bony process in the periphery of the anterior and lateral aspects of the hard palate. Cephalad to the alveolar process are the maxillary sinuses posteriorly and the nasal fossa anteriorly *(Nf* in Fig. 6-16, *C)*. Within the nasal fossa the nasal conchae *(Nc* in Fig. 6-16, *C)* and nasal septum *(Ns* in Fig. 6-16, *C)* are seen. A bony protuberance, the anterior maxillary spine *(As* in Fig. 6-16, *B, C)* is situated just below the nasal fossae in the midline.

Posterior to the maxillary sinus and between it and the pterygoid process *(Pt* in Fig. 6-16, *A, B)* lies the pterygopalatine fossa *(Tp* in Figs. 6-16, *B,* 6-7, *C)*. The maxillary branch *(V2)* of the trigeminal nerve enters the pterygopalatine fossa after exiting the skull base through the foramen rotundum. From here a branch, the pterygopalatine nerve (Fig. 6-13, *B*), travels inferiorly through the pterygopalatine canal to exit the greater (G in Fig. 6-16, *A*) and lesser (L in Fig. 6-16, *A*) palatine foramina as the greater and lesser palatine nerves. In Fig. 6-16, *A*, a white probe, representing the greater palatine nerve, is seen exiting the greater palatine foramen. After exiting, this nerve changes from a craniocaudal direction to run anteromedially (and horizontally) in a groove *(Gg* in Fig. 6-16, *A)* in the hard palate. As it travels in the groove, sensory fibers are given off to supply the posterior two thirds of the hard palate and teeth. The pterygopalatine nerve, represented by the other end of the white probe in Fig. 6-16, *B*, can be traced back into pterygopalatine fossa *(Tp* in Fig. 6-16, *B)*.

Another branch of the pterygopalatine nerve, the superior posterior nasal nerve (Fig. 6-13, *B, C*), enters the posterior nasal cavity through the sphenopalatine foramen. From here it gives off the nasopalatine nerve, a medial branch that runs anteroinferiorly along the nasal septum to enter the nasopalatine canal and incisive foramen (Figs. 6-13, *C,* 6-16, *C)*. The incisive foramen is readily seen as a small, round opening in the hard palate just posterior to the central incisors *(If* in Fig. 6-16, *A)*. Sensory fibers supply the anterior hard palate and along with the anterior superior alveolar nerve (branch of the infraorbital nerve) supply the central teeth. The terminal portions of the nasopalatine nerve anastomose with the terminal portion of the greater palatine nerve. In Fig. 6-16, *A, C*, the black probe represents the course of the nasopalatine nerve. Note how the black probe enters the incisive foramen *(If* in Fig. 6-16, *A)*, travels through the nasopalatine canal *(Np* in Fig. 6-16, *C)*, and then along the nasal septum *(Ns* in Fig. 6-16, *C)* to merge with the superior posterior nasal nerve (Fig. 6-13, *C)*. The right and left nasopalatine canals are situated in the anteroinferior nasal fossa on either side of the nasal septum.

CT Images

Axial Views. The more caudal axial images in Fig. 6-7, *B*, demonstrate the alveolar process *(A)*, incisive foramen *(If)*, and anterior maxillary spine *(As)*. The teeth, which are normally visualized in the alveolar process at this level, are not seen in this edentulous patient. In the more cranial images the maxillary sinus *(Ms)* is visible cephalad to the posterior aspect of the alveolar ridge, and the nasal fossa *(NF)* is seen cephalad to the anterior aspect of this ridge (Fig. 6-7, *B, C*). The nasal septum *(Ns)*, nasal concha *(Nc)*, and nasopharynx *(N)* are visualized on these axial images. Fig. 6-10 illustrates how the right and left nasopalatine canals appear as two separate openings on the more superior cuts but fuse to form a common opening, the incisive foramen, on the inferior images. This is also readily seen on the panoramic view (Fig. 6-7, *D*).

The sutures are identified at the level of the hard palate (Fig. 6-7, *B*). The maxillary bone *(Mb)* is separated from the palatine bone *(Pb)* by the transverse suture *(Ts)*. The median palatine suture *(Mp)* separates the right and left halves of these bones. Also seen at the level of the hard palate is the groove for the greater palatine nerve *(Gg)*. Just cephalad to the hard palate (Fig. 6-7, *C*) the greater *(G)* and lesser *(L)* palatine foramina are seen.

If the greater palatine foramen is followed cephalad, it merges with the pterygopalatine fossa *(Tp)*, which is situated between the posterior wall of the maxillary sinus and the pterygoid process.

Panoramic View. The panoramic view in Fig. 6-7, *D*, illustrates the position of the maxillary sinuses *(MS)* and nasal fossae *(Nf)* just cephalad to the alveolar process *(A)*. On either side of the nasal septum *(Ns)* the right and left nasal palatine canals *(Np)* are clearly visualized merging with the more inferior incisive foramen *(If)*.

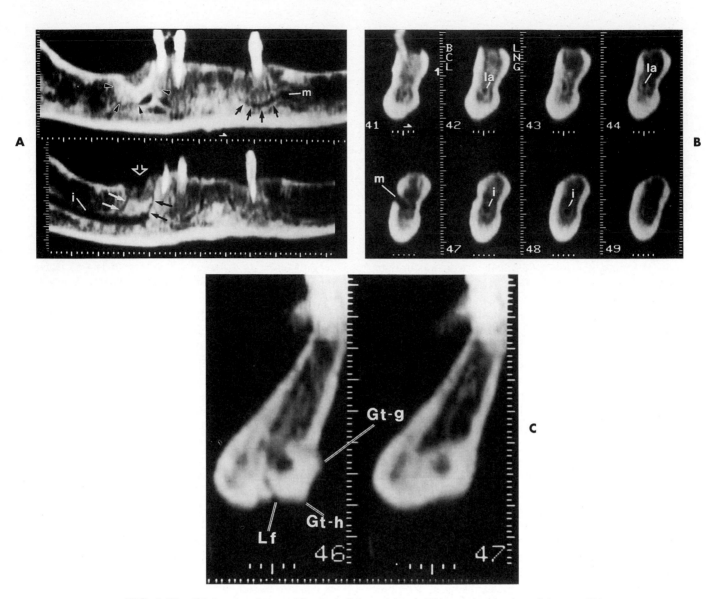

FIG. 6-15   CT showing the canal for the incisive artery. **A,** This panoramic view of the mandible demonstrates a small canal for the incisive artery *(black arrows)*. Note how it extends medial to the mental foramen *(m)* and toward the midline. Also seen are several small nutrient canals *(black and white arrows)* extending from the inferior alveolar canal *(i)* on either side of an extraction socket *(open arrow)*. An area of osteitis condensans surrounds the extraction socket *(arrowheads)*. **B,** Cross-sectional views of the mandible demonstrate the left inferior alveolar canal *(i)* distal to the mental foramen *(m)* and the canal for the incisive artery *(Ia)* medial to it. On the cross-sectional images, caution should be taken not to confuse the inferior alveolar canal with the incisive artery canal. **C,** Midline cross-sectional images in another patient. The incisive artery exits in the midline through the lingual foramen *(Lf)* and an anastomosis with the lingual artery. *Gt-h* indicates genial tubercle (geniohyoid insertion); and *Gt-g,* genial tubercle (genioglossus insertion). (From Abrahams JJ. Anatomy of the jaw revisited with a dental CT software program: Pictorial essay. AJNR 1993; 14:979-990.)

Cross-Sectional Views.   In Fig. 6-7, *E* and *F,* images 1 through 25 correspond to the right half of the maxilla, images 26 and 27 represent the midline with the incisive foramen, and images 28 through 30 represent the more medial aspect of the left maxilla. This may be more readily appreciated by looking at perpendicular lines 1 through 30, which are superimposed on the axial image in Fig. 6-7, *A.* In

the right posterior maxilla (Fig. 6-7, *E*), the greater palatine foramen is visualized (*G* in image 2). As one moves towards the midline, the most proximal portion of the groove (*Gg*) for the greater palatine nerve can be seen in images 3 through 5. The maxillary sinuses (*Ms*) are visualized cephalad to the alveolar process on the more posterior images, and the nasal fossae (*Nf*) are visualized cephalad to the alveolar

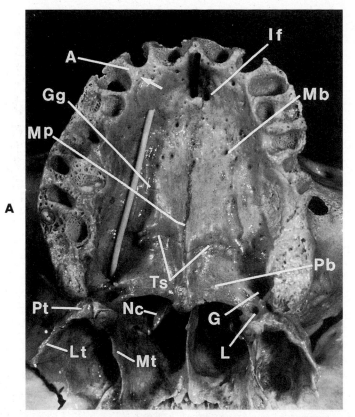

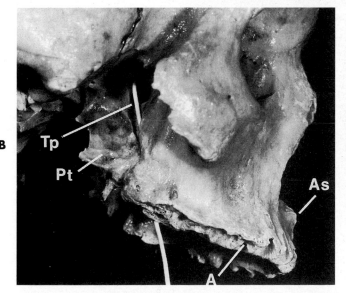

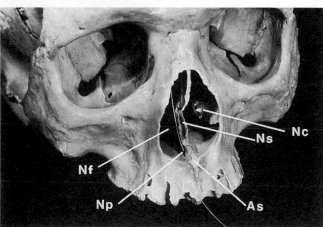

FIG. 6-16   Anatomic specimen demonstrating the inferior (**A**), lateral (**B**), and anterior (**C**) aspects of the maxilla. The *white probe* demonstrates the course of the greater palatine nerve; the *black probe* demonstrates the course of the nasopalatine nerve. *A* indicates alveolar process; *As,* anterior nasal spine; *G,* greater palatine foramen; *Gg,* groove for greater palatine nerve; *If,* incisive foramen; *L,* lesser palatine foramen; *Lt,* lateral pterygoid plate; *Mb,* maxillary bone, palatine process; *Mp,* median palatine suture; *Mt,* medial pterygoid; *Nc,* nasal conchi; *Nf,* nasal fossa; *Np,* nasopalatine canal; *Ns,* nasal septum; *Pb,* palatine bone, horizontal plate; *Pt,* pterygoid process; *Tp,* ptery-gopalatine fossa and *Ts,* transverse suture. (From Abrahams JJ. Anatomy of the jaw revisited with a dental CT software program: pictorial essay. AJNR 1993; 14:979-990.)

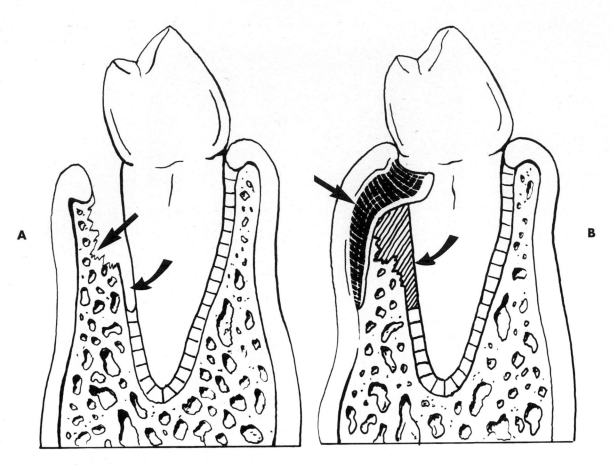

FIG. 6-17   Illustration demonstrating a periodontal pocket and its repair. **A,** Bacterial overgrowth has attacked the periodontal ligament *(curved arrow)* and resorbed bone *(straight arrow),* creating this periodontal pocket. **B,** The periodontal pocket in **A** has now been packed with freeze-dried bone *(curved arrow)* and covered with a Gortex graft *(straight arrow)* to prevent ingrowth of soft tissue while the bone graft heals. The Gortex will be removed in approximately 6 weeks.

process on the more anterior images (Fig. 6-7, *F*). In the midline (image 26 and 27, Fig. 6-7, *F*), the nasopalatine canal *(Np),* incisive foramen *(If),* and anterior maxillary spine *(As)* are seen.

RELATED PATHOLOGY

Most patients being scanned for dental implants have considerable oral pathology, often related to the inflammatory process that caused their edentulism. This inflammatory process starts with the accumulation of bacteria-laden plaque around the teeth. This may harden into tartar or calculus, a tough gritty material that is difficult to remove. The presence of this bacterial overgrowth produces gingivitis, which presents itself clinically with inflammation and swelling of the gums. This is often associated with frequent bleeding secondary to hyperemia from inflammation. If the infection is allowed to persist, the fibers that attach the gingiva to the tooth become involved, allowing bacteria to access the periodontal ligament (periodontitis). Once the periodontal ligament becomes involved, a periodontal pocket forms in which plaque accumulates adjacent to the

root (Fig. 6-17, *A*). Routine dental hygiene at home does not adequately cleanse these infected regions, and the disease progresses. Eventually the periodontal ligament is destroyed, and the adjacent bone surrounding the root is resorbed.[34] On CT this bone loss appears as a radiolucency surrounding the root of the tooth (Fig. 6-18). The chronic inflammatory changes can also cause reactive sclerosis in the adjacent bone, termed *osteitis condensans* (Fig. 6-18).[35]

Another frequently encountered condition in this patient population is an inflammatory cyst surrounding the root apex called a *radicular cyst.*[36] Bacteria gains access to the pulp chamber through dental caries and travels down the root canal to the root apex, where either an acute abscess or a more chronic granuloma forms. Bone loss develops around the root apex, and this appears as a periapical radiolucency on CT (Fig. 6-8). When bacteria enters the pulp chamber through dental caries, it causes pulpitis with inflammation and edema. Because the tooth cannot expand, pressure builds within the pulp chamber and the diminished blood flow causes the tooth to die. Radicular cysts are therefore associated with nonvital teeth. Treatment is to drill through the pulp chamber and drain the abscess (root canal

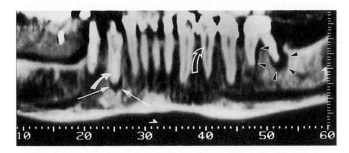

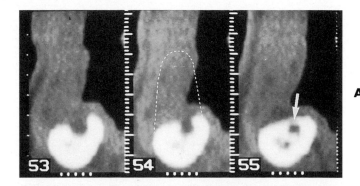

FIG. 6-18 Panoramic CT scan of mandible demonstrating periodontal disease. The radiolucency surrounding the root of the left first molar *(arrowheads)* is due to bone resorption from periodonitis. The periapical lucency around the root apex of the right canine *(long arrows)* is a radicular cyst secondary to a periapical abscess. Note the metal post in the pulp chamber secondary to a prior root canal procedure *(solid curved arrow)* and compare this with the normal radiolucent pulp chamber of the left first premolar *(open curved arrow)*. A zone of relatively dense sclerotic bone (osteitis condensans) is identified surrounding both areas of disease. (From Abrahams JJ. The role of diagnostic imaging in dental implantology. Radiol Clinics of North America 1993; 31(1):163-180.)

procedure). After this drainage is accomplished, a metal post is placed in the pulp chamber to add support to the tooth and prevent it from fracturing. The metal posts from the root canal procedures are readily visualized on CT as a radiodensity, rather than a radiolucency, in the region of the pulp chamber (Fig. 6-18, *curved arrow*).

Periodontal disease may also affect the maxillary sinuses. It is not uncommon to find mounds of inflammatory tissue within the sinus, adjacent to the root apices of diseased teeth. These frequently are misdiagnosed as mucous retention cysts or polyps on axial CT scans. Oroantral fistulas (abnormal communication between the maxillary sinus and oral cavity) have also been identified, particularly after extractions.

Periodontal disease eventually leads to edentulism. The atrophy and resorption of bone, however, continue even after the teeth are lost because the normal vertical stress applied to the bone from the teeth is no longer present. It is believed that the use of dental implants retards this atrophic process. The disuse atrophy affects both the height of the alveolar process (Fig. 6-19, *A*) and the width (Fig. 6-19, *B*). When severe, the mandibular canal, which is normally covered by a considerable amount of bone, may lie just under the gingival surface.

Several augmentation procedures are available for patients who have severe atrophy and have insufficient bone for implants. In the sinus lift procedure the surgeon elevates the periosteum in the floor of the maxillary sinus and packs a freeze-dried bone graft between the elevated periosteum and the bony floor. After this heals, it will increase the height of the alveolar bone available in the maxilla. In both the mandible and maxilla, various bone grafts alone have been used to increase the height and width of the alveolar process. These grafts may be supplemented with freeze- dried bone.

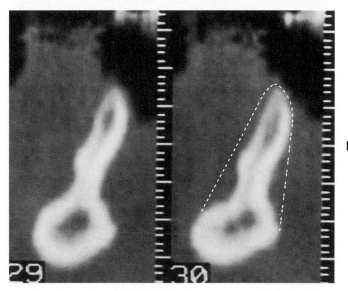

FIG. 6-19 Cross-sectional views of the mandible in two different patients demonstrating bone resorption and atrophy. **A,** Bone loss and atrophy of the height of the mandible in this patient causes the mandibular canal *(arrow)* to sit immediately under the gingival surface. The *dotted line* demonstrates how the bone contour might have appeared before atrophy. The patient has insufficient bone for implants. (From Abrahams JJ. The role of diagnostic imaging in dental implantology. Radiol Clinics of North America 1993; 31(1):163-180.) **B,** The width of the mandible in this patient has been considerably diminished from atrophy. The *dotted line* again demonstrates how the bone might have appeared before atrophy. (From Abrahams JJ. CT assessment of dental implant planning. Oral and Maxillofac Surg Clin North Am 1992;4:1-18.)

Finally, if the implant is placed and either the buccal or lingual surface is exposed and uncovered by bone, a procedure using gortex can be utilized to regenerate the bone adjacent to the implant. Bone graft is packed around the exposed surface of the implant, and then a piece of gortex fabric is placed between the bone graft and soft tissues. The gortex acts as a barrier, preventing the soft tissues from growing into the bone graft, thus allowing time for the graft to take. Typically the gortex remains in place for about 6 weeks. This procedure can also be used when placing an implant in a fresh extraction socket and for filling a periodontal pocket with bone graft as illustrated in Fig. 6-17, *B*.

References

1. Laney WR, Tolman DE, Keller EE et al. Dental implants: tissue-integrated prosthesis utilizing the osseointegrated concept. Mayo Clin Proc 1986; 61:91-97.

2. Abrahams JJ. CT assessment of dental implant planning. Oral and Maxillofac Surg Clin North Am 1992; 4:1-18.

3. Abrahams JJ. The role of diagnostic imaging in dental implantology. Radiol Clin North Am 1993; 31:(1):163-180.

4. Abrahams JJ, Levine B. Expanded applications of DentaScan: (multiplanar CT of the mandible and maxilla). Int J of Periodontics & Restorative Dentistry 1990; 10:464-467.

5. Abrahams JJ, Olivario P. Odonogenic cysts: improved imaging with a dental CT software program. AJNR 1993; 14:367-374.

6. Delbalso AM, Greiner FG, Licata N. Role of diagnostic imaging in evaluation of the dental implant patient. Radiographics 1994; 14:699-719.

7. Fogelman D, Huang AB. Prospective evaluation of lesions of the mandible and maxilla: findings on multiplanar and three-dimentional CT. AJR 1994; 163:693-698.

8. Yanagisawa K, Friedman C, Abrahams JJ. DentaScan imaging of the mandible and maxilla. Head & Neck J 1993; 15:1-7.

9. Albrektsson T, Lekholm W. Osseointegration: current state of the art. Dent Clin North Am 1989; 33:537-544.

10. James R. The support system and perigingival defense mechanism of oral implants. J of Oral Implantology 1975; 6:270-285.

11. Weiss C. Tissue integration of dental endosseous implants: description and comparative analysis of the fibro-osseous integration and osseous integration systems. J of Oral Implantology 1986; 12:169-214.

12. Adell R, Lukholm U, Rockler B et al. A 15-year study of osseointegrated implants in the treatment of the edentulous jaw. Int J Oral Maxillofac Surg 1981; 10:387-416.

13. Branemark PI. Introduction to osseointegration. In: Branemark PI, Zarb G, Albrektsson T, eds. Tissue integrated protheses. Chicago, Ill and Berlin, Germany: Quintessence, 1985.

14. Albrektsson T. A multicenter report on osseointegrated oral implants. J Prosthet Dent 1988; 60(1):75-84.

15. Krauser JT. Hydroxylapatite-coated dental implants. Dent Clin North Am 1989; 33:879-903.

16. Moy PK, Weinlaender M, Kenney EB et al. Soft tissue modifications of surgical techniques for placement and uncovering of osseointegrated implants. Dental Clin of North Am 1989; 4:665-699.

17. McGivney GP, Haughton V, Strandt JA et al. A comparison of computed-assisted tomography and data-gathering modalities in prostodontics. Int J Oral Maxillofac Surg 1986; 1:55-68.

18. Wishan M, Bahat O, Krane M. Computed tomography as an adjunct in dental implant surgery. International Jour of Periodontics and Restorative Dentistry 1988; 8:31-47.

19. Rothman SLG, Chafetz N, Rhodes M et al. CT in the pre-operative assessment of the mandible and maxilla for endosseous implant surgery. Radiology 1988; 168:171-175.

20. Schwarz MS, Rothman SLGM, Chatetz N et al. Computed tomography in dental implantation surgery. Dent Clin North Am 1989; 33:555-597.

21. Schwarz MS, Rothman SLGM, Rhodes ML. Computed tomography. Part I. Pre-operative assessment of the mandible for endosseous implant surgery. Int J Oral Maxillofac Surg 1987; 2:137-141.

22. Schwarz MS, Rothman SLGM, Rhodes ML et al. Computed tomography. Part II. Pre-operative assessment of the mandible for endosseous implant surgery. Int J Oral Maxillofac Surg 1987; 2:143-148.

23. Israelson H, Plemons JM, Watkins P, Crysup S. Barium-coated surgical stints and computer-assisted tomography in the preoperative assessment of dental implant patients. Int J Periodontics & Restorative Dentistry 1992; 11:53-61.

24. Sicher H. The viscera of the head and neck. In: Oral anatomy. 4th edition. St. Louis, Mo: C.V. Mosby Co, 1965; 191-324.

25. Ennis LM, Harrison MB Jr, Phillips JE. Normal anatomical landmarks of the teeth and jaws as seen in the roentgenogram. In: Dental roentgen-ology. 6th edition. Philadelphia, Pa: Lea & Febiger, 1967; 334-407.

26. Gray H. Osteology. In Anatomy of the human body. 28th edition. Philadephia, Pa: Lea & Febiger 1969; 107-293.

27. Gray H. The peripheral nervous system. In: Anatomy of the human body. 28th edition. Philadelphia, Pa: Lea & Febiger, 1969; 907-1042.

28. Gray H. The digestive system. In: Anatomy of the human body. 28th edition. Philadelphia, Pa: Lea & Febiger, 1969; 1161-1263.

29. Gray H. Arteries of the head and neck. In: Anatomy of the human body. 28th edition. Philadelphia, Pa: Lea & Febiger, 1969; 1161-1263.

30. Meschan I. The skull. In: An atlas of anatomy basic to radiology. Philadelphia, Pa: W B Saunders Co, 1975; 209-287.

31. Sicher H. The skull. In: Oral anatomy. 4th edition. St. Louis, Mo: C.V. Mosby Co, 1965, 23-140.

32. Sicher H. The nerves of the head and neck. In: Oral anatomy. 4th edition. St. Louis, Mo: C.V. Mosby Co, 1965; 364-398.

33. Abrahams JJ. Anatomy of the jaw revisited with a dental CT software program: pictorial essay. AJNR 1993; 14:979-990.

34. Burgett F. Periodontal disease. In: Regezi JA, Sciubba JJ eds. Oral pathology: clinical-pathologic correlations. Philadelphia, Pa: W B Saunders Co, 1989; 503-519.

35. Regezi J, Sciubba J. Oral pathology: clinical-pathological correlation. 1st edition. Philadelphia, Pa: W B Saunders Co, 1989; 390-404.

36. Regezi J, Sciubba J. Oral pathology: clinical-pathological correlation. 1st edition. Philadelphia, Pa: W B Saunders Co, 1989; 301-336.

37. Albrektsson T, Dahl E, Enbom L et al. Oseointegrated oral implants: a Swedish multicenter study of 8139 consecutively inserted Nobelpharma implants. J Periodontal 1988; 59:287-296.

7

Temporomandibular Joints

PER-LENNART WESTESSON
RICHARD WIER KATZBERG

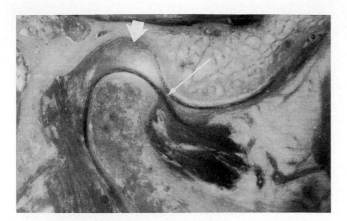

FIG. 7-1 Normal TMJ in sagittal section. Biconcave disk in normal superior position. The posterior band of the disk (*thick arrow*) is lying over the condyle. The simple thin zone of the disk (*thin arrow*) is between the anterior prominence of the condyle and the articular eminence.

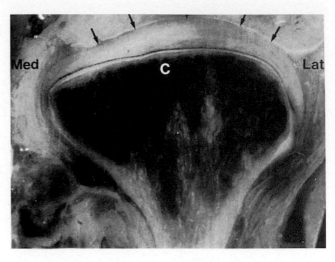

FIG. 7-2 Normal TMJ in coronal section. The disk (*arrows*) is crescent-shaped and located over the condyle. Medially and laterally the disk is attached to the condyle and capsule. The condyle (*C*) is indicated.

The purpose of an imaging assessment of the temporomandibular joint (TMJ) is to depict clinically suspected disorders of the joint. For many years, plain film radiography done mainly in a transcranial projection was the most commonly used method of making this assessment. However, this modality has major limitations because it is sensitive only to changes in the osseous components and depicts just the lateral aspect of the joint. With the evolution of newer imaging modalities such as arthrography, computed tomography (CT), and most importantly, magnetic resonance (MR) imaging, the soft tissues of the joint could be appreciated, and this allowed a better understanding of the anatomy and pathophysiology of internal derangement related to disk displacement.[1]

This chapter begins with descriptions of the anatomy and function of the TMJ and then provides an overview of the various imaging modalities available for evaluating the TMJ. Because most TMJ imaging is directed toward assessment of internal derangements or related degenerative joint changes, the sections addressing imaging methods emphasize the key findings in these important disorders. A variety of miscellaneous diseases that affect the TMJ are then covered, and an algorithm for imaging patients with TMJ problems is given.

ANATOMY OF THE TMJ

Interpreting TMJ imaging studies requires an understanding of the pathophysiology of the joint and a knowledge of both normal and pathologic anatomy of the joint and surrounding structures. Therefore a description of joint anatomy, joint pathology, function and dysfunction is presented in some detail.

The mandible and the temporal bone comprise the osseous components of the TMJ. The mandibular condyle, at the top of the condylar process of the mandible, is the inferior component of the joint, and the temporal bone con-

tributes the glenoid fossa and articular tubercle, which form the superior osseous part of the joint (Fig. 7-1). Unlike most other joints of the body, which have cartilaginous coverings, the articulating surfaces of the TMJ are covered by a thin layer of dense fibrous tissue.

The TMJ disk is a biconcave fibrous structure located between the mandibular condyle and the temporal component of the joint. The disk is round to oval with a thick periphery and a thin central part, and the mediolateral dimension of the disk is approximately 20 mm. In a sagittal section the normal disk appears biconcave, and the anterior and posterior parts of the disk are called the *anterior* and *posterior bands*.[2] In the normal joint the posterior band is located over the condyle, and the central thin zone is located between the condyle and the posterior part of the articular tubercle (Fig. 7-1). The anterior band is located under the articular tubercle. In a coronal plane the disk is crescent-shaped (Fig. 7-2). A joint capsule surrounds the joint, emerging from the temporal bone and extending like a funnel inferiorly to attach to the neck of the condyle. The medial and lateral edges of the disk attach to the capsule and then to the mandible at the inferior edge of the medial and lateral poles of the condyle (Fig. 7-2). Posteriorly the disk is attached to the temporal bone and to the condyle by the posterior disk attachment. This posterior disk attachment is extremely important in internal derangements of the TMJ. This region has also been referred to as the bilaminar zone or the retrodiskal tissue. The bilaminar zone consists of loose fibrous connective and elastic tissue components. It has traditionally been called the bilaminar zone because initial histologic studies indicated that the upper part was elastic tissue and the lower part consisted of more connective tissue. More recent histologic studies have failed to confirm the bilaminar nature of the posterior disk attachment. The term bilaminar zone, however, continues to be used both in

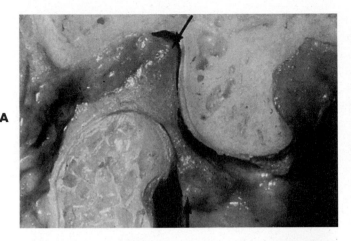

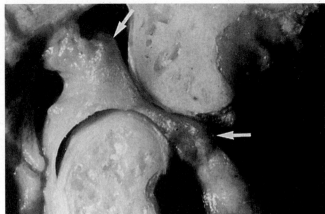

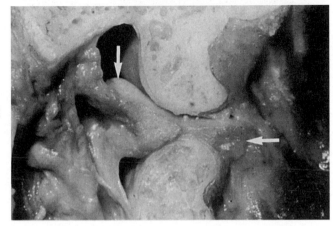

FIG. 7-3 Normal TMJ function. **A,** Normal TMJ in closed mouth position. The anterior and posterior bands of the disk are indicated by arrows. **B,** Normal TMJ in half opened mouth position. Anterior and posterior bands of the disk are indicated by arrows. **C,** Normal TMJ in open mouth position. Anterior and posterior bands of the disk are indicated by arrows.

clinical and scientific work. Anteriorly the disk is attached to the joint capsule, and in the anteromedial portion of the joint the disk also merges with the upper head of the lateral pterygoid muscle.

There are two joint spaces, or compartments. The superior space separates the glenoid and articular eminence of the temporal bone from the disk and its attachments. The inferior joint space separates the disk and its attachments from the condyle of the mandible. The anterior recess is a small space in the inferior joint compartment anterior to the condyle. The posterior recess is the part of the inferior joint space posterior to the condyle. The lower part of the bilaminar zone (posterior disk attachment) curves downward to attach to the condylar neck and thus forms the posterior boundary of the posterior recess of the inferior joint compartment.

FUNCTION OF THE TMJ

The function of the TMJ is complex because the upper and lower joint compartments principally act as two small joints within this same joint capsule. This allows for proportionally greater movement of the TMJ in relation to the actual size of the joint. The principal function of the disk is to permit relatively large movements within a small joint while maintaining stability. Rotation and translation occur in both the upper and lower joint spaces. However, translation predominantly occurs in the upper space, and rotation is more evident in the lower joint space. In the initial phase of jaw opening, the condyle rotates in the lower joint compartment. After this initial rotation, translation occurs in the upper and subsequently in the lower joint space. During translation the condyle and the disk translate together under the articular tubercle. During all mandibular movements, the central thin part of the disk is located between the condyle and the articular tubercle. This suggests that the thick periphery of the disk and the thick posterior and anterior bands act as functional guides for the joint. This normal joint function can be identified in anatomic specimens of the TMJ (Fig. 7-3).

INTERNAL DERANGEMENT RELATED TO DISPLACEMENT OF THE DISK

Internal derangement is a general orthopedic term implying a mechanical fault that interferes with the smooth action of a joint.[3] Internal derangement is thus a functional diagnosis, and for the TMJ the most common cause of internal derangement is displacement of the disk.[4-9] Most often the disk displaces in an anterior, anterolateral, or anteromedial direction. Thus the posterior band of the disk prolapses anteriorly, relative to the superior surface of the condyle (Figs. 7-4 7-5), instead of remaining in position between the

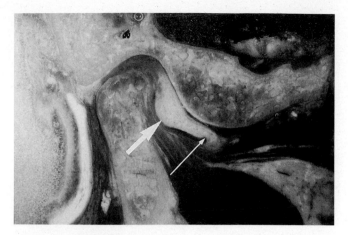

FIG. 7-4 Anterior disk displacement. The disk is anteriorly displaced with its posterior band (*thick arrow*) located forward of the condyle. Note that the central thin zone of the disk (*thin arrow*) is separated from the anterior prominence of the condyle.

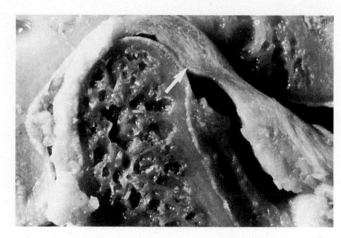

FIG. 7-5 Anterior disk displacement. The disk is anteriorly displaced with its posterior band (*arrow*) located slightly forward of the condyle.

▼

BOX 7-1

TERMINOLOGY FOR DESCRIBING THE POSTION OF THE DISK

Normal	Superior
Abnormal	Anterior, partial or complete
	Anteromedial rotation
	Anterolateral rotation
	Medial sideways
	Lateral sideways
	Posterior

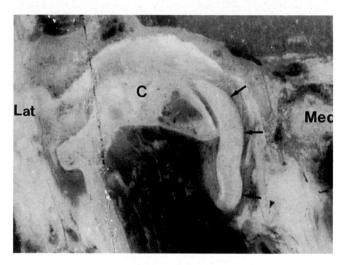

FIG. 7-6 Coronal section of TMJ showing medial disk displacement. The disk is indicated by arrows. The condyle (*C*) is sclerotic.

condyle and glenoid fossa. As a consequence the condyle is positioned under the posterior disk attachment rather than under the disk, and the condyle closes on the posterior attachment (bilaminar zone or retrodiskal tissues) rather than on the disk itself. The central, thin part of the disk lies inferior to the articular tubercle.

Studies have shown that the disk frequently is also displaced in a medial (Fig. 7-6) or lateral direction.[10-13] Posterior disk displacement (Fig. 7-7) does occur, but it is rare. When present, it is frequently seen in combination with medial disk displacement. A general classification of the different types of disk displacement of the TMJ is shown in the Box 7-1. Pure lateral and pure medial sideways displacements of the disk also occur, but not as commonly as in combination with an anterior displacement.[11-13] The combination of anterior and lateral or medial displacement is called rotational displacement, whereas pure lateral or pure medial displacement is called sideways displacement.[11]

The functional aspects of disk displacement include displacement with or without reduction, and the functional categories of internal derangement are illustrated in Fig. 7-8. In disk displacement with reduction (Fig. 7-8, *B*) the anteriorly displaced disk reverts to a normal superior position during opening. In disk displacement without reduction (Fig. 7-8, *C*) the disk lies anterior to the condyle during all mandibular movements and the normal condyle-disk relationship is not reestablished.

Disk Displacement with Reduction

When a displaced disk reduces to a normal position, a click is usually heard. When the jaw closes, the disk again displaces anteriorly, usually during the last phase of the closing movement of the jaw, and again a click is commonly heard. The closing click usually is less prominent than the opening click. The cyclic nature of disk displacement was described by Ireland in 1951.[14] The clicking sound has been shown to

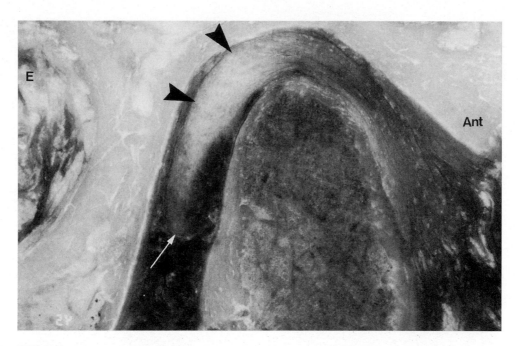

FIG. 7-7 Posterior disk displacement. The disk (*arrowheads*) is posterior to the condyle. The external auditory canal (*E*) and anterior (*Ant*) are indicated for orientation. Inferiorly and posteriorly there is folding of the disk (*thin arrow*) similar to what is seen with anterior disc displacement.

be caused by the impact of the condyle hitting against the temporal component of the articulation after the condyle has passed under the posterior band of the disk.[15,16]

Disk Displacement without Reduction

In disk displacement without reduction (Fig. 7-8, *C*) the disk remains displaced relative to the condylar head, regardless of the jaw position. In the initial stages of this condition, jaw opening is typically limited and the jaw deviates to the side of the affected joint. However, this clinical characteristic is typical only during the initial (early) phase; with time the opening capacity of the TMJ increases and the jaw no longer deviates to the affected side. This is the result of stretching or progressive elongation of the posterior disk attachment and to a lesser extent deformation of the disk itself. In the early stage, disk displacement without reduction is usually not associated with joint sounds.

Disk Deformation

The normal disk is biconcave when viewed in the sagittal plane (Fig. 7-3). In the early stages of internal derangement the disk remains normal in shape. However, the displaced disk begins to deform, as noted by a thickening of the posterior band and shortening of the entire anteroposterior length of the disk (Fig. 7-9).[4,9,17-19] Additionally, both the central thin part and the anterior band decrease in size. The end result is a biconvex disk configuration and a stretched, elongated, and thinned posterior disk attachment. The gross changes of the disk are associated with histologic alterations within the disk that lead to metaplastic hyaline cartilage, hyalinization, and accumulation of foci of calcium deposits and abnormal collagen patterns.[20,21] Changes also occur in the posterior disk attachment itself, leading to fibrosis and narrowing of vessels.[22,23] Histologic studies of the posterior disk attachment in joints with disk displacement have shown narrowing of the arterial lumen, increased density of fibroblasts, and hyalinization of loose connective tissue.[24]

Late-Stage Changes Following Disk Displacement

In the late or chronic stages of disk displacement without reduction, the disk is deformed and has a stretched, torn, or detached posterior attachment and communications between the upper and lower joint spaces (perforation) are often seen.[8,9,19,25] Most commonly the perforations are found in the posterior disk attachment, at its junction with the disk itself (Fig. 7-10). Infrequently, perforations are found in the disk per se.[19] Thus although traditionally this condition has been designated as perforation of the disk, this is not anatomically correct because the perforations are usually found in the posterior disk attachment rather than the disk proper.

Osseous changes involving the condyle and temporal bone often occur as sequelae of disk displacement.[7-9,18,26]

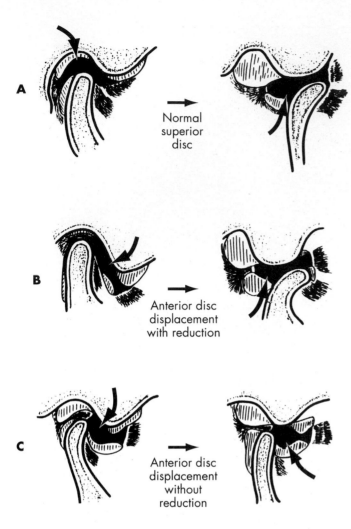

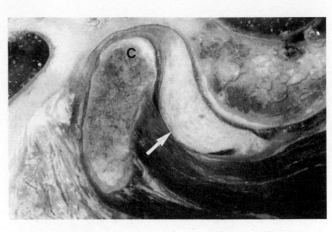

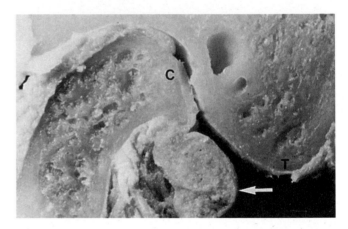

FIG. 7-9 Anterior displacement and deformation of disk. The disk (*arrow*) is biconvex. The condyle (*C*) articulates with the posterior disk attachment.

FIG. 7-8 Schematic drawing of normal TMJ and different categories of internal derangement. The disk is black and is indicated by the curved arrows. **A,** Normal. **B,** Anterior displacement with reduction. **C,** Anterior displacement without reduction.

FIG. 7-10 Anterior displacement and extensive deformation of the disk (*arrow*) with perforation of the posterior disk attachment. The condyle (*C*) is flattened with an anterior osteophyte and surface irregularities.

Osseous changes consist of flattening and osteophytosis of the mandibular condyle and flattening of the temporal component of the articulation. These changes are more commonly observed in the lateral part of the joint and can be detected on plain film imaging. It should be noted that osseous changes are relatively late findings in the disease process, and it is often difficult to radiographically differentiate between advanced remodeling and degenerative joint disease.

Clinical Aspects of Internal Derangement

The preceeding classification of disk position and function is based only on anatomic and functional aspects. In the clinical setting the patient's history, signs, and symptoms must be incorporated into the staging of the disease. Patients may complain of pain or of clicks when opening and closing the mouth. Physical examination may show tenderness on palpation of the joint or associated muscles. Palpable clicks or crepitus on movement of the jaw may be clinically evident, and abnormalities of occlusion or deviation of the jaw on opening may also suggest TMJ abnormality.

However, the clinical assessment of the TMJ has definite limitations. Multiple studies have shown that the accuracy of physical examination in predicting the status of the joint is about 70%.[27-33] The intensity and location of pain in a study of more than 200 patients did not distinguish patients with internal derangement from those without internal derangement, and there was no consistent relationship between occlusion and the status of the joint. These studies indicate that physical examination alone is not reliable in determining the status of the joint.[28-34]

The situation is further complicated by the fact that clinical signs of TMJ internal derangement are relatively common in the general population. An epidemiologic study of

▼

BOX 7-2
CLASSIFICATION OF INTERNAL DERANGEMENT

Early Stage

Clinical   No significant mechanical symptoms other than reciprocal clicking (early in opening movement, late in clos-
                ing movement, and soft in intensity); no pain or limitation in opening motion

Radiologic   Slight forward displacement; good anatomic contour of disk; normal tomograms

Surgical   Normal anatomic form; slight anterior displacement; passive incoordination (clicking) demonstrable

Early-Intermediate Stage

Clinical   First few episodes of pain; occasional joint tenderness and related temporal headaches; beginning major
                mechanical problems; increase in intensity of clicking sounds; joint sounds later in opening movement; and
                beginning transient subluxations or joint catching and locking

Radiologic   Slight forward displacement; slight thickening of posterior edge or beginning anatomic deformity of disk;
                normal tomograms

Surgical   Anterior displacement; early anatomic deformity (slight to mild thickening of posterior edge); well-defined
                central articulating area

Intermediate Stage

Clinical   Multiple episodes of pain, joint tenderness, temporal headaches, major mechanical symptoms: transient catch-
                ing, locking, and sustained locking (closed locks); restriction of motion; difficulty (pain) with function

Radiologic   Anterior displacement with significant anatomic deformity or prolapse of disk (moderate to marked thicken-
                ing of posterior edge); normal tomograms

Surgical   Marked anatomic deformity with displacement; variable adhesions (anterior, lateral, and posterior recesses);
                no hard-tissue changes

Intermediate-Late Stage

Clinical   Characterized by chronicity with variable and episodic pain, headaches, variable restriction of motion;
                undulating course

Radiologic   Increase in severity over intermediate stage; abnormal tomograms; early to moderate degenerative remodeling
                hard-tissue changes

Surgical   Increase in severity over intermediate stage; hard-tissue degenerative remodeling changes of both bearing
                surfaces; osteophytic projections; multiple adhesions (lateral, anterior, and posterior recesses); no perforation
                of disk or attachment

Late Stage

Clinical   Characterized by crepitus on examination; scraping, grating, grinding symptoms; variable and episodic pain;
                chronic restriction of motion; and difficulty with function

Radiologic   Anterior displacement; perforation with simultaneous filling of upper and lower compartments; filling
                defects; gross anatomic deformity of disk and hard tissues; abnormal tomograms; essentially degenerative
                arthritic changes

Surgical   Gross degenerative changes of disk and hard tissues; perforation of posterior attachments; erosions of bearing
                surfaces; multiple adhesions equivalent to degenerative arthritis (sclerosis, flattening, and anvil-shaped
                condyle, osteophytic projections, and subcortical cystic formation).

From Wilkes CH. Internal derangement of the TMJ. Pathologic variations. Arch Otolaryngol Head Neck Surg 1989; 115:469-477.

more than 400 individuals ranging in age from 28 to 73 years showed clinical evidence of internal derangement in 39% of the patients. Most of these individuals had functional symptoms with clicking or limitation of opening, but the majority did not have any pain associated with the dysfunction. Studies of asymptomatic volunteers using both arthrography and MR imaging, have shown disk displacement in approximately 20% to 25% of this population.[35-37] The finding of anatomic abnormalities in the joints of asymptomatic individuals is not unique to the TMJ. Similar observations have been shown in MR studies of the knee, cervical spine, and lumbar spine.[38-42]

The prevalence of disk displacement in symptomatic individuals is much higher (about 80%) than in a "normal" population.[43] However, in view of the high incidence of displacement in asymptomatic patients, the precise relationship of symptoms to the displacement is difficult to define.

Among patients presenting with TMJ symptoms there is a significant prevalence of young females, and in the clinical material the female to male ratio has been between

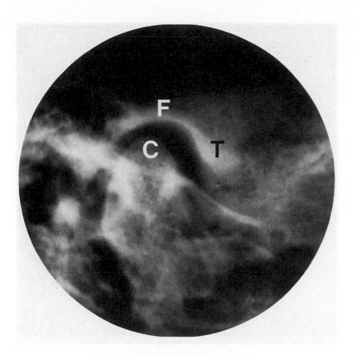

FIG. 7-11 Transcranial radiograph of TMJ. The condyle (*C*), fossa (*F*), and tubercle (*T*) are indicated.

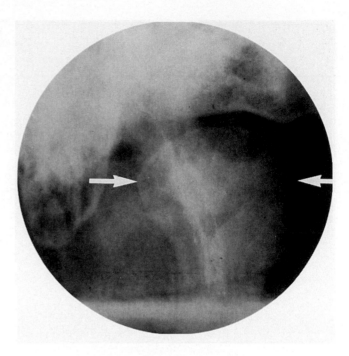

FIG. 7-12 Transmaxillary radiograph of TMJ. The lateral and medial poles of the condyles are indicated by arrows.

5:1 and 10:1. The reason for the female dominance among TMJ patients is not fully understood. Cadaver studies have found that approximately 50% of elderly individuals have an internal derangement with no significant difference between the sexes.[44]

Because of the difficulty in the clinical evaluation of a potential disk displacement, imaging must be done to define the anatomy of the joint and to determine the relationship of the disk to the condyle. The purpose of an imaging study is to identify and characterize the anatomy in a patient who presents with symptoms. Because of the overlap of morphologic abnormalities in symptomatic and asymptomatic individuals, imaging findings should always be interpreted in light of clinical findings. Similarly the choice of imaging studies must depend on the clinical evaluation, and an algorithm for TMJ imaging can be made based upon prior clinical and imaging experience.

An appropriate patient evaluation integrates the imaging and clinical findings, and a workable classification of TMJ disorders, related to internal derangement, is also necessary for communication among clinicians and radiologists. The classification developed by Wilkes[9] encompasses clinical, radiographic, and morphologic observations and categorizes internal derangement into early, intermediate, and late stages. This classification is presented in Box 7-2.

IMAGING
Transcranial and Transmaxillary Projections

The most common and well-established plain film technique for examination of the TMJ is the transcranial projection

(Fig. 7-11). The lateral aspect of the joint is well visualized, but the central and medial parts of the joint are not clearly seen because the x-ray beam is not tangent to these articular surfaces. This disadvantage is partly compensated for because most of the early osseous changes occur laterally in the joint.[45]

It has been recommended that, in addition to the transcranial projection, an anteroposterior projection should be obtained to depict the central and medial parts of the condyle, and a transmaxillary projection (Fig. 7-12) or a transorbital projection also is suggested.[46]

Tomography

Complex motion tomography has been recommended for detection of early osseous changes (Fig. 7-13). Studies have demonstrated that a clearer depiction of the osseous anatomy can be gained from tomography than can be gained from transcranial radiography.[47] Tomography may also be performed in the coronal plane, providing information about the medial and lateral poles of the condyle, which are usually not adequately depicted on the sagittal tomograms. The disadvantage of tomography is the rather large radiation dose delivered to the lens of the eye. To a large extent, tomography has been replaced by CT, and CT probably represents the most effective modality for demonstrating osseous abnormalities.

Arthrography
Development of TMJ Arthrography

Early attempts at TMJ arthrography were undertaken by Nørgaard in the 1940s.[48,49] However, this procedure was not

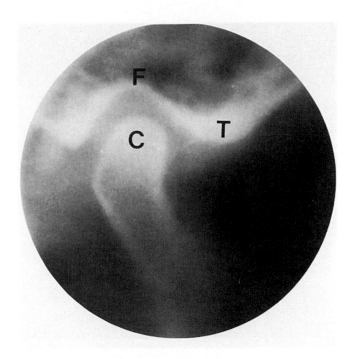

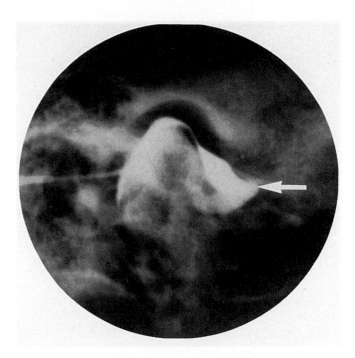

FIG. 7-13 Sagittal tomogram of TMJ. The condyle (*C*), fossa (*F*), and tubercle (*T*) are indicated.

FIG. 7-14 Lower compartment arthrogram of TMJ showing anterior disk displacement. Prominent anterior recess (*arrow*) of the lower joint space is a sign of disk displacement.

adopted by many clinicians. It was considered technically difficult and painful for the patient, and the information gathered was not considered of great value for treatment planning and evaluation of prognosis. Only a few descriptions of TMJ arthrography appeared in the literature over the ensuing 25 years.

Toward the end of the 1970s, several articles appeared, describing the clinical and arthrographic characteristics of internal derangement related to displacement of the disk.[7,8,50-52] These arthrographic studies were actually the first to depict displacement of the disk, a pathologic entity that had been suspected earlier.[14,53-57] During the following years, considerable enthusiasm developed for TMJ arthrography, and a large number of publications describing the usefulness of the technique appeared in the literature. The changed attitude toward TMJ arthrography can be traced to the following factors: (1) use of an image intensifier to facilitate joint puncture and to study and document joint dynamics, (2) identification of disk displacement as a common cause of TMJ pain and dysfunction, and probably most importantly, (3) introduction of new, conservative surgical methods for treating disk displacement.[7,8,50,51,58-62] These newer treatment methods required accurate information about the status and function of the joint. The use of non-ionic contrast medium, which made the examination less painful, and the combination of arthrography and tomography also influenced the increased use of arthrography.[6,25]

Single- and Double-Contrast Arthrography

Injection of contrast medium into only the lower space (Fig. 7-14) is a simplification of the original arthrographic tech-

nique in which contrast medium was injected into both upper and lower joint spaces.[5,50,51] This simplification further popularized the use of arthrography, and currently single-contrast lower compartment arthrography is the most commonly used arthrographic technique.[5,50]

Double-contrast arthrography (Fig. 7-15) is a variant of arthrography in which injection of iodine contrast medium is combined with an injection of air.* The double-contrast technique is superior to the single-contrast study in its demonstration of the configuration of the disk and the posterior disk attachment (Figs. 7-15, 7-16). However, the double-contrast technique is technically more difficult to perform, because it requires cannulation of both upper and lower joint spaces and the injection of both contrast medium and air.

Indications and Contraindications

The most common indication for arthrography is assessment of the position and function of the disk in patients with pain and dysfunction suggesting internal derangement Box 7-3. Arthrography can also be used in patients with TMJ disk displacement with reduction to determine the mandibular position that reestablishes a normal condyle-disk relationship.[50,65] The purpose of this would be to establish the optimum position for initiating protrusive splint therapy (conservative therapy).[50,65] Infrequently, arthrography is performed to delineate loose bodies within the joint spaces, for diagnostic aspiration of joint fluid, for intraarticular injection of cortisone, or for evaluation of the TMJ after trauma.

---

*References 6,17,25,52,63,64.

BOX 7-3
INDICATIONS AND CONTRAINDICATIONS
FOR TMJ ARTHROGRAPHY

Indications

Common	Assess position, function, and configuration of the disk
	Differential diagnosis in patients with diffuse facial and head pain
	Establish a jaw position for protrusive splint therapy
Infrequent	Diagnosis of loose bodies in the joint space
	Evaluation after trauma
	Aspiration of joint fluid
	Intraarticular injections
Contraindications	Infections in the preauricular area
	Allergy to contrast medium
	Bleeding disorder
	Anticoagulation medication

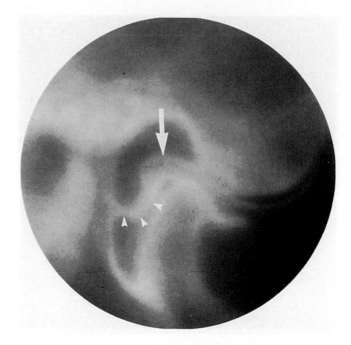

FIG. 7-15 Dual space double-contrast arthrotomogram showing the disk (*arrow*) in a superior position. The mouth was halfway opened and the redundant posterior disk attachment (*arrow heads*) is seen between the disk and the posterior capsule. The upper and lower joint spaces are radiolucent due to the intraarticular injection of air.

There are indications that arthrography occasionally has a therapeutic effect on patient symptomatology.[66] Manipulation and lavage of the joint was shown to improve mobility and decrease pain symptoms in a small clinical study.[66] The mechanism is not fully understood, and the precise indications for therapeutic arthrography must await further studies.

An infrequent contraindication for TMJ arthrography is infection in the preauricular area, which could potentially result in contamination of the joint during the arthrographic procedure. In patients with previous reactions to contrast medium, other modalities such as MR imaging should be considered as alternative imaging techniques. However, arthrography has been performed on such patients without any premedication and there was no untoward reaction. Bleeding disorders and anticoagulation medication also are relative contraindications to arthrography.

Radiologic Equipment and Procedure

A fluoroscopic table or a C-arm unit with an image intensifier is necessary equipment for this study. Because of the small size of the TMJ, it is also useful to be able to magnify the image to about three times its normal size. The capability for spot filming and videotape recording is valuable for documentation and the evaluation of joint dynamics. For double-contrast arthrography, tomography is also needed.

The examination is explained to the patient. The patient is placed on the tabletop in a laterally recumbent position,

and the head is oriented so that the side to be injected faces upward. The head is slightly tilted, the transcranial projection is optimized with fluoroscopy. Opening and closing movements of the jaw, with attention to the condyle and fossa, are recorded on videotape before contrast medium is injected.

Technique for Single-Contrast Arthrography

The superoposterior aspect of the condyle is clinically and fluoroscopically identified and indicated on the skin by a metal marker.[67] The area is marked with a pen, and local anesthesia (1% to 2% lidocaine) is injected. The joint is punctured with a 23-gauge, ¾ to 1 inch scalp vein needle introduced perpendicular to the skin surface, and contrast medium (nonionic, 300 mg iodine/ml) is injected into the lower joint space (Fig. 7-17, *A*). Contrast medium is injected until optimum visualization of the joint space has been achieved as determined by fluoroscopic observation of the joint space. Usually between 0.2 and 0.4 ml of contrast medium is injected. The needle is then withdrawn from the joint space, but the tip of the needle is left in the soft tissue lateral to the joint. The patient is asked to open and close the mouth several times while the image is recorded on videotape. The free flow of contrast medium around the top of the condyle, the anterior aspect of the condylar head, and into the anterior recess of the inferior space indicates a successful injection. Simultaneous filling of the upper joint space indicates a perforation between these spaces. In joints with

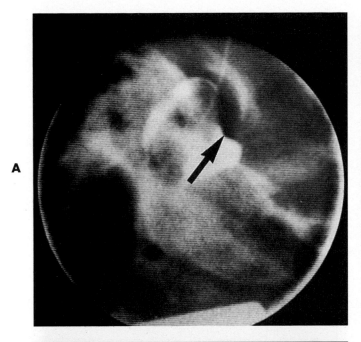

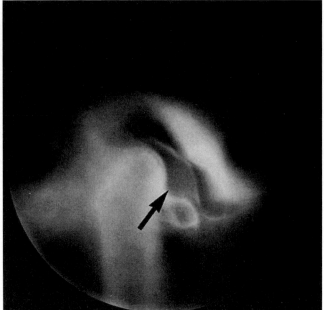

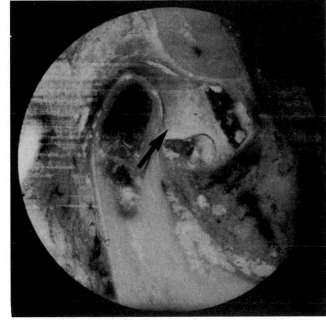

FIG. 7-16 **A** and **B,** Single and dual space double-contrast arthrotomography. **C,** Corresponding cryosection of TMJ with anterior disk displacement. The location of the posterior band is indicated by arrows.

perforation, additional contrast medium usually needs to be injected for optimum image quality. Spot films are obtained in at least the closed and open mouth positions and at additional positions where abnormalities are clearly seen.

If the diagnosis is not clear from these images, it may be helpful to also inject contrast medium into the upper joint space (Fig. 7-17, *B*). This can be done either by withdrawing the needle slightly and then directing the needle superiorly into the upper joint space (if the needle was left in place after the initial injection) or by reinserting the needle while the patient is holding the mouth half open. Injection of the upper joint space allows a clearer delineation of the disk because both its under and upper surfaces are now coated by contrast medium.

Technique for Double-Contrast Arthrography

If double-contrast arthrography is to be performed, the joint spaces are punctured with catheters (Angiocath 0.8 mm in diameter and 25 mm in length) instead of needles.[17,25] Contrast medium is injected via extension tubes and aspirated after the dynamic phase of the study. Room air is then injected via new extension tubes, and images are obtained on an upright tomographic unit such as the Phillips polytome. A book cassette with five films 3 mm apart for simultaneous tomography facilitates the rapid acquisition of multiple sections and is recommended. A complete description of the double contrast technique is given elsewhere.[68]

Arthrographic Findings of the Normal TMJ

In a normal TMJ the posterior band of the disk is located superior to the condyle (Fig. 7-18). The lower joint space has a relatively small anterior recess. However, studies of normal individuals without symptoms have shown a great variation in the size of this recess despite the disk being located in the superior position.[69] At maximum opening the disk is located inferior to the articular tubercle, and the condyle articulates with the central thin zone and the posterior part of the disk (Fig. 7-18).

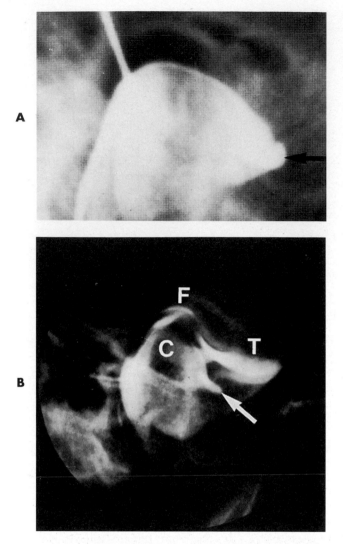

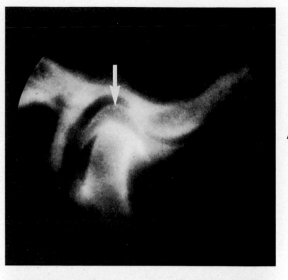

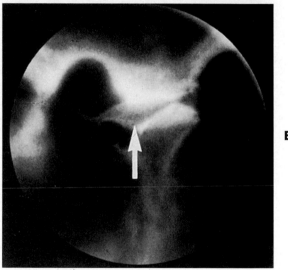

FIG. 7-17 A, Normal TMJ single-contrast arthrogram with contrast injection into the lower joint compartment only. The small anterior recess of the lower joint compartment (*arrow*) suggests a normal superior disk position. **B,** Normal TMJ demonstrated by single-contrast arthrogram with contrast injection into both upper and lower joint spaces. The condyle (*C*), fossa (*F*), and tubercle (*T*) are indicated. The arrow indicates the anterior recess of the lower joint space.

FIG. 7-18 A, Normal TMJ with dual space double-contrast arthrotomography in closed mouth position. The posterior band (*arrow*) of the disk is located over the condyle. **B,** Normal TMJ dual space double-contrast arthrotomography in open mouth position. The posterior band (*arrow*) of the disk is located posterior to the condyle.

Abnormal Findings

Displacement of the disk with reduction (Figs. 7-19) and without reduction (Fig. 7-20) are the most frequent pathologic findings in TMJ arthrography. Principally this means that the posterior thick part (posterior band) of the disk is located anterior to the condyle in the closed mouth position, and the condyle closes on the posterior disk attachment (bilaminar zone). An arthrographic sign of disk displacement in single-contrast lower compartment arthrography is enlargement of the anterior recess of the lower joint space (Fig. 7-21).

In disk displacement with reduction the disk is usually biconcave, although there may be some minor enlargement of the posterior band. This corresponds to the early-interme-

diate stage in the classification scheme described by Wilkes. Box 7-2.[9] In disk displacement without reduction a more extensive deformity of the disk is frequently encountered (Fig. 7-22), and this corresponds to the late stage in the same classification scheme.[9] This is consistent with the deformities observed in pathologic specimens, which include thickening and shortening of the anteroposterior dimension of the disk. Perforation of the posterior disk attachment is another sign of late stage internal derangement. Perforation is indicated by passage of contrast medium from the lower to the upper joint space (Fig. 7-23) when only the inferior space is injected.

Demonstration of pathology other than internal derangement is distinctly uncommon at TMJ arthrography. Patients

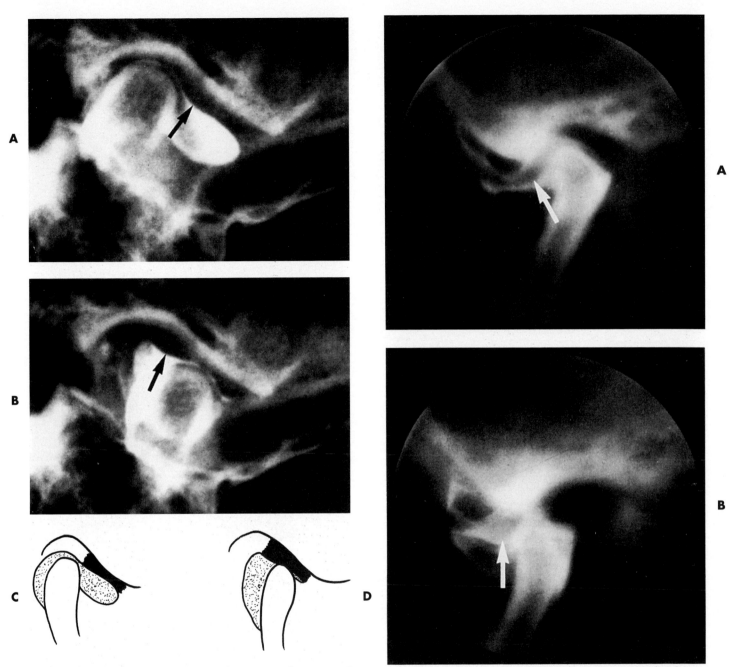

FIG. 7-19 A and **C,** Anterior disc displacement as demonstrated with single-contrast lower compartment arthrography. The posterior band, *(arrow)* of the disk is located anterior to the condyle. **B** and **D,** After reduction the disk is in a normal superior position with the posterior band *(arrow)* posterior to the condyle.

FIG. 7-20 Anterior disk displacement without reduction, double contrast arthrogram. **A** and **B,** In closed mouth and maximum mouth opening the disk is located anterior to the condyle. The position of the posterior band is indicated by arrows.

with symptoms such as clicking and locking may occasionally have one or more loose bodies within the joint space.[70] Synovial chondromatosis, osteoarthrosis, or osteochondritis dissecans are the three principal causes of loose bodies in a joint.

Inflammatory joint disease such as rheumatoid arthritis is another pathologic entity that may affect the TMJ. However, this is usually diagnosed clinically, and patients with these diseases are rarely seen for TMJ arthrography. Osseous

changes associated with rheumatoid arthritis can be clearly demonstrated with tomography or CT.

Complications Following Arthrography

Serious complications after arthrography are rare; no cases of infection following arthrography have been reported in the literature. Transient facial nerve palsy may result from extensive injection of local anesthetic agent around the condyle and condylar neck, and the patient may encounter

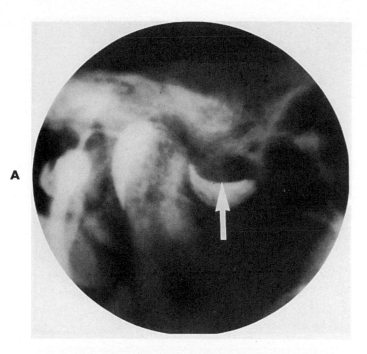

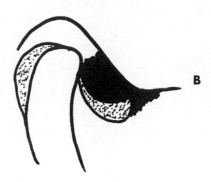

FIG. 7-21 A and **B,** Anterior disk displacement with associated enlargement of the posterior band of the disk (*arrow*).

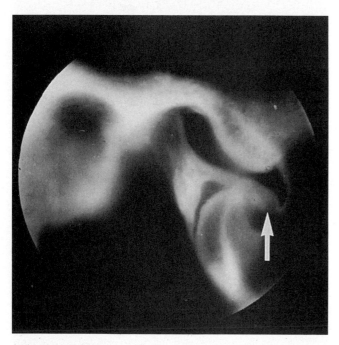

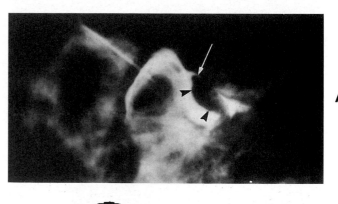

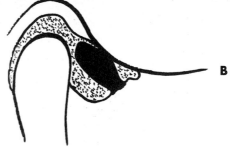

FIG. 7-22 Anterior disk displacement with extensive deformation of the disk. Dual space, double contrast arthrogram. The disk is biconvex (*arrow*).

FIG. 7-23 Perforation. **A,** Contrast material was injected into the lower joint space, and there is an overflow (*arrow*) to the upper joint space indicating perforation. The disk (*arrowheads*) is anteriorly displaced and deformed. **B,** Schematic drawing of **A.**

mild to moderate local discomfort for 1 to 2 days after the procedure. The use of nonionic or low-osmolality contrast media has been helpful in reducing the patient's discomfort.

Computed Tomography

CT scanning of the TMJ can be performed either as direct sagittal scanning (Fig. 7-24) or as axial scanning with sagittal reconstructions.[71,72,73] Both techniques have been reported to be successful in demonstrating internal derangement and osseous disease.[74-76] However, the use of CT for diagnosis of soft-tissue changes in the TMJ has decreased rapidly during the past few years because of the superiority

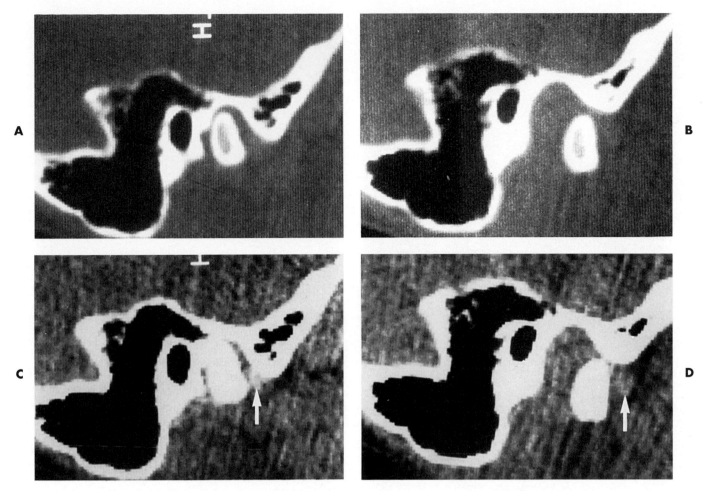

FIG. 7-24 A, Direct sagittal CT of TMJ showing posterior condylar position. **B,** Same joint as in A obtained at maximal mouth opening showing some limitation of anterior condylar translation. **C,** Same joint as in **A** and **B** with soft-tissue setting showing disk (*arrow*) anterior to the condyle. **D,** Same joint as in **A, B,** and **C.** Soft-tissue setting at maximal mouth opening showing the disk (*arrow*) anterior to the condyle, suggesting anterior disk displacement without reduction.

of MR imaging with surface coils (Fig. 7-25).[77] Although CT is not used for visualization of the disk, it still represents the best means of examining the osseous structures of the joint.

The two main reasons to use CT today are for evaluation of fractures and postsurgical changes involving the osseous components of the joint. Thus CT can clearly demonstrate the integrity of the glenoid fossa and note the presence of extensive erosions. Perforation into the middle cranial fossa after alloplastic implants also are shown best on CT.

Technique for Computed Tomography Scanning

Direct sagittal CT scanning is preferred over axial or coronal acquisitions for disk visualization. Coronal scanning is equally good when evaluating the integrity of the roof of the glenoid fossa, and this is a common indication for CT in patients who have received alloplastic TMJ implants. Axial scanning with 1 mm increments is used when the patient cannot be positioned adequately for direct sagittal or coro-

nal scanning, and the sagittal and coronal images are reformatted from the original axial data.

The design of most CT scanners requires an additional stretcher to position the patient in the direct sagittal CT imaging plane.[71,72] The stretcher is placed laterally at an angle with respect to the scanner table and the scanner gantry. Once the patient is in the correct position, scans are performed at 1-to 2-mm intervals from the medial to the lateral poles of the condyle. Additional images are then obtained at maximum mouth opening. Open mouth images are only obtained through the center of the joint. CT scans are reconstructed for both bone detail and soft-tissue detail, and in this way the need for conventional radiography or tomography is eliminated.

Computed Tomography Findings

When the disk is normal and thus positioned superior to the condyle, it is usually relatively difficult to visualize. Indeed the inability to see the disk anterior to the condyle and infe-

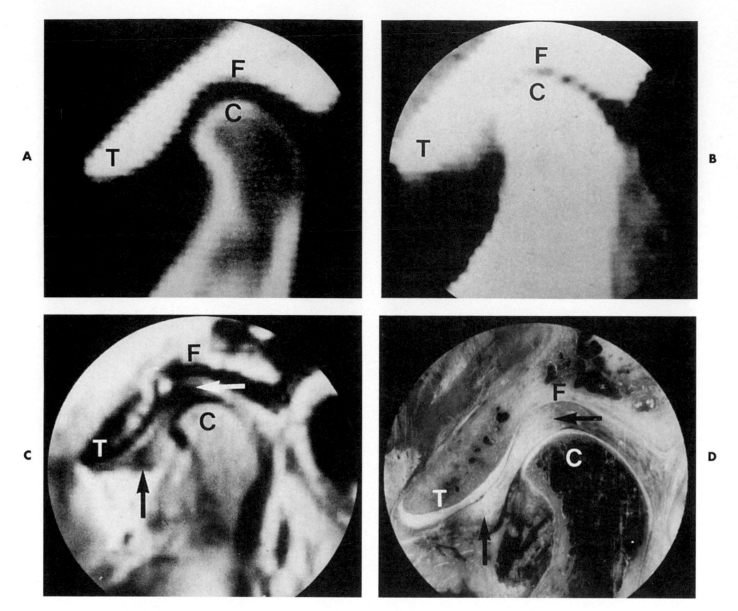

FIG. 7-25 CT in hard-tissue (**A**) and soft-tissue (**B**) settings, MRI (**C**), and corresponding cryosection (**D**) of TMJ with normal superior disk position. The tubercle (*T*), fossa (*F*), and condyle (*C*) are indicated. The anterior and posterior bands of the disk are indicated by arrows.

rior to the tubercle is interpreted as a diagnosis of normal disk position (Fig. 7-25). The lateral pterygoid fat pad refers to the fat around the lateral pterygoid muscle. Some fat is also seen between the two bellies of the lateral pterygoid muscle. This fat is an important landmark used to determine disk displacement. CT scans with wide mouth opening usually produce the optimum images of the disk (Fig. 7-26); however, open mouth images are not diagnostic for disk displacement with reduction.

When the disk is anteriorly displaced, it appears as a high-attenuation small mass anterior to the condyle, inferior to the tubercle, and within the low-attenuation lateral pterygoid fat pad (Fig. 7-26). The configuration of the disk typically cannot be determined by CT because the soft-tissue

separation is not sufficient for this purpose. The depiction of the disk on CT depends on the disk's density and size. Thus if the disk is thin and small, it usually is not identified on CT, leading to a higher incidence of false-negative diagnoses. On the other hand, if the disk is large, it can be demonstrated by CT.

Magnetic Resonance Imaging

MRI has been used to image the TMJ since 1984, and imaging quality has continuously improved since that time.[1,10,78-85] A major advantage of MRI over all other radiographic imaging techniques is the absence of patient radiation. This is especially pertinent for TMJ imaging, because a significant number of the patients are young females.[60] The soft-tissue

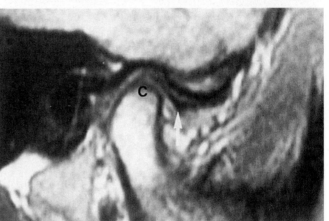

FIG. 7-26 CT scan with soft-tissue setting depicting anterior disk displacement without reduction. The image of the disk is indicated by arrows and has a relatively high CT attenuation.

differentiation of MRI is also superior to all other imaging modalities that have been applied to this joint, and at this time MRI is the primary imaging technique for most clinical presentations.

The objective of MRI of the TMJ is to document soft- and hard-tissue abnormalities of the joint and its surrounding structures. The ability of MRI to visualize the soft-tissue structures around the joint is another advantage of this modality over arthrography, and a comparison of these two imaging modalities on the same joint shows this fact (Fig. 7-27).

Magnetic Field Strength and Comparison with Computed Tomography

One of the most significant characteristics of an MR scanner is probably its magnetic field strength. Scanners with magnetic field strengths from 0.05 to 2 Tesla are currently in clinical use; however, studies that compare the image quality of these scanners with different magnetic field strengths are scarce. One study compared images from two different scanners obtained with equal acquisition time and demonstrated significantly better image quality with the high field system (Fig. 7-28).[86] Although the lower image quality of the 0.3 Tesla scanner could be somewhat compensated for by increasing the acquisition time (the number of excitations) by a factor of about 4, in clinical work this increases the risk for motion artifact.[86]

Some principal advantages and disadvantages of MRI as compared with CT are outlined in Box 7-4. Contraindications for MRI are outlined in Box 7-5.

Surface Coil and Scanning Technique

The oblique sagittal and oblique coronal planes are standard for MRI of the TMJ (Fig. 7-29). A standard imaging protocol is shown in Table 7-1. The use of the dual surface coil technique for imaging of left and right TMJs at the same time has been of great value because the time on the scanner can be significantly shortened for bilateral TMJ imag-

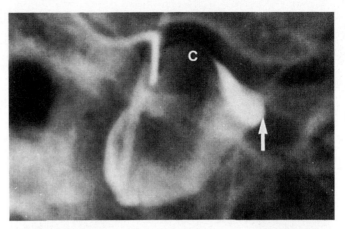

FIG. 7-27 **A,** Arthrogram. **B,** MRI image of the same TMJ showing normal superior disk position. The anterior recess of the lower joint compartment is indicated by an arrow in the arthrogram. In the MR image the disk is located superior to the condyle. The condyle (*C*) is noted in both studies.

ing.[87,88] Bilateral abnormalities are seen in up to 60% of patients with pain and dysfunction who initially present with unilateral symptoms.[89,90]

MRI is performed using the body coil as the transmitter and the two surface coils as the receivers. Surface coils are essential for good image quality and a diameter between 6 and 12 cm provides optimal signal to noise in most patients. The standard imaging protocol obtains oblique sagittal and oblique coronal images perpendicular and parallel to the long axis of the mandibular condyle (Fig.7-29).[91] Sagittal images should be obtained in both closed and open mouth positions to determine the function of the disk. Coronal images are usually obtained only in the closed mouth position. The protocol shown in Table 7-1, may need to be adjusted, depending on the performance of the scanner and the type of surface coils used.

Proton density images are preferable to T1-weighted (T1W) images for outlining morphology because of the "greater latitude" and better visualization of disk tissue relative to the surrounding joint capsule and cortical bone. T2W images are obtained routinely to document the pres-

---

BOX 7-4

ADVANTAGES AND DISADVANTAGES OF MAGNETIC RESONANCE IMAGING COMPARED WITH COMPUTED TOMOGRAPHY

Advantages	No ionizing radiation
	Fewer artifacts from dense bone and metal clips
	Imaging possible in several planes without moving the patient
	Superior anatomic detail of soft tissues
Disadvantages	High initial cost of the scanner
	Special site planning and shielding
	Patient claustrophobia in magnet
	Inferior images of bone

BOX 7-5

CONTRAINDICATIONS FOR MRI

Absolute	Patients with cerebral aneurysm clips
	Patients with cardiac pacemakers
Relative	Ferromagnetic foreign bodies in critical locations (e.g., eyes)
	Metallic prosthetic heart valves
	Claustrophobic or uncooperative patients
	Implanted stimulator wires for pain control
Not contraindications	Metallic prostheses
	Orthodontic fixed appliances

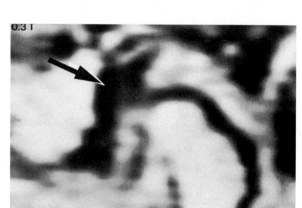

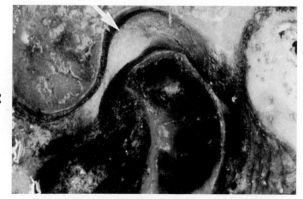

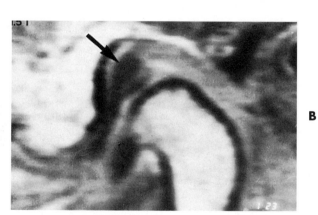

FIG. 7-28 **A** and **B,** MRI scan in 0.3 Tesla and 1.5 Tesla. **C,** Corresponding cryosection showing normal superior disk position (*arrow*). Image quality of 1.5 Tesla scanner is superior to that of 0.3 Tesla scanner, when comparable imaging times are used.

TABLE 7-1
Scanning Parameters for MRI

Image	Scanning Time
Axial Localizer	25 sec
TR/TE = 300 ms; 16 ms	
NEX = 0.5	
FOV = 18 cm	
Slice thickness = 3 mm	
Matrix = 256 × 128	
Sagittal, Closed-mouth	3 min, 52 sec
TR/TE = 2000 ms; $^{19}/_{80}$ ms	
NEX = 0.5-0.75	
FOV = 10-12 cm	
Slice thickness = 3 mm	
Matrix = 256 × 192	
Sagittal, Open-mouth	2 min, 42 sec
TR/TE = 1500 ms; $^{19}/_{80}$ ms	
NEX = 0.75	
FOV = 10-12 cm	
Slice thickness = 3 mm	
Matrix = 256 × 128	
Coronal, Closed-mouth	3 min, 52 sec
TR/TE = 2000 ms; $^{19}/_{80}$ ms	
NEX = 0.5-0.75	
FOV = 10-12 cm	
Slice thickness = 3 mm	
Matrix = 256 × 192	

FOV, field of view; *NEX,* number of excitations

ence of joint effusion and inflammatory changes in the joint capsule. Because of the arthrographic effect created by the high signal intensity of the joint effusion on T2W images, these also may be useful for outlining perforations. T2W images obtained in both sagittal and coronal planes frequently help outline the joint effusion.

Fast spin-echo T2W images provide better signal to noise than standard T2W images. However, the standard proton density images provide superior soft-tissue separation, and many imagers prefer standard spin-echo images because they are sharper than fast spin-echo images. Open mouth images are obtained to determine the function of the disk. Syringes of variable sizes or commercially available bite block devices are used to stabilize the patient's jaw in the open mouth positions (Fig. 7-30). Slice thickness should be 3 mm or less. The gap or interval between slices should be between 0.5 and 1.5 mm for the sagittal images; for the coronal images this should be reduced to about 0.3 mm to obtain at least one good image through the center of the condyle. The anteroposterior dimension of the condyle is usually about 8 to 10 mm, and volume averaging is a greater problem for coronal images than for sagittal images. By angling the coronal images along the horizontal long axis of the condyle, images of both left and right joints can be obtained simultaneously. In the rare instance when the slices of the left and right joints interfere, separate acquisitions of the left and right joints should be obtained.

The coronal images are valuable in identifying medial and lateral displacements of the disk. Additionally the osseous anatomy of the condyle can sometimes be better appreciated in the coronal plane.

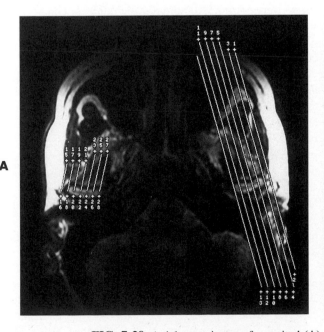
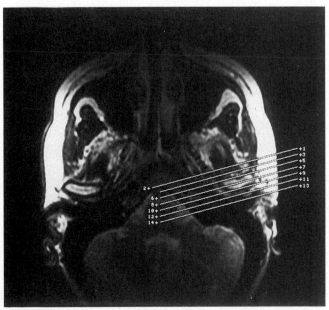

FIG. 7-29 Axial scout images for sagittal (**A**) and coronal (**B**) MR images. The orientation of the sagittal and coronal images are outlined. It is important to cover the area of the lateral and medial poles of the condyle with the sagittal images. For the coronal images, one image should be through the center of the condyle.

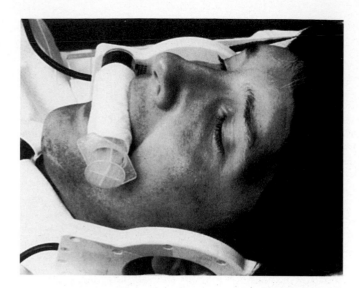

FIG. 7-30 Clinical positioning with dual surface coils and syringe between upper and lower teeth used as a bite block.

If the patient's oral splint is to be assessed, additional oblique sagittal images are obtained with the splint in place. The same scanning parameters are used for the closed mouth sagittal images.

Magnetic Resonance Imaging Findings of the Normal TMJ

MRI nicely shows the normal TMJ anatomy in the sagittal and coronal planes (Fig. 7-31). In the sagittal plane the disk is biconcave with the posterior band (posterior thick part) lying over the condyle. The central thin zone articulates against the anterior prominence of the condyle. Because the fibrous connective tissue of the disk has a low signal intensity, the disk usually can be distinguished from the surrounding tissues, which have a higher signal intensity. The cortices of both the condylar and temporal components of the joint have a low signal intensity, but the articular coverings of the joint have a higher signal intensity. This makes the outline of the osseous components easily visible. The posterior disk attachment has a relatively high signal intensity compared with the posterior portion of the disk itself because of the fatty tissue in the posterior disk attachment. MRI is the only modality that allows the disk to be distinguished from its posterior attachment.

In MRI scans obtained at maximum mouth opening the central thin zone of the disk is visualized between the condyle and the tubercle (Fig. 7-31, B). The posterior band of the disk articulates against the posterior surface of the condyle, as has been demonstrated in anatomic specimens (Fig. 7-3).

In the coronal plane (Fig. 7-31, C) the normal disk has a crescent appearance. The medial aspect of the disk attaches just inferior to the medial pole of the condyle and to the medial capsule. Similarly the lateral part of the disk attaches just inferior to the lateral pole of the condyle and to the lateral capsule (Fig. 7-2). Normally the lateral and medial capsules are visualized and do not bulge outward.

Disk Displacement

Displacements of the disk in the anterior (Fig. 7-32), anteromedial, or anterolateral directions are the most common findings observed when interpreting MR images of patients with clinical signs and symptoms of internal derangement.[43] In the sagittal plane the disk is noted to be displaced when its posterior band is anterior to the condyle (Fig. 7-32).

Disk displacement could be complete or partial. In complete disk displacement the entire mediolateral dimension of the disk is displaced anterior to the condyle. In partial disk displacement, only the medial or lateral part of the disk is displaced anterior to the condyle. Most frequently the lateral part is anteriorly displaced and the more medial part of the disk is still in a normal superior position. Partial disk displacement is frequently seen in joints with disk displacement with reduction (Fig. 7-33); the disk is anteriorly displaced in the lateral part of the joint (Fig. 7-33, A) and is in a normal position in the medial part of the joint (Fig. 7-33, B). This probably results because the displaced part of the disk, being anchored by the normally positioned medial portion of the disk, is allowed to revert into the normal position on opening without being squeezed between the two joint components as much as in cases with a complete anterior disk displacement.

Frequently the anterior disk displacement is combined with either medial or lateral displacement. Initially, when MRI was done in the true coronal plane, medial displacements were considered more prevalent than lateral displacements. This was probably the result of the scanning technique rather than pathologic changes because, with oblique coronal images parallel to the horizontal long axis of the condyle, medial and lateral displacements are seen with approximately the same frequency. In most cases the sagittal images show the anterior component of the displacement, and the coronal images show the medial or lateral component. In approximately 10% of patients presenting with TMJ pain and dysfunction there is a pure lateral or pure medial disk displacement that is not detected on sagittal images (Fig. 7-34).[10] The displacement can be dramatic in both the lateral (Fig. 7-34) and the medial (Fig. 7-35) directions. When the disk is displaced medially or laterally in combination with an anterior displacement it is called rotational disk displacement (Box 7-1).

The empty fossa sign seen in the sagittal images (Fig. 7-36) is an indication of a medial or lateral disk displacement. When the disk displaces in a medial direction, the lateral capsular tissue is pulled between the condyle and glenoid fossa and gives the appearance of an "empty" fossa. Thus when the disk is not clearly seen in the glenoid fossa in the closed mouth position (Fig. 7-36), a medial or lateral disk

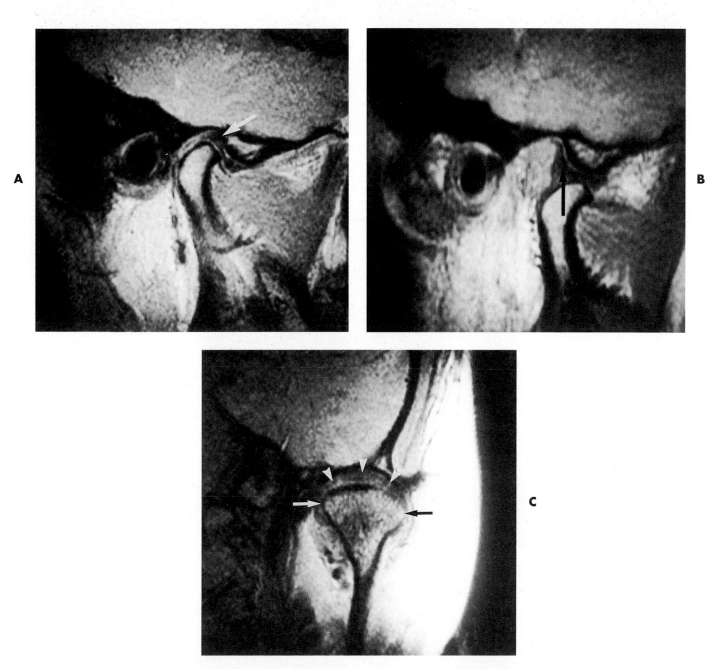

FIG. 7-31 MRI scan of normal TMJ. **A,** Closed jaw position. The posterior band (*arrow*) is superior to the condyle. **B,** Open mouth. Disk (*arrow*) has bow tie configuration and lies between condyle and articular tubercle. **C,** Coronal image. Medial and lateral poles of the condyle (*arrows*) are clearly visualized. The disk (*arrowheads*) is crescent-shaped, superior to the condyle.

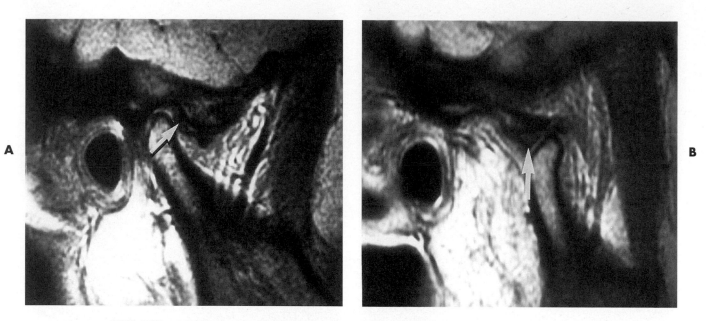

FIG. 7-32 Disk displacement with reduction. **A,** A posterior band of the displaced disk (*arrow*) is anterior to the condyle. **B,** Open mouth image shows the posterior band (*arrow*) in a normal relationship posterior to the condyle. This indicates reduction on opening.

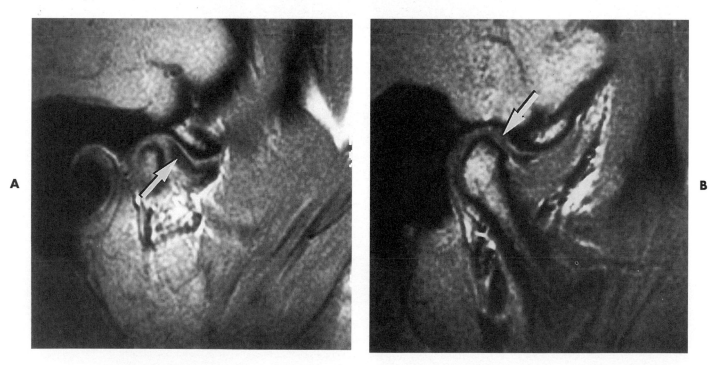

FIG. 7-33 Partial anterior disk displacement. **A,** In the lateral part of the joint the disk (*arrow*) is anteriorly displaced. **B,** In the medial part of the joint the disk (*arrow*) is located in a normal superior position. This indicates a partial anterior disk displacement.

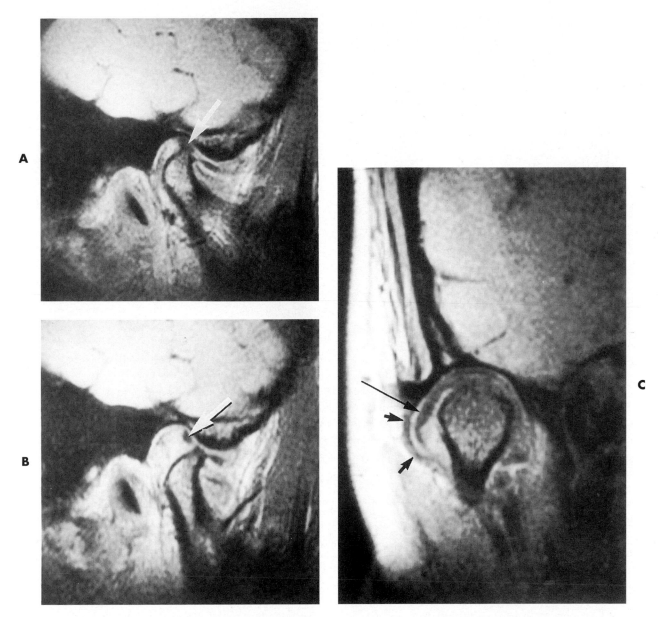

FIG. 7-34 Sideways lateral disk displacement. **A,** In the closed mouth position the disk (*arrow*) is located superior to the condyle. **B,** On opening the disk (*arrow*) functions in a normal fashion. **C,** The coronal image shows a significant lateral disk displacement (*long arrow*). There is also bulging of the lateral capsule (*short arrows*).

displacement should be suspected. The coronal images are examined for verification. Medial and lateral disk displacement may or may not (Fig. 7-36) reduce on opening. The function of the disk with sideways disk displacement is more difficult to evaluate than with anterior displacement because the location of the disk is best seen in the coronal plane at closed position and the sagittal plane at open position.

MR scans obtained at maximum mouth opening determine whether the disk displacement reduces. In displacement with reduction (Fig. 7-32) the disk position normalizes during jaw opening. In disk displacement without reduction (Fig. 7-37) the disk remains anterior to the condyle in all

mandibular positions. Disk displacement with reduction practically always precedes the late-stage disk displacement without reduction.

Disk Deformity

Deformity of the disk (Fig. 7-9) resulting from chronic displacement, can usually be demonstrated by MRI (Fig. 7-38). Initial deformity includes thickening of the posterior band. Late stage deformity may include a rounder, biconvex disk or a severely diminished amount of disk tissue. Disk deformation is significant for the clinical management of patients because a deformed disk cannot usually be surgically repo-

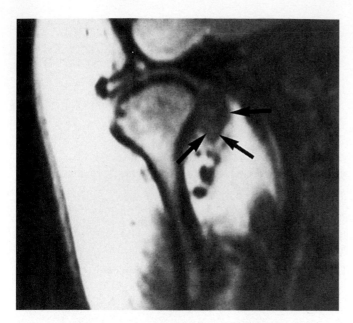

FIG. 7-35 Medial disk displacement. Coronal MR image shows the disk (*arrows*) displaced medial to the condyle.

sitioned, and more aggressive surgical treatment with diskectomy may be necessary. It is therefore important to evaluate the degree of disk deformation and communicate this information to the referring clinician.

Another form of tissue alteration secondary to disk displacement is the formation of the so-called pseudodisk (Fig. 7-39). A pseudodisk appears as a bandlike structure of low signal intensity, replacing the normally bright signal from the posterior disk attachment. Histologically it is thought to represent the fibrotic change that occurs in the posterior disk attachment in response to pressure from the condyle against the loose tissue of the posterior disk attachment (bilaminar zone). It has been suggested that this fibrotic change in the posterior disk attachment is associated with decreasing pain, but this has not been confirmed in systematic studies.[92,93]

Other Findings and Conditions Related to Internal Derangement
Joint Effusion

An assessment of the amount of joint fluid is essential because small amounts are seen outlining the articular surfaces in normal and abnormal individuals (Fig. 7-40).[94] Large accumulations of joint effusion (Fig. 7-41) are seen only in symptomatic patients. There is an association between pain and joint effusion so that joint effusion is significantly more prevalent in painful joints than in nonpainful joints.[94] Not all individuals with pain have joint effusion, but a significant accumulation of joint effusion is likely associated with a painful joint (Fig. 7-41). Joint effusion may also have some diagnostic value for outlining the morphology of the disk and detecting perforations in the posterior disk attachment (Fig. 7-42).

Osteoarthritis

Osteoarthritis is frequently seen in joints with longstanding disk displacement without reduction.[18,26] Disk displacement seems to be a precursor of osteoarthritis. Osteoarthritis is infrequently seen in joints with normal superior disk position, occasionally in disk displacement with reduction, and more frequently when disk displacement without reduction has been present for some time.

Disk displacement and internal derangement is, however, only one cause of osteoarthritis, which is the common final pathway for a multitude of primary joint lesions. Imaging evidence of osteoarthritis can be seen in young individuals (teenagers) with disk displacement without reduction.

Osteoarthritis is radiographically characterized by flattening and irregularities of the articular surfaces, osteophytosis, and erosion (Fig. 7-43). The distinction between early arthritis and advanced remodeling on MRI, as well as on other imaging modalities, is difficult to define, and overlap will exist.

Avascular Necrosis and Bone Marrow Edema

Claims have been made, based on comparison with other joints, that areas within the bone marrow of the condyle, having low signal intensity surrounded by a layer of higher signal intensity, represent avascular necrosis (Fig. 7-44).[85,95] However, other etiologies such as sclerosis or fibrosis of the bone marrow cannot be ruled out based on the MRI appearance.

Bone marrow edema has been suggested to be an early stage or precursor of avascular necrosis. This can be seen on T2W MR images. Thus bone marrow with intermediate signal intensity on the T1W and proton density images and an increased signal intensity on the T2W image (Fig. 7-45) could represent bone marrow edema. It appears that avascular or aseptic necrosis can affect the TMJ condyle (Figs. 7-46, 7-47). Fibrosis, sclerosis, and transient osteoporosis are other etiologies that may cause signal intensity changes in the bone marrow of the condyle.

Avascular necrosis is best characterized in the hip. Predisposing factors include sickle cell disease, alcoholism, and steroid therapy. Avascular necrosis in the mandibular condyle probably has a different etiology and has not been associated with the same systemic factors but rather with local trauma from internal derangement.[85]

Osteochondritis Dissecans

Loose bodies in the TMJ are rare conditions. One loose body in the joint space associated with a defect in the condyle of the same size can be characterized as osteochondritis dissecans.[85] In this condition a small part of the condyle is dislodged into the joint space and acts as a small loose body (Fig. 7-48). The condition has been described as being associated with avascular necrosis, although the relationship between the two conditions is not fully understood.[85] Osteochondritis dissecans in a cadaver joint sagittal section can be well demonstrated (Fig. 7-49).

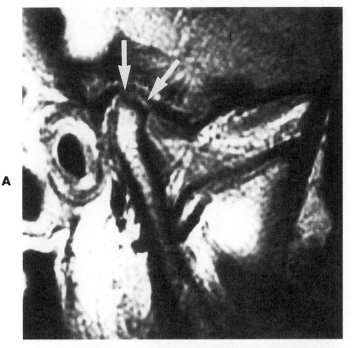

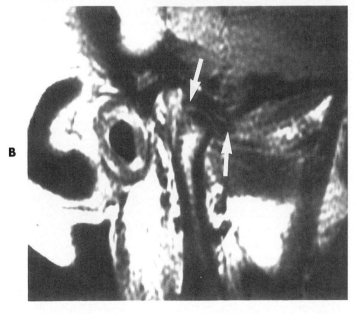

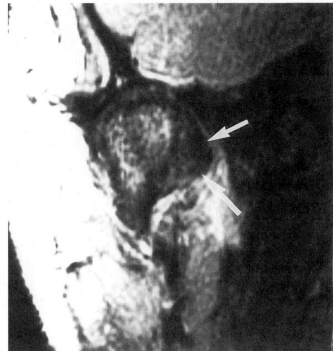

FIG. 7-36 Empty fossa with medial disk displacement. **A,** In the sagittal closed mouth image there is tissue of intermediate signal (*arrows*) in the glenoid fossa. This is termed empty fossa. **B,** On opening, the disk (*arrow*) is seen. **C,** The coronal image (closed mouth) shows the disk (*arrows*) medially displaced. The empty fossa is an indication of medial or lateral disk displacement.

Multiple loose bodies are discussed in the section on synovial chondromatosis.

Stuck Disk

In the normal opening sequence the disk moves both relative to the condyle and the temporal component of the joint. There is both translation and rotation in both joint spaces, but there is more translation or sliding in the upper compartment and there is more rotation in the lower joint space. It has been suggested in the arthroscopic literature that inability of the disk to move, relative to the glenoid fossa, is a significant cause of pain and dysfunction.[28] This observation has not been extensively and systematically documented, but there are indications that MR definition of a stuck disk (Fig. 7-50) could be associated with pain and dysfunction.[96]

Subluxation

The most frequent situation with locking of the TMJ is the inability of the patient to open the mouth. This is most frequently caused by disk displacement without reduction.

Text continued on p. 405.

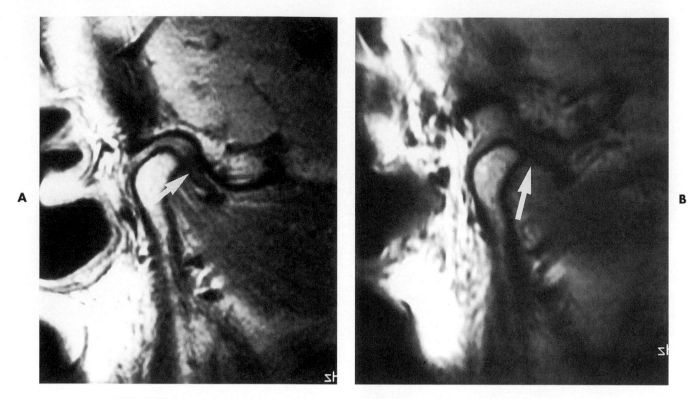

FIG. 7-37 Anterior disk displacement without reduction. **A,** In the closed mouth image the disk (*arrow*) is anterior to the condyle. **B,** On opening, the disk (*arrow*) remains anterior to the condyle, indicating anterior disk displacement without reduction.

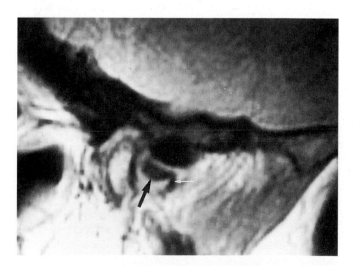

FIG. 7-38 Disk deformation. The disk (*black arrow*) is anteriorly displaced. It is deformed with thickening of the posterior band, which is indicated by the black arrow. The anterior part of the disk (*white arrow*) is folded.

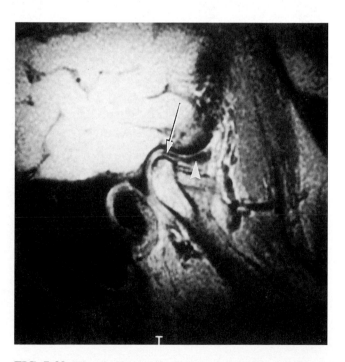

FIG. 7-39 Fibrosis of posterior disk attachment. The disk (*arrow-head*) is anteriorly displaced. There is an area of low signal in the posterior disk attachment (*long arrows*), which indicates fibrosis.

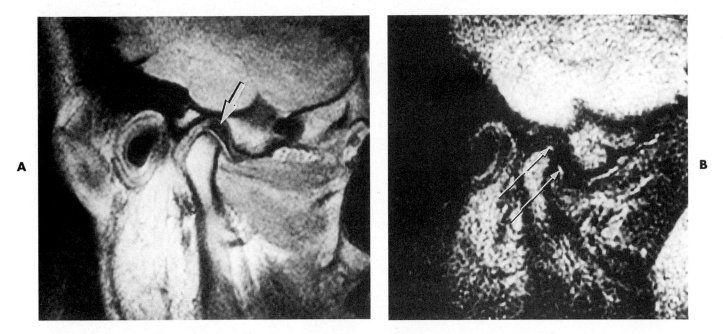

FIG. 7-40 Minimal joint effusion in normal joint. **A,** On proton density the disc (*arrow*) is located in a normal superior position. **B,** In the T2W image there is a minimal amount of high signal (*arrows*) in the lower joint space. This indicates a minimal joint effusion which occurs in normal joints.

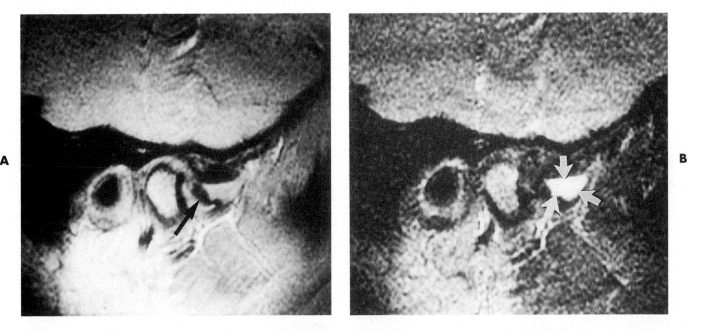

FIG. 7-41 Large joint effusion in painful joint. **A,** Proton density showing anterior disk (*arrow*) displacement. **B,** In the T2W image there is a large effusion in the upper joint space (*arrows*). This was associated with significant joint pain.

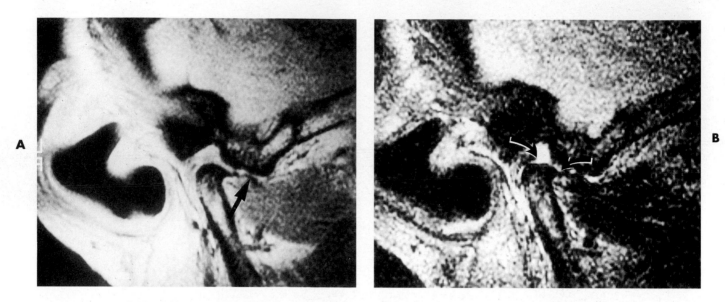

FIG. 7-42 Disk perforation demonstrated with proton density. **A,** The disk *(arrow)* is anteriorly displaced and extensively deformed. There is an anterior osteophyte of the condyle, indicating degenerative changes. Also the component is flattened. **B,** In the T2W image the defect in the posterior disc attachment (arrows) is well outlined by the joint effusion.

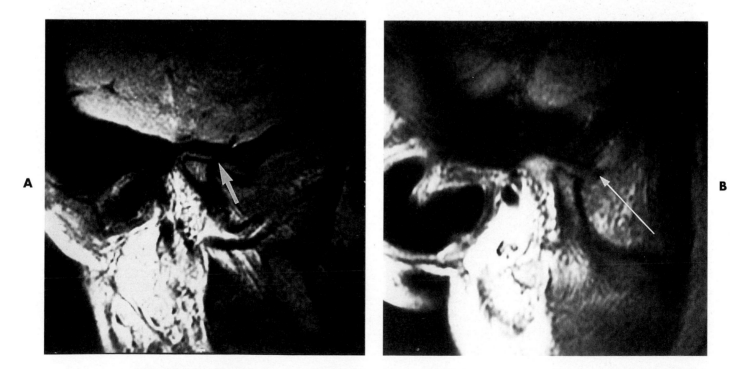

FIG. 7-43 Osteoarthritis. **A,** Proton density closed mouth image shows an anterior osteophyte of the condyle *(arrow)* and a superior flattening. The glenoid fossa is widened, and the articular tubercle is flattened. These changes are consistent with degenerative joint disease. **B,** On opening there is sliding of the two flat articular surfaces against each other, and a small part of the disk remains anterior *(arrow)*.

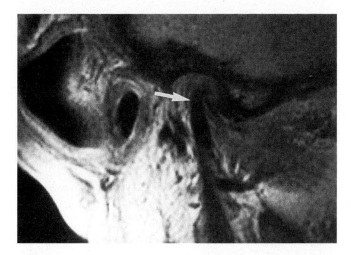

FIG. 7-44 Sclerosis of the condyle and condyle neck. Proton density shows decreased signal from the entire condyle head and condyle neck (*arrow*). This could indicate sclerosis, fibrosis, or possibly avascular necrosis. No histologic proof was available in this case.

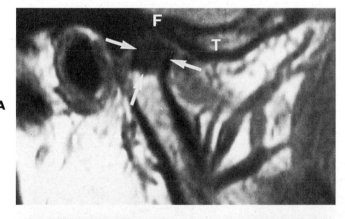

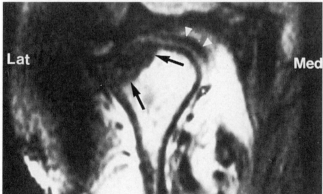

FIG. 7-46 Probable aseptic necrosis. **A,** Sagittal MRI scan showing decreased signal from the bone marrow in the upper part of the mandibular condyle (*arrows*). The fossa (*F*) and tubercle (*T*) are indicated. **B,** Coronal MRI scan of the same joint as in A showing the low signal intensity area (*arrows*) in the lateral part of the joint. In the medial part of the condyle the disk is seen superior to the condyle (*arrow heads*) and laterally the disk is absent, suggesting perforation.

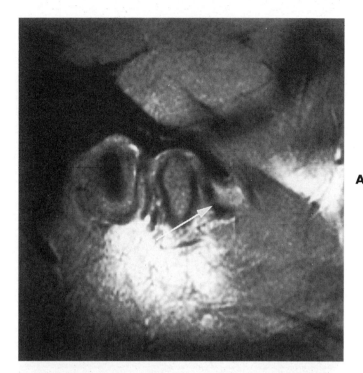

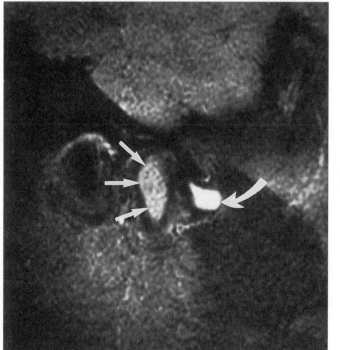

FIG. 7-45 Bone marrow edema. **A,** Proton density sagittal MR image shows anterior displacement of the disk (*arrow*). **B,** T2W image shows increased signal in the bone marrow of the condyle (*arrows*). There is also a large effusion (*arrowheads*) in the upper joint space. The increased signal in the bone marrow indicates bone marrow edema.

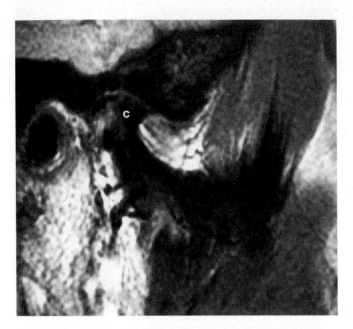

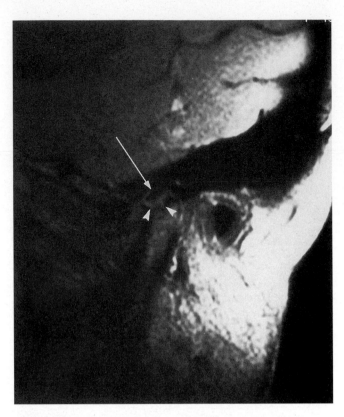

FIG. 7-47 Sagittal proton density MR image showing degenerative changes of the mandibular condyle (*C*). A core biopsy of this condyle showed avascular necrosis.

FIG. 7-48 Osteochondritis dissecans. Sagittal MR image shows a defect in the upper part of the condyle (*arrowheads*) and a corresponding structure in the glenoid fossa, which was interpreted as a loose body (*long arrow*). This condition is consistent with osteochondritis dissecans.

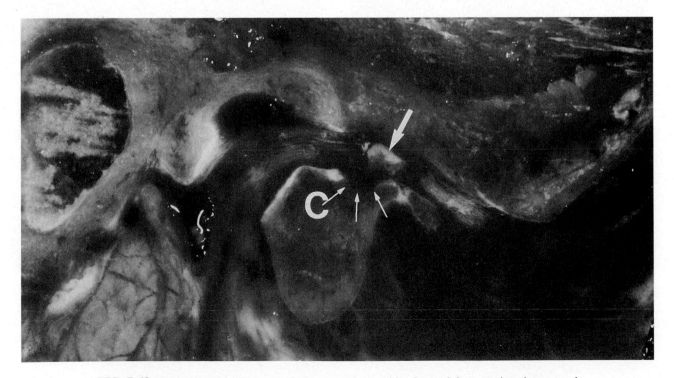

FIG. 7-49 Osteochondritis dissecans. Cadaver specimen with advanced degenerative changes and a loose body (*thick arrow*) in the joint space with a corresponding defect in the mandibular condyle (*thin arrows*).

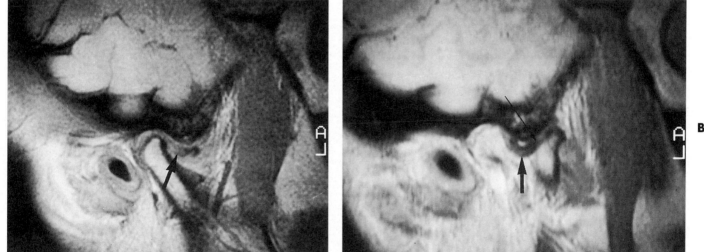

FIG. 7-50 Stuck disk. Sagittal proton density MR images at closed mouth (**A**) and maximal mouth opening (**B**) in a patient with limitation of mouth opening. The disk (*arrow*) is located in normal superior position at closed mouth. On opening the disk does not move out of the glenoid fossa, and the condyle does not translate all the way down to the articular eminence. This is consistent with a stuck disk condition.

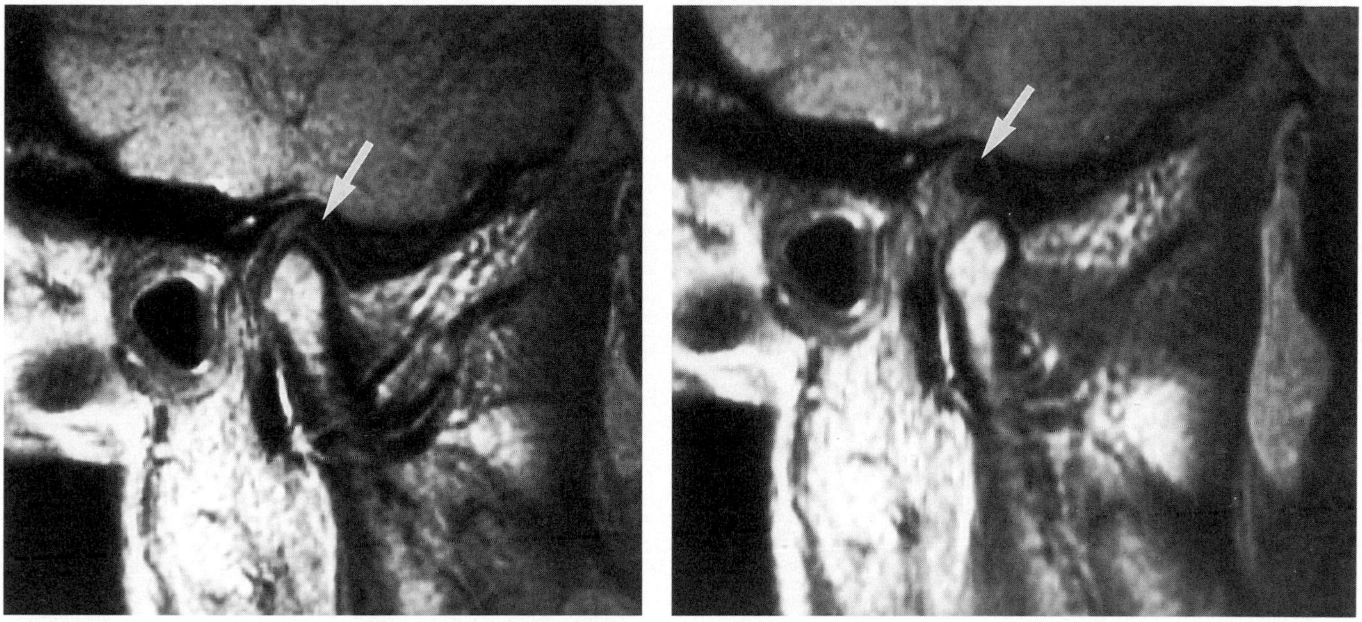

FIG. 7-51 Subluxation in front of the disk. **A,** Proton density sagittal MR image shows the disk (*arrow*) anterior to the condyle. The disk is deformed. **B,** On maximal mouth opening the condyle is in front of the disk (*arrow*), and the disk is preventing the condyle from reverting back into the glenoid fossa. The long arrow indicates the anterior edge of the disk.

Open lock condition is encountered more infrequently. In this condition the patient can open the mouth widely but is temporarily or permanently unable to close the mouth. This condition sometimes requires manipulation of the jaw by the patient or a health care professional to get the mandible into place. These patients frequently present in the emergency room but rarely for imaging assessment.

There are two principally different causes of the open lock condition. The classical situation is where the condyle is luxated in front of the articular eminence, and the articular eminence prevents the condyle from retruding back into the glenoid fossa. The other situation is one in which the condyle translates anterior to the anterior band of the disk, and the disk prevents the condyle from retruding back into

TABLE 7-2
Accuracy of TMJ Imaging Osseous Changes

Imaging	Accuracy (%)	Sensitivity	Specificity
Tomography	63-85	0.47	0.94
CT	66-87	0.28-0.75	0.91-1.0
MRI	60-100	0.50-0.87	0.71-1.0

Modified from Lindvall et al. Radiographic examination of the temporomandibular joint. Dentomaxillofac Radiology 1976; 5:24-32; Bean et al. Comparison between radiologic observations and macroscopic tissue changes in temporomandibular joint. Dentomaxillofac Radiol 1977; 6:90-106; Rohlin et al. Tomography as an aid to detect microscopic changes of the temporomandibular joint. Acta Odontol Scand 1986; 44:131-140; Tanimoto, et al. Comparison of computed with conventional tomography in the evaluation of temporomandibular joint disease: a study of autopsy specimens. Dentomaxillofac Radiol 1990; 19:21-27; Westesson et al. CT and MRI of the temporomandibular joint: comparison using autopsy specimens. Am J Roentgenol 1987; 148:1165-1171; Westesson et al. Temporomandibular joint: comparison of MR images with cryosectional anatomy. Radiology 1987; 164:59-64; Hansson et al. MR imaging of the temporomandibular joint: comparisons of images of specimens made at 0.3T and 1.5T with cryosections. Am J Roentgenol 1989; 152:1241-1244; and Tasaki, Westesson. Temporomandibular joint: diagnostic accuracy with sagittal and coronal MR imaging. Radiology 1993; 186:723-729.

TABLE 7-3
Accuracy of TMJ Imaging for Disk Position

Imaging	Accuracy (%)	Sensitivity	Specificity
Lower space, single-contrast arthrography	84-100	0.95	0.76
CT	40-67	0.45-0.85	0.50-0.87
MRI	73-95	0.86-0.90	0.63-1.0

Modified from Westesson et al. Temporomandibular joint: Correlation between single-contrast videoarthrography and post mortem morphology. Radiology 1986; 160:767-771; Schellhas et al. The diagnosis of temporomandibular joint disease: two-compartment arthrography and MR. Am J Neuro Radiol 1988; 51:341-350; Tanimoto et al. Computed tomography versus single-contrast arthrotomography in evaluation of the temporomandibular joint disc. A study of autopsy specimens. Int J Oral Maxillofac Surg 1989;18:354-358; Westesson et al. Temporomandibular joint: Comparison of MR images with cryosectional anatomy. Radiology 1987; 164:59-64; Hansson et al. MR imaging of the temporomandibular joint: comparisons of images of specimens made at 0.3T and 1.5T with cryosections. Am J Roentgenol 1989; 152:1241-1244; Westesson et al. CT and MRI of the temporomandibular joint: Comparison using autopsy specimens. Am J Roentgenol 1987; 148:1165-1171; and Tasaki, Westesson. Temporomandibular joint: diagnostic accuracy with sagittal and coronal MR imaging. Radiology 1993; 186:723-729.

the glenoid fossa (Fig. 7-51). Characteristically, in this situation the disk is folded behind the condyle (Fig. 7-51). It is usually not possible to differentiate between the two causes on physical examination. Although the acute management with reduction of the subluxation is similar in both situations, if definitive surgery is necessary, it differs depending on the cause of the subluxation. If the disk is blocking the reversion of the condyle, surgery has to be directed to the disk. If the articular eminence is the cause of the patients inability to close the mouth, surgery has to be focused on the bone.

Accuracy of TMJ Imaging

Knowing the diagnostic accuracy of an imaging modality is essential for its clinical use. The accuracy of tomography, arthrography, CT, and MRI has been investigated in several studies on fresh autopsy material (Tables 7-2, 7-3).[77,97-100] All techniques have demonstrated relatively high accuracy in determining osseous conditions and disk position; however, MRI has the highest accuracy and demonstrates both joint structures and the soft tissues surrounding the joint.

The accuracies noted in Tables 7-2 and 7-3 are from investigations performed without the biases of clinical work. The figures are relevant for the comparison between the different techniques because the studies were performed under the same conditions. In a clinical situation, however, additional information about the patient is available that might help further improve the image interpretation. In addition by detecting medially or laterally displaced disks, the multiplanar imaging capability of MRI may provide even greater accuracy rates (Fig. 7-52). A recent study demonstrated the accuracy of MRI in determining disk position and configuration to be more than 90%.[101]

Imaging After Treatment

Imaging after surgical treatment is indicated in patients who continue to have symptoms that might be related to intraarticular pathology such as recurrence of disk displacement, intraarticular adhesions, or inflammatory changes. Although surgery is performed for a variety of pathologies of the jaw and TMJ, most surgery is done for patients with internal derangements. Because of this, the imaging of the postoperative joint is covered in this section.

The primary goal of treatment of TMJ disorders is to eliminate pain and dysfunction. Secondary goals are restoration of normal anatomy and prevention of disease progression. Although the majority of TMJ treatments are successful, if a patient continues to have symptoms after treatment, imaging is frequently helpful in determining the etiology of the problem.

Treatment Modalities for TMJ Internal Derangement

Conservative treatment of TMJ internal derangement includes reassurance, observation, occlusal adjustment, bite splints, nonsteroidal antiinflammatory medications, muscle relaxants, and physical therapy. Arthroscopic surgery includes lysis and lavage of adhesions and disk repositioning. Open joint surgery includes disk repositioning, diskectomy without replacement, diskectomy with autologous implant, and joint reconstruction with rib grafts. The use of alloplastic disk replacement implants has been discontinued.

Imaging Techniques after Surgical Treatment

Before the availability of MRI, plain films (Fig. 7-53), tomography, and arthrography were used to evaluate patients after surgery. Plain films and tomography show

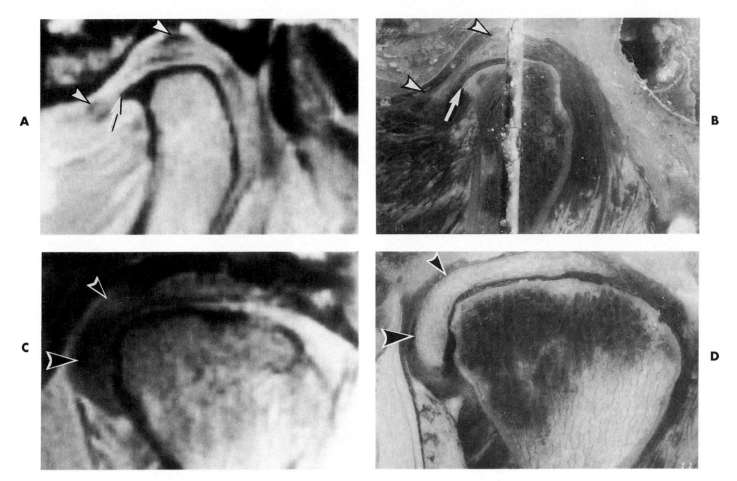

FIG. 7-52 Correlation between MR image and cryosection. **A** and **C,** Sagittal and coronal MR images show the disk (*arrowheads*) superior to the condyle in the sagittal view (A) but medially displaced in the coronal view. **B** and **D,** The corresponding cryosections confirm the MR images. The condyle also demonstrates an anterior osteophyte (*arrow* in **A**).

only the osseous structures, and there is often a need for soft-tissue evaluation as well. Arthrography can be difficult to perform once surgery has been done because the anatomy is altered and the joint spaces are narrowed as a result of peripheral and intraarticular adhesions (Fig. 7-54). For this reason, MRI is a preferable method of examination in most postoperative patients.[1,78,79]

Postoperative MRI is helpful in confirming whether surgical treatment has corrected the position of the displaced disk. Frequently, however, the disk remains anteriorly displaced after disk-repositioning surgery. This is seen in both symptomatic and asymptomatic individuals, and less emphasis should be placed on the position of the disk after surgery because symptoms may be associated more with peripheral adhesions than with disk position per se.

In patients who have undergone diskectomy, there is a soft-tissue interface between the condyle and the glenoid fossa (Fig. 7-55), which is a natural replacement for the extirpated disk.[102] This is a normal post surgical development. On MRI this soft tissue has intermediate to high signal intensity as opposed to fibrous adhesions that have a low signal intensity (Fig. 7-56). The most important imaging

assessment in these patients is to evaluate for peripheral or intraarticular adhesions following diskectomy, because such intraarticular adhesions (Fig. 7-56) frequently are the cause of the patient's limited opening and pain. Thickening of the lateral joint capsule is also frequently seen after surgery (Fig. 7-57) in both symptomatic and asymptomatic individuals and is probably of limited clinical significance as long as the scar tissue does not extend into the joint space. The amount of scar tissue in the lateral capsule wall varies significantly between patients; some scar in asymptomatic patients is quite large but does not extend into the joint space (Fig. 7-57).

A complete fibrous (Fig. 7-56) or bony ankylosis (Fig. 7-58) may occur after surgery in a few instances. Jaw motion is severely restricted, but opening can be up to about 10 mm, even with a heavy fibrous ankylosis. In bony ankylosis (Fig. 7-58) there is no motion, and CT or tomography are preferred over MR imaging.

Alloplastic Implants

During the 1980s and early 1990s alloplastic implants were used to replace the disk. Mainly two types of implants,

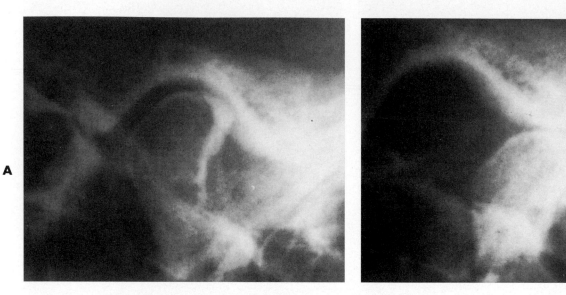

FIG. 7-53 Transcranial plain film in the closed **(A)** and open **(B)** mouth positions 29 years after discectomy. The osseous structures are relatively normal with only a decreased joint space. The outline of the condyle and temporal joint components is smooth without evidence of degenerative joint disease.

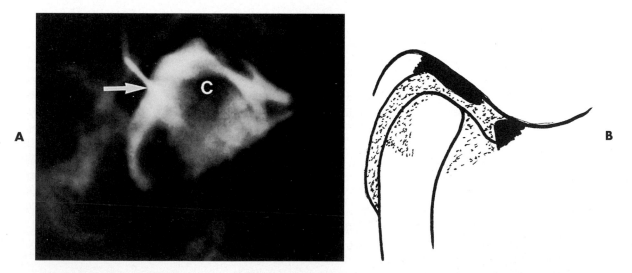

FIG. 7-54 A and **B,** Postsurgical arthrogram and schematic drawing. Contrast medium was injected into the lower joint space (*arrow*), and there is a perforation to the upper joint space. Peripheral adhesions make the joint space smaller than normal. A disk plication had been performed 2 years before this arthrogram.

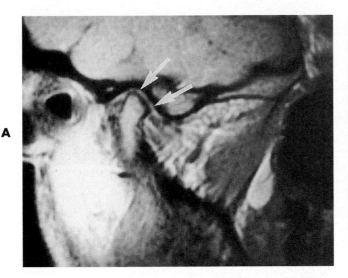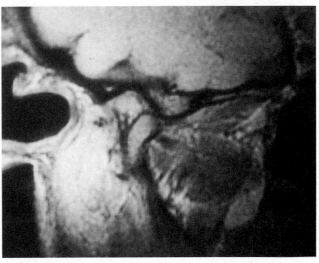

FIG. 7-55 Successful discectomy. **A,** Closed mouth MR image shows an area of intermediate to high signal (*arrows*) in the joint space. This is the normal appearance after a successful diskectomy. **B,** On opening, the condyle translates anteriorly and inferiorly and there is no evidence of fibrous ankylosis.

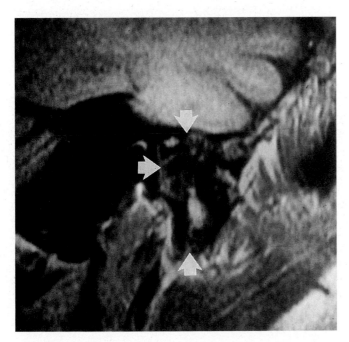

FIG. 7-56 Intraarticular adhesions following discectomy. Sagittal MR image 2 years after discectomy. There is an irregular area of low density in the entire joint region (*arrows*). This is indicative of extensive fibrous adhesions.

Proplast Teflon (Figs. 7-59, 7-60) and silicone rubber material (Silastic) were used. The Proplast implants were intended to be permanent, whereas the silicon implants were used either on a temporary or permanent basis. The initial results were favorable, and these surgical techniques quickly gained popularity, although clinical studies to support long term success were lacking. After about 2 to 4 years, the patients frequently developed gradually increasing pain. These symptoms were later shown to be due to fragmentation of the implant material and a foreign body giant cell reaction to this material. Although the reaction to the particulated material occurred similarly with both silastic and Proplast, the reaction seemed more aggressive with the Proplast. Clinically the patient presented with pain and radiographically erosive changes of the bone have been observed (Fig. 7-61). The long-term prognosis for TMJ alloplastic implants is poor, and probably all implants eventually have to be removed.

While the implants are still in place, imaging evaluation is frequently necessary. The principal findings relate to the extent of erosive change of the glenoid fossa and the mandibular condyle. The integrity of the glenoid fossa is critical since erosions can extend into the middle cranial fossa (Fig. 7-60). For the initial evaluation of a patient with a TMJ alloplastic implant, both MRI (Fig. 7-59) and CT (Figs. 7-60, 7-62) may be necessary. The MR shows the extent of the soft-tissue alteration (Fig. 7-59), fragmentation of the implant material, and the expansion of the joint cap-

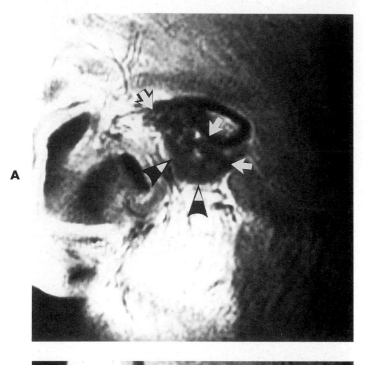

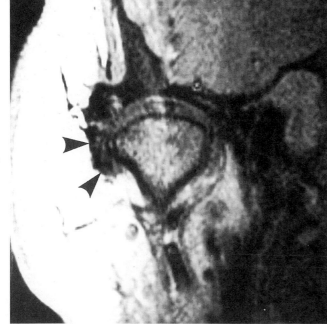

FIG. 7-57 Scar tissue in lateral capsule. Sagittal (**A**) and coronal (**B**) MR images after diskectomy. There is an irregular area of decreased signal in the lateral capsule wall (*arrows*). This is indicative of scar tissue in the lateral capsule wall. Coronal image (**B**) shows the area confined to the capsule wall. This fibrous tissue (*arrowheads*) does not extend into the joint space.

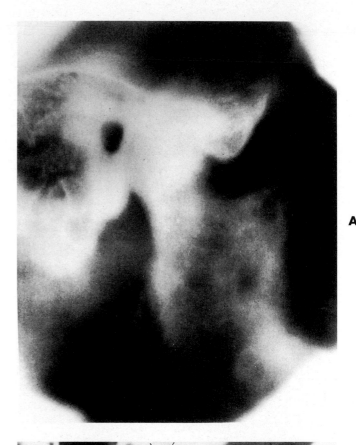

FIG. 7-58 Bony ankylosis. **A,** Sagittal tomogram shows bony ankylosis between condyle and glenoid fossa in a patient with multiple previous surgeries. **B,** Sagittal CT scan confirms the bony nature of the ankylosis (*arrows*).

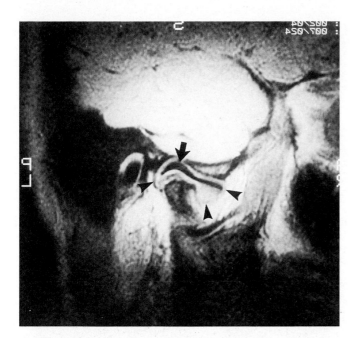

FIG. 7-59 Alloplastic TMJ implant. Sagittal proton density MR image shows an alloplastic TMJ implant (*arrow*). The implant has been in place for 3 years, and there is an expanded capsule (*arrowheads*) surrounding the implant. Degenerative changes of the condyle with an anterior osteophyte.

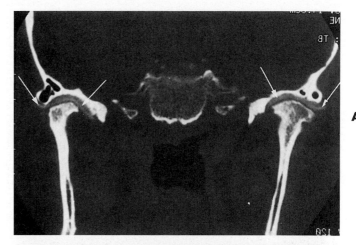

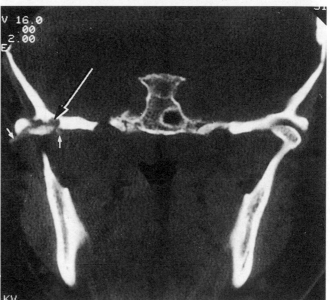

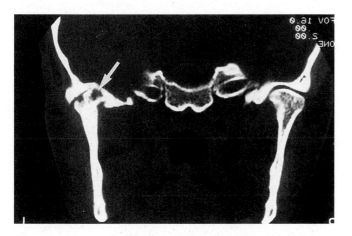

FIG. 7-61 Erosions and bony ankylosis following temporary silastic implant. Coronal CT scans through the TMJ show extensive erosive changes of the right condyle. There is bony ankylosis between the condyle and the glenoid fossa and the medial part of the joint. The patient had a history of a few months use of a temporary silastic implant. These extensive radiographic changes are the sequela from the use of the implant.

FIG. 7-60 A, Bilateral Proplast Teflon implants in good condition. Coronal CT scan of patient with bilateral Proplast Teflon implants (*arrows*) in good condition. There is no evidence of erosions into the middle cranial fossa, and the implants appear intact and in good relationship to condyle and glenoid fossa. **B,** Erosions of glenoid fossa secondary to alloplastic implant. Coronal CT scan of another patient with a Proplast Teflon implant (*short arrows*) and erosions of the glenoid fossa (*long arrow*). Also note that the implant is difficult to outline due to partial fragmentation of the implant.

sule. CT is valuable for assessment of bones, especially the integrity of the glenoid fossa (Fig. 7-60, *B*). For follow-up examination, CT with coronal or direct sagittal scans is the optimal imaging modality. Irregularity of the implant is best appreciated on CT. However, postitioning the patient for imaging in the sagittal plane, which is preferred for examination of the superior and inferior surfaces of the implant, can be quite difficult. Coronal CT may best show extensive

erosive changes of the condyle, following the temporary use of Silastic, as well as bony ankylosis that may occur between the condyle and the glenoid fossa (Fig. 7-61).

Total Joint Replacement

Total replacement of the TMJ has been attempted for many years.[103,104] There continue to be problems with stabilization of both the glenoid and condyle parts of the prosthesis, and

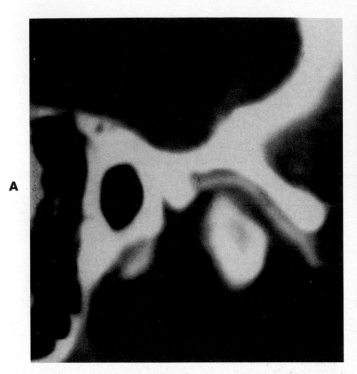
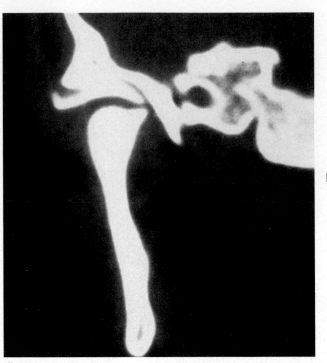

FIG. 7-62 CT scan in sagittal (**A**) and coronal (**B**) planes showing implant in good position.

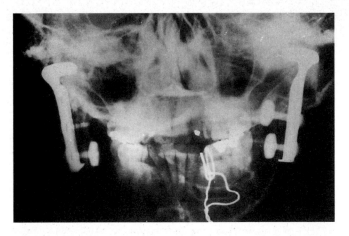

FIG. 7-63 Bilateral total joints. Anterior posterior plain film shows bilateral total replacement. The condyle fragments are attached to the ramus of the mandible. Proplast Teflon fossa implants are attached to the articular eminence and the zygomatic arch with screws. Also note osteosynthesis in left symphysis region from old mandibular fracture.

these patients frequently present for imaging evaluation. In a situation where there are large metallic implants, because of degradation artifacts, neither CT nor MRI is feasible and plain film and tomography are the only imaging modalities available (Fig. 7-63). The assessment should concentrate on motion between the implant and the underlying bone, osteolytic changes of the bone, and evidence of loosening of the implant.

Costochondral Grafts

Costochondral grafts had been used in the past for reconstruction of the TMJ and have recently regained popularity since the alloplastic total joint prostheses have essentially been abandoned.[105] Imaging of costochondral grafts can be done with plain film, tomography, CT, and MRI. Probably the most efficient way to look at the joint is with MRI. CT can be used in an asymptomatic patient to show bilateral costochondral grafts (Fig. 7-64). However, the cartilaginous portion of the grafts are not well visualized. CT imaging with 3D reconstructions allows for a more graphic demonstration of the relationship between the joint components; however, portions of the cartilaginous graft are still not visualized (Fig. 7-65).

Metallic Artifacts

Metallic artifacts are frequently seen in MRI of postoperative osseous structures. The metallic artifact appears as an area of signal void bordered by areas of high signal intensity (Fig. 7-66). Even very small metallic particles can cause significant areas of loss of signal, and thus minuscule pieces shredded from metallic instruments used to scrape or work on the bone could be sufficient to create a significant artifact. These small artifacts are seen in both symptomatic and asymptomatic patients after surgery, and they are probably of no clinical significance.[102] The most important aspect of the metallic artifact is that it may prevent further MR imaging.

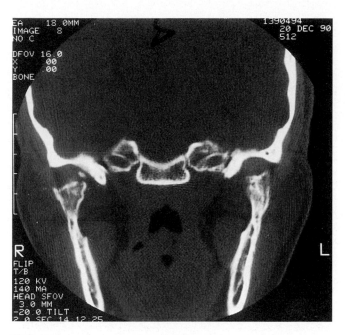

FIG. 7-64 Bilateral costochondral grafts. Coronal CT scan of asymptomatic patient with bilateral costochondral grafts. Note how the grafts are integrated into the ramus of the mandible. The most superior cartilaginous parts of the grafts are not well visualized on CT imaging.

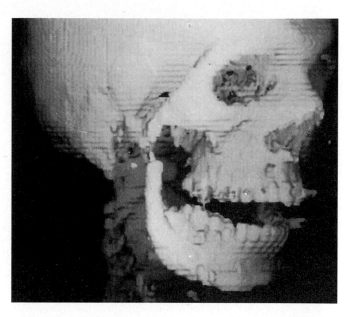

FIG. 7-65 Three-dimensional costochondral graft. Asymptomatic patient with a right-sided costochondral graft. Note that the graft is integrated into the mandible. The superior cartilaginous portion of the graft is not well visualized on the CT scan. The image was obtained in partial open position.

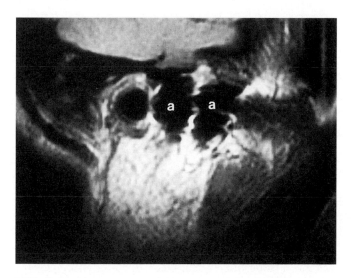

FIG. 7-66 Metal artifact. MR image (proton density) of a joint with metallic wires. These artifacts (*a*) are characterized by irregular areas of signal void bordered by areas of high signal.

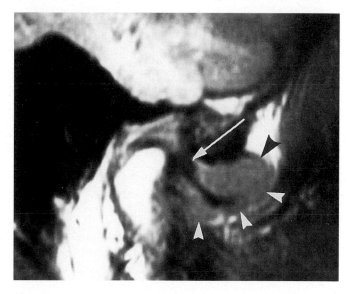

FIG. 7-67 Synovial chondromatosis. Sagittal MR image showing expansion of the upper and lower joint spaces (*arrows*). The disk is anteriorly displaced. The expansion of the joint spaces indicates neoplastic process.

MISCELLANEOUS CONDITIONS INVOLVING THE TMJ

Although most imaging evaluations are done for possible internal derangements and their sequelae, many other types of pathology occasionally affect the TMJ. Tumors, systemic arthritides, and congenital anomalies may be found during an evaluation of the TMJ or during assessment for suspected pathology in the adjacent head and neck region.

Tumors and Tumorlike Conditions of the TMJ
Synovial Chondromatosis

The TMJ is infrequently affected by tumors. The most common neoplastic lesion affecting the TMJ is probably synovial chondromatosis.[106,107] This tumor can be locally aggressive, and cases with intracranial extension have been

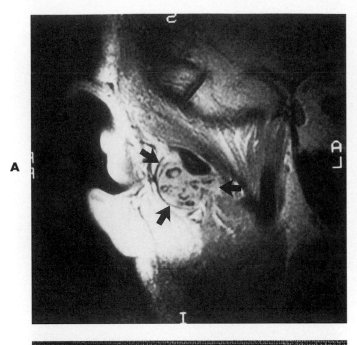

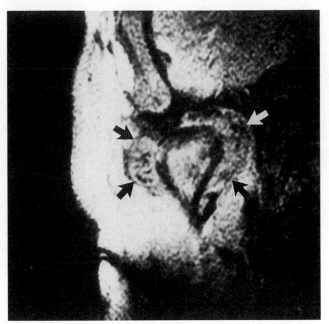

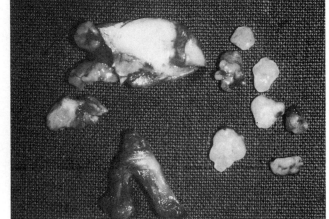

FIG. 7-68 Synovial chondromatosis. **A,** Sagittal proton density MR image from the lateral aspect of the TMJ. There is expansion of the joint capsule (*arrows*) with multiple areas of low signal. **B,** Sagittal proton density MR image. In the coronal image there is expansion of both the lateral and medial capsule walls (*arrows*). This indictes a neoplastic intraarticular process. The finding of multiple areas of low signal within the expanded joint capsule is consistent with synovial chondromatosis. **C,** Small bodies of cartilaginous material removed from a joint (another patient) with synovial chondromatosis.

described.[108,109] This is a benign tumor characterized by formation of multiple small "pearls" of cartilage, usually within the joint space. MRI can show synovial chondromatosis primarily affecting the upper joint space (Fig. 7-67) or both the upper and lower joint spaces (Fig. 7-68). There is often significant joint expansion, and there may be multiple areas of low signal intensity that represent the "pearls" (Fig. 7-68). The clinical presentation of patients with synovial chondromatosis is similar to the general presentation of TMJ pain and dysfunction, and the findings are usually detected with imaging studies or at surgery. Evaluation can be done both with MRI and CT.[110-112]

Osteochondroma

Osteochondroma is probably the second most common neoplastic lesion affecting the TMJ. Osteochondroma (Fig. 7-69), osteoma, or condyle hyperplasia are difficult to differ-

entiate clinically and on imaging studies. MRI can define these conditions in both the sagittal and coronal planes, but CT may more precisely delineate the extension of the tumor and its relationship to anatomic structures medial to the TMJ region.

Chondrocalcinosis

The deposition of crystalline calcium pyrophosphate dehydrate (pseudogout) in the articular cartilage is not uncommon in the semilunar cartilage of the knee and in the triangular ligament of the wrist; however, the TMJ is an unusual location for pseudogout. Cases of this condition have been described with subtle calcifications in the joint space (Fig. 7-70). Clinically the patient presents with pain and dysfunction similar to the symptoms of other TMJ patients. There can be associated swelling. CT is the best imaging modality for demonstration of the minute intraarticular calcifications.

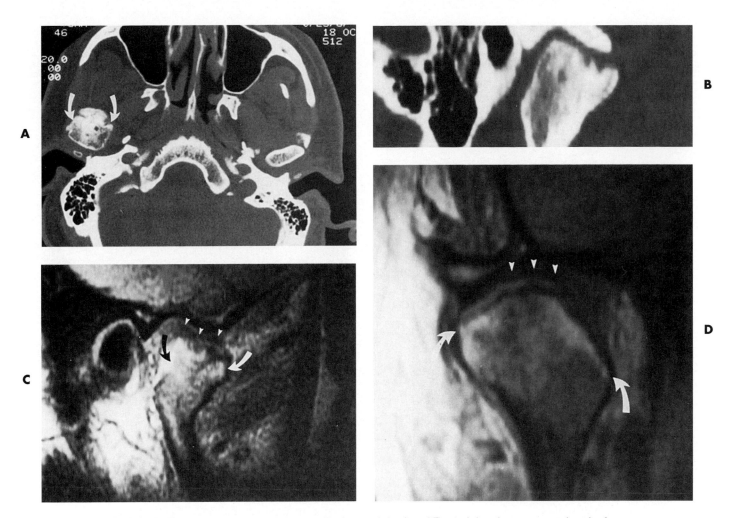

FIG. 7-69 Osteochondroma of the mandibular condyle. **A** and **B,** Axial and reconstructed sagittal CT scans show the right condyle (*arrows*) to be two to three times larger than the left condyle. There is also irregular mineralization in this condyle. **C** and **D,** Sagittal and coronal MRI scans of the same joints show mixed low and high signal from the enlarged parts of the condyle (*curved arrows*). The temporal component is normal. The disk (*arrowheads*) is biconcave and located in a normal superior position. (Courtesy Dr. Donald Macher, Rochester, New York.)

Synovial Cysts and Simple Bone Cysts

Synovial cysts of the TMJ have been reported but are rare (Fig. 7-71).[113,114] They present with unilateral pain and possible enlargement of the condyle head, and there can be associated swelling.

Simple bone cysts are most frequently located in the body of the mandible. However, they may occur in the condyle head (Fig. 7-72), and often the remaining joint components are normal.

Eosinophilic Granuloma

Eosinophilic granuloma may also present as a lytic lesion involving the mandibular condyle and ramus (Fig. 7-73).

Metastatic Disease in the TMJ Region

Fewer than 1% of all tumors metastasize to the maxillofacial area.[115-117] Adenocarcinoma is the most common of all metastatic tumors in the jaw, accounting for 70% of the cases. A review of 115 cases of mandibular metastasis found that 30% were metastasis from breast carcinoma, 16% from kidney, 15% from lung, 8% from colon and rectum, 7% from prostate, 6% from thyroid, 5% from stomach, 4% from skin, 3% from testes, and other sites represented less than 1% each. Most metastases are found in the molar and premolar regions of the mandible, and only a few cases of metastasis to the mandibular condyle have been reported. Most cases with metastasis to the TMJ region have presented with TMJ related symptoms.[116] Lymphoma can also rarely involve the TMJ (Fig. 7-74), and bone regeneration may occur after chemotherapy (Fig. 7-74, *B*).[118]

Arthritides

The TMJ is involved in approximately 50% of patients with rheumatoid diseases such as rheumatoid arthritis, ankylosing spondylitis, and psoriatic arthritis. Imaging is an important adjunct to the clinical diagnosis and is particularly valu-

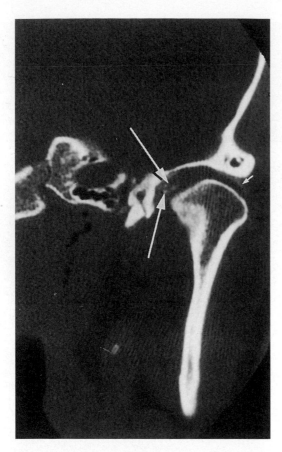

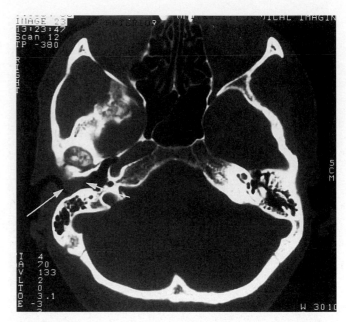

FIG. 7-71 Synovial cyst. Axial CT scan of patient with 1 cm synovial cyst (*arrows*) extending into the external auditory canal. There are extensive degenerative changes of the condyle head. At surgery the cyst extended into the joint through the bony fissure.

FIG. 7-70 Pseudogout. Coronal CT scan of patient with chronic TMJ pain and normal disk position on MR image (not shown). There are subtle calcifications in the joint space (*arrows*). Aspiration showed pyrophosphate crystals.

able for follow-up of patients with these diseases. Plain films and panoramic images are standard, but MR may be indicated to evaluate the soft-tissue involvement of these diseases.[119] Morphologically, inflammatory arthritis is characterized by synovial proliferation and secondary erosive changes of the bone (Fig. 7-75). Studies with MRI have shown potential for accurate evaluation of the soft-tissue components of the joint (Fig. 7-76).[81,82] A study indicated the additional value of contrast-enhanced images for defining the area of inflammatory change within the joint and in the periarticular soft-tissue (Fig. 7-76, *B*).[119] Only limited experience is available with MRI of other inflammatory arthritides such as psoriatic and ankylosing spondylitis.

Acute Trauma

Patients with acute trauma to the jaw rarely present for TMJ imaging other than plain films. However, it is likely that in many instances there is also injury to the TMJ in patients with condyle neck and mandibular fractures. Such TMJ trauma is frequently not recognized until after the acute clinical course. Occasionally, however, symptoms following trauma may not be associated with a fracture detectable on plain film or even CT, and the patient may be evaluated with

MR imaging. MRI may show fractures and effusions not seen on other imaging studies (Fig. 7-77), and thus MRI could be helpful in patients with acute pain following trauma to the face and jaw despite negative plain film or panoramic examinations.

Both CT and MRI might be helpful in cases with intracapsular fractures (Fig. 7-78). Although CT may show the positional relationship of the osseous fragments, MRI (Fig. 7-78) shows any associated disk abnormality. In a situation where reconstructive surgery is contemplated, 3D reconstructions (Fig. 7-78, *D*) may be helpful to evaluate the positional relationships between the joint components.

Penetrating trauma to the TMJ is relatively rare, but it warrants imaging evaluation. It can cause fracture, hematoma, and dislocations. CT is the preferred method of examination, and it is important to obtain both axial and coronal scans if the condition of the patient permits (Fig. 7-79).

Coronoid Hyperplasia

Hyperplasia or elongation of the coronoid process of the mandible can mimic symptoms of TMJ internal derangement with limitation of opening. This condition has been extensively described, and a study has indicated that elongation of the coronoid process may occur in up to 5% of patients with TMJ symptoms and limitation of opening.[120-122] If the coronoid process is significantly elongated, it can impact on the zygomatic process of the maxilla, thus causing limitation of jaw opening. CT in the axial or sagittal plane, acquired at the closed and open mouthed positions, is

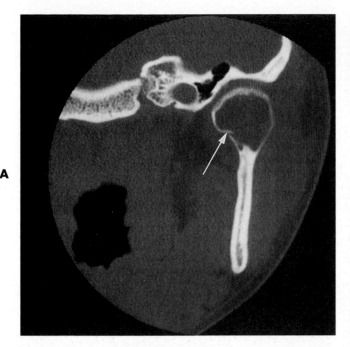

A

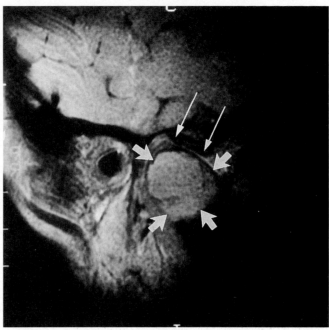

B

FIG. 7-72 Simple bone cyst. **A,** Coronal CT scan shows a large cystic lesion involving the entire condyle head. There is an expansion and enlargement of the condyle and thinning of the cortex. Medially and inferiorly (*arrow*) there is a small pathologic fracture. **B,** Sagittal proton density MR image shows intermediate signal of the expanded bone marrow of the condyle (*thick arrows*). The disk (*long arrows*) is in normal location.

valuable in the imaging assessment of patients with a clinical suspicion of coronoid hyperplasia because it can demonstrate the coronoid impaction on the maxilla (Fig. 7-80). Surgical treatment with removal of the coronoid process usually yields good results.

Congenital Anomalies
Bifid Condyle

Congenital anomalies of the TMJ are relatively rare. The most common congenital anomaly is probably the so-called bifid condyle. This implies a partial or complete separation of the condyle into a lateral and medial half (Fig. 7-81). This is usually of no clinical significance other than in the rare situation in which surgery should be performed and a preoperative knowledge about the morphology is important. The picture of a bifid condyle is characteristic on coronal imaging and should be distinguished from acquired pathologic conditions with remodeling and degenerative joint disease.

Hemifacial Microsomia

The TMJ is affected in other conditions such as hemifacial microsomia with underdevelopment of the TMJ. Frequently there is a flat articular eminence and a small mandibular condyle (Fig. 7-82). The mastoid typically is underdeveloped with no aeration. The disk is usually in a normal loca-

tion in hemifacial microsomia. In advanced cases the entire ramus, condyle, and coronoid process of the mandible are not developed (Fig. 7-83).

Asymmetry of the Mandible

Asymmetry of the mandible is a frequent clinical presentation. The most prominent facial features include a shift of the chin to the short side and prominence of the mandibular angle on the long side. There are several obvious causes of mandibular asymmetry such as trauma with fractures, tumors, and congenital anomalies. In many cases, however, the cause of mandibular asymmetry leading to facial deformities is unclear on physical examination and imaging assessment may be warranted.[123,124]

Mandibular asymmetry can principally result from either enlargement of the condyle head (condylar hperplasia) on the long side (Fig. 7-84) or from decreased condyle growth (condylar hypolasia) (Fig. 7-85) or degenerative joint disease on the short side (Fig. 7-86).[124-126] Imaging studies are done to determine the cause of mandibular asymmetry and for treatment planning. The imaging evaluation of mandibular asymmetry is outlined in Box 7-6. Soft-tissue imaging is important, and MRI should be the first choice in most situations. Condylar hypoplasia is most frequently caused by regressive remodeling secondary to longstanding internal derangement; however, the condyle may have a relatively

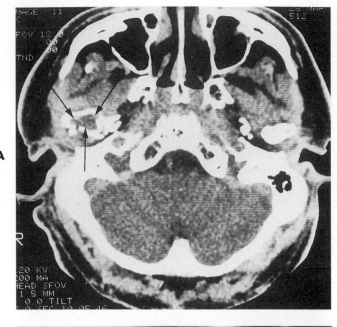

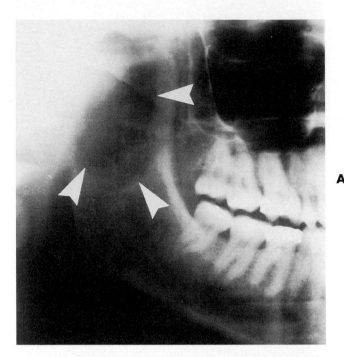

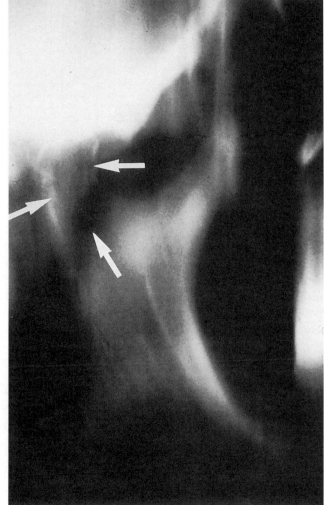

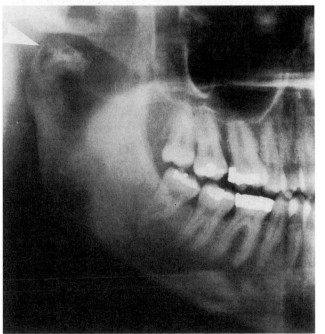

FIG. 7-73 Eosinophilic granuloma. **A,** Axial CT scan through the TMJ shows expansion and lytic changes of the right condyle (*arrows*). **B,** Sagittal tomogram shows the lesion to extend down into the neck of the condyle. (Courtesy Dr. Susan White, Gainesville, Florida.)

FIG. 7-74 Metastatic lymphoma to TMJ. **A,** Large osteolytic defect involving the condyle, condyle neck, coronoid process, and upper half of ascending ramus (*arrowheads*). **B,** Following chemotherapy there was regeneration of the condyle neck and condyle (*arrowhead*). The patient died 1 year later from intracranial and generalized metastasis.

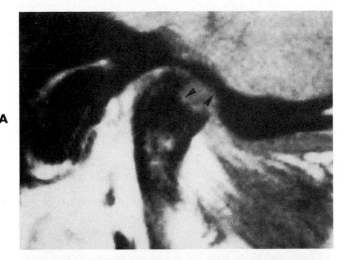

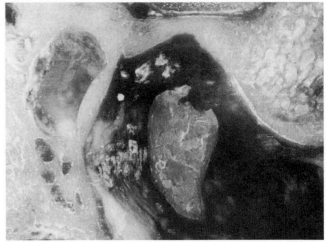

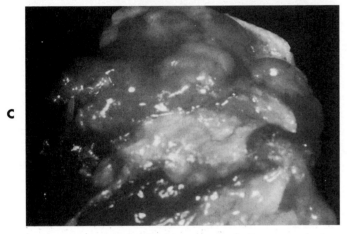

FIG. 7-75 A, Rheumatoid arthritis. T1W MR image showing erosive changes of condyle and articular eminence (*arrowheads*) and decreased signal from the bone marrow of condyle. The disk is absent. (Courtesy Dr. Tore Larheim, Oslo, Norway.) **B,** Rheumatoid arthritis. Corresponding cryosection from different patient shows similar erosive changes of the condyle in this individual with a long history of rheumatoid arthritis. There is extensive granulation tissue in the joint and periarticular area. **C,** Rheumatoid arthritis. Anterior aspect of condyle from another individual with a long history of rheumatoid arthritis shows extensive synovial proliferation overlying the entire condyle head.

normal appearance without evidence of degenerative joint disease. The joint appears to be more sensitive to regressive remodeling if the internal derangement occurs during the growth and development phase. However, mandibular asymmetry and change in occlusion have also been described as occurring in adults.

Atrophy of the Muscles of Mastication

Atrophy of the muscles of mastication is occasionally seen in patients with inability to open their mouth. These atrophic changes in the muscles are most frequently secondary to trauma or orthognathic surgery.[84,127] On MRI the atrophic changes of the muscles of mastication are usually reflected as fatty replacement (Fig. 7-87).

Following orthognathic surgery, there is frequently asymptomatic muscle atrophy (Fig. 7-88).[127] Occasionally this is associated with chewing difficulties and fatigue in the jaw muscles, and in these cases, MRI is the best imaging modality. Electromyography might be of some value when asymmetric recordings of the left and right sides can be documented.

MISCELLANEOUS IMAGING
Radionuclide Imaging

Studies have suggested that radionuclide imaging of the TMJ (Fig. 7-89), using conventional skeletal imaging techniques, may be a valuable screening test for osseous disease.[128,129] The technique can be performed easily, and the radiation dose to the patient is low.[1] An advantage of the technique is that conditions outside the joint also may be easily detected. Radionuclide imaging has not gained popularity for TMJ imaging. This is probably because it is nonspecific, and frequently a second imaging modality is needed to determine the nature of the problem and to form a treatment plan.

Thin Section Magnetic Resonance Imaging

There is a continuously ongoing development in MRI technology. The signal to noise and soft-tissue and spatial resolution are improved each time MR scanners are upgraded. This means that the image quality can be expected to continue to improve, and experimental MR images with improved spatial and soft-tissue resolution (Fig. 7-90) may soon be avail-

Text continued on p. 429

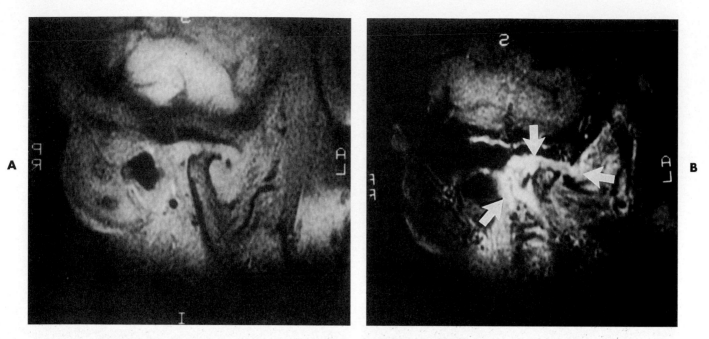

FIG. 7-76 Rheumatoid arthritis with contrast enhancement. A, Sagittal proton density image shows advanced degenerative disease of both condyle and temporal joint component. B, With contrast enhancement there is significant enhancement in the joint and periarticular area (*arrows*). This indicates the area of synovial proliferation. There is also a small area of meningeal enhancement of unclear clinical significance.

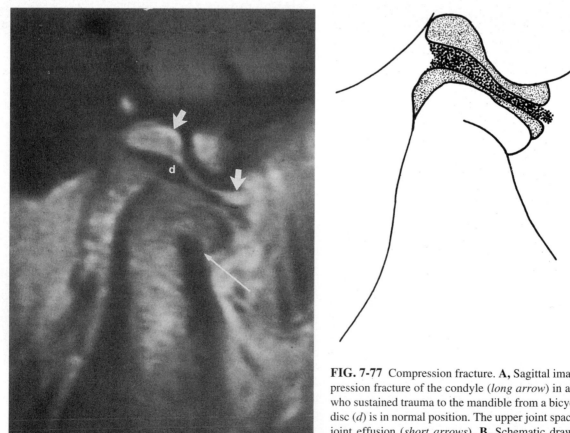

FIG. 7-77 Compression fracture. A, Sagittal image shows a compression fracture of the condyle (*long arrow*) in an 8-year-old boy who sustained trauma to the mandible from a bicycle accident. The disc (*d*) is in normal position. The upper joint space is expanded by joint effusion (*short arrows*). B, Schematic drawing outlines the anatomy. (Courtesy Dr. Richard W. Katzberg, Sacramento, California.)

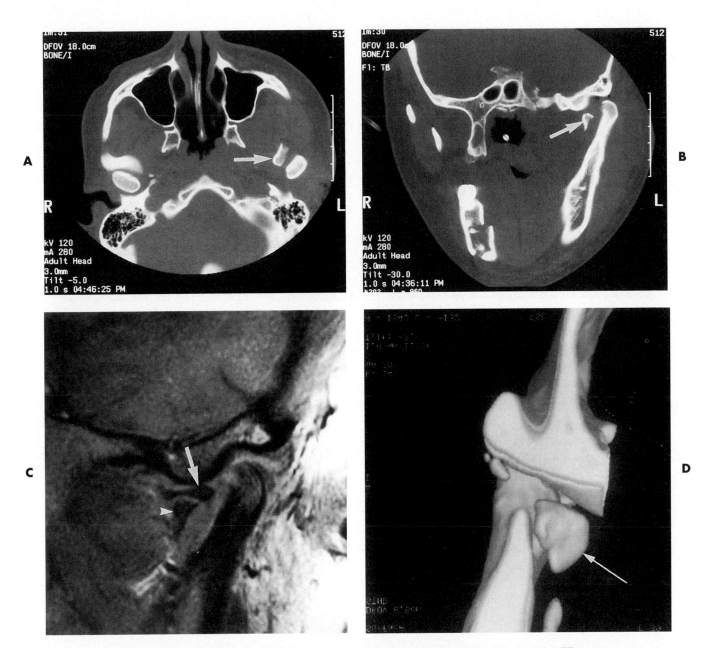

FIG. 7-78 Intracapsular fracture with displacement of condyle fragment and disk. **A,** Axial CT scan shows fracture of the medial part of the condyle (*arrow*) with anterior and medial displacement. **B,** Coronal CT scan confirms the inferior medial displacement of the condyle fragment (arrow) and also shows small intraarticular collections. Note contralateral mandibular body fracture. **C,** Sagittal proton density MR image shows condyle fragment (*arrowhead*) anteriorly and inferiorly displaced. The disk (*arrow*) is located superior to the fragment but is anteriorly and inferiorly displaced relative to the remaining condyle. **D,** Coronal 3D reconstruction of CT image demonstrates the inferior medial location of the displaced fragment (*arrow*).

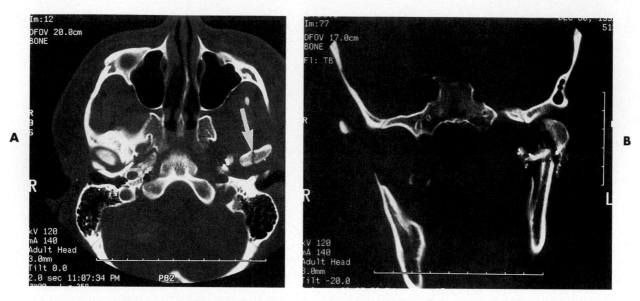

FIG. 7-79 Penetrating trauma to TMJ. **A,** Axial CT scan through the condyle shows a sagittal fracture in the center of the condyle head. **B,** Coronal image through the joint shows comminuted fractures with displacement of the medial fragment. Axial and coronal views are supplementary because the displacement was not well appreciated on the axial image.

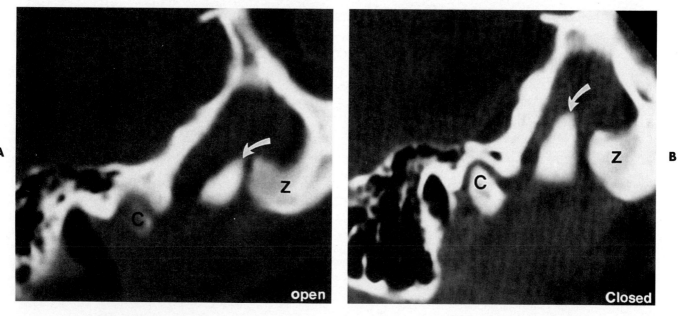

FIG. 7-80 Coronoid hyperplasia restricting mouth opening. **A** and **B,** Direct sagittal CT scan at opened and closed mouth positions showing the elongated coronoid process (*arrows*) to interfere with the zygomatic process (*z*) of the maxilla at the open mouth position. The condyle (*C*) is in the glenoid fossa.

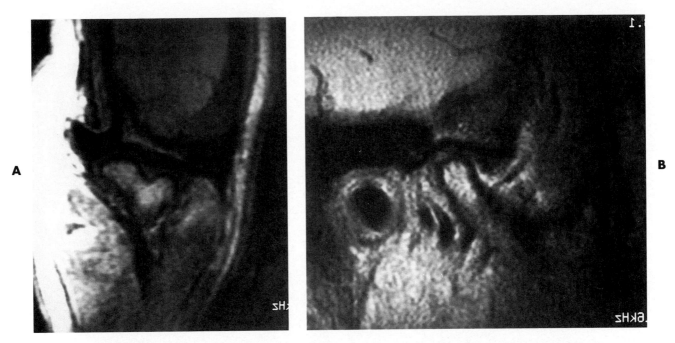

FIG. 7-81 Bifid condyle. **A,** Coronal MR image shows a characteristic appearance of a bifid condyle. **B,** The sagittal MR image shows a normal appearance of the condyle and disk.

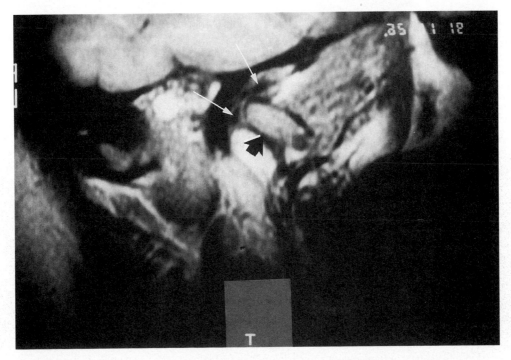

FIG. 7-82 Hemifacial microsomia. Sagittal MR image of a young patient with hemifacial micro-somia. The temporal bone is underdeveloped. The mastoid is not aerated, and instead there is fat fill-ing the mastoid air cells. The mandibular condyle (*thick arrow*) is underdeveloped with a curvature posteriorly. The disc (*thin arrows*) is in normal relationship with the condyle. The articular eminence is absent, and the condyle is essentially articulating against the flat skull base. The lateral pterygoid muscle appears normal.

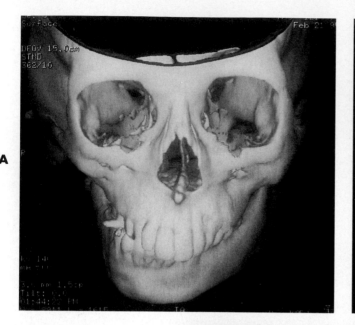

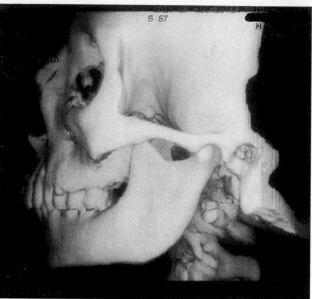

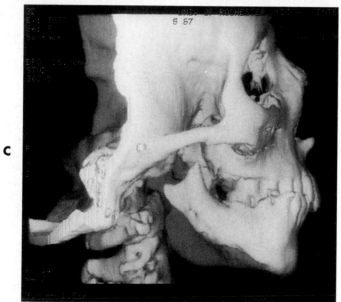

FIG. 7-83 Hemifacial microsomia. Three-dimensional CT scan shows asymmetry of the maxillo-facial and mandibular regions. **A,** The right side of the face is underdeveloped. **B,** The left side of the face is of normal configuration and size. **C,** The right side of the face shows diminished size of the body of the mandible and ramus of the mandible. Also the midface structures are underdeveloped in this 9-year-old female with hemifacial microsomia. Note in the frontal view (*A*) that there is a crossbite on the right side with the mandibular teeth occluding on the buccal side of the maxillary teeth.

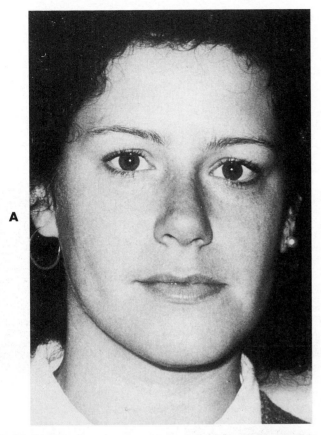

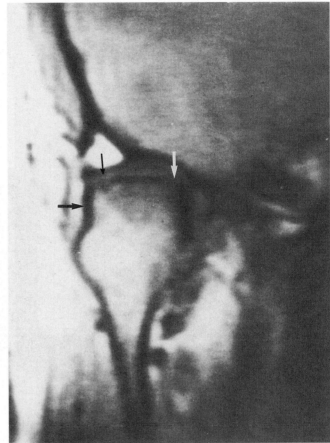

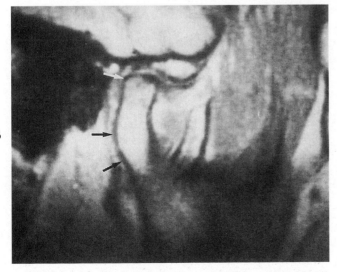

FIG. 7-84 Mandibular asymmetry caused by condyle hyperplasia. **A,** Photograph. **B** and **C,** sagittal and coronal MR images of the left condyle of a patient with deviation of the chin to the right. The MR images show elongation of the condyle and condyle neck (*arrows*) as the cause of mandibular asymmetry.

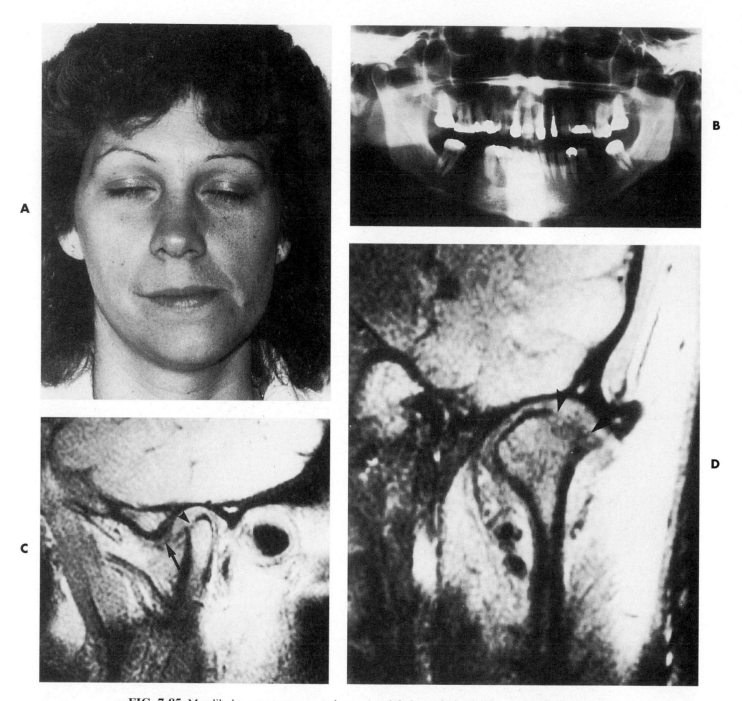

FIG. 7-85 Mandibular asymmetry secondary to condyle hypoplasia. **A,** Photograph. **B,** Panoramic image. **C,** Sagittal MR image. **D,** Coronal MR image. There is deviation of the chin to the left. Panoramic view (**B**) shows a normal configuration on the right side of the mandible. The left side shows shortening of the ramus and regressive remodeling of the left condyle. MR images (**C** and **D**) show erosive changes of the condyle (*arrowheads*) and anterior disk displacement (*arrow*). The diminished size of the left condyle was the cause of the asymmetry in this patient.

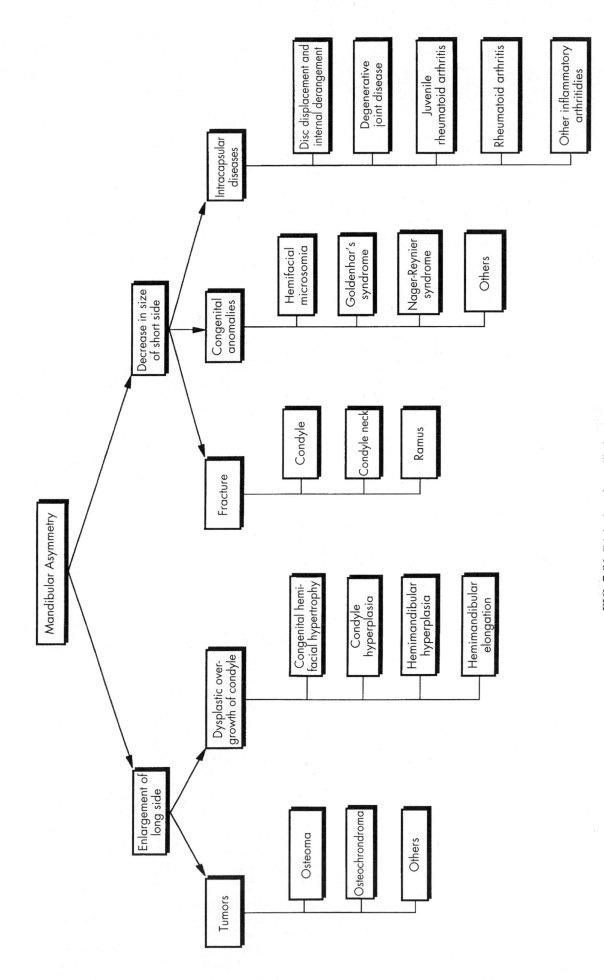

FIG. 7-86 Etiologies of mandibular asymmetry.

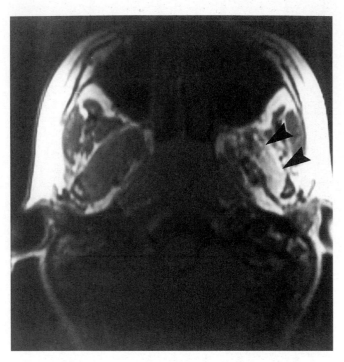

FIG. 7-87 Muscle atrophy. Axial T1W MR image through the level of the muscles of mastication in a young patient with limitation of opening. The lateral pterygoid muscle on the left side is atrophic and shows fatty replacement (*arrowheads*). This condition is most likely secondary to a history of facial trauma.

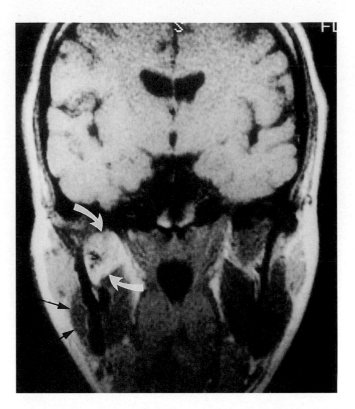

FIG. 7-88 Atrophy of muscles of mastication. Coronal MR image through the ascending ramus of the mandible in a patient who had vertical osteotomy performed on the right ramus 3 years before this image. There is atrophy of the masseter muscle on the right side (*long arrows*) as compared with the left side. Also the lateral pterygoid muscle (*between curved arrows*) is atrophic with fatty replacement as compared with the left side.

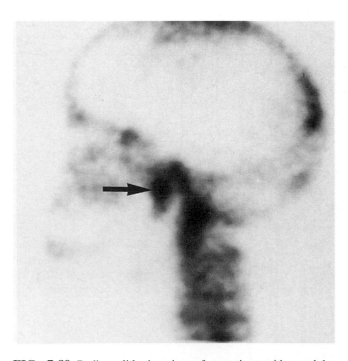

FIG. 7-89 Radionuclide imaging of a patient with condylar hyperplasia of left TMJ (*arrow*).

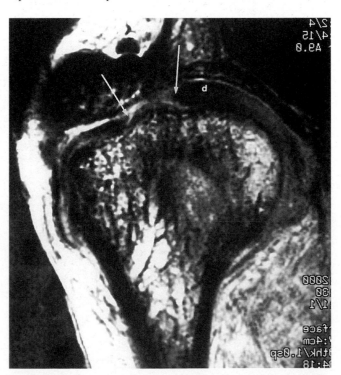

FIG. 7-90 High resolution MR image. This experimental MR image was obtained with slice thickness of 1.5 mm and a field of view of 4 cm. The perforation of the disk (*between long arrows*) and the osteophyte of the condyle filling the perforation are well visualized. The disk (*d*) is indicated for orientation.

able commercially. Fig. 7-90 was obtained on an autopsy TMJ specimen and shows significantly improved spatial and soft-tissue resolution because of thinner slice thickness and a smaller field of view. In this image the trabecular pattern of the condyle can be clearly identified, and the perforation of the disk and the osteophyte of the condyle, protruding into the perforation, can be seen with exquisite detail.

Dynamic Magnetic Resonance Imaging

The time to acquire an image is also rapidly decreasing, and within the next few years, one may be able to obtain real time dynamic MR images. This will make possible the study of joint dynamics without injection of contrast medium or local anesthesia. Pseudodynamic imaging with magnetic resonance is possible today, but its value for diagnostic work is not fully understood.[130] Multiple images are collected with the mouth opened to different widths, and the images are rapidly viewed on a "cine loop." This creates the illusion of a real-time examination even though the images were acquired at separate points in time. However, the position of the disk can be followed, and the snapping of the condyle over the back of the disk can be appreciated.

▼

BOX 7-6
IMAGING STRATEGY FOR PATIENTS WITH
MANDIBULAR ASYMMETRY

1. Lateral and anterior posterior cephalograms
2. Lateral tomograms of TMJs, including entire mandibular ramus
3. MR or arthrography of both left and right TMJs

Magnetic Resonance Spectroscopy

The third area that will probably develop into a more useful clinical tool is MR spectroscopy. This may be helpful in evaluating metabolic and biochemical changes in the joints and muscles. Previous reports have suggested abnormalities of lactate accumulation in the intervertebral peridiskal tissues of the spine in the presence of degeneration and herniation.[131] MR spectroscopy has also been applied to experimental situations and appears capable of showing changes in area of inflammation.[132]

References

1. Katzberg RW. Temporomandibular joint imaging. Radiology 1989; 170:297-307.
2. Rees LA. The structure and function of the mandibular joint. Br Dent J 1954; 96:125-133.
3. Adams JC. Outline of orthopedics, 9th Edition, London, England: Churchill Livingstone Inc, 1981; 61-61.
4. Eriksson L, Westesson P-L. Clinical and radiological study of patients with anterior disc displacement of the temporomandibular joint. Swed Dent J 1983; 7:55-64.
5. Katzberg RW, Dolwick MF, Helms CA et al. Arthrotomography of the temporomandibular joint. Am J Roentgenol 1980; 134:995-1003.
6. Westesson P-L. Double-contrast arthrography and internal derangement of the temporomandibular joint. Swed Dent J Suppl 1982; 13:1-57.
7. Wilkes CH. Arthrography of the temporomandibular joint in patients with the TMJ pain-dysfunction syndrome. Minn Med 1978; 61:645-652.
8. Wilkes CH. Structural and func-

tional alterations of the temporomandibular joint. Northwest Dent 1978; 57:287-294.
9. Wilkes CH. Internal derangements of the temporomandibular joint. Arch Otolaryngol 1989; 115:469-477.
10. Brooks SL, Westesson P-L. Temporomandibular joint: value of coronal MR images. Radiology 1993; 188:317-321.
11. Katzberg RW, Westesson P-L, Tallents RH et al. Temporomandibular joint: magnetic resonance assessment of rotational and sideways disc displacements. Radiology 1988; 169:741-748.
12. Liedberg J, Westesson P-L. Sideways position of the temporomandibular joint disk: coronal cryosectioning of fresh autopsy specimens. Oral Surg Oral Med Oral Pathol 1988; 66:644-649.
13. Liedberg J, Westesson P-L, Kurita K. Sideways and rotational displacement of the temporomandibular joint disk: diagnosis by arthrography and correlation to cryosectional morphology. Oral Surg Oral Med Oral Pathol 1990; 69:757-763.

14. Ireland VE. The problem of the "clicking jaw." Proc R Soc Med 1951; 44:363-372.
15. Isberg-Holm AM, Westesson P-L. Movement of disc and condyle in temporomandibular joints with clicking: an arthrographic and cineradiographic study on autopsy specimens. Acta Odontol Scand 1982; 40:151-164.
16. Isberg-Holm AM, Westesson P-L. Movement of disc and condyle in temporomandibular joints with and without clicking: a high speed cinematographic and dissection study on autopsy specimens. Acta Odontol Scand 1982; 40:165-177.
17. Westesson P-L. Arthrography of the temporomandibular joint. J Prosthet Dent 1984; 51:534-543.
18. Westesson P-L, Rohlin M. Internal derangement related to osteoarthritis in temporomandibular joint autopsy specimens. Oral Surg Oral Med Oral Pathol 1984; 57:17-22.
19. Westesson P-L, Bronstein SL, Liedberg J. Internal derangement of the temporomandibular joint: morphologic description with correlation to function. Oral Surg

Oral Med Oral Pathol 1985; 59:323-331.

20. Bessette RW, Katzberg RW, Natiella JR et al. Diagnosis and reconstruction of the human temporomandibular joint after trauma or internal derangement. Plast Reconstr Surg 1985; 75:192-205.

21. Kurita K, Westesson P-L, Sternby NH et al. Histologic features of the temporomandibular joint disk and posterior disk attachment: comparison of symptom-free persons with normally positioned disks and patients with internal derangement. Oral Surg Oral Med Oral Pathol 1989; 67:635-643.

22. Blaustein DI, Scapino RP. Remodelling of the temporomandibular joint disk and posterior attachment in disk displacement specimens in relation to glycosaminoglycan content. Oral Surg Oral Med Oral Pathol 1986; 78:756-764.

23. Isberg AM, Isacsson G. Tissue reactions associated with internal derangement of the temporomandibular joint: a radiographic, cryomorphologic, and histologic study. Acta Odontol Scand 1986; 44:160-164.

24. Pereira FJ Jr, Lundh H, Eriksson L et al. Histologic characterization of the TMJ in patients and asymptomatic persons. Manuscript in preparation.

25. Westesson P-L. Double-contrast arthrotomography of the temporomandibular joint: introduction of an arthrographic technique for visualization of the disc and articular surfaces. J Oral Maxillofac Surg 1983; 41:163-172.

26. Westesson P-L. Structural hard-tissue changes in temporomandibular joints with internal derangement. Oral Surg Oral Med Oral Pathol 1985; 59:220-224.

27. Paesani D, Westesson P-L, Hatala MP, et al. Accuracy of clinical diagnosis for TMJ internal derangement and arthrosis. Oral Surg Oral Med Oral Pathol 1992:73:360-363.

28. Roberts D, Schenck J, Joseph P et al. Temporomandibular joint: magnetic resonance imaging. Radiology 1985; 155:829-830.

29. Roberts CA, Tallents RH, Espeland MA, et al. Mandibular range of

motion versus arthrographic diagnosis of the temporomandibular joint. Oral Surg Oral Med Oral Pathol 1985; 60:244-251.

30. Roberts CA, Tallents RH, Katzberg RW et al. Clinical and arthrographic evaluation of temporomandibular joint sounds. Oral Surg Oral Med Oral Pathol 1986; 62:373-376.

31. Roberts CA, Tallents RH, Katzberg RW et al. Comparison of internal derangements of the TMJ to occlusal findings. Oral Surg Oral Med Oral Pathol 1987; 63:645-650.

32. Roberts CA, Tallents RH, Katzberg RW et al. Clinical and arthrographic evaluation of the location of TMJ pain. Oral Surg Oral Med Oral Pathol 1987; 64:6-8.

33. Roberts CA, Tallents RH, Katzberg RW et al. Comparison of arthrographic findings of the temporomandibular joint with palpation of the muscles of mastication. Oral Surg Oral Med Oral Pathol 1987; 64:275-277.

34. Anderson GC, Schiffman EL, Schellhas KP et al. Clinical vs. arthrographic diagnosis of TMJ internal derangement. J Dent Res 1989; 68:826-829.

35. Drace JE, Enzmann DR. Defining the normal temporomandibular joint: closed-, partially open-, and open-mouth MR imaging of asymptomatic subjects. Radiology 1990; 177:67-71.

36. Kircos LT, Ortendahl DA, Mark AS et al. Magnetic resonance imaging of the TMJ disk in asymptomatic volunteers. J Oral Maxillofac Surg 1987; 45:852-854.

37. Westesson P-L, Eriksson L, Kurita K. Temporomandibular joint: variation of normal arthrographic anatomy. Oral Surg Oral Med Oral Pathol 1990; 69(4):514-519.

38. Boden SD, Davis DO, Dina TS et al. Abnormal magnetic resonance scans of the lumbar spine in asymptomatic subjects. A prospective investigation. J Bone Joint Surg (Am) 1990; 72; 403-408.

39. Boden SD, Davis DO, Dina TS et al. A prospective and blinded investigation of magnetic resonance imaging of the knee. Abnormal findings in asymptomatic subjects. Clin Orthop 1992; 282:177-185.

40. Kornick J, Trefelner NE, McCarty S et al. Meniscal abnormalities in the asymptomatic population in MR imaging. Radiology 1990; 177:463-465

41. Nagendak WG, Fernandez FR, Halbrun LK et al. Magnetic resonance imaging of meniscal degeneration in asymptomatic knees. J Orthop Res 1990; 8:311-320.

42. Shellock FG, Morris E, Deutsch AL et al. Hematopoietic bone marrow hyperplasia: high prevalence on MR images of the knee in asymptomatic marathon runners. AJR 1992; 158:335-338.

43. Paesani D, Westesson P-L, Hatala M et al. Prevalence of internal derangement in patients with craniomandibular disorders. Am J Orthod Dentofacial Orthop 1992; 101:41-47.

44. Widmalm S-E, Westesson P-L, Kim I-K et al. Temporomandibular joint pathosis related to sex, age, and dentition in autopsy material. Oral Surg Oral Med Oral Pathol 1994; 78:416-425.

45. Oberg T, Carlsson GE, Fajers CM. The temporomandibular joint: a morphologic study of human autopsy material. Acta Odontal Scand 1971; 29:349-384.

46. McCabe JB, Keller SE, Moffet BC. A new radiographic technique for diagnosing temporomandibular joint disorders. J Dent Res 1959; 38:663.

47. Omnell K-A, Peterson A. Radiography of the temporomandibular joint utilizing oblique lateral transcranial projections: comparison of information obtained with standardized technique and individualized technique. Odontol Rev 1976; 26:77-92.

48. Nørgaard F. Artografi av kaebeleddet. Preliminary report. Acta Radiol 1944; 25:679-685.

49. Nørgaard F. Temporomandibular arthrography. Thesis. Copenhagen, Munksgaard, 1947.

50. Farrar WB, McCarty WL Jr. Inferior joint space arthrography and characteristics of condylar paths in internal derangements of the TMJ. J Prosthet Dent 1979; 41:548-555.

51. Katzberg RW, Dolwick MF, Bales DJ et al. Arthrotomography of the temporomandibular joint: new technique and preliminary obser-

vations. Am J Roentgenol 1979; 132:949-955.

52. Westesson P-L, Omnell K-Å, Rohlin M. Double-contrast tomography of the temporomandibular joint. A new technique based on autopsy examinations. Acta Radiol (Diagn) (Stockh) 1980; 21:777-784.

53. Annadale T. Displacement of the inter-articular cartilage of the lower jaw, and its treatment by operation. Lancet 1987; 1:411.

54. Burman M, Sinberg SE. Condylar movement in the study of internal derangement of the temporomandibular joint. J Bone Joint Surg (Br) 1946; 28:351-373.

55. Farrar WB. Diagnosis and treatment of anterior dislocation of the articular disc. NY J Dent 1971; 41:348-351.

56. Pringle JH. Displacement of the mandibular meniscus and its treatment. Br J Surg 1918; 6:385-389.

57. Silver CM, Simon SD, Savastano AA. Meniscus injuries of the temporomandibular joint. J Bone Joint Surg (Am) 1956; 38A:541-552.

58. Bell KA, Walters PJ. Videofluoroscopy during arthrography of the temporomandibular joint. Radio-logy 1983; 147:879.

59. Dolwick MF, Riggs RR. Diagnosis and treatment of internal derangements of the temporomandibular joint. Dent Clin North Am 1983; 27:561-572.

60. Lundh H, Westesson P-L, Kopp S et al. Anterior repositioning splint in the treatment of temporomandibular joints with reciprocal clicking: comparison with a flat occlusal splint and an untreated control group. Oral Surg Oral Med Oral Pathol 1985; 60:131-136.

61. McCarty WL, Farrar WB. Surgery for internal derangements of the temporomandibular joint. J Prosthet Dent 1979; 42:191-196.

62. McCarty WL. Surgery. In: Farrar WB, McCarthy WL, eds. A clinical outline of temporomandibular joint diagnosis and treatment. 7th Edition. Montgomery, Ala: Normandie Publications, 1982.

63. Arnaudow M, Haage H, Pflaum I. Die Doppelkontrastarthrographie des Kiefergelenkes. Dtsch Zahnarztl Z 1968; 23:390-393.

64. Arnaudow M, Pflaum I. Neue Erkenntnisse in der beurteilung bei der Kiefergelenktomographie. Dtsch Zahnarztl Z 1974; 29:554-556.

65. Tallents RH, Katzberg RW, Macher DJ et al. Arthrographically assisted splint therapy: 6-month follow-up. J Prosthet Dent 1986; 56:224-226.

66. Ross JB. The intracapsular therapeutic modalities in conjunction with arthrography: case reports. J Craniomandib Disord 1989; 3:35-43.

67. Katzberg RW, Westesson P-L. Diagnosis of the temporomandibular joint. In: Temporomandibular joint arthrography, Section I. Single contrast arthrography. Philadephia, Pa: WB Saunders, 1993; 101-142.

68. Katzberg RW, Westesson P-L. Diagnosis of the temporomandibular joint. Double contrast arthrography, Philadephia, Pa: WB Saunders, 1993: 143-165.

69. Westesson P-L, Eriksson L, Kurita K. Reliability of a negative clinical temporomandibular joint examination: prevalence of disk displacement in asymptomatic temporomandibular joints. Oral Surg Oral Med Oral Pathol 1989; 68:551-554.

70. Anderson QN, Katzberg RW. Loose bodies of the temporomandibular joint: arthrographic diagnosis. Skeletal Radiol 1984; 11:42-46.

71. Manzione JV, Seltzer SE, Katzberg RW et al. Direct sagittal computed tomography of the temporomandibular joint. AJNR 1982; 3:677-679.

72. Manzione JV, Katberg RW, Brodsky Gl, et al. Internal derangement of the temporomandibular joint: diagnosis by direct sagittal computed tomography. Radiology 1984; 150:111-115.

73. Helms CA, Morrish RB Jr, Kircos LT et al. Computed tomography of the meniscus of the temporomandibular joint: preliminary observations. Radiology 1982; 145:719-722.

74. Manco LG, Messing SG, Busino LJ et al. Internal derangements of the temporomandibular joint evaluated with direct sagittal CT: a

prospective study. Radiology 1985; 157:407-412.

75. Sartoris DJ, Neumann CH, Riley RW. The temporomandibular joint: true sagittal computed tomography with meniscus visualization. Radiology 1984; 150:250-254.

76. Thompson JR, Christiansen EL, Hasso AN et al. The temporomandibular joint: high resolution computed tomographic evaluation. Radiology 1984; 150:105-110.

77. Westesson P-L, Katzberg RW, Tallents RH et al. CT and MRI of the temporomandibular joint: comparison with autopsy specimens. Am J Roentgenol 1987; 148:1165-1171.

78. Harms SE, Wilk RM, Wolford LM et al. The temporomandibular joint: magnetic resonance imaging using surface coils. Radiology 1985; 157:133-136.

79. Katzberg RW, Schenck J, Roberts D et al. Magnetic resonance imaging of the temporomandibular joint meniscus. Oral Surg Oral Med Oral Pathol 1985; 59:332-335.

80. Katzberg RW, Besettte RW et al. Normal and abnormal temporomandibular joint: MR imaging with surface coil. Radiology 1986; 158:183-189.

81. Larheim TA. Imaging of the temporomandibular joint in rheumatic disease. In: Westesson P-L, Katzberg RW, eds. Imaging of the temporomandibular joint. Cranio Clinics International, Williams and Wilkins, Baltimore, Md: 1991; 1:133-153.

82. Larheim TA. Imaging of the temporomandibular joint in juvenile rheumatoid arthritis. In: Westesson P-L, Katzberg RW, eds. Imaging of the temporomandibular joint. Cranio Clinics International, Williams and Wilkins, Baltimore, Md: 1991; 1:155-172.

83. Manzione JV, Katzberg RW, Tallents RH et al. Magnetic resonance imaging of the temporomandibular joint. J Am Dent Assoc 1986; 113:398-402.

84. Schellhas KP. MR imaging of muscles of mastication. Am J Roentgenol 1989; 153:847-855.

85. Schellhas KP, Wilkes CH, Fritts HM

et al. MR of osteochondritis dissecans and avascular necrosis of the mandibular condyle. AJNR 1989; 10:3-12.

86. Hansson L-G, Westesson P-L, Katzberg RW et al. MR imaging of the temporomandibular joint: comparison of images of autopsy specimens made at 0.3 T and 1.5 T with anatomic cryosections. Am J Roentgenol 1989; 152:1241-1244.

87. Hardy CJ, Katzberg RW, Frey RL et al. Switched surface coil system for bilateral MR imaging. Radiology 1988; 167:835-838.

88. Shellock FG, Pressman BD. Dual-surface-coil MR imaging of bilateral temporomandibular joints: improvements in imaging protocol. AJNR 1989; 10:595-598.

89. Isberg A, Stenstrom B, Isacsson G. Frequency of bilateral temporomandibular joint disc displacement in patients with unilateral symptoms: a 5-year follow-up of the asymptomatic joint. A clinical and arthrotomographic study. Dentomaxillofac Radiol 1991; 20:73-76.

90. Sanchez-Woodworth RE, Tallents RH, Katzberg RW et al. Bilateral internal derangements of temporomandibular joint: evaluation by magnetic resonance imaging. Oral Surg Oral Med Oral Pathol 1988; 65:281-285.

91. Musgrave MT, Westesson P-L, Tallents RH et al. Improved magnetic resonance imaging of the temporomandibular joint by oblique scanning planes. Oral Surg Oral Med Oral Pathol 1991; 71:525-528.

92. Manzione JV, Tallents RH.

"Pseudomeniscus" sign: potential indicator of repair or remodeling in temporomandibular joints with internal derangements. Presented at Radiologic Society of North America. Radiology 1992; 185 (suppl) :175.

93. Paesani D, Westesson P-L. MR imaging of the TMJ: decreased signal from the retrodiscal tissue. Oral Surg Oral Med oral Pathol 1993; 76:631-635.

94. Westesson P-L, Brooks SL. Temporomandibular joint: relation between MR evidence of effusion and the presence of pain and disk displacement. Am J Roentgenol 1992; 159:559-563.

95. Schellhas KP, Wilkes CH. Temporomandibular joint inflammation: comparison of MR fast scanning with T1-and T2-weighted imaging techniques. Am J Rentgenol 1989; 153:93-98

96. Rao VM, Lliem MD, Farole A et al. Elusive "stuck" disk in the temporomandibular joint: diagnosis with MR imaging. Radiology 1993; 189:823-827.

97. Westesson P-L, Rohlin M. Diagnostic accuracy of double-contrast arthrotomography of the temporomandibular joint: correlation with postmortem morphology. Am J Roentgenol 1984; 143:655-660.

98. Westesson P-L, Bronstein SL, Liedberg J. Temporomandibular joint: correlation between single-contrast videoarthrography and postmortem morphology. Radiology 1986; 160:767-771.

99. Westesson P-L, Katzberg RW, Tallents RH et al. Temporomandibular joint: comparison of

MR images with cryosectional anatomy. Radiology 1987; 164:59-64.

100. Westesson P-L, Bronstein SL. Temporomandibular joint: comparison of single- and double-contrast arthrography. Radiology 1987; 164:65-70.

101. Tasaki M, Westesson P-L. Temporomandibular joint: diagnostic accuracy with sagittal and coronal MR imaging. Radiology 1993; 186:723-729.

102. Hansson L-G, Eriksson L, Westesson P-L. Temporomandibular joint: magnetic resonance evaluation after diskectomy. Oral Surg Med Oral Pathol 1992; 74:801-810.

103. Kent JN, Misiek DJ, Akin RK et al. Temporomanidbular joint condylar prosthesis: a ten-year report. J Oral Maxillofac Surg 1983; 41:245-254.

104. Kent JN, Block MS, Homsey CA et al. Experience with a polymer glenoid fossa prosthesis for partial or total temporomandibular joint reconstruction. J Oral Maxillofac Surg 1986; 44:520-533.

105. Lindqvist C, Jokinen J, Paukku P, et al. Adaptation of autogenous costochondral grafts used for temporomandibular joint reconstruction: a long-term clinical and radiologic follow-up. J Oral Maxillofac Surg 1988; 46(6):465-470.

106. Heffez LB. Imaging of internal derangements and synovial chondromatosis of the temporomandibular joint. Radiol Clin North Am 1993; 31:149-162.

107. Nomoto M, Nagao, Numata T et al. Synovial osteochondromatosis of

the temporomandibular joint. J Laryngol Otol 1993; 107:742-745.

108. Quinn PD, Stanton DC, Foote JW. Synovial chondroamtosis with cranial extension. Oral Surg Oral Med Oral Pathol 1992; 73:398-402.

109. Sun S, Helmy E, Bays R. Synovial chondromatosis with intracranial extension. a case report. Oral Surg Oral Med Oral Pathol 1990; 70:5-9.

110. Boccardi A. CT evaluation of chondromatosis of the temporomandibular joint. J Comp Assist Tomogr 1991; 15:826-828.

111. Herzog S, Mafee M. Synovial chondromatosis of the TMJ: MR and CT findings. Am J Neuroradiol 1990; 11:742-745.

112. van Ingen JM, de Man K, Bakri I. CT diagnosis of synovial chondromatosis of the temporomandibular joint. Brit J Oral Maxillofac Surg 1990; 28:164-167.

113. Lopes V, Jones JAH, Sloan P et al. Temporomandibular ganglion or synovial cyst? Oral Surg Oral Med Oral Pathol 1994; 77:627-630.

114. McGuirt WF, Myers EN. Ganglion of the temporomandibular joint. Presentation as a parotid mass. Otolaryngol Head Neck Surg 1993; 109:950-953.

115. Bhaskar SN. Synopsis of oral pathology. St. Louis, Mo: CV Mosby Co, 1977; 304-324.

116. Ruben MM, Jui B, Cozzi GM. Metastatic carcinoma of the mandibular condyle presenting as temporomandibular joint syndrome. J Oral Maxillofac Surg 1989; 47:511-513.

117. Zachariades N. Neoplasms metastatic to the mouth, jaws and surrounding tissues. J Craniomaxillofacial Surg 1989; 17:283-291.

118. Ruggiero SL, Donoff RB. Bone regeneration after mandibular resection: report of two cases. J Oral Maxillofac Surg 1991; 49:647-651.

119. Smith HJ, Larheim TA, Aspestrand F. Rheumatic and nonrheumatic disease in the temporomandibular joint: gadolinium-enhanced MR imaging. Radiology 1992; 185:229-234.

120. Isberg A, Isacsson G, Nah KS. Mandibular coronoid process locking: a prospective study of frequency and association with internal derangement of the temporomandibular joint. Oral Surg Oral Med Oral Pathol 1987; 63:275-279.

121. Langenbeck B. Augeborene kleinheit des unterkiefers; kiefersperre verbunden, geheilt durch resection der processus coronoidei, Archiv fur Klin Chir 1860; 1:30.

122. Munk PL, Helms CA. Coronoid process hyperplasia: CT studies. Radiology 1989; 171:783-784.

123. Markey RJ, Potter BE, Moffett BC. Condylar trauma and facial asymmetry: an experimental study. J Maxillofac Surg 1980; 8:38-51.

124. Wang-Norderud R, Ragab RR. Unilateral condylar hyperplasia and the associated deformity of facial asymmetry. Scand J Plast Reconstr Surg Hand Surg 1977; 11:91-96.

125. Lineaweaver W, Vargervik K, Tomer BS et al. Posttraumatic condylar hyperplasia. Ann Plast Surg 1989; 22:163-171.

126. Katzberg RW, Tallents RH, Hayakawa K et al. Internal derangements of the temporomandibular joint: findings in the pediatric age group. Radiology 1985; 154:125-127.

127. Westesson P-L, Dahlberg G, Hansson L-G et al. Osseous and muscular changes after vertical ramus osteotomy. An MRI study. Oral Surg Oral Med Oral Pathol 1991; 72:139-145.

128. Collier DB, Carrera GF, Messer EJ et al. Internal derangement of the temporomandibular joint: detection by single-photon emission computed tomography. Radiology 1983; 149:557-561.

129. Katzberg RW, O'Mara RE, Tallents RH et al. Radionuclide skeletal imaging and single photon emission computed tomography in suspected internal derangements of the temporomandibular joint. J Oral Maxillofac Surg 1984; 42:782-787.

130. Bell KA, Jones JP, Miller KD et al. The added gradient echo pulse sequence technique: application to imaging of fluid in the temporomandibular joint. Am J Neuroradiol 1993; 14:375-381.

131. Diamant B, Karlsson J, Nachemson A. Correlation between lactate levels and pH in disks in patients with lumbar rhizopathies. Experientia 1969; 24:1195-1196.

132. Alder ME, Dove SB, Murrah VA et al. Magnetic resonance spectroscopy of inflammation associated with the temporomandibular joint. Oral Surg Oral Med Oral Pathol 1992; 74:515-523.

PART III

Upper Aerodigestive Tract

8

Pharynx

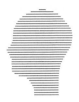

SECTION ONE
SURESH K. MUKHERJI
ROY A. HOLLIDAY

SECTION TWO
JANE L. WEISSMAN
ROY A. HOLLIDAY

SECTION ONE
NASOPHARYNX-OROPHARYNX

The pharynx is a musculomembranous tube that extends from the skull base to the cervical esophagus.[1,2] Historically the pharynx has been divided into three parts: the nasopharynx, which extends from the skull base to the hard palate; the oropharynx, which extends from the hard palate to the level of the hyoid bone; and the hypopharynx, which extends from the hyoid bone to the caudal margin of the cricoid cartilage.

Three overlapping constrictor muscles make up the pharyngeal musculature.[1] All of these muscles insert posteriorly in the midline on a median raphe that is attached to the skull base at the pharyngeal tubercle. The superior pharyngeal constrictor has its origin from the lower posterior edge of the medial pterygoid plate, the pterygomandibular raphe, the alveolar process of the mandible, and the lateral aspect of the tongue. The middle constrictor muscle has its origin along the stylohyoid ligament and the greater and lesser cornua of the hyoid bone. The inferior constrictor muscle has its origin from the oblique line of the thyroid cartilage, the lateral cricoid cartilage, and the posterior border of the cricothyroid muscle. The cricopharyngeus muscle consists of nonraphed, parallel, horizontal fibers that extend from one side of the cricoid cartilage to the other. This sphincter muscle separates the hypopharynx from the cervical esophagus.[1] The pharyngeal constrictor muscles contract the pharynx in an organized, peristoltic manner from superiorly to inferiorly. There are no major pharyngeal dilator muscles. The pharynx is primarily passively dilated by increasing pharyngeal and oral pressure. The salpingopharyngeus, stylopharyngeus, palatopharyngeus, and the tensor and levator veli palatini muscles also contribute to the pharynx and its function. The salpingopharyngeus extends from the eustachian tube cartilage to interdigitate with posterior fascicles of the palatopharyngeus. This muscle helps raise the nasopharynx and open the eustachian tube orifice. The stylopharyngeus extends from the styloid process to the superior and posterior borders of the thyroid cartilage, and some fibers intermingle with the constrictor muscles. This muscle raises and to a minimal degree dilates the pharynx. The palatopharyngeus extends from the soft palate and the pharyngeal wall to the posterior border of the thyroid cartilage, forming the structure of the posterior tonsillar pillar. This muscle narrows the oropharyngeal isthmus, elevates the pharynx, and helps close off the nasopharynx. The tensor veli palatini extends from the scaphoid fossa, sphenoid spine, and the lateral side of the eustacian tube to the soft palate. It is innervated by the third division of the trigeminal nerve. The levator veli palatini muscle extends from the under surface of the petrous temporal bone and the medial side of the eustacian tube to the soft palate. It is innervated by the pharyngeal plexus via fibers of cranial nerve IX. Together these muscles function to elevate the soft palate and maintain patency of the eustacian tube orifice during swallowing.

The arterial supply of the pharynx is from the major branches of the external carotid artery, including the ascending pharyngeal artery, tonsillar branches of the facial artery, and the palantine branches of the maxillary artery.[1,2] The primary venous drainage is via the pharyngeal veins, which communicate with the pharyngeal plexus located in the lateral aspect of the pterygopalatine fossa, and which then drain inferiorly into the internal jugular vein. The pharyngeal musculature, except for the stylopharyngeus muscle, is innervated primarily by the vagus nerve through the pharyngeal plexus.[1] The glossopharyngeal nerve supplies the stylopharyngeal muscle. The primary lymphatic drainage from the nasopharynx and oropharynx is to the retropharyngeal and internal jugular chain lymph nodes.[1,2]

EMBRYOLOGY

The embryology of the branchial apparatus is discussed in detail in Chapters 1, 10, and 14. Only that embryology pertinent to the pharynx will be briefly reviewed here. Derivatives of the first branchial arch that pertain to the pharynx include the muscles of mastication, the tensor veli palatini, the tensor tympani, and the anterior belly of the digastric, all of which receive their innervation from the mandibular division of trigeminal nerve. The first pharyngeal pouch is the precursor to the eustachian tube, tympanic cavity, and the mastoid air cells.[3]

The ventral portion of the second brachial arch (Reichert's cartilage) forms the lesser cornu and superior portion of the hyoid bone. The dorsal portion gives rise to portions of the incus, malleous, stapes, and styloid process. A portion of the cartilage between the hyoid bone and the styloid process forms the stylohyoid ligament. The muscles derived from the mesoderm of the second arch and innervated by the facial nerve include the posterior belly of the digastric, the stylohyoid, stapedius, and the superficial muscles of facial expression.[3] The ventral portion of the second pharyngeal pouch is largely obliterated by the development of the palatine tonsil, and the dorsal portion gives rise to the tonsillar fossa. The endoderm proliferates and forms the surface epithelium and lining of the crypts of the palantine tonsil, and the mesenchyme gives rise to the lymphatic nodules within the palantine tonsil.

The cartilage of the third branchial arch forms the lower body and greater cornu of the hyoid bone. The musculature derived from the the third branchial arch is limited to the stylopharyngeus, which is supplied by the glossopharyngeal nerve. The mucosa covering the posterior third of the tongue (base of tongue) is also a derivative of the third arch. Some authors claim that the palatopharyngeus muscle is also a third arch derivitive.[4]

ANATOMY

Nasopharynx

The nasopharynx is an epithelial-lined cavity that occupies the uppermost aerodigestive tract. It is approximately 2 cm in anteroposterior diameter and 4 cm in height. The roof of the nasopharynx is downward sloping and is formed cranially to caudally by the basisphenoid, basiocciput, and the anterior aspect of the first two cervical vertebra.[1,5] The inferior aspect of the nasopharynx is formed by the hard palate, soft palate, and the ridge of pharyngeal musculature that opposes the soft palate when it is elevated (Passavant's ridge). The lateral nasopharyngeal walls are formed by the margins of the superior constrictor muscle. Anteriorly the nasopharynx is in direct continuity with the nasal cavity via the posterior choanae.[1,5]

The nasopharynx is in direct communication with the middle ear cavity via the eustachian tubes. These tubes gain access into the nasopharynx through the sinus of Morgagni, which is a defect in the anterior portion of the pharyngobasilar fascia above the superior pharyngeal constrictor muscle (Figs. 8-1, 8-2). This natural defect may also allow access for advanced nasopharyngeal carcinoma to spread to the parapharyngeal space and central skull base.[5,6] The opening of the eustachian tube is located along the posterolateral wall of the nasopharynx, and the cartilaginous eustacian tube, the levator veli palatini muscle, and the overlying mucosa form a prominent structure, the torus tubarius. Because of the location of the pharyngeal opening of the eustachian tube, nasopharyngeal masses, including hypertrophic adenoids and tumors, may obstruct the tube and result in eustachian tube dysfunction and serous otitis media.[5,6,9] Located just behind and above the torus tubarius is a mucosal reflection that is the most cranial aspect of the lateral recess of the nasopharynx, the fossa of Rosenmüller. This fossa is just lateral to the flexor muscles of the neck, the longus capitus and coli muscles (Fig. 8-3), and is a common site of origin of nasopharyngeal cancer. When tumors here are small, they are often clinically occult.[5,6]

The mucosa of the nasopharynx is composed of both stratified squamous and columnar epithelium. The later predominates during the first 10 years of life, whereas stratified squamous epithelium is more common with advancing age. The adenoids are lymphatic tissue that are located in the upper posterior aspect of the nasopharynx. Prominent adenoids are typically present in children, and if such adenoids are not present, an immune deficiency syndrome is probably present. Around puberty, gradual involution normally begins, and the majority of individuals have lost most of this adenoidal tissue by 30 years of age.[7] Nonetheless, normal adenoidal tissue may occasionally be seen in adults in their fourth and fifth decades of life.

The buccopharyngeal (visceral) fascia surrounds the nasopharyngeal mucosa and the constrictor muscles. This fascia separates the nasopharynx from the deep fascial spaces and is thought to be a barrier to deep spread of infection and early malignancy (Figs. 8-4, 8-5).[5-9] An extensive lymphatic plexus drains the nasopharynx and explains the high incidence of cervical nodal metastases associated with nasopharygeal carcinoma.[5,9] The primary eschelon drainage is to the retropharyngeal nodes and jugulodigastric nodes (level II). However, there are inconstant lymphatic vessels that pass directly to the spinal accessory and midjugular

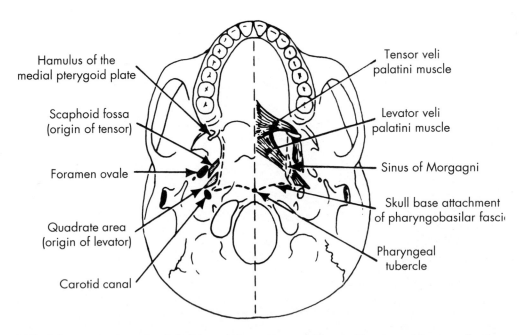

FIG. 8-1 Axial schematic of skull base demonstrates attachment of levator and tensor veli palatini muscles and pharyngobasilar fascia. (Courtesy Dr. Wendy Smoker, University of Utah.)

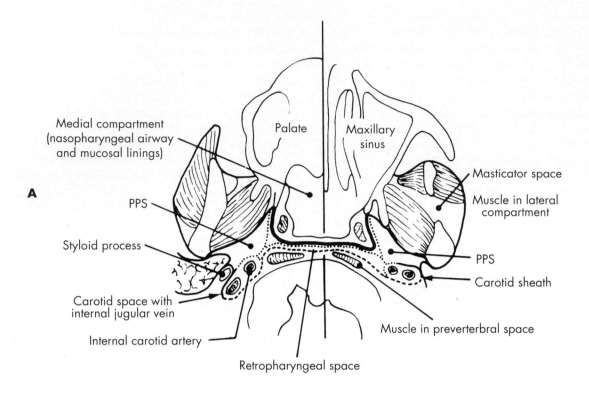

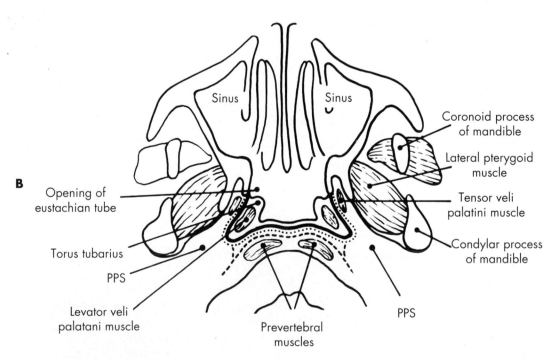

FIG. 8-2 **A,** Axial schematic of upper nasopharynx. Left side of image is at lower level than right side of image. Various deep spaces of head and neck include masticator space, parapharyngeal space *(PPS)*, carotid space, and retropharyngeal and prevertebral spaces. Dense heavy line represents pharyngobasilar fascia; thin dotted line represents buccopharyngeal facia. Note that carotid sheath is made up of components of all fascial layers. **B,** Axial schematic through mid-nasopharynx demonstrating relationship of levator and tensor palatini muscles to pharyngobasilar fascia and torus tubarius. (Courtesy Dr. Wendy Smoker, University of Utah.)

nodes, explaining the occasional isolated involvement of these nodal groups.[5,10]

Oropharynx

The oral portion of the upper aerodigestive tract is divided into two major components: the oral cavity and the oropharynx. The oral cavity contains the anterior two thirds of the tongue, the buccal mucosa, the floor of the mouth, and the supporting mandible and maxillary bones. This component is discussed in Chapter 9. The oropharynx is that region posterior to the circumvallate papilla of the tongue and includes the posterior one third of the tongue (tongue base), the palatine tonsils, the soft palate, and the oropharyngeal mucosa and constrictor muscles from the level of the palate to the hyoid bone. The posterior oropharyngeal wall is related to the second and third cervical vertebrae. Laterally there are two faucial arches, the anterior (palatoglossus muscle) and the posterior arch (palatopharyngeus muscle), and between them is the tonsillar fossa, which harbors the palatine tonsil. The visceral fascia about the mucosa and musculature of the pharynx often acts as a barrier to contain tumor. However, if this fascia is violated, the tumor can become fixed to the prevertebral soft tissues and invade the vertebrae. The lingual tonsil lies at the base of the tongue and is usually more concentrated on the lateral surfaces.

The major arterial supply is from the tonsillar branch of the facial artery, the ascending pharyngeal artery, the dorsal lingual arteries, and the internal maxillary and facial arteries. The venous drainage is in major part through the peritonsillar veins, which pierce the constrictor musculature and drain into the common facial vein and the pharyngeal plexus. The primary lymphatic drainage is to the jugulodigastric nodes, the retropharyngeal nodes, and the posterior cervical nodes.

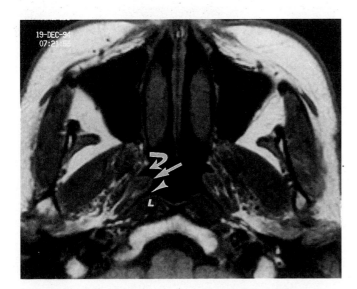

FIG. 8-3 Axial T1W MRI shows the normal superficial landmarks of the nasopharynx. *Curved arrow,* Eustachain tube opening; *straight arrow,* torus tubraius; *arrowhead,* fossa of Rosenmuller (lateral pharyngeal recess); *L,* longus coli muscle.

IMAGING TECHNIQUES
Computed Tomography
Patient Positioning

The pharynx is best examined with the patient supine, the patient's head in a neutral position, and the scan plane parallel to the infraorbital-meatal line. The head should be carefully positioned so that it is not askew along the cephalocaudad axis, since this may result in an appearance that may simulate pathology. Similarly, when positioning the patient for direct coronal examinations, the head must not be turned to one side because the resulting anatomic distortion makes reliable diagnosis difficult. A localizing lateral scout image is obtained, and the study should extend from the external auditory canal to the top of the manubrium. This allows evaluation of the pharynx, as well as all the node-bearing areas. Direct coronal scans should also be performed in any patient suspected to have a nasopharyngeal, skull base, or palatal mass.

The oropharynx and nasopharynx should be studied during suspended respiration. If amalgam artifacts degrade

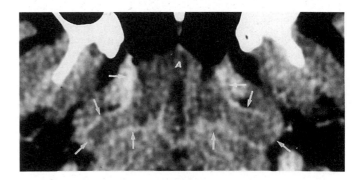

FIG. 8-4 Axial contrast-enhanced CT through the nasopharynx of a 4-year old child shows normal enhancement of the venous plexus and pharyngobasilar fascia *(arrows).* Note the adenoidal tissue normally seen in this age group *(A).*

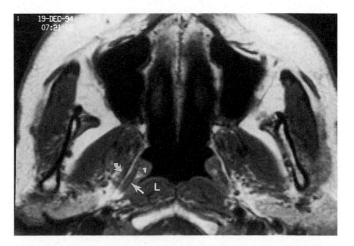

FIG. 8-5 Axial T1W MRI illustrates the normal appearance of the deep muscles of the nasopharynx. *Curved arrow,* Tensor veli palatini; *straight arrow,* levator veli palatini; *arrowhead,* salpingopharyngeus; *L,* longus coli.

some images, additional complementary scans should be obtained at an angle that avoids these artifacts.

Computed Tomography Scanning Parameters

The study should be obtained as contiguous 3 to 5 mm scans, and the field of view should be as small as possible, while still including all essential anatomy. Bone algorithms are essential to evaluate any pathologic bone involvement, and if skull base erosion is suspected, direct coronal scans should be obtained when possible.

Intravenous Contrast

All studies performed to evaluate the nasopharynx and oropharynx should be performed with intravenous contrast because vascular opacification is necessary to best distinguish between vessels and adjacent lymph nodes. The contrast material should be administered using a power injector, usually with a loading bolus of 50 ml administered at 2 ml/second, followed by a continuous infusion at 1 ml/second.

Magnetic Resonance Imaging

To obtain high-quality magnetic resonance images (MRI) of the head and neck, the patient must be instructed that motion (swallowing, talking, or snoring) degrades the images. Scans of the nasopharynx and oropharynx are performed with a head coil. Scans of the neck must utilize a dedicated neck coil of sufficient size to cover the patient from the floor of the mouth to the supraclavicular region.

Selection of pulse sequences depends on the type and extent of the pathology. For routine screening examinations, localization is done from a sagittal T1-weighted (T1W) spin-echo sequence. Axial T2W scans are then obtained through the field of interest. On these T2W scans, fat and muscle have fairly low signal intensities and while lymph nodes and areas of pathology usually have higher signal intensity. Finally a coronal T1W sequence provides an additional orthogonal image of the skull base and superior nasopharynx.

The use of intravenous paramagnetic contrast is essential when evaluating patients with malignancies of the nasopharynx and oropharynx. Before the use of contrast, a noncontrast T1W sequence should be obtained. This approach prevents confusion of areas of high T1W signal intensity (i.e., fat or proteinaceous fluid) with areas of enhancement.

The MRI studies of the oropharynx and oral cavity are performed primarily in the axial plane. Coronal scans may be of use in assessing the anterior tongue or palate but have little role in assessing the tongue base or oropharynx. T2W axial sequences are performed following a T1W sagittal localizing sequence. Scanning coverage should include at least the region between the palate and the hyoid bone. The cervical neck nodes must then be examined with a neck coil. Sections 4 or 5 mm thick are mandatory to prevent volume averaging. Presaturation pulses are extremely useful. They have the effect of saturating the entry-slice signal (produc-

ing signal void) within the vessel lumen and secondarily reducing the phase-encoding flow artifact, which is so often troublesome in neck imaging (Figs. 8-6 to 8-14). Selection of the proper field of view and acquisition matrix (18 to 20 cm, 192 to 256 matrix) are also important to optimize the MR study.

There are three major types of soft tissue present in the oropharynx: muscle, lymphoid tissue, and fat, and they each exhibit different MRI and CT characteristics.[11] On CT, muscle and lymphoid tissues are often difficult to distinguish from neoplastic tissues but are easily differentiated from fat. On MRI, muscle has an intermediate T1W and low T2W signal intensity. By comparison, most cellular tumors have an intermediate T1W and a slightly higher intermediate T2W signal intensity, allowing distinction from muscle.

Lymphoid tissue, present in the palatine and lingual tonsils and on the inferior surface of the soft palate, has a signal intensity similar to muscle and most tumors on T1W images.[11-15] However, lymphoid tissue has a relatively long T2 relaxation time and therefore increases in signal intensity relative to muscle on T2W images. T1W MRI sequences afford the best contrast between fat and muscle, whereas T2W MRI sequences demonstrate the best contrast between muscle and lymphoid tissue.[12,14,15] Because of similar signal intensities, tumor and lymphoid tissue in the palatine fossa and lingual tonsil cannot be reliably differentiated from each other on MRI. The dominant fat plane deep to the airway is the parapharyngeal space, which is best defined on T1W sequences. Infiltration of the parapharyngeal space fat usually indicates deep invasion of a neoplasm.

On CT the tonsils and faucial pillars have a similar density, and they usually appear as bilaterally symmetric soft-tissue densities on either side of the airway.[16,17] Any asym-

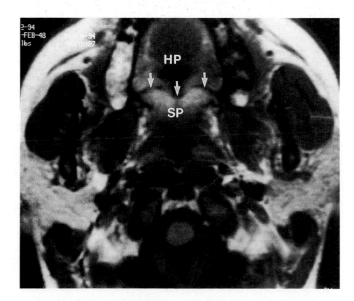

FIG. 8-6 Axial T1W MR demonstrates the normal MR appearance of the soft palate *(SP)*, the mucosa on the oral surface of the hard palate *(HP)*, and the bony margin at the dorsal aspect of the hard palate *(arrows)*.

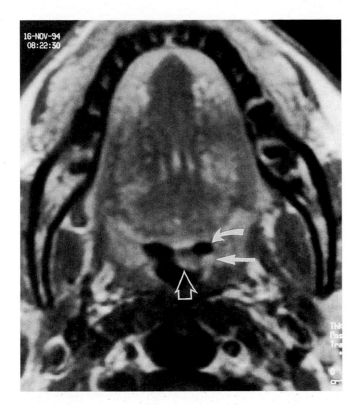

FIG. 8-7 Axial T1W MRI obtained through the oropharynx demonstrates the region of the anterior tonsillar pillar *(curved arrow)* and posterior tonsillar pillar *(straight arrow)*. The tip of the uvula is indicated by the open arrow.

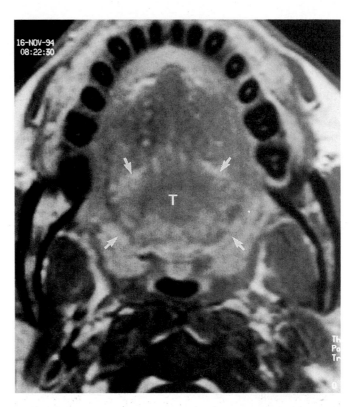

FIG. 8-8 Axial T1W MRI shows the normal appearance of the tongue base *(T)*. Note the margins surrounding the tongue base, which are well visualized with MRI *(arrows)*.

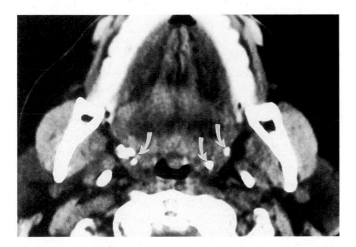

FIG. 8-9 Axial CT demonstraes the characteristic appearance of benign tonsillar calcifications *(curved arrows)*.

metry in the size of the palatine tonsils may indicate that a tumor is present in the larger side. Dystrophic calcification from previous infection is commonly seen within the tonsillar beds (Fig. 8-9). On MRI these lymphoid structures have a slightly more intense signal than muscle on T1W images, and they increase in signal intensity on T2W images.[11] Occasionally, benign retension cysts may occur in areas rich in lymphoid tissue, and these cysts are commonly seen in the nasopharynx (Fig. 8-10) and palatine tonsils (Fig. 8-11).

On CT the soft palate has a density similar to that of muscle. However, on MRI the appearance of the palate reflects the large number of glandular elements that are intermixed with fat,[11] and the palate has a nonhomogeneous appearance on T1W images and a high signal intensity on T2W images.[11]

NEOPLASMS
Nasopharyngeal Carcinomas
Clinical Features

In adults, squamous cell carcinomas (SCCA) accounts for about 70% of the malignancies arising in the nasopharynx.[5,6] Lymphomas account for approximately 20% of the cases; the remaining 10% are due to a variety of lesions that include adenocarcinoma, adenoid cystic carcinoma, rhabdomyosarcoma, melanoma, extramedullary plasmacytoma, fibrosarcoma, and carcinosarcoma.[6] SCCA of the nasopharynx is a relatively rare cancer that accounts for 0.25% of all malignancies in North America. However, this tumor has a high rate of incidence in Asia, where it is the most common cancer in males and the third most common cancer in females, accounting for 18% of all cancers in China.[18] In the United States, SCCA is more common in males than in females, with the majority of cases being diagnosed during the sixth decade of life.[6] The biologic behavior of nasopha-

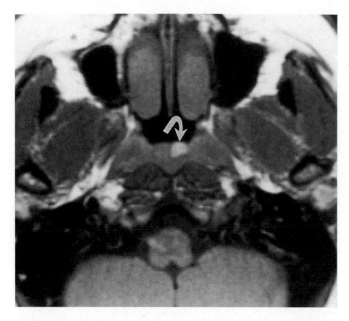

FIG. 8-10 Noncontrast axial T1W MRI demonstrates a high signal intensity, round lesion (arrow), with well-defined margins, located just at and deep to the mucosa of the nasopharynx. This was a rentention cyst, and the increased signal was due to the high protein content of the cyst fluid.

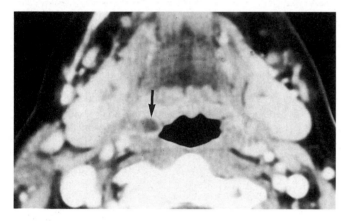

FIG. 8-11 Axial CT shows a well-delineated low-attenuation lesion in the right palatine tonsil (arrow). The patient had no symptoms referable to this lesion, which has an incidental tonsillar retension cyst.

▼
BOX 8-1
AJCC STAGING FOR NASOPHARYNGEAL CANCER

Tis	Carcinoma in situ
T1	Tumor confined to one subsite of the nasopharynx
T2	Tumor invades more than one subsite of the nasopharynx
T3	Tumor invades the nasal cavity or the oropharynx
T4	Tumor invades the skull base or cranial nerve(s)

ryngeal carcinomas is the same, regardless of ethinic origin. The staging of nasopharyngeal cancer is given in Box 8-1.

Several factors have been linked with an increased likelihood of developing SCCA of the nasopharynx. IGA antibodies against the Epstein-Barr virus have been associated with the undifferentiated form of this tumor, and HLA-A2 and HLA-B-Sin histocompatibility loci have been identified as possible markers for genetic susceptibitily to SCCA among the Chinese population.[19] The incidence of this tumor decreases among Chinese born in North America, although the rate is still seven times higher than that in native Americans.[20] Other potential risk factors include nitrosamines (present in dry-salted fish), polycyclic hydrocarbons, poor living conditions, and chronic sinonasal infections.[6]

The most commonly used classification for nasopharyngeal carcinoma has been established by the World Health Organization (WHO), which divides these tumors into three types based on their histopathology: squamous cell carcinoma (type 1), nonkeratinizing carcinoma (type 2), and undifferentiated carcinoma (type 3). Type 1 tumors are keratinized lesions that are similar to other SCCA found in the remainder of the upper aerodigestive tract. Type 2 lesions have little or no keratin production, and because of their resemblance to urinary tract tumors, they are sometimes referred to as transitional cell carcinomas. Type 3 carcinomas often resemble large cell lymphomas and constitute a diverse group of malignancies that include lymphoepitheliomas, anaplastic lesions, and spindle cell and clear cell varieties of SCCA.[21]

The clinical presentation depends on the size and location of the lesion, with most small lesions being asymptomic. The most common presenting complaint is internal jugular or spinal accessory lymphadenopathy. Nasopharyngeal carcinoma is one of the few head and neck primary tumors that has no relationship between primary size and the presence of nodal disease. Large tumors may have no nodal metastasis, and small tumors may present with diffuse, bilateral cervical metastases. Serous otitis media may also be a presenting complaint, which is caused by eustachain tube obstruction by the tumor. Other symptoms include headaches, nasal obstruction, epistaxis, sore throat, trismus, and proptosis. Advanced lesions may spread to the adjacent cranial nerves and present with neurologic symptoms. Tumor extension into the cavernous sinus may result in palsies of cranial nerves II through VI, and tumor in the parapharyngeal space may involve cranial nerves IX through XII and the sympathetic chain. Such tumor extension may result in the patient presenting with otalgia or a unilateral Horner's syndrome.[5,6]

The standard treatment of nasopharyngeal carcinoma is external beam supervoltage irradiation, and brachytherapy may be of some benefit in selected individuals. Surgery plays a limited role in the treatment of nasopharyngeal carcinoma because adequate surgical margins are difficult to obtain However, if neck disease persists or recurs after radiotherapy, a neck dissection is usually performed to con-

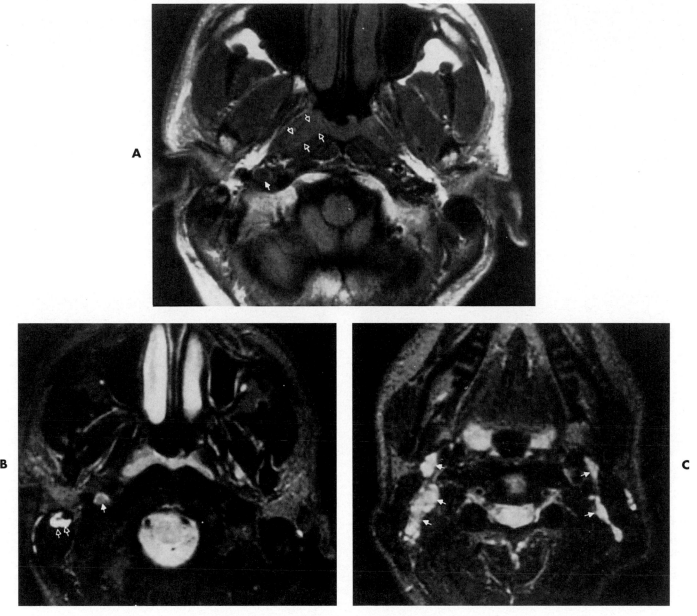

FIG. 8-12   Squamous cell carcinoma of right nasopharynx isolated to fossa of Rosenmüller. 28-year-old male presented with unilateral hearing loss. **A,** Axial T1W MR image through upper nasopharynx demonstrates low-intensity mass occupying right nasopharynx and fossa of Rosenmüller *(open arrows)*. Also present is necrotic retropharyngeal node *(closed arrow)*. **B,** Axial T2W MRI view through same level as **A**. Mass has increased signal intensity similar to that surrounding adenoidal tissue. Note increased signal intensity of retropharyngeal node *(closed arrow)*. Fluid within mastoid *(open arrows)* is due to serous otitis media. **C,** Axial T2W MR image through lower neck demonstrates multiple bilateral posterior triangle and anterior cervical nodes *(arrows)*.

trol the disease.[5,6] The reported 5-year survival rates, for patients treated with radiation therapy at M. D. Anderson Hospital, vary with the histologic type and are as follows: squamous cell carcinoma (42%), lymphoepithelioma (65%), and unclassified carcinomas (14%).[22] However, the overall prognosis is dependent on other factors that include size of the primary lesion, extent of disease, duration and extent of symptoms, the presence of skull base erosion, and nodal involvement at multiple levels.

Imaging Features

CT and MRI play complementary roles for imaging patients with nasopharyngeal carcinoma. Imaging studies are usually unable to differentiate between SCCA and other malignancies, and the primary role of imaging is accurate disease mapping. The most reliable imaging finding of a malignancy is an aggressive, often enhancing mass that infiltrates the deep fascial planes and spaces about the nasopharynx.[9] A noninfiltrating, homogeneously enhancing mass situated

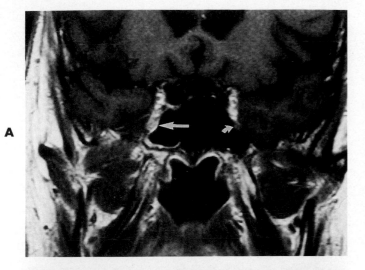

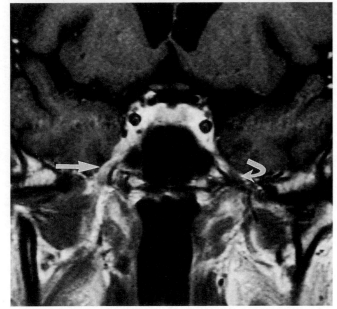

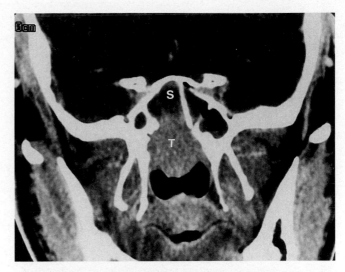

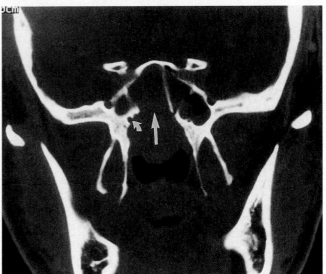

FIG. 8-13 **A,** Coronal-enhanced T1W MRI shows enlargement and enhancement of the second division of the trigeminal nerve *(straight arrow)* caused by perineural spread of squamous cell carcinoma. Note the normal appearance of V2 on the opposite side *(curved arrow).* **B,** Post-gadolinium coronal T1W MRI shows perineural spread of tumor along the third division of the trigeminal nerve *(straight arrow).* Note the normal appearance of V3 on the opposite side *(curved arrow).*

FIG. 8-14 **A,** Coronal CT shows a nasopharyngeal carcinoma that erodes into the sphenoid sinus. Note the difference between the attenuation characteristics of the tumor *(T)* and the retained secretions *(S)* within the obstructed sinus. **B,** Bone window shows the marked destruction *(large arrow)* of the base of the sphenoid sinus and erosion of the bony margin of the vidian canal *(small arrow).*

on the mucosal surface may be prominent adenoidal tissue. When such a mass is identified, clinical correlation should be requested (Fig. 8-12). MRI provides excellent visualization of the soft-tissue plane of the nasopharynx and is superior to CT for detecting perineural spread of tumor (Fig. 8-13). Conversely, although both MRI and CT may detect bone erosion, CT is superior for identifying small areas of bone destruction or seeing tumoral calcification (Fig. 8-14). Skull base erosion is especially important because up to 25% of cases have clinically occult bone disease. In addition, skull base and perineural involvement alter irradiation treatment ports and upgrade the tumor to a T4 stage.

Nasopharyngeal malignancies tend to grow along the path of least resistance, and potential pathways of tumor extension include growth along muscle bundles, neurovascular bundles, fascial planes, and within the mucosa and submucosa. However, the natural spread of tumor may be altered by certain normal structures that are relatively resistent to tumor invasion. In the nasopharynx, such structures are the cartilaginous portion of the eustachian tube and the pharyngobasilar fascia.[8,9]

As mentioned, small lesions are often limited by the surrounding pharyngobasilar fascia (Fig. 8-15). However, once this barrier is breached, the tumor may directly invade the

A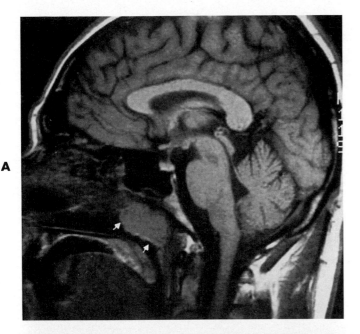

B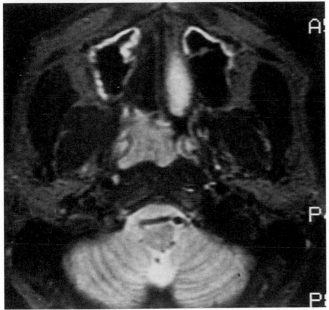

FIG. 8-15 Exophytic squamous carcinoma of nasopharynx. **A,** Sagittal T1W MRI view of nasopharynx demonstrates soft-tissue mass occupying superior aspect of nasopharynx *(arrows)*. This appearance is quite similar to residual adenoidal tissue seen in younger patients. **B,** Axial T2W MR image through nasopharynx. Mass is contained within right nasopharynx and has similar signal intensity to residual adenoidal tissue. Diagnosis cannot be certain based on image intensity; however, appearance of unilateral nasopharyngeal mass in middle-aged or elderly patient should require endocscopic examination and biospy.

skull base; the most common site of intrusion is the region of the petroclinoid fissure and foramen lacerum. Aggressive lesions may then extend into the foramen lacerum, encase the internal carotid artery, and gain access into the cavernous sinus (Fig. 8-16). Skull base erosion is also likely to

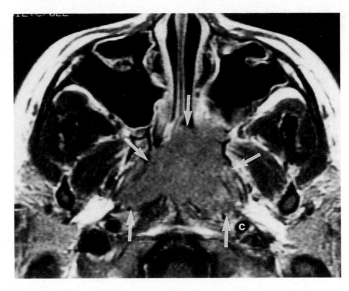

FIG. 8-16 Axial T1W contrast-enhanced MRI better demonstrates the full extent of this lymphoepithioma *(arrows)*. Note the proximity of the tumor to the left carotid artery *(C)*.

occur at sites of musculature attachments, and the levator and tensor veli palatini muscles provide common pathways for cranial tumor spread.[8,9]

The superior and anterior portion of the lateral wall of the nasopharynx is incomplete due to the sinus of Morgagni, which allows passage of the cartilaginous portion of the eustachian tube and the levator veli palatini muscle.[5] However, this natural defect also allows passage of tumor into the parapharyngeal space and carotid sheath. Once in these areas, tumor may also involve V_3 and extend retrograde into the cavernous sinus. Such nerve invasion, or perineural invasion should be suspected when there is enlagement and abnormal enhancement of the nerve with obliteration of the surrounding fat planes (Fig. 8-13). Tumors may also directly invade the skull base at the foramen ovale, and CT and MRI can help identify whether or not tumor has invaded the sphenoid sinus (Figs. 8-14, 8-17).

Continued tumor extension may involve the pterygopalatine fossa or posterior aspect of the nasal cavity; however, invasion of the posterior ethmoids, orbit, and maxillary antrum is unusual. Caudal tumor extension along the lateral pharyngeal walls and the anterior and posterior tonsillar pillars is seen in nearly 33% of patients.[5] This form of spread is often submucosal and may be clinically occult.

Imaging of all of the cervical lymph nodes is essential because 85% to 90% of patients have nodal spread at the time of initial diagnosis, and nearly 50% of patients have bilateral disease.[5, 22, 23] The retropharyngeal nodes are usually the first nodes to become involved; however, level II nodes may be involved without radiographic evidence of retropharyngeal nodal disease. Submental and occipital nodes typically become affected only when there is an obstruction to the primary lymphatic drainage such as that which follows radiation therapy.[5]

Orpharyngeal Carcinomas

The majority of tumors involving the oropharynx are SCCA, followed by other less common lesions such as lymphoma, minor salivary gland tumors, and other rare mesenchymal lesions. The incidence of SCCA of the oropharynx increases in patients with a history of tobacco or alcohol abuse. The staging system for these tumors is given in Box 8-2. Because the spread patterns and lymphatic drainage vary with the site of origin, these sites are discussed separately.

Anterior Tonsillar Pillar

Tumors arising on the anterior tonsillar pillar (arch) ATP tend to spread along the palatoglossus muscle and its fascial attachments. The tumor may spread superiorly to involve the soft palate, and once there, it may extend anteriorly to involve the posterior aspect of the hard palate or extend further superiorly along the tensor and levator veli palatini muscles and the pterygoid muscles.[24, 25] Advanced tumor with this spread pattern may eventually reach and invade the

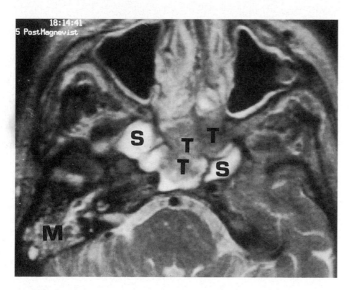

FIG. 8-17   Axial T2W MRI obtained through the skull base in a patient with nasopharyngeal carcinoma shows the intermediate signal intensity tumor *(T)* invading the sphenoid sinus. The high signal *(S)* represents retained secretions within the obstructed sphenoid sinus. Note the increased signal within the mastoid air cells *(M)* caused by tumor obstructing the eustachian tube.

▼

BOX 8-2
AJCC STAGING FOR OROPHARYNGEAL CANCER

Tis	Carcinoma in situ
T1	Tumor is 2 cm or less in greatest diameter
T2	Tumor is more than 2 cm but less than 4 cm in greatest diameter
T3	Tumor is more than 4 cm in greatest diameter
T4	Tumor invades adjacent structures (e.g., through cortical bone, soft tissues of the neck, or deep (extrinsic) muscles of the tongue)

---

skull base. Such large tumors may be difficult to differentiate from nasopharyngeal carcinomas that have spread inferiorly. However, extensive ATP lesions tend to invade and extend into the ipsilateral nasopharynx and masticator space, whereas nasopharyngeal carcinomas that extend inferiorly tend to diffusely involve the nasopharynx. ATP lesions may also spread anteriomedially along the superior constrictor muscle to involve the pterygomandibular raphe, and from there they continue to spread to the buccinator muscle, thereby mimicking the spread pattern of tumors arising in the retromolar trigone. Tongue base invasion may be present in large lesions and is most likely a result of inferior tumor growth along the palatoglossus muscle.[24-26]

The lymphatic drainage of ATP tumors is primarily to the submandibular and internal jugular nodes. However, because the lymphatic drainage is determined by the site of the tumor, a lesion spreading to the soft palate and above will acquire the drainage pattern of this area. The overall likelihood of positive nodes with ATP carcinomas at presentation is 45%, although the incidence is dependent on the stage of the disease as follows: T_1, 11%; T_2, 38%; T_3, 54%; and T_4, 68%.[24, 27] The likelihood of nodal involvement in a clinically negative neck (N0) is 10%; contralateral nodal involvement has been reported to occur in 5% of cases.[24]

Posterior Tonsillar Pillar

Isolated posterior tonsillar pillar (PTP) lesions are rare, and when present, they are usually small. Because the PTP is comprised of the palatopharyngeus muscle, these lesions may spread along the course of this muscle and its overlying mucosal fold. Superior extension may involve the soft palate, and inferior growth may involve the posterior aspect of the thyroid cartilage, the middle pharyngeal constrictor, and the pharyngoepiglottic fold.[24]

Although the primary lymphatic drainage is to the level II nodes, if these tumors spread posteriorly, they can involve the posterior pharyngeal wall and place the retropharygeal and spinal accessory nodal chains at risk.[24]

Tonsillar Fossa

Malignancies of the tonsillar fossa are believed to arise from the mucosa lining the niche between the ATP and PTP, or from remnants of the palatine tonsil (Fig. 8-18).[24] Tumors in this location often are clinically occult and present with cervical nodal metastases. Given the location, these lesions may spread anteriorly or posteriorly to involve the adjacent tonsillar pillars, thereby acquiring the potential spread patterns associated with these sites. These lesions may also extend deeply and invade the superior constrictor muscle, and once they have done so, they may gain access to the paraphayrngeal space and extend to the skull base.[24-26]

The primary lymphatic drainage for the tonsillar fossa is to the internal jugular chain, although the spinal accessory chain and posterior submandibular nodes are also at risk. Tumors arising within the tonsillar fossa have an overall 76% chance of having clinically positive nodal metastases.

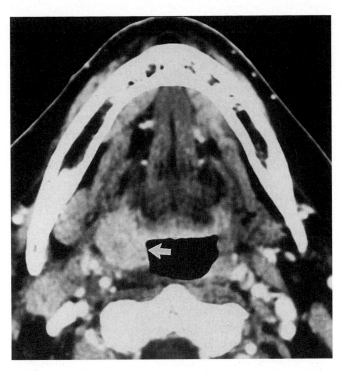

FIG. 8-18 Axial contrast-enhanced CT demonstrates the typical appearance of a squamous cell carcinoma located in the right tonsillar fossa *(arrow)*.

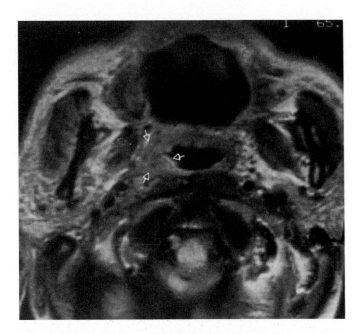

FIG. 8-19 Squamous cell carcinoma of right tonsil. Axial T1W MRI sequence through oropharynx demonstrates soft-tissue mass involving right pharyngeal wall and tonsil *(arrows)*.

Specifically the likelihood of having clinically positive nodes for tonsillar fossa tumors are as follows: T_1, 71%; T_2, 68%; T_3, 70%; and T_4, 89%.[27] The incidence of involved contralateral nodes is 11% and increases if the lesion invades the tongue base or spreads across the midline of the soft palate.[24,25]

Soft Palate

The majority of soft palate malignancies are SCCA (Fig. 8-19); however, minor salivary gland cancers also have their highest frequency in the posterior soft palate. Carcinomas of the palate usually affect the oral aspect, tend to be well differentiated, and have the best prognosis of all of the oropharyngeal carcinomas. The nasopharyngeal side of the soft palate is rarely involved, even when the tumors are extensive. Although tumor extension of palatal cancer can occur in any direction, the tonsillar pillars and hard palate are usually affected first. Deep lateral invasion occurs along the levator or tensor veli palatini muscles and into the parapharyngeal space, nasopharynx, and base of the skull.

At the time of the diagnosis, lymphatic spread is present in 60% of patients with carcinoma of the palate. The incidence of cervical node metastases depends on the size of the primary lesion, with T1 carcinomas (less than 2 cm in diameter) having an 8% incidence, and T4 tumors (greater than 4 cm in diameter with invasion) have a 70% incidence. Palatal carcinomas drain first to the high internal jugular and subdigastric nodes, with subsequent involvement of the lower internal jugular chain or retropharyngeal nodes. Tumor extension up the greater and lesser palatine nerves

can occur, allowing spread into the pterygopalatine fossa and cavernous sinus. The treatment of palatal lesions depends on the stage of the disease. Advanced lesions such as T2 and T3 carcinomas are usually treated with both surgery and radiation to the primary tumor and cervical lymph nodes. However, because surgery requires a wide excision, there may be significant postoperative difficulty with phonation and swallowing.[28]

The CT findings of soft palate carcinomas depend on the size and extent of the lesion. Small lesions along the oral surface of the soft palate may appear as minimal fullness of the soft palate and may be best seen on direct clinical examination. Large lesions may cause unilateral fullness in the region of the tonsil and soft palate, and there may be invasion of the parapharyngeal space.[29] Direct coronal CT must be used to evaluate the soft and hard palates because these structures lie in the axial plane and therefore are poorly examined by axial CT. MRI is ideally suited to evaluate the palate in both the sagittal and coronal planes.[30] In general, T1W images suffice because T2W images provide little additional information. Because the palate has intrinsically high T1W signal intensity, probably caused by the mucous glands and fat that are abundantly present, tumors are usually easily identified because of their lower signal intensity.

Base of Tongue

The tongue base is defined as the area posterior to the circumvallate papilla, and it extends inferiorly to the vallecula. The tongue base contains varying amounts of lingual tonsil, and because of this, it is often difficult to diagnose small tumors on both CT and MRI. Superficial lesions detected by direct visualization may not be seen on imaging studies. In addition the fat planes, which are normally seen in areas such as the floor of the mouth and masticator space and which allow detection of subtle lesions, are not as evident in the base of the tongue. Rather this area consists mostly of dense musculature. Tongue base carcinomas are often clinically silent, and this is a common location of occult malignancies originating in the upper aerodigestive tract. Because of this, these lesions often have progressed to an advanced stage at the time of initial presentation.[24,25] On MRI the T2W images are most helpful to visualize the full extent of these lesions and specifically to help determine whether the tumor has crossed the midline. This is especially important if the patient is a candidate for partial glossectomy.

Malignancies of the tongue base often are limited to one side of the tongue, crossing the midline only when the tumor becomes large. These tumors may also spread to the tonsillar pillar, pharyngeal wall, submucosally under the valleculae into the supraglottic larynx (Fig. 8-20) or anteriorly into the sublingual space (Fig. 8-21).[24] Lesions may also grow inferiorly and laterally to spread into the deep soft tissues of the neck, eventually involving the styloid musculature and the internal carotid artery.[24,25]

The tongue base has a rich lymphatic network with a significant amount of cross-drainage, explaining why nearly 30% of patients have bilateral cervical metastases at initial presentation.[24, 27] The primary lymphatic drainage sites are the internal jugular nodes and to a lesser degree the spinal accessory nodes. Tumor spread to the floor of mouth may also involve the submandibular nodes. Overall, 75% of patients will have positive nodes on clinical examination. When analyzed by tumor stage, the incidence of clinically positive nodes is as follows: T_1, 70%; T_2, 70%; T_3 = 75%; and T_4, 84%.[27] Presumably because of the rich lingual lymphatic network and the often advanced stage at which these tumors are discovered, there is a high incidence (nearly 60%) of nodal metastases in clinically negative necks.[24, 31] In these cases the cervical nodes must be carefully scrutinized on CT or MRI because the identification of clinically occult nodal disease will alter treatment.

Lymphomas
Clinical Features

Lymphoma is the most common lymphoproliferative disorder occurring in the extracranial head and neck.[32] Hodgkin's disease (HD) is a malignancy of the hematopoietic system that predominantly affects adolescents and young adults, with males being affected more frequently than females (2:1). The diagnosis of HD is stongly suggested by the presence of Reed-Sternberg cells on a nodal biopsy. Although extranodal primary sites are unusual, systemic involvement may result from disease progression. The commonly affected organs include the liver, spleen, lungs, bone, and bone marrow. The most common extranodal site is the spleen, and hepatic involvement usually occurs in the presence of splenic disease. Bone marrow involvement is believed to result from hematogenous spread, whereas pulmonary involvement is thought to be secondary to direct extension from hilar and mediastinal lymph nodes.[32, 33] The region of Waldeyer's ring is often uninvolved in patients with HD.

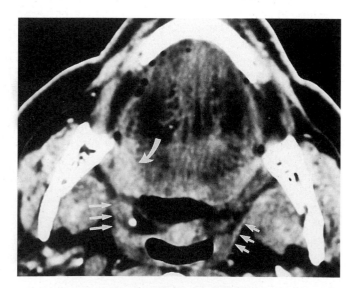

FIG. 8-20   Axial contrast-enhanced CT obtained through the oropharynx demonstrates carcinoma of the tongue base (large curved arrow) extending posteriorly along the superior constrictor muscle (large straight arrows). Compare the involved superior constrictor muscle with its normal appearance seen on the uninvolved left side (small straight arrows).

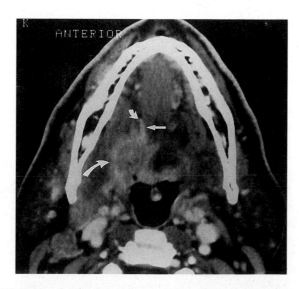

FIG. 8-21   Axial contrast-enhanced CT shows the characteristic appearance of a tongue base carcinoma (large curved arrow). There is extension into the floor of the mouth (small straight arrow), with infiltration and obliteration of the fat surrounding the lingual vessels (small curved arrow), suggesting perineural or perivascular invasion of tumor. This was confirmed at histologic examination of the resected specimen.

Non-Hodgkin's lymphoma (NHL) is most commonly seen in an older age group than in patients with HD, and males are more commonly affected than females. Predisposing conditions include various congenital and acquired immunodeficiency states. There are a variety of classifications that categorize NHL. The most commonly used classification systems are the Rappaport, and the Lukes and Collins. The former system is based on the resemblance of the various types of malignant cells to their benign counterparts, whereas the latter system is based on immunologic markers that separate the cell types into B-cell, T-cell, and histiocytic. Unfortunately, the majority of patients with NHL

have advanced disease at time of presentation. Whereas 98% of HD presents as nodal disease, 60% of NHL presents in extranodal sites, and 60% of all extranodal presentations occur the head and neck.[34] Extranodal areas predisposed for developing lymphoma are those areas normally rich in lymphoid tissue such as Waldeyer's ring. Other primary sites in the extracranial head and neck include the parotid gland (15% of patients have a prior history of Sjögren's syndrome), palate, gingiva, lacrimal gland, eyelid, conjunctiva, and paranasal sinuses.[32]

Typically, patient's with HD present with a painless mass, or complain of sytemic symptoms such as night sweats, fever, and weight loss. The clinical symptoms of patients with extranodal NHL often mimic those of patients with SCCA arising at the same site. Thus patients with lymphoma arising in the nasopharynx may present with nasal obstruction or unilateral serous otitis media, whereas patients with tonsillar or tongue base lymphoma complain of unilateral sore throat, dysphagia, or other obstructive symptoms. Nodal involvement is present in 80% of patients with NHL who present with extranodal primary lesions.[32]

The treatment of HD and NHL must be individualized and depends on the stage of disease and histologic type. Potential treatment modalities include radiation therapy, chemotherapy, and occasionally surgery for a localized extranodal NHL site.[32]

Imaging Findings

The imaging findings of extranodal head and neck lymphomas are essentially indistinguishable from those of the more common SCCA. The diagnosis may be suggested if

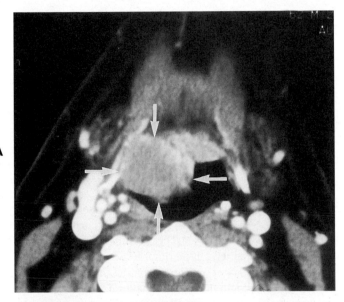

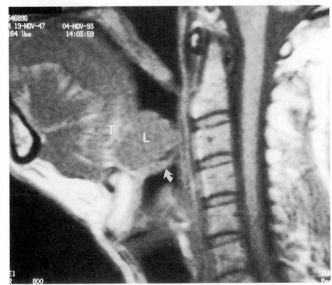

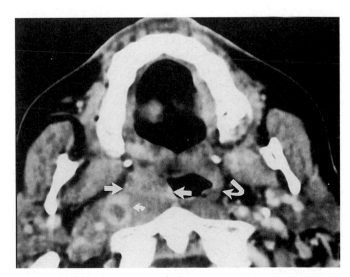

FIG. 8-22 A, Axial contrast-enhanced CT obtained through the base of tongue shows an exophytic soft-tissue mass *(arrows)* bulging into the right valeculla. Histologic examination showed non-Hodgkins lymphoma. **B,** Sagittal T1W MRI demonstrates a primary lymphoma *(L)* arising within the lingual tonsil. Note how the mass is situated anterior to the epiglottis *(curved arrow)* and posterior to the tongue base *(T).*

FIG. 8-23 Axial contrast-enhanced CT shows an aggressive lesion growing along the right pharyngeal wall and the superior constrictor muscle, located at the junction of the right tonsil and soft palate *(straight arrows).* Compare the tumor with the normal appearance on the uninvolved left side *(large curved arrow).* Note the involved retropharyngeal lymph node *(small curved arrow).* Biopsy showed a non-Hodgkin's lymphoma.

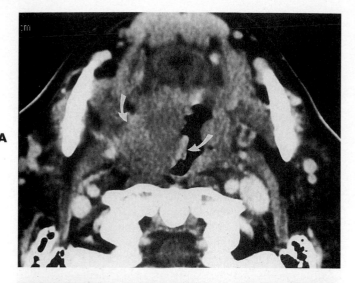

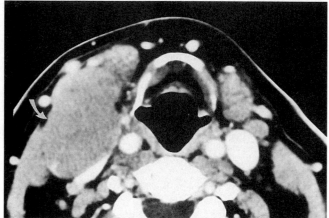

FIG. 8-24 A, Axial contrast-enhanced CT shows a large mass located within the right tonsillar fossa *(arrows)*. The radiographic appearance of this lesion is nonspecific and is most commonly caused by squamous cell carcinoma. The exophytic component of this lesion is suggestive of primary tonsillar lymphoma. Biopsy showed non-Hodgkin's lymphoma. B, This patient also had a palpable right neck mass. Axial CT shows an enlarged homgeneously enhancing lymph node *(arrow)*, which is typical of a lymphomatous lymph node. This appearance, however, is not pathognomic, because it may be mimicked by metastatic moderate to poorly differentiated squamous cell carcimonas.

the pharyngeal lesion is associated with large, homogeneously enhancing lymph nodes that do not have central necrosis. However, this combination of findings may also be seen in poorly differentiated SCCA. As mentioned, the high concentration of lymphoid tissue in the tongue base and palatine tonsil make these areas likely sites for developing lymphoma (Figs. 8-22 to 8-25). Large lesions may infiltrate the deep spaces and radiographically mimick advanced SCCA (Fig. 8-26). Primary nasopharyngeal lesions may also invade the skull base and spread along nerves in a manner similar to SCCA. Ultimately the diagnosis of lymphoma and the other lymphoproliferative disorders is made by histologic examination.

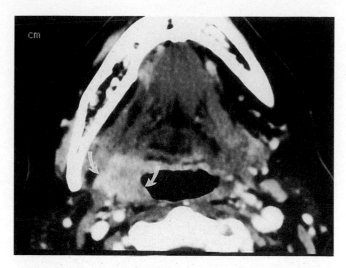

FIG. 8-25 Axial contrast-enhanced CT shows an enhancing mass centered within the right palatine tonsil *(arrows)*. Histologic examination of this lesion was consistent with pseudotumor.

Minor Salivary Gland Tumors
Clinical Features

Minor salivary gland tumors (MSGT) are unusual lesions that account for 2% to 3% of all malignancies of the extracranial head and neck.[35] These tumors most commonly occur in adults, and there is no reported sex prediliction. The MSGT include adenoid cystic carcinoma, mucoepidermoid carcinoma, adenocarcinoma, malignant mixed tumor, acinic cell carcinoma, and pleomorphic adenoma. Approximately 50% of MSGT are malignant, with adenoid cystic carcinoma being the likely histologic type.

The soft palate is the most common site of MSGT. In the soft palate the incidence of tumors of minor salivary gland origin is almost equal to that of SCCA. These tumors are usually off midline in the posterolateral portion of the soft palate, and they are not typically found anterior to a line drawn between the first upper molars.[35] These lesions may spread directly anteriorly to invade the hard palate (Fig. 8-27). Other extracranial sites include the lips, gingiva, buccal mucosa, tongue base, floor of the mouth, paranasal sinuses, nasal cavity, nasopharynx, trachea, and larynx (Figs. 8-28, 8-29).

Imaging Features

The radiographic findings of these tumors are nonspecific, and the diagnosis is based on endoscopy and biopsy. Although CT and MRI play complementary roles for evaluating patients with MSGT, the full extent of the tumor and any perineural spread is best evaluated with MRI. Bone invasion is best seen on CT, and both axial and coronal post-contrast (3 mm contiguous sections) should be taken through the palate. Intraoral films are also recommended for evaluating early bone erosion, if the lesion is adjacent to the lingual surface of the maxillary alveolar ridge.

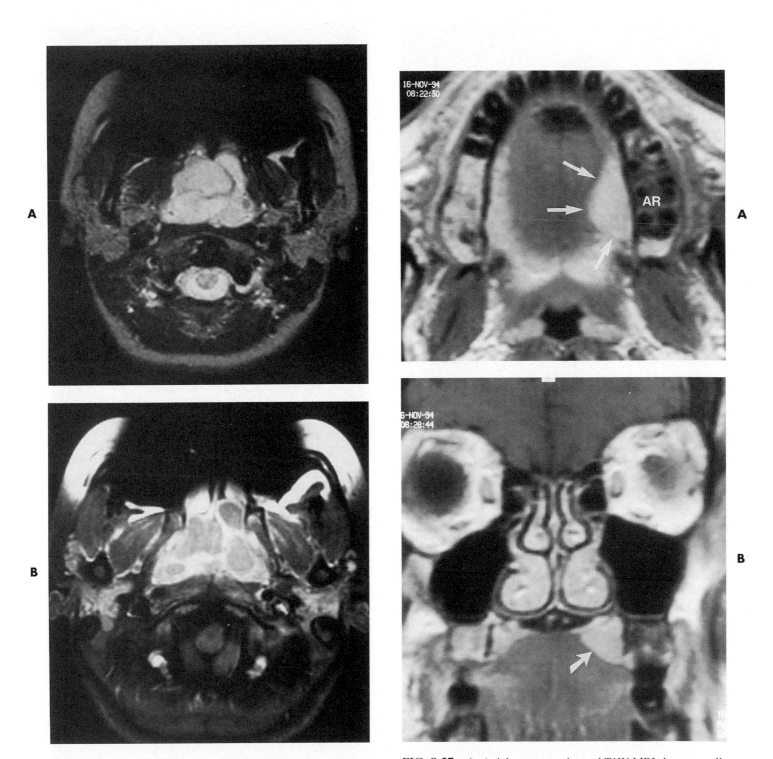

FIG. 8-26 Non-Hodgkin's lymphoma involving the nasopharynx in 14-year-old female with nasal stuffiness and bilateral conductive hearing loss. **A,** Axial T2W MRI sequence. Bulky mucosal mass of increased signal intensity is seen filling nasopharyngeal lumen. Note that there is no deep invasion of soft-tissue structures. **B,** T1W MRI sequence following gadolinium-DTPA. Peripheral enhancement is noted within mass. There is homogeneous appearance to mass without evidence of necrosis. Diagnosis is non-Hodgkins lymphoma.

FIG. 8-27 **A,** Axial contrast-enhanced T1W MRI shows a well-demarcated enhancing lymphoma *(arrows)* situated along the lateral aspect of the hard palate, which abuts the lingual surface of the maxillary alveolar ridge *(AR)*. **B,** Coronal T1W MRI demonstates the lesion situated on the lateral aspect of the hard palate *(arrow)*.

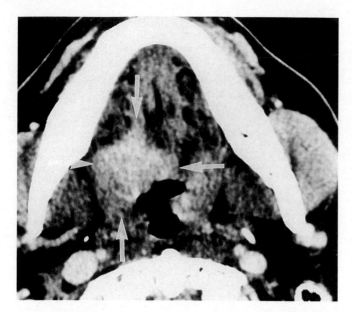

FIG. 8-28 Axial contrast-enhanced CT shows an aggressive mass *(arrows)* invading the right side of the tongue base with extension into the floor of mouth and pharyngeal wall. Biopsy showed a mucoepidermoid carcinoma.

Adenoid cystic carcinoma has a strong predilection to spread along perineural pathways, with such disease being diagnosed histologically in approximately 50% of cases. Continued tumor growth may eventually extend into the skull base and cavernous sinus, and, if unrecognized, it may cause treatment failure. To further complicate matters, perineural spread may occur with skip areas of intervening normal nerve. Recent investigations have suggested that this propensity for perineural spread may be due to the production of a substance that promotes adhesion to neural elements (neural cell adhesion molecule [N-CAM]).[36] The role of mutations in the genome that normally produces the suppressor protein p53, and the relationship to the recurrence of adenoid cystic carcinoma are also currently being investigated.[37] Because of these factors, close imaging attention must be paid to areas adjacent to the tumor that are rich in neurovasculature. This is especially true of lesions that arise in the soft palate because of their proximity to the pterygopalantine fossa. Obliteration of the fat in this fossa or erosion or asymmetrical enlargement of the greater and lesser palantine foramina are highly suggestive findings of perineural tumor spread (Fig. 8-30).

In the oropharynx the risk of nodal involvement is directly related to the size, grade, and location of the primary lesion. The likelihood of cervical metastasis increases in sites that are rich in lymphatic drainage, and the chance of nodal metastasis for nasopharyngeal and oropharyngeal tumors is nearly eight times greater (59% vs. 7%) than for tumors arising in the paranasal sinuses.[35] Thus imaging should always include the entire neck, if such potential nodal metastases are to be identified.

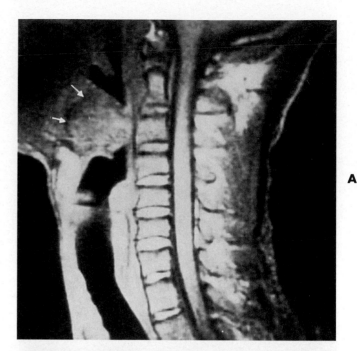

A

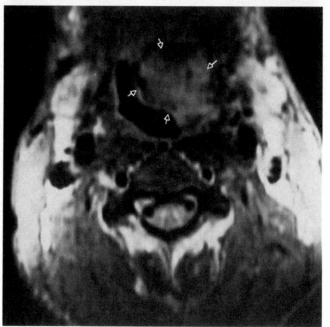

B

FIG. 8-29 Benign mixed cell tumor of tongue base. 38-year-old male presented with dysphasia. **A,** Sagittal T1W MR image. Homogeneous mass fills vallecula and indents base of tongue *(arrows)*. **B,** Proton density axial MRI through tongue base. Mass demonstrates intermediate-signal intensity *(arrows)*. Appearance is nonspecific. On biospy this proved to be benign mixed cell tumor.

Rhabdomyosarcomas

Rhabdomyosarcomas are rare mesenchymal malignant tumors found throughout the body.[38,39] About 30% of these tumors involve the head and neck, with the orbit and nasopharynx being the most frequently involved sites, followed by the paranasal sinuses and the middle ear. These

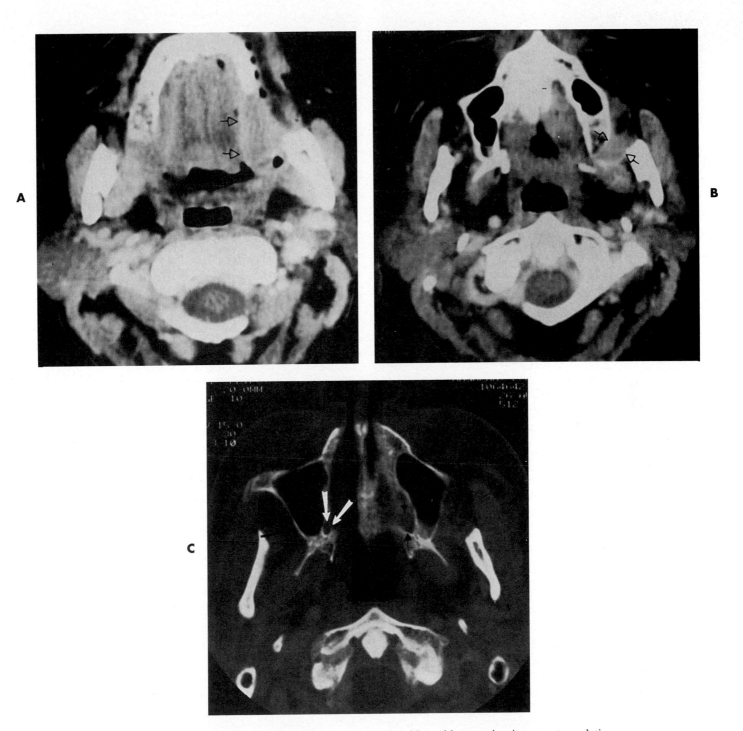

FIG. 8-30   Adenoid cystic carcinoma in left alveolar ridge with extension into greater palatine foramen. **A,** CT scan through upper oropharynx demonstrates subtle isointense mass involving left superior alveolar ridge *(arrows)*. **B,** Axial CT scan at higher level than **A** demonstrates extension of mass through buccinator space *(arrows),* a common finding in patients with lateral palate carcinoma. **C,** Bone window at level of hard palate demonstrates expansion of greater palatine foramen *(black arrows).* Normal greater palatine foramen is seen on right *(white arrow).* Extension up greater palatine foramen is common with palatal carcinomas. This may extend upward to pterygopalatine fossa and into cavernous sinus.

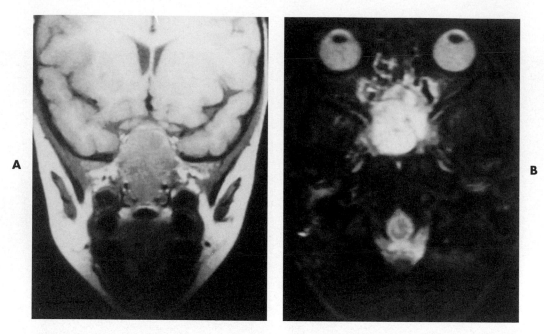

FIG. 8-31 Six-year-old female with rhabdomyosarcoma of nasopharynx invading skull base and sphenoid sinus. **A,** Coronal T1W MRI demonstrates mass extending into sphenoid sinus and posterior ethmoid air cells. Mass extends upward to involve planum sphenoidale. **B,** Axial, T2W MRI sequence demonstrates diffuse homogeneous increased signal intensity. Intensity is nonspecific. Rhabdomyosarcoma must be included in differential diagnosis along with nasopharyngeal lymphoma and squamous carcinoma in young patient with nasopharyngeal mass.

tumors occur primarily in young children, but they may occur in adolescents and rarely present in adults.[40] The tumor is thought to arise from rhabdomyoblasts within the muscles of the nasopharynx, and the initial symptoms may be abrupt or insidious, depending on the location of the tumor. Nasopharyngeal rhabdomyosarcomas usually present with rhinorrhea, sore throat, and serous otitis media. Invasion of the skull base is common and often produces a cavernous sinus syndrome. Local recurrence and distant metastases are also common. Combined therapeutic regimens with chemotherapy, radiation therapy, and surgery have improved response rates to more than 60% to 70%.[41] The 5-year survival rate after recurrence is less than 5%. On CT, nasopharyngeal rhabdomyosarcoma appears as an infiltrating soft-tissue mass that produces destruction of the skull base and posterior maxillary sinus.[42] The MRI features of rhabdomyosarcoma are also similar to SCCA (Fig. 8-31); however, rhabdomyosarcomas are primarily submucosal tumors, and they show a variable amount of enhancement following contrast administration. In children, malignant tumors that may mimic rhabdomyosarcomas of the nasopharymx include neuroblastoma and rhabdoid tumor (Fig. 8-32).

Granular Cell Tumors
Clinical Features

Granular cell tumors (GCT) are unusual benign neoplasms that can be found throughout the body.[1] They occur most often in the fourth decade of life, and they are more common in females than males (2:1) and in African Americans than Caucasians (5:1). Multiple GCT occur in approximately 4% to 10% of patients.

Of GCT, 50% occur within the tongue and approximately 30% arise in the skin. The remaining GCT are seen in the breast, muscle, bronchi, temporal bone, and other areas of the upper respiratory and digestive tract.[43] Most of the GCT found in the upper aerodigestive tract are intraluminal and solitary; however, synchronous lesions do occur and, when present, tend to behave more aggressively.[44] When these lesions occur in the larynx, the most common location is the posterior aspect of the true vocal cords, although GCT have been reported in the subglottic and supraglottic larynx.[44]

GCT of the upper aerodigestive tract occur in two forms. One type occurs in the gingiva of newborns and has been termed congenital epulis. The second type occurs later in life, arises predominately within the submucosa of the upper respiratory and digestive tract, and is referred to as GCT. Although these lesions are similar histologically, the latter form is considered a separate diagnostic entity because of its unique location and the age of the patients.

The histogenesis of GCT is controversial, and this has lead to a diversity of terms including Abrikosov's tumor, congenital epulis, nonchromaffin paraganglioma, granular cell myoblastoma, granular cell neurofibroma, myoblastic myoma, uniform myoblastoma, and embryonal rhabydomyoblastoma.[44] GCT is now believed to be of primitive neuroectodermal origin, and the term *granular cell tumor* is thought to be most appropriate.

Histologically this tumor has a characteristic appearance. Its cells are polymorphic, ranging from a definite polyhedral

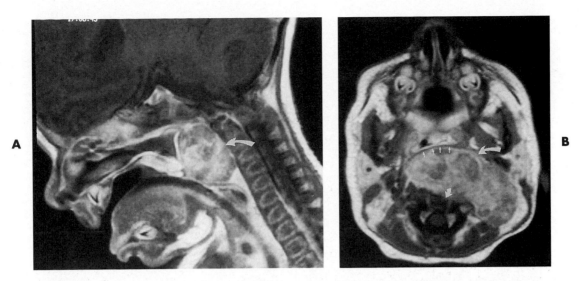

FIG. 8-32 **A,** Contrast-enhanced sagittal T1W MRI demonstrates a large heterogenous mass *(curved arrow)* in the posterior aspect of the nasopharynx. Biopsy showed a rhabdoid tumor. **B,** Axial image shows that the mass *(large curved arrow)* extends into the lateral compartment of the neck. There is erosion of the anterior portion of the vertebral body *(small curved arrow)* and anterior displacement of the posterior pharyngeal wall *(small straight arrows).*

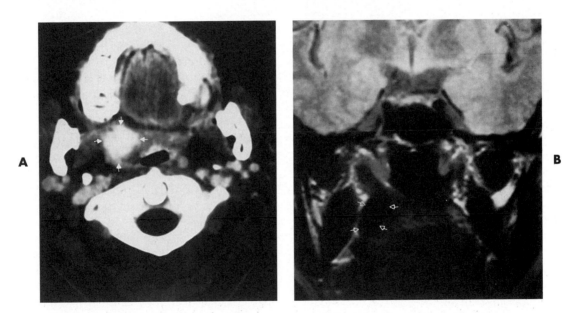

FIG. 8-33 Granular cell of right tonsillar pillar. **A,** Contrast-enhanced axial CT scan demonstrates enhancing mass, which involves right tonsil *(arrows).* **B,** Coronal proton density MR. Mass has decreased signal intensity *(arrows).* This is typical for carcinoma. Low signal is reflection of fibrotic elements within granular cell myoblastoma. (**A** and **B** courtesy Dr. H. Ric Harnsberger, University of Utah.)

shape to a bizarre spindle form, and mitoses are uncommon.[45] The tumor cells are embedded in variable amounts of connective or reticular tissue, and they may extend into the adjacent fibrous stroma. GCT are often circumscribed but not encapsulated.

Imaging Features

The imaging features of a laryngeal lesion are thought to be typical of this lesion occurring anywhere in the upper aerodigestive tract. On MRI, GCT have a slightly low T1W signal intensity, and they homogeneously enhance. On T2W images they may have either increased or decreased signal intensity. On CT these lesions are solid and relatively homogeneously enhancing (Fig. 8-33). Radiographically, GCT may mimic a primary SCCA.

Other Tumors
Rhabdomyomas

Rhabdomyomas are rare benign skeletal tumors that have a predilection for the head and neck. Whereas cardiac rhabdomyomas affect patients with tuberous sclerosis, extracardiac rhabdomyomas have no relationship to this syndrome.

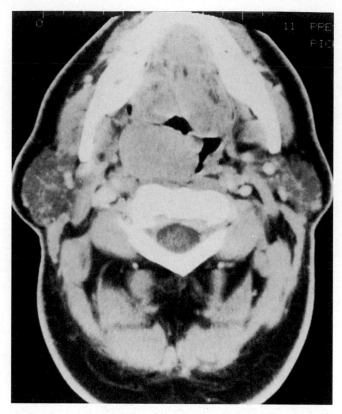

FIG. 8-34 Rhabdomyoma of posterior pharyngeal wall. Contrast-enhanced axial CT scan demonstrates well-circumscribed mass of muscular intensity involving posterior right lateral wall of pharynx. Note sharp interface with surrounding parapharyngeal space, tongue, and prevertebral muscles. Biospy proved this to be benign rhabdomyoma.

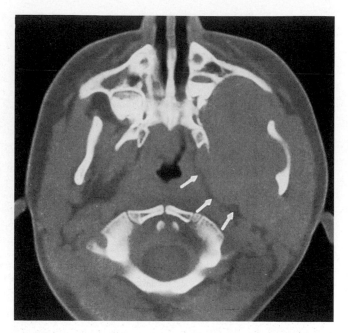

FIG. 8-35 Masticator space mass in a 6-year-old patient with aggressive fibromatosis of masticator space with deviation of left mandible and left maxillary sinuses. This mass compresses parapharyngeal space posteriorly and medially (arrows). This deviation is typical of masticator space masses.

Affected regions include the oropharynx, nasopharynx, larynx, and submandibular triangle. On CT and MRI the tumors are well circumscribed with a density or intensity similar to that of muscle.

A subgroup of rhabdomyomas occur in newborns and children less than 3 years of age. These so-called fetal rhabdomyomas may actually be hamartomatous malformations rather than true neoplasms (Fig. 8-34).[46]

Fibromatoses

Fibrous lesions of the head and neck vary in their biologic activity and histologic appearance. Even though in some cases their histologic appearance is benign, they may be so locally aggressive that they are considered to be low-grade fibrosarcomas. The term desmoid has also been applied to a subgroup of these lesions, which present as well-differentiated but locally infiltrating fibrous masses near the musculoaponeurotic junctions. Of desmoids, 12% involve the region of the head and neck, most commonly the soft tissues of the supraclavicular region and face.[47] Involvement of the oral cavity or nasopharynx is rare in adults, and the CT findings of the fibromatoses are nonspecific. Desmoids involving the head and neck usually encase and infiltrate the

musculature of the supraclavicular region. They may infiltrate fat planes, and on CT they cannot be differentiated from malignant lesions (Fig. 8-35).

Schwannomas and Neurofibromas

Of all schwannomas, 25% are located in the head and neck region, and most involve the cranial nerves. The tongue, palate, and floor of the mouth are the most frequent sites in the oral cavity. Most schwannomas are diagnosed in the second and third decades of life as asymptomatic enlarging masses. On CT they are solitary, ovoid, well-encapsulated masses.[48] Small lesions are usually homogeneous, whereas focal cystic areas are often present in larger masses. These tumors enhance well, despite the fact that they are relatively hypovascular.[48] On MRI, schwannomas have low T1W and high T2W signal intensity, and they enhance with contrast. Neurofibromas of the oral cavity are rare lesions, which are usually associated with von Recklinghausen's syndrome.[49] The tongue is the most frequent oral region affected, and unilateral macroglossia is a characteristic finding (Fig. 8-36).

Hemangiomas

In children, hemangiomas are the most common tumor in the cervical region. They may involve the oropharynx or face, usually as a sessile reddish submucosal mass near the base of the tongue. The cavernous type is most common. CT demonstrates a mass of muscle intensity that may or may not enhance. If present, phleboliths are diagnostic. MRI demonstrates an infiltrative mass of low T1W and high T2W signal intensity (Fig 8-37).[50]

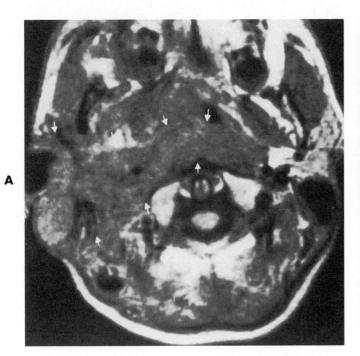

A

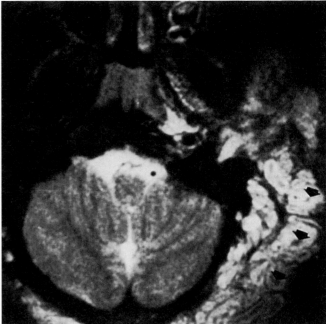

B

FIG. 8-36   Two different patients with neurofibromatosis involving nasopharynx. **A,** Axial T1W MR images through nasopharynx of 16-year-old demonstrates invasive mass that diffusely involves nasopharynx, retropharyngeal space, and carotid space. Mass is homogeneous and infiltrates throughout these spaces, as well as throughout subcutaneous tissue *(arrows)*. **B,** Axial T2W MRI view of upper nasopharynx in another patient with neurofibromatosis. Plexiform neurofibroma involves subcutaneous tissues, as well as parotid and carotid spaces. Note punctate areas of focal hypointensity in centers of these neurofibromas characteristic of neurofibromatosis *(arrows)*. Hypointensity relates to fibrosis at center of neurofibroma.

Unknown Primary Tumors
Clinical Features

Patients with SCCA of the upper aerodigestive tract frequently present with cervical metastases.[51] The majority of these patients have an identifiable primary tumor. However, about 10% of patients have no visible lesion, even following careful endoscopy and multiple blind biopsies. The diagnosis of metastatic SCCA is established by needle biopsy of the cervical adenopathy. These patients are considered to have an unknown primary tumor of the upper aerodigestive tract.

Treatment of patients believed to have an occult malignancy of the upper digestive tract varies from institution to institution. Most physicians favor wide-field external beam radiation to the nasopharynx, tonsil, tongue base, and pyriform sinus.[51, 52] Other physicians favor a more conservative approach consisting of a unilateral neck dissection and close observation to eventually identify a primary site.[53]

Identifying a primary cancer in a patient thought to have an occult or unknown tumor will alter the treatment plan. If the patient is to be treated with primary radiation, a wide-field radiation plan becomes more focused by applying a shrinking-field technique to the primary site. This change potentially increases the total dose delivered to the primary tumor from 5500 cGy to 7440 cGy.[51] The concomitant reduction of the volume of tissue irradiated may decrease

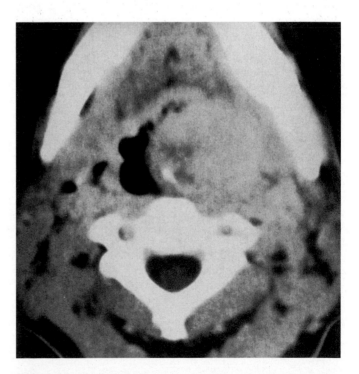

FIG. 8-37   Hemangioma of base of tongue. Axial CT scan following contrast administration in 6-year-old male demonstrates large base of tongue mass with focus of calcification. At resection this proved to be cavernous hemangioma.

both the acute and chronic complications associated with radiation therapy. Thus identification of a primary tumor site results in a higher and more localized tumor dose, reduces treatment morbidity, may increase local tumor control, and may lead to an increase in patient survival.

Detection of a clinically occult lesion is difficult for the otolaryngologist, radiation therapist, and radiologist. "Blind" endoscopic biopsies are often performed in locations known to be of high risk. Some centers perform an ipsilteral tonsilectomy, given the high incidence of occult lesions present in the palatine tonsil. Despite these efforts, the likelihood of detecting an occult lesion from such efforts is only 20%.[51] One thing that has become clear in recent years is that if imaging is to help identify such an unknown tumor, the imaging must be performed before any scoping or biopsy. If the imaging is performed before these clinical manipulations, any site of mucosal thickening is suspect of being a primary tumor and directed biopsies can be obtained. If imaging is performed after scoping, hemorrhage and edema in the pharyngeal wall lessen the sensivity of the study.

Imaging Findings

CT has been shown to be useful for detecting an unknown primary tumor and in experienced hands has a sensitivity of 37%.[54,55] To obtain the maximum information from CT, the study must be of high quality and be performed with 3 mm contiguous sections from the nasopharynx into the thoracic inlet. Involved spinal accessory nodes are suggestive of a nasopharyngeal lesion.[54] The presence of large necrotic nodes have been historically associated with clinically occult tonsilar tumors.[51] Bilateral upper cervical lymph nodes suggest a lesion within the nasopharynx, tongue base, soft palate, supraglottic larynx, or pyriform sinus.[51] The main role of CT is to focus the endoscopic evaluation and guide the otolaryngologist so that a larger biopsy may be obtained from suspicious areas, thus potentially increasing the diagnostic yield over the limited and "undirected" speculative biopsies. Special attention should be paid to areas of asymmetric fullness ipsilateral to the side of nodal involvement. The precise role of MRI for detecting occult lesions has not yet been determined.

Recently, imaging with 2-[F-18] fluoro-2-deoxy-D-glucose (FDG) has shown promise for detecting occult primary lesions of the upper aerodigestive tract.[54] Using FDG with a single photon emission computed tomography (SPECT) unit equipped with specially designed collimators, early experience suggests a sensitivity of 82% for detecting occult lesions (Fig. 8-38). However, larger series are necessary before any conclusions can be reached regarding the eventual role of such FDG imaging. It should be noted that the majority of detected tumors were located in the oropharynx, predominantly in the tonsil and tongue base, lending support for the concept of performing an ipsilateral tonsilectomy at time of endoscopy.[54] The fact that several lesions were present in the tongue base may also suggest that an increase in the depth and number of biopsies in this area may increase the rate of detection of these malignancies.

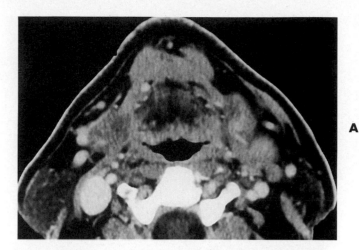

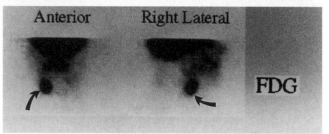

FIG. 8-38 **A,** Axial CT from a contrast enhance study demonstrates a normal-appearing tongue base. **B,** FDG images show a focus of abnormal uptake in the tongue base (*arrows*). Biopsies of this area showed squamous cell carcinoma.

NONNEOPLASTIC PROCESSES
Retropharyngeal Infections
Clinical Features

A retropharyngeal space infection is a potentially life-threatening disease whose incidence has decreased in the antibiotic era. Historically these infections were believed to occur almost exclusively in children less than 6 years of age.[56] However, with the increase in the immunocompromised patient polulation, these infections have become more frequent in adults, being more common in males than in females (2:1). Infections involving the retropharyngeal space usually result from an infection at a site whose primary lymphatic drainage is to the retropharyngeal lymph nodes. These sites include the sinonasal tract, throat, tonsil, oral cavity, and middle ear. Retropharyngeal infections also can result secondary to a direct traumatic innoculation.[57, 58]

The anatomy of the retropharyngeal space is discussed in Chapter 13. It extends from the skull base to the level of the carina, and the contents of this space include fat and lymph nodes. The retropharyngeal lymph nodes are subdivided into lateral and medial groups.[59] The lateral group consists of one to three nodes situated just medial to the carotid sheath on the longus coli and longus capitus muscles behind the posterior pharyngeal wall. These lymph nodes usually extend from the skull base to the level of C3. The medial group is inconstant and is located near the midline. When present, these nodes are usually found at the level of the C2, although they may extend inferiorly as low as the vertebral body of C6. The afferent drainage of the retropharyngeal lymph nodes is from the nasopharynx, oropharynx, palate, nasal cavity, paranasal sinuses, middle ear, and eustachain tube, and the efferent drainage is to the high internal jugular nodes (level II).

The danger space is situated dorsal to the retropharyn-geal space. This space extends from the skull base to the level of the posterior diaphragm, and it is discussed in Chapter 13. Infections that involve the retropharyngeal space may enter the danger space and thus extend into the mediastinum.

Patients with retropharyngeal space infections often present with fever, chills, odynophagia, sore throat, dysphagia, nausea, vomiting, respiratory distress, and neck pain and stiffness; these symptoms may suggest meningitis. On physical examination the patient may be drooling and diaphoretic, and bulging of the posterior oropharyngeal wall is characteristic of infection involving the retropharyngeal space.

Historically a retropharyngeal space abscess was believed to be the ultimate result of efferent spread of infection to the retropharyngeal lymph nodes.[57] These nodes enlarged and underwent suppuration, eventually rupturing into the retropharyngeal space and creating an abscess. With the development of broad spectrum antibiotics, the evolution of this disease has been slowed so that it is diagnosed and treated at an earlier stage, often before the development of a frank retropharygeal abscess.

Today a true retropharyngeal abscess is often the result of penetrating trauma to the oropharynx or nasopharynx, caused by direct spread from an osteomyelitis or diskitis involving the cervical spine or as a complication of spinal surgery.[56] The treatment is surgical drainage, either by an intraoral or open procedure, depending on the size of the lesion and the clinical stability of the patient.

Currently, retropharygeal infections are often diagnosed before the formation of a true retropharyngeal abscess, and recent experience suggests that a retropharyngeal suppurative adenitis, diagnosed on either CT or MRI, may be successfully managed with antibiobitics without the need for surgical exploration and drainage.[60]

The ability to successfully medically manage a retropharyngeal abscess appears to be the result of both sectional imaging and the early use of effective antibiotic therapy. Historically, no more than 10% to 15% of these infections resolved with medical therapy alone. Recent reports suggest that 40% to 50% of patients can be successfully treated without surgical drainage.[56]

Imaging Features

The initial diagnostic evaluation of patients suspected of having retropharyngeal space infections usually consists of a lateral plain film of the neck, taken during quiet breathing. The presence of prevertebral swelling, loss of the normal cervical lordosis, and air in the prevertebral soft tissues are all findings suggestive of an underlying infection. However, the exact location and the extent of the process usually cannot be determined by plain films alone.

CT and MRI permit accurate localization of infections involving the deep neck and help distinguish between suppurative retropharyngeal adenitis with associated retropharyngeal space edema and a true retropharyngeal abcess. CT is the preferred modality because of its high resolution, shorter scan times, lower costs, and overall better evaluation of nodal disease. The reduction in scan time with CT is especially advantageous in the pediatric population and may reduce or eliminate the need for sedation in infants and young children.

A retropharyngeal abscess appears as a low-attenuation mass with an enhancing capsule. These lesions are often associated with a significant mass effect, and the posterior pharyngeal wall may be quite ventrally displaced. Abcesses resulting from an adjacent diskitis are contiguous with the adjacent disk space and are associated with erosion of the neighboring vertebral body endplates (Fig. 8-39).

Suppurative retropharyngeal adenitis is charaterized by an enlarged retropharyngeal lymph node that contains a low-attenuation center (Fig. 8-40).[60] However, this low-attenuation center does not nesessarily imply the presence of pus because the same CT appearance is present in lymph nodes containing early liquefaction (presuppurative phase) and in those that have undergone complete liquefaction necrosis (suppurative phase). Suppurative retropharyngeal adenitis is often associated with edema, which is characterized by a smooth expansion of the retropharyngeal space with "mucoid" density material (10 to 25 HU) without evidence of an enhancing rim.

Previous reports have shown that ultrasound may be used to differentiate solid lesions from complex fluid collections located within the retropharynx.[61] However, ultrasound is often unable to determine whether these collections are within enlarged lymph nodes or involve the entire retropharyngeal space. Because of this, if ultrasound is the only imaging modality, surgical intervention has been recommended in all of these cases. CT and MRI permit localization of areas of liquefaction and in most cases allow accurate differentiation between suppurative adenitis and a retropharyngeal abscess.

Peritonsillar Abscesses

Acute tonsillitis is usually a self-limited febrile disease of adolescents or young adults. The most common offending bacterial organisms include beta-hemolytic streptococcus, staphylococcus, pneumococcus, and hemophilus. Suppurative uncontrolled infection of the tonsils may result in a peritonsillar abscess (quinsy) or rarely in a tonsillar abscess. A peritonsillar abscess is an accumulation of pus around the palatine tonsils, and if this abscess extends outside the tonsillar fossa, it may involve the lateral retropharyngeal or parapharyngeal spaces. A severe sore throat and pharyngeal edema that progress despite antibiotic therapy are the usual clinical presentations of such an abscess. Trismus develops if the medial pterygoid muscle is involved.

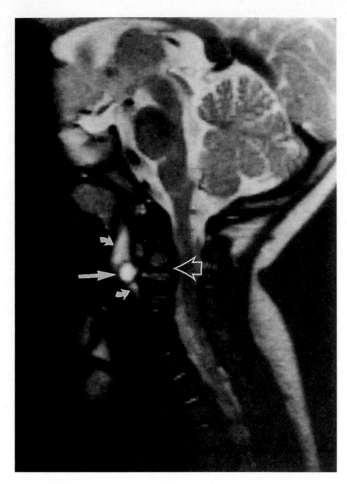

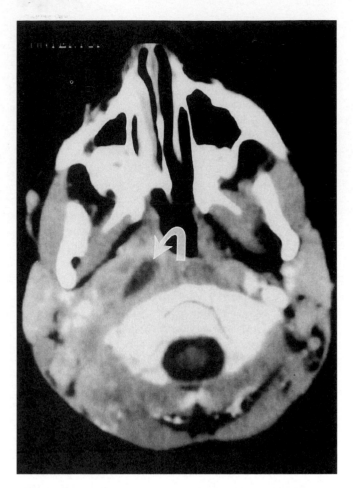

FIG. 8-39 Sagittal T2W MRI shows a fluid-containing mass *(solid straight arrow)* located within the retropharyngeal space with surrounding edema *(curved arrows)* consistent with a retropharyngeal space abscess. The abscess was secondary to a diskitis seen as a loss of height of the adjacent disk space *(open arrow)*. There was erosion of the endplates of the adjacent vertebral bodies on CT (not shown).

FIG. 8-40 Axial contrast-enhanced CT demonstrates an oval-shaped, low-attenuation lesion *(arrow)* in the expected location of a lateral retropharyngeal lymph node. This is the typical finding of a suppurative retropharyngeal adenitis.

On CT the appearance of acute or chronic tonsillitis is nonspecific. There is a focal homogeneous swelling of the palatine tonsil that may simulate a tumor. The inflammatory process may extend laterally into the parapharyngeal space, medial pterygoid muscle, and soft palate, and if mature, the peritonsillar or tonsillar abscess has a low-density center surrounded by an enhanced rim. The abscess may extend from the tonsillar bed superiorly into the retropharyngeal space or inferiorly into the submandibular space (Fig. 8-41).[62]

Tornwaldt's Cysts
Clinical Features

Tornwaldt's cyst is a benign developmental lesion within the midline nasopharynx. Its incidence at autopsy is 4%, the peak age of incidence is 15 to 30 years, and there is no sex predilection. The development of Tornwaldt's cyst is related to the embryogenesis of the notochord. In the early embyo, before the notochord reaches the prechordal plate, it descends and comes into contact with the endoderm of the primitive phar-

ynx. At this level, a small outpouching of the pharyngeal mucosa develops, directed toward the brain. This is called *Seessel's pouch,* and it contributes to the preoral gut.[7] If a focal adhesion develops between the notochord and this endoderm, when the notocord ascends back to the level of the developing skull base, a small portion of the nasopharyngeal mucosa is carried along it. This results in the creation of midline diverticulum that in the adult is lined by normal pharyngeal mucosa. When the patient develops a pharyngitis, the orifice of this diverticulum swells and closes and a cyst is formed. The cyst contents typically have a high protein content and are infected with anaerobic bacteria. In this state these Tornwaldt's cysts are usually asymptomatic, incidental imaging findings. Periodically the pressure within the cysts increases and overcomes the relative stenosis at the orifice. This releases anaerobic secretions into the nasopharynx, and the patient complains of periodic halitosis. Asymptomatic cysts require no treatment, but symptomatic lesions are drained via an intraoral approach.

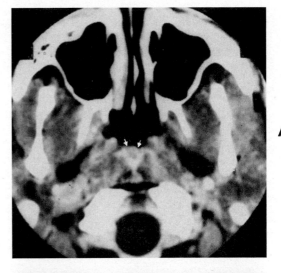

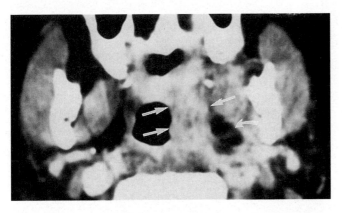

FIG. 8-41 Axial CT obtained through the level of the soft palate shows diffuse enhancement and thickening of the left tonsil *(straight arrows)* associated with a fluid collection within the left parapharyngeal space *(curved arrow)*. This was a peritonsillar abscess.

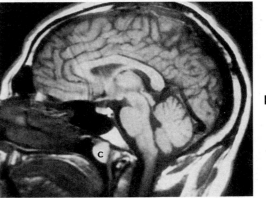

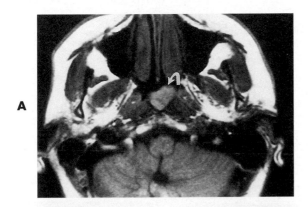

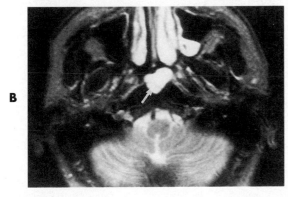

FIG. 8-42 **A,** Axial T1W noncontrast MR shows a well-delineated lesion *(arrow)* with increased signal intensity located within the nasopharynx. This was a Tornwaldt's cyst. **B,** There is increased signal within the lesion on the T2W sequence, which is consistent with the cystic nature of the mass. Note the internal septation present within the lesion *(arrow)*.

FIG. 8-43 Tornwaldt's cyst. **A,** CT scan through upper nasopharynx demonstrates midline Tornwaldt's cyst *(arrows)*. Note that its density is similar to surrounding muscle. High density of this cyst is probably related to high-protein concentration. **B,** Sagittal T1W MRI scan through upper nasopharynx demonstrates high signal intensity Tornwaldt's cyst *(c)*. High intensity is due to high-protein concentration within cyst. This shortens T1 relaxation time sufficiently to produce increase in intensity on T1W images.

Imaging Features

On MRI Tornwaldt's cyst appears as a well-delineated, thin-walled, midline cystic lesion that usually varies between 2 and 10 mm in diameter. The signal characteristics vary as does the protein content of the cyst. The T1W weighted signal intensity can be either low or high, and the T2W signal intensity is high (Fig. 8-42). There usually is no enhance-ment with contrast. On CT these cysts present as midline nasopharygeal cysts, usually of a mucoid attenuation. If the cyst contains a high-protein content, the resulting increased density may, on occasion mimic a soft-tissue mass (Fig. 8-43). In patients with prominent adenoids these cysts may be difficult to identify.

Adenoidal Hypertrophies

Adenoids, or nasopharyngeal tonsils, are located in the roof of the nasopharynx. They start to become prominent by age 2 to 3 years, often filling the entire nasopharynx and extending into the posterior choanae. Regression starts in early adolescence and continues into later life. Most people have little if any identifiable adenoidal tissue by age 30 to 40 years. However, normal adenoids can occasionally be identified in patients 50 to 60 years old. Conversely, if no adenoidal tissue is seen in a young child, the possibility of an immune deficiency syndrome should be considered. On CT,

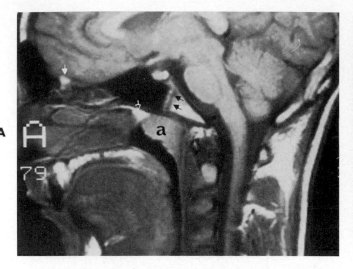
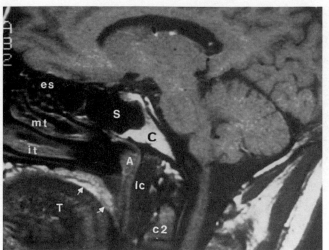

FIG. 8-44   **A,** Sagittal T1W MRI scan through the mid-oropharynx and nasopharynx. Note in this young individual, hypertrophied adenoidal tissue *(a)* occupying superior and lateral recesses of nasopharynx. Its signal intensity is slightly higher than that of surrounding muscle but much higher than that of fat. Also seen are elements of fatty marrow within crista galli *(closed white arrow)* and vomer bone *(open white arrow)*. Occipital sphenoid suture is hypointense line dividing midclivus *(black arrows)*. **B,** Parasagittal T1W MR images through lateral nasopharynx. Demonstrated here are longus colli muscles extending to skull base *(lc)* and lateral aspect of adenoidal tissue *(A)*. Fat and glandular elements within hard and soft palate *(white arrows)* exhibit high signal intensity. *T,* Tongue; *C,* clivus; *S,* sphenoid sinus; *es,* ethmoid sinus; *mt,* middle turbinate; *it,* inferior turbinate; *C2,* second cervical vertebrae.

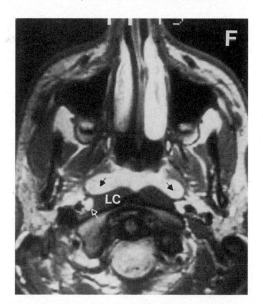

FIG. 8-45   Proton density axial view through nasopharynx demonstrates adenoidal tissue filling recesses of nasopharynx *(arrows)*. Notice sharp contrast between hyperintense adenoidal tissue and longus capitis-colli muscle *(LC)*. Also note reactive lateral retropharyngeal node *(open white arrow)* interposed between longus capitis muscle and internal carotid artery.

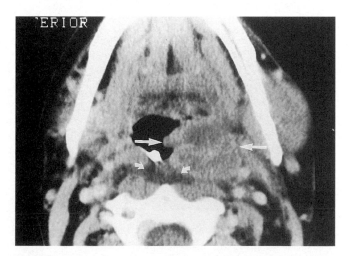

FIG. 8-46   Axial contrast-enhanced CT demonstrates a soft-tissue mass situated in the left tonsil *(straight arrows)* associated with edema in the retropharyngeal space *(curved arrows)*. The patient was involved in a motor vehicle accident and the lesion was due to a hematoma located within the tonsillar fossa.

adenoids appear as homogeneous, superficial soft tissue, filling the superior and upper lateral recesses of the nasopharynx. The adenoids have an attenuation similar to that of muscle, and small superficial cysts and calcifications are often present. After contrast, a thin enhancing line is seen along the deep surface of the adenoids. This mucosal

venous and pharyngobasilar enhancement should be present and intact because violation of this line indicates the presence of an aggressive mass in the nasopharyngeal roof. On MRI the adenoids have a T1W signal intensity similar to that of muscle; however, they have a high T2W signal intensity, distinguishing them from muscle (Figs. 8-44, 8-45).

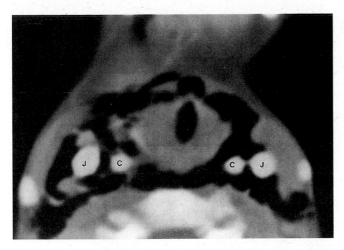

FIG. 8-47   Axial CT shows air dissecting along the fascial planes of the neck following a injury that perforated the posterior wall of the oropharynx. *c*, Carotid; *J*, jugular.

Unfortunately, the signal intensities of the adenoids are similar to those of lymphoma and most cellular tumors, and distinction between normal lymphoid tissue and tumor may be impossible on CT and MRI.[63] Endoscopy with biopsy is the only way to definitively make this distinction. Reactive cervical adenopathy often accompanies prominent adenoidal tissue in children, but it can also be seen in HIV-infected patients and in patients with nasopharyngeal lymphoma.

Trauma

Trauma affecting the oropharynx or nasopharynx is not nearly as common as that affecting the hyopharynx or larynx. Pharyngeal trauma may be due to blunt trauma such as that experienced in a motor vehicle accident and may result in mucosal and retropharyngeal hematoma formation (Fig. 8-46). Penetrating trauma can cause perforation of the pharyngeal wall, resulting in a direct communication between the oral cavity and the retropharyngeal space. Persistent communication results in large amounts of air tracking throughout the deep fascial planes (Fig. 8-47). This communication provides a direct route for spread of organisms that normally colonize the oral cavity to enter the deep neck and place the patient at high risk for developing a retropharyngeal abscess, fascitis, and even mediastinitis.

POSTTREATMENT PHARYNX
Radiation Therapy

Radiation therapy (RT) has proven to be an effective modality for the treatment of a variety of laryngeal and pharyngeal carcinomas, with local control rates similar to that achieved with surgery.[64-68] RT is being given to patients in whom RT is the preferred treatment, as well as patients who refuse surgery or who are poor surgical candidates because of underlying medical conditions.

Histologically, RT results in an acute inflammatory reaction within the deep connective tissues, which is characterized by leukocytic infiltration, histiocyte formation, necro-

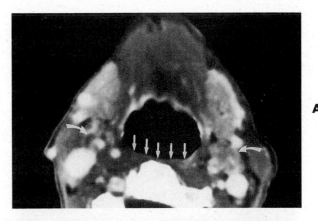
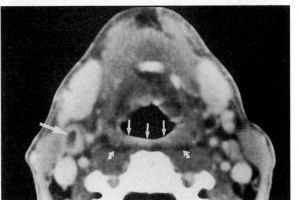
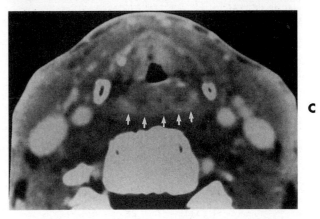

FIG. 8-48   **A,** Axial contast-enhanced CT performed before the initiation of RT demonstrates the normal appearance of the posterior wall of the oropharynx *(straight arrows)*. Note the abnormal level II lymph nodes present on both sides *(curved arrows)*. **B,** Following completion of RT, there is thickening of the posterior wall of the oropharynx *(small straight arrows)* and retropharyngeal space edema *(curved arrows)*. Note the reduction in size of the node in the left neck, but the persistence of a low attenuation lymph node in the right neck *(large straight arrow)*. **C,** More inferiorly there is enhancement of the pharyngeal mucosa *(arrows)* resulting from radiation-induced mucositis.

sis, and hemorrhage.[68-73] Detachment of the lining endothelial cells of small arteries, veins, and lymphatics causes increased permeability resulting in interstitial edema. Within 1 to 4 months after RT, there is deposition of rich collaginous

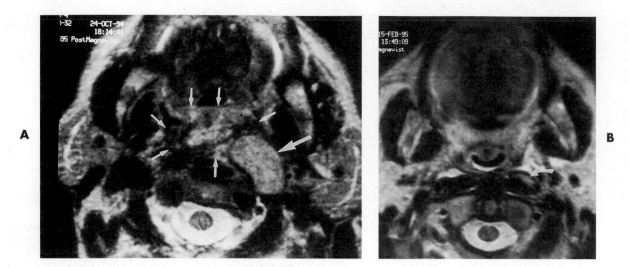

FIG. 8-49 A, Axial T2W MRI shows a tumor involving the posterior wall of the oropharynx *(arrows)* associated with an enlarged retropharyngeal lymph node *(large arrow).* **B,** Following completion of radiation therapy, there is marked reduction in the size of the primary tumor and the previously involved retropharyngeal lymph node *(curved arrow).* Biopsies from these areas were negative for residual disease.

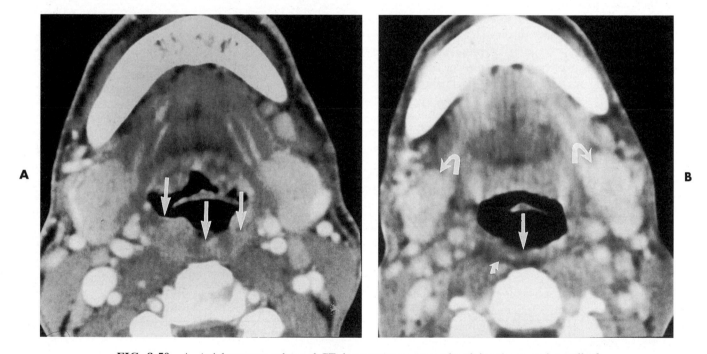

FIG. 8-50 A, Axial contrast-enhanced CT demonstrates a tumor involving the posterior wall of the oropharynx *(arrows)* with bilateral nodal disease. **B,** Following radiation therapy, there is a marked reduction in the size of the tumor with residual thickening of the posterior wall of the oropharynx *(straight arrow).* Retropharyngeal space edema *(small curved arrow)* and mild atrophy of the submandibular glands *(large curved arrows)* are normal changes resulting from radiation therapy.

fibers with sclerosis and hyalinosis of the connective tissues. This inflammatory process eventually results in the obstruction of small arteries, veins, and lymphatics. By 8 months, there is advanced sclerosis, hyalinosis, and fragmentation of the collagen fibers within the connective tissues. Eventually there may be a reduction in interstitial fluid resulting from the formation of collateral neocapillary and lymphatic channels.[69, 72] The extent of the observed changes in the area

included within the radiation port is mainly dependent on the total dose. More advanced and persistent changes may be seen in patients who continue to smoke after RT.

The pharynx is subjected to a high dose of radiation during definitive treatment of cancers and subsequently undergoes predictable changes that should not be confused with tumor. Pharyngeal changes resulting from RT include increased enhancement of the pharyngeal mucosa, which is thought to be due to the formation of telangiectatic vessels that may arise as a sequela of the radiation-induced mucositis.[72] The posterior pharyngeal wall typically thickens from a normal 2 to 3 mm to 6 to 7 mm in the post RT patient. Additionally, patients typically develop 3 to 5 mm of edema in the retropharyngeal space (Fig. 8-48). These reactive changes may persist for many months or years.[72]

As has been previously reported for laryngeal tumors, successfully treated pharyngeal tumors result in a reduction in primary lesion size (Fig. 8-49)[73]. However, the diffuse and residual changes occurring in the pharynx should not be confused with residual tumor (Fig. 8-50). Often this distinction is best made by comparing a present imaging study with a prior examination. Soft-tissue thickening caused by RT will not progressively enlarge, and any such progressive change should be suspected of representing tumor.

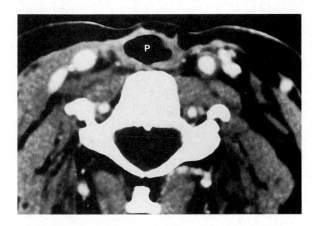

FIG. 8-51 Axial CT shows the normal appearance of the pharynx *(P)* following a total laryngectomy. Because the larynx has been removed, the pharynx is in a more anterior position and is typically situated just deep to the subcutaneous fat.

Surgery

A variety of surgical procedures are available for treatment of malignancies involving the upper aerodigestive tract. However, resection results in marked distortion of the underlying anatomy, making interpretation of postoperative imaging studies difficult. The postoperative pharyngeal wall is typically thin and smooth (Fig. 8-51).

A variety of reconstruction procedures have been developed, which utilize either myocutaneous flaps or free flaps.[74] This topic is discussed further in Chapter 21. When a myocutaneous flap is used, the resulting imaging picture characteristically shows the thin, rotated mucosal surface overlying the fatty bulk of the flap (Fig. 8-52).

The postsurgical neck is difficult to evalaute because of the extensive anatomic alterations caused by the resection. Because granulation and scar tissue normally enhance, the presence of contrast enhancement on CT or MRI does not help differentiate tumor from postoperative change. However, if an area that has reduced T1W signal intensity progressively loses signal intensity on proton density and T2W images, it is likely to be fibrosis rather than tumor. As mentioned, comparison with a baseline, posttreatment CT or MRI is often the best way to evaluate recurrent disease. When there is progressive enlargement of a node or a mass within the original primary site or along the the margins of the surgical resection, tumor recurrence should be diagnosed.[75] If prior studies are unavailable, the most reliable signs of recurrent disease are the presence of an obvious dense, cellular mass at the primary site or an obviously positive lymph node as seen on CT. Tumor invasion of the internal carotid artery is difficult to diagnose on CT and MRI, unless there is obvious narrowing of the vessel caliber. The greater the circumference of vessel surrounded by tumor, the more likely it is that the adventitia is invaded (Fig. 8-53). However, focal tumor adherence to a vessel may be present if the tumor abuts the vessel with loss of the intervening fat planes.

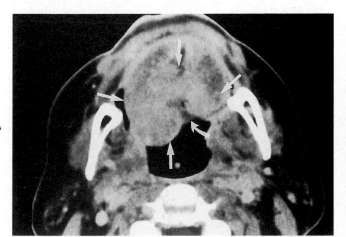
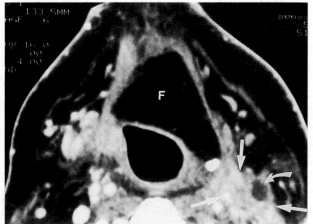

FIG. 8-52 **A,** Axial CT obtained through the tongue base shows a large, ulcerated mass invading and replacing the tongue base. *(straight arrows,* tumor; *curved arrow,* ulceration. **B,** This patient underwent a total glossectomy and myocutaneous flap reconstruction. The flap *(F)* fills in the operative defect and provides a mucosal surface to the pharynx. Note the low-attenuation lymph node *(curved arrow)* and surrounding soft-tissue mass *(straight arrows)* indicating recurrent disease.

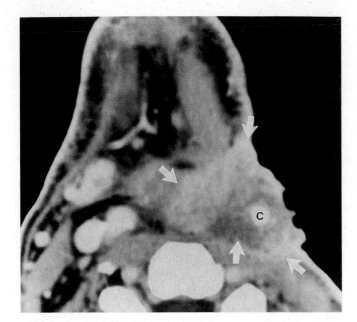

FIG. 8-53 Axial contrast-enhanced CT shows recurrent tumor *(arrows)* encasing the carotid artery *(C)*. This patient had previously undergone a left radical neck dissection.

Because tumors are more metabolically active than nontumorous surrounding tissue, the measurement of the metabolic activity of a potential tumor recurrence may be more beneficial than pure anatomic analysis. Modalities that can evaluate metabolic activity such as FDG, Thallium-201, and MR spectroscopy are currently being investigated (Fig. 8-54).[76,77]

Acquired Immunodeficiency Syndrome

Acquired immunodeficiency syndrome (AIDS) is caused by human T-cell lymphotrophic virus type III (HTLV-III) and is a potentially devastating disease of childhood and adulthood.[78]

Opportunistic infections and certain malignancies have been identified in up to 50% of patients with AIDS.[78-80] A variety of infections involving the oral cavity and oropharynx have been described in AIDS patients, including fungal diseases such as oral candidiasis, cryptococcus, and histoplasmosis; bacterial infections, including those caused by *S. pneumonia, S. aureus,* and *H. influenzae;* and herpes simplex infections, which require treatment with oral acyclovir or intravenous foscarnet (Fig. 8-55).[81,82] Hairy cell leukoplakia is a manifestation of Epstein-Barr virus and presents as a white plaque most often seen on the lateral margin of the tongue.

A variety of neoplasms have been reported to have a predilection to occur in AIDS patients. Because of their rarity in the general population, in the proper clinical setting, these neoplasms are considered AIDS-defining malignancies.[78] These malignancies include Kaposi's sarcoma, small noncleaved B-cell (Burkitt's, non-Burkitt's) and large B-cell

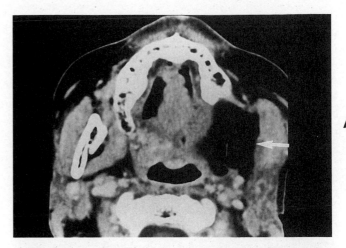

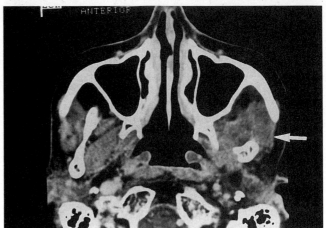

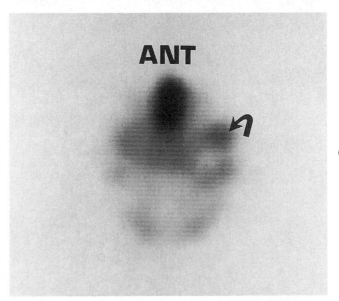

FIG. 8-54 **A,** Axial CT demonstrates the normal appearance of a reconstructive flap placed following a tumor involving the retromolar trigone. **B,** Axial CT obtained through the nasopharynx shows a clinically occult infiltrative mass obliterating the fat planes within the masticator space *(arrow)*. This lesion arose along the superior margin of the flap shown in **A**. **C,** Axial image from a Thallium-201 study shows increased uptake within the suspicious region *(arrow)* consistent with recurrent tumor.

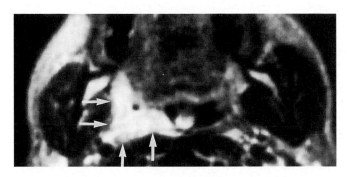

FIG. 8-55 Axial T2W MRI shows thickening and increased signal intensity of the posterior and lateral oropharyngeal walls *(arrows)* consistent with a clinical diagnosis of herpes pharyngitis.

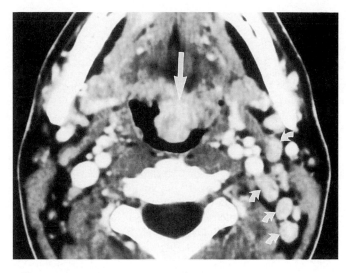

FIG. 8-57 Axial contrast-enhanced CT shows an enhancing mass *(arrow)* in the tongue base, and multiple-enhancing cervical lymph nodes *(curved arrows)*. Biopsy showed Kaposi's sarcoma.

A

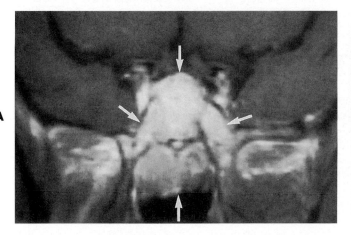

B

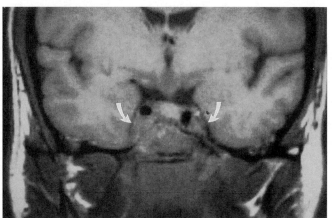

FIG. 8-56 **A,** Coronal-enhanced T1W MRI performed with fat saturation shows a large nasopharyngeal mass *(arrows)* that has invaded the sphenoid sinus in this patient who was HIV-positive. Biopsy showed immunoblastic lymphoma. **B,** Coronal T1W noncontrast MR scan shows that there is abnormal soft tissue present within the cavernous sinuses *(arrows in* **B***)*. This disease homgeneously enhances with contrast.

(immunoblastic) non-Hodgkin'slymphoma (Fig. 8-56). Involvement of the oropharynx has been reported in up to 20% of patients with cutaneous Kaposi's sarcoma, although any portion of the upper aerodigestive tract may be involved (Fig. 8-57).[83,84] Clinically these tumors may present as either small violaceous nodules or lobulated masses that measure several centimeters in diameter. Lymphoma preferentially involves the adenoidal and palatine tonsillar lymphoid tissues, and early nasopharyngeal lesions may mimic the diffuse adenoidal hypertrophy typically seen in immunocompromised hosts.[85] The triad of increased adenoidal tissue, parotid cysts (lymphoepithelial cysts), and diffuse cervical lymph adenopathy is highly suggestive of HIV infection. Large lymphomas may extend into the cavernous sinus, usually along neurovascular channels. On imaging, skull base erosion is rarely demonstrated.[78]

Advanced SCCA have recently been reported in patients under the age of 45 years. In many of these patients the typical risk factors of smoking and alcohol abuse were not present. The prognosis of these patients was poor despite combined therapy. At present, it is unclear whether the immune systems of these patients were normal, and the relationship of HIV infection and squamous cell carcinoma of the upper aerodigestive tract is also unclear.[86]

References

1. Moore KL. The neck. In: Clinically oriented anatomy. 2nd Edition. Baltimore, Md: Williams & Wilkins, 1985; 1033-1050.

2. Wenig BM, Kornblut AD. Pahryngitis. In: Baily BJ, ed. Head and neck surgery - otolaryngology. Philadelphia, Pa: J B Lippincott Co, 1993; 551-553.

3. Moore KL. The branchial apparatus and the head and neck. In: Moore KL, ed. The developing human: clinically oriented embryology. 4th Edition. Philadelphia, Pa: W B Saunders Co, 1988; 170-194.

4. Batsakis JG. Cysts, sinuses and "coeles." In: Tumors of the head and neck. 2nd Edition. Baltimore, Md: Williams & Wilkins; 1979; 514-520.

5. Mendenhall WM, Million RR, Mancuso AA, et al. Nasopharynx. In: Million RR, Cassisi NJ, eds. Management of head and neck cancer: a multidisciniplinary approach. Philadelphia, Pa: J B Lippincott, 1994; 599-626.

6. Neel HB, Slavitt DH. Nasopharyngeal cancer. In: Baily BJ, ed. Head and neck surgery - otolaryngology. Philadelphia, Pa: J B Lippincott, 1993; 1257-1260.

7. Dillon WP. The pharynx and oral cavity. In: Som PM, Bergeron RT. Head and neck imaging. 2nd Edition. St Louis, Mo: Mosby–Year Book, 1991; 407-465.

8. Lederman M. Cancer of the nasopharynx: Its natural history and treatment. Springfield, Ill: Charles C Thomas, Publisher, 1961; 1-50.

9. Mancuso AA, Hanafee WN. Nasopharynx and parapharyngeal space. In: Computed tomography and magnetic resonance imaging of the head and neck. 2nd Edition. Baltimore, Md: Williams & Wilkins, 1985; 428-498.

10. Rouvierre H. Anatomy of the human lymphatic system. (Translated by Tobias MJ) Ann Arbor, Mich: Edwards Brothers, 1938; 10-12.

11. Dillon WP, Mill CM, Kjos B, et al. Magnetic resonance image of the nasopharynx. Radiology 1984; 152:731-735.

12. Unger JM. The oral cavity and tongue: magnetic resonance imaging. Radiology 1986; 155:151-153.

13. Lufkin RB, Larsson SG, Hanafee WN. Work in progress: NMR anatomy of the larynx and tongue base. Radiology 1983; 148:173-175.

14. Lufkin R, Wortham DG, Dietrich RB, et al. Tongue and oropharynx: findings on MR imaging. Radiology 1986; 161:69-75.

15. Larsson SG, Mancuso AA, Hanafee WN. Computed tomography of the tongue and floor of the mouth, Radiology 1982; 143:493-500.

16. Byrd SE, Schoen PJ, Gill G, et al. Computed tomography of palatine tonsillar carcinoma, J Comput Assist Tomogr 1983; 7:976-982.

17. Muraki AS, Mancuso AA, Harnsberger HR. CT of the oropharynx, tongue base and floor of the mouth: normal anatomy and range of variations and applications in staging carinoma. Radiology 1983; 148:725-731.

18. Hsu MM, Huang SC, Lynn TC, et al. The survival of patients with nasopharyngeal carcinoma. Otolaryn Head Neck Surg 1982; 90: 289-290.

19. Simons MJ, Wee GB, Day NE, et al. Immunogenetic aspects of nasopharyngeal carcinoma. I. Differences in HLA antigen profiles between patients and control groups. Int J Cancer 1974; 13:122-124.

20. Dickson RI. Nasopharyngeal carcinomas: an evaluation of 209 patients. Laryngoscope 1981; 91:333-334.

21. Shanmugaratnam K, Sobin LH. Histologic typing of upper respiratory tract tumors. In: International histologic classification of tumors. No. 19. Geneva, Switzerland: World Health Organization, 1978.

22. Mesic JB, Fletcher GH, Goepfert H. Megavoltage irradiation of epithelial tumors of the nasopharynx. Int J Rdaiat Oncol Biol Phys 1981; 7:447-453.

23. Fletcher GH, Million RR. Malignant tumors of the nasopharynx. Am J Roentgenol Radium Ther Nucl Med 1965; 93:44-45.

24. Million RR, Cassisi, NJ, Mancuso AA. The oropharynx. In: Million RR, Cassisi NJ, eds. Management of head and neck cancer: a multidisciniplinary approach. Philadelphia, Pa: 1994; 402-431.

25. Mancuso AA, Hanafee WN. Oral cavity and oropharynx including tongue base, floor of mouth and mandible. In: Computed tomography and magnetic resonance imaging of the head and neck. 2nd Edition Baltimore Md: Williams & Wilkins; 1985; 358-427.

26. Batsakis JG. Tumors of the head and neck: clinical and pathologic considerations 2nd Edition. Baltimore Md: Williams & Wilkins: 1979; 144-176.

27. Lindberg RD. Distribution of cervical lympnode metastases from squamous cell carcinoma of the upper respiratory and digestive tracts. Cancer 1972; 29: 1448-1449.

28. Russ JE, Applebaum EL, Sisson CA. Squamous cell carcinoma of the soft palate. Laryngoscope 1977; 87:1151-1156.

29. Byrd SE, Schoen PJ, Gill G, et al. Computed tomography of palatine tonsillar carcinoma. J Comput Assist Tomogr 1983; 7:976-982.

30. Schaefer SD, Marvilla KR, Suss RA, et al. Magnetic resonance imaging versus computed tomography: comparison in imaging oral cavity and pharyngeal carcinomas. Arch Otolaryngol Head Neck Surg 1985; 111:730-734.

31. Byers RM, Wolf PF, Ballantyne AJ. Rationale for elective modified neck dissection. Head and Neck Surg 1988; 10:106-167.

32. Mendenhall NP. Lymphomas and related diseases presenting in the head and neck. In: Million RR, Cassisi NJ, ed. Management of head and neck cancer: a multidisciniplinary approach. Philadelphia, Pa: J B Lippincott, 1994; 857-878.

33. Myers EN, Cunningham MJ. Tumors of the neck. In: Bluestone CD, Stool SE, Scheetz MD. Pediatric otolaryngology. Vol 2. Philadelphia, Pa: WB Saunders, 1990; 1339-1363.

34. Wong DS, Fuller LM, Butler JJ, et al. Extranodal non-Hodgkin's lymphomas of the head and neck. Am J Radiol 1975; 123:471-481.

35. Million RR, Cassisi, NJ. Minor salivary gland tumors. In: Management of head and neck cancer: a multidisciniplinary approach. Philadelphia, Pa: J B Lippincott Co, 1994; 737-750.

36. Gandour-Edwards R, Kapadia SB, Barnes L, et al. Neural cell adhesion molecule (N-CAM) in adenoid cystic carcinoma of the skull base (abstr). Presented at the North

American Skull Base Society, 1995.

37. Papadaki H, Kournelis S, Bakker A, et al. The role of p53 mutation and protein expression in the recurrence of skull base adenoid cystic carcinoma (abstr). Presented at the North American Skull Base Society, 1995.

38. Lee FA. Rhabdomyosarcoma. In: Parker BR, Castellano RA, eds. Pediatric oncologic radiology. St Louis, Mo: CV Mosby Co, 1977; 33-55.

39. Canalis RF, Jenkens HA, Hemenway WG, et al. Nasopharyngeal rhabdomyosarcoma: a clinical perspective. Arch Otolaryngol Head Neck Surg 1978; 104:122-126.

40. Dito WR, Batsakis JG. Intra-oral, pharyngeal and nasopharyngeal rhabdomyosarcoma. Arch Otolaryngol Head Neck Surg 1963; 77:123-129.

41. McGill T. Rhabdomyosarcoma of the head and neck: an update. Otolaryngol Clin North Am 1989; 22(3):631-636.

42. Scotti G, Harwood-Nash DC. Computed tomography of rhabdomyosarcomas of the skull base in children. J Comput Assist Tomogr 1982; 6(1):33-39.

43. Robb PJ, Girling A. Granular cell myoblastoma of the supraglottis. J Laryngol Otol 1989; 103:328-330.

44. Cree IA, Bingham BJG, Ramesar KCRB. View from beneath: pathology in focus granular cell tumour of the larynx. J Laryngol Otol 1990; 104:159-161.

45. Batsakis JF. Tumours of the head and neck: clinical and pathological considerations. 2nd Edition. Baltimore, Md: Williams & Wilkins, 1979; 313-333.

46. Batsakis JG. Tumors of the head and neck. 2nd Edition. Baltimore, Md. Williams & Wilkins, 1979; 228-289.

47. Masson JK, Soule EH. Desmoid tumor of the head and neck. Am J Surg 1966; 112:615-622.

48. Som PM, Lanzieri CF, Sacher M, et al. Extracranial tumor vascularity: determination by dynamic CT scanning. Radiology 1985; 154:401-412.

49. Das Gupta TK. Tumors of the peripheral nerves. In: Das Gupta TK, ed. Tumors of the soft tissues. East Norwalk, Conn: Appleton-Century-Crofts, 1983; 89-95.

50. Itoh K, Nishimura K, Togashi K, et al. MR imaging of cavernous hemangioma of the face and neck. J Comput Assist Tomogr 1986; 10:831-835.

51. Million RR, Cassisi NJ, Mancuso AA. The unknown primary. In: Million RR, Cassisi NJ, eds. Management of head and neck cancer: a multidisiplinary approach. 2nd Edition. Philadelphia, Pa: J B Lippincott Co, 1994; 311-321.

52. Harper CS, Mendenhall WM, Parsons JT, et al. Cancer in neck nodes with unknown primary site: role of mucosal radiotherapy. Head Neck 1990; 12: 463-469.

53. Templer J, Perry MC, Davis WE. Metastatic cervical adenopathy from an unknown primary tumor: treatment dilemma. Arch Otolaryngol 1981; 107:45-47.

54. Mukherji SK, Drane WE, Mancuso AA, et al. Detection of unknown primary tumors of the head and neck using 2-[F-18] Fluoro-2-Deoxy-D-Glucose (FDG) SPECT (abstr). Presented at the Radiological Society of North America, 1994.

55. Johnson JT, Newman RK. The anatomic location of neck metastases from occult squamous cell carcinoma. Otol Head Neck Surg 1981; 89:54-58.

56. Gianoli GJ, Espinola TE, Guarisco JL, et al. Retropharyngeal space infection: changing trends. Otolol Head Neck Surg 1991; 105:92-100.

57. Grodinsky M. Rctrophayngeal and lateral pharyngeal space abscesses: an anatomical and clinical study with review of the literature. Am J Surg 1979; 110:179-199.

58. Batsakis JG, Sneige N. Parapharyngeal and retropharyngeal sopace disease. Ann Otol Rhinol Laryngol 1989; 98:320-321.

59. Davis WL, Harnsberger HR, Smoker WRK, et al. Retropharyngeal space: evaluation of normal anatomy and disease with CT and MR imaging. Radiology 1990; 174:59-64.

60. Mukherji SK, Mancuso AA, Shook J. Retropharyngeal suppurative lymphadenitis: differentiation from retropharyngeal abcess and treatment implications (abstr). Presented at the Radiological Society of North America, 1994.

61. Glasier CM, Stark JE, Jacobs RF, et al. CT and ultrasound imaging of retropharyngeal abscesses in children. AJNR; 13:1191-1195.

62. Kornbutt AD. Infections of the pharyngeal spaces. In: Paparilla M, Shumrick M, eds. Otolaryngology. Vol 3. Philadelphia, Pa: WB Saunders Co, 1980.

63. Dillon WP, Mills CM, Kjos B, et al. Magnetic resonance image of the nasopharynx. Radiology 1984; 152:731-735.

64. Fein DA, Mendenhall WM, Parsons JT, et al. T1-T2 Squamous cell carcinoma of the glottic larynx treated with radiotherapy: a multivariate analysis of variables potentially influencing local control. Int J Radiation Oncology Biol Phys 1993; 25:605-611.

65. Lee WR, Mancuso AA, Saleh EM, et al. Can pretreatment computed tomography findings predict local control in T3 squamous cell carcinoma of the glottic larynx treated with radiotherapy alone? Int J Radiation Oncology Biol Phys 1993; 25:683-687.

66. Freeman DE, Mancuso AA, Parsons JT, et al. Irradiation alone for supraglottic carcinoma: can CT findings predict treatment results? I Int J Radiation Oncology Biol Phys 1990; 19:485-490.

67. Amdur RJ, Parsons JT, Mendenhall WM, et al. Postoperative irradiation for squamous cell carcinoma of the head and neck: an analysis of treatment results and complications. Int J Rad Onc Biol Phy 1989; 16:25-36.

68. Mukherji SK, Mancuso AA, Mendenhall W, et al. Can pretreatment computed tomography predict local control in T2 glottic carcinomas treated with radiation therapy alone? AJNR In Press.

69. Manara M. Histological changes of the human larynx irradiated with various technical therapeutic methods. Arch Ital Otol 1966; 79: 596-635.

70. Goldman JL, Cheren RV, Zak FG, et al. Histopathology of larynges and radical neck specimens in a combined radiation and surgery for advanced carcinoma of the larynx and hypopharynx. Ann Otol 1966; 75:313-321.

71. Calcaterra TC, Stern F, Ward PH. Dilemma of delayed radiation injury of the larynx. Ann Otol Rhinol Laryngol 1972; 81: 501-507.

72. Mukherji SK, Mancuso AA, Kotzur IM, et al. Radiographic appearance of the irradiated larynx. Part I,

Expected changes. Radiology 1994; 193:141-148.

73. Mukherji SK, Mancuso AA, Kotzur IM, et al. Radiographic appearance of the irradiated larynx. Part II, Primary site response. Radiology 1994; 193: 149-154.

74. Tiwari R, Snow GB. Role of myocutaneous flaps in reconstruction of the head and neck. J Laryngol Otol 1983; 97:441-458.

75. Hudgins PA, Burson JG, Gussak GS, et al. CT and MR appearance of recurrent malignant head and neck neoplasms after resection and flap reconstruction. AJNR 1994; 15:1689-1694.

76. Mukherji SK, Dranc WE, Tart RP, Mancuso, et al. Comparison of SPECT FDG and SPECT Thallium-201 For Imaging of Squamous Cell Carcinoma of the Head and Neck. AJNR 1994; 15:1837- 1842.

77. Mukherji SK, Buejenovich S, Weeks S, et al. Initial experience using Thallium-201 SPECT for imaging patients with squamous cell carcinoma of the upper aerodigestive tract (abstr). ASHNR, 1995.

78. Holliday RA. Manifestations of AIDS in the oromaxillofacial region: the role of imaging. Radiol Clin North Am 1993; 31:45-60.

79. Marcusen DC, Sooy CD. Otolaryngologic and head and neck manifestations of acquired immunodeficiency syndrome (AIDS). Laryngoscope 1985; 95:401-405.

80. Rosenberg RA, Schneider KL, Cohen NL. Head and presentations of acquired immunodeficiency syndrome. Otolaryngol Head and Neck Surg 1985; 93:700-705.

81. Grepp DR, Chandler W, Hyams V. Primary Kaposi's sarcoma of the head and neck. Ann Intern Med 1984; 100:107-114.

82. MacPhail LA, Greenspan D, Schiodt M, et al. Acyclovir-resistant, foscarnet-sensitive oral herpes simplex type 2 lesion in a patient with AIDS. Oral Surg Oral Med Oral Pathol 1989; 67:427-432.

83. Abeymayor E, Calcterra T. Kaposi's sarcoma and community acquired immunodeficiency syndrome: an update with emphasis on its head and neck manifestations. Arch Otolaryngol 1983; 109:536-542.

84. Grepp DR, Chandler W, Hyams V. Primary Kaposi's sarcoma of the head and neck. Ann Intern Med 1984; 100:107-114.

85. Stern JC, Lin PT, Lucente FE. Benign nasopharyngeal masses and HIV infection. Arch Otolaryngol Head Neck Surg 1990; 116:206-208.

86. Roland JT, Rothstein SG, Khushbakhat, RM et al. Squamous cell carcinoma in HIV-positive patients under age 45. Laryngoscope 1993; 103:509-511.

SECTION TWO
HYPOPHARYNX

NORMAL ANATOMY

The hypopharynx, or laryngopharynx, is the most caudal portion of the pharynx that extends from the level of the hyoid bone and valleculae to the cricopharyngeus.[1,2] On imaging this caudal margin can be approximated by the lower level of the cricoid cartilage. Below this level, the gullet becomes the cervical esophagus (Fig. 8-58). Most authors divide the hypopharynx into the following three regions: the pyriform sinuses, the posterior wall, and the postcricoid region (Fig. 8-58).[1-3] Some authors also refer to a fourth or "marginal" area, the hypopharyngeal (lateral) surface of the aryepiglottic folds (Fig. 8-58).[4]

Pyriform Sinus

The pyriform (pear-shaped) sinus is an anterolateral recess of the hypopharynx situated on each side of the pharynx between the inner surface of the thyrohyoid membrane and thyroid cartilage and the aryepiglottic fold. The anterior pyriform sinus mucosa abuts on the posterior paraglottic space.[1] The most caudal portion, or apex, of each pyriform sinus lies at the level of the true vocal cord (Fig. 8-58). The lateral wall of the pyriform sinus is formed above by the thyrohyoid membrane and below by the thyroid cartilage. These two areas have been respectively referred to as the "membranous" and "cartilaginous" portions of this pyriform sinus wall.[1-3]

The lateral aspect of the aryepiglottic fold forms the medial wall of the pyriform sinus, and it is often considered a "marginal" zone. Although the aryepiglottic fold is a part of the supraglottic larynx, it can also be considered part of the hypopharynx. An aryepiglottic fold tumor confined to the laryngeal surface behaves as a supraglottic tumor; however, a tumor involving the lateral wall of the aryepiglottic fold usually behaves more aggressively, like a pharyngeal tumor.

Posterior Hypopharyngeal Wall

The posterior wall of the hypopharynx is considered to start at the level of the valleculae (Fig. 8-58), being continuous above this level with the posterior wall of the oropharynx.[2] Caudally the posterior wall of the hypopharynx merges with the posterior wall of the cricopharyngeus and then the cervical esophagus (Fig. 8-58). The retropharyngeal space lies behind the posterior pharyngeal wall.

Postcricoid Hypopharynx

The postcricoid region is the anterior wall of the lower hypopharynx. This area is the interface between the hypopharynx posteriorly and the larynx anteriorly. The postcricoid portion of the hypopharynx extends from the level of the arytenoid cartilages down to the lower edge of the cricoid cartilage, thus abutting the dorsal surface of the cricoid lamina.[1-3]

Muscles

The inferior pharyngeal constrictor muscle has two components. The upper fibers arise from a posterior midline raphe and insert on the thyroid cartilage. These fibers are obliquely oriented, being highest in the posterior midline.[5] The inferior pharyngeal oblique fibers overlap and interdigitate with the oblique muscle fibers of the middle pharyngeal constrictor muscle.[6] The lowermost portion of the inferior pharyngeal constrictor, the cricopharyngeus, is composed of nonraphed

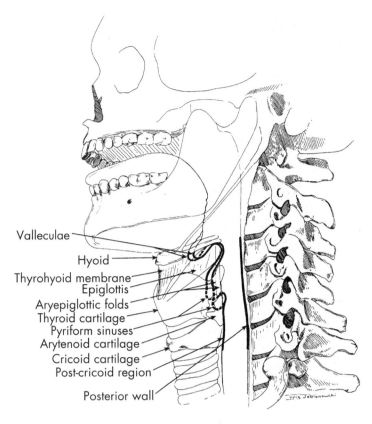

Valleculae
Hyoid
Thyrohyoid membrane
Epiglottis
Aryepiglottic folds
Thyroid cartilage
Pyriform sinuses
Arytenoid cartilage
Cricoid cartilage
Post-cricoid region
Posterior wall

FIG. 8-58 Diagram of the hypopharynx. The heavy black lines indicate the region of the hypopharynx.

muscle fibers that arise from either side of the cricoid cartilage. These fibers are horizontally oriented, and they become continuous with the circular muscles of the cervical esophagus.[5,6] Between the upper border of the cricopharyngeus and the lowermost margin of the oblique fibers of the inferior pharyngeal constrictor muscle is a small triangular space called Killian's dehiscence. It is through this area that the Zenker's diverticulum arises.

The superior, middle, and inferior pharyngeal constrictors contract in a coordinated peristaltic manner with each swallow. The cricopharyngeus, or superior esophageal sphincter, is normally closed as are the other natural sphincters of the body. In response to a minimum specific volume and pressure in the hypopharynx, the cricopharyngeus relaxes, allowing the hypopharyngeal bolus to enter the cervical esophagus. Equally important, the cricopharyngeus then closes to prevent esophagopharyngeal reflux.[6]

Nerves

The pharyngeal plexus of nerves receives contributions from the glossopharyngeal and vagus nerves. The vagus primarily supplies motor innervation to the constrictors.[6] Sensory information from the hypopharynx travels along the glossopharyngeal nerve and the internal laryngeal branch of the superior laryngeal nerve, which arises from the vagus nerve.[1]

Pain referred from a hypopharyngeal tumor may be transmitted up from the pyriform sinus along the internal branch of the superior laryngeal nerve, to the auricular nerve, another branch of the vagus. The auricular nerve (Arnold's nerve) supplies sensory innervation to the external auditory canal and pinna, and because of this, a hypopharyngeal tumor may present with otalgia.[1]

Lymphatics

The lymphatic drainage of the hypopharynx is extensive and complex. The pyriform sinuses are drained by a network of lymphatics, most of which are directed to the upper and mid-jugular nodes (levels II and III) and are directed secondarily to posterior cervical nodes (level V).[1,3,7] The lymphatics of the posterior wall of the hypopharynx drain to these jugular nodes, as well as the retropharyngeal nodes.[3] The postcricoid lymphatics drain to the mid- and lower jugular nodes (levels III and IV), as well as to paratracheal nodes (level VI).[7]

Arterial Supply and Venous Drainage

Branches of the superior and inferior thyroid arteries supply most of the lower pharynx.[6] Venous drainage is into the pharyngeal plexus more superiorly and into the superior and inferior thyroid veins, as well as individual pharyngeal veins that may drain directly into the internal jugular veins.[6]

IMAGING STRATEGIES
Barium Studies

Barium continues to play an important role in the radiographic assessment of benign and malignant abnormalities of the hypopharynx. Unlike CT and MRI, a barium swallow is a dynamic study that can show if the pharyngeal wall is pliable or fixed. Diminished or absent pharyngeal movement suggests, for example, that a neoplasm of the posterior hypopharyngeal wall has invaded through constrictor muscles and is fixed to the prevertebral muscles. This important observation may change the surgical approach because deeply invasive tumors may be deemed unresectable.[1]

A barium swallow is usually the first radiographic study performed in patients with dysphagia and odynophagia. Barium studies detect mucosal abnormalities that are not apparent on CT and MRI, and the diagnosis of traumatic or iatrogenic perforations and postoperative fistulae are also in the province of oral contrast studies.

Barium is suitable for the evaluation of dysphagia and odynophagia and to search for a tumor. However, water-soluble iodinated medium is preferable when a perforation or fistula is suspected because water-soluble contrast such as a solution of diatrizoate meglumine and diatrizoate sodium (Gastrografin; Squibb, Princeton, NJ), is absorbed from the soft tissues of the neck. But the water-soluble contrast mediums are quite hypertonic (1900 mosm/kg water), and they are contraindicated in patients who may have significant aspiration.[8] Aspirated hypertonic contrast medium draws fluid into the lungs and can cause pulmonary edema. For patients who aspirate, in whom the question of a perforation or fistula must be addressed, ideal agents are low-osmolality, iodinated, water-soluble contrast mediums such as metrizamide and iohexol.[8]

Because there is approximately a 10% incidence of a second primary tumor in patients with a SCAA of the upper aerodigestive tract, virtually all of these patients should preoperatively undergo a barium swallow or endoscopy. These second cancers most often arise in the lung and the upper aerodigestive tract.[3]

Barium is also used to evaluate deglutition. Thin and thick liquid barium barium purees, puddings, and solids such as cookies crumbled into barium are all useful approximations of a patient's normal diet. The assessment of the normal and abnormal swallowing mechanism is beyond the scope of this chapter.

Computed Tomography Technique

Most CT studies of the neck are performed with the patient supine and with the head in a neutral postion. The entire neck from the external auditory canal to the manubrium is usually examined by either 3 or 5 mm contiguous scans.

If the patient is suspected of having a tumor, CT of the hypopharynx should delineate the anatomic extent of the lesion, determine whether or not metastatic adenopathy is present, and evaluate any tumor extension into the larynx or the adjacent neck and carotid sheath. Such information is of great clinical importance because it will helps determine therapy. The CT evaluation of the larynx is discussed in Chapter 11.

Intravenous contrast medium is helpful because it may emphasize subtle enhancement differences between the tumor and adjacent normal tissue, and it makes much easier the task of distinguishing between lymph nodes and blood vessels. However, even with rapid (1 to 2 second) scan times, motion artifact can thoroughly degrade an image. Because of this, patients should be instructed to breathe quietly and to refrain from talking, swallowing, and coughing during the examination. When the pyriform sinuses are not seen well on routine CT studies, phonation and Valsalva maneuvers will distend the hypopharynx and may be diagnostically helpful.

Magnetic Resonance Technique

The use of a neck coil gives the best MR images of the hypopharynx.[9] Although a body coil can also be used, neck coil images provide better detail. After a sagittal localizing sequence is obtained, axial T1W, proton density, and T2W images are acquired. Coronal T1W images are also very useful for determining the inferior extent of a hypopharyngeal tumor. After gadolinium administration and fat suppression, T1W images may further differentiate enhancing tumor from adjacent normal tissues.

Although intravenous contrast is useful in MRI, it is not crucial because inherent signal intensity differences between tumor, fat, and muscle often allow an accurate delineation of tumor extent without gadolinium. T2W images often provide more diagnostic information than contrast-enhanced sequences.

NORMAL RADIOGRAPHIC APPEARANCE
Barium Studies

The hypopharynx and pyriform sinuses are seen well on anteroposterior (AP) frontal views of a barium study (Fig. 8-59 A, B), as are the valleculae and aryepiglottic folds. The pyriform sinus apex, often difficult for the clinician to assess endoscopically, is readily seen on barium studies (Fig. 8-59, A). The epiglottis and the postcricoid larynx are usually seen as a "filling defect" in a full barium column (Fig. 8-59, A). Alternately the epiglottis may or may not be coated by barium using air-contrast techniques (Fig. 8-59, B). On a lateral barium study view, the valleculae are seen just beneath the base of the tongue at the level of the hyoid bone. Normal lingual tonsil may also be present at the tongue base, and this tissue normally does not extend onto the floor or posterior wall of the valeculae. If soft tissue is seen in these areas, a tumor should be suspected. The position of the epiglottis varies with swallowing. In the normal patient, barium does not reach the laryngeal vestibule (penetration) or the true vocal cords (aspiration). The pyriform sinuses are not seen optimally on a lateral view.

On the lateral view the postcricoid region (anterior wall) often appears irregular (Fig. 8-59, C). This usually is a normal appearance secondary to a prominent submucosal venous plexus and to redundant, pliable mucosa. However,

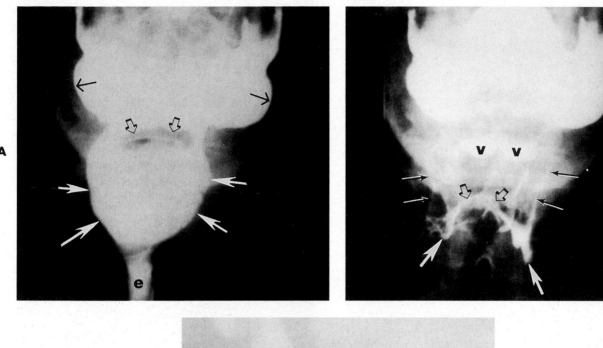

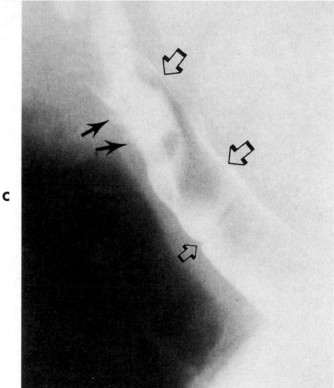

FIG. 8-59 Normal hypopharynx—barium studies **A,** Frontal (AP) view of the hypopharynx, single contrast. The lateral walls of the pyriform sinuses are smooth *(white arrows).* Epiglottis *(open arrows).* Esophagus *(e).* Barium in the oral cavity *(solid black arrows).* **B,** Frontal view, air-contrast. Barium coats the pyriform sinuses *(highlighted arrows)* and epiglottis *(open arrows)* and fills the valleculae *(v).* The apex of the right pyriform sinus is not distended as well as the apex of the left pyriform sinus *(white arrows).* **C,** Lateral view. The posterior wall *(large open arrows)* is smooth and lies close to the vertebral bodies. The irregularity of the post-cricoid region is normal *(solid arrows).* There is an incidental esophageal web *(small open arrow).*

it is sometimes difficult to differentiate this normal postcricoid appearance from tumor, and direct clinical inspection may be necessary.

In patients with large shoulders, oblique projections allow an unobstructed view of the hypopharynx and cervical esophagus, and these oblique views should supplement the standard frontal and lateral views.

Computed Tomography and Magnetic Resonance Studies

The aryepiglottic fold on each side makes up the medial wall of each pyriform sinus (Fig. 8-60, A, B). The hypopharynx may be filled with air (Fig. 8-60, C) or may be collapsed, with its mucosal surfaces touching. In particular, on CT and MRI a collapsed pyriform sinus can mimic a tumor. If this is identified at the time of the study, a modified Valsalva maneuver may distend this region and rule out the presence of a tumor. Superficial mucosal lesions in the hypopharynx are evaluated best by barium studies and by direct clinical inspection.

The paraglottic fat in the larynx is the normal anterior boundary of each pyriform sinus (Fig. 8-61).[9] The low density of this normal fat on CT studies and the high T1W signal intensity on MRI provides inherent contrast to identify anteriorly infiltrating pyriform sinus tumors.

At the level of the cricopharyngeus muscle on axial scans the pharynx is oval, being wider from side to side than from front to back (Fig. 8-62, A, B). During bolus administration of contrast, enhancement of this mucosa is a normal CT finding. On T2W MRI the mucosa is hyperintense and is contrasted well against the lower signal intensity muscular wall of the hypopharynx. Below the cricopharyngeus on axial images, the cervical esophagus has a round cross-sectional configuration (Fig. 8-62, C), and the point at which the oval shape of the pharynx changes into the rounder shape of the esophagus marks the transition from hypopharynx to the cervical esophagus.

SQUAMOUS CELL CARCINOMA

The hypopharynx is lined by stratified squamous epithelium, and more than 95% of the tumors that occur there are SCCA.[1] These tumors are etiologically associated with alcoholism, smoking, and previous radiation therapy.[3]

Patients with the Plummer-Vinson syndrome (named for two American investigators, but also called the Paterson-Brown-Kelly syndrome, for the Europeans who described a similar syndrome) have a high incidence of postcricoid carcinoma.[10] The four components of Plummer-Vinson syndrome are dysphagia, iron-deficiency anemia, weight loss, and webs in the hypopharynx and cervical esophagus.[10] The syndrome is much more prevalent in women, and the carcinomas that develop are usually in the postcricoid area, perhaps related to stasis above the webs.[10]

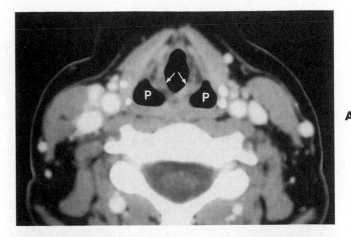

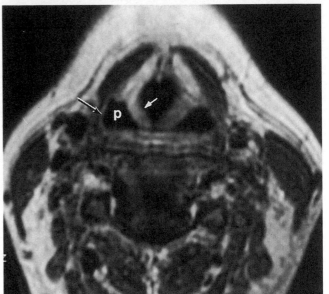

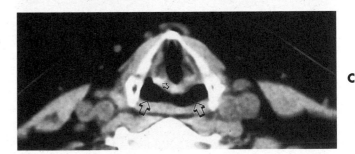

FIG. 8-60 Normal hypopharynx—axial CT and MR studies. **A,** Axial CT through the pyriform sinuses *(P)* and aryepiglottic folds *(arrows).* **B,** T1W MRI after gadolinium shows normal enhancement of the mucosa of the aryepiglottic folds *(white arrow).* The thin, smooth mucosa *(highlighted arrow)* of the pyriform sinuses *(p)* also enhances. **C,** Normal axial CT of another patient shows air distending the hypopharynx *(large open arrows).* Arytenoid cartilage *(small open arrow).*

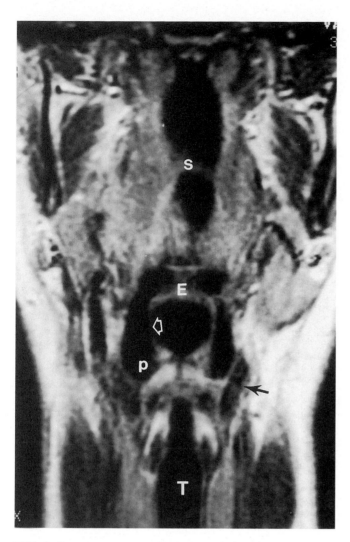

FIG. 8-61 Coronal T1W MRI after gadolinium shows the pyriform sinuses *(p)*, epiglottis *(E)*, and aryepiglottic folds *(open arrow)*, thyroid cartilage *(solid arrow)*, soft palate *(s)*, and trachea *(T)*.

Hypopharyngeal tumors may be indolent and remain relatively asymptomatic for long periods of time.[3] Extensive submucosal growth is common, and although this submucosal spread may not be apparent on direction laryngoscopy, it is often quite conspicuous on CT and MRI.[11]

At the time of diagnosis, up to 75% of patients with hypopharyngeal tumors have metastases to cervical lymph nodes, and 20% to 40% of patients will also develop distant metastases.[1] In addition, between 4% and 15% of patients with SCCA of the hypopharynx have a synchronous or metachronous second primary tumor. Of these, 25% are diagnosed at the time of the hypopharyngeal tumor and 40% are diagnosed 6 months or more after diagnosis of the initial primary tumor.

The American Joint Committee on Cancer's TNM system to stage hypopharyngeal carcinomas is used widely (Box 8-3).[2] CT and MRI of these hypopharyngeal cancers often demonstrate more extensive tumor than was clinically apparent, usually because of submucosal spread. "Upstaging" such a tumor may affect the surgical approach and treatment philosophy. Although it may not be possible to determine the precise site of origin of a large, bulky tumor, this is actually less important in these cases than accurate tumor mapping, and the best mapping is achieved with CT and MRI.

Because hypopharyngeal cancers, especially tumors of the pyriform sinus, tend to invade the larynx, it is impossible to discuss carcinoma of the hypopharynx without considering the larynx. Similarly, laryngeal tumors, especially supraglottic carcinomas, may involve the hypopharynx either by submucosal spread through the paraglottic fat or by direct extension. Further examples of hypopharyngeal tumors are given in Chapter 11.

▼

BOX 8-3
AMERICAN JOINT COMMITTEE ON CANCER STAGING PROTOCOL FOR MALIGNANT TUMORS

Primary Tumor (T)

TX	Primary tumor cannot be assessed
T0	No evidence of primary tumor
Tis	Carcinoma in situ
T1	Tumor limited to one subsite of hypopharynx
T2	Tumor invades more than one subsite of hypopharynx or an adjacent site, without fixation of hemilarynx
T3	Tumor invades more than one subsite of hypopharynx or an adjacent site, with fixation of hemilarynx
T4	Tumor invades adjacent structures (e.g., cartilage, soft tissues of neck)

Regional Lymph Nodes (N)

NX	Regional lymph nodes cannot be assessed
N0	No regional lymph node metastasis
N1	Metastasis in one ipsilateral lymph nodes 3 cm or less in greatest dimension
N2	N2a Metastasis in a single ipsilateral lymph node, more than 3 cm but not more than 6 cm in greatest dimension
	N2b Metastasis in multiple ipsilateral lymph nodes, none more than 6 cm in greatest dimension
	N2c Metastasis in bilateral or contralateral lymph nodes, none more than 6 cm in greatest dimension
N3	Metastasis in a lymph node more than 6 cm in greatest dimension

Distant Metastasis (M)

MX	Presence of distant metastases cannot be assessed
M0	No distant metastases
M1	Distant metastases

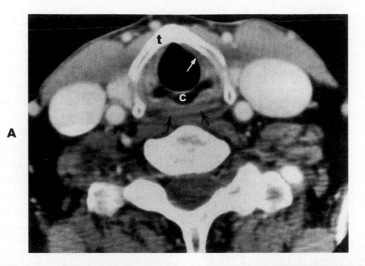

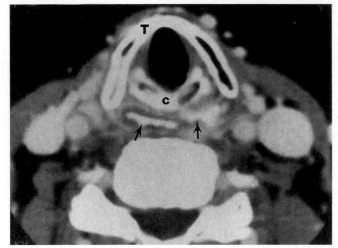

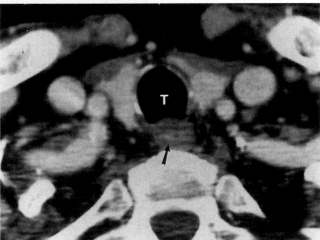

FIG. 8-62   Axial CT images through the normal post-cricoid region. **A,** The post-cricoid mucosa *(black arrows)* is slightly more dense than the wall. This image is at the level of the cricoid cartilage *(c)*, thyroid cartilage *(t)*, and inferior surface of the true vocal cords *(white arrow)*. **B,** Barium shows the location of the lumen of the post-cricoid hypopharynx *(arrows)*. Cricoid cartilage *(c)*. Thyroid cartilage *(T)*. When not distended by air, the shape of the post-cricoid hypopharynx is a flattened oval. **C,** Axial CT through the upper cervical esophagus for comparison. Instead of the flattened oval of the hypopharynx, the cervical esophagus is round *(arrow)*, and indents the membranous posterior wall of the trachea *(T)*.

Pyriform Sinus

A small pyriform sinus tumor may be confined to one wall (Figs. 8-63, *A, B,* 8-64, *A*), and this disease can be seen well on frontal views of a barium study (Fig. 8-63, *A*). As mentioned, the apex of the pyriform sinus may be difficult to clinically evaluate, and the barium studies can often show whether tumor spares (Fig. 8-63, *A*) or involves (Fig. 8-63, *B*) the apex.

A pyriform sinus tumor may spread submucosally into the posterior wall of the hypopharynx (Fig. 8-64, *B*), the postcricoid region, or the aryepiglottic fold (Figs. 8-64, 8-65).[1] Large tumors also extend up into the paraglottic fat (Fig. 8-65, *A*), the preepiglottic fat, and the base of the tongue.[1] These tumors may erode the posterosuperior

cricoid cartilage (Fig. 8-65, *B*) and invade the upper pole of the thyroid gland.[1] Tumors arising from the lower lateral wall or apex of the pyriform sinus often have invaded the thyroid cartilage by the time of diagnosis.[1,10]

Lesions of the medial wall of the pyriform sinus may spread along the aryepiglottic fold into the false vocal cord and arytenoid cartilage.[1] They also may grow posteriorly into the postcricoid region, then cross the midline to involve the contralateral pyriform sinus.[1] Medial wall lesions also can invade the paraglottic and preepiglottic fat.[1]

Postcricoid Hypopharynx

Tumors confined to the postcricoid region are rare (Fig. 8-66, *A, B*).[1] Patients, mostly women, with Plummer-Vinson syndrome are the exception. Often, posterior wall tumors invade the posterior larynx (arytenoid and posterior cricoid cartilages), causing vocal cord paralysis and hoarseness.[1] Large tumors concentrically infiltrate and narrow the lumen of the hypopharynx (Fig. 8-66, *A*).[1]

Posterior Wall

Carcinoma of the posterior wall of the hypopharynx spreads up and down the posterior wall and may infiltrate deeply into the adjacent soft tissues. The submucosal tumor spread at times may become quite bulky (Fig. 8-67, *A-C*).[1] Tumor may extend up into the posterior wall of the oropharynx and

even infiltrate the posterior aspect of the tonsillar pillars.[1] A posterior wall tumor may also extend down into the cervical esophagus. Rarely, aggressive, invasive posterior wall tumors extend through the mucosa into the prevertebral muscles, and they may even invade the vertebrae.[1]

Fixation of a posterior wall tumor to the prevertebral muscles may prevent complete extirpation. CT and MRI may show effacement of the prevertebral fat planes, but distinction between tumor invasion and peripheral edema may not be possible on these sectional imaging studies. In equivocal cases, fixation of the posterior wall to the underlying muscles is not determined best by static CT or MRI or even

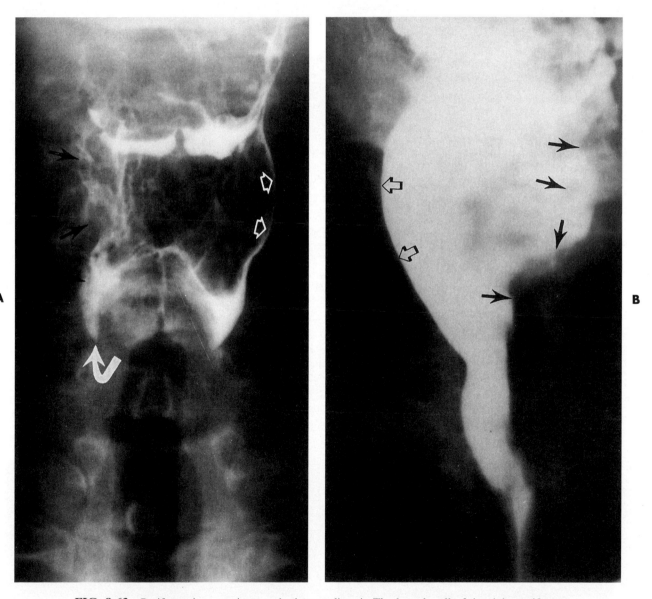

FIG. 8-63 Pyriform sinus carcinoma—barium studies. **A,** The lateral wall of the right pyriform sinus *(black arrows)* is irregular with tumor on this frontal air-contrast study. The tumor spares the apex of the pyriform sinus *(curved arrow)*. The lateral pharyngeal wall on the left is normal *(open arrows)*. **B,** In another patient a frontal view from a single-contrast barium study shows irregularities and filling defects *(solid arrows)* along the lateral wall of the left pyriform sinus. The right pyriform sinus wall is normal *(open arrows)*.

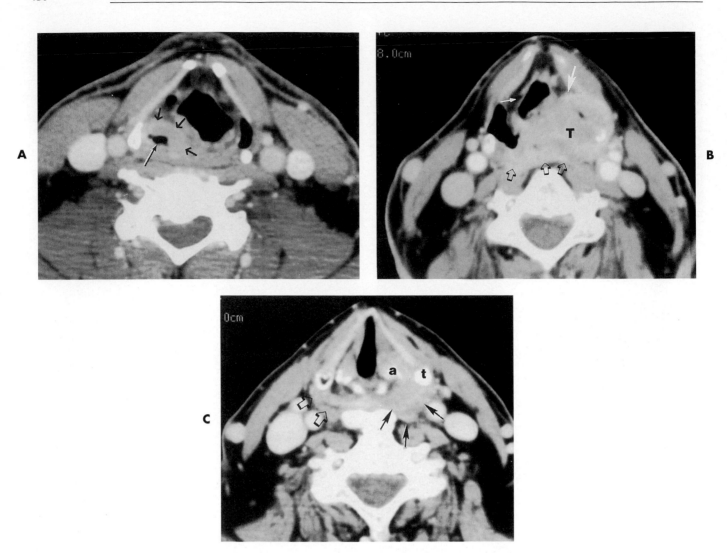

FIG. 8-64 Pyriform sinus carcinoma—CT scans. **A,** Axial CT scan shows tumor infiltrating along the lateral aspect of the right aryepiglottic fold *(black arrows),* narrowing the lumen of the pyriform sinus *(highlighted arrow).* **B,** Axial CT scan of another patient with a larger tumor *(T)* that has effaced the left aryepiglottic fold and pyriform sinus, infiltrated into the paraglottic fat *(large arrow),* and extended along the posterior wall, crossing the midline *(open arrows).* The paraglottic fat on the right is normal *(small arrow).* **C,** At the level of the true vocal cords, a CT image of another patient shows the tumor *(highlighted arrows)* extending out between the thyroid *(t)* and arytenoid *(a)* cartilages. The hypopharynx on the right is normal *(open arrows).*

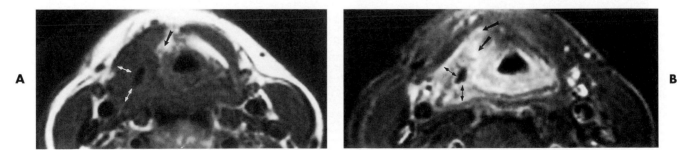

FIG. 8-65 Pyriform sinus carcinoma—MR images. **A,** Axial T1W image of a carcinoma infiltrating the right pyriform sinus *(double-headed arrows)* and the paraglottic (paralaryngeal) fat *(black arrow).* **B,** Axial T1W image after gadolinium and fat suppression shows the pyriform sinus tumor *(double-headed arrows).* The anterior extent of the tumor is apparent *(single black arrows),* but the infiltration of the paraglottic fat is not seen well.

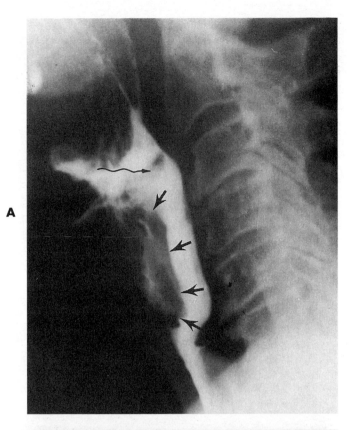

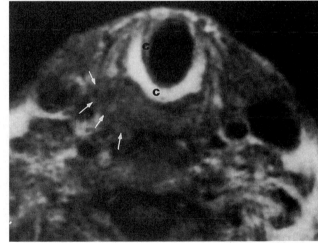

FIG. 8-66 Post-cricoid carcinoma. **A,** Lateral view from a barium study shows post-cricoid irregularity *(straight arrows)* that is much more pronounced and extensive than normal. At fluoroscopy, the irregularity was fixed and not pliable. Epiglottis *(wavy arrow).* **B,** Axial T1W MRI image shows the bulky post-cricoid tumor *(arrows).* The cricoid cartilage is ossified, and the high-signal marrow fat is intact *(c).* The cricoid cartilage was spared at histological examination.

a spot view from a barium swallow; fluoroscopic evaluation of the hypopharynx while the patient ingests barium in the lateral projection will show whether or not the wall moves with respect to the spine. Absence of movement suggests that the tumor has invaded through the posterior wall into the prevertebral muscles.

NONSQUAMOUS CELL NEOPLASMS

Minor salivary glands are located throughout the submucosa of the upper aerodigestive tract. A large variety of salivary gland tumors have been reported in these glands, with the most common ones being pleomorphic adenoma and adenoid cystic, acinic cell, and mucoepidermoid carcinomas. Athough on CT and MRI there is nothing characteristic about these tumors, they do have a tendency to grow more diffusely than SCCA, often spreading submucosally throughout the pharynx. The diagnosis is made by the pathologist, but the imaging studies are important to delineate the extent of the tumor.

On imaging, lymphoma may be identical to SCCA (Fig. 8-68, *A*). It is important to establish this diagnosis, because the primary therapy for lymphoma is chemotherapy and irradiation, whereas SCCA is primarily treated with surgery and irradiation.

Kaposi's sarcoma of the head and neck is seen almost exclusively in patients with AIDS (Fig. 8-68, *B*). In these patients, Kaposi's sarcoma is the most common malignancy, with lymphoma being the next most frequent tumor.[12] Involvement of the hypopharynx is seen much less often than oral cavity disease, and the symptoms reflect the location and vascularity of the tumor including, airway obstruction, dysphagia, and bleeding.[12] Other hypopharyngeal sarcomas (Fig. 8-68, *C*) are rare, and most have no distinguishing imaging characteristics.

Lipomas often occur in the posterior neck, but they are rare in the hypopharynx.[13] In the hypopharynx the most common location is the aryepiglottic fold.[13] They are smooth, compressible, and painless masses, although bulky ones may cause dysphagia or dyspnea, and large retropharyngeal lipomas may compress the hypopharynx.[13,14] Rare hibernomas also have also been reported in the retropharyngeal region. On imaging, all of these fatty tumors can be diagnosed by their low CT density and their fatty MR signal characteristics.

NONNEOPLASTIC PROCESSES

The typical immuno-competent patient with a pharyngitis usually does not have a CT or MRI. The diagnosis is established clinically and by cultures. However, the immuno-compromised patient with pharyngitis may have an opportunistic infection such as candida or cytomegallic virus, with involvement of the hypopharynx and esophagus. In these patients, occasional imaging is performed with the goal of mapping the disease and establishing the presence or abscence of an associated abscess.

Hematoma of the hypopharynx may be iatrogenic either from instrumentation (Fig. 8-69, *A*) or a foreign body such as a chicken bone. Rarely, retropharyngeal hematomas have occurred after minor trauma in hemophiliac patients. The high CT density of a hematoma usually allows the diagnosis to be suggested (Fig. 8-69, *A*). On a barium swallow the

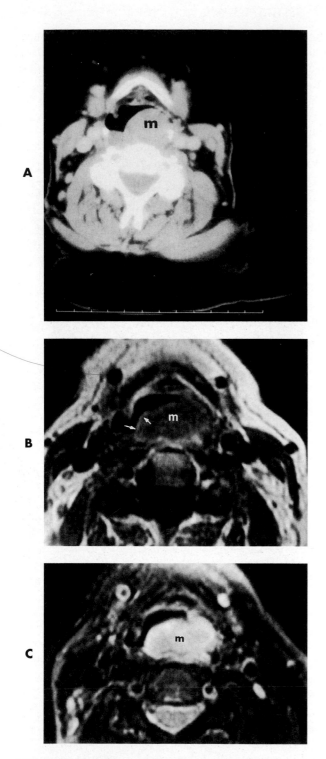

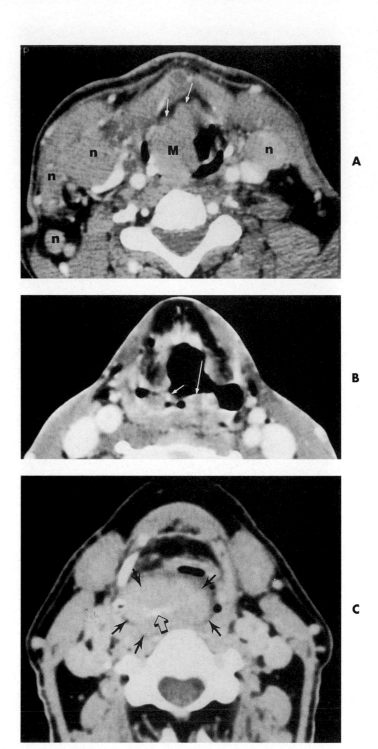

FIG. 8-67 Carcinoma of the posterior wall of the hypopharynx. **A,** Axial CT scan shows a smooth, bulky mass *(m)* arising from the posterior wall of the hypopharynx. **B,** Axial T1W image with gadolinium of the same patient as **A** shows that the tumor *(m)* enhances slightly. The mass is submucosal, and the overlying mucosa is a thin, smooth, enhancing line *(arrows)*. **C,** Axial T2W image shows that the tumor is hyperintense *(m)*.

FIG. 8-68 Non-squamous cell neoplasms—CT images. **A,** Lymphoma. Bulky mass of the right aryepiglottic fold *(M)* infiltrating the paraglottic and pre-epiglottic fat *(arrows)*, with bilateral lymphadenopathy *(n)*, cannot be distinguished radiographically from squamous cell cancer. **B,** Kaposi's sarcoma. Exophytic mass arising from the posterior wall of the hypopharynx *(large arrow)*, extending into the right pyriform sinus *(small arrow)*. **C,** Synovial cell sarcoma. Bulky tumor of the right pyriform sinus and aryepiglottic fold *(solid arrows)*, with calcification *(open arrow)* that is unusual in squamous cell cancer.

smooth narrowing of the lumen may be indistinguishable from the appearance of edema or other submucosal tumors.

On imaging, pharyngeal granulation tissue can mimic carcinoma (Fig. 8-69, *B*), and a biopsy is usually necessary to differentiate between them. "Crack" cocaine burns of the larynx and hypopharynx may also mimic carcinoma, both clinically and radiographically, and the patient may not volunteer the history that would help establish the correct diagnosis.[15]

After radiation therapy, hypopharyngeal and laryngeal edema usually persists for many months or years. These changes probably reflect a radiation-induced obliterative endarteritis (Fig. 8-69, *C*). On CT, enlarged, hypodense pharyngeal and supraglottic mucosa should not be mistaken for residual or recurrent tumor. In addition the subcutaneous fat is thickened and streaky, and the overlying platysma muscle

and skin are thick. These additional findings usually allow one to make the diagnosis of radiation-induced edema.

A retention cyst of a minor salivary gland is a small superficial mass that can occur virtually anywhere in the pharynx and supraglottic larynx. Its CT fluid density and MR signal intensities are fairly diagnostic. The appearance is similar to retention cysts elsewhere in the pharynx.

CONGENITAL ANOMALIES

The topic of the branchial embryology of the neck is discussed in detail in Chapter 14. Germain to the hypopharynx are the rare third and fourth branchial abnormalities that retain a persistent communication with the pyriform sinus.[16] The third pouch has a sinus opening in the upper pyriform sinus, and the fourth pouch sinus enters the lower pyriform

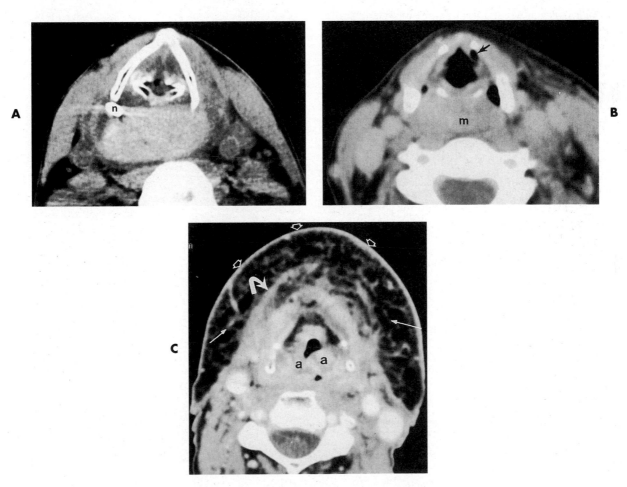

FIG. 8-69   A, Axial CT without contrast shows a large, hyperdense intramural hematoma of the hypopharynx. The patient had been anticoagulated, then required emergency intubation. The nasogastric tube *(n)* is in the right hypopharynx. **B,** Axial CT shows a large post-cricoid mass *(m)* thought to be carcinoma clinically and radiographically. Biopsy showed acute and chronic inflammation and granulation tissue in a patient who had been intubated for long periods of time. There is a small amount of air in the appendix of the left laryngeal ventricle *(arrow)*. **C,** Axial CT with contrast shows diffuse edema secondary to radiation therapy. The aryepiglottic folds are thick *(a)*, the subcutaneous fat is streaky *(thin, straight arrows)*, the platysma muscle *(curved arrow)* and the skin *(open arrows)* are thick.

sinus (Fig. 8-70, *A,B*). These anomalies are far rarer than first or second branchial anomalies. The overwhelming majority of fourth branchial pouch sinuses are on the left side, for reasons that are not known.[16] However, recurrent suppurative (left-sided) thyroiditis in a child or adult should strongly suggest this diagnosis (Fig. 8-70, *A*).[16] A fourth branchial pouch anomaly may present in the neonate as a lateral neck mass that clinically resembles a lymphangioma.[16]

EXTRINSIC MASSES

On a barium swallow, during maximum relaxation of the cricopharyngeus, there normally should be no posterior submucosal mass seen that identifies the level of the cricopharyngeus. If such an impression is identified (Fig. 8-71, *A*), it suggests dyssynergy or cricopharyngeal spasm. Posterior submucosal impressions on the barium column can result from osteophytes (Fig. 8-71, *B*) or rare anterior bulgings of intervertebral disks. Interestingly, even exhuberant anterior osteophytes rarely cause dysphagia unless there is a concomitant reason to limit the range of motion of the larynx (prior surgery, irradiation, etc.). A prominent lobe of the thyroid gland may occasionally cause an extrinsic mass on the anterolateral pharyngeal barium column, especially in older patients. It must be also remembered, that often symptoms of dysphagia reflect an hiatus hernia with reflux.

A tortuous common carotid artery may swing behind the posterior wall of the hypopharynx (Fig. 8-71, *C*), and on clinical inspection a pulsating, submucosal bulge is apparent. Before the CT and MRI era this abnormality was considered rare. However, presently this abnormality is considered relatively common, often seen on a scan as an incidental observation. The importance of imaging is to identify the etiology of this diagnosis, thus stopping an unnecessary and dangerous biopsy.

In patients with neurofibromatosis type I, plexiform neurofibromas may arise within the soft tissues surrounding the hypopharynx, and large neurofibromas can encroach upon the hypopharyngeal airway (Fig. 8-71, *D*).

Perforation of the hypopharynx may result from an ingested foreign body or instrumentation (endoscopy, biopsy). Such perforation of the pharynx may lead to development of a retropharyngeal abscess, and pus and edema can spread throughout the retropharyngeal space (Fig. 8-71, *E*). Suppurative adenitis of a retropharyngeal lymph node can also result in retropharyngeal edema and infection. However, retropharyngeal edema from prior irradiation may persist for many months after the radiation (Fig. 8-69, *C*) and can mimic the imaging appearance of a retropharyngeal infection. These two entities should not be confused, and history in these patients is very important (Fig. 8-71, *E*).

DIVERTICULA

Zenker's diverticulum is a mucosal lined outpouching of the hypopharynx (Fig. 8-72, *A*), and dyssynergy of the cricopharyngeus muscle seems to play a role in the formation of this

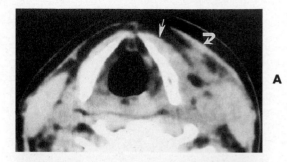

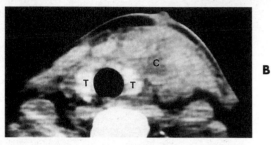

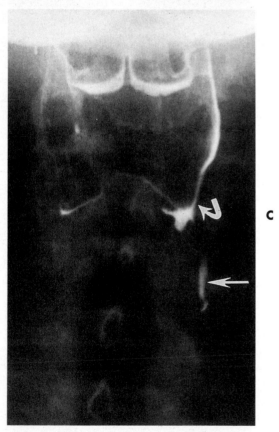

FIG. 8-70 Fourth branchial pouch sinus. **A,** Axial CT at the level of the hypopharynx shows diffuse edema of the left neck; the strap muscles *(straight arrow)* and platysma muscle *(curved arrow)* are enlarged, and the fat is infiltrated. **B,** Axial CT at the level of the thyroid gland *(T)* shows a heterogeneous collection *(C)* deep to the edematous sternocleidomastoid muscle. **C,** Frontal view from a barium swallow shows the sinus tract *(straight arrow)* extending down from the lower pyriform sinus *(curved arrow)*.

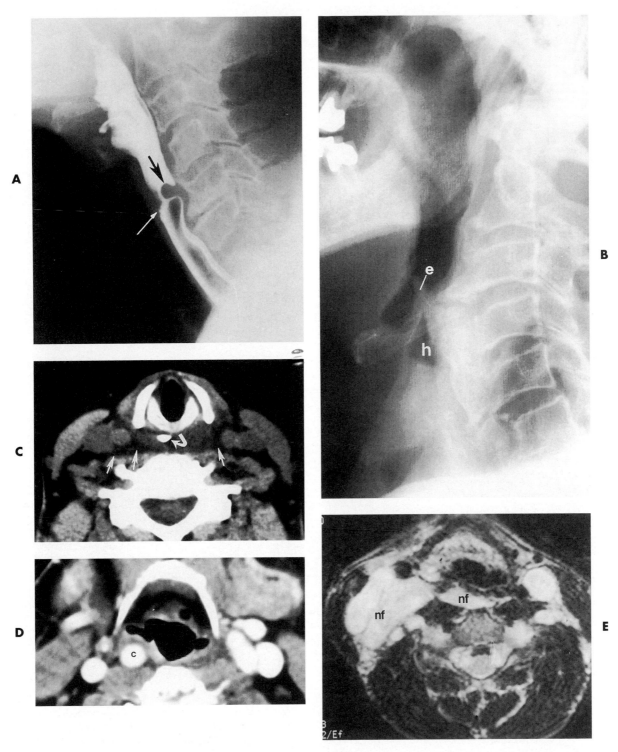

FIG. 8-71 Extrinsic impressions on the hypopharynx. **A,** Lateral view of a barium swallow of a patient with dysphagia shows a prominent cricopharyngeus muscle *(black arrow)* that fails to relax as the bolus passes. The irregularity of the postcricoid region is normal *(white arrow)*. **B,** Lateral view of the cervical spine of a patient who complained of repeated aspiration. Large anterior osteophytes compress the hypopharynx *(h)*. Epiglottis *(e)*. **C,** Axial CT of a patient who ingested a pork bone *(curved arrow)* that perforated the hypopharynx, causing retropharyngeal edema *(straight arrows)*. (Courtesy Dr. Deborah Reede.) **D,** Contrast-enhanced CT shows a tortuous right common carotid artery *(c)* indenting the posterior wall of the pyriform sinus. **E,** Axial T2W image with gadolinium shows an extensive plexiform neurofibroma in the right neck that extends behind the hypopharynx *(nf)*. There are also tumors in the left neck and the neural foramina, in this patient who had neurofibromatosis type 1.

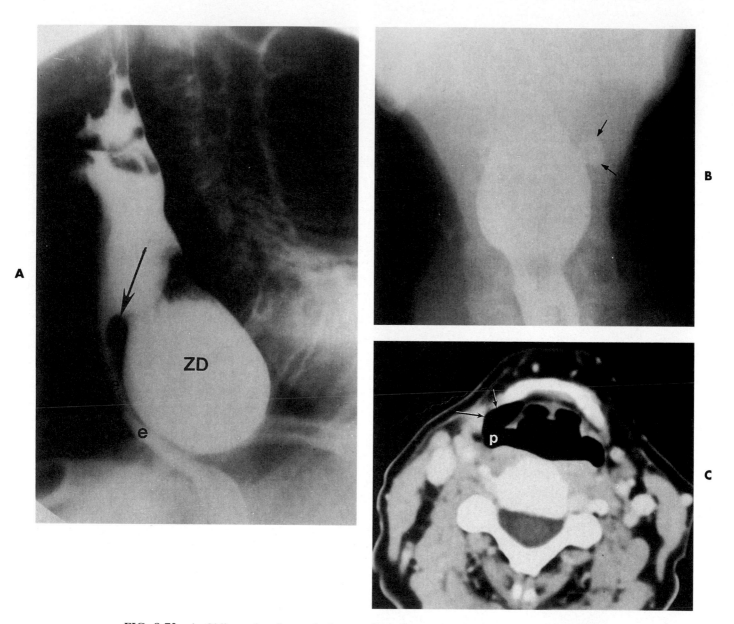

FIG. 8-72   **A,** Oblique view from a barium swallow shows a large Zenker's diverticulum *(ZD)* extending from the hypopharynx above the cricopharyngeus muscle *(arrow)* and extending down into the upper chest behind the cervical esophagus *(e)*. **B,** Frontal view of a barium swallow shows a small pharyngocele *(arrows)* arising from the left pyriform sinus. **C,** Axial CT shows an air-filled pharyngocele *(arrows)* arising from the right pyriform sinus *(p)*.

pulsion diverticulum.[5] Because this muscle fails to relax as a bolus passes, a high "upstream" pressure is created, thus contributing to the development of this diverticulum. The Zenker's diverticulum protrudes through Killian's dehiscence, extends posteriorly and often laterally, usually to the left side.[5]

A pharyngocele is a benign outpouching of the pharyngeal mucosa of the upper pyriform sinus. A frontal barium swallow film best shows the pharyngocele, which fills with barium (Fig. 8-72, *A*) as a broad-based outpouching. These pharyngoceles distend on phonation and with Valsalva maneuvers. An air-filled pharyngocele can occasionally be seen on CT as an incidental finding (Fig. 8-72, *B*).

In a patient with a paralyzed vocal cord or unilateral vagal paralysis, the ipsilateral pyriform sinus may be large. This appearance is described further in Chapter 11.

References

1. Million RR, Cassisi NJ, Mancuso AA. Hypopharynx: pharyngeal walls, pyriform sinus, postcricoid pharynx. In: Million RR, Cassisi NJ, eds. Management of head and neck cancer: a multidisciplinary approach. Philadelphia, Pa: JB Lippincott Company, 1994:505-532.

2. Beahrs OH, Henson DE, Hutter RVP, et al, eds. American Joint Committee on Cancer, manual for staging of cancer. Pharynx (including base of tongue, soft palate, and uvula). 4th Edition. Philadelphia, Pa: JB Lippincott, 1992;33-38.

3. Barnes L, Gnepp DR. Diseases of the larynx, hypopharynx, and esophagus. In: Barnes L, ed. Surgical pathology of the head and neck. New York, NY: Decker, Inc, 1985; 141-226.

4. Muntz H, Sessions DG. Surgery of laryngopharyngeal and subglottic cancer. In: Bailey BT, Hiller HF, eds. Surgery of the larynx. Philadelphia, Pa: WB Saunders Co, 1985; 293-315.

5. Graney DO, Marsh B. Trachea/bronchus/esophagus: anatomy. In: Cummings CW, Fredrickson JM, Harker LA, et al. Otolaryngology-head and neck surgery. St. Louis, Mo: Mosby-Year Book, 1993; 2207-2216.

6. Hollinshead WH. Textbook of anatomy. Hagerstown, Md: Harper and Row, Publishers Inc, 1974; 928-948.

7. Robbins KT. Pocket guide to neck dissection classification and TNM staging of head and neck cancer. Alexandria, Va: American Academy of Otolaryngology-Head and Neck Surgery Foundation, Inc, 1991.

8. Brick SB, Caroline DF, Lev-Toaff AS, et al. Esophageal disruption: evaluation with Iohexol esophagography. Radiology 1988; 169:141-143.

9. Lufkin RB, Hanafee WN, Wortham D, et al. Larynx and hypopharynx: MR imaging with surface coils. Radiology 1986; 158:747-754.

10. Adams GL. Malignant neoplasms of the hypopharynx. In: Cummings CW, Fredrickson JM, Harker LA, et al. Otolaryngology-head and neck surgery. St. Louis, Mo: Mosby-Year Book, 1993; 1955-1973.

11. Aspestrand F, Kolbenstvedt A, Boysen M. Carcinoma of the hypopharynx: CT staging. J Comput Assist Tomogr 1990; 14:72-76.

12. Goldberg AN. Kaposi's sarcoma of the head and neck in acquired immunodeficiency syndrome. Am J Otolaryngol 1993; 14:5-14.

13. Barnes L. Tumors and tumorlike lesions of the soft tissues. In: Barnes L, editor. Surgical pathology of the head and neck. New York, Ny: Decker, 1985; 725-880.

14. Johnson JT, Curtin HD. Deep neck lipoma. Annals Otol Rhinol Laryngol 1987; 96:472-473.

15. Snyderman CH, Weissman JL, Tabor ET, et al. Crack cocaine burns of the larynx. Arch Otolaryngol Head Neck Surg 1991; 117:792-795.

16. Rosenfeld RM, Biller HF. Fourth branchial pouch sinus: diagnosis and treatment. Otolaryngol Head Neck Surg 1991; 105:44-50.

9

Oral Cavity

WENDY R.K. SMOKER

The oral cavity is the most ventral portion of the aerodigestive tract, and it is separated from the oropharynx by a ring of structures that includes the circumvallate papillae, the anterior tonsillar pillars, and the soft palate. From a clinical standpoint this anatomic subdivision is useful because malignancies, especially squamous cell carcinomas, in these two regions differ in their presentations, prognoses, and histologic grades.[1,2] This chapter is primarily confined to the oral cavity, including the oral tongue (anterior two thirds of the tongue), floor of the mouth, lips, gingivobuccal and buccomasseteric regions, and the supporting bones of the maxilla (hard palate) and mandible. The posterior one third of the tongue (base of the tongue), considered a part of the oropharynx, is discussed in Chapter 8.

NORMAL ANATOMY
Oral Tongue

The tongue consists of symmetrical halves separated from each other by a midline septum. It has a "supporting skeleton" composed of the lingual septum and the hyoglossus membrane, a thin, broad sheet suspended between the two minor tubercles of the hyoid bone. The fibrous lingual septum arises from the midline of the hyoglossus membrane and the middle of the hyoid bone. This fibrous lingual septum, referred to by some as the *midline low-density plane* (MLDP), is visible as a hypodense midline structure on virtually every CT scan of the tongue (Figs. 9-1, 9-2).[3,4] Each half of the tongue is composed of muscular fibers arranged in various directions, which can be divided into extrinsic

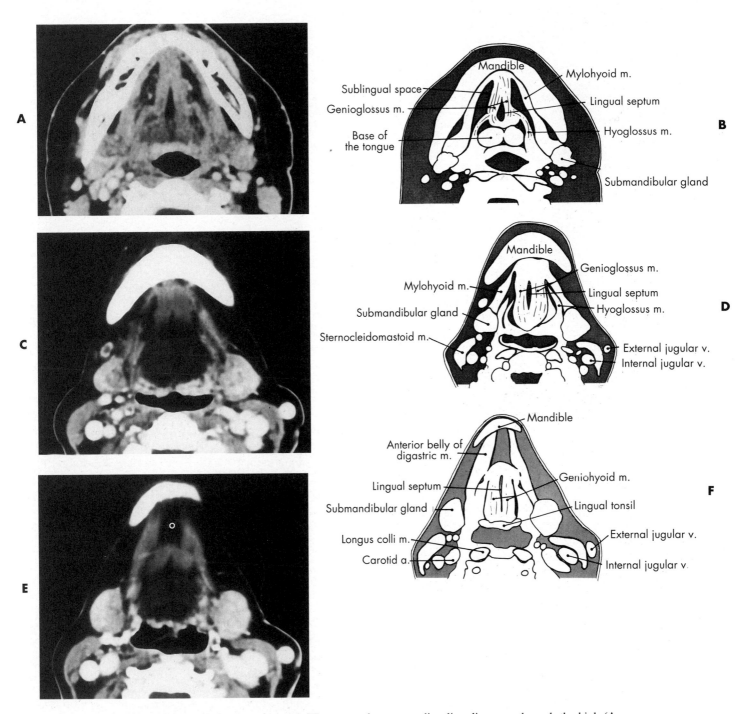

FIG. 9-1 Normal anatomy. Axial CT scans and corresponding line diagrams through the high (**A** and **B**), middle (**C** and **D**), and low (**E** and **F**) floor of the mouth. (*White dot* in **E** represents the fat-filled, midline submental space.)

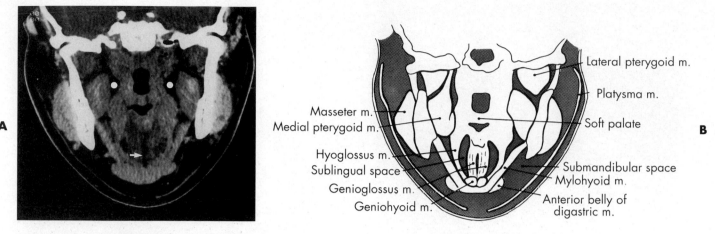

FIG. 9-2 Normal anatomy. Coronal CT (**A**) and corresponding line diagram (**B**) through the floor of the mouth, buccomasseteric regions, and masticator spaces. *Arrow*, Lingual septum; *dots*, parapharyngeal space fat.

and intrinsic muscles. There are four interdigitating intrinsic tongue muscles: the superior and inferior longitudinal, the transverse, and the vertical or oblique muscles, which make up the bulk of the tongue. The extrinsic muscles are those that have their origins external to the tongue itself, yet their more distal fibers interdigitate within the substance of the tongue. The extrinsic muscles provide attachment of the tongue to the hyoid bone, mandible, and styloid process of the skull base. The main extrinsic tongue muscles are the genioglossus, hyoglossus, and styloglossus muscles.[5,6] Some also consider the palatoglossus and superior pharyngeal constrictor muscles in their discussion of the extrinsic tongue muscles.[7]

Intrinsic Muscles of the Tongue

The superior longitudinal muscle consists of a thin layer of oblique and longitudinal fibers that arise from the hyoglossus membrane and the fibrous lingual septum. The fibers fan out into a broad sheet, passing forward and outward to the edges of the tongue, just under the mucosa of the dorsum of the tongue.

The inferior longitudinal muscle has the same origin as the superior longitudinal muscle, but it is divided into two halves by the genioglossus muscle situated in the undersurface of the tongue. The inferior longitudinal muscle extends from the base to the tip of the tongue, lying medial to the hyoglossus and lateral to the genioglossus muscles.

The transverse muscles originate from the fibrous septum and fan outward to insert into the submucosal fibrous layer at the sides of the tongue. Intersecting with these transverse fibers are fibers from the vertical (oblique) muscles that extend from the upper surface to the undersurface of the tongue. Vertical fibers are only encountered at the borders of the anterior portion of the tongue.[7]

The intrinsic muscles are difficult to identify on CT,

and fibers of the superior longitudinal muscle have on occasion been mistaken for a tumor.[4] However, these muscle bundles are easily appreciated on MR because the low signal intensity muscle fibers are surrounded by the higher signal intensity of the fibrofatty tissues.[8] In particular, sagittal MRI will demonstrate the entirety of the longitudinal muscles (Fig. 9-3).[9]

The complex arrangement of the tongue musculature enables enunciation of various consonants. The superior longitudinal muscle tends to shorten the tongue and turn its tip and sides upward to render the dorsum concave. The inferior longitudinal muscle also shortens the tongue but pulls the tip downward to render the dorsum convex. The transverse muscle fibers narrow and elongate the tongue, and the vertical fibers flatten and broaden the tongue. The intrinsic muscles of the tongue receive motor innervation from the hypoglossal nerve (XII).

Extrinsic Muscles of the Tongue

Genioglossus Muscles. The paired genioglossus muscles originate via a short tendon from the superior genial tubercle on the inner surface of the mandible, just above the origin of the geniohyoid muscles. The fibers quickly fan out, the inferior fibers attaching via a thin aponeurosis to the body of the hyoid bone, the middle fibers coursing posteriorly, and the superior fibers directed upward and forward insert into the entire length of the undersurface of the tongue from its base to its apex. Posteriorly the genioglossus muscles are quite distinct from each other, separated by the midline lingual septum and fatty tissue, and they are easily identified on both axial and coronal CT and MRI (Figs. 9-1, 9-2). The two muscles are quite symmetric, measuring 9 to 11 mm in transverse dimension at their intersection with the hyoglossus muscle.[10] More anteriorly, however, the fibers from the two muscles are less distinct and somewhat blended

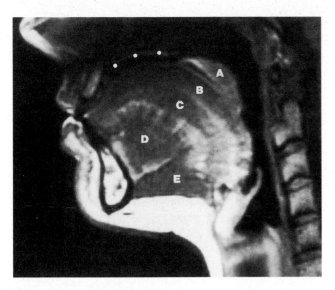

FIG. 9-3 T1W, midsagittal MR scan. *Dots,* Hard palate; *A,* soft palate; *B,* superior longitudinal muscle fibers; *C,* transverse muscle fibers; *D,* genioglossus muscle; *E,* geniohyoid muscle.

together because fascicles from one muscle cross the midline to interdigitate with those of the contralateral muscle.[7]

Hyoglossus Muscle. The hyoglossus muscles are thin, flat, quadrilateral muscles, forming the lateral borders of the tongue. They arise from the greater cornua of the hyoid bone and course vertically, lateral to the genioglossus muscles, to insert into the sides of the tongue. In its posterosuperior aspect, fibers of the hyoglossus interdigitate with fibers of the styloglossus muscle (see next paragraph). The hyoglossus muscle is best evaluated by CT or MRI in the axial plane (Fig. 9-1).[3] The normal transverse diameter of each muscle, measured in the axial plane, is 5 to 7 mm.[10]

Styloglossus Muscle. The styloglossus muscle arises from the anterolateral surface of the styloid process of the temporal bone, near its apex, and from portions of the stylomandibular ligament. Passing downward and forward between the internal and external carotid arteries, it divides at the side of the tongue into two sets of fibers. The longitudinal fibers enter the side of the tongue near its dorsal surface, anterior to the hyoglossus fibers, and the more posterior oblique fibers interdigitate with fibers of the hyoglossus muscle.

Motor and Sensory Innervation of the Tongue

The intrinsic and extrinsic muscles of the tongue all receive motor innervation from the hypoglossal nerve (XII), which courses between the mylohyoid and hyoglossus muscles. Adjacent to the hypoglossal nerve is the lingual nerve, a branch of the trigeminal nerve that carries sensory fibers from the anterior portion of the tongue. Special sensory taste fibers from the anterior two thirds of the tongue (oral tongue) course with the lingual nerve over a short distance before they coalesce to form the chorda tympani nerve, which extends to the lateral skull base, traverses the middle

ear, and joins the facial nerve. Special sensory taste fibers from the posterior one third of the tongue (tongue base) are supplied by the glossopharnygeal nerve (IX).

Floor of the Mouth

The floor of the mouth is a U-shaped structure covered by squamous mucosa. The primary muscles comprising the floor of the mouth are the mylohyoid muscles and their fibrous median raphe. Additional support is provided by the paired anterior bellies of the digastric muscles and the geniohyoid muscles (Fig. 9-2). Surgically the floor of the mouth is considered that space between the mucosa of the floor of the mouth and the mylohyoid muscle sling. Caudal to this muscle but above the hyoid bone, the space is considered the suprahyoid neck.

Mylohyoid Muscle

The mylohyoid muscle is a flat, triangular muscle that arises from the entire length of the mylohyoid ridge on the inner surface of the mandible and extends from the mandibular symphysis anteriorly to the last molar tooth posteriorly.[7] Posterior fibers course inferiorly to insert onto the body of the hyoid bone. The remaining middle and anterior fibers insert into the fibrous median raphe that runs between the mandibular symphysis and the hyoid bone, thus joining with fibers from the opposite side to form a U-shaped muscular floor of the mouth. The mylohyoid muscle sling is best demonstrated by CT and MRI in the coronal plane (Fig. 9-2). The mylohyoid branch of the inferior alveolar nerve (a branch of the mandibular division of the trigeminal nerve [V3]) provides motor innervation to the mylohyoid muscle. Just before entering the mandibular foramen, the inferior alveolar nerve gives off the small mylohyoid nerve, which descends in a groove on the inner surface of the mandible, held in position by a fibrous membrane.[7]

There is a gap at the free posterior border of the mylohyoid muscle, between it and the hyoglossus muscle. It is via this gap that the submandibular gland wraps around the dorsal aspect of the mylohyoid muscle, with the deep lobe of the gland lying medial (cranial) to the muscle fibers and the superficial lobe lying on its external (caudal) surface.

Digastric Muscle

The digastric muscle consists of two bellies. The anterior belly arises from the digastric fossa on the inner surface of the mandible, just below the genial tubercles. The posterior belly arises from the digastric fossa on the inner surface of the mastoid process of the temporal bone. The two bellies terminate in a central tendon that pierces the stylohyoid muscle and runs through a fibrous loop (lined with a synovial membrane) that is attached to the body and greater cornua of the hyoid. The two paramedian anterior digastric muscles lie just below the mylohyoid muscle sling and thus contribute to the muscular floor of the mouth. They are best demonstrated on CT and MRI in the coronal plane. The anterior belly of the digastric muscle is innervated by the mylohyoid branch of the mandibular nerve (V3), and the posterior belly receives its innervation from the facial nerve (VII).

Geniohyoid Muscle

The geniohyoid muscle is a slender muscle that arises from the inferior genial tubercle on the inner surface of the mandible. It passes inferiorly to insert onto the anterior surface of the body of the hyoid bone. Closely approximated, the geniohyoid muscles lie just above the mylohyoid sling; this is best appreciated on CT and MRI obtained in the coronal plane. Because the geniohyoid muscles do not have interspersed fibrofatty tissue, as do the extrinsic muscles of the tongue, they may occasionally appear more dense than the genioglossus muscles on CT. Motor innervation to the geniohyoid muscles is variably described as being from the hypoglossal nerve (XII) by a few fibers from C1 that course with the hypoglossal nerve until it crosses the internal carotid artery or by motor fibers from both C1 and C2.[5-7,11]

Sublingual Region

Superomedial to the mylohyoid muscle, lateral to the genioglossus-geniohyoid muscles, and below the mucosa of the floor of the mouth is the primarily fat-filled sublingual region, referred to by some authors as the *lateral low-density plane (LLDP)*.[3,4,12] This region, also known as the *sublingual space*, or *compartment of the submandibular space*, is continuous with the submandibular region at the posterior margin of the mylohyoid muscle (Fig. 9-4, *A*). Contents of this sublingual "space" include the sublingual gland and ducts, the submandibular gland duct (Wharton's duct), and occasionally a portion of the hilum of the submandibular gland, the anterior fibers of the hyoglossus muscle, and the lingual nerve, artery, and vein. The hyoglossus muscle is an important surgical landmark to the anatomy of the sublingual region because it separates Wharton's duct and the hypoglossal and lingual nerves, which lie lateral to the muscle, from the lingual artery and vein, which course medial to this muscle (Fig. 9-4, *B*).[3] The submandibular gland duct arises from the deep portion of the gland and runs anteriorly, in contact with the hypoglossal and lingual nerves. Initially it lies between the hyoglossus and mylohyoid muscles, and more anteriorly it lies between the genioglossus and mylohyoid muscles. The duct drains into the floor of the mouth, just lateral to the frenulum of the tongue.

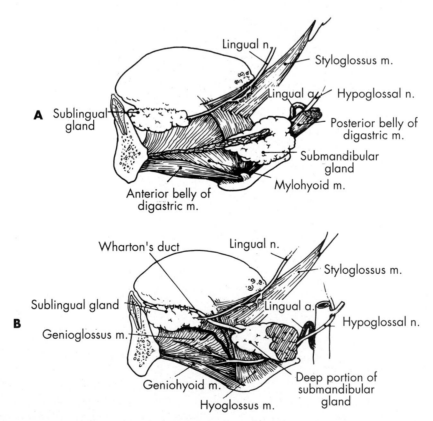

FIG. 9-4 Line diagram demonstrating normal structure relationships. **A,** Lateral view with mylohyoid muscle in place. The mylohyoid muscle separates the anterior belly of the digastric muscle, which lies superficial, from the geniohyoid muscle, which lies on a deeper plane. The submandibular gland wraps around the posterior margin of the mylohyoid muscle, and its deep lobe enters the posterior aspect of the sublingual space. Note the fibrous loop that anchors the common digastric tendon to the hyoid bone. **B,** Lateral view of the oral cavity with the mylohyoid and digastric muscles removed. Note that Wharton's duct, along with the hypoglossal and lingual nerves, lies superficial to the hyoglossus muscle and the facial vessels lie on a plane deep to the muscle.

Lips and Gingivobuccal Region

The lips are composed primarily of the orbicularis oris muscle, which consists of multiple strata of muscular fibers with different directions that surround the orifice of the mouth. The orbicularis oris is not a sphincter muscle, but it is composed of muscle fibers derived from multiple facial muscles that insert into the lips and some additional fibers proper to the lips themselves. Muscles that contribute to the orbicularis oris include the levator labii superioris alaeque nasi, levator labii superioris, levator anguli oris, zygomaticus major, depressor anguli oris, platysma, risorius, and buccinator muscles.[7] Motor innervation to the lips is supplied by the facial nerve (VII), and lymphatic drainage is primarily to the submental and submandibular lymph nodes. The external surface of the lips is covered by keratinizing stratified squamous epithelium, and the internal surface is lined by nonkeratinizing stratified squamous mucosa.

The vestibule of the mouth separates the lips and cheeks, which are lined by buccal mucosa, from the teeth and gums. It is essentially a cleft into which drain the ducts of the parotid glands and mucous glands of the lips and cheeks. The vestibule is bounded superiorly and inferiorly by reflection of buccal mucosa of the lips and cheeks onto the mandible and maxilla and is continuous posteriorly with the oral cavity proper through an interval between the last molar tooth and the ramus of the mandible.

The gingiva is the mucosal covering, overlying both the medial (lingual) and lateral (buccal) aspects of the mandible and maxilla. The junction of the gingiva with the buccal mucosa is termed the *gingivobuccal sulcus* and is a common location for squamous cell carcinoma of the oral cavity. There is, in addition, a triangular area of mucosa posterior to the last mandibular molar tooth, termed the retromolar trigone, which covers the ascending ramus of the mandible. The retromolar trigone is another area in which squamous cell carcinomas commonly arise.

Buccomasseteric Region

The term *buccomasseteric region* refers to the masseter and buccinator muscles, the buccal space situated lateral to the buccinator muscle and anterior to the masseter muscle, and the inferior body of the mandible (Fig. 9-5).[13] The masseter, one of the four muscles of mastication, is innervated by the masticator nerve, a branch of the mandibular division of the trigeminal nerve (Table 9-1). Posteriorly the muscle is largely covered by the superficial lobe of the parotid gland, and buccomasseteric pathology is not infrequently initially mistaken as parotid disease.

The buccinator (*buccina*, a trumpet) muscle, the major muscle of the cheek, is located external to the buccal mucosa. It is a deep muscle of facial expression that is innervated by a branch of the facial nerve (VII) (see Table 9-1). Its main function is to compress the cheeks (i.e., during mastication, playing the trumpet, etc.). The origin of this muscle is from the alveolar process of the maxilla and mandible opposite the sockets of the molar teeth and the anterior bor-

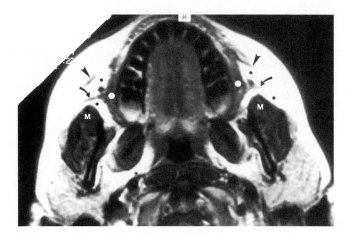

FIG. 9-5 Buccomasseteric region, normal anatomy. Axial T1W MR scan demonstrates the buccal spaces bilaterally *(black dots)*, lying between the fibers of the zygomaticus major muscles *(arrowheads)* and the masseter muscles *(M)*. The parotid gland ducts are identified bilaterally *(curved arrows)*, crossing the buccal space fat pads to pierce the buccinator muscles *(white dots)* and open into the vestibule of the mouth opposite the second maxillary molars. The facial arteries are well visualized bilaterally, just anterior to the parotid gland ducts.

der of the pterygomandibular raphe. The fibers of the buccinator muscle converge toward the angle of the mouth, where they blend and insert into the orbicularis oris muscle. One origin of the buccinator muscle is from the pterygomandibular raphe, a thick fascial band that extends between the hamulus of the medial pterygoid plate and the mylohyoid ridge of the mandible. The pterygomandibular raphe, forming the line of attachment for the buccinator and superior pharyngeal constrictor muscles, is the junction of the oropharynx and oral cavity, lying between the anterior tonsillar pillar and the retromolar trigone.[14] Malignancies may extend cephalad along this raphe into the upper buccinator space or the suprazygomatic portion of the masticator space, or they may reach caudally to the mylohyoid muscle and along the floor of the mouth. The pterygomandibular raphe delimits the pterygomandibular space, a fat-filled region medial to the mandible and medial pterygoid muscle and anterior to the deep lobe of the parotid gland. The significance of this space lies in the fact that the lingual and inferior alveolar branches of the trigeminal nerve traverse it.

The buccal space, limited by the superior and inferior attachments of the buccinator muscle, is located lateral to the buccinator muscle, deep to the zygomaticus major muscle, and anterior to the mandibular ramus and masseter muscle. It contains primarily the buccal fat pad, a usually well-circumscribed mass of fat with prolongations that may extend between the muscles of mastication.[15] The superior extent of the buccal fat pad is continuous with the retroantral fat behind the posterior wall of the maxillary antrum in the infratemporal fossa. The duct of the parotid gland (Stenson's duct) crosses the masseter muscle, courses through the buccal fat pad, pierces the buccinator muscle opposite the second maxillary molar, and drains into the vestibule of the

TABLE 9-1
Muscles Associated with the Oral Cavity

Intrinsic Muscles of the Tongue	Origin	Insertion	Motor Innervation	Action
Superior longitudinal constrictor muscles	Hyoglossal membrane and fibrous lingual septum	Edges of the tongue under dorsum mucosa, fanning out to a broad sheet	Hypoglossal nerve (XII)	Shortens the tongue and turns the tip and sides up to render the dorsum concave
Inferior longitudinal constrictor muscles	Hyoglossal membrane and fibrous lingual septum but divided by genioglossus muscles and situated on undersurface of the tongue	From base to the tip of the tongue medial to hyoglossus and lateral to genioglossus muscles	Hypoglossal nerve (XII)	Shortens the tongue but pulls tip downward to render the dorsum convex
Transverse muscles	Fibrous lingual septum	Fan out to insert into the submucosal fibrous layer at sides of tongue	Hypoglossal nerve (XII)	Narrows and elongates the tongue
Vertical/ oblique muscles	Upper surface of the tongue	Undersurface of the tongue	Hypoglossal nerve (XII)	Flattens and broadens the tongue
Genioglossus muscle	From the upper mental spines of the genial tubercles	Contacts its counterpart in the median plane and fans vertically into the tongue, inserted throughout its length; some inferior fibers reach the hyoid bone	Hypoglossal nerve (XII)	Acting together, the two muscles protrude the tongue; one muscle is paralyzed, the tip of the tongue deviates toward the inactive side
Hyoglossus muscle	Body and greater horn of hyoid bone	Posterior one half of the side of the tongue	Hypoglossal nerve (XII)	Depresses the sides of the tongue and enlarges the cavity of the mouth
Styloglossus muscle	From tip of styloid process of temporal bone and adjacent part of stylohyoid ligament	Entire length of the side of the tongue, interdigitating with fibers of the hyoglossus muscle	Hypoglossal nerve (XII)	Pulls the tongue postero-superiorly during swallowing
Mylohyoid muscle	Entire length of the mylohyoid line on inner surface of the mandible	Into a fibrous median raphe extending from the symphysis of the mandible to the body of the hyoid bone	Mylohyoid nerve branch of the inferior alveolar branch of the mandibular division of the Trigeminal nerve (V_3)	Raises the hyoid bone and tongue during swallowing and forms the muscular floor of the mouth.
Anterior belly of the digastric muscle	Digastric fossa of the mandible just below the genial tubercles	United by an intermediate tendon with the posterior belly, bound to the upper border of the hyoid bone by a loop of fibrous tissue	Mylohyoid nerve branch of the inferior alveolar branch of mandibular division of Trigeminal nerve (V_3) (*Note*: The posterior belly is innervated by the facial nerve [VII])	Acting with its posterior belly, it raises the hyoid bone during swallowing; acting with the infrahyoid strap muscles, it fixes the hyoid bone to form a stable base on which the tongue can move
Geniohyoid muscles	From the lower mental spines of the genial tubercles, on inner surface of mandible near midline	The paired muscles course side by side on the superior surface of the mylohyoid muscle to insert onto the anterior body of the hyoid bone	Fibers from C1	Pulls the hyoid bone anterosuperiorly

TABLE 9-1
Muscles Associated with the Oral Cavity —cont'd

Intrinsic Muscles of the Tongue	Origin	Insertion	Motor Innervation	Action
Buccinator muscle	Outer surface of the alveolar processes of the mandible and maxilla corresponding to the three molar teeth; anterior margin of the pterygomandibular raphe	Fibers coverge toward the angle of the mouth where central fibers intersect each other, being continuous with the orbicularis oris, and upper and lowermost fibers continuing into corresponding segments of the lip without decussation	Facial nerve (VII)	Used during mastication to press cheek against the teeth, thus preventing food from escaping into vestibule of the mouth
Masseter muscle	Inferior margin and deep surface of zygomatic arch from tubercle at its root posteriorly to the junction with the zygomatic process of the maxilla anteriorly	Lateral surface of the ramus and coronoid process of the mandible	Branch of the mandibular division of Trigeminal nerve (V_3)	Raises the mandible, clenches the teeth, and superficial fibers help protract mandible
Medial pterygoid muscle	Superficial head arises from maxillary tuberosity; deep head arises from medial surface of the lateral pterygoid plate, deep to the lateral pterygoid muscle	Rough area between the mandibular foramen and angle of the mandible; its fibers essentially parallel those of the anterior masseter fibers	Branch of the mandibular division of Trigeminal nerve (V_3)	Raises the mandible, assists in protrusion, and slews the chin to the opposite side; acting alternately, the muscles produce a grinding movement
Lateral pterygoid muscle	Upper head arises from infratemporal ridge and infratemporal surface of greater wing of sphenoid bone; lower head arises from lateral surface of lateral pterygoid plate	Into front of the neck of the mandible and the articular disk through the capsule of the temporomandibular joint	Branch of the mandibular division of the Trigeminal nerve (V_3)	Together, the two muscles protrude the mandible and depress the chin, drawing the head of the mandible and the disk forward onto articular tubercle; when one acts alone, the head of the mandible on that side is drawn forward, the mandible pivots around the joint and the chin is slewed to the opposite side
Temporalis muscle	Floor of the temporal fossa and from temporal fascia	Summit and anterior margin of coronoid process and anterior margin of ramus; medial side of coronoid process down to junction of ramus with body of mandible behind the third molar tooth	Deep temporal branches of the mandibular division of the Trigeminal nerve (V_3)	Raises the mandible; posterior fibers retract the mandible after protraction

mouth (Fig. 9-5). The facial artery also courses through the buccal fat pad, typically seen in cross section on axial images. When involved by tumor or infection, the buccal space may serve as a route of spread between the mouth and the parotid gland.[16]

The buccomasseteric region is also commonly involved by disease processes involving the masticator space, a fas-cially defined region that contains the muscles of mastication, including the masseter muscle, portions of the mandible, the maxillary artery, and branches of the mandibular division of the trigeminal nerve (Fig. 9-6).[17,18] Pathology of the masticator space most commonly results from dental infections involving the second or third mandibular molars.

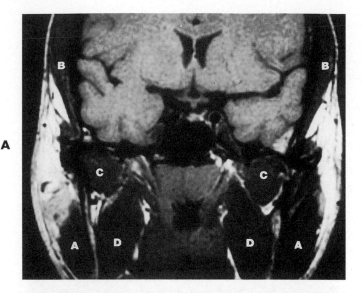

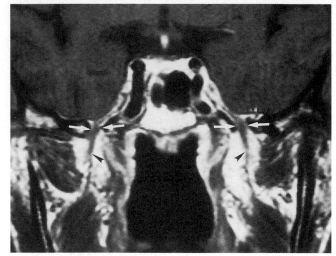

FIG. 9-6 Masticator space, normal anatomy. **A,** Coronal T1W MR demonstrates normal muscles of mastication bilaterally. *A,* Masseter muscles; *B,* temporalis muscles; *C,* lateral pterygoid muscles; *D,* medial pterygoid muscles. **B,** Coronal T1W MR following contrast administration optimally demonstrates the mandibular nerves bilaterally *(black arrowheads)* as they traverse the foramen ovale bilaterally *(white arrows).*

PATHOLOGY
Congenital Anomalies
Congenital Absence of the Tongue

Extremely rare, congenital absence of the tongue has been reported in only a single instance.[19]

Accessory Parotid Tissue

In approximately 20% of the population, accessory parotid tissue is present, usually just anterior to the parotid gland hilum, lying over the anterior margin of the masseter muscle. The accessory parotid tissue may be unilateral (Fig. 9-7) or bilateral, drains into Stenson's duct, and usually is situated cranial to this duct. Accessory parotid tissue is histologically and physiologically identical to the main parotid gland and

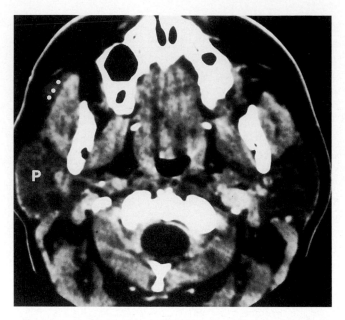

FIG. 9-7 Accessory parotid tissue. Contrast-enhanced CT scan demonstrates unilateral accessory parotid tissue *(white dots)* on the right, overlying the right masseter muscle. The accessory parotid tissue is of similar density to the tissue of the main parotid gland *(P).* (From Tryhus MR, Smoker WRK, Harnsberger HR. The normal and diseased masticator space. Seminars in Ultrasound CT and MR 1990; 11:476-485.)

is affected by the same pathology.[20] Although neoplastic involvement of accessory parotid tissue is uncommon, it is significant that more than 50% of tumors are reported to be malignant.[21] Among the benign lesions, pleomorphic adenomas are most common.[22]

Digastric Muscle Anomalies

Anomalies of the anterior belly of the digastric muscle are uncommon, ranging from discrete findings of interdigitating fibers between the two anterior digastric muscles or between the anterior digastric and mylohyoid muscles to four separate digastric muscle bundles.[23,24] Both bilateral and unilateral accessory anterior digastric muscles have been described, with a unilateral muscle being most common.[23,24] Hypoplasia or aplasia of one anterior belly of the digastric muscle has also been recorded.[24,25] The importance of being familiar with the various anterior digastric muscle anomalies was highlighted in Larsson and Lufkin's paper that emphasized the risk of confusing these anomalies with masses in the floor of the mouth or enlargement of submental lymph nodes.[23] Hypoplasia or aplasia may also be mistaken for denervation atrophy of the mylohyoid nerve; however, the identification of a normal ipsilateral mylohyoid muscle bundle makes a distal V_3 injury highly unlikely.

Vascular Lesions

The nomenclature concerning vascular lesions of the head and neck has been confusing, based neither on their cellular kinetics nor on their clinical behavior. In an attempt to address these issues, Mulliken and Glowacki proposed a biologic classification for these lesions that lends some insight into their natural history and management.[26] Two major types of lesions are recognized: hemangiomas and vascular malformations. Vascular malformations are further subdivided into capillary, venous, arteriovenous, and lymphatic malformations.

Hemangiomas. Hemangiomas are neoplastic and exhibit increased proliferation and turnover of endothelial cells, mast cells, fibroblasts, and macrophages.[27] They are the most common tumors of the head and neck in infancy and childhood, accounting for approximately 7% of all benign soft-tissue tumors.[28] Using the classification proposed by Mulliken and Glowacki, the term *hemangioma* should be reserved for those lesions that present in early infancy, rapidly enlarge, and ultimately involute by adolescence.[26]

Although they are rarely present at birth, hemangiomas typically become apparent during the first month of life.[28] Eighty percent occur as single lesions, and females are more commonly affected (4:1). One half of all hemangiomas resolve completely by 5 years of age, and 70% resolve by 7 years of age.[29]

Previously termed "strawberry" hemangiomas, these lesions are most often superficial (cutaneous hemangiomas) and easily diagnosed clinically.[30] Occasionally, however, they may extend deeply through the skin to infiltrate the underlying muscles (subcutaneous hemangiomas), presenting as nonspecific soft-tissue masses, making clinical diagnosis difficult. Osseous deformity or skeletal hypertrophy may be associated with these lesions, but intraosseous invasion is extremely uncommon.[31]

Hemangiomas are classified as high-flow lesions that are well circumscribed and angiographically exhibit a lobular pattern of intense persistent tissue staining.[32] The frequent arteriovenous shunting and high flow in these lesions may not permit distinction from vascular malformations. On MRI the solid component of the hemangioma demonstrates signal intensity isointense or slightly hyperintense to muscle on T1-weighted (T1W) images, higher signal intensity on progressively more heavily T2W scans, and enhancement following contrast administration (Fig. 9-8).[33]

Vascular Malformations. As opposed to hemangiomas, vascular malformations are not tumors but are true congenital vascular anomalies that are present at birth, although they may not manifest clinically until late infancy or early childhood. The proliferation and turnover characteristics of the endothelial cells are normal. These lesions demonstrate slow, steady growth commensurate with the growth of the child, and they neither regress nor involute. Skeletal changes are more commonly associated with vascular malformations (35%) than with hemangiomas.[34] Rapid enlargement of these lesions is reported to occur in association with trauma, infection, or endocrine changes (i.e., puberty and pregnancy).[35] Vascular malformations are classified, based on the predominant type of anomalous vessel, into capillary, venous, arterial, and lymphatic malforma-

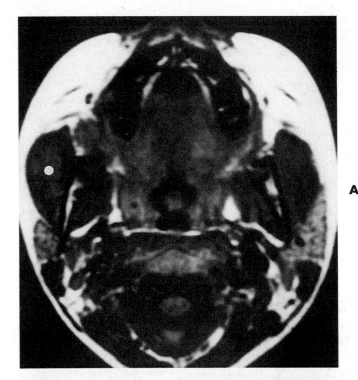

A

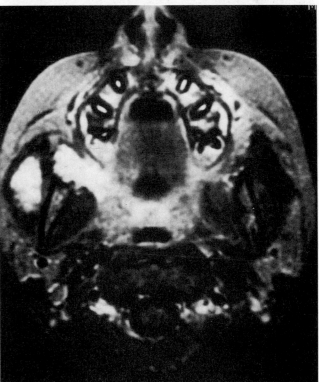

B

FIG. 9-8 Hemangioma. **A,** T1W MR without contrast demonstrates a lesion within the right masseter muscle *(white dot),* slightly hyperintense to the surrounding muscle fibers. **B,** T1W MR following contrast administration performed with fat suppression technique demonstrates intense enhancement of this deep hemangioma. (Courtesy Dr. Patricia Hudgins.)

tions.[27,30] A variety of therapies have been employed for the treatment of vascular malformations and rapidly enlarging hemangiomas, with varying degrees of success. These include steroid administration, laser photocoagulation, sclerotherapy, embolization, and surgical resection.[36-46]

Capillary malformations. These lesions have been referred to as port-wine stains, capillary hemangiomas, and nevus flammeus.[47] They are low-flow lesions and may be associated with the distribution of the trigeminal nerve as one component of the Sturge-Weber syndrome, which also involves an underlying vascular anomaly of the choroid plexus and leptomeninges. Other syndromes associated with capillary malformations include ataxia telangiectasia (Louis-Barr) and Osler-Weber-Rendu (hereditary hemorrhagic telangiectasia).[27] The underlying cheek, lip, and gingiva may be affected, and gingival hypertrophy or chronic hemorrhage may be associated with capillary malformations.

Venous malformations. These lesions, occasionally erroneously termed cavernous hemangiomas, unlike true hemangiomas may involve bone and do not involute.[47] These lesions are the most common ones to affect the oral cavity and share many imaging features with subcutaneous hemangiomas. Venous malformations may attain enormous size and cause airway compromise when located in the extracranial head and neck. Although they are predominantly soft-tissue masses, they may infiltrate deeply along fascial planes and rarely may be entirely intramuscular.[48,49] Of all skeletal muscle hemangiomas-venous malformations, approximately 14% occur in the head and neck region, with the masseter muscle being most commonly affected, followed by the trapezius, and sternocleidomastoid muscles.[50,51] These lesions typically present as muscle-density masses on CT and manifest variable patterns of enhance-

ment.[16] Like their capillary counterparts, venous malformations are low-flow lesions supplied by small arteries. As a consequence of their slow blood flow, on CT they may not demonstrate sufficient enhancement to enable separation of their margins from surrounding muscles, and angiographically one may not be able to identified their arterial supply.[52] On MRI these lesions may appear very similar to deep hemangiomas because they are isointense or hyperintense to muscle on T1W images, become hyperintense on T2W images, and typically enhance following the administration of contrast (Fig. 9-9). The identification of discrete areas of homogeneous high signal intensity, representing venous lakes, or the presence of phleboliths may be extremely helpful in suggesting the diagnosis of a venous malformation (Fig. 9-10).[29,52,53]

Arterial malformations. These lesions are high-flow malformations that result from abnormal blood vessel morphogenesis. Arteriovenous malformations and fistulae are included in this category. The head and neck region is considered one of the more common sites for congenital arterial malformations, although they are uncommonly encountered within the oral cavity itself.[1] Angiographically, arterial malformations are characterized by rapid flow and enlarged, tortuous arteries and draining veins. Parenchymal staining is unusual. On MRI the enlarged arterial components appear as flow voids on T1W and T2W images.

A subgroup of patients demonstrates combined vascular malformations that share features of both high- and low-flow lesions.[31] These lesions may be highly invasive, become enormous in size, and be resistant to all forms of therapy, tending to involve the deep musculature and subcutaneous tissues.[30] On MRI these lesions demonstrate serpiginous flow voids characteristic of an arterial malformation, as well as a soft-tissue, infiltrating component typical of venous malformations (Fig. 9-11).[30]

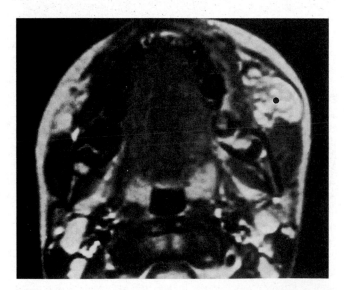

FIG. 9-9 Venous malformation. Proton density-weighted MR demonstrates a discrete, mildly heterogeneous, high signal intensity mass *(dot)* within the left buccal space, immediately anterior to the left masseter muscle.

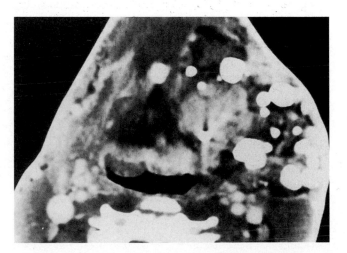

FIG. 9-10 Venous malformation. Contrast-enhanced CT scan demonstrates multiple phleboliths within an extensive venous malformation involving the buccomasseteric region and oral cavity on the left.

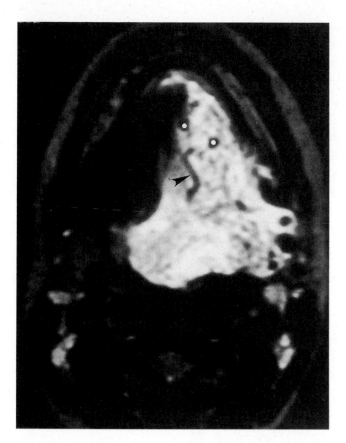

FIG. 9-11 Combined vascular malformation. Proton density-weighted MR demonstrates a large, invasive, vascular malformation, possessing features consistent with both arterial and venous components. Vessels are seen as serpinginous signal voids *(arrowhead)*. Circular signal voids *(white dots)* may represent vessels or phleboliths. A large solid mass component demonstrates high signal intensity and marked heterogeneity involving the left half of the tongue, crossing the midline. (Courtesy Dr. Edward Kassel.)

Lymphatic malformations (lymphangiomas). These lesions are believed to arise from sequestrations of the primative embryonic yolk sac. They enlarge either because of failure of the tumor to communicate with central lymphatic channels and veins, leading to inadequate drainage, or from excessive secretion of lining cells.[54] Although the vast majority of lymphatic malformations are congenital in origin, some instances of acquired lesions, presenting later in life, have been reported in association with tumors, trauma, infection, or previous surgical procedures (iatrogenic).[55,56] They are classified, based on their clinical and histologic findings, into four categories: (1) capillary lymphangiomas, (2) cavernous lymphangiomas, (3) cystic (hygromas) lymphangiomas, and (4) lymphangioma-hemangiomas.[55,57]

Capillary lymphangiomas are cutaneous lesions that commonly affect the oral region, appearing as small wart like excrescences on the skin or mucous membranes. The simplex variety is confined to the epidermis and superficial dermis, and the circumscriptum variety can extend into the deeper layers of the dermis.[55,57]

Cavernous lymphangiomas affect the subcutaneous tissues and may extend deeply into the underlying muscles. They are usually diagnosed within the first months of life and commonly affect the oral cavity, neck, and tongue.[55,57] The loose variety is most often encountered in the mucous membranes of the lips, cheeks, and floor of the mouth, and the compact form more commonly affects the tongue, where the surrounding structures are more muscular.[55] There are isolated reports of lymphangiomas, probably of the cavernous variety, involving the masseter muscle.[58] Diffuse lymphangiomas of the tongue are usually bilateral, may produce macroglossia, and lead to a variety of dentoalveolar complications, although respiratory problems seem to be rare.[59]

Cystic lymphangiomas (hygromas) are the lesions that most often present for imaging. The vast majority of these lesions are encountered in the cervical region, with a predilection for the left posterior triangle. This location corresponds to the more complex and extensive lymphatic system in this region, as compared with other areas of the body.[55] Of these lesions, 75% are present at birth and 90% manifest by 3 years of age. When they extend to involve the floor of the mouth, sublingual and submandibular regions, or the tongue, cystic hygromas may displace the soft tissues sufficiently posteriorly into the oropharynx to obstruct both breathing and swallowing.[55] On imaging studies, cystic hygromas appear as large, single or multiseptated, heterogeneous, fluid-filled masses. They are of low density on CT (Fig. 9-12) and demonstrate variable enhancement of the septations following contrast enhancement.[60] At times on CT it may be difficult to separate the lesion from surrounding soft-tissue structures of similar attenuation.[61] On MRI, cystic hygromas typically manifest a signal hypointense or isointense to muscle on T1W images, and a high signal intensity, greater than that of fat, on T2W images (Fig. 9-13).[61,62] Focal inhomogeneities, corresponding to fibrous

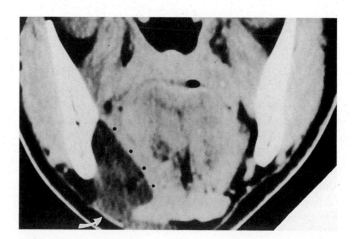

FIG. 9-12 Lymphangioma. Coronal contrast-enhanced CT scan demonstrates a lymphangioma in the right submandibular space, elevating and displacing the right mylohyoid muscle *(black dots)*. The lesion is contained by fibers of the platysma muscle *(white arrow)*.

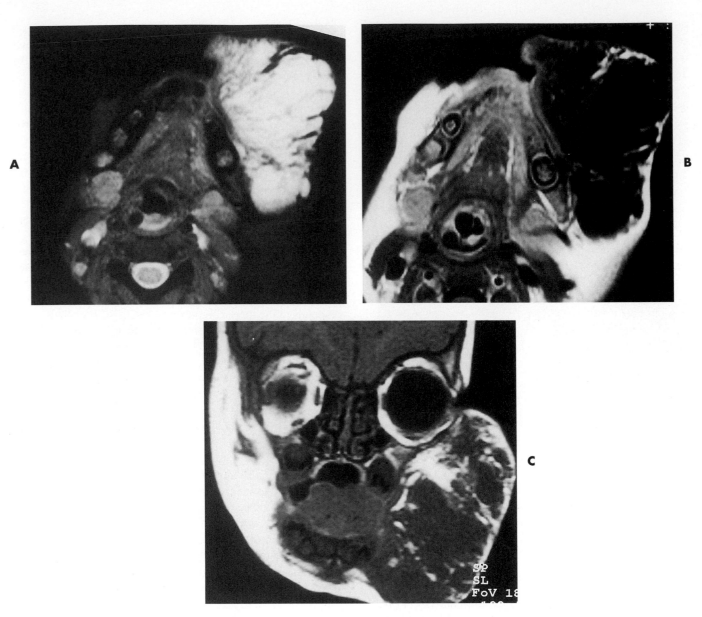

FIG. 9-13 Lymphangioma. **A,** Axial T2W image. **B,** T1W image following contrast enhancement. These images demonstrate a large, subcutaneous lymphangioma involving the left buccal region. The lesion is isointense to muscle on the T1W image **(B),** is markedly hyperintense on the T2W image **(A),** and demonstrates no enhancement following contrast administration **(B). C,** Coronal T1W MR image demonstrates the marked craniocaudad extent of this large lymphangioma.

septae, are identified in many patients. Most cystic hygromas have a signal intensity greater than that of CSF on both T1W and T2W sequences, suggesting the presence of proteinaceous fluid that may contain subacute blood or lipid components.[62] Multiple fluid-fluid levels are common. Contrast-enhanced MRI usually demonstrates enhancement of the cyst wall and septae, providing clearer definition of the capsule and septae than the noncontrast images.[62]

Lymphangioma-hemangiomas (diffuse systemic lymphangiomas) are rare and not well described in discussions of lymphatic malformations.[55] They have not been reported in the oral cavity.

Dermoid Cysts

Dermoid cysts are the most uncommon of all congenital neck lesions, accounting for only 7% of all cysts in this location.[63] Despite Meyer's detailed classification of these lesions into epidermoid, dermoid, and teratoid forms, the term dermoid cyst continues to be used commonly in reference to all three types of lesions, without regard to their differing histologies.[64] Epidermoid cysts consist of simple squamous cell epithelium with a fibrous wall. Dermoid cysts have, in addition, a variable number of skin appendages such as hair follicles and sebacceous glands, and teratoid cysts contain any number of diverse tissues derived from all three germ cell layers.[65] All three varieties may be filled with a cheesy keratinaceous material. The most popular theory regarding the etiology of these lesions suggests that they are derived from epithelial rests that become enclaved during midline closure of the first and second branchial arches.[66] This theory may help explain the simultaneous occurance of sublingual and submental cysts. A case of a dermoid cyst of the floor of the mouth and a coexisting gastric choristoma has also been reported.[67]

When they occur in the oral cavity, dermoid cysts most commonly involve the floor of the mouth (sublingual, submental, or submandibular regions), although other sites have been reported, including the lips, tongue, and buccal mucosa.[66,68-73] Extracapsular excision of cysts in the floor of the mouth is performed by either an intraoral or an external approach, depending on the relationship of the cyst to the mylohyoid muscle.[74] For those cysts that lie above the mylohyoid muscle (sublingual), an intraoral approach is preferable because it avoids a conspicuous scar, preserves the mylohyoid muscle, and is associated with a shorter recovery time. Those lesions that lie inferior to the mylohyoid muscle (submental and submandibular cysts) must usually be removed via an external approach. Therefore the imaging identification of the cyst in relationship to the mylohyoid muscle is extremely helpful in surgical planning. Axial and especially coronal imaging are useful in this regard.[74]

On CT, dermoid cysts typically appear as low-density, well-circumscribed, unilocular masses, less dense than muscle, that may or may not contain fat (Figs. 9-14 to 9-16). The wall of the cyst usually enhances following contrast. In the absence of fat globules, epidermoid and dermoid cysts are indistinguishable.[75] On MRI, epidermoid cysts are of low-signal intensity on T1W images and are of high signal intensity on T2W images, reflecting their fluid content. Dermoid lesions present a more variable appearance, depending on their fat content being either hypointense or hyperintense to muscle on T1W images (Figs. 9-17, 9-18).[74] They are typically hyperintense on T2W sequences. The use of contrast permits determination of the thickness of the cyst wall (2 to 6 mm).[74]

Thyroglossal Duct Cysts

Thyroglossal duct cysts (TGDC) are the most common non-odontogenic cysts occurring in the neck, and they account for 70% of congenital neck abnormalities.[1,76] They most often present in the young-adult age-group, 50% occurring before age 20, and 70% occurring before age 30.[77] However, they can be encountered in the adult population, even into the eighth decade.[78,79] These lesions may occur anywhere along the course of the thyroglossal duct, from the base of the tongue to the thyroid gland. Approximately 65% are infrahyoid in location, in the region of the thyrohyoid membrane, 15% are at the level of the hyoid bone, and the remaining 20% are suprahyoid.[1] As opposed to the typically paramedian infrahyoid TGDC, suprahyoid TGDC are commonly midline, located between the bellies of the anterior

digastric muscles (Fig. 9-19). They are frequently embedded within or lie below the mylohyoid sling in the submental region, and rarely they may present as masses within the floor of the mouth.[80] One to 2% of TGDC are reported to be intralingual.[77] On CT, TGDC are usually well circumscribed, occasionally septated, cystic lesions, 2 to 4 cm in diameter, that exhibit capsular enhancement.[81] On MRI, TGDC exhibit low to intermediate signal intensity on T1W images, depending on the protein content of the cyst, and are of high signal intensity on T2W images. The adjacent soft tissues and fascial planes are normal unless infection, which is reported in approximately 60% of patients, is present.[82] In the presence of infection, thickening of the overlying skin or platysma muscle and induration of the subcutaneous fat may be demonstrated.[81] Less than 1% of thyroglossal duct abnormalities are associated with coexisting carcinoma, papillary carcinoma being the most common, although follicular, adenocarcinoma, and squamous cell carcinoma have also been reported.[83-87]

Lingual Thyroid

Failure of the thyroid gland to descend from the foramen cecum to the lower neck results in residual thyroid tissue along the thyroglossal duct track. In autopsy studies, ectopic thyroid tissue less than 3 mm in size has been reported in 10% of the normal population.[1] Ectopic thyroid tissue, which may or may not be functioning, has a high female to male preponderance (7:1), which is attributed to hormonal disturbances in females during puberty and pregnancy.[88] The tongue is the most common location, accounting for 90% of ectopic thyroid tissue, most of which occurs in the midline dorsum of the tongue, although rare cases of involvement of the entire tongue have been reported.[89,90] Ectopic thyroid tissue is typically asymptomatic and discovered incidentally; however, symptoms of dysphagia, dysphonia, stridor, dyspnea, hemorrhage, and hoarseness may occur.[91-94] Hypothyroidism and cretinism have both been reported in patients with lingual thyroid tissue.[95,96] Malignancy in lingual thyroid is rare.[97] In a high percentage of patients (70% to 80%), no other functioning thyroid tissue is present, and surgical excision would subsequently render the patient permanently hypothyroid. For this reason, if surgery is contemplated, Iodine-123 radionucide scanning should be performed to establish the presence or absence of normally functioning thyroid tissue within the neck. This study will also establish the presence of functioning lingual thyroid tissue.

On noncontrast CT, lingual thyroid tissue usually presents as a hyperdense mass within the instrinsic musculature of the tongue and enhances avidly, typically in a homogeneous fashion (Fig. 9-20).[3,94] Markedly heterogenous contrast enhancement has been reported in a patient with goitrous changes and thyroiditis affecting the lingual thyroid tissue.[93] On MRI, lingual thyroid tissue is isointense to hyperintense to the tongue musculature on both T1W and T2W sequences and strongly enhances following contrast injection.[92] The imaging characteristics of pathologic lin-

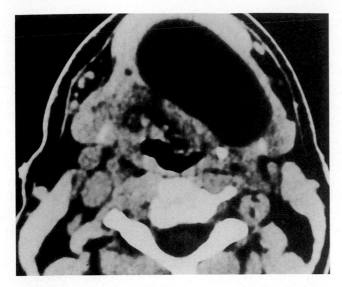

FIG. 9-14 Epidermoid cyst. Axial CT scan reveals a large, unilocular, hypodense cystic lesion in the floor of the mouth. From an imaging standpoint this appearance would be consistent with either an epidermoid or a dermoid cyst.

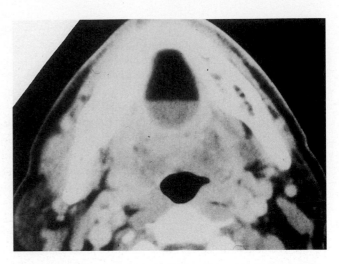

FIG. 9-15 Dermoid cyst. Axial contrast-enhanced CT scan demonstrates a midline cystic lesion with a fat-fluid level and peripheral rim enhancement. The presence of fat is virtually pathognomonic for a true dermoid cyst.

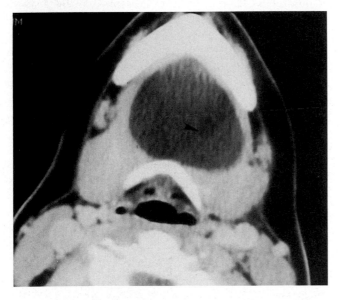

FIG. 9-16 Axial dermoid cyst. Contrast-enhanced CT scan demonstrates a large, unilocular cystic lesion in the floor of the mouth, superior to the mylohyoid muscle. A single fat globule *(arrowheads)* is contained within this lesion, assuring the diagnosis of a true dermoid cyst. (Courtesy Dr. Deborah Reede.)

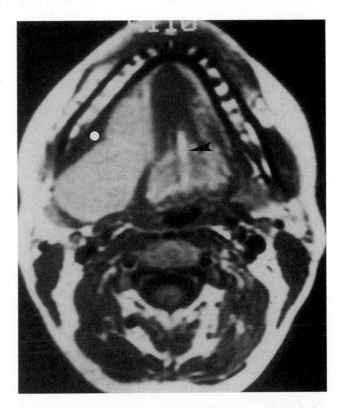

FIG. 9-17 Dermoid cyst. Axial, T1W MR scan reveals the lesion to be of high signal intensity on this T1W scan but of slightly less intensity than that of the subcutaneous fat. The relationship of this lesion to the right mylohyoid muscle *(white dot)* is clearly established on the MR image. The fatty lingual septum *(arrowhead)* is well defined, displaced slightly to the left of midline. This lesion involves much of the right sublingual space, dissecting posteriorly to involve the deep aspect of the right submandibular space.

gual thyroid tissue are similar to those of pathology involving the thyroid gland (multinodular goiter, thyroiditis, carcinoma, etc.) (Fig. 9-21).

Lingual Artery Aneurysm

Aneurysms of the external carotid artery branches are distinctly uncommon, with the superficial temporal artery being most often affected as a result of trauma.[98] Aneurysms of the lingual artery, on the other hand, are uncommon.[99-104] Rare reports of presumed congenital lingual artery aneurysms

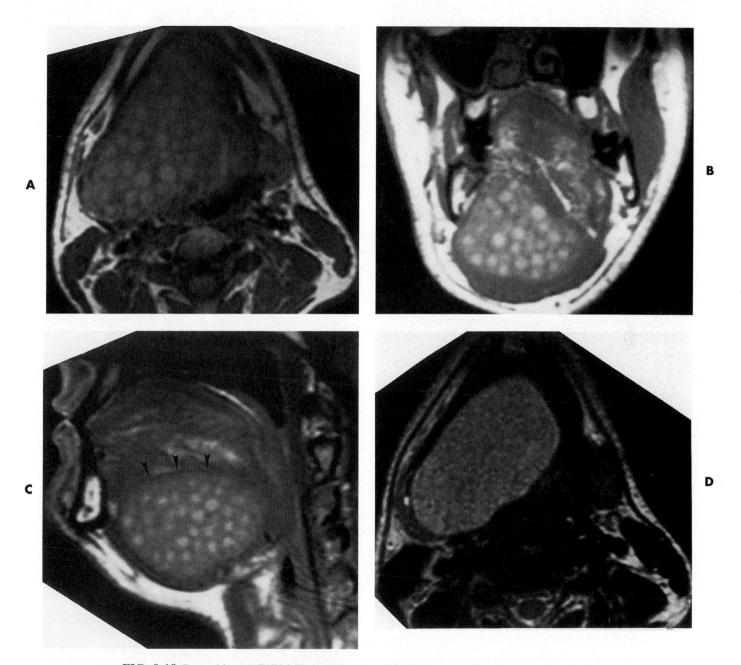

FIG. 9-18 Dermoid cyst. T1W MR scans in the axial **(A)**, coronal **(B)**, and sagittal **(C)** planes demonstrate a large, sublingual dermoid cyst characterized by the presence of multiple fat globules, easily identified by their high signal intensity on these T1W images. The relationship of this lesion to the floor of the mouth musculature is well demonstrated on the sagittal image **(C)**, on which it lies between the fibers of the mylohyoid muscle inferiorly and those of the geniohyoid muscle *(arrowheads)* superiorly. Axial T2W MR study **(D)** reveals a very heterogeneous signal to the contents of this dermoid cyst, without definition of the individual fat globules so easily visualized on the T1W scans (Courtesy Dr. Walter Rose).

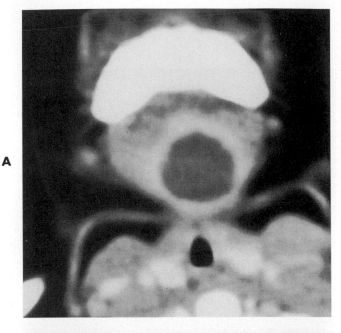

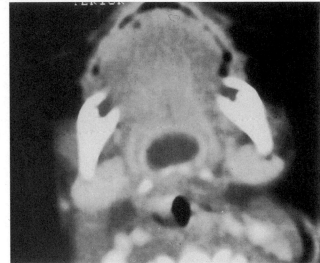

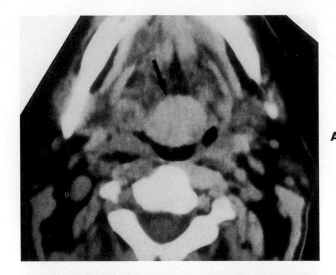

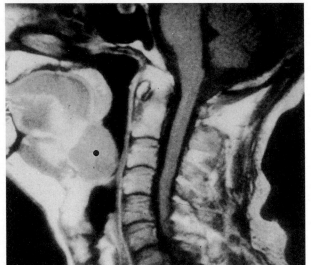

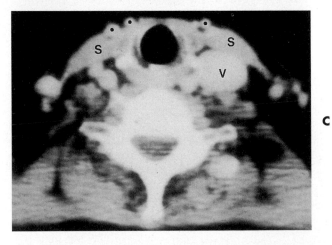

FIG. 9-19 Thyroglossal duct cyst. **A** and **B,** Contrast-enhanced axial CT scans demonstrate a midline thyroglossal duct cyst lying between the anterior bellies of the digastric muscle. On the more superior plane **(B)** the cyst is identified in the region of the foramen cecum, at the base of the tongue. It is unilocular and exhibits capsular enhancement.

(absence of previous trauma) exist.[100] In one report a patient with bilateral lingual artery aneurysms presented with ecchymosis of the neck, following spontaneous rupture of one of the aneurysms.[102] CT may suggest the diagnosis but may not be able to distinguish an aneurysm from other vascular lesions.[102] The aneurysm's appearance is variable, depending on the degree of thrombosis (Fig. 9-22). Although the use of MR has not been reported, its ability to demonstrate vascular structures as flow voids may prove useful in the evaluation of these lesions, as might MRA.

FIG. 9-20 Lingual thyroid. **A,** Contrast-enhanced axial CT scan reveals a well-delineated, enhancing, midline lesion at the tongue base *(arrow).* **B,** Midsagittal, T1W MR scan demonstrates a sharply defined tongue-base mass *(dot),* with signal intensity isointense to tongue musculature. **C,** Axial CT scan with contrast at the level of the lower neck reveals complete absence of normal thyroid tissue in its expected location. *V,* Large left internal jugular vein; *black dots,* anterior jugular veins; *S,* sternocleidomastoid muscles.

Infections and Inflammatory Lesions

Infections within the oral cavity, including the sublingual and submandibular regions, most commonly result from either stenosis or calculi within the salivary gland ductal systems or from dental infections or manipulation. In many cases, infections may primarily involve the masticator space and secondarily spread to involve the oral cavity. The relationship of the apices of the mandibular teeth to the mylohyoid ridge may determine which region of the floor of the mouth is primarily involved by dental infections. The roots of the second and third molars lie below the mylohyoid ridge, and apical infections of these teeth directly involve the submandibular region. By comparison the apices of the first molar and premolar root apices are located above the mylohyoid ridge, and infections of these teeth preferentially involve the sublingual region.[103]

For evaluation of oral cavity infections in adults, CT with contrast enhancement is preferred to MRI because CT is superior for demonstrating small calculi and for assessing the integrity of the mandibular cortex. In addition, total examination times are typically shorter, an important consideration for the acutely ill patient.[104] For patients in the pediatric age group and for adults in whom the use of iodinated contrast is contraindicated, MRI is the study of choice. The ability of MR to image in multiple planes and the decreased susceptibility to artifacts from dental amalgams are distinct advantages over CT.

On CT an abscess appears as a single or multiloculated low-density area, with or without gas collections, that usually conforms to fascial spaces and demonstrates peripheral rim enhancement (Figs. 9-23 to 9-25). On MRI an abscess typically has low T1W and high T2W signal intensities. Rim enhancement following contrast is identified in mature abscesses (Fig. 9-26). In addition to the abscess cavity, cutaneous and subcutaneous manifestations of infection are typically present, including myositis (adjacent muscle enlargement), thickening of the overlying skin, "dirty" edematous fat, and enhancement of fascial planes (Figs. 9-27, 9-28). These cutaneous manifestations are not as obvious on MRI as they are on CT, which is one limitation of MRI when scanning for infections.[104] The presence of these cutaneous and subcutaneous manifestations, without a definite low-density collection, is consistent with cellulitis.

Inflammatory processes involving the submandibular gland most often result from obstructing intraductal calculi. This may lead to dilatation of the submandibular gland duct

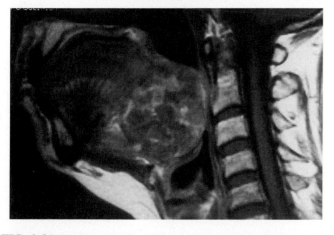

FIG. 9-21 Lingual thyroid with goiter. **A** and **B,** Axial and midsagittal T1W MR images following contrast administration reveal marked heterogeneous enhancement of this multinodular goiter affecting lingual thyroid tissue. Note severe compromise of the oropharyngeal airway on all images. (Courtesy Dr. Jan Casselman.)

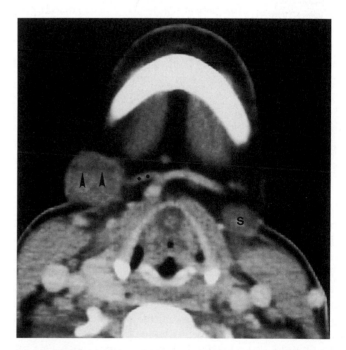

FIG. 9-22 Lingual artery aneurysm. Axial contrast-enhanced CT scan, in a 23-year-old female with a right submandibular region mass clinically, demonstrates a well-circumscribed lesion on the right, clearly separate from the submandibular gland *(s)*. There is a fluid level visible within the lesion *(arrowheads),* and a branch of the right lingual artery can be seen entering this lesion *(black dots).*

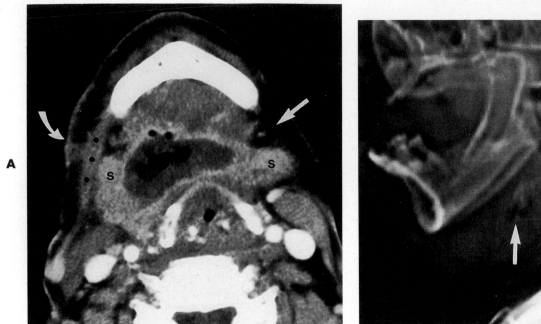
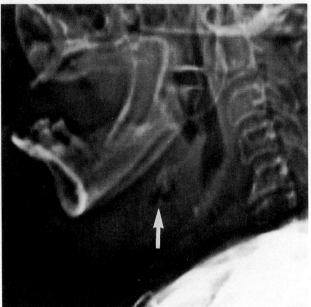

FIG. 9-23 Floor of the mouth abscess. **A,** Contrast-enhanced axial CT scan through the floor of the mouth reveals a large abscess containing gas. The margins of the abscess exhibit peripheral rim enhancement. Both submandibular glands *(s)* are identified on this plane. In addition to the abscess, marked cellulitis of surrounding soft tissues is identified; this is manifested by thickening of the right platysma muscle *(black dots),* when compared with the left platysma muscle *(white straight arrow).* There is thickening of the skin on the right *(white curved arrows)* and dirty edematous fat in the subcutaneous soft tissues between the thickened skin and thickened platysma muscle on the right. **B,** The location of the abscess in a craniocaudad dimension is well illustrated on the lateral scanogram (the patient was too ill to undergo coronal scanning). Air within the abscess is well demonstrated *(arrow)* as is marked edema of the submandibular soft tissues.

and if protracted, may result in a submandibular gland abscess (Fig. 9-29). Visualization of the submandibular gland ducts is common on both CT and MRI. Whenever a salivary duct is greater than 3 mm in diameter, whether intraglandular or extraglandular, there should be a thorough evaluation to exclude small calculi, and obstructing floor of mouth tumors (Fig. 9-30).[105] When large, calculi may be visualized on MR, as well as CT (Fig. 9-31).

Ludwig's Angina

Ludwig's angina is a term used to refer to an extensive infection of the floor of the mouth, typically caused by oral flora (especially streptococcal and staphylococcal bacteria). Specifically, infections of the mandibular molars account for up to 90% of the reported cases.[106] Before the antibiotic era, infections in this region dissected inferiorly along fascial planes into the mediastinum and the patient presented with angina-like chest pain. As early as 1939, Grodinsky established strict clinical criteria to diagnose this entity.[107] Ludwig's angina is a cellulitis, not a focal abscess, that (1) always involves both the sublingual and submandibular spaces and is frequently bilateral, (2) produces gangrene or serosanguinous phlegmon but little or no frank pus, (3) involves connective tissue, fascia, and muscle but not glan-

dular structures, and (4) is spread by contiguity not lymphatics. The main role of imaging is to evaluate the integrity of the airway and document the presence of gas-forming organisms, underlying dental infection, and possibly drainable neck abscesses (Fig. 9-32).[106]

Reactive or suppurative adenopathy involving the submandibular and submental lymph nodes is commonly seen in association with oral cavity infections or as part of a more systemic process involving multiple lymph node chains. The submandibular and submental lymph node chains receive drainage from the chin, lips, cheeks, floor of the mouth, and oral tongue, and foci of infection within these regions should be sought.

Ranulas

Ranulas, also termed *mucoceles,* or *mucous retention cysts* of the floor of the mouth, are of two varieties. The simple variety occurs in the floor of the mouth above the mylohyoid muscle in the region of the sublingual gland and is a true epithelial-lined cyst. These simple ranulas are usually due to obstruction of a minor salivary gland or obstruction of the sublingual gland. A "diving" or "plunging" ranula results following rupture of the simple ranula's wall. As such, these ranulas are not true epithelial-lined retention cysts but are

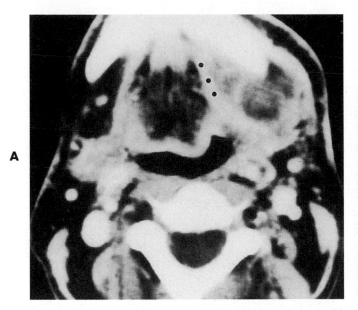
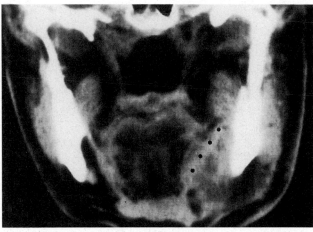

FIG. 9-24 Submandibular space abscess. **A** and **B,** Axial and coronal contrast-enhanced CT scans demonstrate a large submandibular space abscess on the left, limited externally by the fibers of the platysma muscle. The abscess displaces the left mylohyoid muscle *(black dots)* medially and superiorly. (Courtesy Dr. Deborah Reede.)

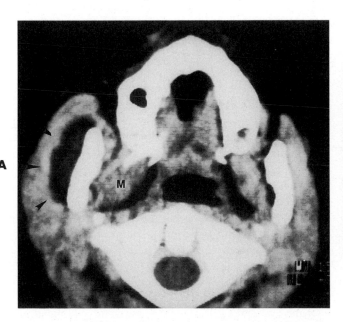
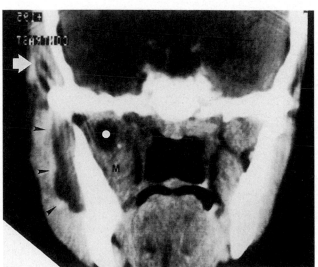

FIG. 9-25 Masticator space abscess. **A** and **B,** Axial and coronal contrast-enhanced CT scans reveal an abscess involving the right masticator space. The large intramasseteric component exhibits faint peripheral rim enhancement *(arrowheads).* The coronal scan also demonstrates an abscess cavity within the lateral pterygoid muscle *(white dot)* and extension above the zygoma to involve the right temporalis muscle in the suprazygomatic masticator space *(white arrow).* Note that the medial pterygoid muscle *(M),* although not involved by an abscess cavity, is edematous and enlarged on the right, when compared with the normal muscle on the left.

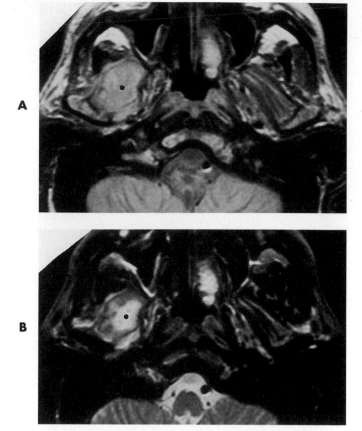

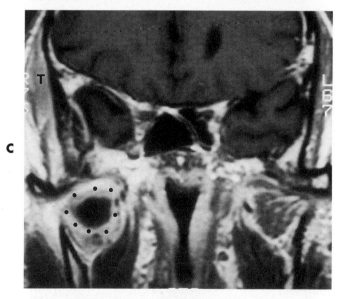

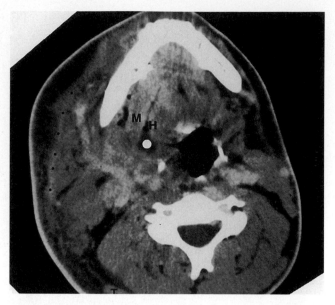

FIG. 9-27 Abscess or cellulitis. Axial contrast-enhanced CT scan demonstrates a small abscess cavity *(white dot)* at the posterior aspect of the right tongue, between the mylohyoid *(M)* and hyoglossus *(H)* muscles, both of which are enlarged due to associated myositis. Small collections of gas can be seen to dissect between the muscle fibers. Marked cellulitis involving multiple fascial spaces is identified. The right platysma muscle *(black dots)* is markedly thickened, and the left muscle is affected much less. There is marked edema and a "dirty" appearance to the subcutaneous fat involving the right face. The skin overlying this edematous fat is slightly thickened as well. This edema and cutaneous thickening extends posteriorly in the superficial space to at least the margin of the right trapezius muscle *(T)*.

FIG. 9-26 Masticator space abscess. Proton-density weighted **(A)**, and T2W MR **(B)**, images demonstrate an abscess cavity centered within the right lateral pterygoid muscle *(dot)*. The abscess cavity was hypointense on the T1W image and very hyperintense on the heavily T2W image **(B)**. Note that the cavity becomes isointense to the surrounding capsule on the proton density-weighted image **(A)**. Coronal T1W **(C)** MR following the administration of contrast reveal thick enhancement of the abscess cavity *(dots)*. The coronal image also demonstrates extension of edema above the zygomatic arch to involve the temporalis muscle *(T)* in the suprazygomatic masticator space.

pseudocysts lined by dense connective or granulation tissue.[108,109] The extravasated mucus is directed posteriorly into the submandibular region and occasionally into the adjacent upper cervical soft tissues. These lesions may therefore present as a mass either in the submental or submandibular region.

Although there are a diversity of proposed etiologies, ranulas most commonly result from trauma (including surgical) or obstruction to the sublingual salivary gland or its ductal elements. Ranulas are reported in approximately 5% to 12% of patients undergoing submandibular duct relocation for management of uncontrolled sialorrhea, presumably because during this procedure, there is invariably surgical trauma to the sublingual gland components.[108,110] Treatment of ranulas is primarily directed toward the transoral drainage of the cyst and excision of the ipsilateral sublingual gland. The more surgically difficult complete dissection of the ranula's lining or the exteriorizing of the cyst have been shown to be unnecessary.[108,109,111,112]

On CT, ranulas are usually thin-walled, unilocular, well-defined, nonenhancing, cystic-appearing lesions of low attenuation (Fig. 9-33).[113,114] They have homogeneously low T1W and high T2W MR signal intensities (Fig. 9-34).[115,116] When simple, they are confined to the sublingual region.

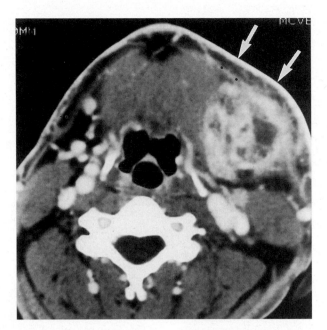

FIG. 9-28 Abscess or cellulitis. Axial contrast-enhanced CT scan demonstrates a large, heterogeneous, multiloculated abscess involving the left submandibular space. Associated with this abscess is marked thickening of the overlying skin *(white arrows)*, thickening of the left platysma muscle *(black dots)*, and a "dirty" stranded appearance to the subcutaneous fat. Note that there is significantly more cellulitis associated with this abscess as compared with the abscess illustrated in Fig. 9-24.

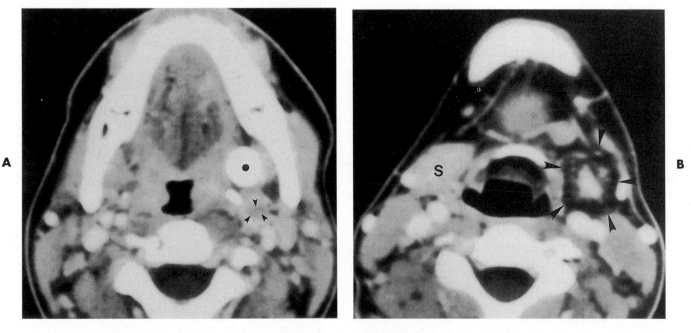

FIG. 9-29 Submandibular gland duct calculus. **A,** Axial CT scan with contrast demonstrates a large calculus *(black dot)* along the course of the submandibular gland duct. The most superior extent of the resulting abscess involving the left submandibular gland may be identified on this image *(arrowheads)*. **B,** Axial CT scan with contrast at a lower level reveals a normal right submandibular gland *(S)*. An extensive abscess involves the majority of the left submandibular gland *(arrowheads)*.

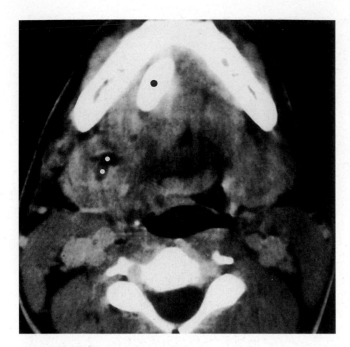

FIG. 9-30 Submandibular gland duct calculus. Axial CT scan performed with contrast enhancement reveals a very large calculus *(black dot)* situated in the distal aspect of the right submandibular gland duct. Marked dilatation of the intraglandular ducts *(white dots)* is identified.

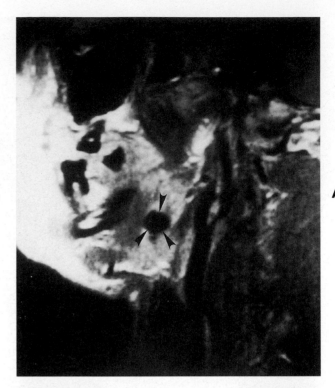

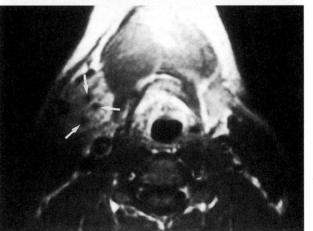

FIG. 9-31 Submandibular gland duct calculus with obstruction. **A,** T1W right parasagittal MR scan demonstrates a large signal void *(arrowheads)* produced by the submandibular gland duct calculus. **B,** Axial T1W MR through the submandibular glands demonstrates marked dilatation of multiple intraglandular ducts *(arrows).*

When diving, the bulk of the ranula is typically identified in the submandibular region, although a portion of the lesion is also identified in the sublingual region, suggesting the diagnosis (Fig. 9-35).[113] Rarely, ranulas may dissect across the midline between the mylohyoid and geniohyoid muscles and present clinically as bilateral masses (Fig. 9-36). A completely intralingual ranula has also been reported (Fig. 9-37).[116] Differential considerations of cystic-appearing lesions in the sublingual and submandibular regions include dermoid cysts, thyroglossal duct cysts, and lymphangiomas.

Benign Lesions
Pleomorphic Adenomas

Pleomorphic adenomas (benign mixed tumors) are the most common benign glandular tumors of the oral cavity and are characterized by the presence of both mesodermal and glandular tissue. Although the majority of pleomorphic adenomas occur in the parotid gland, 8% arise within the submandibular gland, 0.5% involve the sublingual gland, and 6.5% occur in the minor salivary glands situated throughout the upper aerodigestive tract. Only the gingiva and anterior-most portion of the hard palate are relatively devoid of these glands.

On CT, pleomorphic adenomas are usually well-demarcated, homogeneous, and slightly hyperdense to muscle on noncontrast images (Fig. 9-38). Typically there is no significant enhancement. Occasionally the medial margin of a sublingual or submandibular pleomorphic adenoma may be poorly defined, suggesting a more aggressive lesion (Fig. 9-38).[117] When the hard palate is involved, there usually is a surrounding rim of well-defined cortical bone produced by the slow tumor growth and adjacent bone remodeling (Fig. 9-39). Large lesions may be inhomogeneous and have areas of necrosis, cystic change, and amorphous calcification.

On MRI, pleomorphic adneomas are usually isointense to muscle on T1W images and become hyperintense on progressively more T2W sequences.[117] Varying signal intensities within these tumors reflect their heterogeneous composition and cystic change, necrosis, and hemorrhage. These lesions are discussed in greater detail in Chapter 17.

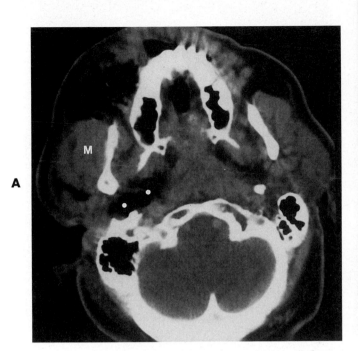
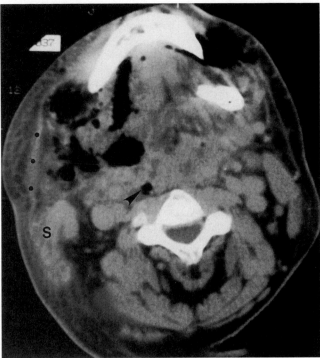

FIG. 9-32 Gas-forming infection. **A,** Axial contrast-enhanced CT scan at the level of the maxilla reveals extensive infection with gas collections involving multiple spaces of the suprahyoid neck. These include the buccal spaces bilaterally and the right parapharyngeal space *(white dots)*. Myositis involving the right masseter muscle *(M)* is easily appreciated. Involvement of the subcutaneous fat on the right is also identified at this level. **B,** Axial CT scan with contrast at a lower level demonstrates gas collections within the right sublingual space, the submandibular spaces bilaterally, the right parapharyngeal space, and the right retropharyngeal space *(arrowhead)*. Note the myositis involving the right sternocleidomastoid *(S)* and platysma *(black dots)* muscles. Extensive subcutaneous infection is manifested by edema and a dirty appearance of the fat. Although this is most prominent on the right, it is also identified on the left, anteriorly. Note the absence of a patent airway at this level.

Aggressive Fibromatosis

Tumors of fibrous origin include a variety of histologies, ranging from simple keloids to fibrosarcomas. In between these extremes is aggressive fibromatosis, an extraabdominal desmoid "tumor." Termed *juvenile fibromatosis* by Stout and aggressive infantile fibromatosis by Enzinger, this entity represents one of the most complex problems in the classification of fibrous lesions.[118,119] Several patterns are identified microscopically that essentially reflect progressive stages of fibroblast differentiation. Distinction between the more cellular varieties of fibromatosis and well-differentiated infantile fibrosarcoma may be extremely difficult, perhaps impossible.[120] Terms such as *aggressive fibromatosis, differentiated fibrosarcoma,* and *fibrosarcoma-like fibromatosis* have all been applied to these lesions.[120]

Approximately 11% of desmoid tumors occur in the extracranial head and neck, frequently in children and young adults. The neck and supraclavicular regions are most commonly affected.[121] The oral cavity, nasal cavity, paranasal sinuses, nasopharynx, and larynx are involved much less fre-

quently.[122] Rare reports of fibromatosis involving the tongue also exist.[123-125] As a group these lesions tend to manifest a much more aggressive behavior than those that originate from the anterior abdominal wall because they infiltrate muscles, encase adjacent nerves and vessels, and may even extend into the spinal canal.[1,126] Although aggressive fibromatosis has no malignant potential and does not metastasize, it manifests innate local aggressiveness and has a high rate of recurrence after incomplete surgical resection. Recurrences after a delay of many years have also been reported.[127]

Aggressive fibromatosis arises as a solitary mass within skeletal muscle or in the adjacent fascia, aponeurosis, or periosteum. It has a fairly homogeneous density on unenhanced CT, may enhance slightly after contrast, and may be inseparable from adjacent muscles (Fig. 9-40).[17,128,129] On MRI, aggressive fibromatosis has variable signal intensity, typically isointense or slightly hypointense to muscle on T1W sequences and hypointense to hyperintense on T2W sequences.[123,130] There is usually some degree of enhancement following contrast administration (Fig. 9-41). It is

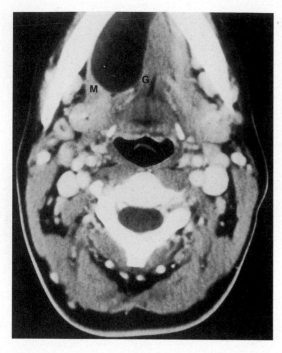

FIG. 9-33 Simple ranula. Contrast-enhanced axial CT scan reveals a large, unilocular cystic mass in the right sublingual space, between the fibers of the mylohyoid *(M)* and genioglossus *(G)* muscles. No enhancement is associated with this simple ranula.

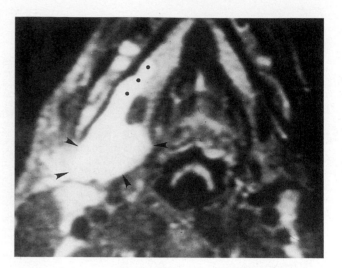

FIG. 9-35 Plunging ranula. T2W axial MR scan reveals a hyperintense lesion that appears primarily centered in the right submandibular space *(arrowheads)*. A tail is seen extending anteriorly into the sublingual space *(black dots)*. The lesion is very homogeneously hyperintense, consistent with fluid. (Courtesy Dr. Deborah Reede.)

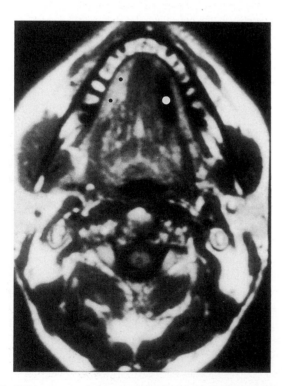

FIG. 9-34 Simple ranula. T1W MR scan reveals a hypointense, cystic-appearing lesion within the left sublingual space *(white dot)*. The normal sublingual space fat, easily appreciated on the right *(black dots)*, is not visible on the left, having been replaced by the ranula. Note the lack of significant mass effect on surrounding structures. (Courtesy Dr. William Kelly.)

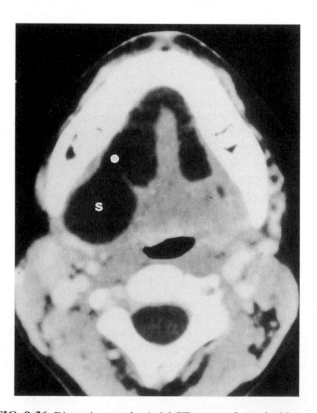

FIG. 9-36 Dissecting ranula. Axial CT scan performed with contrast demonstrates a diving ranula on the right; the bulk of the ranula is centered within the deep aspect of the right submandibular space *(S)*, with a tail extending anteriorly into the right sublingual space *(white dot)*. The ranula has dissected across the midline, between the fibers of the mylohyoid and geniohyoid muscles, to be visualized within the confines of the left sublingual space.

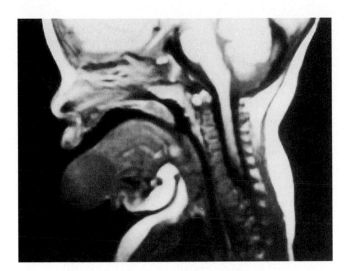

FIG. 9-37 Intralingual ranula. Midsagittal T1W image demonstrates a cystic lesion replacing the distal half of the oral tongue. The lesion is hypointense on T1W images, and it became markedly hyperintense in a very homogeneous fashion on the heavily T2W image, suggesting the fluid nature of the mass. (From Silverstein MI, Castillo M, Hudgins PA et al. MR imaging of intralingual ranula in a child. J Comput Assist Tomogr 1990; 14:672-673.)

probable that the spectrum of appearances on MRI is related to the relative amounts of fibroblast proliferation, fibrosis, and collagen contained within the lesion.[131]

Rhabdomyomas

Rhabdomyomas are rare, benign tumors of striated muscle, most of which occur in the extracranial head and neck. In contrast to cardiac rhabdomyomas, considered to be hamartomatous lesions and often associated with tuberous sclerosis, extracardiac rhabdomyomas bear no association with this syndrome. Extracardiac rhabdomyomas are subdivided clinically and morphologically into two histologic types: adult and fetal.[132] Adult rhabdomyomas occur predominantly in middle-aged men and have a predilection for the base of the tongue, floor of the mouth, larynx, and pharynx. For this reason, it has been suggested that these lesions arise from the striated muscles of the third and fourth branchial arches.[133] Fetal rhabdomyomas usually occur in children under the age of 3 years and also have a predilection for the extracranial head and neck. These fetal lesions may actually be hamartomatous malformations rather than true neoplasms. The preferred treatment for rhabdomyomas is complete surgical excision, which is often easily accomplished because these lesions tend to be well encapsulated.[134]

Rhabdomyomas are of muscle density on unenhanced CT and demonstrate enhancement following the administration of contrast.[135] On MRI, rhabdomyomas are isointense or slightly hyperintense to muscle on T1W images, hyperintense on T2W images, and enhance slightly following contrast (Fig. 9-42).

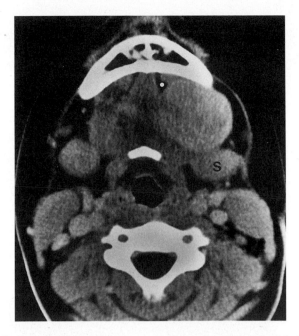

FIG. 9-38 Pleomorphic adenoma. Contrast-enhanced axial CT scan demonstrates a large mass anterior to the left submandibular gland *(S)*, displacing the gland slightly posteriorly. Although, (because of the size of this lesion) the exact epicenter is difficult to ascertain, the fact that the anterior aspect of the left sublingual space *(white dot)* is widened suggests that the lesion arises within this space. Pathologically this proved to be a pleomorphic adenoma of the left sublingual gland. Note that the lesion is extremely homogeneous in its appearance, as well as being very well circumscribed. The lesion abuts the cortex of the mandible; however, the mandible appears intact on this soft-tissue window scan. (Courtesy Dr. Patricia Hudgins.)

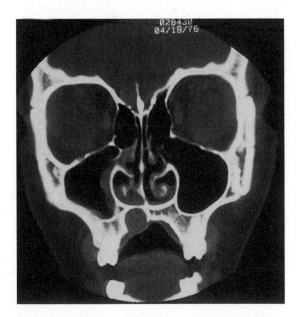

FIG. 9-39 Pleomorphic adenoma. Coronal CT scan demonstrates a well-defined soft-tissue mass replacing much of the right aspect of the hard palate. The mass has characteristics of a benign lesion because the hard palate is remodeled and well margined, rather than being destroyed. (Courtesy Dr. Nicole Freling.)

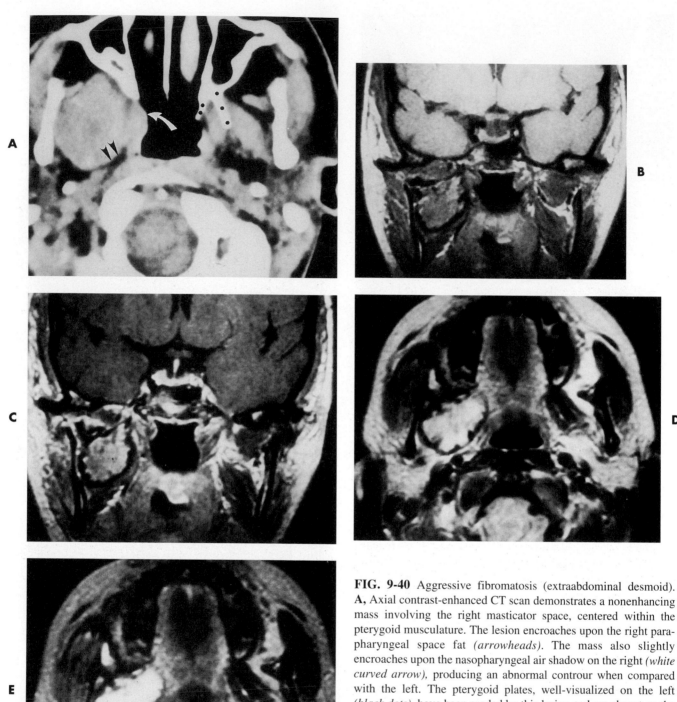

FIG. 9-40 Aggressive fibromatosis (extraabdominal desmoid). **A,** Axial contrast-enhanced CT scan demonstrates a nonenhancing mass involving the right masticator space, centered within the pterygoid musculature. The lesion encroaches upon the right parapharyngeal space fat *(arrowheads)*. The mass also slightly encroaches upon the nasopharyngeal air shadow on the right *(white curved arrow),* producing an abnormal controur when compared with the left. The pterygoid plates, well-visualized on the left *(black dots),* have been eroded by this lesion and are absent on the right. Coronal T1W MR scans without **(B)** and, with **(C)** contrast demonstrate the lesion is slightly hyperintense to muscle on the noncontrast image. Mild enhancement is noted following contrast **(C).** This desmoid tumor is noted to become progressively more hyperintense on the proton density **(D)** and heavy T2W **(E)** MR axial images.

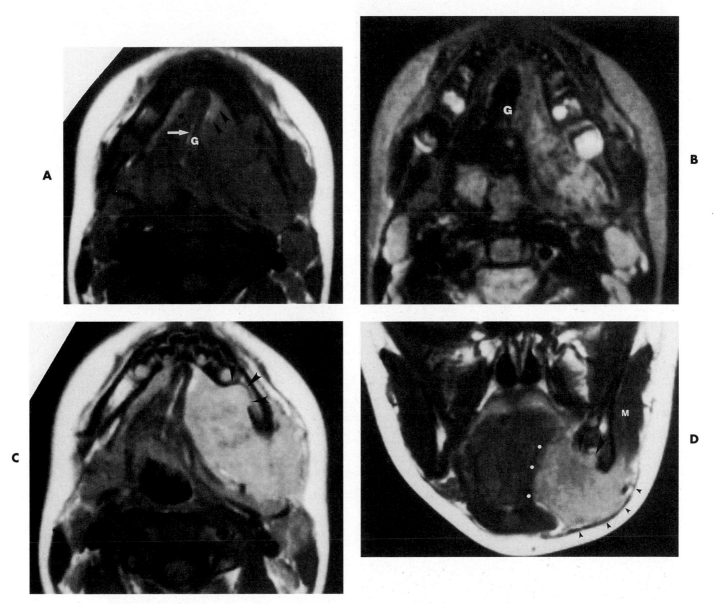

FIG. 9-41 Aggressive fibromatosis. Axial T1W **(A)**, and T2W MR images **(B)** demonstrate a left submandibular space lesion that is minimally hyperintense to muscle on the T1W image **(A)** becoming progressively more hyperintense on the T2W image. Although the lesion can be separated anteriorly from the fat-filled sublingual space on the T1W image *(arrowheads* in **A)**, separation on the T2W **(B)** image is not possible. Note compression of the left genioglossus muscle *(G)* and displacement of the midline lingual septum to the right *(arrow)*. Contrast-enhanced T1W MR images in the axial **(C)** and coronal **(D)** planes demonstrate marked enhancement of this desmoid lesion. Erosion of the lingual surface of the left mandible is well appreciated on the axial image **(C)** with an enhancing mass invading the mandible *(arrowheads)*. Note that the anterior margin of this mass cannot be separated from the sublingual space on the contrast-enhanced axial image **(C)** nearly as well as it could on the noncontrast image **(A)**. Localization of the lesion to the submandibular space is most easily appreciated on the coronal image **(D)** because displacement of the left mylohyoid muscle *(dots)* is well seen. Again noted is involvement of the mandible *(arrowheads)*. This process wraps around the inferior margin of the mandible and ascends in the masticator space, involving the inferior fibers of the left masseter muscle *(M)*. At this time the lesion is well contained by the left platysma muscle, within the submandibular space *(arrowheads)*. (Courtesy Dr. Jan Casselman.)

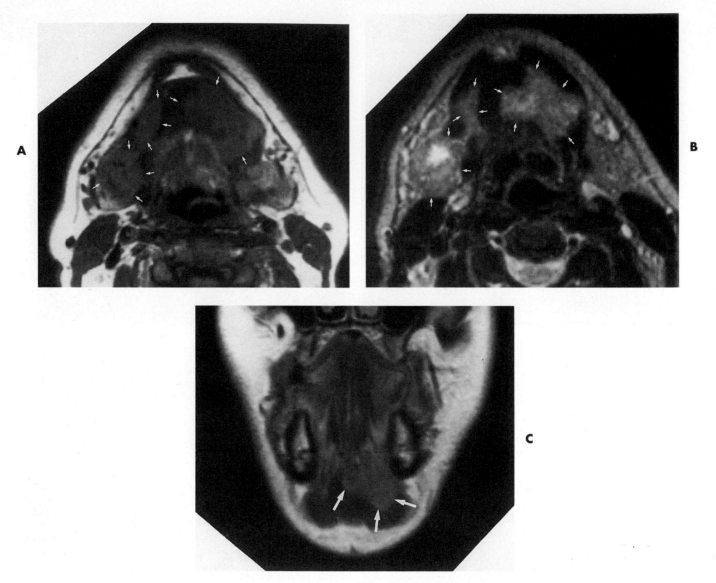

FIG. 9-42 Rhabdomyomas. **A** and **B,** Axial T1W and T2W MR images demonstrate multiple rhabdomyomas involving the oral tongue on the left, the right sublingual space, and the right submandibular region. The lesions are slightly hyperintense to muscle on the T1W image **(A),** becoming more hyperintense to muscle on the T2W image **(B).** **C** , Coronal T1W MR scans following the administration of contrast reveal faint enhancement of these lesions when compared with the noncontrast T1W study **(A).** The lesions on all images are indicated by the arrows. (Courtesy Dr. Jan Casselman.)

Lipomas

The ordinary lipoma is the most common tumor of mesenchymal origin. Only 13% arise in the extracranial head and neck; most are located in the posterior cervical region.[136] The remaining lesions as a group are rare, occuring primarily in the oral cavity, pharynx, parotid gland, and larynx. Within the oral cavity, lipomas represent only 1% to 4% of benign oral tumors and 1% of benign tongue tumors. These lesions are composed of mature fat cells arranged in lobules, separated by fibrous-tissue septae, usually surrounded by a thin fibrous capsule.[137] Some variants have

been classified histologically, according to the kind and amount of tissue, other than fat, that may also be present.[138] Most common is the fibrolipoma, containing an increased amount of fibrous connective tissue between the fat cells. Other variants include the angiolipoma, containing an excess of capillaries, the myxolipoma, with wide areas of myxoid change, and the most uncommon of the variant lipomas, with osseous or cartilaginous change.[137]

Lipomas are more common in overweight individuals and tend to increase in size during periods of rapid weight gain, being most common below the clavicle in obese women over 40 years of age. In contrast, lipomas in men tend to occur after the seventh decade, primarily in the head and neck region.

Within the oral cavity, lipomas, in decreasing order of frequency, are encountered in the cheek, tongue, floor of the mouth, buccal sulcus, palate, lip, and gingiva, with one third to one half occuring in the cheek.[120,138] Of those lesions that occur within the tongue, most arise within the oral tongue, as opposed to the tongue base.

These lesions have a virtually pathognomonic, homogeneous, nonenhancing, low CT attenuation, ranging from -65 to -125 HU (Figs. 9-43, 9-44). The most common differential diagnostic lesions include suprahyoid thyroglossal duct cysts, ranulas, and dermoid lesions, none of which have a typical low fat attenuation. Lipomas often displace and compress adjacent structures but rarely infiltrate them.[139] MRI of a typical lipoma demonstrates high signal intensity, consistent with fat, on T1W images and a lower T2W signal intensity.

Nerve Sheath Tumors

The terminology used to classify nerve sheath tumors has been somewhat confusing. Schwannomas have been variously termed *neurilemmomas, neuromas, neurinomas,* and *perineural fibroblastomas.*[1] Additionally, some have applied the term schwannoma to encompass both neurilemmomas and neurofibromas, while others include schwannomas and neuromas in discussions of neurilemmomas.[140] However, schwannomas (neurilemmomas) and neurofibromas can be distinguished on a histologic basis.[1] Neither should be confused with neuromas, which represent an exaggerated repair response to neuronal injury in which a tangle of regenerating axons, fibrous tissue, and Schwann cells form at the site of a severed nerve.[141]

Approximately 13% of schwannomas occur in the extracranial head and neck; most are encountered in the lateral cervical region, with the sympathetic chain being the most common site of origin.[142,143] In 1977, Gallo et al. reported 152 cases of oral schwannomas, 71 of them lingual.[144] In general, schwannomas tend to be somewhat more common in females and typically occur in the 30 to 40 year-old age-group.[142] Most schwannomas appear as well-circumscribed, homogeneous, soft-tissue density masses on unenhanced CT and exhibit contrast enhancement. Larger lesions may contain one or more cystic areas and present a more variable CT appearance.[145] Schwannomas tend to be isointense to muscle on T1W images and hyperintense on T2W images.[140] The cystic components of larger schwannomas may be difficult to distinguish from the solid components on T2W MR images because both manifest high signal intensity.[145] Enhancement following administration of contrast is the rule.

Neurofibromas involving the oral cavity are rare, and most are associated with neurofibromatosis. They are of similar density to muscle on unenhanced CT studies and enhance following contrast. They are typically isointense to muscle on T1W images and hyperintense on T2W scans.

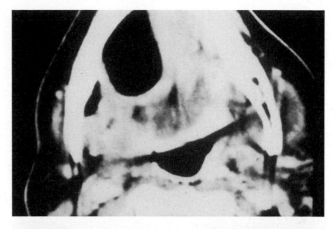

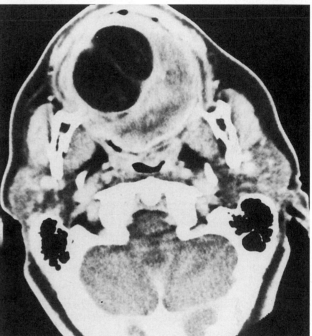

FIG. 9-43 Lipoma. **A,** There is a large, unilocular, very hypodense lesion within the right sublingual space, similar in density to the subcutaneous fat. The characteristics are compatible with a sublingual space lipoma. **B,** Axial CT shows a fat attenuation, slightly lobulated mass in the anterior right tongue. Lipoma of tongue.

Exostoses

Torus palatinus is an exostosis of the hard palate. These lesions typically occur in the middle of the hard palate, reaching a peak incidence before 30 years of age. Women are more commonly affected than men, and the exact cause of these lesions is unknown, although some theories suggest that they may be hereditary.[146] On CT these lesions appear as solid, dense cortical bone (Fig. 9-45) or as cortical bone surrounding areas of cancellous bone, often with a midline fissure.

Miscellaneous Benign Lesions

There are a variety of rare lesions involving the tongue and other regions of the oral cavity that have not been described

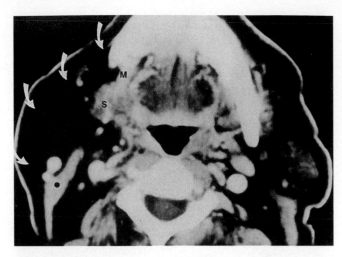

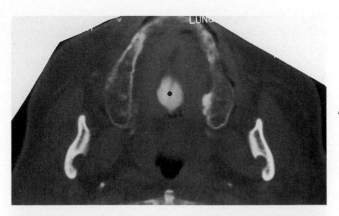

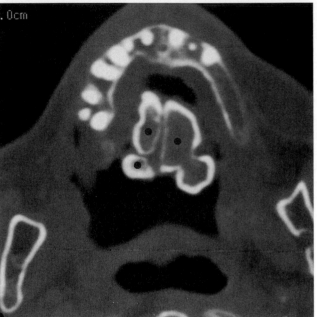

FIG. 9-44 Lipoma. Contrast-enhanced CT scan reveals a large lipoma within the confines of the right submandibular space. The fat-density lesion is virtually impossible to distinguish from the subcutaneous fat, although it is separated by thin fibers of the platysma muscle *(arrows)*. The lesion insinuates among the normal structures of this region. *S,* Submandibular gland; *black dot,* sternocleidomastoid muscle; *M,* mylohyoid muscle.

FIG. 9-45 Torus palatinus. **A,** Axial CT scan obtained at bone-window settings reveals a large calcified mass *(black dot)*. The density of the calcified mass is consistent with cortical bone, without the presence of cancellous bone. (Courtesy Dr. Deborah Reede). Torus palatinus **(B)**. Axial CT scan obtained at bone window setting reveals the presence of a large torus palatinus projecting from the hard palate inferiorly into the upper aspect of the oral cavity. The torus is multilobulated, with multiple, well-corticated areas of cancellous bone *(dots)*. (Courtesy Dr. Deborah Reede.)

on cross-sectional imaging. Some of the more common rare lesions include chondromas, osteomas, and epithelioid hemangioendotheliomas.

Chondroma. Uncommon within the oral cavity, most chondromas occur in the hard palate, alveolar ridge, or involve the condyle or coronoid process of the mandible. Only a few extraskeletal oral chondromas have been recorded, the tongue being the most common site.[147] These lesions most often affect the lateral borders or the dorsum of the oral tongue, occur equally in both sexes, and patients have a mean age at presentation of 31 years.

Osteomas. Osteomas are rare within the soft tissues of the extracranial head and neck, especially the tongue. In a review of the English-language literature in 1989, Nash et al. reviewed 31 previously reported cases of tongue osteomas and added one of their own.[148] These lesions predominate in the third decade of life, and 75% occur in females. The majority of reported lingual osteomas occur at the junction of the anterior two thirds and posterior one third of the tongue, in the region of the circumvallate papillae or foramen cecum (Fig. 9-46). Because of its location, a lingual osteoma may be mistaken clinically for lingual thyroid tissue.[149]

Epithelioid Hemangioendothelioma. Only five cases of these rare lesions involving the oral cavity have been reported.[150-153] Three tumors involved the gingiva, one involved the tongue, and one involved the palate. These lesions are soft-tissue vascular neoplasms characterized by proliferation of endothelial cells with an epithelioid morphology. Their biologic behavior is considered borderline in that they manifest an indolent course with a potential for recurrence but rarely metastasize.

Granular Cell Myoblastomas. These lesions are considered to be of neurogenic origin, although they also contain skeletal muscle and histiocytes. Of these tumors, 50% involve the tongue or floor of the mouth, primarily occuring in young adults. The lateral tip or dorsum of the tongue are most often affected, with infiltration of the surrounding tissues being common. The CT appearance is nonspecific, similar to that of squamous cell carcinoma. The MR features, however, may be somewhat more specific because these lesions tend to exhibit low signal intensity on both T1W and T2W images, most likely reflecting their fibrous or skeletal components.[154]

Malignant Lesions

Only 7% of oral cavity lesions are malignant, but among these lesions squamous cell carcinoma accounts for 90% of the tumors.[155] Other malignancies encountered in this region include minor salivary gland tumors (adenoid cystic carcinoma, adenocarcinoma, and mucoepidermoid carcinoma), lymphomas, and a variety of other rare tumors, including sarcomas (liposarcoma, rhabdomyosarcoma). Most masses within the oral cavity, both benign and malignant, are amenable to direct clinical examination, which is the best means by which to detect mucosal involvement. The primary purpose of imaging these lesions is to detect their deep or submucosal extent. Staging of primary malignancies of the oral cavity is uniformly based on the TNM system developed by the American Joint Commission on Cancer Staging (Box 9-1).[156]

Squamous Cell Carcinoma

Squamous cell carcinoma (SCCa) typically affects middle-aged males with a long history of alcohol and tobacco abuse.[151,75] Approximately two thirds of the tumors are moderately or far advanced at the time of initial presentation. The behavior of SCCa of the oral cavity differs somewhat from SCCa of the oropharynx. The mucosa of the orophar-

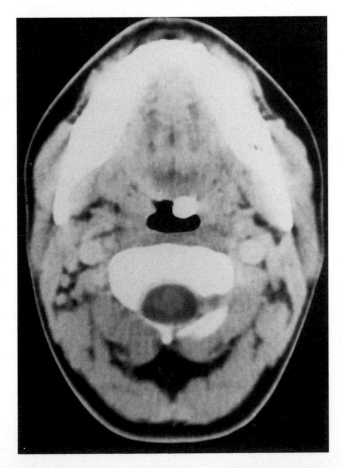

FIG. 9-46 Lingual osteoma. Axial CT scan shows a bone-density mass near the midline of the base of the tongue.

ynx, posterior to the circumvallate papillae, is derived from endoderm and has a tendency to be affected by less well-differentiated, aggressive carcinomas. The squamous epithelium within the oral cavity, however, is derived from ectodermal elements and tends to be affected by less aggressive lesions.[1,158] Differences in lymphatic drainage also exist.

Although SCCa may arise from any mucosal surface, it has a tendency to affect the dependent portions of the oral cavity (lower lip, oral tongue, and floor of the mouth). Frequency according to site of occurrence, as reported by Lederman from a study of 14,253 patients, is listed in Table 9-2.[159] The observation that the vast majority of oral cavity SCCa arises from a relatively limited, dependent portion of the oral cavity mucosa may be due to a variety of factors. These dependent regions are continuously bathed in a pool of saliva, which may serve as a reservoir of exogenous carcinogens, primarily derived from tobacco or the irritating effects of alcoholic beverages. In addition, in contrast to the relatively thick layer of squamous cell epithelium containing well-developed rete pegs and a prominent superficial keratin layer that lines most of the oral cavity, the floor of the mouth and ventral and lateral surfaces of the tongue are lined by thin, relatively atrophic mucosa with shallow or nonexistent rete pegs and little surface keratin.[157]

It is estimated that 30% to 65% of patients with oral cavity SCCa have nodal involvement at the time of initial presentation, and the presence or absence of such metastatic cervical adenopathy is the single most important prognostic indicator in these patients.[2,160-163] For this reason, all of the cervical lymph node chains should be imaged at the same time the primary tumor is imaged.[164] This may be accomplished by either CT or MRI, although currently, MRI is probably not as accurate as CT in its ability to demonstrate either extranodal tumor spread or central nodal necrosis.[165,166] On CT, SCCa has a density similar to that of muscle and enhances to a variable degree following administration of contrast. These tumors are also identified by their distortion of the normal structures and the surrounding fat planes. These lesions possess increased signal intensity on T2W MRI and frequently enhance to some degree with gadolinium.

SCCa of the Floor of the Mouth. Three basic categories of information must be provided when evaluating

TABLE 9-2
Frequency of Oral Cavity Cancer By Location

Location	Frequency (%)
Lower lip	38
Oral Tongue	22
Floor of the mouth	17
Gingiva	6
Palate (hard/soft)	5.5
Upper lip	4
Buccal mucosa	2
Other	5.5

From Lederman M. The anatomy of cancer. J Laryngol Otol 1964; 78:181-208.

▼

BOX 9-1
ORAL CAVITY: OROPHARYNGEAL SCCA

TNM Staging

TX	Primary tumor cannot be evaluated
T0	No evidence of primary tumor
Tis	Carcinoma in situ
T1	Tumor 2 cm or less in greatest diameter
T2	Tumor more than 2 cm but less than 4 cm in greatest diameter
T4	Tumor invades adjacent structures (skin, cortical bone, etc.)
NX	Regional lymph nodes cannot be assessed
N0	No regional lymph node metastases
N1	Metastasis to a single ipsilateral lymph node, less than 3 cm in greatest diameter
N2a	Metastasis to a single ipsilateral lymph node, greater than 3 cm but less than 6 cm in greatest diameter
N2b	Metastasis to multiple ipsilateral lymph nodes, all less than 6 cm in greatest diameter
N2c	Metastases to bilateral or contralateral lymph nodes, all less than 6 cm in greatest diameter
N3	Metastases to any lymph nodes greater than 6 cm in greatest diameter
MX	Presence of distant metastases cannot be assessed
M0	No distant metastases
M1	Distant metastases present
Stage 0	Tis N0 M0
Stage 1	T1 N0 M0
Stage 2	T2 N0 M0
Stage 3	T3 N0 M0
	T1, 2, 3 N1 M0
Stage 4	All T4 lesions
	All N2, N3 lesions
	All M1 lesions

SCCa of the floor of the mouth: (1) the status of the mandible and related teeth, (2) the deep extent of the primary tumor, and (3) the status of regional lymph nodes. Contrast-enhanced CT is the preferred modality for these lesions due to its availability, its better demonstration of cortical bone invasion, and its superior detection of lymph node metastases.[165] MRI, however, is more sensitive than CT for evaluating bone marrow involvement and perineural tumor spread.[4,167,168] T1W images in particular, which normally display mandibular marrow fat as high signal intensity, easily demonstrate marrow replacement, even in the absence of cortical destruction (Fig. 9-47). SCCa of the floor of the mouth is virtually free to spread in all directions, including (1) medial spread across the midline either directly across the genioglossus muscle and lingual septum or via the potential space between the genioglossus and geniohyoid muscles, (2) lateral spread typically contained by the mylohyoid muscle along the periosteum of the mandible, (3) posterior spread along the mylohyoid muscle, usually within the sublingual space, into the deep fascial spaces of the upper neck, (4) inferior spread along the mylohyoid and hyoglossus muscles to their inferior attachments on the hyoid bone, (5) posteroinferior spread to involve the base of the tongue, and (6) spread directly to involve the oral tongue (Fig. 9-48). The ostia of the submandibular ducts may become obstructed by tumors in this region, resulting in duct dilatation or obstructive inflammatory enlargement of the sub-

mandibular gland (Fig. 9-49). Similarly, obstruction or inflammatory involvement of the sublingual salivary glands may also occur. Encasement of the lingual artery is common, but life-threatening hemorrhage is infrequent. The major lymph node drainage from SCCa of the floor of the mouth is to the submental, submandibular, and internal jugular nodes (Fig. 9-50).[2] The depth of tumor invasion in the floor of the mouth is more closely related to the presence of cervical nodal metastasis than is the surface size of the tumor. Thus careful attention should be made to identify this tumor depth on imaging.

SCCa of the Oral Tongue. SCCa of the oral tongue typically invades the tongue musculature, spreading easily along the bundles of the intrinsic muscles deeper into the tongue or along extrinsic tongue muscles to their sites of attachment (hyoid bone, mandible, styloid process, etc). These tumors may also extend submucosally to involve the floor of the mouth, tonsils, mandible, and pharyngeal walls.[2] The lymphatic drainage is primarily to the submandibular and internal jugular nodes, often with bilateral involvement. When evaluating oral tongue SCCa, it is extremely important to assess the extent of the tumor in relation to the midline (Fig. 9-51). Total glossectomy is rarely performed because it is poorly tolerated, and demonstration of tumor extension across the midline will typically preclude a hemiglossectomy. Only recently have more extensive partial glossectomies been performed, usually with a free flap

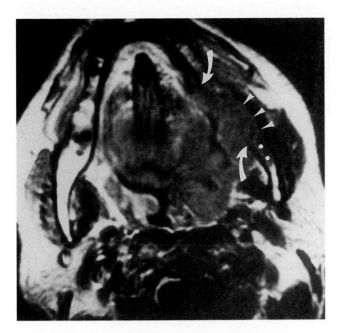

FIG. 9-47 Squamous cell carcinoma invading the left mandible. Axial T1W image demonstrates a large mass centered in the region of the tongue base and left tonsillar fossa with obvious erosion of a large portion of the lingual surface of the left mandible *(curved white arrows).* Tumor is visualized extending to the buccal cortex of the mandible *(arrowheads).* In addition, however, there is tumor extension into the posterior aspect of the mandible, replacing the normal high-signal fat, in an area where no lingual cortical mandibular destruction is identified *(white dots).*

reconstruction, and there is promise that these more advanced procedures may be better tolerated by patients.

SCCa of the Lip. Squamous cell carcinomas of the lip typically arise from the vermillion border and spread to involve the orbicularis oris muscle and adjacent skin. More advanced lesions may extend to directly involve the buccal mucosa, mandible, and rarely the mental nerve, permitting access to the mandibular marrow and potential perineural extension along the inferior alveolar nerve. The lymphatic drainage of these tumors is to the submental, submandibular, and internal jugular nodes (Fig. 9-50).[2]

SCCa of the Gingiva, Buccal Mucosa, and Hard Palate. Overall, squamous cell carcinoma affecting these regions requires a similar evaluation and management as carcinoma in the floor of the mouth and oral tongue. In addition, mandibular invasion is of special concern for these lesions and may be either of a perineural or intramedullary type (Figs. 9-52 to 9-55). When evaluating an uncommon primary SCCa of the hard palate, it is important to assess possible extension to the floor of the nasal cavity, the maxillary sinus, or the soft palate. This is best done by imaging in the coronal plane, and for this reason, due to its direct coronal capabilities, MRI may be preferred over CT (Fig. 9-56).

SCCa of the Retromolar Trigone. Retromolar trigone lesions may extend superiorly, deep to the maxillary tuberosity, and invade the infratemoral fossa fat, posterolat-

eral to the maxillary antrum. This spread, not detected clinically, is seen on imaging as obliteration of the normal fat planes. Involvement of the pterygopalatine fossa and masticator space may also occur, allowing invasion of neurovascular bundles and permitting continued cephalad extension to involve the cavernous sinus via the maxillary and mandibular nerves (Fig. 9-57). Posterolateral spread of retromolar trigone SCCa may reach the ascending ramus of the mandible, masseter muscle, and even the cheek. Medial extension typically affects the medial pterygoid muscle, in which case trismus will almost always be present. Inferomedial spread may reach the mylohyoid muscle and the posterior aspect of the floor of the mouth.

Lymphoma

Both Hodgkin's and non-Hodgkin's lymphomas occur in the head and neck region, with lymph node enlargement being the most common presenting symptom for both types of lymphoma. Although Hodgkin's lymphoma tends to be predominantly nodal with extranodal involvement only uncommonly encountered, non-Hodgkin's lymphoma frequently involves extranodal sites.[169,170]

Although the internal jugular (deep cervical) chain nodes are most often affected, involvement of submandibular nodes occasionally occurs. Involved lymph nodes range in size from one to several centimeters, some have been reported to exceed 10 cm.[170] They exhibit striking homogeneity, may manifest peripheral rim-enhancement, and central necrosis is distinctly uncommon, reported to occur only after the patient has undergone treatment (Fig. 9-58).[169] It is not possible to differentiate lymph nodes involved by Hodgkin's lymphoma from those affected by non-Hodgkin's lymphoma or metastatic disease solely on the basis of CT or MRI. Imaging of the lymph nodes is discussed more thoroughly in Chapter 15.

Adenoid Cystic Carcinoma

Adenoid cystic carcinoma (ACCa) accounts for only 5% of major salivary gland neoplasms, but it comprises more than 25% of the malignancies occurring in the minor salivary glands.[171] More than 1000 minor salivary glands are distributed throughout the upper aerodigestive tract. They are especially concentrated in the buccal, labial, palatal, and lingual regions. Only the gingiva and anterior hard palate have few or none of these glands. Adenoid cystic carcinoma has been reported to involve the minor salivary glands in the maxillary sinuses and nasal cavity, the hard and soft palates, buccal mucosa, floor of the mouth, tongue, lip, and retromolar trigone.[172] These lesions typically occur in the fifth or sixth decade of life, and although some authors report a male predominance, others report a female predominance or no sexual predominance at all.[173-176]

Three histologic subtypes of ACCa exist: tubular, cribriform, and solid. The degree of cellularity increases from the tubular to the solid form, and in general the greater the cellularity, the worse the prognosis.[177] Most tumors manifest

Text continued on p. 526.

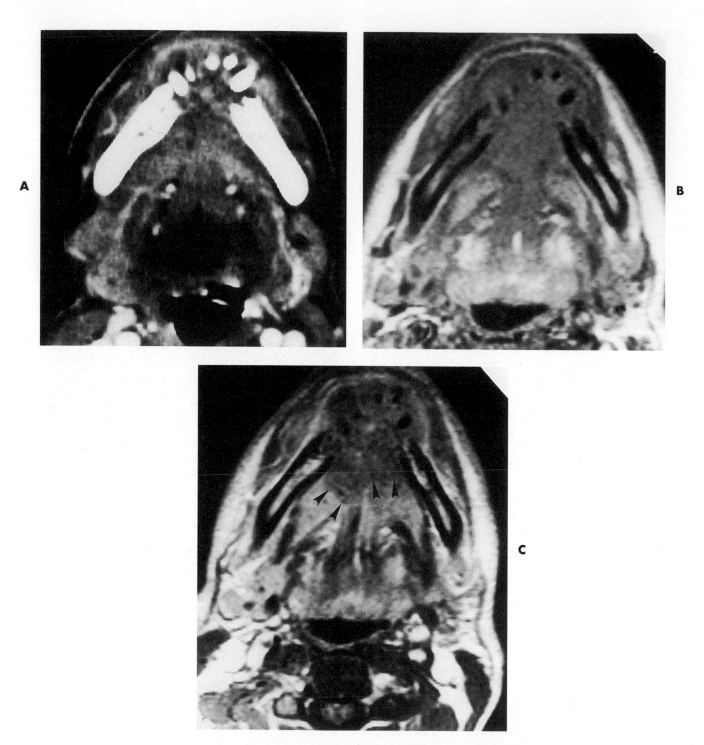

FIG. 9-48 Squamous cell carcinoma of the floor of the mouth. Contrast-enhanced CT scan (**A**) and axial T1W MR scans without (**B**) and with (**C**) contrast enhancement demonstrate a large floor of the mouth lesion, which extends anteriorly to destroy the mandible and involve the soft tissues external to the mandible. The margins of this lesion are extremely difficult to identify on the CT scan. They are somewhat better delineated on the MR performed without contrast (B). However, the best delineation results following the administration of contrast (C) on which the tissues surrounding the carcinoma enhance, although the tumor itself does not enhance. The lesion extends posteriorly to involve the anterior aspect of the oral tongue *(arrowheads)*.

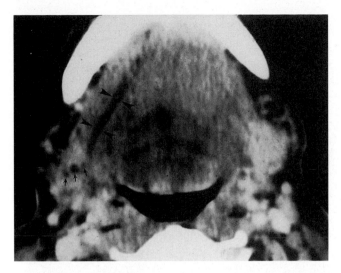

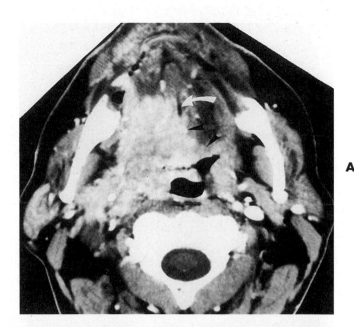

FIG. 9-49 Squamous cell carcinoma of the floor of the mouth. Contrast-enhanced axial CT scan reveals a poorly defined lesion involving the floor of the mouth anteriorly. The lesion has resulted in submandibular gland duct obstruction on the right *(arrowheads)*. In addition to the dilated main duct, dilated intraglandular ducts are also identified *(arrows)*.

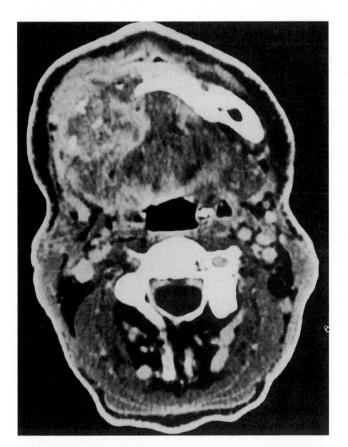

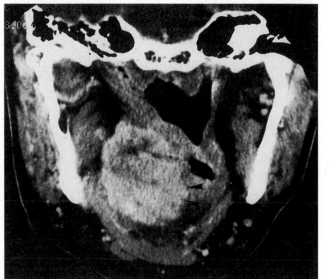

FIG. 9-51 Squamous cell carcinoma. **A** and **B,** Axial and coronal contrast-enhanced CT scans demonstrate a large tumor involving the oral tongue, oropharynx, and tonsillar fossa, with extension to the region of the right carotid space and medial aspect of the right parapharyngeal space. Clear demonstration of extension to the left of midline is identified on both views *(arrowheads)*. The lingual septum is well visualized on the axial image *(white arrow* in **A).**

FIG. 9-50 Squamous cell carcinoma. Axial contrast-enhanced CT scan demonstrates a large destructive lesion involving the right floor of the mouth, destroying the right aspect of the mandible, projecting into the oral tongue, and extending anteriorly into the soft tissues external to the mandible. (Courtesy Dr. Nicole Freling.)

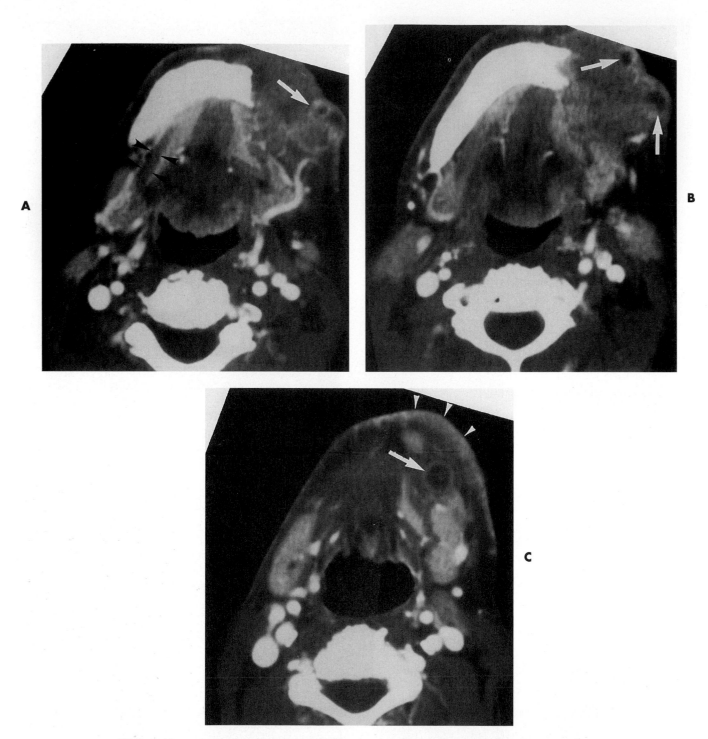

FIG. 9-52 Squamous cell carcinoma probably arising from the gingiva-buccal mucosa. **A, B** and **C,** Axial contrast-enhanced CT scans reveal a large tumor on the left, extending to the skin, destroying the left portion of the mandible, and invading the left mylohyoid muscle. Fibers of the right mylohyoid muscle are well defined *(black arrowheads* in **A**). Metastatic disease to left submandibular nodes is identified in all three sections *(white arrows)*. Thickening and involvement of the skin is easily seen on **C** *(white arrowheads)*.

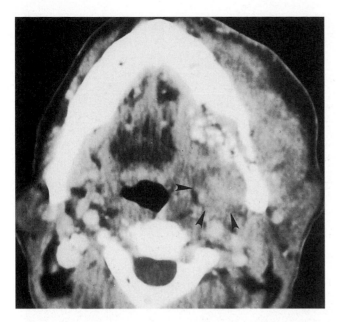

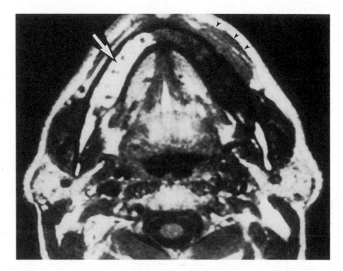

FIG. 9-53 Squamous cell carcinoma of the buccal mucosa. Axial contrast-enhanced CT scan demonstrates a large mass on the left, with its epicenter located in the left gingiva-buccal mucosa. There is obvious destruction of the posterior aspect of the left mandible. Medial to the mandible the tumor appears to be extending along the mylohyoid muscle to involve the deep aspect of the sub-mandibular space *(arrowheads).*

FIG. 9-54 Squamous cell carcinoma of the gingiva-buccal mucosa. Axial T1W MR scan demonstrates a soft-tissue mass lateral to the mandible, on the left *(arrowheads).* Although both the buccal and lingual aspects of the mandibular cortex appear intact, there is replacement of a large portion of the marrow within the mandible, manifested as replacement of the normal high signal intensity fat. Normal fat in the right aspect of the mandible is indicated by the arrow. It is most probable that this has resulted from perineural tumor extension via the mental nerve with retrograde involvement of the inferior alveolar nerve. (Courtesy Dr. Edward Kassel.)

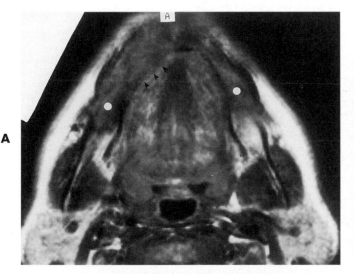

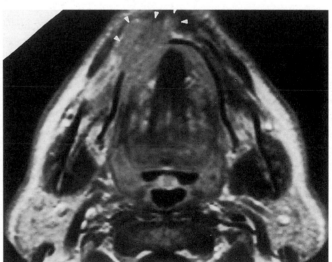

FIG. 9-55 Squamous cell carcinoma of the gingiva-buccal mucosa. Axial T1W MR scans without **(A)** and with **(B)** contrast demonstrate a mass involving the anterior aspect of the right mandible. Both the buccal and lingual cortices are destroyed, and tumor extends into the soft tissues of the face anteriorly and into the anterior aspect of the oral tongue posteriorly *(black arrowheads* in **A**). The anterior extension is somewhat better-defined on the postcontrast image *(arrowheads* in **B**), and separation from the heterogeneous sublingual space is better appreciated on the noncontrast image *(arrowheads* in **A**). Extensive replacement of the high-signal marrow within the mandible is best appreciated on the noncontrast image *(white dots* in **A**), because the lesion enhances slightly postcontrast, somewhat obscuring this separation.

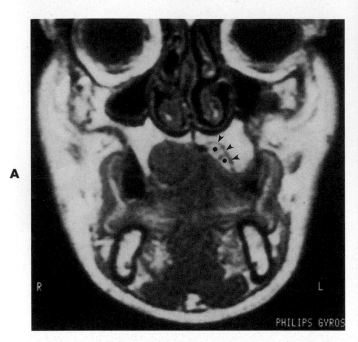

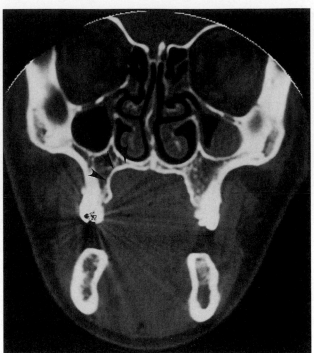

FIG. 9-56 Squamous cell carcinoma of the hard palate. **A,** Coronal T1W MR scan demonstrates a fairly well-defined lesion involving the right hard palate, which appears to be centered within the minor salivary glands. The glandular tissue of the left hard palate is indicated by the dots. A good cortical margin to the left hard palate can be identified *(arrowheads)*. The cortical margin on the right is not, however, appreciated. There is no apparent infiltration or replacement of the marrow. There is no evidence of extension to involve the maxillary sinus or nasal cavity. **B,** Coronal CT scan obtained at bone window levels demonstrates an intact cortical margin to the hard palate on the right *(arrowheads)*. There is slight fossa formation when compared with the left. From an imaging standpoint this squamous cell carcinoma exhibits features of a relatively benign process. (Courtesy Dr. Nicole Freling.)

more than one subtype, making accurate staging difficult. In addition, transformation from one subtype to another suggests that this malignancy may represent a morphologic continuum.

Adenoid cystic carcinoma is characterized by slow, relentless growth and a tendency for extensive local invasion. A particular feature of this tumor is its propensity for perineural tumor extension, and for primary lesions that occur within the oral cavity, this extension mainly affects the maxillary and mandibular branches of the trigeminal nerve because of involvement of the masticator space or the pterygomaxillary fissure. Regional lymph node metastases, however, are uncommon and are primarily associated with more poorly differentiated lesions (solid subtype).[178] Adenoid cystic carcinoma is reported to have a worse prognosis when it involves minor salivary glands compared with the major salivary glands.[174,179] This may be due to the fact that minor salivary gland tumors have a greater opportunity to infiltrate and invade the surrounding soft tissues and bone (Fig. 9-59).[173] In one large series the medium relapse-free interval for patients with major salivary gland adenoid cystic carcinoma was 83 months compared with 52 months for patients with minor salivary gland tumors.[173] Overall, ACCa

carries a grave prognosis, regardless of treatment, as evidenced by the decline in survival of all patients from 58% at 5 years to 16% at 15 years.[180]

On CT and MRI, ACCa cannot be distiguished from squamous cell carcinoma or other malignancies on the basis of density or signal intensity (Figs. 9-60, 9-61). However, signal intensity on T2W images has been shown to correlate well with the degree of tumor cellularity.[181] Lesions with higher signal intensities correspond to tumors with low cellularity and the best prognosis, and tumors with low signal intensity on T2W imaging have dense cellularity and a poor prognosis.

Among patients with extracranial head and neck malignancies, those with ACCa are at greatest risk for perineural tumor extension.[182] Although perineural tumor spread has been reported equally or more commonly in association with SCCa in some literature, this is most likely a reflection of the more frequent overall occurence of SCCa.[183,184]

Although CT and MRI are reported to be virtually identical in demonstrating perineural tumor below the skull base (provided that direct coronal, thin-section CT scans are obtained), MRI is superior to CT in demonstrating involve-

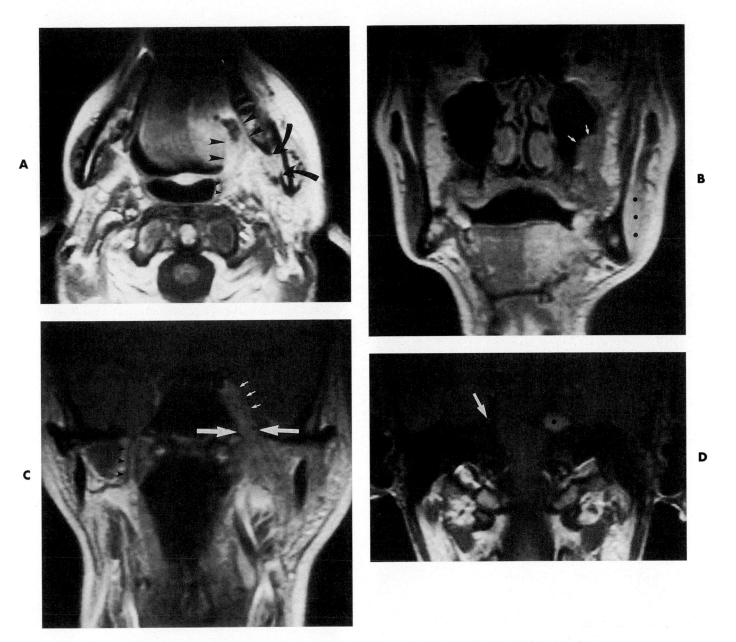

FIG. 9-57 Squamous cell carcinoma of the retromolar trigone in a 48-year-old woman who presents with left trismus and decreased sensation in the distribution of the left maxillary nerve. **A,** Axial contrast-enhanced T1W MR demonstrates an enhancing mass centered in the region of the left retromolar trigone or tonsillar fossa. The exact limits of the tumor are not able to be defined, although extension anteriorly along the mylohyoid muscle into the tongue can be appreciated *(large arrowheads),* as can medial extension to abut the pharyngeal constrictor muscle *(small arrowheads),* and lateral extension as a small knuckle of tumor widens and grows into the inferior alveolar canal *(curved arrows).* **B** through **D,** Coronal T1W MR scans following contrast administration. At the level of the maxillary sinus **(B)** tumor extension through the floor of the left maxillary sinus with a small soft-tissue mass within the inferior aspect of the sinus can be identified *(arrows).* Note the denervation atrophy and fatty infiltration of the left masseter muscle *(dots),* as well as the left hemitongue. Further posteriorly **(C),** perineural tumor extension along the left mandibular nerve, widening the left foramen ovale *(large white arrows)* and extension into the cavernous sinus *(small white arrows)* are identified. The normal mandibular nerve within the masticator space on the right is indicated by the arrowheads. Far posteriorly **(D),** enhancement and marked enlargement of the left trigeminal nerve at its root entry zone is appreciated *(dot).* The normal sized, nonenhancing right trigeminal nerve is indicated by the arrow.

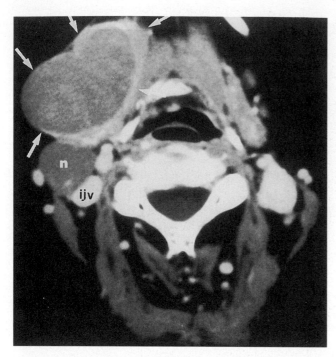

FIG. 9-58 Non-Hodgkin's lymphoma. Contrast-enhanced CT scan reveals a large submandibular space nodal mass *(white arrows)*. Although the margin enhances, the center remains homogeneous and isointense to muscle. A carotid space node *(n)*, compressing the internal jugular vein *(ijv)* is also identifed. (From Fruin ME, Smoker WRK, Harnsberger HR. The carotid space in the suprahyoid neck. Seminars in Ultrasound CT and MR 1990; 11:504-519.)

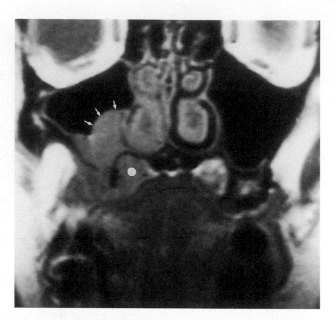

FIG. 9-59 Adenoid cystic carcinoma of the hard palate. Coronal T1W MR demonstrates replacement of the normal high signal intensity of the minor salivary gland tissue in the right aspect of the hard palate *(white dot)*. Normal salivary glands are identified on the left. This tumor has eroded the inferior aspect of the right maxillary sinus and has an intrasinus component *(arrows)*.

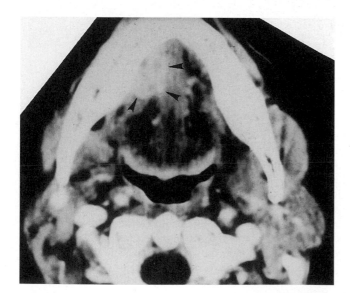

FIG. 9-60 Adnoid cystic carcinoma of the right sublingual gland. Axial contrast-enhanced CT scan reveals an enhancing mass in the anterior aspect of the right tongue, obliterating the normally fat-filled right sublingual space *(arrowheads)*. On the basis of imaging characteristics, this lesion cannot be distinguished from squamous cell carcinoma originating within the oral tongue.

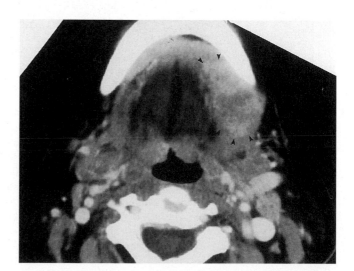

FIG. 9-61 Adnoid cystic carcinoma of the left sublingual gland. Contrast-enhanced axial CT scan demonstrates a heterogeneous mass involving the left lateral aspect of the oral tongue, which appears to obliterate the left sublingual space *(arrowheads)*.

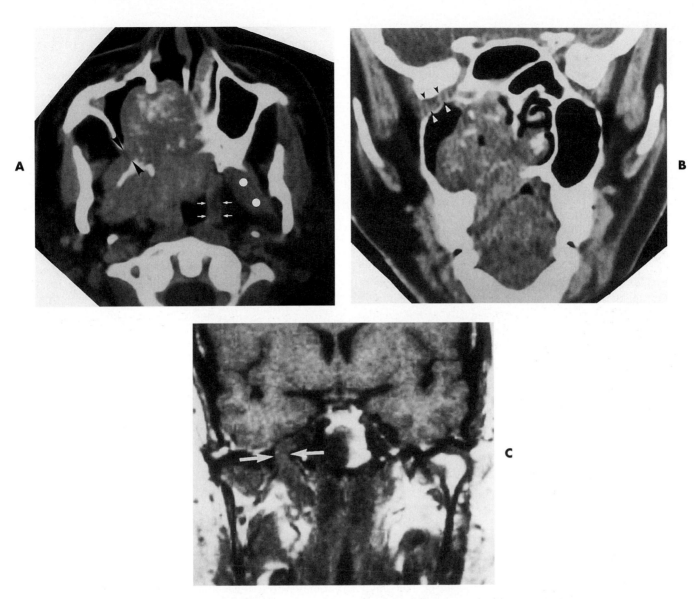

FIG. 9-62 Adenoid cystic carcinoma of the hard palate. **A** and **B**, Axial and coronal contrast-enhanced CT scans demonstrate a destructive lesion of the right hard palate. There is erosion of the medial wall of the right maxillary sinus with extension of tumor into the sinus, as well as destruction of the posterior aspect of the nasal septum with involvement of the nasal cavity bilaterally. There is widening of the pterygomaxillary fissure on the right (*arrowheads* in **A**) and the inferior orbital fissure (*arrowheads* in **B**), which is highly suggestive of perineural tumor involvement. Involvement of the right masticator space musculature is probable, on the basis of enlargement of the right medial pterygoid muscle, when compared with the normal left (*white dots* in **A**). The normal configuration of the right parapharyngeal space fat is lost on the right, when compared with the normal left. Extension of the tumor along the pharyngeal constrictor muscle on the right is identified by enlargement and poor definition of this muscle. The normal contour of the left pharyngeal constrictor muscle is indicated by the white arrows in **A**. **C,** Coronal T1W MR demonstrates perineural tumor extension along the right mandibular nerve as it courses through an enlarged right foramen ovale *(white arrows)* into the inferior aspect of the right cavernous sinus.

ment of the cisternal segments and cavernous sinus portions of the cranial nerves.[184] Thin-section axial and coronal T1W images, both before and after contrast administration, are considered the optimal studies. Because of the high T1W signal intensity of fat, and the possibility of chemical mis-registration artifacts, tumor enhancement may be obscured under the skull base. The addition of fat suppression in combination with contrast enhancement has been shown to be extremely useful in these situations.[185,186]

Perineural tumor may be seen on CT by identifying enlargement of skull base foramina and fissures such as the foramen ovale (V3), foramen rotundum (V2), and the ptery-gomaxillary fissure (and pterygopalatine fossa) (V2). Only rarely can a diffusely enlarged nerve be seen on CT. MRI may demonstrate increased thickness of the affected nerve(s) (Fig. 9-62) and diffuse or marginal enhancement following administration of contrast. Unfortunately, enlargement or enhancement is not pathognomonic for perineural tumor, but may also be caused by edema, neuritis, primary neural tumor, and in the cisternal segments, by meningeal inflammatory conditions.[181,184] False positive perineural tumor spread in patients with ACCa has been reported, producing a false overestimation of the severity of disease.[181]

Mucoepidermoid Carcinoma

Mucoepidermoid carcinomas arise from glandular ductal epithelium, and approximately 30% of these tumors arise from the minor salivary glands that are primarily in the buccal mucosa and palate. These tumors may be classified as low-, intermediate-, or high-grade lesions. The lower grade

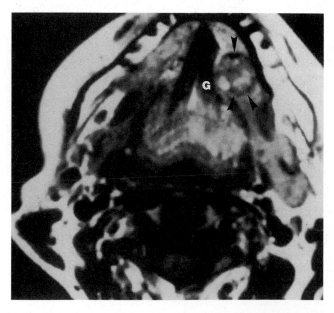

FIG. 9-63 Mucoepidermoid carcinoma of the left sublingual gland. Axial T1W MR demonstrates a fairly well-circumscribed, heterogeneous lesion centered within the left sublingual space (*arrowheads*). The lingual aspect of the adjacent mandibular cortex appears intact, as does the lateral margin of the left genioglossus muscle (*G*).

lesions tend to behave in a fashion similar to benign lesions with an overall 5-year survival of 90%. They have a "benign" imaging appearance with fairly well-delineated, smooth margins. Cystic areas may be present, and rarely calcifications may be encountered (Fig. 9-63). High-grade lesions are poorly circumscribed with indistict, infiltrating margins and an overall 5-year survival of only 42%. These high-grade tumors tend to be solid and demonstrate low to intermediate signal intensity on both T1W and T2W MRI.[187] These lesions are discussed further in Chapter 17.

Liposarcoma

Liposarcomas are rare in the extracranial head and neck, although they are common in the retroperitoneum and peripheral soft tissues. Within the oral cavity, these lesions have been reported in the cheek, lip, palate, floor of the mouth, and the submental regions.[188] They originate from lipoblasts, within or adjacent to fascia and do not originate from preexisting lipomas.[1] They are more common in males than in females and predominately occur in the fourth to sixth decades of life.[188] Histologic tumor type correlates closely with clinical behavior. The 5-year survivals for myxoid and well-differentiated tumors are 77% and 85% respectively, and those for round-cell and pleomorphic lesions are 18% and 21%, respectively.[189]

On CT, liposarcomas are inhomogenous, demonstrating a combination of fat and soft-tissue elements. The density of the fat is greater than that of subcutaneous fat, and these lesions tend to infiltrate adjacent structures. On MRI, liposarcomas primarily appear as fatty lesions but display signal intensities lower than those of subcutaneous fat on short TR sequences.[190]

Rhabdomyosarcoma

Rhabdomyosarcomas are rare malignant mesenchymal tumors, 36% of which involve the head and neck.[191] In spite of a head and neck predilection, rhabdomyosarcoma involving the tongue is rare, representing only 0.34% of cases reported by the Intergroup Rhabdomyosarcoma Studies.[192] These tumors most often involve the base of the tongue, but they have also been reported within the oral tongue.[193] Oral rhabdomyosarcomas are more common in males and predominate within the first 2 decades of life.[194]

Rhabdomyosarcomas appear as muscle density masses on CT and muscle signal intensity masses on MRI, although they often have higher T2W signal intensities than does normal muscle. These tumors tend to infiltrate the surrounding structures. They may exhibit a variable amount of enhancement following contrast administration.

Miscellaneous Malignancies

Cases of other, less common sarcomas involving the oral cavity may be found in isolated reports. These include fibrosarcomas, angiosarcomas, myosarcomas, and leiomyosarcomas.[120,195] Because the buccal space is in intimate contact with the mandible and fascially contained within the masticator space, malignant lesions involving these regions of the oral cavity not infrequently secondarily involve structures within the mandible and the masticator space. Similarly, lesions in the mandible such as chondrosarcomas (Fig. 9-64), osteosarcomas, metastases, and malignant schwannomas of the inferior alveolar nerve (Fig 9-65) can extend into the oral cavity, as can giant cell granulomas (Fig. 9-66) and eosinophic granulomas (Fig. 9-67).[18] Mandibular pathology is discussed in Chapter 5.

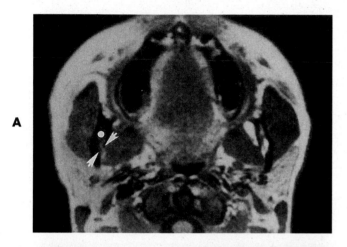

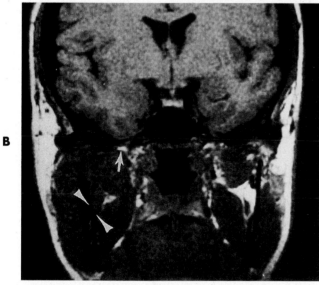

FIG. 9-64 Mandibular chondrosarcoma. **A** and **B,** Axial and coronal T1W MR scans demonstrate a right masticator space mass with involvement of the lateral pterygoid, medial pterygoid, and masseter muscles. There is antegrade perineural tumor extension along the inferior alveolar nerve with widening of the inferior alveolar foramen *(white arrowheads).* Replacement of the normal, high signal fatty marrow is best appreciated on the axial image *(white dot).* At this time there is no evidence of retrograde perineural tumor because the margins of the right foramen ovale are intact and normal fat is identified just inferior to the foramen *(white arrow* in **B).** (From Tryhus MR, Smoker WRK, Harnsberger HR. The normal and diseased masticator space. Seminars in Ultrasound CT and MR 1990; 11:476-485.)

Miscellaneous Pathology
Denervation Muscle Atrophy

The motor innervation to the musculature of the tongue and floor of the mouth is derived from the hypoglossal nerve, the mylohyoid nerve, and fibers from C1. Damage to these nerves anywhere along their course may produce denervation, muscle wasting, fatty infiltration, and atrophy of the involved muscles.[196,197] These changes are easily appreciated on both CT and MRI in either the axial or coronal planes. Various patterns of motor denervation are presented in Fig. 9-68.

Insult to the hypoglossal nerve may produce muscle wasting after only 2 to 3 weeks.[197] The first clinical sign of

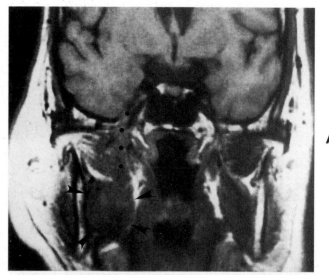

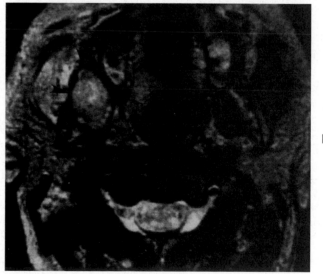

FIG. 9-65 Right mandibular nerve malignant schwannoma. **A,** Coronal T1W MR demonstrates a mass centered within the right medial pterygoid muscle *(arrowheads),* extending along the masticator nerve through the foramen ovale and into the cavernous sinus *(dots).* **B,** Axial T2W MR demonstrates the mass is hyperintense to muscle on the T2W image *(arrowheads).*

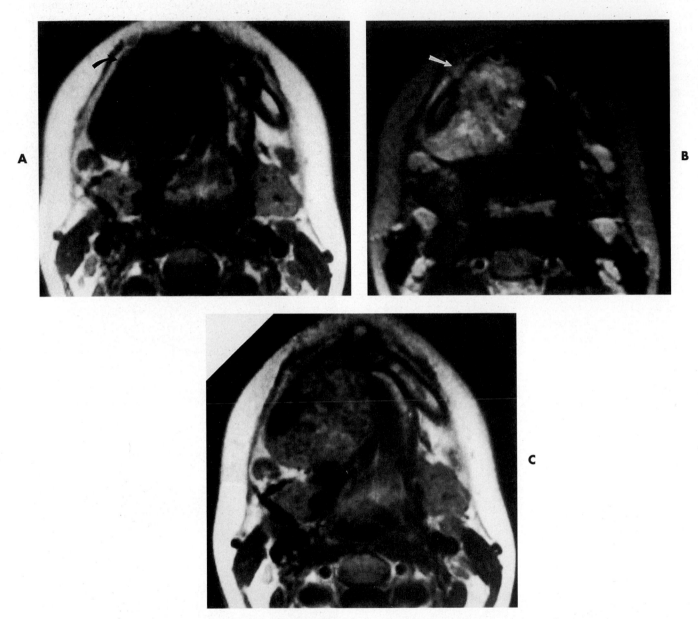

FIG. 9-66 Giant cell granuloma. **A** and **B,** proton-density weighted, and T2W axial MR images demonstrate a large, heterogeneous, well-defined lesion that appears to have its epicenter in the anterior floor of the mouth or alveolar ridge on the right. The lesion is isointense to muscle on the T1W image **(A)** and becomes progressively more hyperintense on the more heavily T2W images. The lesion has extended to erode a large portion of the lingual surface of the right mandible and break through into the soft tissues on the buccal surface of the mandible *(arrows).* **C,** Following the administration of contrast, very heterogeneous mild enhancement is identified. Although in some respects this lesion might be difficult to differentiate from squamous cell carcinoma, the very clear, well-defined margins and the high signal intensity on the T2W images are against this diagnosis. (Courtesy Dr. Jan Casselman.)

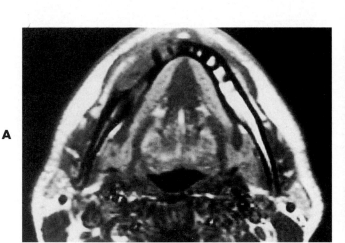
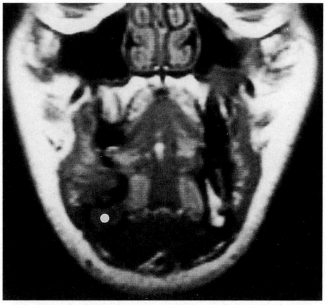

FIG. 9-67 Eosinophilic granuloma. **A** and **B,** Axial and coronal T1W MR scans demonstrate a destructive lesion involving much of the buccal cortex of the mandible on the right and extending into the soft tissues anteriorly. Marrow replacement is identifed, and is most easily appreciated on the coronal study *(white dot)*. Note the similar appearance of this eosinophilic granuloma compared with the buccal squamous cell carcinoma with mandibular invasion presented in Fig. 9-54.

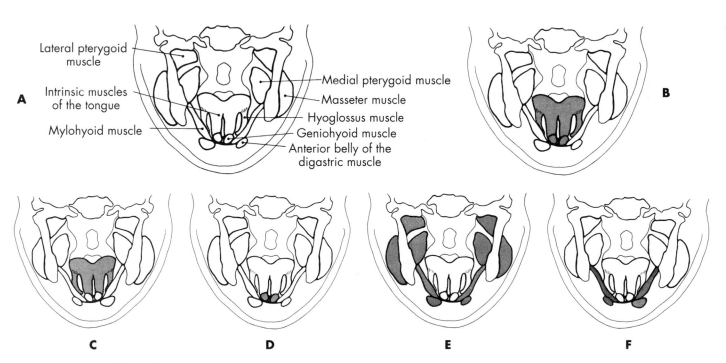

FIG. 9-68 Denervation atrophy patterns. **A,** Line diagram illustrating the muscles of the masticator space, oral tongue, and floor of the mouth. **B** through **F,** Line diagrams illustrating muscles affected by denervation atrophy from injury to **(B)** the hypoglossal nerve and fibers from C1; **(C)** the hypoglossal nerve proper, without C1 fiber involvement; **(D)** selective involvement of C1 fibers, distal to the exit of the main hypoglossal nerve fibers; **(E)** the mandibular division of the trigeminal nerve, involving both the masticator and mylohyoid nerves; **(F)** selective involvement of the mylohyoid nerve (arising from the inferior alveolar nerve).

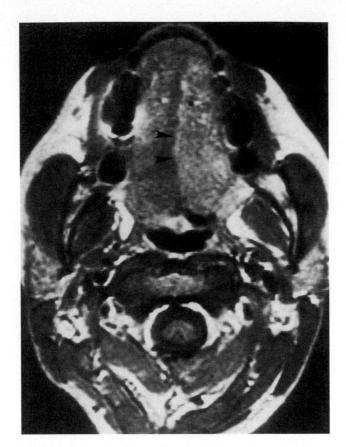

FIG. 9-69 Hypoglossal nerve motor atrophy. Axial T1W MR in a 17-year-old female status post left tonsillectomy 2 weeks earlier. The examination reveals the earliest changes of denervation atrophy of the left hemitongue, which because it is imaged relatively acutely manifests positive mass affect (arrowheads). Early fatty infiltration is identified by high-signal replacement of the intrinsic tongue musculature. (From Smoker WRK. The hypoglossal nerve. Neuroimaging Clin North Am 1993; 3:193-206.)

peripheral hypoglossal nerve palsy is deviation of the tongue on protrusion toward the side of the lesion. Initially the affected side of the tongue may be slightly enlarged, bulging into the oropharynx, and if imaged at this time, the affected side of the tongue may be mistaken as harboring a mass (Fig. 9-69). This early clinical finding is primarily the result of genioglossus muscle paralysis, the muscle that controls protrusion of the tongue. More commonly, however, imaging is not performed until the hypoglossal paralysis has become more permanent, at which time the affected hemitongue is replaced by variable amounts of fat (Fig. 9-70). With long-standing paralysis, the muscle bundles will no longer be recognizable and only the arteries and veins remain intact. At this time the atrophic side of the tongue will prolapse posteriorly into the oropharynx (Fig. 9-71). It is thus important to recognize the varible appearance of hypoglossal motor atrophy. On occasion, a patient may be referred for imaging without prior knowlegde of any hypoglossal nerve injury. If atrophy is identified, the entire course of the hypoglossal nerve back to its origin in the

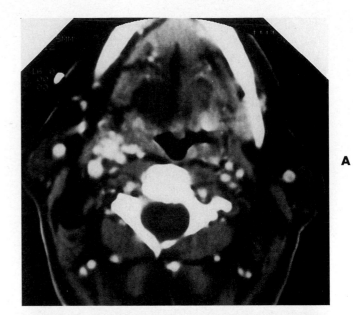

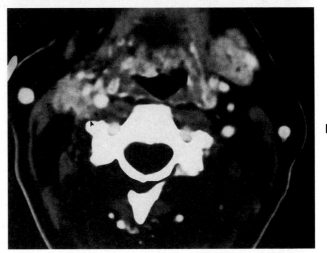

FIG. 9-70 Hypoglossal nerve motor atrophy. **A** and **B,** Axial CT scans in a 46-year-old woman who is 8 years status post mastectomy for breast carcinoma and now presents with right cranial nerve XII palsy. At the level of the mandible (**A**), fatty replacement and loss of muscle fibers involving the intrinsic musculature and genioglossus muscles of the right hemitongue is identified by its lower density compared with the left. On a more inferior plane (**B**) an extranodal mass is visible within the right carotid space (arrowheads), which proved to be metastatic breast carcinoma. This case highlights the importance of imaging the most inferior loop of the hypoglossal nerve, inferior to the mandible, so as to visualize those fibers coursing in the low oropharyngeal carotid space.

medulla must be imaged in an attempt to identify the site of pathology (Fig. 9-72).

The motor portion of the mandibular division of the trigeminal nerve supplies the muscles of mastication (medial and lateral pterygoid, masseter, and temporalis muscles), via its masticator branch, the tensor tympani, and tensor palatini muscles, and via the mylohyoid branch of the inferior alveolar nerve, the mylohyoid, and anterior belly of

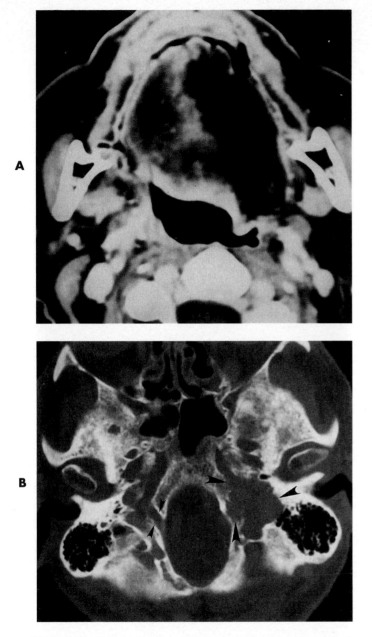

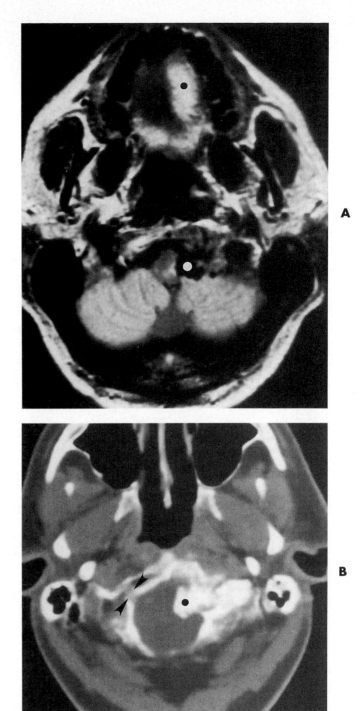

FIG. 9-71 Glomus jugulare with hypoglossal nerve atrophy. **A,** Axial contrast-enhanced CT scan of the oral tongue reveals complete atrophy and fatty replacement of all of the left hemitongue muscular structures, both intrinsic and extrinsic. There is prolapse of the left hemitongue into the oropharynx, producing contour abnormality. **B,** Axial CT scan at the level of the hypoglossal canal with a bone window setting reveals extensive skull base destruction on the left. The cortical margins of the normal right hypoglossal canal are well identified *(small arrowheads).* The large area of skull base destruction on the left *(large arrowheads)* clearly involves the region of the left hypoglossal canal. (From Smoker WRK. The hypoglossal nerve. Neuroimag Clin North Am 1993; 3:193-206.)

FIG. 9-72 Hypoglossal nerve motor atrophy caused by a skull base meningioma. **A,** Axial T1W MR scan demonstrates fatty infiltration of the left hemitongue *(black dot).* Posteriorly, in the region of the left hypoglossal canal, there is a large irregular signal void *(white dot)* producing deformity of the medulla. This markedly hypointense "mass" (signal void) has the characteristics of cortical bone. **B,** Axial CT scan at bone window setting demonstrates the calcific nature of this meningioma *(black dot)* centered at the level of the left hypoglossal canal. The margins of the normal right hypoglossal canal are indicated by the arrowheads. (From Smoker WRK. The hypoglossal nerve. Neuroimag Clin North Am 1993; 3:193-206.)

the digastric muscles. Proximal injury to the nerve will result in denervation and atrophic patterns, as described for the hypoglossal nerve, involving all of these muscles. The mandibular division of the trigeminal nerve is most commonly affected by perineural tumor extension or retrogasserian rhizotomy.[183,184] Atrophy of the muscles of mastication, within the masticator space, is easily appreciated on both axial and coronal CT or MRI (Fig. 9-73). If the injury occurs more distally, involving the mylohyoid branch of the inferior alveolar nerve after it arises from the main motor trunk, selective atrophy of the mylohyoid and anterior belly of the digastric muscles will result (Figs. 9-74,

9-75). As with the hypoglossal nerve, identification of atrophy involving the muscles innervated by the mandibular division of the trigeminal nerve should prompt an exhaustive search along the entire course of the nerve back to the brainstem for identification of the offending lesions. In such cases the nonatrohpic muscles should not be mistaken as harboring a mass (Fig. 9-76).

Isolated pathology of the motor fibers of C1, producing selective atrophy of the geniohyoid muscle, is rare (Fig. 9-68). More often a lesion will involve both the C1 motor fibers and the hypoglossal nerve in the region of the skull base or upper cervical area, thus affecting both the intrin-

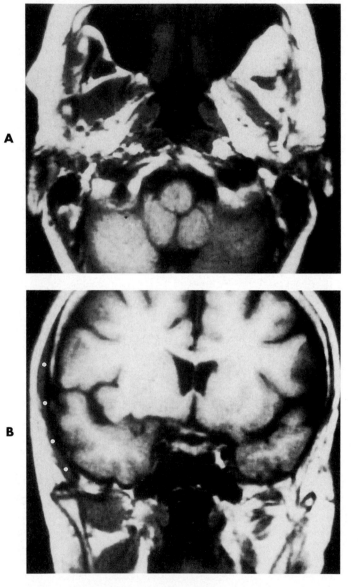

FIG. 9-73 Denervation atrophy of the muscles of mastication. A and B, Axial and coronal T1W MR scans demonstrate marked atrophy and fatty replacement of the muscles of mastication on the left. On the coronal scan (B), note involvement of the suprazygomatic left temporalis muscle fibers. The right temporalis muscle fibers are indicated by the white dots.

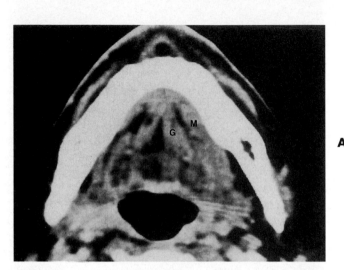

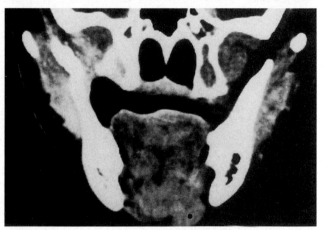

FIG. 9-74 Combined atrophy. A, Axial contrast-enhanced CT scan at the level of the mandible reveals atrophy of the right genioglossus, right hyoglossus, and right mylohyoid muscles, indicating injury to both the hypoglossal and the mylohyoid nerve. G, Left genioglossus muscle; M, Left mylohyoid muscle. B, Coronal CT scan reveals a normal left anterior belly of the digastric muscle (black dot). The corresponding muscle on the right is absent.

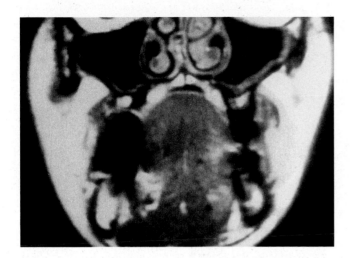

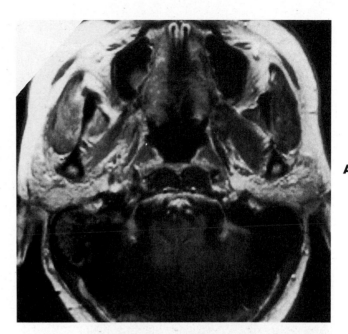

FIG. 9-75 Mylohyoid nerve denervation atrophy. Coronal T1W MR scan reveals a normal right mylohyoid muscle *(small black dots)* and right anterior belly of the digastric muscle *(large black dot).* The corresponding structures on the left are extremely diminutive.

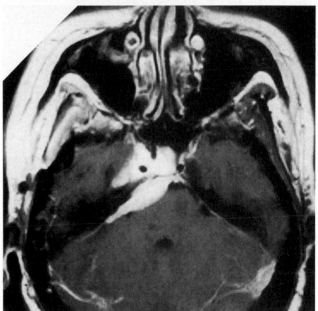

FIG. 9-76 Mandibular nerve denervation atrophy. **A,** Axial T1W MR following the administration of contrast demonstrates mild fatty infiltration and diminutive size of the right muscles of mastication when compared with those on the left. Note the opacification of right mastoid air cells produced by eustation tube dysfunction, secondary to paresis of the right tensor tympani muscle. **B,** Axial contrast enhanced T1W MR at a higher level reveals the causative meningioma affecting the trigeminal nerve in its cisternal and cavernous sinus segments.

sic and extrinsic tongue musculature, as well as the geniohyoid muscle.

Möbius syndrome is a rare syndrome manifested by congenital absence of both V3 and the facial (VII) nerve. In addition to V3 atrophy, there is associated atrophy involving the muscles innervated by the facial nerve including the muscles of facial expression, the platysma, the stylohyoid, and the posterior belly of the digastric (Fig. 9-77).

Benign Masseteric Hypertrophy

Benign masseteric hypertrophy (BMH) refers to idiopathic enlargement of the masseter muscle. Although uncommon, this condition is important in that it must be taken into consideration in the differential diagnosis of masses in the parotid region.[16] Males outnumber females 2:1, and approximately 50% of cases are bilateral. The etiology of BMH is uncertain, although a variety of theories have been suggested. Both familial and acquired forms are likely, with the acquired form most often associated with dental malocclusion or bruxism (teeth grinding).[18] CT or MRI demonstrate homogeneous enlargement of the involved muscle(s), with preservation of the muscle margins and surrounding fascial planes, and the hypertrophic muscle(s) look otherwise the same as the noninvolved normal muscles. In some patients an area of hyperostosis is present at the mandibular insertion of the masseter muscle, probably representing a secondary manifestation of muscle hypertrophy. In addition to isolated BMH, diffuse hypertrophy involving all muscles of mastication in patients with bruxism may occur (Fig. 9-78).[18,198]

Macroglossia

Macroglossia, or tongue enlargement, is for the most part a clinical diagnosis. In addition to occuring in any number of tumoral conditions, macroglossia may occur in a vari-

ety of congenital, endocrine, and metabolic conditions (Box 9-2). From their study of 40 normal patients and 12 patients with systemic primary amyloidosis involving the tongue, Larsson, Benson, and Westermark suggested that macroglossia can be suspected if (1) the base of the tongue is greater than 50 mm in transverse diameter, (2)

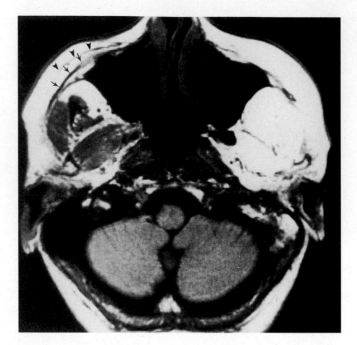

FIG. 9-77 Mobius syndrome. T1W MR scan reveals complete atrophy of the muscles of mastication, the zygomaticus major muscle (one of the muscles of facial expression), and the platysma muscle on the left. The right platysma muscle is indicated by the arrowheads and the right zygomaticus major muscle fibers are indicated by the small black arrows. (From Tryhus MR, Smoker WRK, Harnsberger HR. The normal and diseased masticator space. Seminars in Ultrasound CT and MR 1990; 11:476-485.)

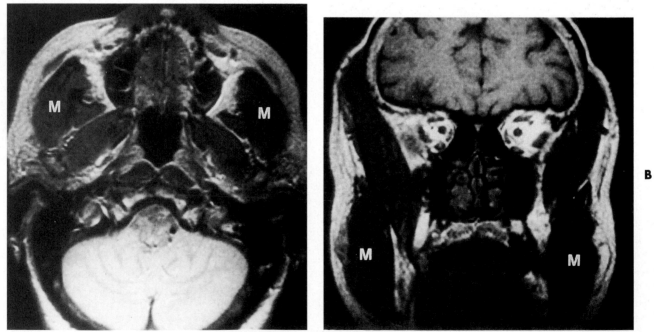

FIG. 9-78 Hypertrophy of the muscles of mastication. **A** and **B,** Axial and coronal T1W MR scans demonstrate marked enlargement of the muscles of mastication in this 65-year-old woman with Parkinson's disease. The masseter muscles *(M)* are notably prominent. The patient presumably had extrapyramidal bruxismlike movements. (From Tryhus MR, Smoker WRK, Harnsberger HR. The normal and diseased masticator space. Seminars in Ultrasound CT and MR 1990; 11:476-485.)

▼

BOX 9-2
Conditions Associated with Tongue Enlargement

Congenital Disorders
    Beckwith-Wiedermann syndrome
    Down's syndrome
    Robinow's syndrome
Endocrine and Metabolic Disorders
    Mucopolysaccharidosis
    Acromegaly
    Cretinism and myxedema
    Amyloidosis
    Lipoid proteinosis
Tumorlike Disorders
    Hemangioma
    Lymphangioma
    Lymphangioendotheliomatosis

the genioglossus muscle measures more than 11 mm in its transverse diameter, (3) the surface of the tongue base has a midline cleft, and (4) despite being normal in size, the submandibular glands are displaced laterally, producing an outward bulging of the overlying platysma muscles.[10]

With regard to amyloidosis of the tongue, scattered CT reports indicate symmetrical enlargement of both the extrinsic and intrinsic tongue musculature. Obliteration of the normal fascial planes caused by increased muscle bulk, is typically present without identification of any focal mass.[10,12] This is in sharp contrast to tumors, which until well advanced usually present as a focal mass that does not typically involve both the intrinsic and extrinsic tongue muscles but does displace the normal fascial planes. In amyloidosis the abnormally enlarged, infiltrated musculature does not exhibit pathologic enhancement.[12] Usually the T1W and T2W signal intensities are similar to those of normal muscle.

References

1. Batsakis JG. Tumors of the head and neck: clinical and pathological considerations. 2nd Edition. Baltimore, Md: Williams & Wilkins, 1979.

2. Million RR, Cassisi NJ. Management of head and neck cancer. 2nd Edition. Philadelphia, Pa: Lippincott, 1994.

3. Larsson SG, Mancuso A, Hanafee W. Computed tomography of the tongue and floor of the mouth. Radiology 1982; 143: 493-500.

4. Muraki AS, Mancuso AA, et al. CT of the oropharynx, tongue base, and floor of the mouth: normal anatomy and range of variations, and applications in staging of carcinoma. Radiology 1983; 148:725-731.

5. Hollinshead W. Anatomy for surgeons. Vol 1. The head and neck. 3rd edition. Hagerstown, NJ: Harper & Row, Publishers Inc, 1982.

6. Last RJ. Anatomy: regional and applied. 6th Edition. Edinburgh, London, and New York, NY: Churchill Livingstone Inc, 1978.

7. Gray H. Anatomy, descriptive and surgical. In: Pick TP, Howden R, eds. Philadelphia, Pa: Running Press, Book Publishers, 1974.

8. Lufkin RB, et al. Tongue and oropharynx: findings on MR imaging. Radiology 1986; 161:69-75.

9. Lufkin RB, Larsson SG, Hanafee WN. NMR anatomy of the larynx and tongue base. Radiology 1983; 148: 173-175.

10. Larsson SG, Benson L, Westermark P. Computed tomography of the tongue in primary amyloidosis. J Comput Assist Tomogr 1986; 10:836-840.

11. Smoker WRK. The hypoglossal nerve. Neuroimag Clin North Am 1993; 3:193-206.

12. Manco LG, Hanafee WN. Computed tomography of macroglossia secondary to amyloidosis. J Comput Assist Tomogr 1984; 8:659-661.

13. Braun IF, Hoffman JC. Computed tomography of the buccomasseteric region. I. Anatomy. AJNR Am J Neuroradiol 1984; 5:605-610.

14. Mancuso AA, Harnsberger HR, Dillon WP. Workbook for MRI and CT of the head and neck. 2nd Edition. Baltimore, Md: Williams & Wilkins, 1989; 163.

15. Paonessa DB, Goldstein JC. Anatomy and physiology of head and neck infections (with emphasis on the fascia of the face and neck). Otolaryngol Clin North Am 1976; 3:562-580.

16. Braun IF, Hoffman JC Jr, Reede D, et al. Computed tomography of the buccomasseteric region. II. Pathology. AJNR Am J Neuroradiol 1984; 5:611-616.

17. Hardin CW, Harnsberger HR, Osborn AG, et al. Infection and tumor of the masticator space: CT evaluation. Radiology 1985; 157:413-417.

18. Tryhus MR, Smoker WRK, Harnsberger HR. The normal and diseased masticator space. Semin Ultrasound CT and MR 1990; 11:476-485.

19. Ardran GM, Becket JM, Kemp FH. Aglossia congenita. Arch Dis Childhood 1964; 39:389-391.

20. Frommer J. The human accessory parotid gland: its incidence, nature, and significance. Oral Surg 1977; 43:671-676.

21. Johnson FE, Spiro RH. Tumors arising in accessory parotid tissue. Am J Surg 1979; 138:576-579.

22. Kakulas EG, Smith AC, Sormann G. Pleomorphic adenoma of the accessory parotid gland: case report. J Oral Maxillofac Surg 1994; 52:867-870.

23. Larsson SG, Lufkin RB. Anomalies of digastric muscles: CT and MR demonstration. J Comput Assist Tomogr 1987; 11:422-425.

24. Traini M. Bilateral accessory digastric muscles. Anat Clin 1983; 5:199-201.

25. Norton MR. Bilateral accessory digastric muscles. Br J Oral Maxillofac Surg 1991; 29:167-168.

26. Mulliken JB, Glowacki J. Hemangiomas and vascular malformations in infants and children: a

classification based on endothelial characteristics. Plast Reconstr Surg 1982; 69:412-420.

27. Chen JW, et al. Hemangiomas and vascular malformations. BNI Quart 1994; 10:19-25.

28. Watson WL, McCarthy WD. Blood and lymphatic vessel tumors: report of 1056 cases. Surg Gynecol Obstet, 1940; 71:569-588.

29. Bowers RE, Graham EA, Tomlinson KM. The natural history of the strawberry nevus. Arch Dermatol 1960; 82:667-673.

30. Baker LL, Dillion Wp, Hieshima GB, et al. Hemangiomas and vascular malformations of the head and neck: MR characterization. AJNR Am J Neuroradiol 1993; 14:307-314.

31. Kaban L, Mulliken JB. Vascular anomalies of the maxillofacial region. J Oral Maxillofac Surg 1986; 44:201-213.

32. Burrows PE, Mulliken JB, Fellowes KE, et al. Childhood hemangiomas and vascular malformations: angiographic differentiation. AJR 1983; 141:483-488.

33. Meyer JS, Hoffer FA, Barnes PD, et al. Biological classification of soft-tissue vascular anomalies: MR correlation. AJR 1991; 157:559-564.

34. Boyd JB, Mulliken JB, Kaban LB, et al. Skeletal changes associated with vascular malformations. Plast Reconstr Surg 1984; 74:789-795.

35. Mulliken JB. Vascular malformations of the head and neck. In: Mulliken JB, Young AE, eds. Vascular birthmarks, hemangiomas and malformations. Philadelphia, Pa: W B Saunders Co, 1988; 301-342.

36. Bartlett JA, Riding KH, Salkeld LJ. Management of hemangiomas of the head and neck in children. J Otolaryngol 1988; 17:111-120.

37. Edgerton MT. The treatment of hemangiomas. Ann Surg 1976; 183:517-530.

38. Sasaki GH, Pang CY, Wittliff L. Pathogenesis and treatment of infant skin strawberry hemangiomas: clinical and in vitro studies of hormonal effects. Plast Reconstr Surg 1984; 73:359-368.

39. Apfelberg DB, Maser MR, White DN, et al. A preliminary study of the combined effect of Neodymium: YAG laser photocoagulation and direct steriod instillation in the treatment of capillary/cavernous hemangiomas of infancy. Ann Plastic Surg 1989; 22:94-104.

40. Waner M, Suen JY, Dinehart S. Treatment of hemangiomas of the head and neck. Laryngoscope 1992; 102:1123-1132.

41. Berthelsen B, Fogdestam I, Svendsen P. Venous malformations in the face and neck: radiologic diagnosis and treatment with absolute ethanol. Acta Radiol 1986; 27:149-155.

42. Yakes WF, Haas DK, Parker SH, et al. Symptomatic vascular malformations: ethanol embolotherapy. Radiology 1989; 170:1059-1066.

43. Forbes G, Earnest F, Jackson IT, et al. Therapeutic embolization angiography for extra-axial lesions in the head. Mayo Clin Proc 1986; 61:427-441.

44. Leikensohn JR, Epstein LI, Vasconez LO. Superselective embolization and surgery of noninvoluting hemangiomas and A-V malformations. Plast Reconstr Surg 1981; 68:143-152.

45. Biller HF, Krespi YP, Som PM. Combined therapy of vascular lesions of the head and neck with intra-arterial embolization and surgical excision. Otolaryngol Head Neck Surg 1982; 90:37-47.

46. Persky MS. Congenital vascular lesions of the head and neck. Laryngoscope 1986; 96:1002-1015.

47. Mulliken JB. Classification of vascular birthmarks. In: Mulliken JB, Young AE, eds. Vascular birthmarks, hemangiomas and malformations. Philadelphia, Pa: WB Saunders Co, 1988; 24-37.

48. Elahi MM, Parnes L, Fox A. Hemangioma of the masseter muscle. J Otolaryngol 1992; 21:177-179.

49. Ott JES: Hemangiomata in skeletal muscle. Br J Surg 1957; 44:496-501.

50. Ingalls GK, Bonnington GJ, Sisk AL. Intramuscular hemangioma of the mentalis muscle. Oral Surg Oral Med Oral Pathol 1986; 60:476-481.

51. Wolf GT, Daniel F, Krause CJ, et al. Intramuscular hemangioma of the head and neck. Laryngoscope 1985; 95:210-213.

52. Itoh K, Nishimura K, Togashi K, et al. MR imaging of cavernous hemangiomas of the face and neck. J Comput Assist Tomogr 1986; 10:831-835.

53. Gelbert F, Riche MC, Reizine D, et al. MR imaging of head and neck vascular malformations. JMRI 1991; 1:579-584.

54. Som PM, Zimmerman RA, Biller HF. Cystic hygroma and facial nerve palsy: a rare association. J Comput Assist Tomogr 1984; 8:110-113.

55. Kennedy TL. Cystic hygroma-lymphangioma: a rare and still unclear entity. Laryngoscope 1989; 99:1-10.

56. Yuh WTC, Gleason TJ, Tali ET, et al. Traumatic cervical cystic lymphangioma in an adult. Ann Otol Rhinol Laryngol 1993; 102:564-566.

57. Stal S, Hamilton S, Spira M. Hemangiomas, lymphangiomas, and vascular malformations of the head and neck. Otolaryngol Clin North Am 1986; 19:769-796.

58. Chisin R, Fabian R, Weber AL, et al. MR imaging of a lymphangioma involving the masseter muscle. J Comput Assist Tomogr 1988; 12:690-692.

59. Postlethwaite KR. Lymphangiomas of the tongue. Br J Oral Maxillofac Surg 1986; 24:63-68.

60. Caro PA, Mahboubi S, Fearber EN. Computed tomography in the diagnosis of lymphangiomas in infants and children. Clin Imag 1991; 15:41-46.

61. Siegel MJ, Glazer HS, St. Amour TE, et al. Lymphangiomas in children: MR imaging. Radiology 1989; 170:467-470.

62. Yuh WTC, Buehner LS, Kao SC, et al. Magnetic resonance imaging of pediatric head and neck cystic hygromas. Ann Otol Rhinol Laryngol 1991; 100:737-742.

63. New GB. Congenital cysts of the tongue, the floor of the mouth, the pharynx and the larynx. Arch Otolaryngol 1947; 45:145-158.

64. Meyer I. Dermoid cysts (dermoids) of the floor of the mouth. Oral Surg Oral Med Oral Pathol 1955; 8:1149-1164.

65. Hunter TB, Paplanus SH, Chernin MM, et al. Dermoid cyst of the floor of the mouth: CT appearance. AJR 1983; 141:1239-1240.

66. Worley CM, Laskin DM. Coincidental sublingual and submental epidermoid cysts. J Oral Maxillofac Surg 1993; 51:787-790.

67. Arcand P, Granger J, Brochu P. Congenital dermoid cyst of the oral cavity with gastric choristoma. J Otolaryngol 1988; 15:219-222.

68. Black EE, Leathers RD, Youngblood D. Dermoid cyst of the floor of the mouth. Oral Surg Oral Med Oral Pathol 1992; 75:556-558.

69. Mathur SK, Menon PR. Dermoid cyst of the tongue: report of a case. Oral Surg Oral Med Oral Pathol 1980; 50:217-219.

70. Quinn JH. Congenital epidermoid cyst of anterior half of tongue. Oral Surg Oral Med Oral Pathol 1960; 13:1283-1285.

71. Rajayogeswaran V, Eveson JW. Epidermoid cyst of the buccal mucosa. Oral Surg Oral Med Oral Pathol 1989; 67:181-183.

72. Ruggieri M, Tine A, Rizzo R, et al. Lateral dermoid cyst of the tongue: case report. Internat J Pediatr Otorhinolaryngol 1994; 30:79-84.

73. Rule DC. Dermoid cyst of the lower lip: a case report. Br J Oral Surg 1976; 131:543-545.

74. Vogl TJ, Steger W, Ihrer S, et al. Cystic masses in the floor of the mouth: value of MR imaging in planning surgery. AJR 1993; 161:183-186.

75. Hardin CW, et al. CT in the evaluation of the normal and diseased oral cavity and oropharynx. Semin Ultrasound CT and MR 1986; 7:131-153.

76. Thomas JR. Thyroglossal duct cysts. Ear Nose Throat J 1979; 58:512-514.

77. Allard RHB. The thyroglossal cyst. Head and Neck Surg 1982; 5:134-146.

78. Shanmugham MS, Todd GB. Thyroglossal cyst in the elderly patient. Ear Nose Throat J 1983; 62:67-70.

79. Topf P, Fried MP, Strome M. Vagaries of thyroglossal duct cysts. Laryngoscope 1988; 98:740-742.

80. Dolata J. Thyroglossal duct cyst in the mouth floor: an unusual location. Otolaryngol Head Neck Surg 1994; 110:580-583.

81. Reede DL, Bergeron RT. CT of thyroglossal duct cysts. Radiology 1985; 157:121-125.

82. Nachlas NE. Thyroglossal duct cysts. Ann Otol Rhinol Laryngol 1950; 59:381-390.

83. Gardner DJ. Unusual CT appearance of a thyroglossal duct cyst carcinoma. J Otolaryngol 1989; 18:258-259.

84. Lustmann J, Benoliel R, Zeltser R. Squamous cell carcinoma arising in a thyroglossal duct cyst in the tongue. J Oral Maxillofac Surg 1989; 47:81-85.

85. McNicoll MP, Hawkins DB, England K, et al. Papillary carcinoma arising in a thyroglossal duct cyst. Otolaryngol Head and Heck Surg 1988; 99:50-54.

86. Silverman PM, Degesys GE, Ferguson BJ, et al. Papillary carcinoma in a thyroglossal duct cyst: CT findings. J Comput Assist Tomogr 1985; 9:806-808.

87. Yildiz K, Koksal H, Ozoran Y, et al. Papillary carcinoma in a thyroglossal duct remnant with normal thyroid gland. J Laryngol Otol 1993; 107:1174-1176.

88. Elprana D, Manni JJ, Smals AGH. Lingual thyroid: case report and review of the literature. ORL Otorhinolaryngol Relat Spec 1984; 46:147-152.

89. Douglas PS, Baker AW. Lingual thyroid. Br J Oral Maxillofac Surg 1994; 32:123-124.

90. Wertz ML. Management of undescended lingual and subhyoid thyroid glands. Laryngoscope 1974; 84:507-521.

91. Chan FL, Low LC, Yeung HW, et al. Case report: lingual thyroid, a cause of neonatal stridor. Br J Radiol 1993; 66:462-464.

92. Johnson JC, Coleman LL. Magnetic resonance imaging of a lingual thyroid gland. Pediatr Radiol 1989; 19:461-462.

93. Shah HR, Boyd CM, Williamson M, et al. Lingual thyroid: unusual appearance on computed tomography. Comput Med Imag and Graphics 1988; 12:263-266.

94. Willinsky RA, Kassell EE, et al. Computed tomography of lingual thyroid. J Comput Assist Tomogr 1987; 11:182-183.

95. Liauba R, Kennedy TL. Lingual thyroid. Trans Pa Acad Ophthalmol Otolaryngol 1983; 36:204-208.

96. Little B, et al. Cryptothyroidism: the major cause of sporadic "athyreotic" cretinism. J Clin Endocrin Metab 1965; 25:1529-1536.

97. Okstad S, Mair IW, Sundsfjord JA, et al. Ectopic thyroid tissue in the head and neck. J Otolaryngol 1986; 15:52-55.

98. Peick AL, Nichols WK, Curtis JJ, et al. Aneurysms and pseudoaneurysms of the superficial temporal artery caused by trauma. J Vasc Surg 1988; 8:606-610.

99. DiStefano JF, Maimon W, Mandel MA. False aneurysm of the lingual artery. J Oral Surg 1977; 35:918-920.

100. Gomori JM, Dermer R, Shifrin E. Aneurysm of the lingual artery. Neuroradiology 1983; 25:111-112.

101. Orron DE, Greenberg JJ, Kim D, et al. Pseudoaneurysm of the lingual artery. Comput Med Imag Graph 1988; 12:349-352.

102. Adib A, Gluckman JL, Mendelson D. Bilateral idiopathic aneurysms of the lingual arteries. Otolaryngol Head and Neck Surg 1993; 108:87-90.

103. Tschiassny K. Ludwig's angina: an anatomic study of the lower molar teeth in its pathogenesis. Arch Otolaryngol 1943; 38:485-496.

104. Holliday RA, Prendergast NC. Imaging inflammatory processes of the oral cavity and suprahyoid neck. Oral Maxillofac Surg Clin North Am 1992; 4:215-240.

105. Aasen S, Kolbenstvedt A. CT appearances of normal and obstructed submandibular gland duct. Acta Radiologica 1992; 33:414-419.

106. Nguyen VD, Potter JL, Hersh-Schick MR. Ludwig angina: an uncommon and potentially lethal neck infection. AJNR Am J Neuroradiol 1992; 13:215-219.

107. Grodinsky MD. Ludwig's angina: an anatomical and clinical study with review of the literature. Surgery 1939; 5:678-696.

108. Crysdale WS, Mendelsohn JD, Conley S. Ranulas-Mucoceles of the oral cavity: experience in 26 children. Laryngoscope 1988; 98:296-298.

109. Galloway RH, et al. Pathogenesis and treatment of ranula: report of three cases. J Oral Maxillofac Surg 1989; 47:299-302.

110. Balakrishnan A, Ford GR, Bailey CM. Plunging ranula following bilateral submandibular duct transposition. J Laryngol Otol 1991; 105:667-669.

111. Barnard NA. Plunging ranula: a bilateral presentation. Br J Oral Maxillofac Surg 1991; 29:112-113.

112. Mizuno A, Yamaguchi K. The plunging ranula. Int J Oral Maxillofac Surg 1993; 22:113-115.

113. Charnoff SK, Carter BL. Plunging ranula: CT diagnosis. Radiology 1986; 158:467-468.

114. Coit WE, et al. Ranulas and their mimics: CT evaluation. Radiology 1987; 263.211-216.

115. Matt BH, Crockett DM. Plunging ranula in an infant. Otolaryngol Head and Neck Surg 1988; 99:330-333.

116. Silverstein MI, Castillo M, Hudgins PA, et al. MR imaging of intralingual ranula in a child. J Comput Assist Tomogr 1990; 14:672-674.

117. Mirich DR, McArdle CB, Kulkarni MV. Benign pleomorphic adenomas of the salivary glands: surface coil MR imaging versus CT. J Comput Assist Tomogr 1987; 11:620-623.

118. Enzinger FM. Fibrous tumors of infancy. In: Tumors of bone and soft tissue: a collection of papers. Eighth Clinical Conference on Cancer. Chicago, Ill: Year Book Medical Publishers, 1965; 375-396.

119. Stout AP. Juvenile fibromatosis. Cancer 1954; 7:953-978.

120. Enzinger FM, Weiss SW. Soft tissue tumors. St Louis, Mo: CV Mosby Co, 1983.

121. Das Gupta TK, Brasfield RD, O'Hara J. Extra-abdominal desmoids: a clinicopathological study. Ann Surg 1969; 170:109-121.

122. Fu YS, Perzin KH. Nonepithelial tumors of the nasal cavity, paranasal sinuses, and nasopharynx: a clinicopathological study. VI. Fibrous tissue tumors (fibroma, fibromatosis, fibrosarcoma). Cancer 1976; 37:2912-2928.

123. Chen PC, Ball WS, Towbin RB. Aggressive fibromatosis of the tongue: MR demonstration. J Comput Assist Tomogr 1989; 13:343-345.

124. Shah AC, Katz RL. Infantile aggressive fibromatosis of the base of the tongue. Otolaryngol Head and Neck Surg 1988; 98:346-349.

125. Swartz HE, Ward PH. Aggressive fibromatosis of the tongue. Am J Otol 1979; 88:12-15.

126. Smoker WRK, Lusk RP, Menezes AH. Supraclavicular fibromatosis with intraspinal extension. Ann Otol Rhinol and Laryngol 1986; 95:319-320.

127. Masson JK, Soule EH. Desmoid tumors of the head and neck. Am J Surg 1966; 112:615-627.

128. El-Sayed Y. Fibromatosis of the head and neck. J Laryngol Otol 1992; 106:459-462.

129. Yang WC, Shah V, Mussbaum M, et al. Desmoid tumor of the neck: CT and angiographic findings. AJNR Am J Neuroradiol 1984; 5:478-480.

130. Aisen AM, Martel W, Braunstein EM, et al. MRI and CT evaluation of primary bone and soft tissue tumors. AJR 1986; 146:49-56.

131. Sundaram M, McGuire MH, Schajowicz F. Soft-tissue masses: histologic basis for decreased signal (short T2) on T2W MR images. AJR 1987; 148:1247-1250.

132. Di Sant'Agnese PA, Knowles DM. Extracardiac rhabdomyoma: a clinicopathological study and review of the literature. Cancer 1980; 46:780-789.

133. Batsakis JG, Manning JT. Soft tissue tumors: unusual forms. Otolaryngol Clin North Am 1986; 19:664-673.

134. Balatsouras DG, Eliopoulos PN, Economou CN. Adult-type rhabdomyoma of the submandibular region. J Otolaryngol 1993; 22:14-17.

135. Boysen M, et al. Rhabdomyoma of the tongue: report of a case with light microscopic, ultrastructural amd immunohistochemical observations. J Laryngol Otol 1988; 102:1185-1188.

136. Som PM, et al. Rare presentations of ordinary lipomas of the head and neck: a review. AJNR Am J Neuroradiol 1986; 7:657-664.

137. Fujimura N, Enomoto S. Lipoma of the tongue with cartilaginous changes: a case report and review of the literature. J Oral Maxillofac Surg 1992; 50:1015-1017.

138. Hatziotis JC. Lipomas of the oral cavity. Oral Surg 1971; 31:511-524.

139. Reede DL, Bergeron RT. The CT evaluation of the normal and diseased neck. Semin Ultrasound CT and MR 1986; 7:181-201.

140. Flickinger FW, et al. Neurilemoma of the tongue: MR findings. J Comput Assist Tomogr 1989; 13:886-888.

141. Abramowitz J, et al. Angiographic diagnosis and management of head and neck schwannomas. AJNR Am J Neuroradiol 1991; 12:977-984.

142. Al-Ghamdi S, Black MJ, Lafond G. Extracranial head and neck schwannomas. J Otolaryngol 1992; 21:186-188.

143. Gore DO, Rankow R, Hanford JM. Parapharyngeal neurilemmoma. Surg Gynecol Obstet 1956; 103:193-199.

144. Gallo WJ, Moss M, Shapiro DN, et al. Neurilemoma: review of the literature and report of five cases. J Oral Surg 1977; 35:235-236.

145. Sutay S, Tekinsoy B, Ceryan K, et al. Submaxillary hypoglossal neurilemmoma. J Laryngol Otol 1993; 107:953-954.

146. Weber AL. The mandible. In: Som PM, Bergeron RT, eds. Head and neck imaging. 2nd Edition. St Louis, Mo: Mosby-Year Book, 1991; 394-395.

147. Tani Y, Azuma T, Nagayama M. Chondroma of the tongue. J Oral Maxillofac Surg 1989; 47:91-92.

148. Nash M, Harrison T, Lin PT, et al. Osteoma of the tongue. Ear Nose Throat 1989; 68:63-69.

149. Lutcavage GJ, Fulbright DK. Osteoma of the tongue. J Oral Maxillofac Surg 1993; 51:697-699.

150. de Araujo VC, Marcucci G, Sesso A, et al. Epithelioid hemangioendothelioma of the gingiva, case

report and ultrastructural study. Oral Surg Oral Med Oral Pathol 1987; 63:472-477.

151. Ellis GL, Kratochvil FJ. Epithelioid hemangioendothelioma of the head and neck, a clinicopathologic report of twelve cases. Oral Surg Oral Med Oral Pathol 1986; 61:61-68.

152. Marrogi AJ, Boyd D, el-Mofty S, et al. Epithelioid hemangioendothelioma of the oral cavity: report of two cases and review of the literature. J Oral Maxillofac Surg 1991; 49:633-638.

153. Moran, WJ, Dobleman TJ, Bostwick DG. Epithelioid hemangioendothelioma (histoid hemangioma) of the palate. Laryngoscope 1987; 97:1299-1302.

154. Dillon WP. The pharynx and oral cavity. In: Som PM, Bergeron RT, eds. Head and neck imaging. 2nd Edition St Louis, Mo: Mosby–Year book, 1991; 407-466.

155. Yarington CT. Pathology of the oral cavity. In: Paparella MM, Shumrick M, eds. Otolaryngology. Philadelphia, Pa: W B Saunders Co, 1980.

156. American Joint Commission on Cancer. Beahrs OH, et al, eds. Manual for staging of cancer. 3rd Edition. Philadelphia, Pa: Lippincott, 1988.

157. Crissman JD, Gluckman J, Whiteley J, et al. Squamous-cell carcinoma of the floor of the mouth. Head neck surg 1980; 3:2-7.

158. Paparella MM, Shumrick DA. Otolaryngology. Vol. 3. Head and neck. Philadelphia, Pa: W B Saunders Co, 1980.

159. Lederman M. The anatomy of cancer. J Laryngol Otol 1964; 78:181-208.

160. Harnsberger HR. Head and neck imaging, Chicago, Ill: Year Book Medical Publishers, 1990.

161. Johnson JT. A surgeon looks at cervical lymph nodes. Radiology 1990; 175:607-610.

162. Lindberg R. Distribution of cervical lymph node metastases from squamous cell carcinoma of the upper respiratory and digestive tracts. Cancer 1972; 29:1446-1449.

163. Som PM. Lymph nodes of the neck. Radiology 1987; 165:593-600.

164. Madison MT. Radiologic diagnosis and staging of head and neck squamous cell carcinoma. Radiol Clin North Am 1994; 32:163-181.

165. Som PM. Detection of metastases in cervical lymph nodes: CT and MR criteria and differential diagnosis. AJR 1992; 158:961-969.

166. Yousem DM, Som PM, Hackney DB, et al. Central nodal necrosis and extracapsular neoplastic spread in cervical lymph nodes: MR imaging versus CT. Radiology 1992; 182:753-759.

167. Mancuso AA. The oropharynx and oral cavity. Proceedings from the 26th Annual Conference and Postgraduate Course of the American Society of Head and Neck Radiology, 1993; 51-60.

168. Takashima S, Ikezo J, Harada K, et al. Tongue cancer: correlation of MR imaging and sonography with pathology. AJNR Am J Neuroradiol 1989; 10:419-424.

169. Harnsberger HR, Bragg DG, Osborn AG, et al. Non-Hodgkin's lymphoma of the head and neck: CT evaluation of nodal and extranodal sites. AJNR Am J Neuroradiol 1987; 8:673-679.

170. Lee YY, Van Tassel P, Nauert C, et al. Lymphomas of the head and neck: CT findings at initial presentation. AJNR Am J Neuroradiol 1987; 8:665-671.

171. Lucas RB. Pathology of tumors of the oral tissues. 3rd Edition. London: Churchill Livingstone, 1976; 329-334.

172. Suei Y, Tanimoto K, Taguchi A, et al. Radiographic evaluation of bone invasion of adenoid cystic carcinoma in the oral and maxillofacial region. J Oral Maxillofac Surg 1994; 52:821-826.

173. Kim KH, Sung MW, Chung PS, et al. Adenoid cystic carcinoma of the head and neck. Arch Otolaryngol Head Neck Surg 1994; 120:721-726.

174. Nascimento AG, Amaral AI, Prado LA, et al. Adenoid cystic carcinoma of salivary glands: a study of 61 cases with clinicopathologic correlation. Cancer 1986; 57:312-319.

175. Spiro RH, Huvos AG, Strong EW. Adenoid cystic carcinoma: factors influencing survival. Am J Clin Pathol 1979; 138:579-583.

176. Waldron CA, El-Mofty SK, Gnepp DR. Tumors of the intraoral minor salivary glands: a demographic and histologic study of 426 cases. Oral Surg Oral Med Oral Pathol 1988; 66:323-330.

177. Perzin K, Gullane P, Clairmont A. Adenoid cystic carcinoma arising in salivary glands: a correlation of histologic features and clinical courses. Cancer 1978; 42:265-282.

178. Stell PM, et al. Lymph node metastases in adenoid cystic carcinoma. Am J Otol 1985; 6:433-436.

179. Maso MD, Lippi L. Adenoid cystic carcinoma of the head and neck: a clinical study of 37 cases. Laryngoscope 1985; 95:177-181.

180. Friedman M, Levin B, Grybauskas V, et al. Malignant tumors of the major salivary glands. Otolaryngol Clin North Am 1986; 19:625-636.

181. Sigal R, et al. Adenoid cystic carcinoma of the head and neck: Evaluation with MR imaging and clinical-pathologic correlation in 27 patients. Radiology 1992; 184:95-101.

182. Castillo M. MRI of perineural tumor spread along the trigeminal nerves. Imag Decisions May/June 15-20, 1994.

183. Laine FJ, Braun IF, Jensen ME, et al. Perineural tumor extension through the foramen ovale: evaluation with MR imaging. Radiology 1990; 174:65-71.

184. Parker GD, Harnsberger HR. Clinical-radiologic issues in perineural tumor spread of malignant diseases of the extracranial head and neck. Radiographics 1991; 11:383-399.

185. Barakos JA, Dillon WP, Chew WM. Orbit, skull base, and pharynx: contrast-enhanced fat suppression MR imaging. Radiology 1991; 179:191-198.

186. Tien RD. Fat-suppression MR imaging in neuroradiology: techniques and clinical application. AJR 1992; 158:369-379.

187. Som PM. Salivary glands. In: Som PM, Bergeron RT, eds. Head and neck imaging. 2nd Edition. St. Louis, Mo: Mosby-Year Book, 1991; 334-335.

188. McCulloch TM, Makielski KH, McNutt MA. Head and neck liposarcoma: a histopathologic reevaluation of reported cases.

Arch Otolaryngol Head Neck Surg 1992; 118:1045-1049.

189. Enzinger FM, Winslow DJ. Liposarcoma: a study of 103 cases. Virchows Arch 1962; 335:367-388.

190. Dooms GC, Hricak H, Sollitto RA, et al. Lipomatous tumors and tumors with fatty component: MR imaging potential and comparison of MR and CT results. Radiology 1985; 157:479-482.

191. Maurer HM, Moon T, Donaldson M, et al. The intergroup rhabdomyosarcoma study: a preliminary report. Cancer 1977; 40:2015-2026.

192. Kodet R, Fajstavr J, Kabelka Z, et al. Is fetal cellular rhabdomyosarcoma an entity or a differentiated rhabdomyosarcoma? A study of patients with rhabdomyoma of the tongue and sarcoma of the tongue enrolled in the Intergroup Rhabdomyosar-coma Studies I, II, and III. Cancer 1991; 67:2907-2913.

193. Doval DC, Kannan V, Acharya RS, et al. Rhabdomyosarcoma of the tongue. Br J Oral Maxillofac Surg 1994; 32:183-186.

194. Peters E, Cohen M, Altini M, et al. Rhabdomyosarcoma of the oral and paraoral region. Cancer 1989; 63:963-966.

195. Schwetschke O, Heppt W, Born JA. Leiomyosarkom von mundboden und oropharynx. HNO 1992; 40:277-279.

196. Harnsberger HR, Dillon WP. Major motor atrophic patterns in the face and neck: CT evaluation. Radiology 1985; 155:665-670.

197. Larsson SG. Hemiatrophy of the tongue and floor of the mouth demonstrated by computed tomography. J Comput Assist Tomogr 1985; 9:914-917.

198. Schellhas KP. MR imaging of muscles of mastication. AJR 1989; 153:847-855.

10

Pediatric Airway Disease

PATRICIA A. HUDGINS
IAN N. JACOBS
MAURICIO CASTILLO

SECTION ONE
EMBRYOLOGY

The components of the pediatric airway develop from the branchial arches, which give rise to the palate, ear, tongue, pharynx, larynx, trachea, bronchi, lungs, tonsils, thyroid, parathyroid, and thymus gland (Fig. 10-1).[1] The pinnae, the tympanic membranes, the ossicles (up to the footplate of the stapes), the styloid processes, the hyoid bone, the trigeminal and facial nerves, and the muscles of mastication and facial expression all derive from the first and second branchial arches (Table 10-1; Fig. 10-2).[2] The third, fourth, and sixth branchial arches form structures located in the lower neck, including portions of the hyoid bone, the larynx, the thyroid gland, and the thymus. Therefore anomalies involving the development of these arches are manifested as a combination of middle and external ear, mandibular, and neck abnormalities. Because the arches are paired (bilateral), anomalies may be unilateral (hemifacial microsomia [Goldenhar's syndrome]) or bilateral. Although the embryology of the face and neck is described in detail in Chapters 1 and 14 respectively, this chapter reviews the pertinent embryology as it applies to the airway.

FACE

The face may be separated into two distinct compartments (superior and inferior) by the oral opening, which will form the mouth and buccal cavity (Fig. 10-3). Inferior to the oral opening lies the mandibular arch, a derivative of the first branchial arch.[2] The mandibular arch is separated from the lower neck by the hypomandibular cleft, and lateral to this cleft lie the ear tubercles. The superior compartment of the face develops partly from the first branchial arch but mostly from the frontonasal process. The first branchial arch contributes to the formation of the paired maxillary processes. The nasooptic groove separates the maxillary processes from the superiorly located nasomedial and nasolateral processes. These two processes are themselves separated by the nasal pits, which later become the nostrils. The nasooptic grooves extend laterally from the nasal pits to the orbits. The frontal prominence is a single midline structure located in the superior aspect of the embryonic face. Between the fourth and eighth week of gestation, all of these facial processes undergo a series of complex fusions and migrations that eventually give rise to the external characteristics of the adult face.

At 6 weeks of gestation, the nasomedial processes merge in the midline with the frontal prominence. The merging is critical because it gives origin to the frontonasal process, from which the following midline structures arise: the nasal bones and the nasal vault cartilaginous capsule, the frontal bones, the central one third of the upper lip and superior alveolar ridges, the central incisors, and the primary palate.[3] Overgrowth of the nasal medial processes produces stenosis of the anterior (pyiform) aperture of the nose.[4]

The formation of the nasal cavity depends mainly on the inferior migration of the primitive nasal septum and the medial migration of the palatal shelves (Fig. 10-4). At approximately 7 weeks of gestation, the nasomedial processes merge with the maxillary processes giving origin to the upper lip, philtrum, and columella.[4] At this same time, the nasolateral processes fuse with the maxillary processes, giving origin to the nasal alae. Hypoplasia of the nasal alae results in respiratory obstruction in the newborn.

Structures that are located slightly off the midline such as the lateral third of the upper lip, lateral third of the superior alveolar ridges, and the palatal shelves, develop from the fusion of the maxillary processes with the frontal prominence. The nasooptic grooves deepen and become the nasolacrimal ducts (lack of canalization may produce nasolacrimal duct mucoceles). The maxillary processes extend inferiorly and merge with the mandibular arches to produce the cheeks and lateral margins of the mouth. Anomalies at

TABLE 10-1
Pharyngeal Arch Derivatives

Arch	Bone	Ligaments	Muscles	Nerves
1 (mandibular)	Meckel's cartilage, maxilla, mandible, malleous, incus	Sphenomandibular, mallear	Muscles of mastication, tensor veli palatini, tensor tympani, digastric (anterior), mylohyoid	Trigeminal
2 (hyoid)	Reichert's cartilage, hyoid*, styloid process, stapes	Stylohyoid	Muscles of facial expression, stapedius digastric (posterior), stylohyoid	Facial
3	Hyoid*		Stylopharyngeus pharyngeal constrictors†	Glossopharyngeal
4	Thyroid, laryngeal		Pharyngeal constrictors,† laryngeal	Recurrent laryngeal of vagus

* Different portions formed by second and third arches
† Different portions formed by third and forth arches

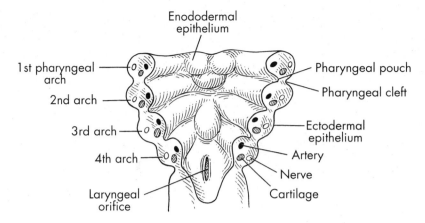

FIG. 10-1   The branchial arch system. Drawing shows that the arch system appears in the fourth and fifth gestational weeks as four prominant arches, each consisting of muscular and cartilaginous components, a nerve, and an artery. (From Langman J. Medical embryology. 4th Edition. Baltimore, Md: Williams & Wilkins, 1981; 270.)

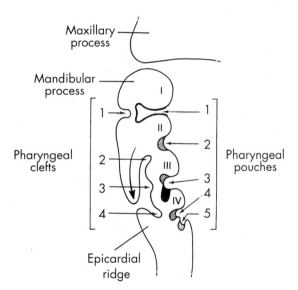

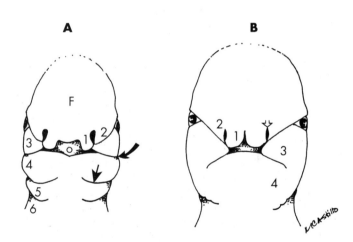

FIG. 10-2   Overgrowth of the second arch. Diagram of a 6-week-old fetus shows that the second arch overgrows the third and fourth arches, and the epicardial ridge develops to oppose it. This creates a cavity, the cervical sinus of His, which covers the second, third, and fourth pharyngeal arches and clefts. Failure of obliteration of the cervical sinus of His, the pharyngeal clefts, or pouches results in branchial cleft sinuses, fistulae, or cysts. (From Langman J. Medical embryology. 4th Edition. Baltimore, Md: Williams & Wilkins, 1981; 274.)

FIG. 10-3   Development of the face. **A,** Frontal drawing of a 5-week-old fetus shows the oral placode *(o),* which divides the face into superior and inferior compartments. Superiorly and centrally is the massive frontal eminence *(F).* The nasal medial processes *(1)* are separated from the nasal lateral processes *(2)* by the nasal pit. The nasooptic groove *(small arrows)* separates the nasal lateral process from the maxillary process *(3).* The inferior compartment of the face is formed by the mandibular arches *(4)* that are separated from the lower hyoid arches *(5)* by the hypomandibular clefts (arrowhead). The third branchial arches *(6)* are present inferiorly. Curved arrow indicates position of ear tubercules. **B,** Frontal drawing of a 7-week-old fetus shows that the face has acquired a more recognizable pattern. The nasal medial *(1)* and lateral *(2)* processes are separated by the rudimentary nostrils *(open arrow)* and are delineated laterally by the nasal alae. The midface is mainly constituted by the maxillary processes *(3).* The inferior face is formed by the mandibular processes *(4).* The orbits are better developed and have migrated inferiorly and medially to a more midline position. The nasooptic grooves *(small arrows)* deepen and eventually canalize to form the nasolacrimal ducts.

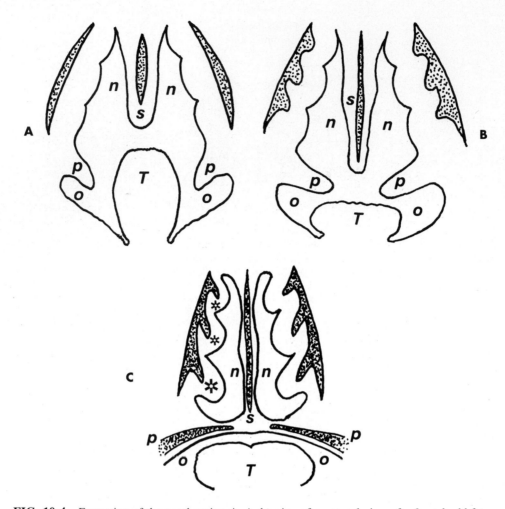

FIG. 10-4 Formation of the nasal cavity. **A,** A drawing of a coronal view of a 6-week-old fetus shows that the oral *(o)* and nasal *(n)* cavities communicate with each other. The superior nasal cavity is divided by the midline septum, which contains cartilage *(shaded area)*. The palatal shelves *(p)* are short and are located posterior to the primary palate. The palatal shelves are separated by a space that contains a relatively large tongue *(T)*. **B,** A drawing of a coronal view of an 8-week-old fetus shows that the nasal septum *(s)* has elongated and extended inferiorly. The rudimentary nasal *(n)* and oral *(o)* cavities remain joined. The palatal shelves *(p)* are larger and begin to migrate medially. The tongue *(T)* is relatively smaller. **C,** A drawing of a coronal view of a 10-week-old fetus shows that the palatal shelves *(p)* and the inferior border of the nasal septum *(s)* have fused, creating a separation between both nasal cavities *(n)* and the oral *(o)* cavity. The tongue *(T)* is now confined to the oral cavity. Rudimentary nasal conchae *(*)* are present. The configuration of this region now approximates that of the adult.

this stage result in transverse facial clefts and macrostomia. Simultaneously the nose descends and the orbits migrate medially to their normal positions.

The orbit and its contents, which are located laterally to the nasooptic groove, develop in concert with the face. The closure of the optic vesicle (globe) occurs during this same period.[3] Therefore abnormalities involving the closure of the midface (medial cleft syndromes) may be accompanied by failure of the globe to close (coloboma), a poorly developed globe (microphthalmos), or an absent globe (anophthalmos).

Midline to the processes that form the external fetal face lies the oral placode, which eventually forms the oral opening and cavity. The oral placode contains a shallow depres-

sion lined with ectoderm, which enlarges and becomes a cavity, the stomodeum, which is separated from the cephalic portion of the pharyngeal gut by the buccopharyngeal membrane. By the fourth week of gestation, the buccopharyngeal membrane is resorbed and a communication between the oral cavity and pharynx is established. Waldeyer's ring appears to be the remnant of this membrane.[3] At approximately the same stage of development, the nasal pits become deeper. They are separated from the stomodeum and the pharynx by the bucconasal plate, which later becomes a membrane that eventually disappears. Persistence of this structure produces bucconasal atresia, which is characterized by lack of communication between the nasal and buccal cavities.

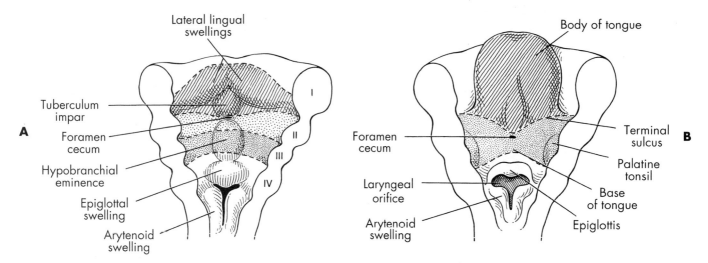

FIG. 10-5 Development of the tongue. **A,** Drawing of a 5-week-old fetus shows that one medial (tuberculum impar) and two lateral lingual swellings have appeared, originating from the mesenchyme of the first pharyngeal arch. **B,** Drawing of a 5-month-old fetus shows that the terminal sulcus divides the anterior two thirds of the tongue from the posterior third. The foramen cecum is the site of origin of the thyroid gland. (A and B From Langman J. Medical embryology. 4th Edition. Baltimore, Md: Williams & Wilkins, 1981; 277.)

The nasal pits also develop dorsal openings termed *primitive posterior choanae.*[3] As the nasal cavity is separated into right and left compartments by the septum, the "secondary" or "permanent" posterior choanae are formed (Fig. 10-4, *B*). Fusion of the palatal shelves with the anterior three fourths of the nasal septum establishes the hard palate. The posterior palatal shelves are devoid of cartilage and give origin to the soft palate.

The exact mechanism responsible for choanal atresia remains unclear. Incomplete formation of the posterior choanae may give rise to stenosis and bony, or membranous, atresias.[4] Lack of canalization of the epithelial plugs that later fill the nasal cavities may also play a role. Because these two hypotheses may not account for this complex anomaly, a more recent explanation proposes a misdirection in the flow of mesodermal elements.[5] This latter hypothesis favors abnormal development, migration, and fusion of all elements (which originate from pluripotential neural crest cells) that are involved in the formation of the nasal and pharyngeal cavities.

TONGUE AND THYROID GLAND

The tongue starts to form in the fourth gestational week. Two lateral and one medial (tuberculum impar) lingual swellings appear, originating from the mesenchyme of the first pharyngeal arch (Fig. 10-5, *A*). The two lateral lingual swellings overgrow the tuberculum impar and merge to form the anterior two thirds of the tongue. Because it is a first arch structure, the anterior portion of the tongue is innervated by the mandibular branch of the trigeminal nerve.

The posterior third of the tongue starts with two struc-

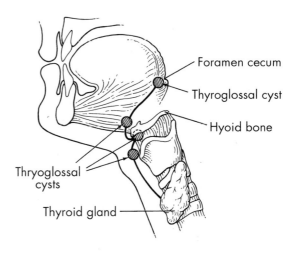

FIG. 10-6 Course of the thyroglossal duct. Drawing of the lateral neck shows the course of the thyroglossal duct and the path of descent of the thyroid anlage. The foramen cecum marks the location of the origin of they thyroid anlage. Thyroglossal duct cysts, remnants of the duct that fail to involute, and ectopic thyroid tissue can occur anywhere along the course of this duct. (From Langman J. Medical embryology. 4th Edition. Baltimore, Md: Williams & Wilkins, 1981; 280.)

tures caudal to the foramen cecum. The copula is formed by the fusion of the ventromedial portion of the second branchial arch, and the hypobranchial eminence, which develops from the mesoderm of the third and fourth branchial arches. The large hypobranchial eminence overgrows the copula, which eventually disappears. The terminal sulcus separates the anterior from the posterior third of the tongue (Fig. 10-5, *B*).

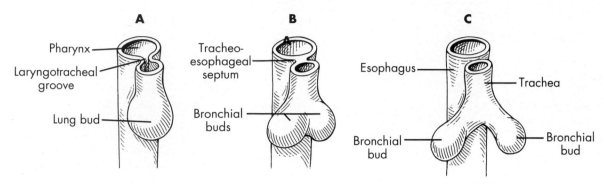

FIG. 10-7 Development of the respiratory system. **A,** Drawing of a 4-week-old fetus shows the laryngotracheal groove developing from the ventral wall of the primitive pharynx. The proximal portion will be the future laryngeal aditus. **B,** Drawing of a 4- to 5-week-old fetus shows that the tracheoesophageal septum now separates the laryngotracheal tube from the primordium of the esophagus. The bronchial buds will become the bronchi. **C,** Drawing at a slightly later stage of development shows that the esophagus and the trachea are now completely separate. A tracheoesophageal fistula is an abnormal persistence of the original communication between the trachea and the esophagus (**A**). (From Moore KL, Persaud TVN. The developing human. 5th Edition. Philadelphia, Pa: WB Saunders Co, 1993; 227.)

The thyroid gland starts as a proliferation of endodermal epithelium just caudal to the medial tongue swelling. This thickening forms the thyroid diverticulum, which may start as a single diverticulum but divides very early into two lateral lobes.[6,7] As the embryo elongates, the thyroid diverticulum descends caudally in the neck and passes ventral to the hyoid bone and the laryngeal cartilages. By the seventh week, the developing thyroid gland is located just below the cricoid cartilage, where it is usually composed of one median isthmus and two lateral lobes. In the tongue the site of origin of the thyroid gland remains as the foramen cecum.

As the thyroid gland descends, it forms a tract known as the thyroglossal duct, which usually passes ventral to the hyoid bone but which may also pass dorsal to or even through the hyoid bone. The rostral and caudal ends of the thyroglossal duct normally degenerate. A thyroglossal duct cyst may occur when portions of this tract persist, and if the entire tract persists, a thyroglossal duct fistula results (Fig. 10-6). Furthermore, ectopic thyroid tissue may be found anywhere along the pathway of this tract's descent.

THYMUS

The thymus is a derivative of the ventral portion of the third branchial pouch. After the fifth gestational week, the tissue loses its connection with the pharyngeal wall (thymopharyngeal duct) and the thymic anlage migrates in a caudal and medial direction, pulling the lower parathyroid gland (also derived from the third pouch) with it. Eventually the main portion of the thymic anlage moves caudally and medially into the thorax, where it fuses with its contralateral component to form the body of the thymus. Thymic rests may develop anywhere along the course of the thymopharyngeal ducts.[8]

PHARYNX, LARYNX, AND TRACHEA

The respiratory primordium begins at about the fourth week of gestation with the formation of the laryngotracheal groove (Fig. 10-7). Lateral furrows develop on each side of the diverticulum, and the gradual elongation of this structure forms the primitive laryngotracheal tube. The distal end of the tube eventually develops into the lung buds, and the proximal end forms the primitive laryngeal aditus. A tracheoesophageal septum develops from caudally to rostrally and separates the respiratory system from the esophagus.[9]

At the end of the fourth week of gestation, a single lung bud appears at the caudal end of the laryngotracheal tube, which soon divides into right and left bronchial buds (Fig. 10-7). These grow caudally and laterally into the pericardioperitoneal cavities. The primitive lung buds then subdivide into secondary and tertiary bronchi. Throughout fetal development, the surrounding pulmongenic mesoderm continues to develop into the lung parenchyma.[10]

The larynx develops on the proximal end of the laryngotracheal groove. Between the fifth and sixth gestational week, three swellings appear at the laryngeal aditus. The anterior swelling, which is the future epiglottis, is probably a derivative of the hypobranchial eminence, from the fourth arch. The two lateral masses give rise to the future arytenoids, also probably from the fourth arch. These two lateral swellings migrate cranially and medially to oppose each other. At this stage, the laryngeal aditus appears as a T-shaped slit (Fig. 10-8).[1,11] The laryngeal lumen becomes occluded at 8 weeks of gestation as a result of epithelial proliferation. If normal recanalization does not occur during the tenth gestational week, a laryngeal web results. The formation of the vocal and vestibular folds (true and false vocal cords) is related to the condensation of mesenchyme and the outpouching of the laryngeal sinus (ventricle). The two vocal folds separate during the third gestational month. Failure of this recanalization process results in congenital atresia of the larynx.

The laryngeal cartilages develop from the branchial arches. The thyroid cartilage develops from the fourth arch as two lateral plates that fuse in the midline. This is almost completed by the ninth gestational week. The cricoid carti-

lage begins as two cartilaginous centers of the sixth arch. First the centers grow and unite in the ventral midline, and then by the seventh gestational week, they fuse dorsally. The rostral advancement of the tracheoesophageal septum results in the fusion of the dorsal cricoid lamina. Failure of advancement of the tracheoesophageal septum results in a laryngotracheal cleft. At first the cricoid lumen is slitlike in shape, but eventually the ventral and lateral walls of the cricoid cartilage condense, and there is progressive enlargement of the lumen. Failure of this condensation process results in congenital subglottic stenosis. The arytenoid cartilages develop from the arytenoid swellings, most likely derivatives of the sixth arch but possibly arising from the fourth arch. They are initially fused to the cricoid cartilage, but they eventually separate from it and form the cricoarytenoid joints. The intrinsic laryngeal muscles develop from the mesoderm of the fourth and sixth arches.[1]

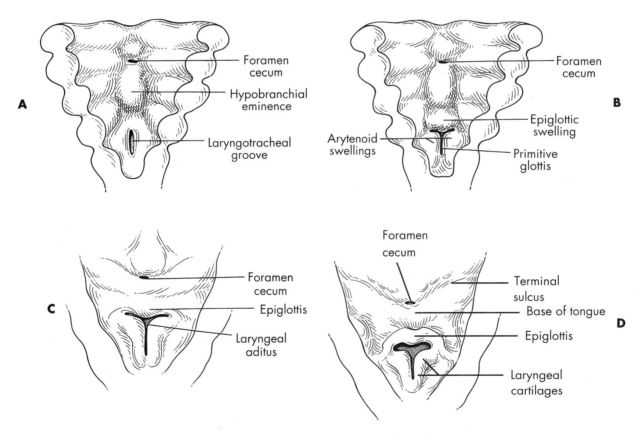

FIG. 10-8   Development of the larynx. **A,** Drawing of 4- to 5-week-old fetus shows that the larynx develops on the proximal end of the laryngotracheal groove. **B,** Drawing of a 5-week-old fetus shows that the paired arytenoid swellings are found lateral to the laryngeal aditus. The anterior midline swelling, the future epiglottis, is a derivative of the hypobranchial eminence. **C,** Drawing of a 6-week-old fetus shows that the arytenoid swellings have migrated medially and toward the tongue, and the laryngeal aditus has become T-shaped. The laryngeal lumen is only a slit. **D,** Drawing of a 10-week-old fetus shows that the laryngeal cartilaginous and muscular structures have formed from the fourth and sixth branchial arches. (From Moore KL, Persaud TVN. The developing human. 5th Edition. Philadelphia, Pa: WB Saunders Co, 1993; 228.

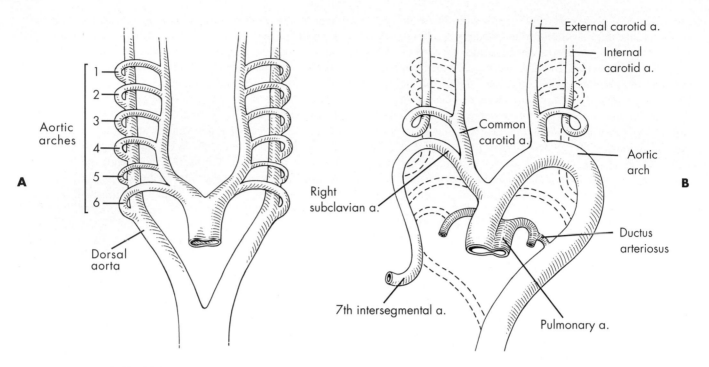

FIG. 10-9 Development of the great vessels. **A,** Diagram of the paired dorsal and ventral aortas, which are connected by six pairs or aortic arches. Each of the six paired aortic arches is the arterial component of a branchial arch. **B,** Diagram at a later stage of development shows that the first, second, and fifth arches have disappeared *(broken lines)*. Errors in the obliterative process result in vascular rings. (From Langman J. Medical embryology. 4th Edition. Baltimore, Md: Williams & Wilkins, 1981; 186.)

GREAT VESSELS

The great cervical and thoracic arteries develop from the paired dorsal and ventral aortas, which are connected by six pairs of branchial aortic arches. The first, second, and fifth vascular arches involute. The third arch pair becomes the common carotid artery, the right fourth arch becomes the innominate artery, and the left fourth arch becomes the aortic arch. The right sixth arch becomes the pulmonary artery, and the distal portion of the left sixth arch persists as the ductus arteriosus (Fig. 10-9).[12,13]

Errors in this embryologic process may result in vascular malformations that can cause impressions on the trachea. Of particular note are the following two situations: the persistence of the entire right dorsal aorta, which results in a double aortic arch forming a complete vascular ring, and the incomplete obliteration of the proximal right dorsal aortic arch with persistence of the distal portion, which results in a retroesophageal subclavian artery.

References

1. Hast MH. Developmental anatomy of the larynx. In: Hinchcliffe R, Harrison D, eds. Scientific foundations of otolaryngology. London, England: Heinemann Medical, 1976.
2. Hiatt JL, Gartner LP. Embryology of the head and neck. In: Gardner J, ed. Textbook of head and neck anatomy. New York, NY: Appleton-Century-Crofts, 1982.
3. Naidich TP, et al. Embryology and congenital lesions of the midface. In: Som PM, Bergeron RT, eds. Head and neck imaging. St. Louis,

   Mo: Mosby–Year Book, Inc. 1991.
4. Castillo M. Congenital abnormalities of the nose: CT and MR findings. AJR 1994; 162:1211-1217.
5. Hengerer AS, Strome M. Choanal atresia: a new embryological theory and its influence on surgical management. Laryngoscope 1982; 92:913-921.
6. Skandalakis JE, Gray SW, Todd NW. The pharynx and its derivatives. In: Skandalakis JE, Gray SW, eds. Embryology for surgeons. Baltimore, Md: Williams & Wilkins, 1994.

7. Weller GL Jr. Development of the thyroid, parathyroid, and thymus gland in man. Contrib Embryol Carnegie Inst Wash 1933; 24:93-142.
8. Langman J, ed. Medical embryology. 4th Edition Baltimore, Md: William & Wilkins, 1981.
9. Moore KL. The developing human-clinically oriented embryology. 3rd Edition. Philadelphia, Pa: WB Saunders, 1982.
10. Spooner BS, Wessels NK. Mammalian lung development: interac-

tions in primordium formation and bronchial morphogenesis. J Exp Zool 1970; 175:445-454.

11. Spector GJ. Developmental anatomy of the larynx. In: Ballenger JJ, ed. Diseases of the ear, nose, and throat.

Philadelphia, Pa: Lea & Febiger, 1984.

12. DeVries PA, DeVries CR. Embryology and development. In: Gans SI, ed. The pediatric airway. Philadelphia, Pa: WB Saunders, 1991.

13. Bisset GS, et al. Vascular rings: magnetic resonance imaging. AJR 1987; 149:251-256.

SECTION TWO
RADIOGRAPHIC TECHNIQUES

The upper airway extends from the nose to the mainstem bronchi, and in the infant or child it can be obstructed at any point. The arbitrary anatomic divisions of the upper airway are the nasopharynx, oropharynx, hypopharynx, supraglottis, glottis, subglottis, and trachea to the level of the carina. When investigating a possible upper airway obstruction, the imaging modality of choice depends on the suspected location of the lesion and whether the airway compromise is acute or chronic. The importance of plain radiographs and fluoroscopy in imaging the pediatric airway cannot be overemphasized. An impending, or progressive, airway obstruction necessitates rapid, efficient workup, often including same day operative endoscopy.

Commonly the first examinations obtained are plain soft-tissue film radiographs of the sinuses, neck, and chest. Tightly coned, high-kilovoltage (to optimize soft-tissue detail and thus maintain resolution of the airway), twice magnified views of the airway are obtained in the lateral projection, and frontal airway films are recommended when the symptoms are not emergent or life-threatening.[1,2] The radiographic appearance of the pediatric airway is affected by position, crying, swallowing, and phase of respiration.[3,4] The lateral film should be obtained with the child upright when possible, with the neck in a neutral position or slightly extended, during deep inspiration. If the neck is flexed or the examination is obtained during expiration or crying, the retropharyngeal soft tissues may appear abnormally prominent, simulating retropharyngeal pathology (Fig. 10-10), or the trachea may buckle to the right on the anteroposterior (AP) examination, suggesting a neck, or mediastinal, mass.

When life-threatening airway obstruction is suspected, as in acute epiglottitis, some clinicians believe that a plain film is not initially needed because the time spent obtaining the examination is time not spent initiating treatment. However, if a film is to be obtained, a single lateral film of the airway may be all that is necessary to confirm the diagnosis. Additional frontal views only delay the workup and treatment and usually contribute little new information. A clinician should accompany the child to the radiology suite, and the radiologist should supervise the appropriate examinations, remaining in the department until the radiographic portion of the workup is completed. The child with acute airway obstruction should not be placed in the supine position or be immobilized because either may exacerbate the airway compromise.[5]

Normal air-filled structures seen on the lateral plain film are the nasopharyngeal, oropharyngeal, hypopharyngeal, and supraglottic airways, as well as the valleculae, laryngeal ventricle, and infraglottic trachea (Fig. 10-11). Soft-tissue structures routinely visualized on the lateral examination are the hard and soft palate, base of tongue, adenoids, epiglottis, aryepiglottic folds, and retropharyngeal and prevertebral soft tissues (Fig. 10-11). The AP film displays the laryngeal and tracheal airway. Specifically the false and true vocal cords, the laryngeal ventricles, the subglottic region, and the trachea can be identified.

On plain films, standard measurements for normal soft-tissue structures have been determined, and soft tissues exceeding the normal values may indicate an airway lesion. However, all measurements should be used with caution because tremendous variability is seen in the normal pediatric airway, especially with dynamic structures such as the epiglottis, pharyngeal soft tissues, and trachea. The retropharyngeal and prevertebral soft-tissue thickness is one of the most commonly measured regions, and the most often used measurement is the distance between the posterior pharyngeal air column and the anterior portion of the third or fourth cervical vertebral body. Normally in children, on a properly positioned film this distance should not exceed one half to three fourths the diameter of the vertebral body.[4]

Chest radiographs often are obtained when evaluating the child with airway obstruction, and the entire trachea to the level of the bifurcation should be evaluated with respect to diameter, position, and patency.

Plain films of the airway provide a relatively large field of view and high resolution, but they are limited because dynamic structures are seen at only one point in the respiratory cycle. On the other hand, fluoroscopy of the airway provides a dynamic study. Video fluoroscopy with 105 mm spot films obtained at 3 to 4 frames per second allows fast imaging, and is useful for evaluating the child with chronic airway obstruction. Changes in airway caliber during inspiration and expiration can be assessed over several respiratory cycles. The tracheal diameter increases during inspiration and decreases during expiration, and any paradoxical changes can be appreciated with dynamic fluoroscopy.[6,7] Dynamic examination of vocal cord movement, during quiet breathing and phonation (crying in the infant), also can be performed using fluoroscopy. The cords should abduct symmetrically during inspiration and adduct with expiration. On such a study an unsuspected vocal cord paralysis can be diagnosed. However, fluoroscopy is limited by its inability to image the soft-tissue structures surrounding the airway.

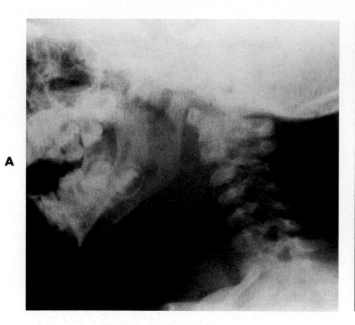
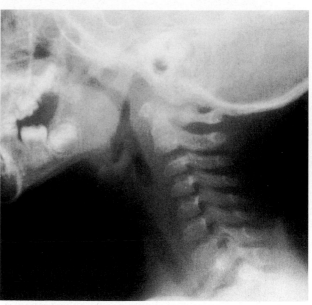

FIG. 10-10   Importance of radiographic technique. Child with fever and drooling. **A,** Lateral plain film of the neck obtained while child is swallowing shows retropharyngeal soft-tissue thickening, simulating abscess or mass in retropharynx. **B,** Repeat film, 5 min later while child is quiet shows normal retropharyngeal soft tissues. (**A** and **B,** From B Gay. Chapter 11, Radiology for anesthesia and critical care. New York, NY: Churchill Livingstone Inc, 1987.)

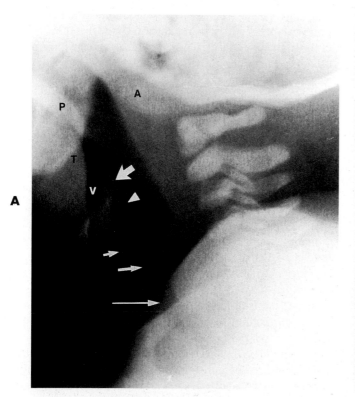
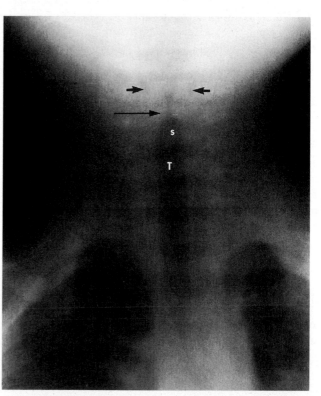

FIG. 10-11   Normal lateral and AP radiographs, 2-month-old infant. **A,** Lateral film obtained during inspiration, with neck in neutral position. Normal soft-tissue structures include adenoidal tissue *(A),* free edge of the epiglottis *(thick white arrow),* aryepiglottic fold *(white arrowhead),* soft palate *(P),* tongue base *(T),* and calcified hyoid bone *(H).* Air-filled structures include the vallecula *(V),* laryngeal ventricle *(short white arrow),* subglottic airway *(white arrow),* and trachea *(long white arrow).* **B,** Normal AP radiograph shows air-filled pyriform sinuses *(short arrows),* true vocal cord *(long arrow),* subglottic airway *(s),* and trachea *(T).*

For example, narrowing of the tracheal airway by a neck mass can be seen, but the characteristics of the mass are determined better on cross-sectional imaging.

A barium esophagogram, performed under fluoroscopic control, is often part of the workup of the pediatric patient with an airway problem, and this study is usually performed in conjunction with airway fluoroscopy. Lesions that may be detected on barium swallow studies include esophageal foreign bodies, congenital vascular rings and slings, mediastinal masses, bronchopulmonary foregut anomalies, and patient aspiration.

Computed tomography (CT) and magnetic resonance imaging (MRI) add important information about the soft tissues surrounding the airway. However, children often require sedation for these studies, and sedation routinely results in a decrease of the AP diameter of the pharynx at the level of the palatine tonsils and soft palate, and at the level of the epiglottis.[8] When general anesthesia is used, there is distortion of the airway as a result of the endotracheal tube (Fig. 10-12).[8]

Lesions within the airway or involving the function of the airway such as subglottic stenosis or tracheomalacia are often best evaluated by fluoroscopy or endoscopy. Conversely, extraluminal disease is best studied with CT or MRI. Because the region of interest is limited, scans should be obtained using axial thin-slice collimation, usually 3-mm contiguous images. Direct coronal MRI or coronal CT reformations are recommended for lesions of the skull base and nasopharynx, as well as the larynx and trachea, because clinicians often find the coronal plane facilitates evaluation of the cranio-caudal extent of disease. When a focal mass or an inflammatory lesion is suspected, intravenous nonionic iodinated CT contrast should be used.

Older children who cooperate can be scanned with conventional CT using a breath-hold technique. This helps assure that the serial scans are performed during the same phase of respiration with similar lung volumes, thus decreasing the potential for respiratory misregistration artifacts. In younger or sedated children who cannot voluntarily suspend respiration, scanning is performed during quiet respiration. Because of the relatively long scan times necessary for a conventional CT study, this examination is a static one and the images are obtained at variable times in the respiratory cycle. Early experience with airway measurements on cine or ultrafast CT suggested that cross-sectional airway areas were reduced in patients with obstructive sleep apnea and tracheomalacia and that dynamic CT could show changes in these areas during different phases of the respiratory cycle.[9-11] However, the cine CT technique was not widely clinically available, and most radiologists had little or no experience with this technique.

Current spiral CT technology, with cable coupling to allow for volume scanning at a rapid speed, is now widely available. In older children this technique allows the neck to be scanned during a single breath-hold. In infants the entire airway can be scanned during a single 10 to 15 second acquisition, often obviating the need for sedation. Sections that are 1-mm thin can routinely be obtained with the spiral technique, and these thin sections are necessary when evaluating a newborn or infant with a suspected small subglottic web, cyst, stenosis, hemangioma, or papilloma. Experience with cine CT has shown that the optimum technique may be to obtain both high-resolution images through the entire airway and cine CT images at areas of localized airway narrowing.[12] Thus the neck is first scanned with the volume technique, and the scan is immediately reviewed with the

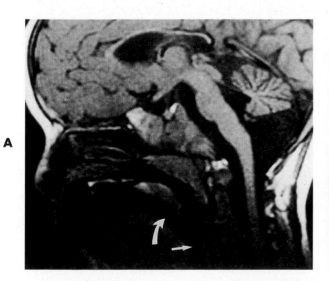 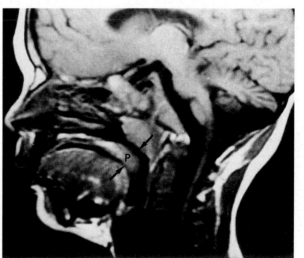

FIG. 10-12   Effect of orotracheal intubation and sedation on airway diameter. **A,** T1W sagittal image of an infant with complex congenital intracranial abnormalities. Orotracheal intubation results in apparent increase of the airway size at the level of the tongue base *(curved arrow)* and epiglottis *(straight arrow).* **B,** Same infant, imaged several months later with oral sedation. T1W sagittal image shows narrowing of the oronasopharyngeal airways *(black arrows)* at the level of the soft palate *(P).*

patient still on the table. If a localized area of narrowing is identified, the patient can then be rescanned with little or no table incrementation during several respiratory cycles. To further aid the clinician, the region of narrowing should be described as being a certain distance from a fixed anatomic landmark such as the glottis, inferior cricoid, or carina. Thus within a short time, both a static and dynamic airway studies can be performed, and lesions that change diameter with the respiratory cycle may be studied, complementing airway fluoroscopy.

When MRI of the pediatric neck and airway is performed, it is recommended that surface coils, multiplanar acquisitions, and both T1- and T2-weighted (T1W and T2W)

images are performed.[13-15] Indications for MRI of the trachea include an abnormal chest x-ray and barium swallow suggesting a vascular ring, a "pulsatile mass" or extrinsic airway compression seen on bronchoscopy, or airway compromise seen on plain films. Cardiac gating and respiratory compensation are useful if the airway lesion is in the thoracic trachea.[16] Coronal T1W images are especially useful to display a paratracheal mass that is causing extrinsic tracheal compression. Any region of airway narrowing should be confirmed with a second acquisition in an orthogonal plane. When imaging neck masses, Gadolinium may be useful, but it is not essential. MR studies are lengthy, and most younger children and virtually all infants require sedation.

References

1. Slovis TL. Noninvasive evaluation of the pediatric airway: a recent advance. Pediatrics 1977; 59:872-880.
2. Joseph PM, Berdon WE, Baker DH, et al. Upper airway obstruction in infants and small children: improved radiographic diagnosis by combining filtration, high kilovoltage and magnification. Radiology 1976; 121:143-148.
3. Macpherson RI, Leithiser RE. Upper airway obstruction in children: an update. Radiographics 1985; 5(3):339-376.
4. Ardran GM, Kemp FH. The mechanism of changes in form of the cervical airway in infancy. Medical Radiography and Photography 1968; 44:26-54.
5. Hedlung GL, Kirks DR. Respiratory system. In: Kirks DR, ed. Practical pediatric imaging: diagnostic radiology of infants and children. Boston, Mass: Little, Brown & Co Inc, 1991.

6. Griscom NT. Diseases of the trachea, bronchi, and smaller airways. Radiol Clin North Am 1993; 31:605-615.
7. Wittenborg MH, Gyepes MT, Crocker D. Tracheal dynamics in infants with respiratory distress, stridor, and collapsing trachea. Radiology 1967; 88:653-662.
8. Shorten GD, Opie NJ, Graziotti P, et al. Assessment of upper airway anatomy in awake, sedated and anaesthetized patients using magnetic resonance imaging. Anaesth Intens Care 1994; 22:165-169.
9. Ell SR, Jolles H, Keyes WD, et al. Cine CT technique for dynamic airway studies. AJR Am J Roentgenol 1985; 145:35-36.
10. Frey EE, Smith WL, Grandgeorge S, et al. Chronic airway obstruction in children: evaluation with cine-CT. AJR Am J Roentgenol 1987; 148:347-352.
11. Brasch RC, Gould RG, Gooding RA, et al. Upper airway obstruction in

infants and children: evaluation with ultrafast CT. Radiology 1987; 165:459-466.
12. Brody AS, Kuhn JP, Seidel FG, et al. Airway evaluation in children with use of ultrafast CT: pitfalls and recommendations. Radiology 1991; 178:181-184.
13. Vogl T, Wilimzig L, Bilaniuk LT, et al. MR imaging in pediatric airway obstruction. J Comput Assist Tomogr 1990; 14:182-186.
14. Dietrich RB, Lufkin RB, Kangarloo H, et al. Head and neck MR imaging in the pediatric patient. Radiology 1986; 159:769-776.
15. Fletcher BD, Dearborn DG, Mulopulos GP, et al. MR imaging in infants with airway obstruction: preliminary observations. Radiology 1986; 160:245-249.
16. Simoneaux SF. MR imaging of the pediatric airway. Radiographics 1995; 15:298-299.

SECTION THREE
NORMAL ANATOMY

NASAL CAVITY

Because babies are obligate nasal breathers, the nasal cavity, from the nostrils to the posterior choanae, is an important component of the pediatric airway. The nasal cavities should be air-filled, and the lateral nasal walls should be straight or slightly concave medially (Fig. 10-13). The normal nasal septum is in the midline, thicker anteriorly, with a clear column of air separating it from the turbinates. The mean width of the posterior choanal airspace in the newborn is 0.67 cm, increasing to 0.86 cm at 6 years and 1.13 cm by 16 years of

age.[1] In patients less than 8 years of age the vomer generally measures less than 0.23 cm in width and should not exceed 0.34 cm, but in children over 8 years of age the mean vomer width should not exceed 0.55 cm.[1]

NASOPHARYNX AND OROPHARYNX

The craniocaudal level of the hard palate separates the nasopharynx from the oropharynx. The pediatric hard palate ranges from 3 to 5 cm in length, and the soft palate is shorter, ranging from 2 to 3 cm in length.[2] On CT and MRI the marrow within the bony hard palate is usually clearly identified. By comparison, the soft palate is primarily muscular, and the junction between the soft and hard palates is

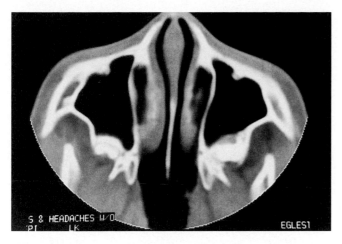

FIG. 10-13   Normal nasal cavity, 13-year-old child. Axial CT scan of a normal nasal cavity in a child is similar in appearance to that of an adult, with the nasal septum wider at its anterior portion, slightly concave lateral nasal walls, and a patent posterior choanae.

seen well on CT and especially well on MRI (Fig. 10-14). The soft palate in the infant and child is a prominent structure on plain radiographs, separating the nasopharyngeal airway from the oropharyngeal airway. During quiet breathing, the soft palate is down, opposing the tongue base. However, during swallowing and phonation, the soft palate elevates and moves posteriorly, closing the nasopharyngeal airway, opening the oropharynx, and respectively preventing nasal regurgitation or nasal speech.[3]

The nasopharynx and oropharynx of the child differ from the adult in that they are smaller and normally have more lymphoid tissue within the mucosa and extending into the airway. The vertical height and depth of the nasopharynx increases during childhood, but the width, or distance between the eustachian tubes, does not significantly increase.[4] The adenoids, or nasopharyngeal tonsils, are situated in the posterior nasopharyngeal roof and upper posterior wall. They appear confluent with the prevertebral soft tissues, and they are separated from the upper surface of the soft palate by the nasopharyngeal airway (Fig. 10-11, *A*) The adenoids are not routinely seen at birth, but they are 1 to 5 mm thick in the normal 3-month old, and if no adenoidal soft tissue is seen by 6 month of age, hypogammaglobulinemia or an immune deficiency syndrome should be suspected.[5,6] The adenoids normally begin to involute in adolescence, and in most people these tissues have completely involuted by middle age. However, in some normal people the adenoids can be identified into the fifth and sixth decades of life.

On CT the adenoidal tissue fills the posterior nasopharynx, is isodense to muscle on noncontrast CT, but clearly enhances with iodinated contrast. Occasional small calcifications, which represent concretions in small lymphoid clefts, can be seen on or just deep to the surface. A thin line of enhancement, most probably being the submucosal veins, is usually seen between the adenoids and the nasopharyn-

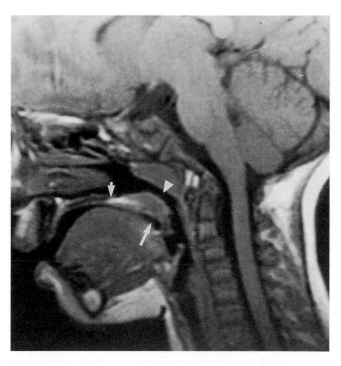

FIG. 10-14   Normal palate and nasooropharyngeal airway, 4-year-old child. T1W sagittal image shows junction of hard and soft palates *(small arrow)*. Soft palate separates nasopharyngeal *(arrowhead)* from oropharyngeal *(large arrow)* airway. During quiet breathing, the soft palate opposes the tongue base.

geal mucosa (Fig. 10-15). Ventrally the adenoidal tissue is usually flat but can appear asymmetrically lobular or full. On T1W images the adenoids are isointense to slightly hyperintense with respect to muscle, and they are decreased in intensity compared with fat. On T2W images they are homogeneously hyperintense with respect to muscle (Fig. 10-16). Occasionally, focal regions of hyperintensity within the adenoids may be seen on both T1W and T2W images, probably representing small proteinaceous cysts. The adenoidal tissue enhances slightly with gadolinium contrast agents (Fig. 10-16, *C*).

The remaining prominent lymphatic tissues in the oropharynx are the bilateral palatine tonsils and the lingual tonsils, the latter being found at the base of the tongue, usually just above the valleculae. The palatine tonsils can be identified radiographically by about 1 year of age, are greatest in size at about 4 years of age, and begin to involute after the age of 10 years.[7] The palatine tonsils may normally be obscured by the tongue base and mandibular angle on a lateral plain film. However, if the airway is distended (as occurs when the child cries) or if there is significant tonsillar hypertrophy, these tonsils can be identified on a lateral plain film (Fig. 10-17). The CT density and MR signal intensities of lingual and palatine lymphatic tissue are similar to those of the adenoidal tissues (Figs. 10-18, 10-19). The median and lateral retropharyngeal lymph nodes are the primary drainage nodes for the sinonasal cavities and pharynx. These nodes are seen on MRI in most infants and chil-

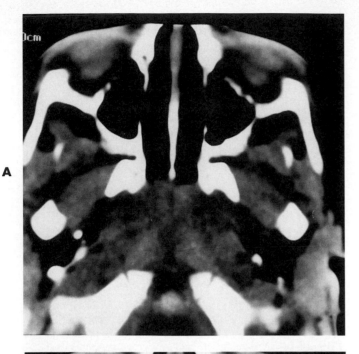

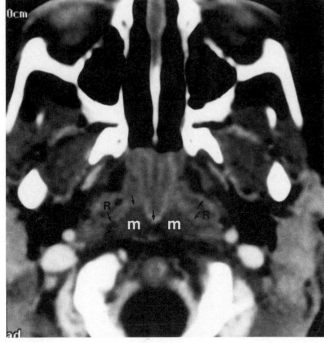

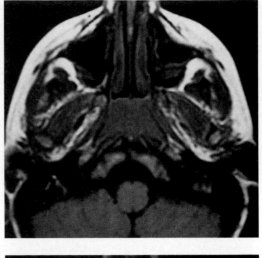

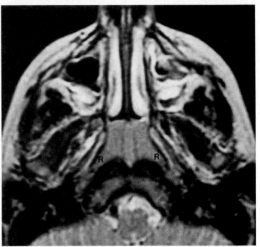

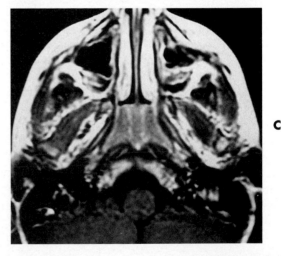

FIG. 10-15 Normal adenoids on CT, 14-month-old child. **A,** Axial noncontrast CT shows adenoidal tissue, nearly isodense to prevertebral muscles, filling nasopharynx. **B,** Same child, scanned following intravenous iodinated contrast using a spiral technique. The adenoidal tissue enhances, but prevertebral muscles *(m)* do not. Notice the thin linear enhancement at the interface between adenoids and muscle *(black arrows).* The adenoidal tissue characteristically fills the lateral pharyngeal recesses *(R),* is flat ventrally, and does not extend into the deep pharyngeal spaces. (Courtesy Dr. John J. Alarcon, Scottish Rite Children's Medical Center, Atlanta, Georgia.)

FIG. 10-16 Normal adenoids on MR. The volume of adenoidal tissue in this normal 7-year-old child is more prominent than in the previous infant (Fig. 10-15). **A,** Adenoidal tissue is isointense to muscle on this axial T1W image. **B,** On this fast-spin echo (FSE) T2W image, adenoidal tissue is homogeneously hyperintense with respect to muscle. Adenoidal tissue fills the lateral pharyngeal recesses *(R)* but does not extend into deep spaces. **C,** After gadolinium, adenoidal tissue enhances homogeneously.

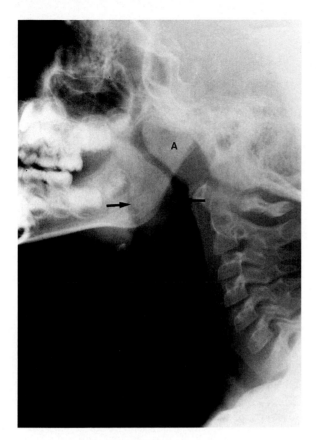

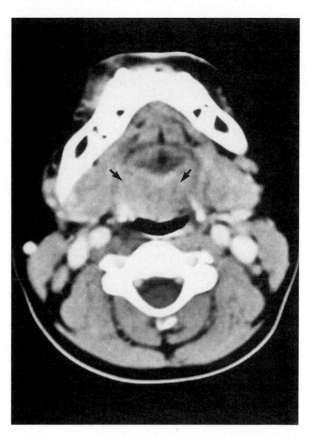

FIG. 10-17 Palatine tonsillar hypertrophy, 5-year-old child. Lateral plain film reveals prominent palatine tonsils *(black arrows)* and adenoidal tissue *(A)* in this child with obstructive sleep apnea.

FIG. 10-18 Lingual tonsillar hypertrophy. Young child with obstructive sleep apnea. Axial CT shows prominent symmetric soft tissue at the tongue base *(arrows),* filling the valleculae bilaterally. Surgically proved hypertrophy of the lingual lymphoid tissue.

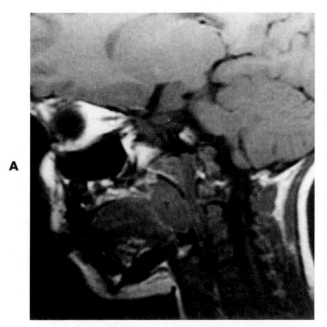

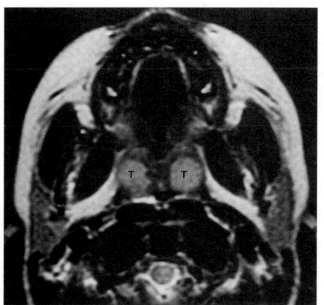

FIG. 10-19 Palatine tonsillar hypertrophy, 4-year-old child with no airway symptoms. **A,** T1W sagittal image shows prominent palatine tonsil, with airway narrowing caused by the tonsillar hypertrophy and oral sedation. **B,** Same child, T2W FSE image shows palatine tonsils are prominent, symmetric, contained within the tonsillar fossae, and nearly touching in the midline.

dren (Figs. 10-19, 10-20). Because they are isodense to muscle on CT, they are only appreciated when enlarged or necrotic. However, because of the numerous normal childhood infections, the efferent lymph vessels to these nodes usually become obstructed by the second decade of life, and these nodes are not commonly seen in the normal adult.

LARYNX AND TRACHEA

The pediatric larynx and trachea differ dramatically in appearance from their adult counterparts. The following four major anatomic factors account for the differences in appearance: size, shape, location, and consistency.[8,9]

Compared with that of an adult, the relative size of the pediatric larynx is smaller in comparison with overall body size.[8] Thin contiguous sections, no greater than 3 mm, are required to adequately image the pediatric larynx. The small size of the pediatric laryngeal airway explains why, with only minimal mucosal edema or swelling as occurs with laryngotracheobronchitis, dramatic symptoms such as stridor and respiratory distress may occur. The glottis in the newborn and infant is only 7 to 9 mm in anteroposterior dimension.[9] The infant subglottic region, which is the smallest area of the pediatric airway, measures only 5 to 7 mm in diameter, and this airway is reduced to 32% of normal size with only 1 mm of mucosa edema.[10,11]

The larynx rapidly increases in size during the first 6 years of life and then gradually slows its growth until adolescence, when it reaches adult proportions. In the adult, only the male thyroid cartilage continues to change shape and grow on its external anterior aspect.[12] The change in voice character normally noted during puberty is secondary to growth of the vocal cords, histologic changes in the vocal folds (as the fibers change in density), and a change in the angle of the thyroid cartilage.[10,12] Of these, the most important change appears to be the thyroid cartilage angle, which until puberty is 100° to 120° open posteriorly. In the male this angle then narrows to about 90°, and in the female it widens to 120°.[10] The larynx of the male at puberty and in adulthood is larger than that of the female, and the thyroid eminence is more prominent.[13]

The pediatric larynx also changes dramatically in shape during early life. In adults the glottis is the narrowest portion of the airway. However, in the infant the larynx has a characteristic funnel shape, which results in the subglottic region being the narrowest portion of the larynx and upper airway as described earlier in this chapter (Fig. 10-21). Below the subglottis, the pediatric airway again widens to a fairly uniform diameter that is maintained down to the level of the carina.

The epiglottis is omega-shaped and is more angular in the infant than in the adult. This contour may be exaggerated in infants who have congenital laryngeal stridor. This characteristic shape and the resultant stridor disappear in most cases by the second year of life.[14] The glottic airway is elliptical in shape with the greatest length in the anteroposterior

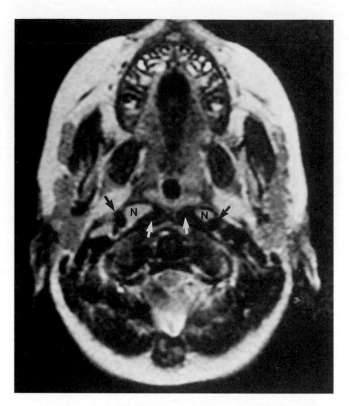

FIG. 10-20 Retropharyngeal lymph nodes. FSE T2W axial image shows normal retropharyngeal lymph nodes *(N)*, medial to the internal carotid arteries *(black arrows)* and lateral to the longus capitus muscles *(white arrows)*. These nodes are a normal finding in the asymptomatic pediatric patient.

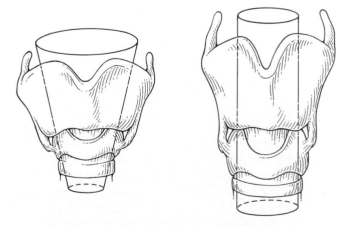

FIG. 10-21 The infantile larynx is funnel shaped. As a result, the narrowest portion of the larynx is the subglottic region, which is 5 to 7 mm in the newborn. The adult larynx is wider at the base, and the glottis is the narrowest portion of the airway. (From Cotton RT. Pediatric otolaryngology. Bluestone, Stool, eds. 1990; 1194.)

dimension, the subglottis is round, and the trachea is ovoid and slightly flatter posteriorly (Fig. 10-22, *C, D, E*). The tracheal shape is consistent between girls and boys.[15]

During the first several years of life, the pediatric larynx changes its position in the neck. Thus the normal radiographic landmarks are different from those in the adult. The free edge of the epiglottis in the neonate is found at or near the C1 level, and the cricoid cartilage, representing the most caudal portion of the larynx, is at C4-C5 level.[16] The epiglottis can be visualized in the oral cavity in most infants, and because of the early rostral position of the larynx, the infant is an obligate nasal breather. By adolescence the epiglottis is found at the C2-C3 level, and the cricoid is at the C6 level. The adult epiglottis is usually seen at the C3 level, with the cricoid at C6-C7 level.[8] The arytenoid cartilage, a radiologic landmark that helps localize the true vocal cord, is found at the C4-C5 level in children.[17]

Although the cartilaginous framework for the larynx is established in the infant, the structures are not calcified at birth. The larynx is softer and the ligaments have greater laxity than they do in the adult larynx. The hyoid bone, the first laryngeal structure to ossify, is partially calcified at birth and completely ossified by the second year of life.[10] Plain films of the airway usually show little or no calcification in the remaining laryngeal cartilaginous structures until about age 20.[10,18] Premature calcification of the laryngeal cartilages in infancy is abnormal and may be associated with stridor.[19-21]

The cricoid cartilage is a complete cartilaginous ring, and it is the narrowest portion of the infantile larynx (Fig. 10-23). The anterior and lateral portions of the cricoid cartilage arch are narrow, and the posterior portion forms a thick lamina. The cricothyroid articulation is on the superolateral portion of the cricoid arch. This small depression articulates with the inferior horn of the thyroid cartilage. The cricothyroid ligament spans the gap between the cricoid and the thyroid cartilages.

The paired arytenoid cartilages sit on the superior rounded surface of the posterior lamina of the cricoid cartilage (Fig. 10-23, *B*). The vocal ligament is attached to the anterior vocal process of the arytenoid cartilage, which is at the level of the cricoarytenoid joint. The primary muscles of the larynx include the cricothyroideus (CT), the posterior cricoarytenoideus (PCA), the lateral cricoarytenoideus (LCA), the interarytenoideus, the thyroarytenoideus (TA), and the vocalis muscles (Fig. 10-24). The PCA muscle originates on the posterior lamina of the cricoid cartilage and inserts into the lateral aspect of the muscular process of the arytenoid. The PCA is the main abductor of the vocal cords. The LCA muscle arises from the upper border and outer surface of the cricoid cartilage and inserts on the anterior surface of the muscular process of the arytenoid cartilage. The LCA adducts the vocal cords. The TA muscle arises on the inner surface of the thyroid cartilage and inserts on the lateral surface of the arytenoid cartilage. The TA muscle draws the arytenoid forward and medial, thereby adducting the true

vocal cord. The vocalis muscle is really the parallel muscle fibers of the TA muscle, and it extends along the length of the free edge of the true vocal cord. The interarytenoid muscle spans the posterior surface of the arytenoids and closes the posterior glottis. The CT muscle arises from the anterior surface of the cricoid arch and has two portions—a superior one that inserts on the inferior external surface of the thyroid cartilage and an inferior tendon that inserts on the inferior horn and the inner surface of the thyroid cartilage. The CT muscle tilts the cricoid lamina backward, thereby lengthening, tensing, and adducting the vocal cords. The individual laryngeal muscles are not usually seen well in the pediatric larynx on either CT or MR.

The CT appearance of the pediatric larynx reflects the anatomic characteristics discussed. Children under the age of about 7 years may require sedation, so scans are obtained during quiet respiration, without breath-hold maneuvers. Therefore respiratory motion artifact is common. The hyoid bone and free edge of the epiglottis are seen at a higher level than in the adult, usually at the C1-C2 level or just at the level of the mandible (Fig. 10-22). The preepiglottic space is fat density and only several millimeters thick, and the paraglottic fat is not as prominent as it is in the adult larynx. The aryepiglottic folds are thin, and the pyriform sinuses are usually air-filled. The thyroid cartilage is occasionally seen as a thin linear high-density structure, despite the fact that calcification is not seen on plain radiographs until the third decade (Fig. 10-22, *B, C*). The ossified, or calcified, arytenoid cartilages, landmarks for the true vocal cords on CT of the adult larynx, are not seen in the pediatric larynx as discrete structures. Therefore the level of the true vocal cords is determined primarily by the contour of the glottis, which has a characteristic oval shape (rather than the adult anteriorly narrowed thin triangular shape). The glottis also can be localized by the location of the air-containing laryngeal ventricle, which is immediately cranial to the true cord, is at the level of C3 in the pediatric larynx, and can often be seen on lateral scout or plain films.[7] Most of the endolaryngeal structures, including the true vocal cords and intrinsic laryngeal muscles, are otherwise featureless on imaging (Figs. 10-22, 10-25). In the subglottis a circumferential rim of soft tissue surrounds the airway. This is the noncalcified cricoid cartilage. The CT appearance of the pediatric larynx also dramatically differs from that of the adult because the cartilaginous structures, although fully formed, are not calcified, or ossified (Fig. 10-26).

High-resolution MRI of the pediatric larynx is difficult to obtain because of the infant's relatively short, fat neck, the high position of the larynx, and respiratory artifact. On MRI there is little paraglottic fat. Whatever fat is present has the characteristic high T1W and lower T2W signal intensity of adult fat (Fig. 10-27).

The nonossified cartilaginous laryngeal structures are hyperintense on T2W images. On T1W images, except for the thyroid cartilage, which is hyperintense to muscle, the cartilaginous structures of the larynx are isointense to soft

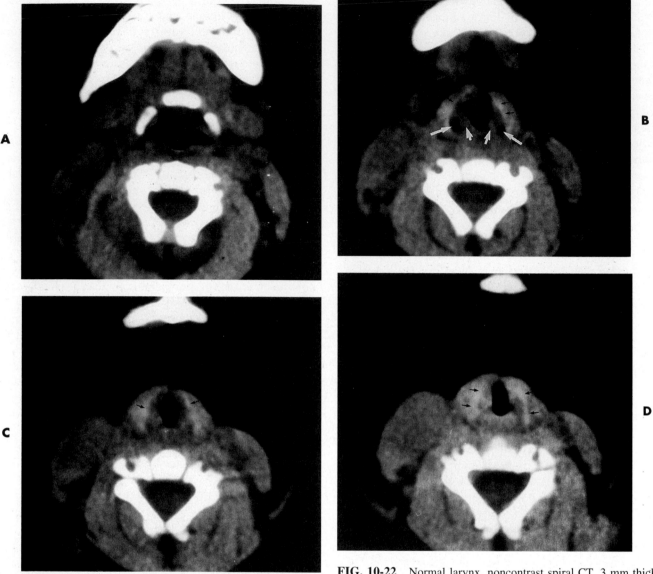

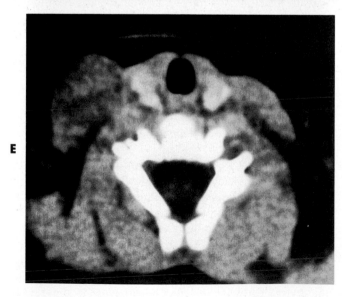

FIG. 10-22 Normal larynx, noncontrast spiral CT, 3 mm thick slice collimation. Oral sedation, quiet respiration, 53-day-old child with mild swelling in right strernocleidomastoid muscle, no airway disease. **A,** The hyoid bone, seen at the level of the mandible, is densely ossified. **B,** Two slices caudal, at the level of the aryepiglottic folds *(small white arrows)* and pyriform sinuses *(large white arrows).* There is little paralaryngeal fat. Notice the thin rim of high density, presumably the noncalcified thyroid cartilage *(black arrows).* **C,** True vocal cords, 3 mm caudal to **B,** just behind the mandible. The airway contour is oval. Seen again is the high-density but nonossified thyroid cartilage *(black arrows),* paucity of paraglottic fat, and lack of calcification of the arytenoid cartilages, the CT landmark for the true vocal cords in the adult. **D,** Subglottic level, 3 mm caudal to **C.** Notice the airway contour remains oval but is narrower than at the glottis. The thyroid cartilage is seen again, but the soft tissue surrounding the airway, presumably the cricoid cartilage, appear noncalcified and entirely featureless. **E,** Trachea, 6 mm caudal to **D.** The airway contour is rounded and is flattened posteriorly. Circumferential featureless soft tissue surrounding the airway is the noncalcified tracheal cartilage. (Courtesy Dr. John J. Alarcon, Scottish Rite Children's Medical Center, Atlanta, Georgia.)

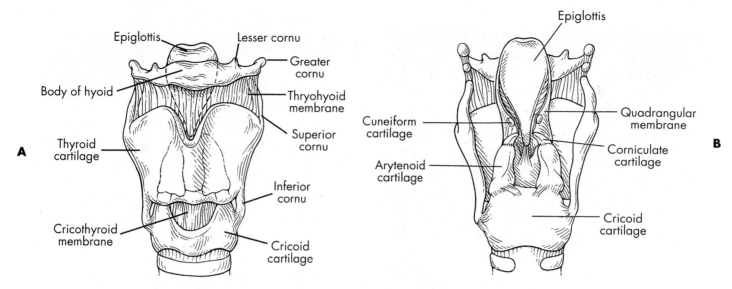

FIG. 10-23 Normal larynx, cartilaginous and ligamentous components. The laryngeal cartilages are calcified or ossified in the adult, and each can be discretely seen on radiographs or CT. However, only the hyoid bone is calcified in the pediatric larynx, and the cartilaginous components cannot be visualized as separate structures on plain radiographs or CT. **A,** Anterior view. The hyoid bone, thyroid cartilage, and anterior ring of the cricoid cartilage are the anterior structures of the larynx. **B,** Posterior view. The laryngeal surface of the epiglottis, the arytenoids, and the posterior portion of the cricoid ring are the important cartilaginous portions of the larynx in this view.

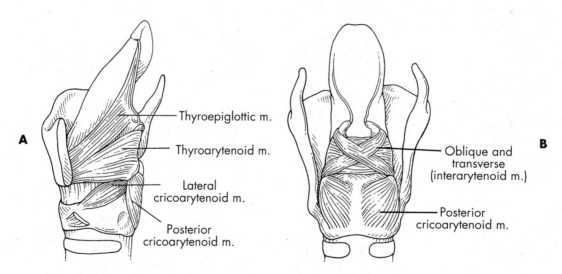

FIG. 10-24 Intrinsic muscles of the larynx. **A,** Lateral view looking into the larynx, with half of the thyroid cartilage removed. **B,** Posterior view. Despite the complexity of the intrinsic laryngeal muscles, they cannot be routinely individually visualized on even high-resolution CT or MRI, but they appear as confluent soft tissue surrounding the airway.

tissue and are featureless. High-resolution MRI of the cadaveric larynx, using a 512 matrix and 4 signal averages, shows that the laryngeal cartilages are hyperintense to muscle on T2W images, with a thin rim of low signal intensity around the cartilage (Fig. 10-27). However, such high-resolution imaging often is not possible or clinically necessary. As with CT, the airway contour indicates airway level.

The cartilaginous trachea in children is uncalcified, smooth, and featureless on CT. Cartilage detail is, however,

seen well on T2W MRI. The tracheal contour is round anteriorly and flat posteriorly, at the membranous portion of the tracheal wall (Fig. 10-22, *E*). Generally the diameter of the normal infant trachea is slightly larger than that of the subglottis. The anteroposterior dimension is slightly greater than the lateral dimension, except at the level of the innominate artery, where normal physiologic AP narrowing can occur. Absolute tracheal measurements on radiographs, fluoroscopic studies, CT, and MRI should be qualified with

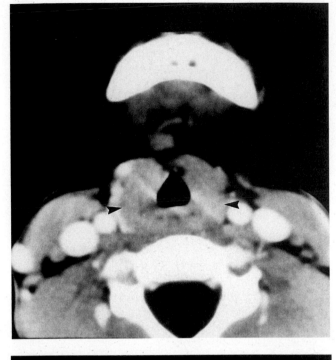

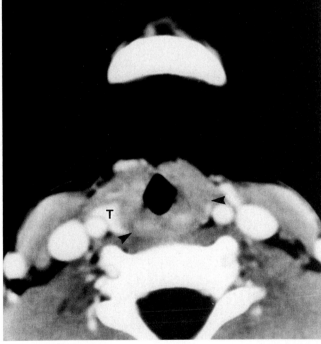

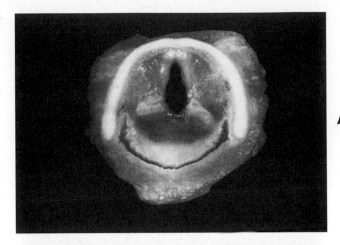

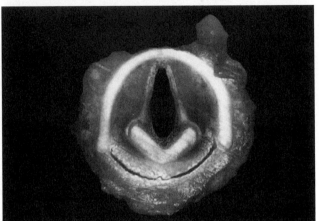

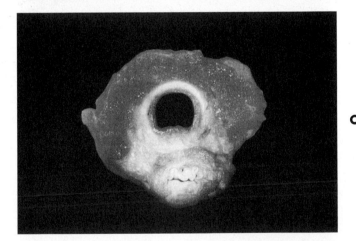

FIG. 10-25 Normal larynx, 5-year-old child with no airway disease. **A,** Supraglottic larynx. Prominent circumferential soft tissue *(arrowheads)* surrounds the airway, but lack of calcification in laryngeal cartilages makes more precise identification of level difficult. **B,** glottic level. Airway contour is oval. Thyroid gland *(T)* is separated from airway by noncalcified laryngeal cartilages *(arrowheads).*

FIG. 10-26 Normal larynx, gross specimen, 9-month-old child who died from complications of complex congenital heart disease, no airway disease. Normal laryngeal anatomy contrasts dramatically with featureless pediatric larynx on CT. **A,** True vocal cords. Notice the thyroid and arytenoid cartilage, vocal cords, and cervical esophagus. **B,** 3 mm caudal to **A,** reveals thyroid and cricoid cartilage and undersurface of true vocal cords. Notice oval contour to airway. **C,** Trachea. 9 mm caudal to **B.** The trachea is round anteriorly, and flat at the posterior membranous portion. Tissue surrounding trachea is thyroid gland.

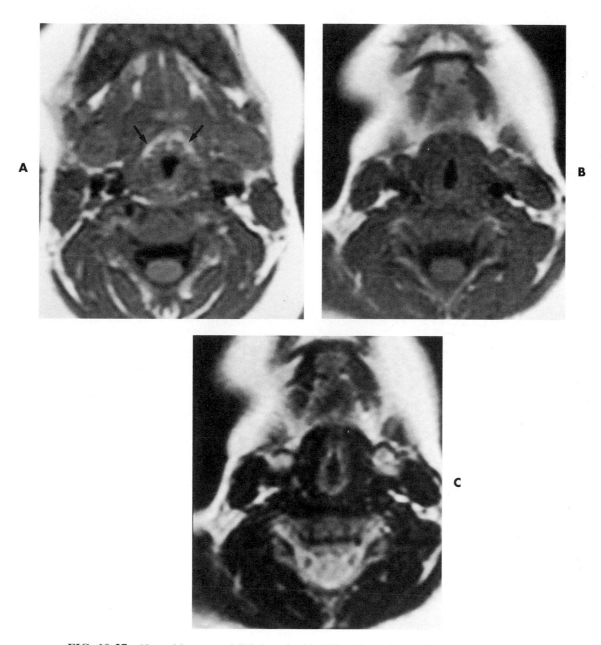

FIG. 10-27   Normal larynx on MRI 4-week-old child with no airway disease. **A,** T1W image of the supraglottic region shows endolaryngeal structures that are isointense to muscle. Notice thin rim of high signal intensity *(arrows),* probably representing the thyroid cartilage. **B,** The glottic-sub-glottic level is relatively high in the pediatric larynx, immediately behind the mandible. The larynx is featureless on this T1W image. **C,** Laryngeal structures are hyperintense on T2W images (compare to C).

respect to phase of respiration because the trachea is a dynamic structure that changes shape and size during the respiratory cycle. The trachea is greatest in diameter during full inspiration and narrows slightly during expiration.[22] In normal infants the AP tracheal diameter may vary from 20% to 50% after breath-holding or crying.[22] Although in one series, as measured on lateral plain films, the anteroposterior tracheal diameters in normal children ranged from 2 to 7 mm, a 5.1-mm outer-diameter endoscope usually passes through the normal newborn airway, including the trachea.[23]

Therefore in the newborn and infant, a tracheal diameter of 5 mm or more is considered normal. Normal tracheal measurements obtained on plain films or CT at maximal inspiration in children older than 10 years of age show coronal tracheal dimensions ranging from 0.9 to 1.8 cm and anteroposterior dimensions ranging from 1.1 to 1.8 cm.[24,25] An abrupt change in tracheal diameter and configuration may be a more significant finding than any single measurement in the airway diameter.

References

1. Slovis TL, Renfro B, Watts FB, et al. Choanal atresia: precise CT evaluation. Radiology 1985; 155:345-348.

2. Brodsky L, Koch J. Anatomic correlates of normal and diseased adenoids in children. Laryngoscope 1992; 102:1268-1274.

3. Rubesin SE, Rabischong P, Bilaniuk LT, et al. Contrast examination of the soft palate with cross sectional correlation. Radiographics 1988; 8:641-665.

4. Scheerer WD, Lammert F. Morphology and growth of the nasopharynx from three years to maturity. Archives Oto-Rhino-Laryngology 1980; 229:221-229.

5. Swischuk LE, Smith PC, Fagan CJ. Abnormalities of the pharynx and larynx in childhood. Seminars in Roentgenology 1974; 9:283-300.

6. Capitanio MA, Kirkpatrick JA. Nasopharyngeal lymphoid tissue. Radiology 1970; 96:389-391.

7. Ardran GM, Kemp FH. A function of adenoids and tonsils. Am J Roentgenology, Radium, Ther and Nucl Med 1972; 114:268-281.

8. Wilson TG. Some observations on the anatomy of the infantile larynx. Acta Oto-Laryngologica 1953; 43:95-99.

9. Tucker G. The infant larynx: direct laryngoscopic observations. 1932; 99:1899-1902.

10. Spector GJ. Developmental anatomy of the larynx. In: Ballenger JJ, ed. Diseases of the nose, throat, ear, head and neck. 13th Edition. Philadelphia, Pa: Lea & Febiger, 1985.

11. Holinger PH, Kutnick SL, Schild JA, et al. Subglottic stenosis in infants and children. Ann Otol Rhinol Laryngol 1976; 85:591-599.

12. Kahane JC. Growth of the human prepubertal and pubertal larynx. J Speech Hear Res 1982; 25:446-455.

13. Kahane JC. A morphological study of the human prepubertal and pubertal larynx. Am J Anat 1978; 151:11-20.

14. Holinger PH, Brown WT. Congenital webs, cysts, laryngoceles and other anomalies of the larynx. Ann Otol Rhinol Laryngol 1967; 76:744-752.

15. Griscom NT. Cross-sectional shape of the child's trachea by computed tomography. AJR Am J Roentgenol 1983; 140:1103-1106.

16. Noback GJ. The developmental topography of the larynx, trachea and lungs in the fetus, new-born, infant and child. American Journal of Diseases of Children 1923; 26:515-533.

17. Koppel HJ, Kendrick GS, Moreland JE. The vertebral level of the arytenoid cartilages. Anat Rec 1968; 160:583-586.

18. Hately BW, Evison G, Samuel E. The pattern of ossification in the laryngeal cartilages: a radiographical study. Br J Radiol 1965; 38:585-591.

19. Goldbloom RB, Dunbar JS. Calcification of cartilage in the trachea and larynx in infancy associated with congenital stridor. Pediatrics 1960; 26:669-673.

20. Russo PE, Coin CG. Calcification of the hyoid, thyroid and tracheal cartilages in infancy, AJR Am J Roentgenol 1958; 80:440-442.

21. Nabarro S. Calcification of the laryngeal and tracheal cartilages associated with congenital stridor in an infant. Arch Dis Child 1952; 27:185-186.

22. Wittenborg MH, Gyepes MT, Crocker D. Tracheal dynamics in infants with respiratory distress, stridor and collapsing trachea. Radiology 1967; 88:653-662.

23. Donaldson SW, Tompsett AC Jr. Tracheal diameter in the normal newborn infant. AJR Am J Roentgenol 1952; 67:785-787.

24. Griscom NT. Computed tomographic determination of tracheal dimensions in children and adolescents. Radiology 1982; 145:361-364.

25. Breatnach E, Abbott GC, Fraser RG. Dimensions of the normal human trachea, AJR Am J Roentgenol 1984; 142:903-906.

Section Four
CLINICAL EVALUATION

Stridor, which is defined as *noisy breathing,* is the audible result of turbulent airflow (Fig. 10-28). Stridor may be either acute or chronic and may result from obstruction anywhere in the airway from the nasal cavity to the distal bronchi. Acute stridor is commonly caused by acquired conditions such as infection, trauma, or a foreign body.[1] The most common causes of chronic stridor in the infant are congenital laryngeal or tracheal anomalies such as laryngomalacia or tracheomalacia and vocal cord paralysis. Stridor may be associated with respiratory distress, and the degree of distress dictates the urgency of the situation and the need for immediate clinical intervention. Labored and rapid respiratory movements, costal retractions, nasal flaring, and fatigue indicate severe respiratory distress. Significant respiratory compromise mandates immediate endoscopy or intubation.[2]

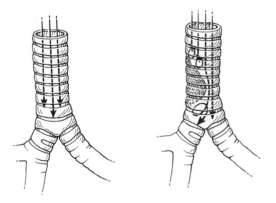

FIG. 10-28 Normal airflow is nonturbulent. Diagram on the left side shows the normal nonturbulent air flow. The diagram on the right side shows the turbulence created by a tracheal mass along the tracheal wall. At the area of obstruction, airflow is most turbulent and noisy. (From Handler SD. Otolaryngology-head and neck surgery. St. Louis, Mo: Mosby–Year Book, 1986; 2220.)

The phase of respiration in which the stridor occurs is the most important characteristic for localizing the site of airway obstruction. Stridor during inspiration indicates obstruction at or above the glottis. Biphasic stridor suggests subglottic or high tracheal obstruction, and expiratory stridor is characteristic of tracheal or bronchial obstruction.[1] The intensity of the stridor correlates with the degree of airway obstruction. Low-pitched stridor indicates nasal or oropharyngeal obstruction. High-pitched sounds usually indicate laryngeal obstruction.

There are other clinical characteristics that may suggest the etiology of the stridor. Fever or cough suggests croup, and drooling or odynophagia is often a presenting sign of epiglottitis. Laryngomalacia causes stridor that is more pronounced in the supine position. Tracheobronchomalacia often exacerbates the respiratory distress during crying or in the agitated child, and feeding may bring on cyanosis in the infant with a vascular ring. Obstructive sleep apnea is worse during sleep. A history of prematurity and prior intubation in a child with stridor suggests the possibility of acquired subglottic stenosis.[2]

Additional workup of the infant or child with stridor includes physical examination of the nasopharynx, oropharynx, neck, larynx, and auscultation of the chest. The nasal airway should be inspected for patency, and a no. 8 French suction catheter should readily pass through the normal nasal cavity. The tongue and tonsils should be examined, and the position of the larynx and trachea should be noted. The chest should be auscultated for rhonchi or wheezing. Depending on the clinical situation and the urgency of the stridor, plain films may be performed. However, if the diagnosis is uncertain or if immediate intervention is required, endoscopy, both flexible fiberoptic and rigid telescopic, should be performed. This is usually done in the operating room, where appropriate equipment and personnel are present. Airway dynamics, including vocal cord motion, tracheal wall motion, and changes in luminal diameter can be appreciated on flexible endoscopy.[2] The structural aspects of the airway are best examined with rigid Storz-Hopkins telescopes.[3] Manipulations such as extraction of foreign bodies can be performed only through the rigid endoscope. Endoscopy is more sensitive than radiographic examination in detecting airway lesions caused by laryngomalacia, subglottic stenosis, and tracheal stenosis, but the two methods are comparable for other common pediatric airway lesions.[4]

Obstructive sleep apnea (OSA) in children results from airway obstruction and cessation of airflow for a finite period of time during sleep. Pharyngeal tone is reduced during sleep, thus exaggerating the obstructive problems. The most common cause of OSA in children is adenotonsillar hypertrophy, which is treated by tonsillectomy and adenoidectomy.[5,6] Less common causes of OSA in children include neuromuscular disorders such as cerebral palsy, macroglossia, nasopharyngeal masses, craniofacial syndromes, obesity, and pharyngeal flaps following cleft palate repair.[5] Certain genetic syndromes may present with OSA. For example, children with Prader-Willi syndrome present with short stature, obesity, gonadal hypodevelopment, and severe OSA.

The diagnosis of OSA is usually established by clinical history alone. Most parents can vividly describe loud snoring, obstructive pauses, retractions, and mouth breathing. When the diagnosis is uncertain, studies such as polysomnography (sleep studies), sleep sonography, physical examination, and radiographs may confirm the diagnosis of OSA. Lateral plain films are useful for evaluating the size of the adenoids and tonsils and for excluding the presence of other obstructing lesions. Additional radiologic evaluation usually is not needed. If the diagnosis remains uncertain after the physical examination and plain films, airway fluoroscopy may determine the actual site of obstruction during quiet respiration or during sleep.[7] Ultrafast, or cine, CT performed during quiet breathing in patients with OSA shows smaller oropharyngeal and nasopharyngeal airways than in control subjects and provides direct data of the airway diameter during sleep.[8,9] Spiral CT with the capacity to scan during several respiratory cycles may prove useful in diagnosing the site of obstruction in children with a questionable diagnosis of OSA.

References

1. Holinger LD. Etiology of stridor in the neonate, infant and child. Ann Otol Rhinol Laryngol 1980; 89:397-400.
2. Handler SD. Diagnosis and management of stridor in children. In: Cummings CW, et al, eds. Otolaryngology-head and neck surgery. Chicago, Ill: Mosby–Year Book, 1986.
3. Benjamin BNP. Indications and techniques. In: Benjamin BNP, ed. Diagnostic laryngology. Philadelphia, Pa: WB Saunders, 1990.
4. Gyepes MT, Nussbaum E. Radiographic-endoscopic correlations in the examination of airway disease in children. Pediat Radiol 1985; 15:291-296.
5. Potsic WP, Wetmore RF. Sleep disorders and airway obstruction in children. Otolaryngol Clin North Am 1990; 23:651-663.
6. Brouillette RT, Fernbach SK, Hunt CE. Obstructive sleep apnea in infants and children. J Pediatr 1982; 100:31-40.
7. Fernbach SK, Brouillette RT, Riggs TW, et al. Radiologic evaluation of adenoids and tonsils in children with obstructive sleep apnea: plain films and fluoroscopy. Pediatr Radiol 1983; 13:258-265.
8. Galvin JR, Rooholamini SA, Stanford W. Obstructive sleep apnea: diagnosis with Ultrafast CT. Radiology 1989; 171:775-778.
9. Crumley RL, Stein M, Gamsu G, et al. Determination of obstructive site in obstructive sleep apnea. Laryngoscope 1987; 97:301-308.

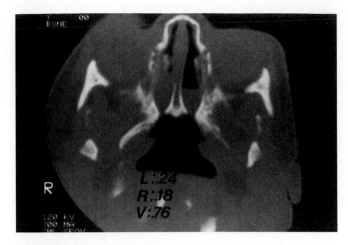

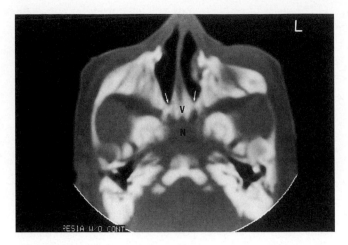

FIG. 10-29 Bilateral bony choanal stenosis with retained secretions in an infant. Axial CT section showing fluid levels in both nasal passages, before suctioning. The left posterior choana measures 0.24 cm and the right side is 0.18 cm, thus they are severely stenotic. The posterior vomer is 0.76 cm, more than twice the normal size.

FIG. 10-30 Bilateral bony choanal atresia in an infant. Axial CT section shows marked thickening of posterior vomer (V), which is fused with the prominent medial aspect of the posterior maxilla, giving rise to complete bony atresia (arrows). The posterior nasopharynx (n) does not contain air. There are no secretions in the nasal passages because this patient was suctioned immediately before the study. (From Castillo M. Congenital abnormalities of the nose: CT and MR findings. AJR 1994; 162:1211-1217.)

SECTION FIVE
CONGENITAL AIRWAY DISEASES

NASAL AIRWAY OBSTRUCTION

Because the infant is an obligate nasal breather, bilateral nasal airway disease often results in severe airway obstruction. Grunting, snorting, low-pitched stridor, and rhinorrhea are common presenting signs of nasal airway obstruction in the neonate or infant.[1] Congenital nasal airway obstruction most commonly occurs in the posterior nasal cavity, secondary to choanal atresia.[2] Nasal airway obstruction may also result from rhinitis, turbinate hypertrophy, congenital syphilis ("snuffles"), and nasal cavity stenosis in association with craniofacial anomalies.[1,2]

Choanal Atresia and Stenosis

Atresia or stenosis of the posterior nasal cavity (choanae) is the most common congenital abnormality of the nasal cavity, occurring in approximately one of every 5000 to 8000 live births, and it is slightly more common in females than in males.[2,3] Stenosis of the posterior choanae is probably more common than true atresia.[4] Although bony atresia is more common than membranous atresia, most cases have elements of both components. Most atresias, or stenoses, are unilateral and may remain undetected until later in life. Patients with unilateral choanal atresia usually present with chronic unilateral purulent rhinorrhea, and the main differential diagnosis in these older children is a unilateral nasal cavity foreign body.

Because the infant is an obligate nasal breather, bilateral choanal atresia may result in severe respiratory compro-

mise, generally aggravated by feeding and alleviated by crying.[3] Severe respiratory difficulty and the inability to insert a nasogastric tube more than 3 to 4 cm into the nose, despite the presence of air in the trachea and the lungs, suggest the diagnosis.

Approximately 75% of children with bilateral choanal atresias have other congenital abnormalities.[5,6] These include facial dysmorphism, Apert's syndrome, Treacher Collins syndrome, fetal alcohol syndrome, CHARGE syndrome (colobomas, heart disease, atresia of choanae, retarded growth, genital abnormalities, and ear anomalies), ventricular septal defects, and gut malrotations.[3]

Surgical correction of bilateral choanal atresia is performed as soon as possible after the diagnosis is made. Before surgery the initial management includes placement of an oral airway. The surgical approach is determined by the type of atresia and the thickness of the bony atresia plate as determined on CT.

CT is the imaging method of choice for the evaluation of these children.[3,7,8] The examinations are obtained with patients supine, after the nasal passages are suctioned free of secretions and topical vasoconstriction is applied (Fig. 10-29). The gantry is angled approximately 5° cephalad to a plane parallel to the hard palate, and contiguous 1 to 1.5 mm scans are obtained. Prospective high-resolution (edge enhancement) bone filters may be helpful because the skull base is only partially ossified at birth and conventional bone window settings may not permit adequate visualization of bone margins. Intravenous contrast is not necessary.

On the CT scans the width of both posterior choanae at maximum stenosis and the maximum width of the infero-posterior vomer are measured. The major component of all

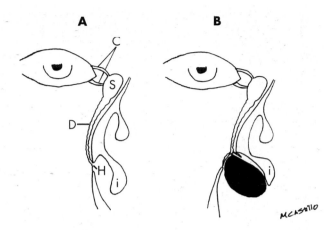

FIG. 10-32 Normal anatomy and distal nasolacrimal duct cyst. **A,** The normal lacrimal apparatus begins at the eyelid puncta, which opens into the superior and inferior canaliculi *(C).* The canaliculi empty into the lacrimal sac *(S),* which drains into the duct *(D).* The distal opening of the duct, the valve of Hasner *(H),* is located under the inferior turbinate *(i)* in the inferior meatus. **B,** The valve of Hasner fails to open secondary to incomplete canalization or inflammation, and accumulated secretions *(dark zone)* form a mucocele. The inferior turbinate *(i)* is displaced superiorly. (From Castillo M, Merten DF, Weissler MC. Bilateral nasolacrimal duct mucocele, a rare cause of respiratory distress: CT findings in two newborns. AJNR 1993; 14:1011-1013.)

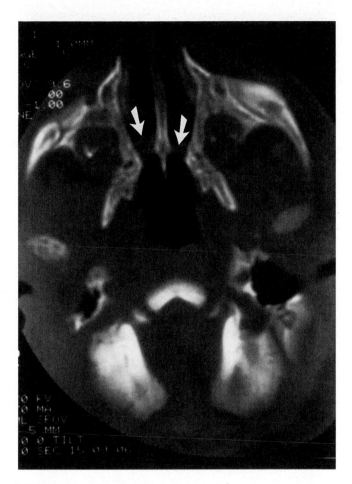

FIG. 10-31 Bilateral membranous choanal atresia in an infant. Axial CT shows soft-tissue membranes *(arrows)* extending from the lateral aspects of the vomer to the medial and posterior maxilla. The width of the vomer and the diameter of the posterior choanae are normal in this patient.

bony atresias is an abnormal widening of the vomer (Figs. 10-29, 10-30). Typically the posteromedial maxilla is bowed medially and touches or is fused with the lateral margin of the vomer (Fig. 10-30). The mean width of the posterior choanal airspace in the newborn is 0.67 cm, increasing to 0.86 cm at 6 years and 1.13 cm by 16 years of age.[8] In patients less than 8 years of age, the vomer generally measures less than 0.23 cm in width and should not exceed 0.34 cm; in children over 8 years, the mean vomer width is 0.28 cm and should not exceed 0.55 cm.[8] The thickness of the bony atretic plate should be reported because this may impact the surgical approach. In general the thicker the plate, the more difficult the surgical repair.

Membranous atresias are characterized by soft tissue filling the posterior choanae, as well as narrowing of the posterior choanae just anterior to the pterygoid plates (Fig. 10-31). The obstructing choanal membranes may be either thin and strandlike or thick plugs. In patients with choanal abnormalities the nasal cavities may contain air, soft tissue, fluid secretions, or hypertrophied inferior turbinates. Topical

vasoconstriction helps differentiate reversible changes from fixed obstructing lesions.

Postsurgical persistent or recurrent choanal stenosis, usually caused by a postoperative scar or an incompletely resected bony atresia plate, also is evaluated best with CT.[7]

Nasolacrimal Duct Mucocele

Nasolacrimal duct mucoceles, or retention cysts, are rare lesions that present in early neonatal life with nasal obstruction and respiratory distress. They may be clinically indistinguishable from bilateral choanal atresia.[9] They may occur anywhere along the path of the nasolacrimal ducts, and they are believed to be caused by failure of canalization of the distal lacrimal ducts (Fig. 10-32). Chronic inflammatory changes may be found in the walls, suggesting the possibility of an intrauterine inflammation.[9] Retained secretions extend downward into the nose under the inferior turbinate. Occasionally, mucoceles may extend upward into the proximal lacrimal duct and protrude into the medial orbital canthus.

Bilateral mucoceles present in early life with nasal obstruction. Unilateral mucoceles are rare. This may be because unilateral distal nasolacrimal duct mucoceles are inadvertently perforated when passing a nasogastric tube in a newborn who has respiratory distress.

CT evaluation should be performed using a technique similar to that described for choanal atresia. CT shows rounded, bilateral or unilateral, homogeneous soft-tissue density structures in the anterior and inferior nasal cavities

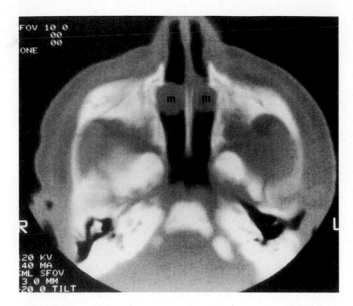

FIG. 10-33 Bilateral nasolacrimal duct cysts in an infant. Axial CT section (bone windows) shows bilateral distal nasolacrimal duct mucoceles *(m)*. The lateral wall of the nasal cavity adjacent to the cysts is remodeled. The nasal septum is midline. (From Castillo M, Merten DF, Weissler MC. Bilateral nasolacrimal duct mucocele, a rare cause of respiratory distress: CT findings in two newborns. AJNR 1993; 14:1011-1013.)

(Fig. 10-33).[9] When bilateral, mucoceles are generally slightly asymmetric in size. The inferior turbinates may be thin and may be displaced medially. Unilateral cysts result in deviation of the thinned nasal septum. There is usually air in the nasal passages and nasopharynx. Nasolacrimal duct cysts may be associated with other abnormalities such as choanal atresia. Treatment is surgical, either by endoscopic marsupialization of the base of the cyst or by fenestration of the walls.

Pyriform Aperture Stenosis

Stenosis of the pyriform (anterior) nasal apertures is a rare anomaly that produces respiratory distress immediately after birth. The main differential diagnosis is bilateral choanal atresia. However, in congenital pyriform aperture stenosis a nasogastric tube cannot be inserted into the nose. Pyriform aperture stenosis may be associated with a lobar and semilobar holoprosencephaly, facial hemangiomata, clinodactyly, endocrine dysfunction, and upper teeth anomalies.[10] Congenital stenosis of the pyriform aperture without a central megaincisor is generally an isolated anomaly with no intracranial defects.[10]

CT should be performed as described for choanal atresia, but the scans should be extended through the maxillary alveolar ridge to evaluate for possible dental abnormalities. Associated intracranial malformations are evaluated better with MRI, but CT is useful screening procedure. CT of a patient with nasal aperture stenosis shows thickening of the nasal process of the maxilla, which results in narrowing of

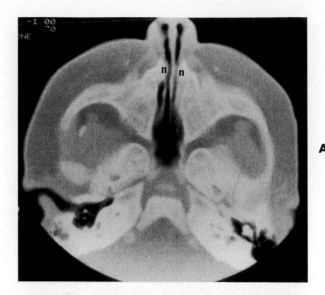

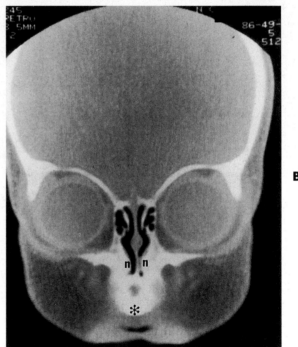

FIG. 10-34 Stenosis of the pyriform aperture in a neonate. **A,** Axial CT shows overgrowth of the medial maxilla *(n)* with medial bowing and anterior pointing. The nasal septum is thin. The inferior nasal passages are severely narrowed. **B,** Coronal CT in the same patient shows medial bowing of the maxilla *(n),* producing severe narrowing of the anteroinferior nasal passages. A central megaincisor *(*)* is present. There were no intracranial abnormalities in this child.

the pyriform aperture, the narrowest portion of the nasal airway.[11-13] The adjacent anterior nasal septum may be thinned. CT also may show a hypoplastic triangular-shaped hard palate with anterior pointing and a central (fused) megaincisor (Fig. 10-34).[13] Patients with a central megaincisor have an increased incidence of endocrine abnormalities

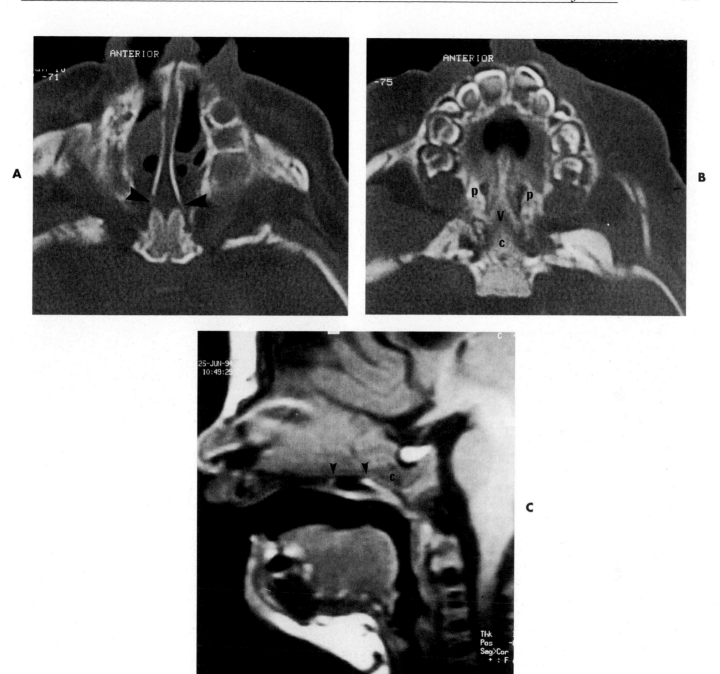

FIG. 10-35   Bucconasal atresia in a newborn. **A,** Axial CT shows absence of the nasopharynx and fusion of the nasal septum to the clivus *(arrowheads).* **B,** Axial CT shows fusion of the vomer *(V)* and hard palate *(p)* with the clivus *(c).* The soft palate and nasopharynx are absent. Left zygomatic arch is hypoplastic. **C,** The T1W midsagittal MR shows fusion of the hard palate *(arrowheads)* with the clivus *(c).* An oral airway is in place. Note the absence of the nasopharynx and soft palate.

referable to the pituitary-adrenal axis and to holoprosencephaly.[10] Therefore imaging of the entire brain is recommended in these patients.

Bucconasal Atresia

Bucconasal atresia is an extremely rare malformation that results in complete isolation of the nasal cavity from the oropharynx.[14] Patients present early in life with severe res-

piratory obstruction. Diagnosis is made when a nasogastric tube cannot be passed more than 3 to 4 cm, and the most important differential diagnosis is that of posterior choanal atresia or stenosis. On CT there is no air in the posterior nasal cavity or nasopharynx. The posterior choanal passages end blindly, the posterior vomer is wide, and both the vomer and the hard palate are fused to the clivus (Fig. 10-35). The soft palate is absent. Soft-tissue density material (probably

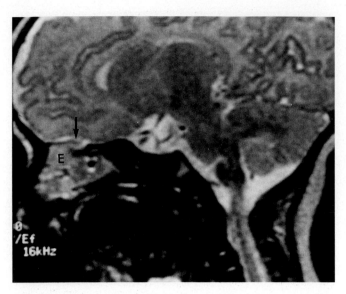

FIG. 10-36 Transethmoidal basal encephalocele, 3-week-old infant with respiratory distress. Sagittal T2W image reveals an anterior skull base defect *(arrow)* and portions of frontal lobes *(E)* herniating through the defect into the nasal cavity.

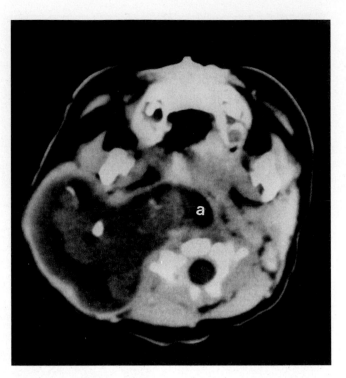

FIG. 10-37 Skull base encephalocele extending through a widened stylomastoid foramen. Newborn with a soft neck mass and respiratory distress. A complex right neck mass with regions of both high and low density is seen on this axial CT. Note marked effacement of the oropharyngeal airway *(a)*.

the primitive nasal plugs incompletely reabsorbed) occupies the nasal cavities. Imaging on conventional CT may not clearly delineate the abnormality, and therefore sagittal T1W MRI should be performed. This study shows absence of the uvula and nasopharynx, confirming the diagnosis. This complex anomaly is managed by tracheotomy and subsequent reconstruction. Other abnormalities associated with bucconasal atresia are facial hemangiomata, cleft lip, and clinodactyly.

Meningocele, Encephalocele, and Nasal Glioma

Nasal obstruction by meningoceles, encephaloceles, or nasal glioma is uncommon. These congenital lesions occur when brain or meninges extend through a cranial defect, resulting in a mass in the nasopharynx or nasal cavity. Nasal meningoceles contain only cerebrospinal fluid (CSF) in a dural sac. Encephaloceles or meningoencephaloceles contain brain tissue and/or CSF, and nasal gliomas are heterotopic foci of neural tissue and meninges in the nose.

Two types of cephaloceles—the basal and sincipital—can involve the nasal or nasopharyngeal airway. Basal cephaloceles are not visible externally, and sincipital cephaloceles result in a visible nasal or forehead mass.[15] The skull base defects of basal cephaloceles are classified as ethmoidal, sphenoethmoidal, transsphenoidal, or frontosphenoidal, depending on the location of the defect. Sincipital cephaloceles are either frontoethmoidal or interfrontal in type.[16]

Basal and sincipital cephaloceles are more common in Southeast Asia than they are in the United States or Europe.[16,17] The infant or child presents with unilateral nasal obstruction, chronic nasal discharge, and an intranasal or nasopharyngeal mass.[18,19] A history of repeated surgeries for "nasal polyps" may precede the correct diagnosis and treatment.[18,20] Associated congenital abnormalities include midface anomalies, hypertelorism, orbital malformations, or hydrocephalus.[16,17]

Although coronal CT is best at showing the bony defect in the skull base, MRI is best at characterizing the soft tissue in the nasal cavity and differentiating between a CSF-containing mass and a lesion containing CSF and brain tissue.[21,22] Bony skull base findings include widening of the foramen cecum, an ipsilateral osseous defect in the cribriform plate, and a bifid or eroded crista galli.[22,23] The nasal mass may be polypoid and small, or it may fill the nasopharynx or nasal cavity (Fig. 10-36). Unlike a benign nasal polyp, the cephalocele presenting in the nasal cavity is located between the middle turbinate and the nasal septum, and it originates from a defect in the skull base.[20] The precise connection between the intranasal mass and the intracranial structures should be sought on coronal and sagittal MRI. Rarely an encephalocele may herniate through the skull base or temporal bone (Fig. 10-37).[24] Treatment consists of surgical excision and repair of the dural defect. The surgical approach to cephaloceles may be endoscopic, intranasal, extranasal, or intracranial, depending on the size of the lesion and skull base defect.

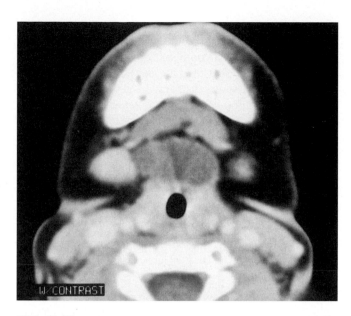

FIG. 10-38 Thyroglossal duct cyst, 1-year-old with a soft midline neck mass. Contrast-enhanced CT shows a low-density nonenhancing unilocular midline mass in the midline floor of the mouth.

The intranasal form of nasal glioma is a nonneoplastic heterotopic mass of neural tissue, usually isolated from the CNS and subarachnoid space. As with cephaloceles, the infant may present with nasal obstruction by a mass that occupies the nasal cavity either medial to the middle turbinate or attached to the nasal septum.[25,26] Imaging findings are similar to meningoceles and encephaloceles, although a stalk or connection between the nasal mass and the intracranial compartment usually is not seen. Treatment is surgical excision.

Miscellaneous

Midface anomalies such as cleft lip and palate and hypoplastic midface anomalies, especially those seen with Crouzon's syndrome or Apert's syndrome, may have airway obstruction at the nasopharyngeal level. Of all the cleft syndromes, unilateral cleft lip and palate has the most severe reduction in nasal airway area.[27,28] Nasal septal deformities and spurs and turbinate hypertrophy associated with cleft syndromes also result in nasal airway encroachment. Although the nasal airways are accessible to direct clinical inspection, CT should always be obtained before craniofacial surgery because size, asymmetry between sides, septal abnormalities such as lateral deviation or spurs, and turbinate anomalies or hypertrophy are details that should be conveyed to the surgeon.

OROPHARYNGEAL OBSTRUCTION
Thyroglossal Duct Cyst and Ectopic Thyroid

A thyroglossal duct cyst is a remnant of the embryologic thyroid primordium and is one of the most common congenital anomalies of the neck.[29] During the first trimester,

the thyroid gland originates at the foramen cecum and then migrates caudally. Failure to completely migrate results in ectopic thyroid tissue. The gland remains connected to the foramen cecum by the thyroglossal duct, which normally involutes by the end of the first trimester. If portions of the thyroglossal duct fail to involute and the epithelial cells maintain secretory activity, a thyroglossal duct cyst results.[29,30]

A thyroglossal duct cyst most commonly presents in the first decade of life as a soft, doughy infrahyoid neck mass without a sinus tract.[31] The cyst may enlarge after an upper respiratory tract infection, but airway obstruction is uncommon. In most cases, ultrasound of the neck demonstrates a cystic structure and confirms that a normal thyroid gland is in the thyroid bed. In such a case, no other imaging is necessary.

Of thyroglossal duct cysts, 20% occur at the base of tongue (foramen cecum) or vallecula, and these are more likely to present with airway obstruction.[32] CT or MRI is performed to characterize the mass, define the extent of the cyst and its relationship to the larynx, and to exclude other lesions such as dermoid cyst, cervical adenopathy, hemangioma, lipoma, or lymphangioma. On CT, suprahyoid thyroglossal duct cysts are typically midline, rarely occurring more than 2 cm laterally (Fig. 10-38).[30] Simple thyroglossal duct cysts are low density, with a thin rim that does not enhance significantly. If infected or if there is a history of infection, the cyst may have a higher density with internal septations and rim enhancement.[33] On MRI the cysts have either low or high T1W signal intensity, high T2W signal intensity, and their rim usually enhances.

If a solid mass is seen in association with a presumed thyroglossal duct cyst, two entities should be considered: (1) ectopic thyroid tissue, which rarely may be seen within the cyst wall or tract, or (2) carcinoma, either papillary thyroid or squamous cell.[30,34] An ^{123}I thyroid scan may differentiate the two lesions. If ectopic thyroid tissue coexists within a thyroglossal duct cyst and if this tissue is the patient's only functioning thyroid tissue, its resection with the cyst will render the patient permanently hypothyroid.[29]

Malignancy, usually papillary adenocarcinoma, is a rare occurrence in a thyroglossal duct cyst. Most patients with thyroglossal duct cysts and associated malignancy are adults, but there are reports of carcinomas occurring in children as young as 6 years.[35,36]

The treatment of thyroglossal duct cysts is surgical excision using the Sistrunk procedure, in which the entire cyst, tract, and central body of the hyoid bone are resected en bloc.[37] If this procedure is not used, the recurrence rate is higher.

Ectopic thyroid tissue at the base of the tongue, known as lingual thyroid, is the most common location for ectopic thyroid to occur, yet it is a rare cause of stridor in the infant.[38-40] Of these patients, 70% have no other functioning thyroid tissue, and complete surgical resection may result in permanent hypothyroidism.[41,42] Congenital hypothyroidism and stridor suggest the diagnosis of lingual thyroid.[39] An ^{123}I scan, the diagnostic test of choice, shows uptake in the tongue base mass and can identify the presence of other thyroid tissue, usually in its normal location (Fig. 10-39). In most cases this is the only imaging test needed. If other imaging is required, ultrasound shows a solid mass, differentiating the ectopic thyroid from a thyroglossal duct cyst. Noncontrast-enhanced CT shows high-density mass at the tongue base.[41,43] Iodinated contrast should not be used in this setting if it is anticipated that radionuclide imaging will be needed to confirm the diagnosis. On MRI the lingual thyroid is hyperintense with respect to the intrinsic tongue muscles on both T1W and T2W images (Fig. 10-40).[44] Regardless of the test performed, imaging should include the thyroid bed in an attempt to identify thyroid tissue in its normal location.[43,44] Airway obstruction mandates surgical excision. Otherwise, hormonal suppression with thyroid hormone is the treatment of choice.

Miscellaneous

Various other cysts may occur in the tongue base and vallecula, including mucous retention cysts, vallecular cysts, or dermoids. A vallecular cyst, also known as mucous retention cyst, often has to be differentiated from ectopic thyroid or a thyroglossal duct cyst on imaging studies (Fig. 10-41). The vallecular cyst may be similar in appearance to a thyroglossal duct cyst or even a dermoid cyst, but it is easily distinguished from a solid mass such as ectopic thyroid.

The dermoid cyst is a rare benign congenital lesion, usually of epidermoid origin, which presents in infants as a midline neck mass or a lesion in the oral cavity. At surgery,

the dermoid cyst may be filled with a cheesy, white material containing skin, skin appendages, hair, or desquamated epithelium. Like the thyroglossal duct cyst, dermoid cysts usually are midline, but they are not adherent to the hyoid bone. CT or MRI shows an encapsulated mass in the floor of the mouth, similar in appearance to the thyroglossal duct cyst (Fig. 10-42). If focal regions of fat density (CT) or fat signal intensity (MRI) are seen within the cyst, the lesion is a dermoid.[45] Treatment is surgical excision.

Obstruction of a salivary gland duct may lead to an enlarging floor of the mouth or a tongue mass, known as a ranula. Imaging shows a cystic mass in the floor of the mouth or tongue (Fig. 10-43).

Oropharyngeal airway obstruction may result from hypoplasia of the mandible with resultant glossoptosis, or posterior displacement of the tongue.[46] Micrognathia, glossoptosis, and cleft palate are part of the Pierre Robin sequence, and respiratory obstruction is common because of glossoptosis.[47,48] Mandibular hypoplasia is also seen in Goldenhar's syndrome, mandibulofacial dysostosis, the cri du chat syndrome, and Treacher Collins syndrome (Fig. 10-44).

Cephalometrics are commonly obtained in patients with midface and mandibular anomalies. These plain radiographs, usually obtained in the surgeon's office with stan-

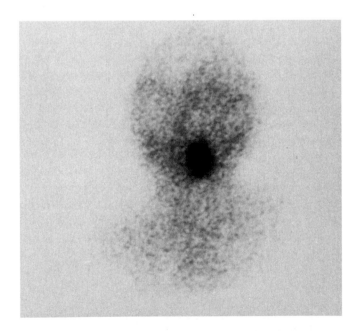

FIG. 10-39 Lingual thyroid, with no functioning thyroid gland in the thyroid bed. [123]I nuclear medicine scan, 1-year-old child with dysphagia. Notice uptake in the floor of the mouth, slightly eccentric to the left, with no radionuclide in the expected location of the thyroid gland. (Courtesy Dr. John Alarcon, Scottish Rite Children's Medical Center, Atlanta, Georgia.)

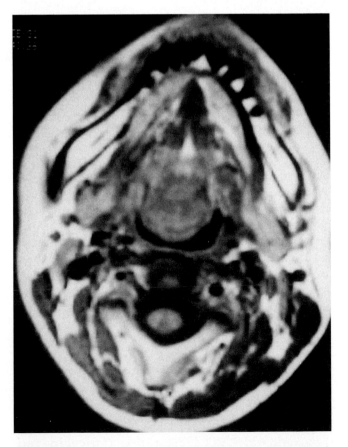

FIG. 10-40 Ectopic lingual thyroid. Adolescent with dysphagia and hypothyroidism. T1W MR image shows a tongue base mass that is isointense to hyperintense to tongue muscles. Notice flattening of the airway.

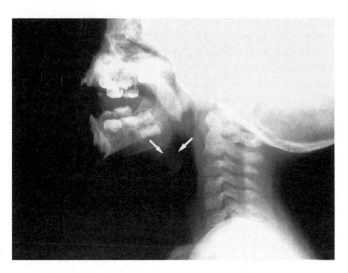

FIG. 10-41   Vallecular cyst in a young child with dysphagia. Lateral plain film reveals a smooth mass *(arrows)* anterior to the epiglottis.

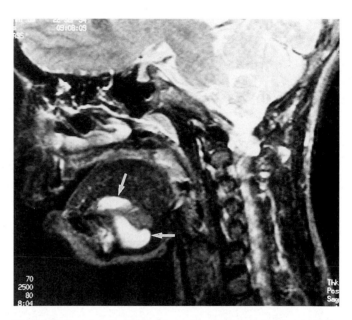

FIG. 10-43   Ranula, floor of mouth and tongue, 9-year-old child with macroglossia and progressive airway obstruction. T2W sagittal image shows a multiloculated high signal intensity mass *(arrows)* in the tongue, with obliteration of the oropharyngeal airway.

dard positioning and x-ray tube-film distances, are used to analyze the facial proportions based on specific osseous landmarks. Thin section high-resolution CT also may be obtained, and two-dimensional (2D) and 3D reformations can help contribute to the preoperative planning. Specific measurements usually are made by the clinician, depending on the clinical problem and planned corrective procedure. The mandible may be symmetrically small, pointed at the mental portion, or asymmetric with unilateral hypoplasia, which is known as hemifacial microsomia. The oropharyngeal airway may be narrowed by posterior displacement of the tongue (Fig. 10-44). Prominence of the adenotonsillar tissue should be noted because obstructive symptoms may be secondary to a combination of glossoptosis and adenotonsillar hypertrophy.[49]

Macroglossia can cause airway obstruction, especially in the supine position. The condition may be seen with cretinism, or congenital hypothyroidism, and the Beckwith-Wiedemann syndrome.[50-52]

LARYNGEAL OBSTRUCTION
Laryngomalacia

Laryngomalacia is the most common cause of stridor in the newborn and infant. The stridor is characteristically high-pitched and inspiratory and is most severe in the supine position.[53] the etiology is thought to be related to delayed development of neuromuscular control of the airway.[54] On direct laryngoscopic examination, laryngomalacia appears as floppy, immature laryngeal cartilaginous structures that are prolapsed or telescoped into the airway with inspiration.[55] Laryngomalacia is a benign, self-limited condi-

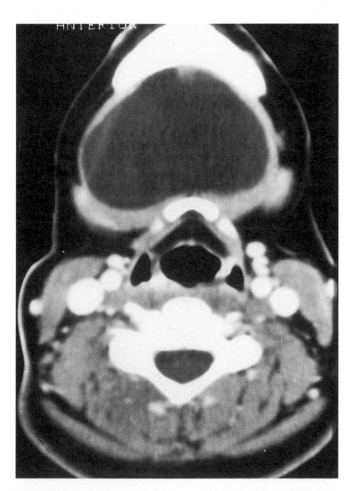

FIG. 10-42   Dermoid cyst, floor of the mouth. Young child with palpable neck mass. The midline neck mass is low density, nonenhancing, and indistinguishable from the more common thyroglossal duct cyst. If fat globules are seen within such a mass, the diagnosis of dermoid cyst can be made preoperatively.

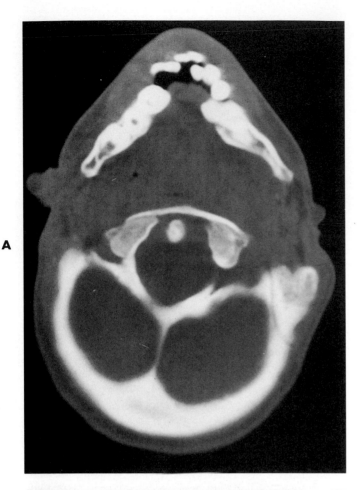

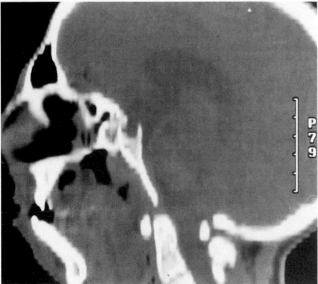

FIG. 10-44   Treacher-Collins syndrome, 16-year-old boy with retromicrognathia and airway obstruction. **A,** Axial CT shows symmetric mandibular hypoplasia, decreased mandibular angle, and complete obliteration of the oropharyngeal airway caused by retromicrognathia. **B,** Midsagittal CT reformation confirms the airway compromise and glossoptosis.

tion, and usually resolves by 18 months of age. Surgery is not indicated.

Flouroscopy or plain radiographs obtained during inspiration show inferior and medial bowing of the arytenoids, aryepiglottic folds, and epiglottis, with ballooning of the laryngeal ventricle and hypopharynx.[55,56] The diagnosis is confirmed with endoscopy.

Vocal Cord Paralysis

Vocal cord paralysis is the second most common cause of stridor in infancy.[57] A general rule is that bilateral vocal cord paralysis is often central in origin, and unilateral paralysis usually has a peripheral cause.[55]

Bilateral vocal cord paralysis is rarely seen in an otherwise normal child.[53] Brainstem malformations, particularly the Arnold-Chiari malformation, are the most common cause of vocal cord paralysis in children. These children present with nonprogressive airway obstruction and usually have bilateral paralysis. The most likely explanations for the paralysis are mechanical stretching of the vagus nerve from the brainstem herniation, congenital dysplasia of the brainstem, and lack of afferent information from the carotid bodies.[57]

Unilateral vocal cord paralysis is most commonly left-sided and is seen in children with congenital cardiac anomalies, following tracheoesophageal fistula repair or corrective surgery for congenital heart disease, and following trauma, particularly traumatic delivery.[54]

Airway fluoroscopy shows limited abduction with respiration or crying. With unilateral paralysis, the AP film shows the paralyzed cord is thinner and lower than the normal cord, the ventricle is usually capacious, and the ipsilateral pyriform sinus may be larger than the normal side. If the lateral plain film is obtained during phonation, two separate air-filled laryngeal ventricles may be seen; the ventricle on the paralyzed side being lower and usually larger than the ventricle on the normal side.[58] MRIs of the brain, posterior fossa, and skull base are important in the evaluation of bilateral paralysis because hydrocephalus, posterior fossa tumors with cerebellar tonsillar herniation, and dysmorphic structural changes of the Chiari II malformation are seen best on this examination. Chest radiographs and a barium swallow may show anomalies of the heart, mediastinum, or great vessels to explain unilateral vocal cord paralysis, and CT or MRI of the neck may be required to trace the entire course of the vagus nerve from the skull base to the larynx, thus excluding a neoplasm as a source of vagal nerve dysfunction.

Laryngoceles and Laryngeal Cysts

A laryngocele is an air-or fluid-filled dilation of the laryngeal ventricle, and it is a rare cause of airway obstruction in infants.[59-61] An internal laryngocele remains within the boundaries of the supraglottic laryngeal superstructure, and an external laryngocele, or combined laryngocele, the most common type, extends through the thyrohyoid membrane and has both an internal and external component. Plain films are often nonspecific, showing a supraglottic airway mass. However, an air collection in the lateral neck, projected over the supraglottic larynx is a highly suggestive finding. The external or combined laryngocele may present as a fluctuating, soft, lateral neck mass, and cross-sectional imaging shows the internal component submucosally filling the paraglottic space and obliterating the fat, and the external component, extending through the thyrohyoid membrane into the lateral neck (Fig. 10-45). The CT density or the MR signal intensity of the laryngocele is variable, depending on whether the cyst is filled with air, fluid, or proteinaceous debris.

The laryngeal or congenital cyst is also a laryngeal mass, but without communication with the airway. These benign lesions are fluid-filled, may be congenital or acquired, and are probably due to obstruction of mucous glands. The clinical presentation and radiographic appearance depends on the size and location of the mass within the airway. Saccular cysts may arise anywhere in the supraglottic larynx, the valleculae, or the tongue base. Plain films show a smooth mass projecting into the airway (Fig. 10-46).[62,63] Typically on CT, laryngeal cysts are well-circumscribed, submucosal, low-density, nonenhancing masses. On MR the signal intensities vary. The T1W signal intensity is usually low (water) but may be high (infection or hemorrhage), and the T2W signal intensity is high. Treatment for both laryngoceles and laryngeal cysts is surgical resection.[55]

Laryngeal Webs and Atresia

A laryngeal web is a membrane that partially occludes the airway lumen and results from failure of recannulation during embryogenesis.[55,62] Although laryngeal webs may occur anywhere in the larynx, most are at the glottic level, usually involving the anterior commissure. Presenting signs depend on the location and the degree of airway obstruction, and they include stridor, hoarseness, weak voice, or feeding difficul-

ties.[56] Endoscopy is the mainstay of diagnosis, but plain films may occasionally show a web of tissue within the airway.

Laryngeal atresia may occur at the supraglottic or glottic level and is extremely rare. The etiology is probably failure of recanalization of the larynx in the first trimester.[55] Unless the lesion is recognized and an immediate tracheotomy is performed, survival is unlikely. Imaging plays little role in the management of this lesion.

SUBGLOTTIC OBSTRUCTION
Congenital Subglottic Stenosis

Congenital subglottic stenosis is the third most common congenital laryngeal abnormality and is the most common lesion requiring tracheotomy in infants under 1 year of age.[56] Infants may present with stridor or recurrent "laryngotracheobronchitis," without a history of prior intubation or other cause of acquired subglottic stenosis. Congenital subglottic stenosis may be isolated or may be associated with congenital syndromes, especially trisomy 21, in which case the entire larynx is small.[62] Of infants with congenital sub-

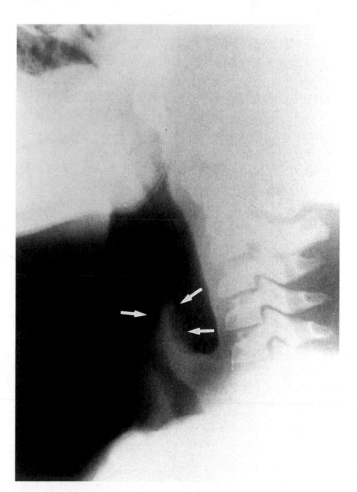

FIG. 10-46 Cyst of the aryepiglottic fold in an infant with respiratory distress. A smooth, well-circumscribed mass *(arrows)* is seen projecting into the supraglottic airway.

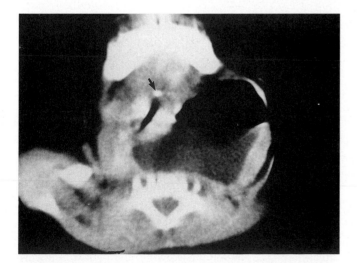

FIG. 10-45 External laryngocele. Full-term infant developed a neck mass and respiratory distress within the first week of life. Axial CT scan shows a large left neck mass with an air-fluid level and compression of the airway at the level of the hyoid bone *(arrow).*

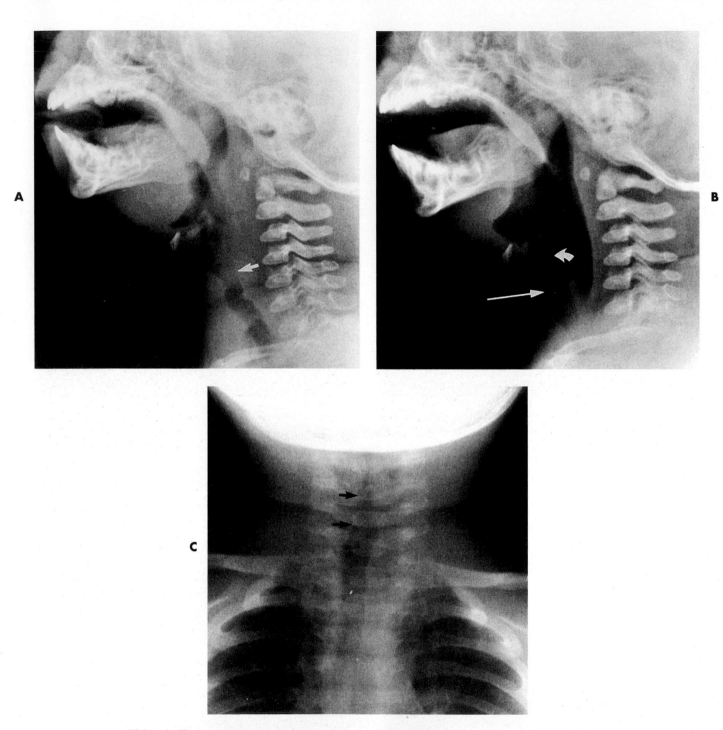

FIG. 10-47   Subglottic hemangioma, 6-month-old girl with recurrent bouts of "laryngotracheo-bronchitis." **A,** Expiratory film reveals a mass in the subglottic airway *(arrow).* **B,** With inspiration, there is distention of the pharynx due to the laryngeal obstruction. This is a nonspecific appearance seen with any obstructing laryngeal lesion. Notice the laryngeal ventricle *(long arrow)* and aryepiglottic folds *(curved arrow).* **C,** AP plain film shows mild asymmetric narrowing of the sub-glottic airway on the right *(arrows).*

glottic stenosis, 7% to 10% have other laryngotracheal anomalies such as tracheoesophageal fistula, vocal cord paralysis, or tracheal stenosis.[64]

The diagnosis of congenital subglottic stenosis is made on plain films and endoscopy. Plain films show symmetric circumferential subglottic narrowing, the typical hourglass appearance. This narrowing extends for 1 to 1.5 cm and is fixed, not changing with the phase of respiration.[65] The diagnosis is confirmed with endoscopy when the subglottic lumen is less than 3.5 mm in a newborn.[55]

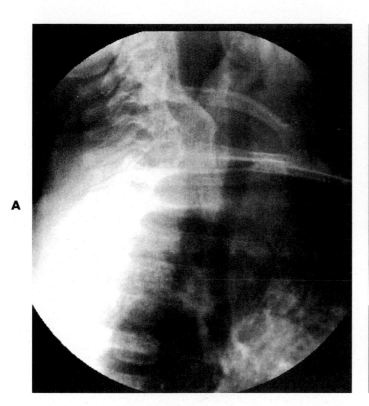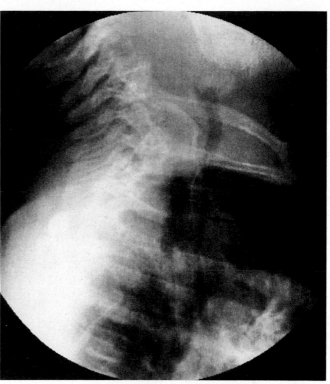

FIG. 10-48 Tracheobronchomalacia with innominate artery compressing the trachea, 5-month-old infant with stridor. **A,** Inspiratory oblique fluoroscopic film shows normal tracheal diameter. **B,** Same projection, obtained during end expiration. Noted marked collapse of the entire trachea *(arrow)* most severe at the expected location of the innominate artery.

The lesion is generally self-limited, resolving with laryngeal growth.[66] However, tracheotomy is often required. Laryngotracheal reconstruction may be necessary if the subglottic airway does not enlarge enough to allow decannulation.

Subglottic Hemangioma

Hemangiomas are congenital vascular malformations, which are commonly found in the head and neck, that can usually be treated conservatively. However, a hemangioma located in the subglottis may cause stridor and airway obstruction.[67] Like congenital subglottic stenosis, before the correct diagnosis is made, the patient may have repeated episodes of "viral laryngotracheobronchitis." Most lesions present within the first 6 months of life. Growth of the hemangioma over 6 to 18 months followed by spontaneous regression is characteristic.[55] Females are affected twice as often as are males, and 50% of affected infants also have cutaneous hemangiomas.[68]

The AP radiograph shows subglottic narrowing, which is classically asymmetric, unlike the concentric symmetric narrowing of congenital subglottic stenosis.[62,69] However, 50% of the time the subglottic narrowing may be symmetric.[70] The lateral film shows a subglottic mass (Fig. 10-47).

The lesion may regress during the second or third year of life. Treatment modalities include steroids, interferon, tracheotomy, and endoscopic ablation with the CO_2 laser.

TRACHEAL OBSTRUCTION
Tracheobronchomalacia

Tracheobronchomalacia (TBM) is an inherent weakness in the structural integrity of the tracheobronchial tree that results in partial or total collapse of the airway and respiratory embarrassment. Patients may experience stridor, wheezing, chronic cough, anoxic spells, and failure to thrive. TBM is often associated with prematurity and prolonged ventilation and may be considered an acquired condition.[71] Because of extrinsic tracheal compression, certain congenital conditions result in secondary TBM. These include aortic vascular rings, aberrant innominate artery compression, and the pulmonary artery sling in which the left pulmonary artery arises aberrantly from the posterior aspect of the right pulmonary artery and passes over the right mainstem bronchus. Secondary congenital TBM may also result from mediastinal masses, esophageal atresia with a dilated pouch, and tracheoesophageal fistula.[65,72] The vascular compression may be alleviated by aortopexy, but complete resolution of respiratory symptoms may be delayed by persistent tracheocartilage deformity.[73] Primary congenital TBM as an isolated lesion is a rare disorder that is due to congenital immaturity of the tracheobronchial cartilages. It usually resolves spontaneously by the second year of life, without surgery.[73] The most severe cases of TBM require tracheotomy or aortopexy to maintain a patent airway.

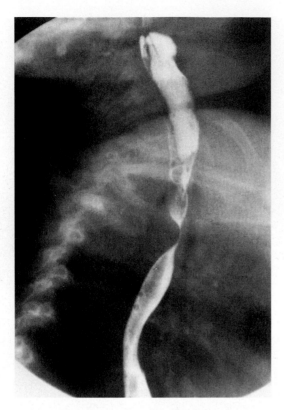

FIG. 10-49 Tracheobronchomalacia resulting from a double aortic arch 11-month-old child with stridor. Extrinsic compression on the posterior esophagus suggests a vascular ring. This was a double aortic arch, confirmed at surgery.

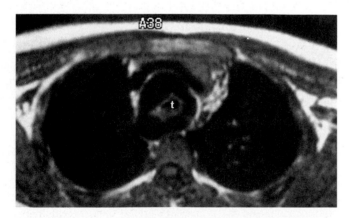

FIG. 10-50 Tracheal compression resulting from a double aortic arch, 10-year-old child with chronic airway obstuctive symptoms. T1W axial image obtained with respiratory compensation shows a vascular structure, the double aortic arch, encircling the trachea (t).

The innominate artery syndrome deserves special mention. The anterior tracheal wall may be compressed by the innominate artery as it crosses from the left to the right, ventral to the trachea, usually 1 to 2 cm above the carina.[74] The artery normally arises just to the left of or in front of the trachea.[75] The diagnosis is controversial because normal children without clinical evidence of airway compromise may

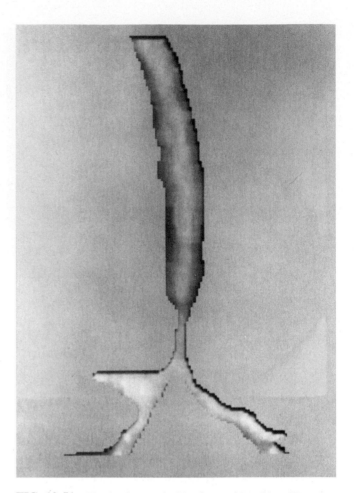

FIG. 10-51 Tracheal stenosis. Newborn with stridor. 3D reconstruction images of the trachea and carina were performed using a segmentation technique. T1W axial images were obtained of the airway, and then coronal reformations confirmed the tracheal narrowing and best showed the cranial-caudal extent of the lumen compromise. The length of narrowing was not appreciated at endoscopy because the endoscope could not pass the narrowed segment.

have, on fluoroscopy or plain films, prominent anterior tracheal impression at the level of the innominate artery.[76] Treatment usually involves aortopexy where the aortic arch is suspended to the undersurface of the sternum.

Although bronchoscopy is the mainstay in diagnosis, airway fluoroscopy can also confirm TBM. In a symptomatic child, when the tracheal diameter decreases more than 50% during expiration as compared with the diameter during inspiration, the diagnosis of congenital tracheomalacia can be made (Fig. 10-48).[77,78] The change in diameter during a respiratory cycle helps differentiate tracheomalacia from a fixed stenotic lesion. Barium swallow can suggest a compressive vascular ring by showing a persistent impression on the posterior esophagus (Fig. 10-49).[79] MRI or CT can show the narrowing in multiple planes, but MRI is the preferred test if plain films or barium swallow suggest that the TBM is due to a vascular ring or sling (Fig. 10-50).[80] MRI is obtained using respiratory compensation techniques, and

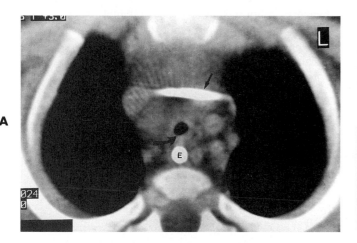

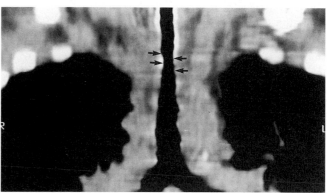

FIG. 10-52 Congenital tracheal stenosis. This 2½-year-old boy had stridor. **A,** Axial spiral CT scan obtained immediately below the endotracheal tube shows a central venous line *(arrow)* and a nasogastric tube in the esophagus *(E)*. The posterior membranous portion of the trachea is not flat but has a rounded contour *(curved arrow)*. **B,** Coronal reformation shows the extent of the tracheal narrowing.

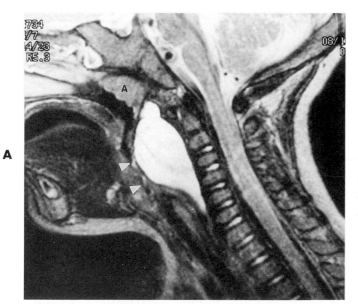

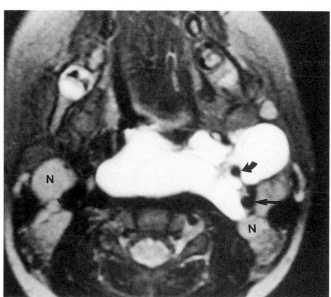

FIG. 10-53 Cystic hygroma. Child with chronic stridor and a neck mass. **A,** T2W FSE image shows the boundaries of the hyperintense mass and the airway narrowing *(arrowheads)*. Adenoids *(A)*. **B,** On this T2W FSE axial image the diffuse infiltrative nature of the mass is displayed, with the lesion insinuating between the internal *(straight arrow)* and external *(curved arrow)* carotid arteries. The cystic hygroma is markedly hyperintense compared with reactive cervical lymph nodes *(N)*.

data are acquired primarily during expiration.[77] 3D reconstruction images may illustrate the degree of compression and the relationship of the extrinsic structures to the trachea (Fig. 10-51).

Tracheal Stenosis

Congenital tracheal stenosis is due to one or more complete cartilaginous tracheal rings. In these rings the normal membranous posterior wall is lacking, and the tracheal airway has a circular shape rather than the normal horseshoe-shaped, cross-sectional configuration.[74,81] The caliber of the distal tracheal airway is reduced, resulting in severe respiratory symptoms. The newborn with congenital tracheal stenosis may be relatively symptom free. However, symptoms worsen as the child outgrows the capacity of the stenotic airway to maintain ventilation.[82]

Plain films either may be normal and underestimate the narrowing or may show a narrowed tracheal air column.[83] Cross-sectional imaging shows a rounded appearance to the trachea, instead of the normal posterior membranous flattening (Fig. 10-52).

Prognosis and treatment depend on the degree and extent of stenosis, with the more severely affected infants requiring early surgical intervention.[84] Surgical options include balloon dilatation, tracheotomy, resection and primary anastomosis, or pericardial patch tracheoplasty.[85-87]

NECK
Cystic Hygroma or Lymphangioma

Lymphangiomas are congenital malformations that may present with airway obstruction, although more commonly they present as soft, mobile, compressible external neck masses, usually in the first 2 years of life.[88-91]

Lymphangiomas probably occur when the embryonic lymph sacs are sequestered and fail to develop normal drainage into the venous system, specifically the jugular vein.[92] Histopathologically, lymphangiomas may be classified based on the size and extent of the abnormal lymphatic channels, and in increasing order of complexity they are as follows: the lyphangioma simplex, the cavernous lymphangioma, and the cystic hygroma.[93] Cystic hygroma, the most complex form of lymphangioma, is composed of lymphatic tissue with large multiloculated cystic spaces.

Most lymphangiomas are found in the posterior triangle of the neck. Less commonly they occur in the anterior triangle or submandibular space. When lymphangiomas occur in the floor of the mouth tongue, oropharynx, hypopharynx, or larynx, they may lead to upper airway obstruction. Typically these lesions follow no predictable pattern but insinuate themselves throughout normal structures in the neck.[29]

The CT and MR appearance is variable, ranging from a small unilocular cyst to an extensive, multiloculated septated mass. The margins may be discrete, or poorly circumscribed. Extension to the retropharyngeal space is seen often, making cystic hygroma the most common mass in the retropharyngeal space in childhood.[50] Characteristically the mass does not displace normal structures but may itself be effaced by the surrounding structures. Peripheral enhancement generally is not seen unless there is a history of infection or surgery. On CT, lymphangiomas are low or water density.[94,95] MR signal intensities may be variable on T1W images, ranging from low to high (if the lesion is proteinaceous or hemorrhagic). Usually there is a high T2W signal intensity. Fluid-fluid levels also may be seen in the cystic hygroma (Fig. 10-53).

Treatment of lymphangiomas, especially when airway obstruction occurs, is surgical. CT and MRI are important in the preoperative evaluation to show the complete extent of the lesion. Incomplete resection or recurrence is common and may be partially obviated by accurate preoperative mapping of the lesion.

References

1. Derkay CS, Grundfast KM. Airway compromise from nasal obstruction in neonates and infants. Int J Pediatr Otorhinolaryngol 1990; 19:241-249.
2. Chinwuba C, Wallman J, Strand R. Nasal airway obstruction: CT assessment. Radiology 1986; 159:503-506.
3. Hengerer AS, Strome M. Choanal atresia: a new embryologic theory and its influence on surgical management. Laryngoscope 1982; 92:913-921.
4. Freng A. Congenital choanal atresia. Scand J Plast Reconstr Surg 1978;

12:261-265.
5. Castillo M. Congenital abnormalities of the nose: CT and MR findings. AJR 1994; 162:1211-1217.
6. Wetmore RF, Mahboubi S. Computed tomography in the evaluation of choanal atresia. Int Pediatr Otorhinolaryngol 1986; 11:265-274.
7. Crockett DM, Healy GB, McGill TJ, et al. Computed tomography in the evaluation of choanal atresia in infants and children. Laryngoscope 1987; 97:174-183.
8. Slovis TL Renfro, B, Watts FB, et al.

Choanal atresia: precise CT evaluation. Radiology 1985; 155:345-348.
9. Castillo M, Merten DF, Weissler MC. Bilateral nasolacrimal duct mucocele, a rare cause of respiratory distress: CT findings in two newborns. AJNR Am J Neuroradiol 1993; 14:1011-1013.
10. Arlis H, Ward RF. Congenital nasal pyriform aperture stenosis. Arch Otolaryngol Head Neck Surg 1992; 118:989-991.
11. Brown OE, Myer CM III, Manning SC. Congenital nasal pyriform aper-

ture stenosis. Laryngoscope 1989; 99:86-91.

12. Bignault A, Castillo M. Congenital nasal piriform aperture stenosis. AJNR AM J Neuroradiol 1994; 15:877-878.

13. Ey EH, Han BK, Towbin RB, et al. Bony inlet stenosis as a cause of nasal airway obstruction. Radiology 1988; 168:477-479.

14. Smith JK, et al. Imaging of bucconasal atresia. Submitted to AJNR, 1994.

15. Mood GF. Congenital anterior herniations of brain. Ann Otol Rhinol Laryngol 1938; 47:391-401.

16. Suwanwela C, Hongsaprabhas C. Fronto-ethomoidal encephalomeningocele. J Neurosurg 1966; 25:172-182.

17. Rapport RL, Dunn RC Jr, Alhady F. Anterior encephalocele. J Neurosurg 1981; 54:213-219.

18. Schmidt PH, Luyendijk W. Intranasal meningoencephalocele. Arch Otolaryngol 1974; 99:402-405.

19. Ziter FMH, Bramwit DN. Nasal encephaloceles and gliomas. Br J Radiol 1970; 43:136-138.

20. Choudhury AR, Taylor JC. Primary intranasal encephalocele. J Neurosurg 1982; 57:552-555.

21. Lusk RP, Lee PC. Magnetic resonance imaging of congenital midline nasal masses. Otolaryngol Head Neck Surg 1986; 95:303-306.

22. Paller AS, Pensler JM, Tomita T. Nasal midline masses in infants and children. Arch Dermatol 1991; 127:362-366.

23. Barkovich AJ, Vandermarck P, Edwards MS, et al. Congenital nasal masses: CT and MR imaging features in 16 cases. AJNR Am J Neuroradiol 1991; 12:105-116.

24. Larson C, Hudgins PA, Hunter SB. Skull base meningoencephalocele presenting as a unilateral neck mass in a neonate. Am J Neuroradiol 1995; 16:1161-1163.

25. Whitaker SR, Sprinkle PM, Chou SM. Nasal glioma. Otolaryngol 1981; 107:550-554.

26. Gorenstein A, Kern EB, Facer GW, et al. Nasal gliomas. Arch Otolaryngol 1980; 106:536-540.

27. Warren DW, Hairfield WM, Dalston ET, et al. Effects of cleft lip and palate on the nasal airway in children. Arch Otolaryngol Head Neck Surg 1988; 114:987-992.

28. Drake AF, Davis JU, Warren DW. Nasal airway size in cleft and non-cleft children. Laryngoscope 1993; 103:915-917.

29. Todd NW. Common congenital anomalies of the neck. Embryology and surgical anatomy. Surg Clin North Am 1993; 73:599-610.

30. Telander RL, Deane SA. Thyroglossal and branchial cleft cysts and sinuses. Surg Clin North Am 1977; 57:779-791.

31. Hawkins DB, Jacobsen BE, Klatt EC. Cysts of the thyroglossal duct. Laryngoscope 1982; 92:1254-1258.

32. Lofgren RG. Respiratory distress from congenital lingual cysts. Am J Dis Child 1963; 106:610-612.

33. Reede DL, Bergeron RT, Som PM. CT of thyroglossal duct cysts. Radiology 1985; 157:121-125.

34. Solomon JR, Rangecroft L. Thyroglossal-duct lesions in childhood. J Pediat Surg 1984; 19:555-561.

35. Butler EC, Dickey JR, Shill Os Jr, et al. Carcinoma of the thyroglossal duct remnant. Laryngoscope 1969; 79:264-271.

36. Bhagavan BS, Rao DRG, Weinberg T. Carcinoma of thyroglossal duct cyst: case reports and review of the literature. Surgery 1970; 67:281-292.

37. Sistrunk WE. The surgical treatment of cysts of the thyroglossal tract. Ann Surg 1920; 71:121.

38. Maddern BR, Werkhaven J, McBride T. Lingual thyroid in a young infant presenting as airway obstruction: report of a case. Int J Pediatr Otorhinolaryngol 1988; 16:77-82.

39. Chan FL, Low LC, Yeung HW, et al. Case report: lingual thyroid, a cause of neonatal stridor. Br J Radiol 1993; 66:462-464.

40. Mahboubi S, Tenore A, Kirkpatrick JA. Diagnosis of ectopic thyroid: value of pretracheal soft-tissue measurements. AJR Am J Roentgenol 1981; 137:717-719.

41. Kansal P, Sakati N, Rifai A, et al. Lingual thyroid: diagnosis and treatment. Arch Intern Med 1987; 147:2046-2048.

42. Radkowski D, Arnold J, Healy GB, et al. Thyroglossal duct remnants: preoperative evaluation and management. Arch Otolaryngol Head Neck Surg 1991; 117:1378-1381.

43. Guneri A, Ceryan K, Igci E, et al. Lingual thyroid: the diagnostic value of magnetic resonance imaging. J Laryngol Otol 1991; 105:493-495.

44. Johnson JC, Coleman LL. Magnetic resonance imaging of a lingual thyroid gland. Pediatr Radiol 1989; 19:461-462.

45. Hunter TB, Paplanus SH, Chernin MM, et al. Dermoid cyst of the floor of the mouth: CT appearance. AJR Am J Roentgenol 1983; 141:1239-1240.

46. Puckett CL, Pickens J, Reinisch JF. Sleep apnea in mandibular hypoplasia. Plast Reconst Surg 1982; 70:213-216.

47. Heaf DP, Helms PJ, Dinwiddie R, et al. Nasopharyngeal airways in Pierre Robin syndrome. 1982; 100:698-703.

48. Jeresaty RM, Huszar RJ, Basu S. Pierre Robin Syndrome. Cause of respiratory obstruction, cor pulmonale, and pulmonary edema. Am J Diseased Child 1969; 117:710-716.

49. Crysdale WS. Malformations and syndromes. In: Bluestone CD, Stool SE, eds. 2nd Edition. Pediatric otolaryngology. Vol. 1. Philadelphia, Pa: WB Saunders, 1990.

50. Swischuk LE, Smith PC, Fagan CJ. Abnormalities of the pharynx and larynx in childhood. Seminars in Roentgenology 1974; 9:283-300.

51. Lodeiro JG, Byers JW, Chuipek S, et al. Prenatal diagnosis and perinatal management of the Beckwith-Wiedeman syndrome: a case and review. Am J Perinatol 1989; 6:446-449.

52. Pettenati MJ, Haines JL, Higgins RR, et al. Beckwith-Wiedemann syndrome: presentation of clinical and cytogenetic data on 22 new cases and review of the literature. Human Genetics 1986; 74:143-154.

53. Holinger PH, Brown WT. Congenital webs, cysts, laryngoceles and other anomalies of the larynx. Ann Otol Rhinol Laryngol 1976; 76:744-752.

54. Belmont JR, Grundfast K. Congenital laryngeal stridor (laryngomalacia): etiologic factors and associated disorders. Ann Otol Rhinol Laryngol 1984; 93:430-437.

55. Cotton RT, Reilly JS. Congenital malformations of the larynx. In: Bluestone CD, Stool SE, eds. Pediatric otolaryngology. 2nd Edition. Philadelphia, Pa: WB Saunders, 1990; 1121-1128.

56. Smith RJH, Catlin FL. Congenital anomalies of the larynx. Am J Diseased Child 1984; 138:35-39.

57. Grundfast KM. Vocal cord paralysis. Otolaryngol Clin North Am 1989; 22:569-597.

58. Bachman AL. Benign, non-neoplastic conditions of the larynx and pharynx. Radiol Clin North Am 1978; 16:273-290.

59. Chu L, Gussack GS, Orr JB, et al. Neonatal laryngoceles: a cause for airway obstruction. Arch Otolaryngol Head Neck Surg 1994; 120:454-458.

60. Donegan JO, et al. Internal laryngocele and saccular cysts in children. Ann Otol Rhinol Laryngol 1980; 89:409-413.

61. Holinger LD, Barnes DR, Smid LJ, et al. Laryngocele and saccular cysts. Ann Otol 1978; 87:675-685.

62. Cotton RT, Richardson MA: Congenital laryngeal anomalies. Otolaryngol Clin North Am 1981; 14:203-218.

63. Shackelford GD, McAlister WH. Congenital laryngeal cyst. AJR Am J Roentgenol 1972; 114:289-292.

64. Marshak G, Grundfast KM. subglottic stenosis. Pediatr Clin North Am 1981; 28-941-947.

65. John SD, Swischuk LE. Stridor and upper airway obstruction in infants and children. Radiographics 1992; 12:625-643.

66. Holinger LD, Oppenheimer RW. Congenital subglottic stenosis: the elliptical cricoid cartilage. Ann Otol Rhinol Laryngol 1989; 98:702-706.

67. Benjamin B, Carter P. Congenital laryngeal hemangioma. Ann Otol Rhinol Laryngol 1983; 92:448-455.

68. Leikensohn JR, Benton C, Cotton R. Subglottic hemangioma. Otolaryngol 1976; 5:487-492.

69. Sutton TJ, Nogrady MB. Radiologic diagnosis of subglottic hemangioma in infants. Pediatr Radiol 1973; 1:211-216.

70. Cooper M, Slovis TL, Madgy DN, et al. Congenital subglottic hemangioma: frequency of symmetric subglottic narrowing on frontal radiographs of the neck. AJR Am J Roentgenol 1992; 159:1269-1271.

71. Jacobs IN, Wetmore RF, Tom LW, et al. Tracheobronchomalacia in children. Arch Otolaryngol Head Neck Surg 1994; 120:154-158.

72. Schwartz M, Filler R, et al. Tracheal compression as a cause of apnea following repair of tracheoesophageal fistula: treatment by aortopexy. J Pediatr Surg 1980; 15:842-848.

73. Schild JA. Congenital malformations of the trachea and bronchi. In: Bluestone CD, Stool SE, eds. Pediatric otolaryngology. Philadelphia, Pa: WB Saunders, 1990; 1129-1151.

74. Chen J-C, Holinger LD. Congenital tracheal anomalies: pathology study using serial macrosections and review of the literature. Pediatr Pathol 1994; 14:513-537.

75. Strife JL, Baumel AS, Dunbar JS. Tracheal compression by the innominate artery in infancy and childhood. Radiology 1981; 139:73-75.

76. Swischuk LE. Anterior tracheal indentation in infancy and early childhood: normal or abnormal? Am J Roentgenol Radium Ther Nucl Med 1971; 112:12-17.

77. Simoneaux SF, et al. MR imaging of the pediatric airway. Radiographics 1994 (in press).

78. Wittenborg MH, Gyepes MT, Crocker D. Tracheal dynamics in infants with respiratory distress, stridor, and collapsing trachea. Radiology 1967; 88:653-662.

79. Macpherson RI, Leithiser RE. Upper airway obstruction in children: an update. Radiographics 1985; 5(3):339-376.

80. Fletcher BD, Dearborn DG, Mulopulos GP. MR imaging in infants with airway obstruction: preliminary observations. Radiology 1986; 160:245-249.

81. Loeff DS, Filler RM, Vinograd I, et al. Congenital tracheal stenosis: a review of 22 patients from 1965-1987. J Pediatr Surg 1988; 23:744-748.

82. Cosentino CM, Backer CL, Idriss FS, et al. Pericardial patch tracheoplasty for severe tracheal stenosis in a child: intermediate results. J Pediatr Surg 1991; 26:879-884.

83. Hedlund GL, Kirks DR. Respiratory system. In: Kirks DR, ed. Practical pediatric imaging: diagnostic radiology of infants and children. Boston, Mass: Little, Brown & Co Inc, 1991.

84. Campbell DN, Lilly JR. Surgery for total congenital tracheal stenosis. J Pediatr Surg 1986; 21:934-935.

85. Longaker MT, Harrison M, Adzick NS. Testing the limits of neonatal tracheal resection. J Pediatr Surg 1990; 25:790-792.

86. Nakayama DK, Harrison MR, de Lorimier AA, et al. Reconstructive surgery for obstructing lesions of the intrathoracic trachea in infants and small children. J Pediatr Surg 1982; 17:854-868.

87. Hebra A, Powell DD, Smith CD, et al. Balloon tracheoplasty in children: results of a 15 year experience. J Pediatr Surg 1991; 26:957-961.

88. Barrand KG, Freeman NV. Massive infiltrating cystic hygroma of the neck in infancy. Arch Dis Child 1973; 48:523-531.

89. Barnhart RA, Brown AK Jr. Cystic hygroma of the neck. Arch Otolaryngol 1967; 86:74-78.

90. Kennedy TL. Cystic hygroma-lymphangioma: a rare and still unclear entity. Laryngoscope 1989; 99 (Suppl):1-10.

91. Singh S, Baboo ML, Pathak IC. Cystic lymphangioma in children: report of 32 cases including lesions at rare sites. Surgery 1971; 69:947-951.

92. Chervenak FA, Isaacson G, Blakemore KJ, et al. Fetal cystic hygroma: cause and natural history. N Engl J Med 1983; 309:822-825.

93. Landing BH, Farber S. Tumors of the cardiovascular system. Atlas of Tumor Pathology. Washington, DC: Armed Forces Institute of Pathology, 1956.

94. Silverman PM, Korobkin M, Moore AV. CT diagnosis of cystic hygroma of the neck. Journal of Computed Axial Tomography 1983; 7:519-520.

95. Zadvinskis DP, Benson MT, Kerr HH, et al. Congenital malformations of the cervico-thoracic lymphatic system: embryology and pathogenesis. Radiographics 1992; 12:1175-1189.

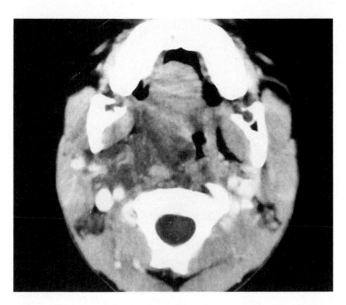

FIG. 10-54 Peritonsillar abscess in a child with fever, trismus, and dysphagia. Axial contrast-enhanced CT shows inflammatory process in right oropharynx, obliterating parapharyngeal space and deviating carotid artery and jugular vein posterolaterally. Although a discrete peripherally enhancing rim was not seen, surgery revealed a parapharyngeal space abscess.

SECTION SIX
INFECTIOUS AND INFLAMMATORY CONDITIONS

TONSILLITIS, PERITONSILLAR AND RETROPHARYNGEAL ABSCESS

Tonsillitis, or adenotonsillitis, is usually a self-limited infection that may be viral or bacterial in origin. Bacterial organisms responsible for tonsillitis include beta-hemolytic streptococcus, *Staphylococcus aureus, Haemophilus influenzae* and bacteroides.[1] Mononucleosis is a disease of adolescence characterized by tonsillitis, cervical adenopathy, and hepatosplenomegaly. Imaging is rarely performed for uncomplicated tonsillitis. Severe tonsillitis may occasionally suppurate, with infection and pus extending between the tonsillar capsule and the anterior and posterior tonsillar pillars, resulting in the peritonsillar abscess. It is usually unilateral, presenting with displacement of the tonsil medially and deviation of the uvula to the opposite side. Uncomplicated peritonsillar abscesses are often surgically drained without preoperative imaging because the clinical presentation is classic.

A peritonsillar abscess may spread around or through the superior constrictor muscle, into the parapharyngeal space, leading to a parapharyngeal space abscess. This results in more severe symptoms that may include torticollis, trismus, and a lateral neck mass. When a parapharyngeal space

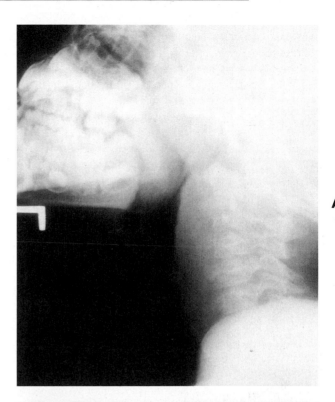

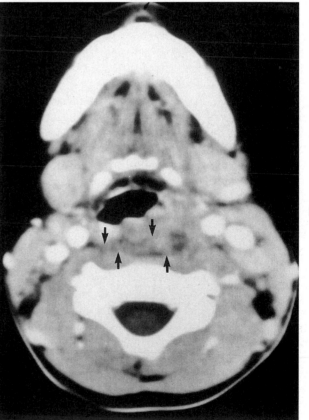

FIG. 10-55 Retropharyngeal abscess secondary to suppurative lymphadenitis of the retropharyngeal nodes, young child with fever and dysphagia. **A,** Lateral plain film reveals diffuse widening of the retropharyngeal soft tissues. **B,** On this axial contrast-enhanced CT obtained the same day as **A,** note the enhancing inflammatory debris *(arrows)* in the retropharyngeal space. Pus was found at surgery.

abscess is clinically suspected, contrast-enhanced CT is obtained primarily to differentiate cellulitis from an abscess.[2] CT shows distortion and increased density of the fat in the parapharyngeal space, distortion of the normal structures in the masticator space, and the mass may displace the carotid artery and jugular vein posterolaterally (Fig. 10-54). A frank abscess shows peripheral enhancement around a low-density central collection.[3] The pharyngeal wall on the affected side is displaced toward the midline, possibly causing airway obstruction.

However, most deep-space neck infections in children are secondary to suppurative lymph nodes. Infections of the nasopharynx or tonsil may involve the lymph nodes, which can suppurate and perforate into the parapharyngeal or retropharyngeal spaces. Clinically the child or young adult has pharyngeal pain, dysphagia, opisthotonus, drooling, and appears toxic. Plain films or CT scans are indicated when a deep-space abscess is suspected.

Lateral plain films show widening of the prevertebral soft tissues if the infection has perforated into the retropharyngeal space or involves the retropharyngeal lymph nodes (Fig. 10-55). CT and MR show that the involved node is enlarged and often has a low-density center with a peripheral enhancing rim (Fig. 10-56). If a deep-neck cellulitis has developed, CT and MRI show phlegmonous changes with fullness and distortion of the soft tissues in the lateral and posterior pharyngeal regions and the deep spaces, including the parapharyngeal and masticator spaces. There may be spasm of the ipsilateral internal carotid artery, which appears smaller in diameter than the contralateral artery on contrast-enhanced CT or MR (Fig. 10-57). Intravenous contrast is helpful for differentiating phlegmon from abscess. As with the abscessed lymph node, a neck abscess has a low-density center surrounded by an enhancing rim.[3] However, it may be difficult to differentiate edema within the retropharyngeal space from pus. The scan should be extended to the mediastinum to cover the full extent of the retropharyngeal space.

Adenitis without abscess may occasionally appear on CT as a hypodense mass, and in one series, ultrasound has been reported to be more sensitive than contrast-enhanced CT in differentiating a mature abscess from adenitis.[4] Surgical incision and drainage is indicated in a child with imaging findings of a deep-neck abscess. The extent of suppuration, the epicenter of the infection, the status of the internal carotid artery and jugular vein, and the degree of airway compromise are critical observations for the radiologist to urgently relay to the clinician.

SUPRAGLOTTITIS OR EPIGLOTTITIS

Supraglottitis, also known as *epiglottitis*, is an acute, potentially fulminant *Haemophilus influenzae* infection that occurs most commonly, though not exclusively, in children between 3 and 6 years of age. The infection typically presents with the rapid development of drooling, fever, sore

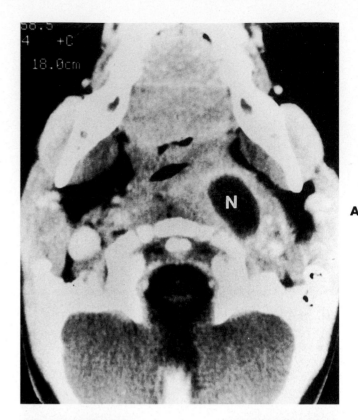

A

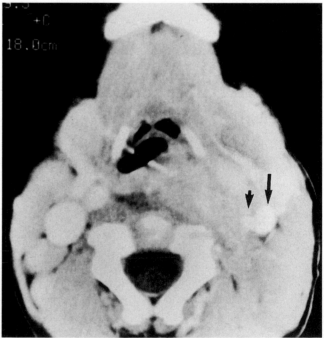

B

FIG. 10-56 Suppurative retropharyngeal lymphadenitis in an adolescent with severe sore throat and fever. **A,** Left retropharyngeal lymph node *(N)* is low density, with a peripheral enhancing rim, consistent with suppurative lymphadenitis. Note effacement of the airway. **B,** Axial scan at the level of the hyoid bone shows fluid in the retropharyngeal space and inflammatory changes in the deep neck, with lateral displacement of the carotid artery *(small arrow)* and jugular vein *(large arrow)*.

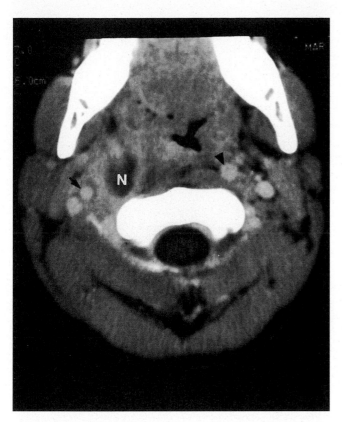

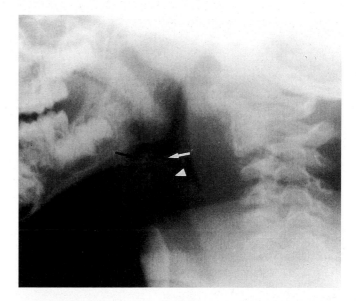

FIG. 10-58   Bacterial supraglottitis (epiglottitis) in a 2-year-old boy with respiratory distress and fever. Lateral plain film shows marked thickening of the epiglottis *(arrows)* and aryepiglottic folds *(arrowhead).*

FIG. 10-57   Suppurative retropharyngeal lymphadenitis, with spasm of the internal carotid artery in an adolescent with fever and dysphagia. Suppurative adenitis of the right retropharyngeal lymph node *(N)* and effacement of the airway are seen. Note that the right internal carotid artery *(arrow)* is displaced posterolaterally and is smaller in diameter than the left internal carotid artery *(arrowhead).* The patient had no neurologic dysfunction and was treated with surgical incision and drainage of the node and antibiotics. (Courtesy Dr. John Alarcon, Scottish Rite Children's Medical Center, Atlanta, Georgia.)

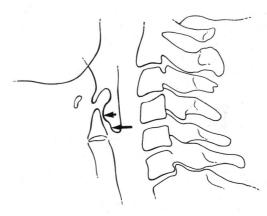

FIG. 10-59   Aryepiglottic fold width should be assessed at the midpoint *(short arrow)* of the folds. The base of the aryepiglottic folds *(large arrow)* may normally appear wider because of overlap with the arytenoid cartilage. (From John SD, et al. Aryepiglottic fold width in patients with epiglottitis: where should measurements be obtained? Radiology 1994; 190: 123-125.)

throat, and respiratory distress that may progress to complete airway obstruction.[5] Bacterial supraglottitis must be clinically differentiating from viral laryngotracheobronchitis (croup), an infection that is less severe because total airway obstruction is less likely. The diagnosis is based on clinical findings, lateral neck films, and endoscopic examination in the operating room. Treatment in children involves intravenous antibiotics, humidification, and possibly intubation.

Swelling of the epiglottis, aryepiglottic folds, false vocal cords, and arytenoids is characteristically seen in epiglottitis. Lateral radiographs may be obtained to help confirm the diagnosis and to exclude viral croup or an aspirated foreign body as the cause of airway compromise.[6,7] The child should be accompanied to the radiology department by personnel who are capable of intubation. The typical plain film findings include thickening of the free edge of the epiglottis, known as the "thumb sign," increased width of the aryepiglottic folds and arytenoids, and overdistention or ballooning of the hypopharynx (Fig. 10-58).[5,8] The aryepiglot-

tic fold width should be evaluated just behind the epiglottis or at the upper half of the folds because measurements taken at the base of the folds where they overlap with the arytenoids may overestimate the degree of swelling (Fig. 10-59).[9] Various ratios have been described to facilitate making a diagnosis. The most useful ratio is the aryepiglottic width to the third cervical vertebral body AP width (AEW/C3W), which, when 0.35 or greater, has been reported to be highly predic-

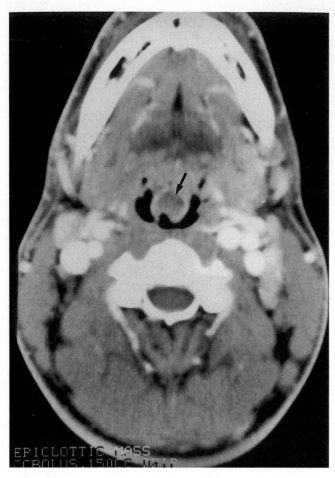

FIG. 10-60 Epiglottic abscess in an adolescent with severe sore throat. Axial contrast-enhanced CT shows a mass in the epiglottis *(arrow),* with partial airway obstruction. At surgery this was an epiglottic abscess.

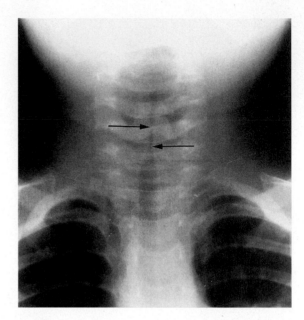

FIG. 10-61 Laryngotracheobronchitis in an 18-month-old boy. AP radiograph reveals the classic "steeple sign," with a long segment of airway narrowing at the glottic and subglottic level *(arrows)* and loss of the normal angle between the vocal cords and subglottic airway. Normally the craniocaudal height of the glottic narrowing is less than 1 cm.

tive of epiglottitis.[10] However, other series report that the sensitivity of lateral plain films for diagnosing epiglottitis is variable, ranging from 38% to nearly 100%.[9-12] The AP film is not routinely obtained if the lateral film is positive. The AP radiograph may be normal or may show narrowing of the subglottic region, a plain film finding similar in appearance to viral laryngotracheobronchitis.[13]

Bacterial epiglottitis is the most common cause of epiglottic enlargement in the pediatric population, but other considerations include angioneurotic edema, epiglottic trauma, caustic laryngeal burns, abscess or hemorrhage within the epiglottis (Fig. 10-60), radiation therapy, benign epiglottic lesions such as cysts or lymphangiomas, or chronic epiglottitis, a rare persistent inflammatory process.[14,15] The clinical presentation should aid in differentiating other lesions from acute bacterial epiglottitis.

LARYNGOTRACHEOBRONCHITIS, OR CROUP

Laryngotracheobronchitis, also known as croup, is an acute viral infection of the subglottic larynx that differs from epiglottitis in that it occurs in younger children (3

months to 3 years of age), and it has a less fulminant course with resolution of airway compromise within days, rarely requiring intubation.[16,17] The onset is gradual, with several days of upper or lower respiratory tract symptoms, followed by development of a classic barking, brassy cough and inspiratory stridor. Drooling and odynophagia are uncommon. Measles, which has not been eradicated but has reemerged as a significant pediatric pathogen, may also cause laryngotracheobronchitis.[18]

Mucosal edema has a dramatic effect in the subglottic larynx. The loosely attached mucosa at this level and the narrowed complete cricoid ring contribute to making this portion of the airway especially vulnerable to compromise. The radiographic appearance of laryngotracheobronchitis is variable, depending on the amount of edema and the phase of respiration during which the film is acquired. Plain films should be interpreted within the context of the clinical setting because the sensitivity and specificity of radiographs in croup has been reported to be low and may be more valuable in excluding other causes of airway obstruction such as a foreign body or bacterial epiglottitis.[19,20] Inspiratory plain films show ballooning and overdistention of the hypophar-

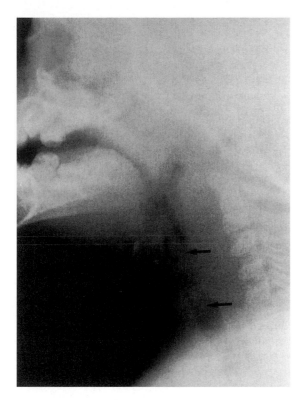

FIG. 10-62   Bacterial tracheitis in an infant. Lateral radiograph shows inflammatory debris and pseudomembranes *(arrows)* in the subglottic airway and cervical trachea. (From Gay, BR. Radiographic anatomy and pathology of the child's airway, Chapter 11. Murphy CH, Murphy MR, eds. Radiology for anesthesia and critical care. New York, Ny: Churchill Livingstone Inc, 1987.)

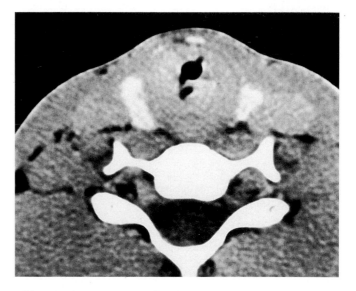

FIG. 10-63   Wegener's granulomatosis in a 17-year-old boy with stridor. Axial noncontrast-enhanced spiral CT scan shows a tracheal web and compromise of the airway lumen.

ynx, with narrowing of the subglottic region and collapse of the cervical trachea.[21] During expiration, overdistention of the cervical trachea, probably secondary to laryngeal obstruction, may be seen.[22] The vocal cords and larynx appear poorly defined. On the AP examination the subglottic region is narrowed for 1 to 2 cm (the "steeple sign"), a finding that does not vary significantly between inspiration and expiration (Fig. 10-61).[22] The epiglottis and aryepiglottic folds are normal, excluding epiglottitis.[23]

MISCELLANEOUS

Hereditary angioneurotic edema, a rare autosomal dominant disease, is due to a deficiency of C1 esterase inhibitor. Lack of this inhibitor leads to vascular damage, and the child presents with recurrent urticaria, subcutaneous soft-tissue swelling, and airway obstruction secondary to edema of the epiglottis and aryepiglottic folds.[15,14] The clinical setting helps differentiate this cause of airway obstruction from acute epiglottitis.

Thickening of the epiglottis and aryepiglottic folds may occur following radiation therapy for head and neck neoplasms, and it is due to mucositis or laryngeal edema.[24] The laryngeal structures are symmetrically thickened, and the paraglottic fat may be "dirty."

Bacterial tracheitis, usually caused by *Staphylococcus aureus*, is a rare cause of airway obstruction in children, but it is associated with high morbidity and mortality.[25] It may follow bronchopneumonia or viral laryngotracheitis, and it can progress to bacterial tracheitis, probably because of secondary bacterial invasion of the diseased tracheal mucosa.[26] Thick purulent tracheal secretions, pseudomembranes, and ulcerated mucosa are characteristic. Lateral plain films, although nonspecific, show narrowing of the subglottic airway with a normal epiglottis and aryepiglottic folds (Fig. 10-62).[27,28] Widespread vaccination has nearly eradicated diphtheria, a common organism responsible for supraglottitis and laryngotracheitis in the early 1900s.

Mucocutaneous candidiasis, parotid enlargement, and cervical adenopathy have been reported in pediatric patients with AIDS, but imaging of the airway is not usually necessary.[29,30]

Wegener's granulomatosis is a necrotizing vasculitis that causes inflammatory lesions, usually granulomas or areas of necrosis, is the respiratory tract and kidneys. Subglottic stenosis is a well-known manifestation of Wegener's in the pediatric population.[31] Tracheal stenosis causing stridor also may occur (Fig. 10-63).[32,33] Differential diagnosis includes sarcoidosis, amyloidosis, and relapsing polychondritis, all uncommon pediatric lesions.[34]

References

1. Shemen LJ. Diseases of the oropharynx. In: Lee KJ, ed. Textbook of otolaryngology and head and neck surgery. New York, NY: Elsevier Science Publishing Co Inc, 1989.

2. Patel KS, Ahmad S, O'Leary G, et al. The role of computed tomography in the management of peritonsillar abscess. Otolaryngol Head Neck Surg 1992; 107:727-732.

3. Nyberg DA, Jeffrey RB, Brant-Zawadzki M, et al. Computed tomography of cervical infections. Comput Assist Tomogr 1985; 9:288-296.

4. Glasier CM, et al. CT and ultrasound imaging of retropharyngeal abscesses in children. AJNR 1992; 13:1191-1195.

5. Poole CA, Altman DH. Acute epiglottitis in children. Radiology 1963; 80:798-805.

6. Rapkin RH. The diagnosis of epiglottitis: simplicity and reliability of radiographs of the neck in the differential diagnosis of the croup syndrome. J Pediatr 1972; 80:96-98.

7. Curtin HD. The larynx. In: Som PD, Bergeron RT, eds. Head and neck imaging. St. Louis, Mo: Mosby–Year Book, Inc. 1991.

8. Macpherson RI, Leithiser RE. Upper airway obstruction in children: an update. Radiographics 1985; 5(3):339-376.

9. John SD, Swischuk LE, Hayden CK Jr, et al. Aryepiglottic fold width in patients with epiglottitis: where should measurements be obtained? Radiology 1994; 190:123-125.

10. Rothrock SG, Pignatiello GA, Howard RM. Radiologic diagnosis of epiglottitis: objective criteria for all ages. Ann Emerg Med 1990; 19:978-982.

11. Stankiewicz JA, Bowes AK. Croup and epiglottitis: a radiologic study. Laryngoscope 1985; 95:1159-1160.

12. Jones JL, Holland P. False positives in lateral neck radiographs used to diagnose epiglottitis, Letter to the editor. Ann Emerg Med 1983; 12:797.

13. Shackelford GD, Siegel MJ, McAlister WH. Subglottic edema in acute epiglottitis in children. AJR Am J Roentgenol 1978; 131:603-605.

14. McCook TA, Kirks DR. Epiglottic enlargement in infants and children: another radiologic look. Pediatr Radiol 1982; 12:227-234.

15. Watts FB, Slovis TL. The enlarged epiglottis. Pediatr Radiol 1977; 5:133-136.

16. Myer CM III, Cotton RT. Pediatric airway and laryngeal problems. In: Lee KJ, ed. Textbook of otolaryngology and head and neck surgery. New York, NY: Elsevier Science Publishing Co Inc, 1989.

17. Fearon B. Acute laryngotracheobronchitis in infancy and childhood. Pediatr Clin of North Am 1962; 9:1095-1112.

18. Manning SC. An epidemic of upper airway obstruction. Otolaryngol Head Neck Surg 1991; 105:415-418.

19. Stankiewicz JA, Bowes AK. Croup and epiglottitis: a radiologic study. Laryngoscope 1985; 95:1159-1160.

20. Kushner DC, Clifton Harris GB. Obstructing lesions of the larynx and trachea in infants and children. Radiol Clin North Am 1978; 16:181-194.

21. Swischuk LE, Smith PC, Fagan CJ. Abnormalities of the pharynx and larynx in childhood. Seminars in Roentgenology 1974; 9:283-300.

22. Currarino G, Williams B. Lateral inspiration and expiration radiographs of the neck in children with laryngotracheitis (Croup). Radiology 1982; 145:365-366.

23. Rapkin RH. The diagnosis of epiglottitis: simplicity and reliability of radiographs of the neck in the differential diagnosis of the croup syndrome. J Pediatr 1972; 80:96-98.

24. Yousefzadeh DK, Tewfik HH, Franken Jr EA. Epiglottic enlargement following radiation treatment of head and neck tumors. J Pediatr Radiol 1981; 10:165-168.

25. Donaldson JD, Maltby CC. Bacterial tracheitis in children. J Otolaryngol 1989; 18:101-104.

26. Manning SC, Ridenour B, Brown OE, et al. Measles: An epidemic of upper airway obstruction. Otolaryngol Head Neck Surg 1991; 105:415-418.

27. Liston SL, Gehrz RC, Jarvis CW. Bacterial tracheitis. Arch Otolaryngol 1981; 107:561-564.

28. Jones R, Santos JI, Overall JC Jr. Bacterial tracheitism. JAMA 1979; 242:721-726.

29. Williams MA. Head and neck findings in pediatric acquired immune deficiency syndrome. Laryngoscope 1987; 97:713-716.

30. Rubinstein A, Sicklick M, Gupta A, et al. Acquired immunodeficiency with reversed T4/T8 ratios in infants born to promiscuous and drug-addicted mothers. JAMA 1983; 249:2350-2356.

31. Lebovics RS, Hoffman GS, Leavitt RY, et al. The management of subglottic stenosis in patients with Wegener's Granulomatosis. Laryngoscope 1992; 102:1341-1345.

32. Bohlman ME, Ensor RE, Goldman SM. Primary Wegener's Granulomatosis of the trachea: radiologic manifestations. South Med J 1984; 77:1318-1319.

33. McDonald TJ, Neel HB, DeRemee RA. Wegener's Granulomatosis of the subglottis and the upper portion of the trachea. Ann Otol Rhinol Laryngol 1982; 91:588-592.

34. Prasad S, Grundfast KW, Lipnick R. Airway obstruction in an adolescent with relapsing polychrondritis. Otolaryngol Head Neck Surg 1990; 103:113-116.

SECTION SEVEN
TRAUMA

DIRECT

The high position of the pediatric larynx, its mobility, and its flexibility make it less vulnerable or susceptible to blunt nonpenetrating trauma than the adult larynx.[1] The mechanism of injury is often a direct blow to the child's extended neck, for example, against the dashboard of the car or against the handlebars of a bicycle. The laryngeal injury may not be recognized initially during the posttraumatic period, and delay in recognition and treatment may result in chronic stenosis.[2]

Acutely, the injury may result in contusion, hematoma, edema, or airway laceration. Endoscopy and emergent tracheotomy are performed if complete or severe airway obstruction results. Endoscopic findings of laryngeal trauma include mucosal tears, hematomas, edema, immobile vocal cords, or cartilaginous fractures or dislocation, including cricoarytenoid disarticulation.[2] Partial airway obstruction, odynophagia, or hoarseness may be evaluated with plain films and CT in conjunction with endoscopy because endoscopy is limited when there is severe edema or blood in the endolaryngeal structures. The advantage of CT in this setting is its ability to display the soft-tissue structures, and it is considered the definitive radiographic method for evaluating the injured larynx.[3,4]

Edema, contusion, or laryngeal hematoma appears radiographically as swelling of the involved portion of the airway. Cervical or mediastinal emphysema suggests an esophageal or laryngeal laceration or a laryngeal fracture (Fig. 10-64).[5] In the unusual instance that MRI is performed, edema of the injured laryngeal structure has a high T2W signal intensity (Fig. 10-65). The degree and level of airway obstruction should be noted. Hyoid bone fracture can be detected on plain films and on CT. In the traumatized patient the epiglottis may be displaced posteriorly by edema or hematoma.[5] Other cartilaginous fractures are difficult to detect in the noncalcified pediatric larynx, but they may be clinically suspected because of an abnormal thyroid eminence or an abnormal endoscopic airway contour.

Tracheal transection is a life-threatening injury and carries a high mortality. If the transection occurs at the thyrohyoid ligament, the supraglottic muscles pull the hyoid bone superiorly, and this can be seen on plain films.[6-8] Transection or avulsion of the recurrent laryngeal nerves is a complication of laryngotracheal transection, and vocal cord paralysis may be a chronic problem if the patient survives the initial injury.[3] Plain films or coronal CT reformations show an increase in the craniocaudal extent of the larynx, as well as disruption of the tracheal air column.

Tracheal injuries or rupture from blunt trauma is not common but should be suspected with severe injury to the neck or chest.[5,9] Persistent pneumomediastinum or pneumothorax that is not relieved by thoracotomy tube may be

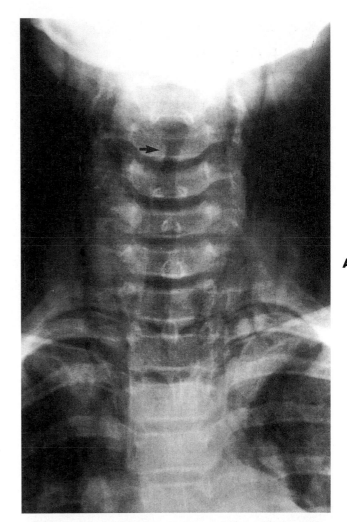

A

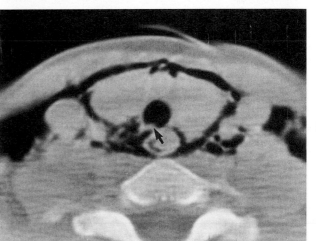

B

FIG. 10-64   Laryngeal trauma, with endotracheal laceration in a 12-year-old boy who sustained a direct blow to the neck. **A,** AP radiograph displays massive subcutaneous emphysema, suggestive of an esophageal or laryngeal tear or laceration. The airway is slightly irregular on the right side *(arrow),* due to submucosal hematoma or edema. **B,** Axial CT performed without intravenous contrast confirms massive emphysema throughout the neck. At endoscopy, a small laceration of the right posterolateral tracheal wall was seen, corresponding to the level of the arrow.

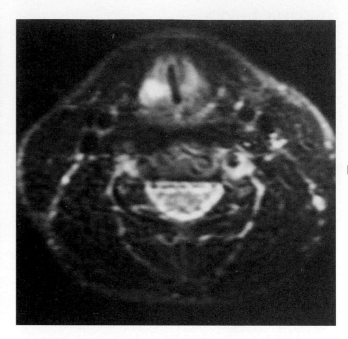

FIG. 10-65   Contusion of the right true vocal cord in a 17-year-old girl who sustained a direct blow to the larynx in an automobile accident complained of hoarseness. **A,** T1W axial image shows mild fullness in the right true vocal cord. Note the normal high signal intensity in the thyroid and cricoid cartilages and the oval contour of the airway. **B,** T2W image obtained at the same level shows high-signal edema in the true vocal cord.

the only sign. Rupture of the anterior portion of the cervical trachea after severe coughing with the neck in extension has been described as "subcutaneous rupture" and results in extensive cervical emphysema (Fig. 10-66).[5]

Penetrating oropharyngeal injury, or the "lollipop" injury, is not common in children, but it may have devastating neurologic sequelae as a result of injury to the high cervical internal carotid artery or jugular vein. The injury occurs when the child falls with a foreign body (toothbrush, pencil, lollipop, popsicle stick, or chopstick) in the mouth. The mechanism of injury is a blow to the lateral soft palate, which can compress the internal carotid artery between the foreign object and the spine. The oropharyngeal injury ranges from a palatal hematoma to a severe palatal or posterior pharyngeal wall laceration.

Radiographic evaluation is not necessary for the mucosal injury, but if the carotid artery has been injured, cerebral angiography may show internal carotid artery dissection, intraluminal thrombus, or complete occlusion resulting in neurologic manifestations.[10-15] Because the neurologic deficit is often delayed by as much as 48 hours, angiography should be considered even in the child who is neurologically intact at presentation. Today, magnetic resonance angiography (MRA) is preferred over invasive angiography in the study of these patients. MRA can detect thrombosis or dissection of the internal carotid artery or the internal jugular vein. If CT is performed, IV contrast should be administered to better display the vascular structures at the skull base (Fig. 10-67).

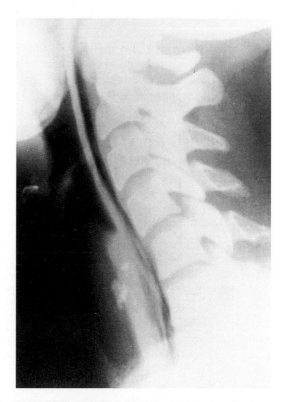

FIG. 10-66   Spontaneous subcutaneous emphysema following paroxysmal coughing in a 19-year-old girl. Lateral radiograph shows massive air in the retropharyngeal space and soft tissues of the neck. The patient noted crepitus in the neck following a paroxysm of coughing during an upper respiratory tract infection. The air gradually resolved.

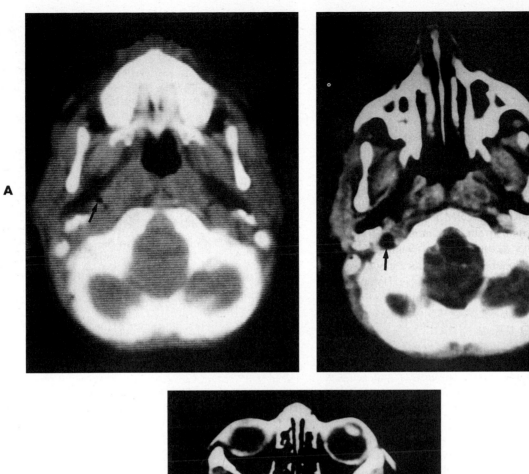

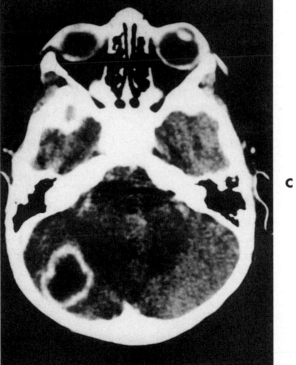

FIG. 10-67   Direct pharyngeal injury, with internal jugular vein thrombosis and cerebellar abscess in a 4-year-old boy who fell while holding a chopstick in his mouth. **A,** Axial nonconstant-enhanced CT obtained hours after the injury shows swelling in the right lateral and posterior pharyngeal region and air immediately anterior to the carotid space *(arrow)*. Oral examination showed a pharyngeal wall laceration. **B,** Several days later the child became ataxic. This contrast-enhanced CT shows thrombosis of the right internal jugular vein *(arrow)* and poor visualization of the right internal carotid artery. **C,** Axial scan slightly higher than **B** shows a peripheral cerebellar abscess. This is an unusual complication of the "lollipop" injury; the more common injury involves the internal carotid artery.

THERMAL TRAUMA AND CAUSTIC INGESTION

Laryngeal edema and obstruction can result from accidental inhalation of steam, hot particles such as ash, or scalding liquids.[16-18] Caustic ingestions of both acidic or basic substances may cause significant injury to the airway. The most severe injuries result from ingestion of large quantities of industrial strength alkali or direct aspiration of caustic substances. Usually the degree of oral mucosal injury does not reflect the severity of the laryngeal burn.

Because of its greater exposure to thermal or caustic substances, the supraglottis is the most commonly injured region of the pediatric airway. Microwave heated liquids are especially dangerous because the outer temperature of the liquid may be much lower than the core temperature.[19-21] In most cases the injury is mild supraglottic edema, which resolves with conservative therapy.

Plain films in children with thermal trauma or caustic ingestion are nonspecific and may show thickening of the laryngeal structures, simulating epiglottitis or croup (Fig. 10-68). In more severe cases, pharyngeal stenosis may occur because of scarring and fixation of the soft palate.[22] If aspiration occurs, significant glottic, subglottic, and tracheal injury may result, with the potential for permanent subglottic or tracheal stenosis.

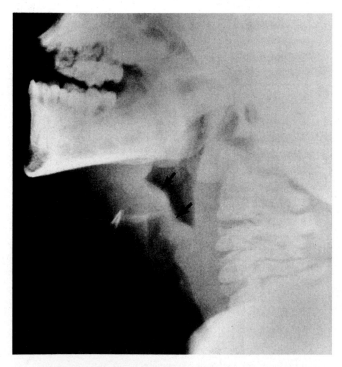

FIG. 10-68 Thermal inhalation injury in a 3-year-old boy who aspirated hot ashes through a straw. Severe perioral burns and respiratory distress were noted on presentation. Lateral radiograph in hyperextension shows marked thickening of the epiglottis and aryepiglottic folds *(arrows)*.

INTUBATION TRAUMA

Complications of intubation most commonly occur at the glottic or subglottic level. Acute intubation injuries occur at predictable locations, including the medial surface of the arytenoids, the cricoarytenoid articulation, the posterior commissure, and the anterior surface of the cricoid lamina.[23] Acute changes, which may be visualized endoscopically, include edema and hyperemia, mucosal erosion, and ulceration. Granulation tissue, intubation granulomas, glottic webs, submucosal cysts, and vocal cord immobility may eventually develop. A traumatic intubation may also dislocate one of the arytenoids or may fracture the cricoid. Prolonged intubation may also result in the formation of subglottic stenosis. Endotracheal intubation is the most common cause of acquired subglottic stenosis.[24,25] However, there are other important etiologic risk factors, including gastroesophageal reflux, sepsis, low birth weight, and frequent self-extubations, and the exact role of each of these risk factors is unknown.[26,27]

Stridor or hoarseness after extubation suggests a complication of intubation. Although imaging may be used to help localize the problem, endoscopy is the mainstay of diagnosis.

An intubation granulation may be focal or nodular, and it occurs most commonly at the vocal process of the arytenoid.[23] Airway fluoroscopy shows a focal mass projecting into the airway at the glottic level. Ischemic pressure necrosis from an endotracheal tube may result in posterior wall granulation tissue, which may lead to glottic stenosis. On imaging this will appear as airway narrowing at the glottic level.

Subglottic cysts are rare acquired retention cysts that usually follow long-term intubation in neonates (Fig. 10-69). The mechanism of formation is fibrosis and obstruction of the mucous glands and subsequent cyst formation.[28] Asymmetric subglottic narrowing may be seen on AP plain films and may be similar in appearance to a subglottic hemangioma.[28]

The severity or extent of acquired subglottic stenosis may be determined on plain films or fluoroscopy of the airway.[29] CT and MRI are usually not performed to evaluate intubation-related complications. Imaging is important, however, when there is complete or severe laryngeal stenosis and it is difficult endoscopically to determine the length of the stenosis. Coronal CT reformations and direct coronal MRI are particularly helpful in evaluating severe grades of laryngotracheal stenosis because the length of stenosis is well demonstrated (Fig. 10-70).[30] The cross-sectional airway area can be readily obtained on either CT or MRI.[31] In this clinical setting, intravenous contrast is not necessary for either CT or MRI.

A tracheotomy often results in similar acquired lesions in the airway, including stomal and distal tracheal granulomas, subglottic stenosis, and collapse of the anterior tracheal wall.[32] The radiographic appearance of these lesions is similar to that of the postintubation lesions (Fig. 10-71).

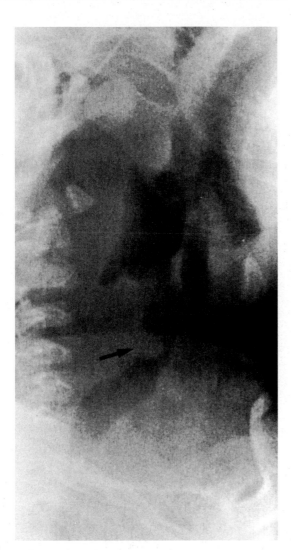

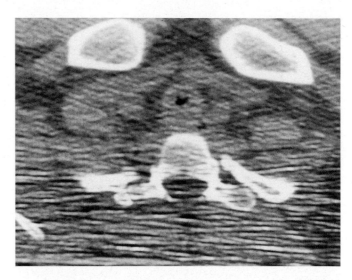

FIG. 10-70 Circumferential granulation tissue causing tracheal stenosis in an 18-year-old boy with Down's syndrome, and a history of long-term intubation following cardiac surgery. Now with intermittent respiratory distress. Spiral 1 mm thick axial noncontrast-enhanced CT shows circumferential endotracheal soft tissue causing marked airway compromise. The scan was performed during quiet nonlabored respiration.

FIG. 10-69 Acquired subglottic cyst caused by long-term intubation in a 7-month-old boy who was born prematurely and required intubation for several months, now with intermittent respiratory distress. Oblique film obtained during airway fluoroscopy shows mass *(arrow)* projecting from the posterior wall at the subglottic level. Endoscopy showed a benign subglottic cyst.

ASPIRATED FOREIGN BODY

Laryngotracheal inhaled foreign bodies are less common than bronchial foreign bodies, accounting for fewer than 20% of all aspirations.[33] However, because of the potential for complete airway obstruction, laryngotracheal foreign bodies are more hazardous than the bronchial ones. The clinical presentation is usually obvious, with severe airway obstruction and stridor. Plain films of the neck help detect foreign bodies that are radiopaque and help exclude croup, although subglottic edema and swelling may be seen with laryngotracheal foreign bodies.[34] Coins, pen caps, screws, pins, including open safety pins, and small toy objects are common radiopaque foreign bodies that may lodge in the larynx, trachea, or bronchi (Fig. 10-72). However, a signifi-

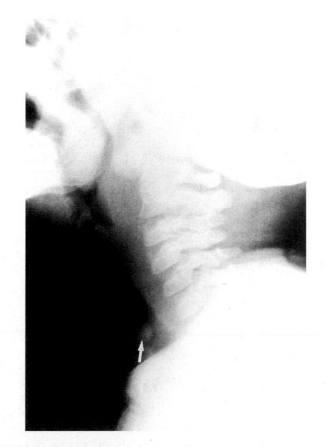

FIG. 10-71 Tracheal granuloma after a tracheostomy tube in a 20-month-old boy with respiratory distress following decannulation. Lateral plain film shows a smooth mass in the cervical trachea *(arrow).*

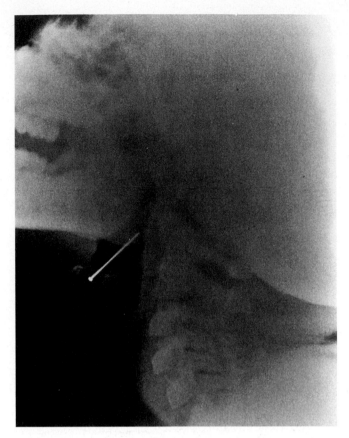

FIG. 10-72 Aspirated foreign body. Young child with respiratory distress and dysphagia. Straight pin lodged obliquely in the vallecula is seen well on this lateral radiograph. AP examination should always follow the lateral film, to lateralize and determine the width of the foreign body.

cant proportion of foreign bodies, especially food particles such as peanuts or small vegetable matter, may not be seen, even with magnification views.[34-36] Because some foreign bodies may be radiolucent, indirect signs of aspiration such as subglottic swelling or airway narrowing should be reported.[37] Both AP and lateral neck films should be obtained to localize the object to the larynx or the esophagus and to determine the contour of the foreign body (Fig. 10-73).

In contrast, bronchial foreign bodies may present more insidiously. Usually smaller objects and particulate matter lodge in the distal bronchi. If the symptoms are mild, diagnosis may be delayed by weeks to months. Because the aspiration is often not witnessed and physical findings are subtle, radiographs are an important part of the workup.

In most cases, radiographic diagnosis is based upon changes secondary to unilateral obstruction of the airway. "Air trapping" occurs because of a ball-valve mechanism from partial occlusion of the bronchus.[38] Air enters on inspiration but does not escape from the obstructed side on expiration. This results in unilateral emphysema, mediastinal shift, and a decrease in pulmonary blood flow to the affected side. In the uncooperative child, lateral decubitus views usually suffice. Bronchial foreign bodies that have been present

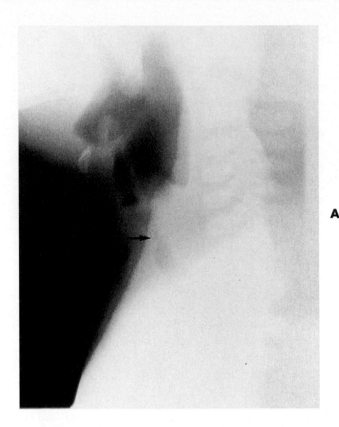

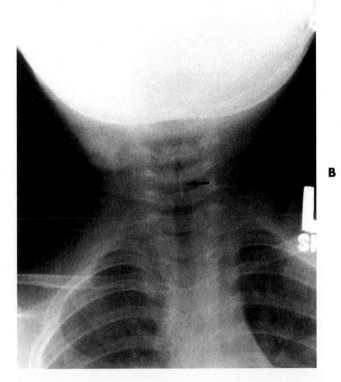

FIG. 10-73 Aspirated foreign body (eggshell) in a 10-month-old girl with respiratory distress. **A,** Lateral radiograph shows poor visualization of the subglottic airway *(arrow)*. **B,** The AP film clearly shows a subglottic foreign body that is narrow and approximately 1 cm in length.

for longer periods may cause chronic inflammation in the bronchial lumen and complete bronchial obstruction, resulting in atelectasis, infiltrates, or effusions. However, in this situation it is also possible to have minimal radiographic findings. For instance, bilateral bronchial foreign bodies may not result in mediastinal shift or signs of air-trapping. endoscopy should be performed whenever clinical suspicion is high.

An esophageal foreign body may also present with airway obstruction secondary to direct pressure on the posterior larynx or trachea.[39,40] Impaction most commonly occurs at or just below the level of the cricopharyngeus muscle.[41] If the foreign body ulcerates and perforates the esophagus, the edema and inflammatory response may compromise the airway. Plain films are important for evaluating esophageal foreign bodies because most are coins. A barium swallow usually is performed to show the site of perforation and extravasation, and if perforation is likely, this study should be performed with water-soluble nonionic contrast (Fig. 10-74).[42,43] An esophageal stricture following a surgical repair for a congenital lesion such as esophageal atresia predisposes to obstructing an esophageal foreign body.[44] A barium swallow helps delineate the location and extent of the stricture.

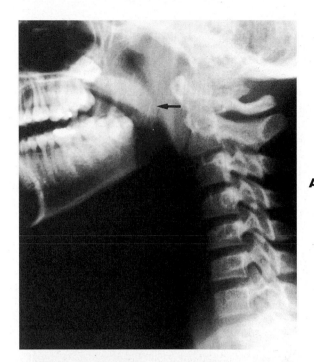

A

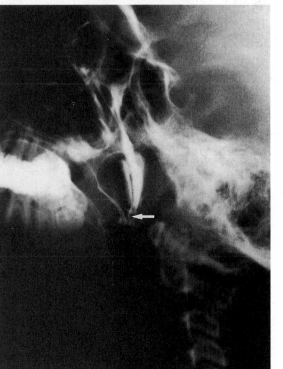

B

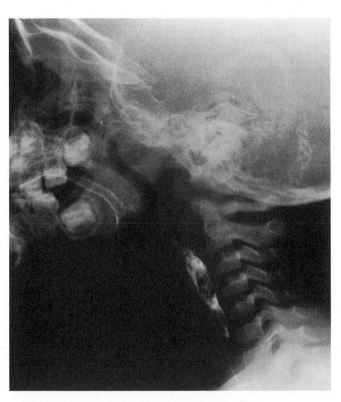

FIG. 10-74 Esophageal foreign body, with perforation and abscess formation. Young child who presented with respiratory distress. Lateral film from a barium swallow examination shows marked prevertebral soft-tissue swelling. A collection of barium is seen extending five vertebral bodies in length, which was caused by posterior esophageal wall perforation by a foreign body. The edema and collection caused mass effect on the airway, resulting in the presenting symptoms of airway compromise.

FIG. 10-75 Nasooropharyngeal stenosis. Young child with respiratory distress, several months following tonsillectomy and adenoidectomy. **A,** Lateral radiograph obtained during quiet breathing shows the soft palate abutting the posterior pharyngeal wall *(arrow),* with no air within the oropharynx at that level. This was a fixed finding on multiple films. **B,** Lateral radiograph, supine position, obtained after a small amount of barium was instilled into the nasal cavity. In addition the patient has swallowed barium, coating the undersurface of the palate. Note that the palatal position is the same as in **A,** and there is pooling of barium above the scarred and fixed posterior palate.

MISCELLANEOUS

Nasopharngeal stenosis, a rare cause of airway compromise, usually results from scarring and cicatration after tonsillectomy and adenoidectomy, especially when surgery included aggressive circumferential cauterization of the nasopharyngeal tissues. Before the widespread availability of antibiotics, nasopharyngeal stenosis was a complication of syphilis or tuberculosis of the pharynx. Fusion of the soft palate and tonsillar pillar to the posterior pharyngeal wall causes complete or partial obstruction. Patients present with respiratory distress and nasal obstruction weeks to months after surgery. The diagnosis is usually made by clinical history and endoscopy. Plain films may demonstrate narrowing or complete nasopharyngeal obstruction (Fig. 10-75). Treatment involves pharyngoplasty with laterally based pharyngeal flaps.[45]

References

1. Fitz-Hugh GS, Powell JB. Acute traumatic injuries of the oropharynx, laryngopharynx, and cervical trachea in children. Otolaryngol Clin North Am 1970; 3:375-393.

2. Stanley RB. Value of computed tomography in management of acute laryngeal injury. J Trauma 1984; 24:359-362.

3. Snow JB Jr. Diagnosis and therapy for acute laryngeal and tracheal trauma. Otolaryngol Clin North Am 1984; 17:101-106.

4. Schild JA, Denneny EC. Evaluation and treatment of acute laryngeal fractures. Head and Neck 1989; 11:491-496.

5. Greene R, Stark P. Trauma of the larynx and trachea. Radiol Clin North Am 1978; 16:309-320.

6. Ardran GM, Kemp FH. The mechanism of changes in form of the cervical airway in infancy. Medical Radiography and Photography 1968; 44:26-38.

7. Polansky A, Resnick D, Sofferman RA, et al. Hyoid bone elevation: a sign of tracheal transection. Radiology 1984; 150:117-120.

8. Curtin HD. The larynx. In: Som PM, Bergeron RT, eds. Head and neck imaging. 2nd Edition. St. Louis, Mo: Mosby–Year Book, Inc, 1991.

9. Symbas PN, Justicz AG, Ricketts RR. Rupture of the airways from blunt trauma: treatment of complex injuries. Ann Thorac Surg 1992; 54:177-183.

10. Radkowski D, McGill TJ, Healy GB, et al: Penetrating trauma of the oropharynx in children. Laryngoscope 1993; 103:991-994.

11. Hengerer AS, DeGroot TR, Rivers RJ, et al. Internal carotid artery thrombosis following soft palate injuries: a case report and review of 16 cases. Laryngoscope 1984; 94:1571-1575.

12. Pitner SE. Carotid thrombosis due to intraoral trauma. N Engl Med 1966; 274:764-767.

13. Mains B, Nagle M. Thrombosis of the internal carotid artery due to soft palate injury. 1989; 103:796-797.

14. Higgins GL III, Meredith JT. Internal carotid artery thrombosis following penetrating trauma of the soft palate: an injury of youth. J Fam Pract 1991; 32:316-322.

15. Braudo M. Thrombosis of internal carotid artery in childhood after injuries in region of soft palate. Br Med J 1956; 1:665-667.

16. Greene R, Stark P. Trauma of the larynx and trachea. Radiol Clin North Am 1978; 16:309-320.

17. Dye DJ, Milling MA, Emmanuel FR, et al. Toddlers, teapots, and kettles: beware intraoral scalds. Br Med J 1990; 300:597-598.

18. Kulick RM, Selbst SM, Baker MD, et al. Thermal epiglottitis after swallowing hot beverages. Pediatrics 1988; 81:441-444.

19. Garland JS, Rice TB, Kelly KJ. Airway burns in an infant following aspiration of microwave-heated tea. Chest 1986; 90:621-622.

20. Goldberg RM, Lee S, Line WS Jr. Laryngeal burns secondary to the ingestion of microwave-heated food. J Emerg Med 1990; 8:281-283.

21. Sando WC, Gallaher KJ, Rodgers BM. Risk factors for microwave scald injuries in infants. J Pediatr 1984; 105:864-867.

22. Scott JC, Jones B, Eisele DW, et al. Caustic ingestions of the upper aerodigestive tract. Laryngoscope 1992; 102:1-8.

23. Benjamin BNP. Special Laryngoscopy techniques. In: Benjamin BNP, ed. Diagnostic laryngology. Philadelphia, Pa: WB Saunders, 1990.

24. Holinger PH, Kutnick SL, Schild JA, et al. Subglottic stenosis in infants and children. Ann Otol Rhinol Laryngol 1976; 85:591-599.

25. Parkin JL, Stevens MH, Jung AL. Acquired and congenital subglottic stenosis in the infant. Ann Otol 1976; 85:573-581.

26. Dankle SK, Schuller DE, McCleod RE. Risk factors for neonatal acquired subglottic stenosis. Ann Otol Rhinol Laryngol 1986; 95:626-630.

27. Grundfast KM, Morris MS, Bernsely C. Subglottic stenosis: retrospective analysis and proposal for standard reporting system. Ann Otol Rhinol Laryngol 1987; 96:101-105.

28. Holinger LD, Toriumi DM, Anadappa EC. Subglottic cysts and asymmetrical subglottic narrowing on neck radiographs. Pediatr Radiol 1988; 18:306-308.

29. Kushner DC, Harris GB. Obstructing lesions of the larynx and trachea in infants and children. Radiol Clin North Am 1978; 16:181-194.

30. John SD, Swischuk LE. Stridor and upper airway obstruction in infants and children. Radiographics 1992; 12:625-643.

31. Faw K, Muntz H, Siegal M, et al. Computed tomography in the evaluation of acquired stenosis in the neonate. Laryngoscope 1982; 92:100-105.

32. Tom LWC, Miller L, Wetmore RF, et al. Endoscopic assessment in children with tracheotomies. Arch Otolaryngol Head Neck Surg 1993; 119:321-324.

33. Daniilidis J, Symeonidis B, Triaridis K, et al: Foreign body in the airways. Arch Otolaryngol 1977; 103:570-573.

34. Esclamado RM, Richardson MA. Laryngotracheal foreign bodies in children. Am J Dis Child 1987; 141:259-262.

35. Kero P, Puhakka H, Erkinjuntti M, et al. Foreign body in the airways of children. Int J Pediatr Otorhinolaryngology 1983; 6:51-59.

36. Blazer S, Naveh Y, Friedman A. Foreign body in the airway. Am J Dis Child 1980; 134:68-71.

37. Morioka WT, Maisel RH, Smith TW, et al. Unexpected radiographic findings related to foreign bodies. Ann Otol 1975; 84:627-630.

38. Macpherson RI. Radiologic aspects of airway obstruction. In: Othersen HB Jr, ed. The pediatric airway. Philadelphia, Pa: WB Saunders, 1991.

39. Newman DE. The radiolucent esophageal foreign body: an often-forgotten cause of respiratory symptoms. Pediatrics 1978; 92:60-63.

40. Tauscher JW. Esophageal foreign body: an uncommon cause of stridor. Pediatrics 1978; 61:657-658.

41. Smith PC, Swischuk LE, Fagan CJ. An elusive and often unsuspected cause of stridor or pneumonia (the esophageal foreign body). AJR 1974; 122:80-89.

42. Kushner DC, Harris GB. Obstructing lesions of the larynx and trachea in infants and children. Radiol Clin North Am 1978; 16:181-194.

43. John SD, Swischuk LE. Stridor and upper airway obstruction in infants and children. Radiographics 1992; 12:625-643.

44. Macpherson RI, Leithiser RE. Upper airway obstruction in children: an update. Radiographics 1985; 5(3):339-376.

45. Cotton RT. Nasopharyngeal stenosis. Arch Otolaryngol 1985; 111:146-148.

SECTION EIGHT
BENIGN TUMORS AND TUMORLIKE CONDITIONS

TONSILLAR AND ADENOIDAL HYPERTROPHY

Hypertrophy of the adenoids and palatine tonsils is common in the pediatric population. Adenoidectomy or tonsillectomy is indicated if the hypertrophy results in nasopharyngeal airway obstruction or chronic otitis medial or serous effusions secondary to eustacian tube obstruction.[1-6]

Although various measurements and ratios have been described to determine the normal adenoidal size, correlation of preoperative radiographic adenoidal size with surgical observations and specimens varies from being excellent to poor.[7,8] The lateral radiograph should be obtained during inspiration through the nose, with the mouth closed. The adenoid to nasopharyngeal (AN) ratio may aid in diagnosing prominent, clinically significant adenoids (Fig. 10-76).[9]

Using this method, adenoids can be reliably diagnosed in a symptomatic patient when the AN ratio is 0.8 or greater (Fig. 10-77).[9] Obstructive secretions generally are not seen in patients with an AN ratio less than 0.5.[10] Because tremendous variation in adenoidal size exists in the normal pediatric patient, any measurement should be used with caution and clinical symptoms must always be considered. Furthermore, in certain craniofacial syndromes such as trisomy 21, because of the smaller nasopharyngeal size, a lower AN ratio may be clinically significant.[11]

Airway compromise or dysphagia caused by palatine tonsillar hypertrophy in the child is also common.[5,11] Less commonly, lingual tonsillar hypertrophy may be associated with airway obstruction.[12-14]

Palatine tonsillar hypertrophy appears as smooth, rounded or oval soft-tissue masses on either side of the oropharynx, bulging into the pharyngeal column (Fig. 10-17). Sagittal MRI, obtained just off the midline, shows similar findings, with the fullness in the tonsillar fossa being isointense to pharyngeal musculature on T1W images and hyperintense to muscle on T2W images (Fig. 10-19). On CT,

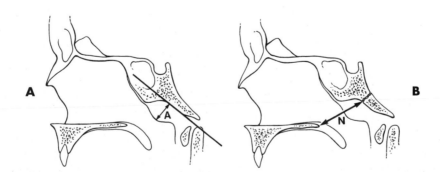

FIG. 10-76 The adenoidal-nasopharyngeal (AN) ratio may be helpful in determining adenoidal size on the lateral radiograph. In the symptomatic child (obstructive sleep apnea or recurrent otitis media) a ratio greater than 0.8 is considered abnormal. **A,** Adenoidal measurement. The distance *(A)* between the maximum convexity of the adenoids and a line drawn along the basiocciput is measured. **B,** Nasopharyngeal measurement. The distance *(N)* between the posterior hard palate and the sphenooccipital synchondrosis is determined. (From Fujioka M, et al. Radiographic evaluation of adenoidal size in children: adenoidal-nasopharyngeal ratio. AJR 1979; 133:401-404.)

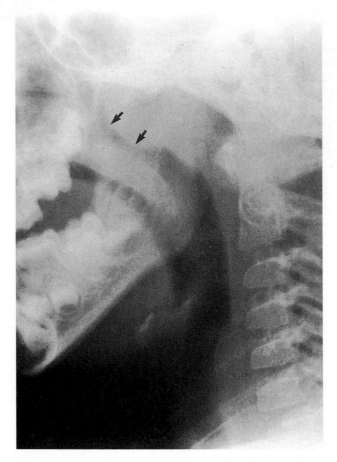

FIG. 10-77 Adenoidal hypertrophy in a 5-year-old boy with obstructive sleep apnea. Lateral plain film shows prominent adenoidal tissue *(arrows)*, filling the posterior nasopharynx and narrowing the airway.

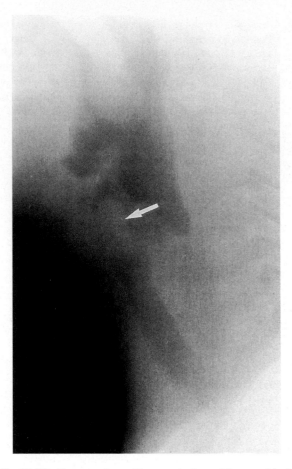

FIG. 10-78 Laryngeal papillomatosis in a 2½-year-old child with stridor. Lateral plain film shows a glottic and supraglottic lobulated mass *(arrow)*.

palatine tonsillar tissue is isodense to the surrounding musculature. On MRI and CT, hypertrophic lingual tonsils are similar in appearance to palatine tonsils, but they occur at the tongue base, often filling the vallecula (Fig. 10-18).

Recurrent Respiratory Papillomatosis

Recurrent respiratory papillomatosis, also known as *juvenile laryngeal papillomatosis*, is a benign neoplasm of the larynx and aerodigestive tract. Although the lesion does occur in adults, it is more common and displays more aggressive behavior in the pediatric population. The disease is caused by the human papilloma virus (HPV), is probably transmitted by an infected mother to the infant during childbirth, and the papillomas have a high tendency to recur, either at the primary site or elsewhere in the airway.[15-17]

Most children present by 3 years of age with hoarseness, stridor, or a change in voice.[15,18] Because growth of the papillomas is gradual, acute airway obstruction is rare. Papillomas are often multiple and most commonly occur at the glottic level, but they can be found virtually anywhere in the aerodigestive tract.[19] Recurrent disease is often subglottic.[16] Plain films show small pedunculated nodular masses within the airway (Fig. 10-78).[20,21] CT and MRI may show small nodules adherent to the airway wall and projecting into the lumen. Larger recurrent lesions may have transbronchial spread, with formation of lung masses and cavities.[22] Malignant transformation may occur, but it is rare.[23,24]

The preferred treatment is laser resection. Nonsurgical treatment such as hormonal therapy or antiviral agents such as interferon also has been used.[15]

Juvenile Nasopharyngeal Angiofibroma

Juvenile nasopharyngeal angiofibroma is a benign but aggressive vascular lesion found exclusively in young boys between 5 and 25 years of age. Unilateral nasal obstruction and recurrent spontaneous epistaxis are the most common presenting symptoms.[25] The lesion usually arises at the sphenopalatine foramen on the lateral nasopharyngeal wall. It extends locally to the pterygopalatine fossa, infratemporal fossa, sphenoid sinuses, posterior nasal fossa, maxillary and ethmoid sinuses, orbit, cheek, and central skull base.[25,26]

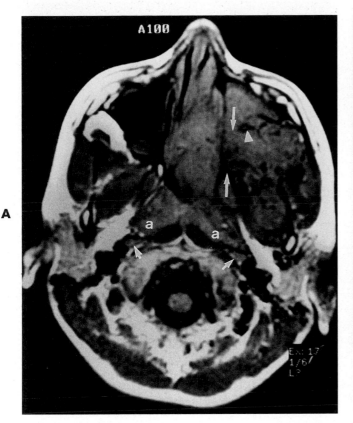

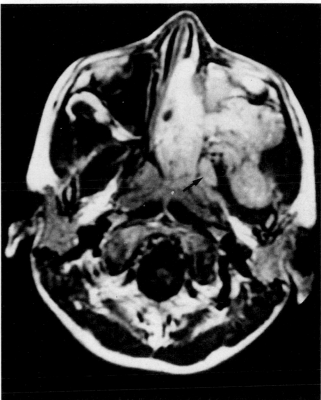

FIG. 10-79 Juvenile nasopharyngeal angiofibroma in a 12-year-old boy with chronic nasal obstruction and epistaxis. **A,** T1W axial image shows a large mass filling the left nasal cavity and nasopharynx, widening the pterygopalatine fossa *(large white arrows)* resulting in anterior displacement of the posterior wall of the maxillary sinus *(arrowhead),* and extending into the masticator space. The mass is slightly hyperintense with respect to normal muscle on this sequence. Soft tissue or fluid fills the left maxillary sinus. On this sequence it is impossible to differentiate tumor within the sinus from retained secretions. Notice the normal adenoidal tissue *(a)* and small retropharyngeal lymph nodes *(small arrows).* **B,** There is intense enhancement within the lesion on this non-fat-suppressed T1W postgadolinium enhanced image. The punctate regions of signal void are seen well on this sequence. Note that tumor fills the pterygoid fossa *(arrow).*

Intracranial extension usually occurs via the superior orbital fissure. Although the lesion is benign, it is extremely vascular, being primarily supplied by the ipsilateral internal maxillary artery, the ascending pharyngeal, and the palatine arteries. It also may recruit supply from the sphenoidal and ophthalmic branches of the internal carotid artery.[26]

The classic plain film findings include an ipsilateral nasal cavity and nasopharyngeal mass, widening of the pterygopalatine fossa, anterior displacement of the posterior wall of the maxillary sinus, erosion of the medial pterygoid plate, and a mass in the sphenoid sinuses. Bone destruction is best seen on thin section direct axial and coronal CT.[27] Central skull base foramen and fissures that may be enlarged by the tumor include the sphenopalatine foramen, the foramen rotundum, and the inferior and superior orbital fissures.[28-30]

On CT there is immediate intense tumor enhancement. On MRI the mass is generally heterogeneous, with prominent vascular flow voids (Fig. 10-79). Intense enhancement with gadolinium is typical. One advantage of MRI over CT is the increased ability to differentiate obstructed secretions from intrasinus tumor. Conventional angiography shows the prominent vascular supply, usually from the ipsilateral external carotid artery branches but often involving the contralateral vessels as well. Internal carotid artery supply may be seen when the lesion has extended intracranially. A dense homogeneous blush persisting into the venous phase is typical.[27] Early draining veins are not common.

Treatment consists of surgical resection, often with preoperative embolization.[27,31,32] Radiation generally is not the primary treatment, but it may be considered in some cases.[33]

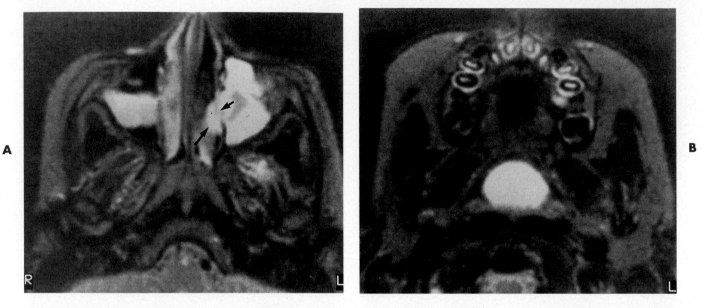

FIG. 10-80   Antrochoanal polyp in an 8-year-old boy with chronic left nasal obstruction. **A,** T2W image shows a hyperintense mass *(large arrow)* extending through the medial wall *(small arrow)* of the left maxillary sinus. **B,** At a level slightly below **A,** note the smooth, round distal portion of the mass filling the posterior nasopharynx.

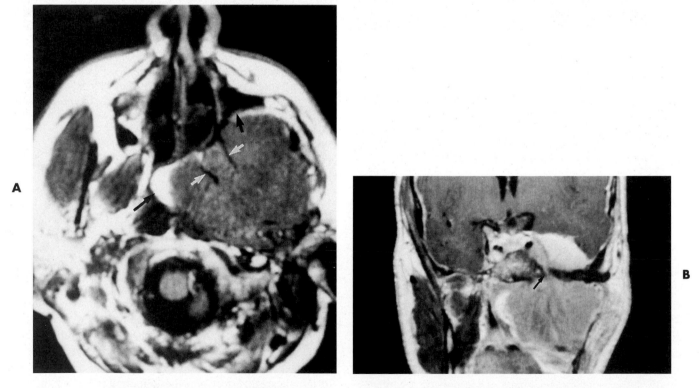

FIG. 10-81   Large neurofibroma in a teenage boy with neurofibromatosis type II and chronic nasopharyngeal obstruction. **A,** Axial T1W image shows a homogeneous mass filling the masticator space, obliterating the parapharyngeal fat, and filling the nasopharynx. The medial portion of the mass is hyperintense *(large black arrow)*, probably because of a recent biopsy. Note that the posterior wall of the maxillary sinus has been displaced anteriorly *(small black arrow)*, as in Fig. 10-79, but the lesion is more homogeneous, with no regions of signal void. Pterygoid plates *(white arrows)*. **B,** Coronal postgadolinium T1W image shows the foramen ovale is widened *(arrow)*, and there is involvement of the cavernous sinus.

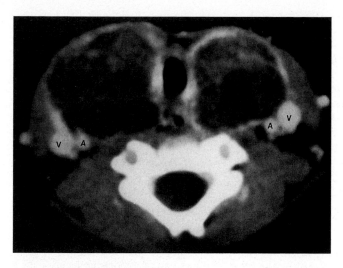

FIG. 10-82 One-year-old with congenital hypothyroidism and stridor. Axial contrast-enhanced CT shows symmetric enlargement of the thyroid gland. Note that the gland does not enhance normally. The common carotid arteries *(A)* and internal jugular veins *(V)* are deviated posterolaterally, and the trachea is compressed.

MISCELLANEOUS

Antrochoanal polyps and inflammatory sinonasal polyps, especially in the child with cystic fibrosis, may cause nasal airway obstruction. Imaging findings are similar to those described in adults (Fig. 10-80).

Large neurofibromas may occasionally cause airway obstruction (Fig. 10-81). These lesions are typically well circumscribed, with bone remodeling rather than frank bone destruction.

The larynx is the most common site for isolated amyloid, a rare benign condition in children.[34,35] On CT the solid laryngeal mass is similar in attenuation to muscle, and on MRI the signal intensities of the amyloid disease are the same as those of muscle. The process enhances with gadolinium.[35]

Congenital hypothyroidism may be caused by dyshormonogenesis, resulting in a large thyroid gland that is in the normal thyroid bed.[36] The mass may be extensive, extending retropharyngeally and causing airway compromise (Fig. 10-82).[37,38]

References

1. Gates GA, Avery CA, Prihoda TJ, et al. Effectiveness of adenoidectomy and tympanostomy tubes in the treatment of chronic otitis media with effusion. N Engl J Med 1987; 317:1444-1451.
2. Gates GA, Avery CA, Prihoda TJ. Effect of adenoidectomy upon children with chronic otitis media with effusion. Laryngoscope 1988; 98:58-63.
3. Levy AM, Tabakin BS, Hanson JS, et al. Hypertrophied adenoids causing pulmonary hypertension and severe congestive heart failure. N Engl J Med 1967; 277:506-511.
4. Cayler GG, Johnson EE, Lewis BE, et al. Heart failure due to enlarged tonsils and adenoids. Am J Dis Child 1969; 118:708-717.
5. Brodsky L, Kock RJ. Anatomic correlates of normal and diseased adenoids in children. Laryngoscope 1992; 102:1268-1274.
6. Lind MG, Lundell BPW. Tonsillar hyperplasia in children. Arch Otolaryngol 1982; 108:650-654.
7. Cohen LM, Koltai PJ, Scott JR. Lateral cervical radiographs and adenoid size: do they correlate? Ear Nose Throat 1992; 71:638-642.
8. Hibbert J, Whitehouse GH. The assessment of adenoidal size by radiological means. Clin Otolaryngol 1978; 3:43-47.
9. Fujioka M, Young LW, Girdany BR. Radiographic evaluation of adenoidal size in children: adenoidal-nasopharyngeal ratio. AJR 1979; 133:401-404.
10. Fernbach SK, Brouillette RT, Riggs TW, et al. Radiologic evaluation of adenoids and tonsils in children with obstructive sleep apnea: plain films and fluoroscopy. Pediatr Radiol 1983; 13:258-265.
11. Potsic WP. Assessment and treatment of adenotonsillar hypertrophy in children. Am J Otolaryngol 1992; 13:259-264.
12. Willatt D, Youngs R. The value of soft tissue radiography in the assessment and treatment of lingual tonsillar hypertrophy. J Laryngol Otol 1984; 98:1217-1219.
13. Epstein BS, Sternberg J, Shapiro E. Acute respiratory distress in an infant produced by hypertrophied tonsils, Am J Radiol 1964; 91:571-572.
14. Fitzgerald P, O'Connell D. Massive hypertrophy of the lingual tonsils: an unusual cause of dysphagia. Br J Radiol 1987; 60:505-506.
15. Pransky SM, Seid AB. Tumors of the larynx, trachea and bronchi. In: Bluestone CD, Stool SE, eds. Pediatric otolaryngology. Philadelphia, Pa: WB Saunders, 1990.
16. Doyle DJ, Gianoli GJ, Espinola T, et al. Recurrent respiratory papillo-matosis: juvenile versus adult forms. Laryngoscope 1994; 104:523-527.
17. Abramson AL, Steinberg BM, Winkler B. Laryngeal papillomatosis: clinical, histopathologic and molecular studies. Laryngoscope 1987; 97:678-685.
18. Irwin BC, Henrickse WA, Pincott Jr, et al. Juvenile laryngeal papillomatosis. J Laryngol Otol 1986; 100:435-445.
19. Benjamin B, Parsons DS. Recurrent respiratory papillomatosis: a 10 year study. Laryngol Otol 1988; 102:1022-1028.
20. Macpherson RI, Leithiser RE. Upper airway obstruction in children: an update. Radiographics 1985; 5:339.
21. Kushner DC, Harris GB. Obstructing lesions of the larynx and trachea in infants and children. Radiol Clin North Am 1978; 16:181-194.
22. Hedlund GL, Kirks DR. Respiratory system. In: Kirks DR, ed. Practical pediatrics imaging: diagnostic radiology of infants and children. Boston, Mass: Little, Brown & Co Inc, 1991.
23. Solomon D, Smith RR, Kashima HK, et al. Malignant transformation in non-irradiated recurrent respiratory papillomatosis. Laryngoscope 1985; 95:900-904.
24. Schnadig VJ, Clark WD, Clegg TJ, et al. Invasive papillomatosis and

squamous carcinoma complicating juvenile laryngeal papillomatosis. Arch Otolaryngol Head Neck Surg 1986; 112:966-971.

25. Gullane PJ, Davidson J, O'Dwyer T, et al. Juvenile angiofibroma: a review of the literature and a case series report. Laryngoscope 1992; 102:928-933.

26. Harrison DFN. The natural history, pathogenesis, and treatment of juvenile angiofibroma. Arch Otolaryngol Head Neck Surg 1987; 113:936-942.

27. Davis KR. Embolization of epistaxis and juvenile nasopharyngeal angiofibromas. AJNR Am J Neuroradiol 1986; 7:953-962.

28. Lloyd GAS, Phelps PD. Juvenile angiofibroma: imaging by magnetic resonance, CT and conventional techniques. Clin Otolaryngol 1986; 11:247-259.

29. Chrys RA, Pribram HF, Strelzow V, et al. Juvenile angiofibroma: a unique case presenting with intracranial air. Otolaryngol Head Neck Surg 1987; 97:572-575.

30. Jacobsson M, Petruson B, Svendsen P, et al. Juvenile nasopharyngeal angiofibroma. Acta Otolaryngol 1988; 105:132-139.

31. Garcia-Cevigon E, Bien S, Rufenacht D, et al. Pre-operative embolization of naso-pharyngeal angiofibromas. Neuroradiol 1988; 30:556-560.

32. Roberts JK, Korones GK, Levine HL, et al. Results of surgical management of nasopharyngeal angiofibroma. Cleve Clin J of Med 1989; 56:529-533.

33. Robinson ACR, Khoury GG, Ash DV, et al. Evaluation of response following irradiation of juvenile angiofibromas. Br J Radiol 1989; 62:245-247.

34. Hurbis CG, Holinger LD. Laryngeal amyloidosis in a child. Ann Otol Rhinol Laryngol 1990; 99:105-107.

35. O'Halloran LR, Lusk RP. Amyloidosis of the larynx in a child. Ann Otol Rhinol Laryngol 1994; 103:590-594.

36. Wells RG, Sty JR, Duck SC. Technetium 99m pertechnetate thyroid scintigraphy: congenital hypothyroid screening. Pediatric Radiol 1986; 16:368-373.

37. Hayden CK, Swischuk LE. Head and neck lesions in children. In: Bergeron RT, Osborn AG, Som PM, eds. Head and neck imaging. St. Louis, Mo: The CV Mosby Co, 1984.

38. Optican RJ, White KS, Effmann EL. Goitrous cretinism manifesting as newborn stridor: CT evaluation. AJR 1991; 157:557-558.

SECTION NINE
MALIGNANT TUMORS AND TUMORLIKE CONDITIONS

LYMPHOMA

In the pediatric population, lymphoma is the most common malignancy occurring in the head and neck.[1] Boys are affected more commonly than girls for all lymphoma types. Non-Hodgkin's lymphoma primarily affects children between 2 and 12 years of age, and Hodgkin's lymphoma, rarely seen before age 5 years, is most common in adolescence. Because of improved detection and staging and multimodality treatment regimens, the 5-year survival rate has improved over the past two decades and is now 88% for Hodgkin's lymphoma and 54% for non-Hodgkin's lymphoma.[2]

The presence of the Reed-Sternberg cell, a multinucleate giant cell, differentiates Hodgkin's lymphoma from other types of lymphoma. In children, Hodgkin's lymphoma is primarily nodal, and at initial presentation, extranodal disease is rare.[3] Unilateral or asymmetric nontender, rubbery cervical or supraclavicular nodes are the most common presenting signs of disease. Because inflammatory lymphadenitis in children is common, delay in the diagnosis of lymphoma may occur.[4] During childhood, airway obstruction is not a common presenting symptom of Hodgkin's lymphoma.

Non-Hodgkin's lymphoma is subtyped into B-cell, T-cell, and true histiocytic types. In children, although cervical adenopathy may be the presenting sign of disease, extranodal involvement in the nasopharynx, oropharynx, orbit, or the lymphoid tissue of Waldeyer's ring is common.[1,3,5] When disease involves the airway, symptoms of airway obstruction occur. Non-Hodgkin's lymphoma occurs with a higher incidence in patients with acquired or congenital immune disorders, including acquired immunodeficiency syndrome (AIDS).[6]

Burkitt's lymphoma is a type of non-Hodgkin's lymphoma with a unique epidemiology. The disease occurs both as an endemic African form and a nonendemic American form.[1] Antibody titers to Epstein-Barr virus are high in the African type, but only 15% to 20% of American children have elevated viral titers.[7,8] The African type commonly involves the oral cavity and jaw, and the American type more commonly presents as an abdominal mass. Involvement of the cervical lymph nodes, nasopharynx, and oropharynx are less common than in the other lymphomas.[9] However, Burkitt's lymphoma has an extremely short doubling time and is the fastest growing human tumor. As a result, it may present with rapidly progressive airway obstruction.[7,8]

CT and MRI cannot differentiate nodal disease caused by Hodgkin's lymphoma from that of non-Hodgkin's lymphoma. Lymphadenopathy, sometimes only 1 cm in diameter, is seen in multiple locations, usually with a dominant larger node or group of nodes. However, because prominent hyperplastic nonneoplastic lymphadenopathy is common in the pediatric population, it occasionally may be impossible to differentiate lymphomatous from reactive nodes.[10] Lymphomatous adenopathy is not commonly necrotic or calcified, although focal calcifications may be seen in treated nodes. Nodal biopsy is required to establish a diagnosis and disease subtype.

Non-Hodgkin's lymphoma involving Waldeyer's ring is usually bilateral and fills or obliterates the airway. On CT the tumor is isodense to the pharyngeal musculature, and on

MRI the tumor is isointense to muscle on T1W images and generally hyperintense to muscle on T2W images (Fig. 10-83). Lytic bone destruction in the central skull base and associated cervical lymphadenopathy also may be seen.[11] Infectious mononucleosis, with prominence of Waldeyer's ring lymphoid tissue and cervical adenopathy, may be impossible to differentiate from non-Hodgkin's lympholma.[12] In children, extranodal lymphoma is nonspecific in appearance, but because lymphoma is one of the most common lesions in the head and neck, it should be included in the differential for any large neck mass with malignant characteristics on CT or MRI (Fig. 10-84). Non-Hodgkin's lymphoma is associated with AIDS (Fig. 10-85).

On follow-up CT or MRI, after successful treatment, extranodal disease should appear smaller, or it should completely resolve. Lymphomatous nodes should decrease in size and number, although small nodes may remain. A new nodal or nonnodal mass following treatment for childhood lymphoma may represent recurrent disease or a new primary tumor because these patients are at risk for secondary malignant disease.[13]

RHABDOMYOSARCOMA

In the pediatric population, rhabdomyosarcoma is the most common soft-tissue sarcoma, and the second most frequent head and neck malignancy.[14,15] The disease has a peak age presentation at 2 to 5 years and again at 15 to 19 years.[16] White children are affected most often, and there is a slight male predominance. Approximately 50% of children with rhabdomyosarcoma have a chromosomal translocation.[17] There is also an association between bilateral retinoblastoma of the orbit and rhabdomyosarcoma.[18]

Three main histopathologic types of rhabdomyosarcoma have been described: (1) embryonal, which accounts for 75% of tumors and is most common in younger children, (2) alveolar (20%), which has the worst prognosis and is seen in older children, and (3) pleomorphic, which accounts for 5% of the cases. Head and neck disease is further divided into three categories based on site of occurrence: (1) orbital, which carries the best prognosis, (2) parameningeal, which has the poorest prognosis, and (3) other sites. Parameningeal disease arises primarily in the middle ear, posterior nasopharynx, and nasal cavity and commonly involves the meninges, with intracranial spread.[19] The incidence of metastatic cervical adenopathy at the time of presentation ranges from 3% to 25%.[16,20] As with other head and neck malignancies in children, presenting signs and symptoms may initially be innocuous, resulting in a delay in diagnosis. Large nasopharyngeal, oropharyngeal, or laryngeal lesions may present with airway obstruction (Fig. 10-86).[18,21] The prognosis, as reported by the Intergroup Rhabdomyo-sarcoma Study (IRS), is best with complete surgical resection (Box 10-1).

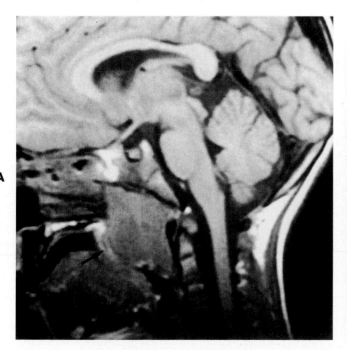

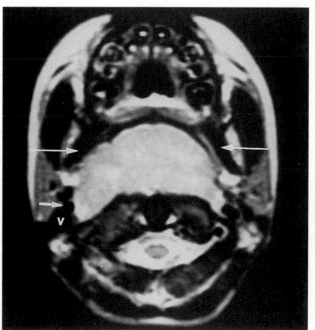

FIG. 10-83 Non-Hodgkin's lymphoma in a 6-year-old boy with severe airway obstruction. **A,** T1W sagittal image shows a large nasooropharyngeal mass obliterating the airway. The soft palate (*arrow*) is pushed anteroinferiorly by the mass. **B,** On this FSE T2W axial image the mass has pushed the vessels (*arrow,* internal carotid artery; *v,* internal jugular vein) and the pterygoid muscles (*long arrow*) laterally. Despite the large size, there is no skull base destruction and no cervical adenopathy.

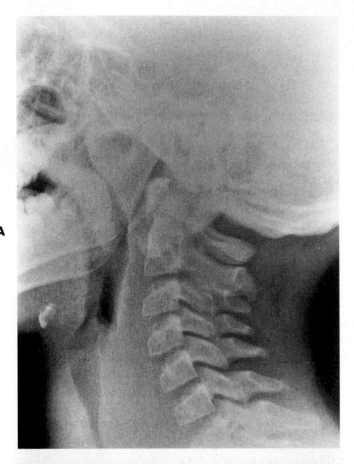

A

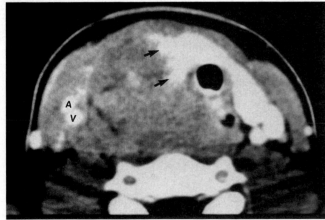

B

FIG. 10-84 Non-Hodgkin's lymphoma involving the thyroid gland in a 10-year-old boy with airway obstruction. **A,** Lateral plain film shows that the retropharyngeal soft tissues are prominent and the airway is narrowed. **B,** Axial contrast-enhanced CT shows a large right nonenhancing neck mass involving the right lobe of the thyroid *(arrows)* and extending behind the trachea and esophagus. The common carotid artery *(A)* and internal jugular vein *(V)* are pushed laterally.

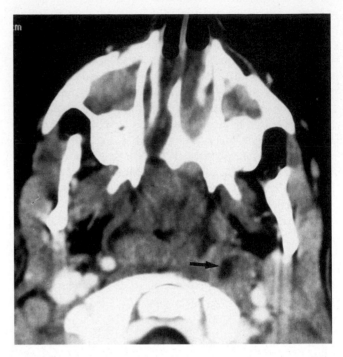

FIG. 10-85 Six-month-old boy with prenatally acquired AIDS and non-Hodgkin's lymphoma. Axial spiral contrast-enhanced CT shows a nasopharyngeal mass obliterating the airway. Note the necrotic left retropharyngeal lymph node *(arrow)*. (Courtesy Dr. John Alarcon, Scottish Rite Children's Medical Center, Atlanta, Georgia.)

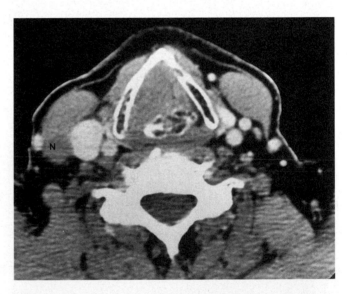

FIG. 10-86 Laryngeal rhabdomyosarcoma in an adult presenting with stridor. Although this spiral-enhanced CT scan is from an adult patient (notice laryngeal cartilaginous calcification), the characteristics of a nonenhancing laryngeal lesion are similar to those reported in the pediatric population. Note the ipsilateral metastatic internal jugular chain node *(N)*.

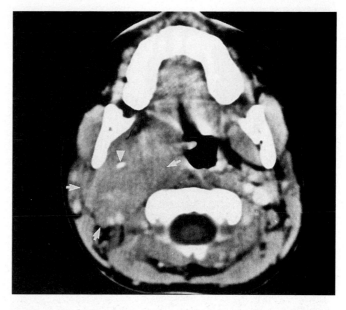

FIG. 10-87 Embryonal rhabdomyosarcoma in a young girl. There is little enhancement within this large skull base mass *(arrows),* arising in the retrostyloid space. Styloid process *(arrowhead).*

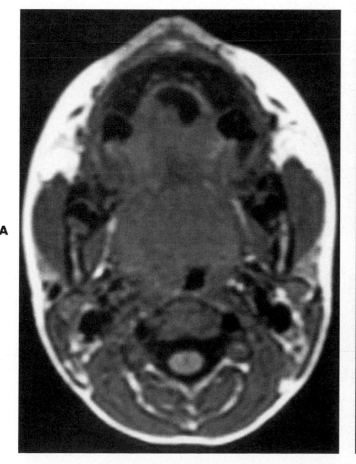

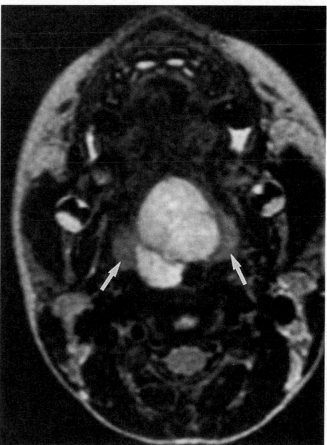

FIG. 10-88 Rhabdomyosarcoma in a young boy who presented with obstructive sleep apnea and difficulty swallowing. **A,** Axial T1W image shows a mass nearly obliterating the airway, but the borders of the mass are poorly seen on this sequence. **B,** The borders of the lesion are better appreciated on this T2W sequence. Note that the lesion is arising from the tongue. The normal palatine tonsils *(arrows)* are slightly lower in signal intensity than the tumor.

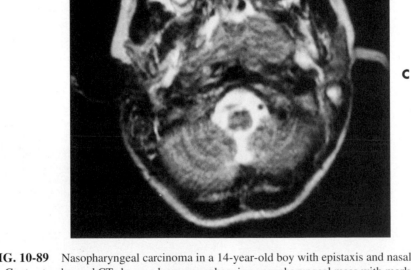

FIG. 10-89 Nasopharyngeal carcinoma in a 14-year-old boy with epistaxis and nasal obstruction. **A,** Contrast-enhanced CT shows a large nonenhancing nasopharyngeal mass with marked encroachment on the airway. Soft-tissue fullness *(N)* medial to the internal carotid arteries suggests retropharyngeal lymph node enlargement. **B,** After gadolinium, little enhancement is seen in the tumor, which has clearly infiltrated the prevertebral muscles on the left *(white arrows),* but a clear plane between the tumor and the soft tissues persists on the right *(black arrow).* Pretreatment imaging should determine the extent of disease, specifically skull base, intracranial, or prevertebral soft tissue involvement, in addition to nodal metastases. **C,** The mass is hypointense on this FSE T2W image, in contrast to the hyperintense benign secretions in the maxillary sinuses and the posterior nasopharynx. (Courtesy Dr. John Alarcon, Scottish Rite Children's Medical Center, Atlanta, Georgia.)

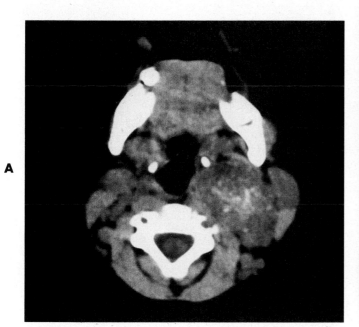
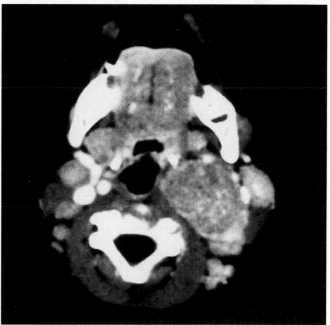

A

B

FIG. 10-90 Metastatic neuroblastoma to a cervical node in an 11-month-old boy. **A,** Axial non-contrast-enhanced CT shows a large left neck mass with mild effacement on the left airway. Note the punctate calcifications within the tumor, a characteristic of neuroblastoma. **B,** Contrast-enhanced bolus spiral CT shows minimal enhancement within the nodal mass, as compared with A. The vessels are splayed anterolaterally by the lesion. (Courtesy Dr. John Alarcon, Scottish Rite Children's Medical Center, Atlanta, Georgia.)

Imaging shows a soft-tissue mass, often with bone destruction. The tumor is usually heterogeneous, may be hemorrhagic, and has poorly defined infiltrating borders.[19,22] On CT, tumors mildly enhance (Fig. 10-87), whereas on MRI, most rhabdomyosarcomas markedly enhance (Fig. 10-88).[22] The presence of parameningeal involvement is important to detect preoperatively because combined craniofacial surgery may be performed.[15] MRI is the preferred modality when skull base disease is present because parameningeal involvement in these cases is common. A survey of the cervical lymph node chain also should be performed to detect metastatic adenopathy. The diagnosis is confirmed by excisional biopsy.

Treatment involves surgery, radiation, and chemotherapy. Posttreatment resolution of the tumor is a good indicator of prognosis, but disease may recur at a later date, and serial scans are recommended to detect early disease recurrence.[19]

NASOPHARYNGEAL CARCINOMA

Nasopharyngeal carcinoma, previously called lymphoepithelioma, is an uncommon malignancy in children. Nasopharyngeal carcinoma may be similar in presentation, imaging appearance, and even histology to the more common tumors, lymphoma and rhabdomyosarcoma.[1] As in the adult population with this disease, children commonly have elevated titers to the Epstein-Barr virus, suggesting an infectious etiology.[1] Unilateral nasal obstruction and otitis media, epistaxis, and rhinorrhea are common presenting findings.[3,23] Headache and cranial neuropathy imply skull base and intracranial extension. Most children have metastatic cervical adenopathy at the time of presentation.[1]

CT and MRI of nasopharyngeal carcinoma show a large, inhomogeneous mass filling the nasopharyngeal airway, often with skull base erosion and intracranial extension (Fig. 10-89).[24] Necrotic cervical adenopathy, particularly involving the retropharyngeal and high jugular chain nodes, is common.

The primary treatment modality is radiation, with a 5-year survival of 60% in some series.[25]

MISCELLANEOUS

There is a variety of miscellaneous rare malignancies in the head and neck, which may have airway involvement. Neuroblastoma of the head and neck is most commonly metastatic from neural crest sympathetic precursor cells in the adrenal gland. There usually is disease in the cervical lymph nodes, the orbit, or the skull.[1,14] CT or MRI of the tumor is nonspecific, showing either a large cervical node or a mass in the orbit or skull, sometimes with dystrophic calcification and often with extensive bone destruction (Fig. 10-90). Imaging of the primary lesion, especially the adrenal

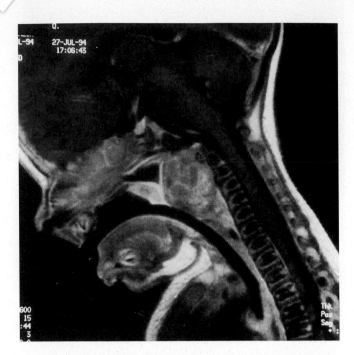

FIG. 10-91 Malignant rhabdoid tumor in an infant. Sagittal postgadolinium T1W sequence show an inhomogeneously enhancing mass in the retropharyngeal and precervical soft tissues. (Courtesy Dr. Suresh Mukerji.)

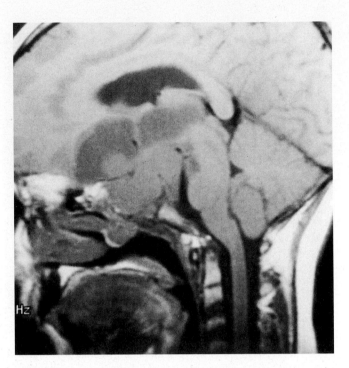

FIG. 10-92 Sagittal T1W MRI shows a primitive neuroectodermal tumor. This complex mass arose intracranially, extending through the skull base and sphenoid sinus and into the posterior nasal cavity. This 10-year-old boy presented with headaches.

gland, should be performed.[1] Malignant rhabdoid tumor is a rare aggressive pediatric neoplasm that originates either from the kidney or from extrarenal sites, including the head and neck.[26] The radiographic appearance is nonspecific (Fig. 10-91). Thyroid carcinoma is rare in children and is strongly associated with a prior history of radiation.[1] This tumor also may be increased in incidence in long-term survivors of acute lymphoblastic leukemia.[27] Patients present with a palpable neck mass, hoarseness, or dysphagia.[27] Ultrasound or ^{123}I thyroid scan are often used to image the lesion and determine if the mass is "cold." Cold nodules in children have a higher incidence of malignancy, up to 29% in some series,[28,29] than in adults. The definitive diagnosis is made by fine needle aspiration or surgical biopsy.

Laryngeal carcinoma, also a rare pediatric neoplasm, is associated with recurrent respiratory papillomatosis or juvenile laryngeal papillomatosis and is similar in CT and MR appearance to adult laryngeal carcinoma.[30-32] Chondrosarcomas, other sarcomas, malignant teratomas, and other carcinomas have been reported in the head and neck in children, but they rarely cause airway compromise. Skull base lesions, when large, may affect the airway (Fig. 10-92).

Airway neoplasms in children with AIDS include non-Hodgkin's lymphoma, bronchial leiomyomata, a benign smooth muscle tumor, and bronchial leiomyosarcomas.[1,33] Inflammatory disease such as chronic sinusitis and otitis media are more common in pediatric AIDs patients.

References

1. Myers EN, Cunningham MJ. Tumors of the neck. In: Bluestone CD, Stool SE, eds. Pediatric otolaryngology. Philadelphia, Pa: WB Saunders, 1990.
2. Silverberg E, Lubera J. Cancer statistics. CA - A Cancer Journal for Clinicians and the American Cancer Society, Inc 1988; 38:5-22.
3. Cunningham MJ, Myers EN, Bluestone CD. Malignant tumors of the head and neck in children: a twenty-year review. Int J Pediatr Otorhinolaryngol 1987; 13:279-292.
4. Bonilla JA, Healy GB. Management of malignant head and neck tumors in children. Pediatr Clin North Am 1989; 36:1443-1450.
5. Hoppe RT, Burke JS, Glatstein E, et al. Non-Hodgkin's lymphoma: involvement of Waldeyer's Ring. Cancer 1978; 42:1096-1104.
6. Balsam D, Segal S. Two smooth muscle tumors in the airway of an HIV infected child. Pediatr Radiol 1992; 22:552-553.
7. Ziegler JL. Burkitt's lymphoma. N Engl J Med 1981; 305:735-745.
8. Kearns DB, Smith RJH, Pitcock JK. Burkitt's lymphoma. Int J Pediatr Otorhinolaryngol 1986; 12:73-84.
9. Levine PH, Kamaraju LS, Connelly RR, et al. The American Burkitt's lymphoma registry: eight years' experience. Cancer 1982; 49:1016-1022.
10. Murphy SB. Classification, staging and end results of treatment of childhood Non-Hodgkin's lymphomas: dissimilarities from lymphomas in adults. Seminars in Oncology 1980; 7:332-339.
11. Harnsberger HR, Bragg DG, Osborn AG, et al. Non-Hodgkin's lymphoma of the head and neck: CT evaluation of nodal and extranodal sites. AJNR Am J Neuroradiol 1987; 8:673-679.
12. Reede DL, Som RM. Lymph nodes. In: Som PM, Bergeron RT, eds. Head and neck imaging. Philadelphia, Pa: Mosby–Year Book, Inc, 1991.
13. Sullivan MP. Hodgkin's disease in children. Hematology/Oncology Clin North Am 1987; 1:603-620.
14. Jaffe BF, Jaffe N. Head and neck tumors in children. Pediatrics 1973; 51:731-740.
15. MacArthur CJ, McGill TJI, Healy GB. Pediatric head and neck rhabdomyosarcoma. Clinical Pediatrics 1992; 31:66-70.
16. Anderson GJ, Tom LW, Womer RB, et al. Rhabdomyosarcoma of the head and neck in children. Arch Otolaryngol Head Neck Surg 1990; 116:428-431.
17. McGill T. Rhabdomyosarcoma of the head and neck: an update. Otolaryngol Clin North Am 1989; 22:631-636.
18. Brookes CN, van Velzen D. Rhabdomyosarcoma, presenting as a facial swelling in a child. A case report and review of the literature. Br J Oral and Maxillofacial Surg 1990; 28:117-121.
19. Latack JT, Hutchinson RJ, Heyn RM. Imaging of rhabdomyosarcomas of the head and neck. AJNR Am J Neuroradiol 1987; 8:353-359.
20. Coene IJ, Schouwenburg PF, Voute PA, et al. Rhabdomyosarcoma of the head and neck in children. Clin Otolaryngol 1992; 17:291-296.
21. Dodd-o JM, Wieneke KF, Rosman PM. Laryngeal rhabdomyosarcoma. Cancer 1987; 59:1012-1018.
22. Yousem DM, Lexa FJ, Bilaniuk LT, et al. Rhabdomyosarcomas in the head and neck: MR imaging evaluation. Radiology 1990; 177:683-686.
23. Huang T. Cancer of the nasopharynx in childhood. Cancer 1990; 66:968-971.
24. Bass IS, Haller JO, Berndon WE, et al. Nasopharyngeal carcinoma: clinical and radiographic findings in children. Radiology 1985; 156:651-654.
25. Fearon B, Forte V, Brama I. Malignant nasopharyngeal tumors in children. Laryngoscope 1990; 100:470-472.
26. Schmidt D, Leuschner I, Harms D. Malignant rhabdoid tumor: a morphological and flow cytometric study. Path Res Pract 1989; 184:202-210.
27. DeKeyser L, Van Herle A. Differentiated thyroid cancer in children. Head Neck Surg 1985; 8:100-114.
28. White AK, Smith RJH. Thyroid nodules in children. Otolaryngol Head Neck Surg 1986; 95:70-75.
29. Desjardins JG, Khan AH, Montupet P, et al. Management of thyroid nodules in children: a 20-year experience. J Pediatr Surg 1987; 22:736-739.
30. Schwartz DA, Katin L, Lesser RD, et al. Juvenile laryngeal carcinoma: correlation of computed tomography and magnetic resonance imaging with pathology. Ann Clin Lab Science 1990; 20:225-226.
31. Schnadig VJ, Clark WD, Clegg TJ, et al. Invasive papillomatosis and squamous carcinoma complicating juvenile laryngeal papillomatosis. Arch Otolaryngol Head Neck Surgery 1986; 112:966-971.
32. Solomon D, Smith RR, Kashima HK, et al. Malignant transformation in non-irradiated recurrent respiratory papillomatosis. Laryngoscope 1985; 95:900-904.
33. Balsam D, Segal S. Two smooth muscle tumors in the airway of an HIV infected child. Pediatr Radiol 1992; 22:552-553.

11

Larynx

HUGH D. CURTIN

Technologic advances in computed tomography (CT) and magnetic resonance imaging (MRI) have had a definite effect on our ability to image the larynx.[1-10] The quality of laryngeal images always has been related to the acquisition speed and the degradation motion artifacts from breathing, swallowing, and carotid artery pulsations. Today with spiral CT scanning and fast MR techniques, excellent images can be achieved. Using these techniques, the radiologist can visualize and assess the deeper laryngeal structures, and combined with the surface visualization of modern laryngoscopy, the referring clinician now can have an excellent understanding of the extent of a lesion.

In most cases the otolaryngologist has evaluated the mucosal surface and, in the case of carcinoma, has no question about the diagnosis. The radiologist's role, as is so often the case in head and neck radiology, is to show the deeper disease extent, defining the tumor margins in relationship to precise anatomic landmarks. Because these determinations

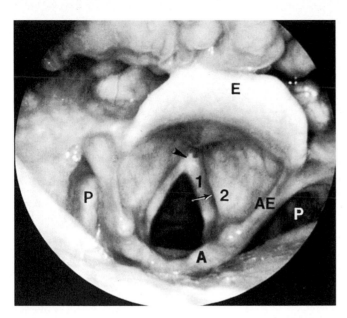

FIG. 11-1 Endoscopic view of the larynx. *1,* True vocal cord; *2,* false vocal cord; *E,* epiglottis; *AE,* aryepiglottic fold; *A,* arytenoid prominence; *P* pyriform; *arrowhead,* anterior commissure. Arrow points to the entrance of the ventricle. (From Hanafee W. Hypopharynx and larynx. In: Valvassori GE, et al. Head and neck imaging. New York, NY: Thieme Medical Publishers, 1988.)

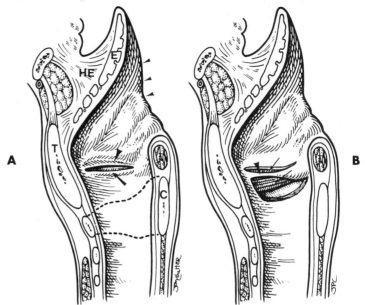

FIG. 11-2 **A,** Lateral wall of the airway. The larynx has been sectioned sagittally in the midline. True cord *(arrow)* and false cord *(large arrowhead)* are separated by the slitlike ventricle. *Small arrowheads,* AE fold; *T,* thyroid cartilage; *C,* lamina of the cricoid cartilage (the projection of the arch of the cricoid is seen as a *dashed line); HE,* hyoepiglottic ligament; *E,* epiglottis. **B,** The mucosa of the true cord has been excised showing the thyroarytenoid muscle *(arrow)* paralleling the margin of the true cord *(arrowhead).*

can make the difference between a total laryngectomy and a voice-sparing partial resection, to best communicate with the surgeon, the radiologist must know the anatomy from an otolaryngologist's perspective.

This chapter begins with the normal anatomy as seen using various imaging modalities. The discussion of the alterations of this anatomy as a result of various types of pathology follows. For completeness, some processes in which imaging is seldom helpful are included. The laryngopharynx is included because of its intimate relationship with the posterior aspects of the larynx.

SECTION ONE
ANATOMY

The larynx is composed of a mucosal surface and a supporting cartilaginous skeleton. The mucosal surface, which is familiar to any otolaryngologist, has typical landmarks, including the epiglottis, true and false cords, aryepiglottic folds, and pyriform sinuses (Figs. 11-1, 11-2). Between the mucosal surface and the cartilaginous skeleton lie the paraglottic and preepiglottic spaces, which contain loose areolar tissues, lymphatics, and key muscular structures.

The skeleton of the larynx is made up of cartilage and fibrous bands (Figs. 11-3, 11-4). The foundation is the cricoid cartilage, which is the only complete cartilaginous ring in the respiratory system. The cricoid is shaped like a signet ring, with the larger "signet" part facing posteriorly.

This broader signet segment is called the *quadrate lamina.* The narrower arch extends anteriorly from the margins of the lamina to complete the ring. The complete arch is only at the caudal margin of the cricoid cartilage, and it will define the caudal aspect of the larynx. On each side, at the junction of the arch and lamina, is a small facet for the articulation of the inferior horn of the thyroid cartilage.

On the upper margin of the lamina are two paired facets, on which are situated the arytenoid cartilages (Figs. 11-3, 11-5). Each arytenoid is pyramidal in shape and is important as a surgical landmark and as a radiologic guide to help determine the level of an axial scan within the larynx. The base of the arytenoid has a posterolateral mass called the *muscular process* and an anterior caudal vocal process to which the vocal ligament attaches (Figs. 11-3, 11-5). The cricoarytenoid joint is at the base of the arytenoid and at the level of the vocal process.

The largest cartilage is the double-winged thyroid cartilage, with prominant superior and inferior cornua projecting from the posterior margin of each side of the thyroid ala (wings). The lower cornu articulates with the lateral facets of the cricoid cartilage, forming the cricothyroid joint. The superior thyroid cornu is connected to the dorsal tip of the greater cornu of the hyoid bone by the thyrohyoid ligament, and the remaining gap between the upper surface of the thyroid cartilage and the hyoid bone is filled by the tough thyrohyoid membrane. Similarly the gap between the lower surface of the thyroid cartilage and the cricoid cartilage is filled by the cricothyroid membrane. The anterior thyroid

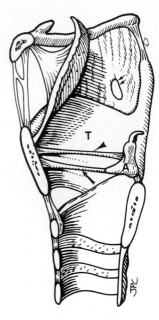

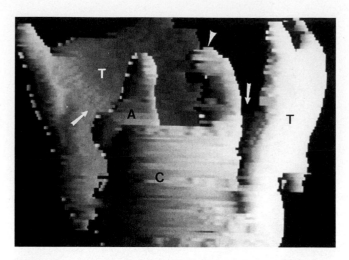

FIG. 11-3   Lateral diagram of the larynx with the mucosa, laryngeal muscles, and paraglottic fat removed to show the skeleton of the larynx. The vocal ligament *(arrow)* stretches from the vocal process of the arytenoid *(A)* to the anterior thyroid cartilage. The ventricular ligament *(arrowhead)* stretches from the upper arytenoid to the thyroid cartilage. The small structure at the upper tip of the arytenoid is the corniculate cartilage. The lamina of the thyroid cartilage is represented by the letter *T*. The small hole *(double small arrows)* in the thyrohyoid membrane transmits the internal branch of the superior laryngeal nerve and the accompanying vessels. The posterior thyrohyoid ligament *(open arrow)* represents the posterior margin of the thyrohyoid membrane.

FIG. 11-4   Computer reconstruction of the larynx, from axial CT scans, is viewed from posteriorly and slightly to the right. The arytenoid *(A)* is perched on the lamina of the cricoid cartilage *(C)*. Thyroid cartilage is represented by the letter *T*. Arrows show the thyroarytenoid gap representing the position of the apex of the pyriform sinus. Arrowhead shows the corniculate cartilage.

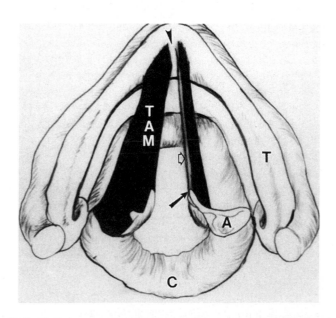

FIG. 11-5   Larynx viewed from above; the mucosa and most of the soft tissues of the larynx have been removed to show the relationship of arytenoid *(A)*, cricoid ring *(C)*, and thyroid cartilage *(T)*. The vocal ligament *(open arrow)* stretches from the vocal process *(arrow)* of the arytenoid to the anterior commissure *(arrowhead)*. *TAM,* Thyroarytenoid muscle. Only the medial muscle bundle *(vocalis)* is seen on the right.

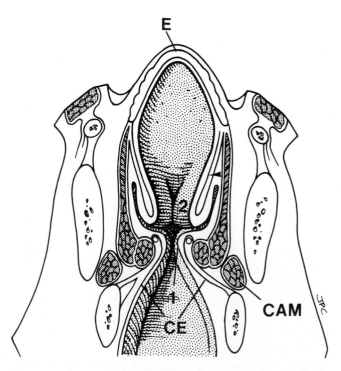

FIG. 11-6   Diagram of a coronal section through the larynx. The thyroarytenoid muscle forms the mass of the cord. The lateral cricoarytenoid muscle *(CAM)* is also seen slightly laterally and inferiorly. The conus elasticus *(CE)* extends from the vocal ligament at the cord level to the upper margin of the cricoid. On the right side of the diagram, the conus terminates at the upper margin of the cricoid cartilage. On the left side of the diagram, some fibers of the conus continue along the medial surface of the cricoid as described by some authors. *E,* Epiglottis; *1,* true cord; *2,* false cord; *arrowhead,* quadrangular membrane.

cartilage has a deep notch in its upper surface called the *superior thyroid notch*. Where the thyroid alae join at the bottom of this notch there is a prominence that forms the "Adam's apple." The thyroid and cricoid cartilages act as the external protective shield for the inner larynx. The cricoid, thyroid, and arytenoid cartilages are all hyaline cartilages, which ossify to varying degrees. On the outer surface of the thyoid cartilage is the oblique line, which extends downward and anteriorly from the root of the superior thyroid cornu to the lower border of the thyroid ala. The sternothyroid, thyrohyoid, and inferior pharyngeal constrictor muscles attach to this line.

The epiglottis is formed by yellow elastic fibrocartilage that, unlike the thyroid, cricoid, and arytenoid cartilages, seldom shows significant calcification. The epiglottis is extremely flexible and has a "memory" that allows it to return to its normal shape after being bent nearly at right angles. The epiglottis has a flattened teardrop shape that tapers to an inferior point called the petiole of the epiglottis. Although the major portion of the epiglottis extends down behind the protective shield of the thyroid cartilage, a small portion, often referred to as the *suprahyoid epiglottis* extends above the hyoid bone. The epiglottic cartilage is held in place by the hyoepiglottic and thyroepiglottic ligaments.

Three smaller pairs of cartilage are found in the upper larynx. They are less significant radiologically, but they are occasionally visualized. The corniculate cartilages are small structures sitting immediately superior to the arytenoids (Fig. 11-3). Slightly lateral and above the corniculate cartilages, buried in the aryepiglottic folds, are the thin cuneiform cartilages, which are almost never visualized on sectional imaging. The triticeous cartilage (cartilaginous triticea) is found in the thyrohyoid ligament.

The hyoid bone is the "rafter" from which the larynx is suspended. Muscles acting on the hyoid elevate the larynx, and thus provide the primary protection from aspiration. The hyoid bone is U shaped, having an anterior body and two large (greater) cornua that project posteriorly. Two small (lesser) cornua project superiorly from the hyoid body, and the stylohyoid ligaments attach to these lesser cornua.

Together the hyoid bone, thryoid and cricoid cartilages, and the cricothyroid and thyrohyoid membranes complete the external supportive architecture of the larynx and define the external anatomic limits of the larynx.

Two parallel ligaments extend anteriorly from the arytenoid cartilages, reaching and attaching to the inner lamina of the thyroid cartilage (Fig. 11-3). The more inferior vocal ligament stretches from the vocal process of the arytenoid cartilage to the middle third of the anterior fused portion of the thyroid cartilage. This vocal ligament forms the medial support of the true vocal cord, and the point of its attachment to the thyroid cartilage is called the *anterior commissure*. The ventricular ligament, on the other hand, attaches to the superior aspect of the arytenoid cartilage and stretches across the larynx (parallel to the vocal ligament) to attach to the inner lamina of the thyroid cartilage just above the attachment of the vocal ligament. This ligament is actually

the lower free margin of the quadrangular membrane, and it forms the free edge of the false cord, or plica ventricularis.

The quadrangular membrane attaches posteriorly to the upper arytenoid and corniculate cartilages, then sweeps across the upper larynx to attach to the lateral margin of the epiglottis (Fig. 11-6). The lower margin is free and is the ventricular ligament, and the upper margin forms the support of the aryepiglottic fold, which is the upper lateral wall of the supraglottic larynx.

A second membrane or fibrous layer, the conus elasticus, stretches downward from the vocal ligament of the true cord to attach to the upper inner margin of the cricoid cartilage (Fig. 11-6). Although some fibers of the conus may reflect along the inner margin of the cricoid to its lower surface, for the purposes of this discussion it will be considered that the conus attaches to the superior cricoid margin. The conus elasticus is a thicker, more clearly defined membrane than the quadrangular membrane, and anteriorly the conus fuses with the inner surface of the anterior cricothyroid membrane.

As was previously mentioned, the epiglottis is partially supported by the quadrangular membrane. However, the primary supports of the epiglottis are the hyoepiglottic and thyroepiglottic ligaments. The hyoepiglottic ligament is a definite fibrous structure that extends from the ventral vertical midline of the epiglottis to the dorsal margin of the body of the hyoid bone (Fig. 11-2). The midline (or median) glossoepiglottic fold and the more lateral pharyngoepiglottic folds are more mucosal reflections than they are true ligaments. They define the margins of the valleculae. Inferiorly the thyroepiglottic ligament extends from the petiole to the midline inner surface of the thyroid cartilage, just above the attachment of the vocal ligaments (anterior commissure).

The laryngeal muscles are described in terms of their origins and insertions. To the radiologist, the most important muscle is the thyroarytenoid muscle because of its role as a landmark defining the level of the true vocal cord (Figs. 11-2, 11-5, 11-7).

Each thyroarytenoid muscle stretches from the anterior lower surface of the arytenoid cartilage to the inner aspect of the thyroid cartilage, paralleling the vocal ligament. The thyroarytenoid muscle is responsible for most of the bulk of the true cord. Each muscle can be separated into two bellies—medial and lateral—that run roughly parallel to each other. The medial portion is often called the *vocalis muscle*. The mass of the lateral portion of the muscle is at the level of the true cord, but a few fibers can extend superiorly to insert high on the thyroid cartilage. Thus a narrow slip of the thyroarytenoid muscle may be present above the level of the true cord.

Of equal importance to the function of the larynx but not as crucial to the radiologist are the cricoarytenoid muscles (Fig. 11-8). The lateral cricoarytenoid muscle stretches from the muscular process of the arytenoid to the upper lateral cricoid cartilage. The posterior cricoarytenoid muscle stretches from the muscular process of the arytenoid to the posterior surface of the cricoid. These small antagonistic muscles occasionally can be identified on CT and MRI. The

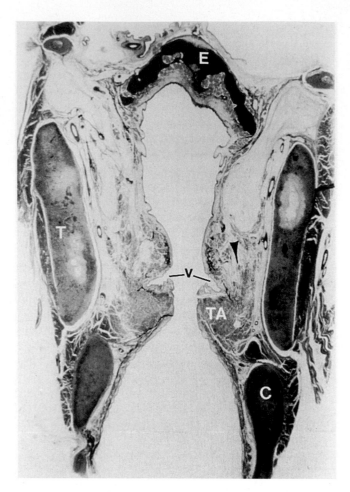

FIG. 11-7   Coronal section of the larynx. The bulk of the true cord is made up of the thyroarytenoid muscle *(TA)*. The ventricle *(v)* is seen between true and false cords. The paraglottic space *(arrowhead)* at the level of the false cord contains small slips of muscle but is filled predominantly with fat. *T,* Thyroid cartilage; *C,* cricoid cartilage; *E,* epiglottic cartilage.

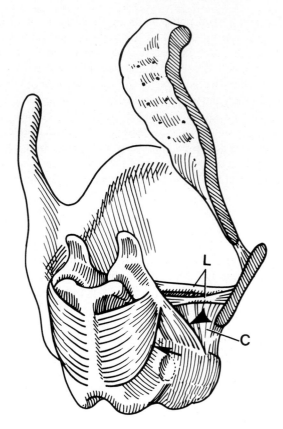

FIG. 11-8   Diagram of a postero-right lateral view of the laryngeal skeleton (right thyroid lamina has been removed) showing the posterior *(arrow)* and lateral *(arrowhead)* cricoarytenoid muscles. The posterior cricoarytenoid muscle is totally responsible for abduction of the true cord as the muscle pulls posteriorly on the lateral muscular process of the arytenoid. *C,* Conus elasticus; *L,* vocal ligaments.

posterior cricoarytenoid muscle is the only muscle that directly swings the vocal cord laterally (abduction). The interarytenoid muscles stretch from one arytenoid to the other, completing the midline posterior wall of the larynx above the cricoid. The lateral cricoarytenoid and the interarytenoid muscle both adduct the true cords. The interarytenoid muscles are the only laryngeal muscles to have bilateral innervation from the recurrent laryngeal nerves; all the other intrinsic muscles are innervated either by the left or right recurrent laryngeal nerves. The cricothyroid muscle, which extends from the lower thyroid cartilage to the upper cricoid cartilage, is the only extrinsic laryngeal muscle. It is also the only laryngeal muscle supplied by the external branch of the superior laryngeal nerve (X).

The pharyngeal constrictors attach posteriorly to a midline raphe and then sweep obliquely downward around the lumen of the pharynx to attach to the hyoid bone above and more inferiorly to the sides of the cricoid and thyroid cartilages. Notably the more inferior fibers attach to the lateral ala of the thyroid cartilage, not along the posterior margin of the cartilage, but along the oblique line on the lateral surface

of this cartilage. This becomes important when evaluating tumors, as described in a later section. The pharyngeal constrictors are innervated by the pharyngeal plexus, which has major contributions from the vagus nerve (X) and lesser contributions from the glossopharyngeal nerve (IX).

The most caudal oblique fibers of the inferior constrictor muscle are separated from the top of the lowermost parallel, nonraphed fibers of the inferior constrictor muscle by a triangular space referred to as Killian's dehiscence. It is through this area that a Zenker's diverticulum extends. These parallel, nonraphed muscle fibers are usually referred to as the *cricopharyngeus muscle,* which acts as a sphincter between the pharynx and the esophagus, stretching continuously from each lateral surface of the cricoid cartilage circumferentially around the gullet.

The inner surface of the larynx has two prominent parallel horizontal bands—the true and false cords (Figs. 11-1, 11-2). The true cord is the more inferior and is separated from the false cord by a slitlike lateral outpouching, the laryngeal ventricle. Each true cord attaches anteriorly just off of the midline, leaving a small "bare" area in the precise midline where the mucosa of the larynx is immediately adjacent to the thyroid cartilage. This region is called the anterior commissure, and it is slightly caudal to the thyroid attachment of the petiole (Fig. 11-3).

Above the false cords, the laryngeal mucosa reflects upward toward the free edges of the aryepiglottic folds. These aryepiglottic folds form the lateral margins of the vestibule, or supraglottic airway. Each aryepiglottic fold stretches from the upper margin of the arytenoid to the lateral margin of the epiglottis. Within the aryepiglottic fold are the small corniculate and cuneiform cartilages that help support the edge of each fold.

The epiglottis projects superiorly toward the oropharynx, causing several small folds and recesses to be defined. The valleculae are small recesses between the free margin of the epiglottis and the base of the tongue. As described above, the valleculae are separated in the midline by a small fold, the median glossoepiglottic fold, and laterally on each side the pharyngoepiglottic folds form the posterior aspect of each valleculae.

The cranial margin of the larynx is considered to be the fold of mucosa that extends anteriorly across the upper surface of the epiglottis, then posteriorly along the free edge of each aryepiglotiic fold, to the posterior margin at the interaryentoid notch.

The preepiglottic space is the space between the epiglottis (posteriorly) and the lowermost hyoid bone, thyrohyoid membrane, and thyroid cartilage (anteriorly). The cranial limit of this space is the thryohyoid ligament, and the caudal limit is the thyroepiglottic ligament. This space is primarily filled with fat; however, there is a rich lymphatic and microvascular network within this fat and the adjacent paraglottic spaces, which communicate on either side with the preepiglottic space.

The paraglottic space (occasionally referred to as the paralaryngeal space) is the fat-containing space between the mucosal surface of the larynx and the thyrohyoid membrane, thyroid cartilage, and upper surface of the croid cartilage (Figs. 11-6, 11-7). Thus the paraglottic space is the region deep to the mucosal surface of the true and false cords. At the false cord level, the paraglottic space is almost entirely composed of the fat lying between the quadrangular membrane and the thyroid cartilage. As previously stated, although small slips of thyroarytenoid muscle may cross the space, there is no bulky muscle present. The laryngeal ventricle extends laterally into each space; however, the ventricle does not reach the inner surface of the thyroid cartilage. Thus a narrow band of paraglottic fat is present lateral to each ventricle. At the level of the true cord, the thyroarytenoid muscle fills almost all of the paraglottic space (Fig. 11-7). Thus the paraglottic space is continuous from the false cord to the true cord levels, passing along the lateral aspect of the ventricle.

At the level of the false cord, a small recess projects superiorly from the anterior ventricle into the paraglottic fat. This recess is called the *laryngeal saccule,* or *appendix,* and it lies between the quadrangular membrane and the thyroid

cartilage. Dilatation of the saccule causing a submucosal supraglottic mass is called a laryngocele.

Lateral to the aryepiglottic fold is the pyriform sinus of the pharynx (Fig. 11-9). This anterior mucosal recess pushes between the posterior third of the thyroid cartilage and the aryepiglottic fold. The extreme lower aspect of the pyriform sinus, called the apex, is actually situated between the mucosa-covered arytenoid and the mucosa-covered thyroid cartilage and is at the level of the true vocal cord. Anteriorly the pyriform sinus protrudes into the paraglottic space.

INNERVATION AND BLOOD SUPPLY

The larynx is innervated primarily by the vagus nerve. Each recurrent laryngeal nerve, after looping around the aortic arch on the left side and the subclavian artery on the right side, travels in the tracheoesophageal groove at the lateral margin of the esophagus. Each nerve then passes medial to the lower margin of the cricopharyngeus muscle, and enters the larynx in the sulcus between the thyroid cartilage and the cricoid cartilage, just above the cricothyroid joint. The recurrent laryngeal nerve innervates all of the intrinsic muscles of the larynx. As mentioned, the only extrinsic laryngeal muscle, the cricothyroid muscle, is innervated by the

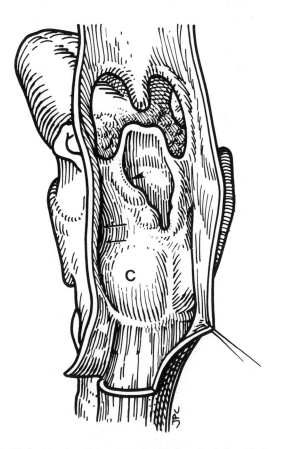

FIG. 11-9 A view from posterior and to the left with the pharynx open. The arrows show the pyriform sinus. *Arrowhead,* aryepiglottic fold; *C,* cricoid. (Modified from Berman JM. Surgical anatomy of the larynx. In: Bailey BJ, Biller HF. Surgery of the larynx. Philadelphia, Pa: WB Saunders Co, 1985; 20.)

external branch of the superior laryngeal nerve, which never enters the inner larynx. The internal branch of the superior laryngeal nerve does perforate the posterior lateral portion of the thyrohyoid membrane, and it provides sensation to the laryngeal mucosa.

The blood supply to the larynx accompanies the nerves. The superior laryngeal artery is a branch of the superior thyroid artery and follows the internal branch of the superior laryngeal nerve. The inferior laryngeal artery is a branch of the inferior thyroid artery, which in turn is a branch of the thyrocervical trunk. The inferior laryngeal artery accompanies the recurrent laryngeal nerve into the larynx.

LYMPHATIC DRAINAGE

The lymphatic drainage of the larynx follows the embryological derivation of the larynx, which means that the supraglottic larynx can be considered a derivative of the pharynx and the subglottic larynx can be considered a derivative of the trachea. Thus the mucosal lymphatics of the supraglottic larynx drain to the upper jugular nodes. Those of the subglottic larynx drain into the paratracheal and pretracheal nodes and eventually into the lower jugular nodes. The mucosal surface of the true cord has almost no lymphatic drainage. As mentioned, the preepiglottic and paraglottic spaces are particularly rich in lymphatics, and the greater the tumor infiltration into these areas, the more likely it is that there will be cervical metastatic nodal disease. The Delphian node is situated anterior to the cricothyroid membrane, and tumor can reach this node either by direct extension or by lymphatic drainage from the region of the anterior commissure and subglottic larynx. Enlargement of this node may be the first clinical manifestation of the presence of subglottic tumor.

The lymphatics of the paraglottic space drain superiorly, again to the upper jugular nodes. According to Pressman, Simon, and Monell, an injection of dye into the deep cord (thyroarytenoid muscle) also drains superiorly, past the ventricle and through the thyrohyoid membrane, into the upper jugular nodes along with the lymphatics of the upper larynx.[11] Thus the drainage of the deep larynx (as opposed to the mucosal surface) flows only in a superior direction.

REGIONS

Certain anatomic terms are important when describing the larynx, and this is especially true when discussing tumors. The larynx is subdivided by two theoretical horizontal (axial) planes; one extends through the apex of the two laryngeal ventricles, and the second parallel plane is 1 cm caudal to the first plane. The supraglottic larynx is that portion of the larynx cranial to the first plane, and the upper margin of the supraglottic larynx, as described previously, is the free edge of the epiglottis and the aryepiglottic folds. The upper arytenoid cartilages are included in the supraglottic larynx. The glottis is the region between the two planes and includes the anterior and posterior commissures. The subglottis is the region between the lower plane and the caudal margin of the cricoid cartilage.

The suprahyoid portion of the epiglottis is often called the *free segment,* and the anterior surface of the free segment of the epiglottis, as well as the valleculae, are often included in discussions of the base of the tongue and the pharynx. The postcricoid region is the mucosal covering of the posterior surface of the cricoid, representing the anterior wall of the pharynx at this level. A prominent venous plexus is present in this region, often being confused with a tumor on barium studies. Because of its relationship to both the pharynx and the larynx, the free edge of the aryepiglottic fold is at times referred to with the terms junctional or marginal.

References

1. Castelijns JA, Gerritesen GJ, Kaiser MC, et al. Invasion of laryngeal cartilage by cancer: comparison of CT and MR imaging. Radiology 1987; 166:199-206.
2. Castelijns JA, Kaiser MC, Valk K, et al. MR imaging of laryngeal cancer. JCAT 1987; 11(1):134-140.
3. Curtin HD. Current concepts of imaging of the larynx. Radiology 1989; 173:1-11.
4. Giron J, Joffre P, Serres-Cousine O, et al. [Magnetic resonance imaging of the larynx: its contribution compared to x-ray computed tomography in the pre-therapeutic evaluation of cancers of the larynx. Apropos of 90 surgical cases]. [French]. Original Title: L'imagerie par resonance magnetique du larynx. Apport comare a celui de la tomodensitometrie dans le bilan pre-therapeutique des cancers du larynx. A propos de qauatre-vingt dix cas operes. Ann Radiol (Paris) 1990; 33(3):170-184.
5. Hanafee WN. Hypopharynx and larynx. In: Valvassori GE, et al. Head and neck imaging. New York, NY: Thieme Medical Publishers Inc, 1988; 311-338.
6. Lufkin RB, Hanafee WN. Application of surface coil to MR anatomy of the larynx. AJR 1985; 145:483-492.
7. Lufkin RB, Hanafee WN, Wortham D, et al. Larynx and hypopharynx: MR imaging in surface coils. Radiology 1986; 158:747-754.
8. Mancuso AA, Hanafee WN. Larynx and hypopharynx. In: Computed tomography and magnetic resonance of the head and neck. 2nd Edition. Baltimore, Md: Williams & Wilkins, 1985; 241-357.
9. McArdle CB, Bailey BJ, Amparo EG. Surface coil magnetic resonance imaging of the normal larynx. Arch Otolaryngol Head Neck Surg 1986; 112:616-622.
10. Stark DD, Moss AA, Gamsu G, et al. Magnetic resonance imaging of the neck. I. Normal anatomy. Radiology 1984; 150:447-452.
11. Pressman JJ, Simon MB, Monell C. Anatomic studies related to the dissemination of cancer of the larynx. Trans Am Acad Ophthalmol Otolaryngol 1960; 64:628-644.

SECTION TWO
IMAGING

In this section the various imaging modalities are discussed, along with the normal anatomy visible on each examination. A review of certain respiratory movements is included also because these maneuvers can be used to accentuate different areas in the larynx during imaging. Although these respiratory maneuvers were used extensively with laryngography and multidirectional tomography, they have proved less useful with CT and MRI. Initially the patient could not maintain the respiratory maneuver for the length of time required to perform the CT or MR scan. However, with today's faster imaging, examinations in different respiratory phases may be possible again. The coronal plane is ideal for appreciating these movements, so tomography is used for illustration.

RESPIRATORY MANEUVERS

In quiet respiration the vocal cords are abducted off of the midline but not completely effaced against the lateral laryngeal wall. In the coronal plane the cord has a flat upper surface, and the lower surface has a downward slope to the lateral wall of the subglottic larynx. This slope is best seen in phonation, and it is often called the *subglottic arch*. With slow inspiration the true cords and false cords further abduct, disappearing as they flatten against the now smooth lateral wall of the larynx. When the patient holds his or her breath and "bears down" (Valsalva's maneuver), the cords go to the midline (adduct), squaring off the subglottic arch. No airway is seen at the true cord level, and the false cords may also approximate in the midline. The modified Valsalva's maneuver is done with the cheeks puffed and the patient allowing the slow escape of air. This maneuver puffs not only the cheeks but also dilates the pyriform sinuses and all the airway structures above the true cords. With phonation (the patient makes a high-pitched "eeee" sound), the cords tense and approach the midline, leaving a narrow airway. The ventricle may be expanded or collapsed in any maneuver. The reverse, or inspiratory *eeee* maneuver, usually dilates the ventricle. Although this maneuver may be difficult for many patients, usually any noise made while breathing in will suffice.

Although these maneuvers are expected to produce the described effects, many times the particular structure the radiologist is trying to visualize shows up on the "wrong" maneuver. Thus the typical examination usually takes the patient through all of these maneuvers (Figs. 11-10, 11-11).

PLAIN RADIOGRAPHS

The soft-tissue technique uses a lower kilovolt (kV) than that used for cervical spine films. The soft-tissue films of the neck are a good survey study, using the air as natural contrast to visualize the lumen of the larynx and trachea (Figs. 11-12, 11-13). The retropharyngeal soft-tissue thickness

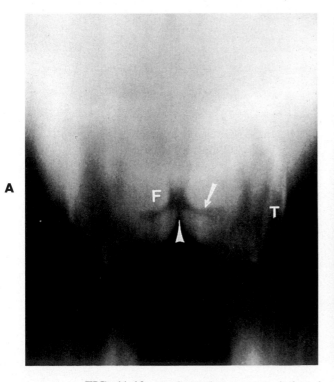
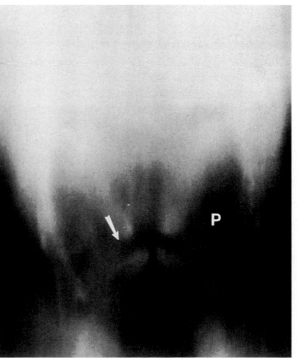

FIG. 11-10 **A,** Coronal tomograms during phonation. The true cords approximate with only a small residual airway *(arrowhead)*. The ventricle *(arrow)* is partially filled with air. *T,* Thyroid cartilage; *F,* false cord. **B,** Reverse phonation shows more dilatation of the ventricles *(arrow)*. *P,* Pyriform sinus.

also can be appreciated on lateral films. The epiglottis and the aryepiglottic folds usually are well visualized, and air in the ventricle often marks the position of the upper margin of the true cord. The tracheal air column extends below the larynx. Some information about the cartilages can be determined, depending on the degree of ossification.

The variability of calcification (actually ossification) of the laryngeal cartilage makes prediction of a pathologic condition from the plain films hazardous. Frequently the partly calcified cartilages create a diagnostic problem for the radiologist examining for foreign bodies. Because of this, the radiologist should be familiar with the most common "pitfalls" or false foreign bodies.

The superior margin of the cricoid lamina often calcifies early, before the remainder of the signet portion of the cricoid does so (Fig. 11-12). This linear calcification is often mistaken for a foreign body. The triticeous cartilage in the posterior thyrohyoid ligament is another foreign body mimic (Fig. 11-13). Less commonly the calcified arytenoid and the cornua of the thyroid cartilage may be mistaken for a foreign body.

Diagnosis on the frontal film is severely limited because of superimposition of the cervical spine. High kV-filtered radiographs can be used to make the bony structures less obvious. Tomography blurs the image of the spine such that the airway contour can be better appreciated.

HIGH-KILOVOLT FILTERED RADIOGRAPH

High-kV films are used to "soften" the spine, allowing visualization of the airway in the frontal projection; 140 kV is used with 1 mm of copper filter placed between the tube and the patient to give a lowered film contrast.[1,2]

XERORADIOGRAPHY

Xeroradiography uses edge enhancement to clearly show the anatomy of the airway, cartilages, and even muscle and fat planes (Fig. 11-14).[3] This technique is ideal for visualizing foreign bodies and for evaluation of the trachea (e.g., for subglottic stenosis, granuloma, etc.). However, xeroradiography has an exposure 3 to 5 times that of the standard soft-tissue film, and its usefulness in imaging soft tissues and cartilage has been superseded by CT and MR.

TOMOGRAPHY

Today, conventional linear or multidirectional tomography seldom is used for the evaluation of the larynx. Tomography does allow the frontal view anatomy to be seen without the problems of the superimposed spine (Fig. 11-10). However, the lateral tomographic view offers little more information than plain film radiography. The exposure can be made in several seconds, rapidly enough that the various maneuvers

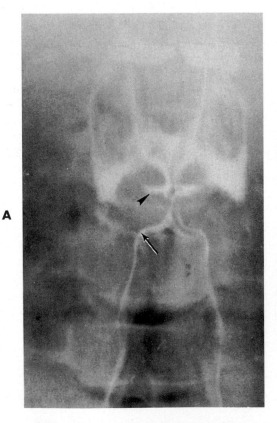
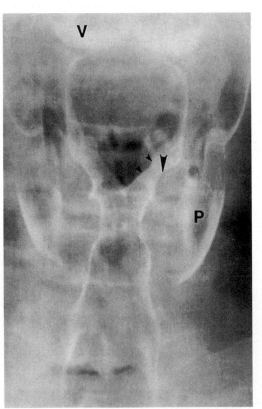

FIG. 11-11 **A,** Laryngogram, frontal views, Valsalva maneuver. Note squaring of the subglottic arch *(arrow),* and collapse of the ventricle *(arrowhead).* **B,** Laryngogram, puffed cheek, modified valsalva. Pyriform sinuses *(P)* are distended. The AE fold *(small arrowheads)* and the inner wall of the larynx *(large arrowhead)* are well demonstrated. *V,* Valleculae.

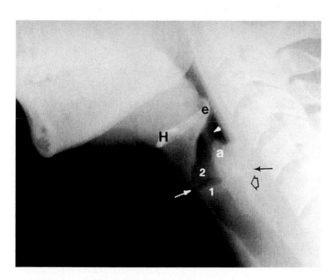

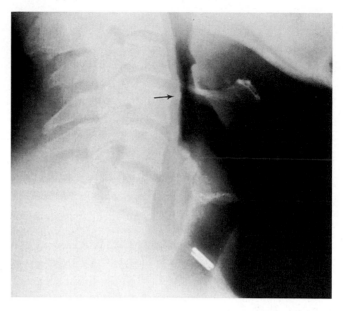

FIG. 11-12 Lateral plain film of the neck shows the true cord *(1)* and the false cord *(2)* separated by the black air-filled linear ventricle. The white arrow points to the anterior ventricle. The anterior commissure (junction of the true cords) is just inferior to this point. The black arrow shows the calcified superior margin of the cricoid lamina, which is often mistaken for a foreign body. The open black arrow shows the calcified lower horn of the cricoid. *H,* Hyoid; *a,* arytenoid prominence; *e,* epiglottis; *arrowhead,* AE fold.

FIG. 11-13 Lateral soft tissue film with calcification of the cartilages, including the triticeous cartilage *(arrow)* in the posterior margin of the thyrohyoid membrane *(thyrohyoid ligament).*

(e.g., phonation, Valsalva, etc.) can be used to show specific anatomic landmarks in the coronal plane. However, only the surface deformity can be visualized by this technique. The deep extent of a tumor can be estimated by the degree of distortion of the false and true cords. Because the pyriform sinus protrudes between the thyroid cartilage and the inner wall of the larynx, the width of this wall can be estimated in an attempt to show tumor extending through the paraglottic space toward the true cord. Subglottic extension can usually be well seen by the flattening of the subglottic arch.

Because tomography requires multiple slices and multiple maneuvers, the examination has a fairly high radiation exposure. Every attempt should be made to place the airway in the plane of section that is parallel to the tabletop. Placing a bolster under the buttocks, with additional support of the knees, allows positioning without forcing the patient to straighten the natural angle between the thoracic and cervical spines.

FLUOROSCOPY

Because some patients will not tolerate direct clinical visualization of the larynx without anesthesia and some patients may have a tumor blocking the clinician's view, fluoroscopy can be helpful in assessing vocal cord mobility. This process requires that the patient be awake and be able to follow verbal commands. The examination is recorded on videotape to allow review without additional patient exposure.

CONTRAST EXAMINATIONS

Contrast laryngography was developed to better define the mucosal irregularities of the larynx and to visualize areas that were poorly seen by the laryngologist.[4-6] The procedure

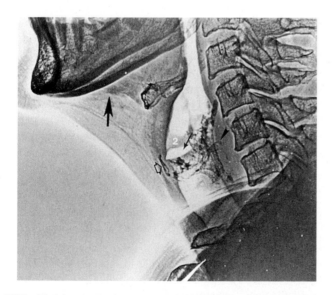

FIG. 11-14 Xeroradiogram lateral view shows the true cord, false cord, and ventricle with better definition of the fat planes. Note the calcified upper margin of the cricoid lamina *(arrowhead)* is more obviously seen here than in Fig. 11-12. Note how the muscles in the floor of the mouth *(large arrow)* can be seen against the fat. *2,* False cord; *small arrow,* ventricle; *open arrow,* partially calcified anterior thyroid cartilage.

is rarely done today because most of the information derived from the laryngogram is obtainable by endoscopy, and the submucosal regions can be better visualized with CT and MRI. Contrast laryngography is difficult for many patients to tolerate, and this examination is contraindicated in those patients that the clinician most often would like to have this study, namely, patients in whom a tumor causes significant airway obstruction, thus limiting direct visualization. The examination is contraindicated in these patients because there is always some element of mucosal edema in response to the topical anesthetic and the contrast material, further narrowing an already compromised airway.

If no contraindication exists, the patient may be given atropine (0.4 mg) and codeine (60 mg). The atropine decreases secretions and dries the mucosa, enabling better contrast coating, but it should not be given to patients with glaucoma or prostate enlargement. Codeine limits coughing.

The anesthesia of the larynx is the most important part of the contrast laryngogram. Initial anesthesia can be done with a spray or gargle using topical anesthetic. After initial anesthesia is achieved, a curved cannula is placed over the back of the tongue and 2% xylocaine is dripped into the pyriform sinus and larynx as the patient is told to breathe in and out. Alternatively a soft rubber tube can be passed through the nose and directed over the larynx.

Some radiologists have used 4% xylocaine, but this must be done with extreme caution because xylocaine is rapidly absorbed through the mucosa. This can precipitate cardiac arrhythmias, hypotension, or an excited or depressed central nervous system state. In addition to airway compromise a contraindication to anesthesia is patient allergy to xylocaine. If atropine is contraindicated, it simply is not used.

Initially the patient will cough as the xylocaine drips into the laryngeal lumen, but as anesthesia occurs, the coughing stops. The procedure can then continue, with administration of the contrast medium. In the United States, oily propyliodone (Dionosil) is the most common contrast agent used. The contrast is warmed and mixed well, then it is dripped by syringe and laryngeal cannula or nasal tube into the larynx. The patient is asked to breathe in slowly as the contrast is administered. The patient coughs lightly to distribute the contrast. Administration can be monitored in the lateral projection with intermittent fluoroscopy. When sufficient coating has occurred, the patient is placed in frontal, lateral, and oblique positions and is asked to perform the various maneuvers described (Figs. 11-11).

Historically the laryngogram has been considered especially helpful in certain important areas of the larynx. The ventricle and anterior commissure can be obscured from the clinician's view by overhanging tumor. On a lateral view, if contrast fills the ventricle and the thin opaque contrast line reaches the anterior junction of the ventricle and epiglottis, this is presumptive evidence that the region is clear of tumor. Phonation or inspiratory *eeee* may distend the ventricle. Because the two ventricles are superimposed on the lateral projection, frontal films also must be obtained to determine that the ventricle fills on both sides. With modern endoscopy, these areas usually can be visualized. The subglottic angle can be clearly defined with laryngography, but as stated this region is more easily assessed by CT or MRI.

The pyriform sinus and postcricoid area can be seen when coated with contrast. However, this area can be evaluated without anesthetizing the larynx, merely by having the patient swallow thick barium. After coating is accomplished, the patient does a modified Valsalva's maneuver to distend the pyriform sinuses. Often the relationship of the tumor to the apex of the pyriform sinus can be shown.

BARIUM SWALLOW

The barium swallow is used to evaluate the pharyngeal wall. The barium column is followed through the pharynx into the esophagus. The motility and pliability of the pharyngeal wall and the mucosal surfaces are assessed. Demonstration of normal pliability of the pharyngeal wall suggests normal tissue. Tumor infiltration causes a lack of pliability or distensibility, as well as mucosal irregularity.

In the frontal view the pyriform sinuses fill as the epiglottis deflects the barium column to either side, around rather than over the vestibule of the larynx (Fig. 11-15). As the larynx elevates, the pyriform sinuses lose their sharply curved lower borders, become continuous with the remaining hypopharynx, and drain through the cricopharyngeus into the esophagus. As the barium column splits to pass through the pyriform sinuses, the larynx becomes a "filling defect" in the barium column and should not be mistaken for a mass.

On the lateral view, the cricopharyngeus opens as the pharynx propels the bolus toward the pharyngoesophageal junction. The cricopharyngeus is inspected for late or incomplete relaxation and for the formation of an outpouching such as a Zenker's diverticulum. On the lateral film, some irregularity is often seen on the anterior wall of the lower pharynx and the postcricoid area. This is due to a venous plexus and some degree of normal mucosal redundancy. However, at times differentiation from a tumor may be impossible. The relationship of the posterior pharyngeal wall to the cervical spine and possible anterior vertebral osteophytes is well seen in the lateral view.

COMPUTED TOMOGRAPHY SCANNING

CT scanning allows evaluation of the laryngeal structures deep to the mucosa.[5,7,8] A lateral scout view is performed and the slice orientation is selected parallel to the ventricle, which is seen as a dark air line in the laryngeal airway. If the ventricle is not seen well or if the airway is obscured by the shoulders in a patient with a short or thick neck, the slice orientation is estimated to be perpendicular to the axis of the spine at the level of the larynx. The axial images are made with a field of view corresponding to the size of the neck. Rapid scans (1 to 2 seconds) decrease respiratory and swal-

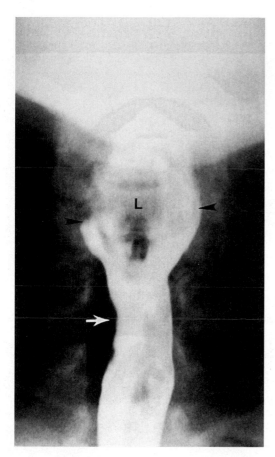

FIG. 11-15 Frontal view of a barium swallow, normal. The barium *(arrowheads)* is deflected around the larynx with an apparent filling defect caused by the larynx *(L)*. The impression on the upper esophagus *(white arrow)* is caused by osteophytes.

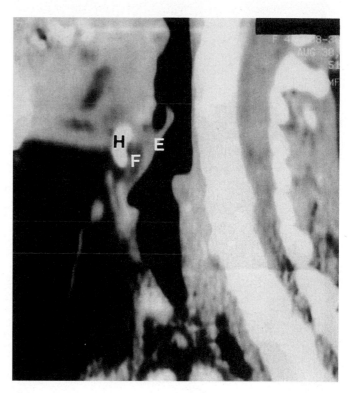

FIG. 11-16 Normal larynx. Reformatted image from spiral CT. Sagittal reformat shows preepiglottic fat *(F)*, hyoid *(H)*, and epiglottis *(E)*.

lowing artifacts. The choice of slice thickness is arbitrary. Some clinicians use 1 mm every 3 mm, and some survey the larynx with 3 mm slices every 3 or 5 mm. If the relationship of the lesion to the ventricle is still in question, once the area of the ventricle is identified, thin slices (1 mm) can be taken.

Spiral scanning rapidly acquires a complete data set through the larynx. The images then can be reconstructed to give overlapping slices at any level, and this is particularly helpful at the level of the ventricle. Coronal, sagittal, and even three-dimensional (3D) images can be generated from the same data set (Fig. 11-16). The real advantage of spiral scanning is that the entire larynx can be examined in less than 10 seconds. This allows the patient to remain motionless during the examination and thus minimizes or eliminates motion artifact. In addition with spiral CT scanning, examination of the larynx during respiratory maneuvers is possible. This may be done to optimize visualization of a particular region of the larynx or the margin of a tumor. More clinical experience is necessary before the usefulness of these techniques is accepted.

The region covered should extend below the level of the cricoid cartilage. The starting point can be the tip of the epiglottis or the hyoid bone, depending on the origin of the lesion (see following discussions on squamous cell carcinoma, other malignancies, and benign tumors). If nodal regions are to be studied, the scan should start at the external auditory meatus. The examination can be done with the patient breathing quietly or breath-holding for each slice. Before the actual scan is started, the patient should practice any breathing maneuver, and the technologist should be confident that motion can be minimized during the scan. If the scan is done during quiet breathing, the patient should attempt as much as possible to breathe with the abdominal muscles. Intravenous contrast helps distinguish lymph nodes from blood vessels and thus is used in tumor cases, but it is not necessary in laryngeal trauma evaluation.

In the upper axial slices, the epiglottis and connecting ligaments and folds are seen (Fig. 11-17). More inferiorly the lateral edges of the epiglottis merge with the aryepiglottic folds, which converge toward the midline and unite posteriorly at a more caudal level. At the upper levels of the larynx, the preepiglottic space is filled with fat, and the hyoepiglottic ligament can be seen crossing the fat in the midline. At the level of the false cord, the paraglottic region, lateral to the airway, is also predominantly fat density. As the axial slice passes the ventricle, the paraglottic space

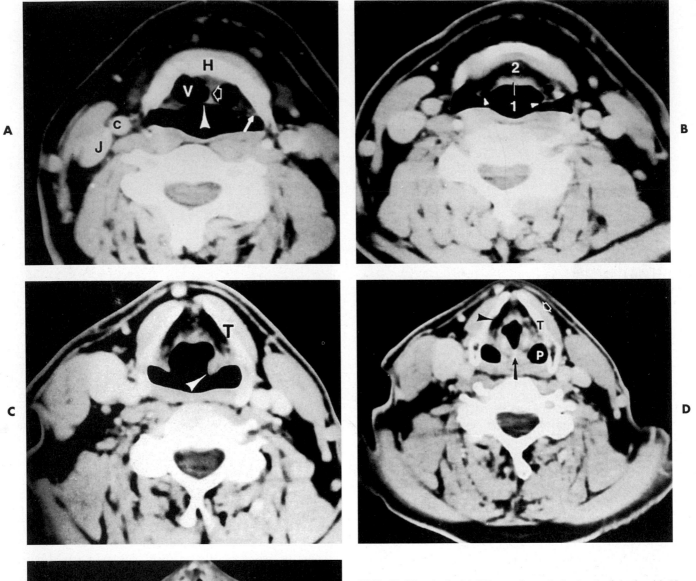

FIG. 11-17 **A,** Axial CT scan through the level of the hyoid. *H,* Hyoid; *V,* valleculae; *C,* carotid; *J,* jugular; *arrowhead,* epiglottis; *open arrow,* glossoepiglottic fold; *arrow,* pharyngoepiglottic fold. **B,** Slightly lower scan through upper AE fold *(arrowheads).* *1,* Epiglottic cartilage; *2,* preepiglottic space. **C,** CT scan, supraglottic larynx slightly lower than in **B.** *T,* Thyroid cartilage; *arrowhead,* aryepiglottic fold. Note the fat in the preepiglottic space. **D,** Slightly lower scan through the supraglottic larynx of a man. The aryepiglottic folds have converged *(arrow).* *T,* Thyroid cartilage; *P,* pyriform sinus; *arrowhead,* fat in the paraglottic space; *open arrow,* strap muscles. **E,** Slightly lower scan, close to the ventricle. Still fat in the supraglottic-paraglottic fat *(arrowhead).* *T,* Thyroid cartilage; *A,* arytenoid cartilage; *C,* upper margin of the cricoid cartilage.

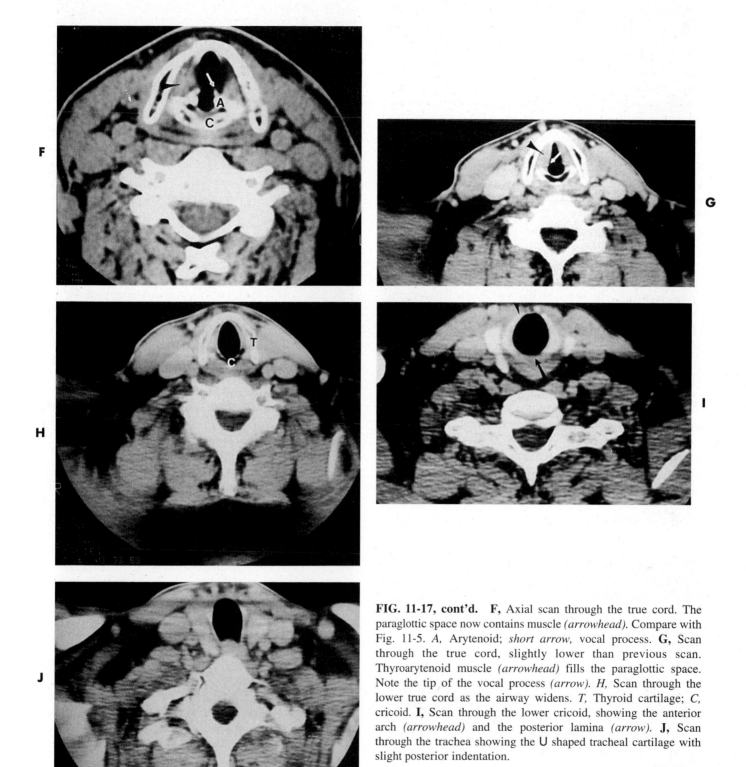

FIG. 11-17, cont'd. **F,** Axial scan through the true cord. The paraglottic space now contains muscle *(arrowhead)*. Compare with Fig. 11-5. *A,* Arytenoid; *short arrow,* vocal process. **G,** Scan through the true cord, slightly lower than previous scan. Thyroarytenoid muscle *(arrowhead)* fills the paraglottic space. Note the tip of the vocal process *(arrow)*. **H,** Scan through the lower true cord as the airway widens. *T,* Thyroid cartilage; *C,* cricoid. **I,** Scan through the lower cricoid, showing the anterior arch *(arrowhead)* and the posterior lamina *(arrow)*. **J,** Scan through the trachea showing the U shaped tracheal cartilage with slight posterior indentation.

changes from predominantly fat density to muscle density. Here the slice has entered the thyroarytenoid muscle. The shape of the airway narrows at the cord level, becoming more slitlike, but then widening to a rounder appearance at the level of the subglottis. The paraglottic space, limited by the conus elasticus, stops at the upper margin of the cricoid. Thus there should be no soft tissue within the ring of the cricoid cartilage.

The appearance of the cartilage can vary considerably, depending on the degree of ossification and the amount of fatty marrow in the ossified medullary region. Both thyroid and cricoid cartilages are easily identified. The thyroid cartilage spans the level of true and false cords. The axial slices are ideal for evaluating the thyroid and cricoid cartilages, displaying them in perfect cross-section. The arytenoid cartilages are important landmarks that can help identify the cord, ventricle, and false cord relationships. Approached from superiorly, the upper arytenoid is seen first at the level of the false cord as a square- or triangular-shaped density. At more caudal levels, the anteriorly pointed vocal process can be identified projecting from the arytenoid base. The vocal process identifies the level of the true cord. Because the level of the vocal process is also at the level of the cricoarytenoid joint, the posterior commissure can be identified when the arytenoid cartilages are seen on the same axial scan as the top of the cricoid lamina. Unfortunately there is no definite landmark on any of the cartilages that defines the exact level of the laryngeal ventricle.

The appearance of the vocal cords varies with the phase of respiration. In quiet breathing the airway is open and the cords are slightly abducted. If the patient is breath-holding for each scan, the cords usually come together (Fig. 11-18). This may actually give a slightly clearer visualization of paraglottic fat.

The anterior commissure should have air closely approximating the cartilage. If this appearance is seen, the radiologist can confidently exclude disease at this site. On CT, obliteration of the anterior commissure can be seen secondary to tumor, but it may also be an artifact resulting from minor cord position changes or cord edema. Repeating the scans at different phases of respiration may help, but reproducing the exact scan level is difficult because the larynx moves slightly during the different phases of respiration.

At the lower margin of the cricoid cartilage, the appearance of the posterior pharyngeal musculature changes from a flat, elongated appearance to a rounder shape (Fig. 11-19). This signifies the change from the hypopharynx to the cervical esophagus and documents the level of the cricopharyngeus. The flatter shape of the pharyngeal musculature is the result of its attachment to the lateral aspect of the thyroid and cricoid cartilages.

In general the angle made by the two thyroid alae is wider in women than in men.

MAGNETIC RESONANCE IMAGING

Because of motion artifact, the larynx has been difficult to image well with MRI, but this modality does have the capability of multiplanar high-resolution imaging, and when compared with CT, MRI has an increased ability to separate various soft tissues.[7,9-16]

The actual pulse sequences used by different radiologists vary considerably and certainly will change with the continued evolution of this technology. As with CT, for MRI the patient is positioned with the airway as parallel to the tabletop as possible. Currently a sagittal T1-weighted (T1W) localizer series is obtained to identify the axis of the larynx. This sequence covers from one sternocleidomastoid muscle to the other, to include the major lymph node groups.

A coronal T1W series is performed with thin sections (3 to 5 mm), extending from the anterior vocal cords to the posterior larynx, in a plane perpendicular to the cords. This may necessitate oblique off-axis imaging. An axial thin section T1W sequence is then done covering the larynx from the upper epiglottis to the lower cricoid. Because short TR sequences are limited in the number of MR slices available in each study, the anatomic level is chosen to cover the area of maximum interest (usually the true cord, ventricle, and false cord). Finally an axial T2W sequence is performed, usually with a TR of 2000 and TEs of 30 and 90 msec. The long TR allows multiple slices to be obtained, and thus the primary node-bearing areas can be covered. If there is a supraglottic lesion, the region from the midmandible to below the cricoid is imaged. With lower cord or subglottic lesions, the lower neck is evaluated.

Fast spin-echo (FSE) imaging has made a significant difference in the ability of MR to image the larynx with long TR sequences. Because the images are obtained much faster than conventional spin-echo images, motion artifacts are less of a problem and excellent images with valuable T2 information are now obtainable. Fat suppression is used to lower the signal of the fat, which is high on FSE images

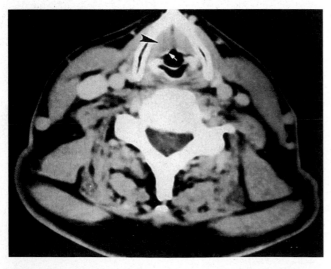

FIG. 11-18   Axial CT with breath-holding. The true cords are apposed. *Arrowhead,* Thyroarytenoid muscle; *arrow,* vocal process.

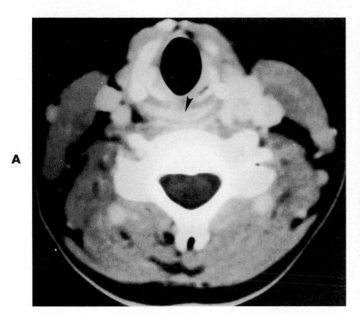 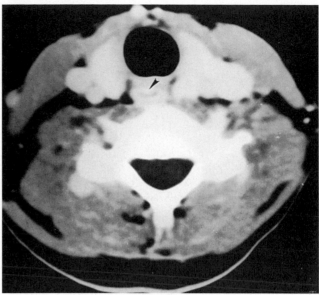

FIG. 11-19 A, Axial scan with bolus contrast showing enhancement of the mucosa of the pharynx at the level of the lower pharynx. Note its flattened configuration *(arrowhead)* caused by the attachment of the pharyngeal musculature at the lateral aspect of the cricoid and thyroid. **B,** Lower scan showing the esophageal wall *(arrowhead)* with a rounder and narrower appearance than the wall of the pharynx.

even when a long TR is used. This allows better appreciation of the higher signal intensity coming from abnormal soft tissues that may be bordered by fat. At this time, FSE T1W images are becoming available (Fig. 11-20).

The use of gadolinium in laryngeal imaging is still controversial. Some feel that by using gadolinium, important information can be obtained regarding the interface of tumor with muscle. Often axial postcontrast images are the most useful. However, FSE T2W images may generate very similar information, obviating the need for gadolinium.

Motion artifacts from breathing, swallowing, and even the pulsatile flow in the carotid arteries are major imaging problems. A number of flow compensation techniques, respiratory and cardiac gating, and presaturation pulses have all been tried with varying results. Phase-encoding gradients are placed in the anteroposterior direction to move flow artifact away from the larynx in the axial images. Patient education is even more important with MRI than with CT. The patient is instructed to breathe quietly and to practice doing so without moving the neck. Abdominal rather than chest breathing is encouraged, and the patient is instructed not to swallow or at least to swallow as seldom as possible during the sequence. The neck should not be hyperextended because this makes swallowing more difficult. The neck is kept in a more relaxed position.

A surface coil is used as a receiver.[13,14] Because the coil should move as little as possible, the technologist should take care to separate the coil from the chest wall while maintaining close approximation to the neck.

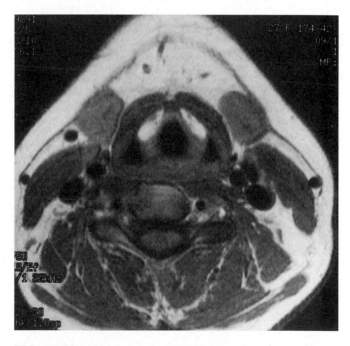

FIG. 11-20 Fast spin-echo T1W image through the larynx. Axial 512 × 256 matrix shows excellent detail in the paraglottic space and pyriform sinuses.

Sagittal images show the epiglottis, valleculae, and base of the tongue well (Fig. 11-21). The laryngeal surface of the epiglottis can be followed down to the petiole and anterior commissure. The postcricoid area is seen well, and the arytenoid cartilage often can be visualized perched atop of the

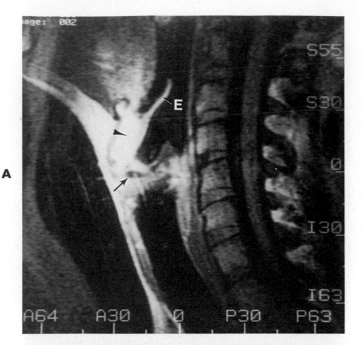

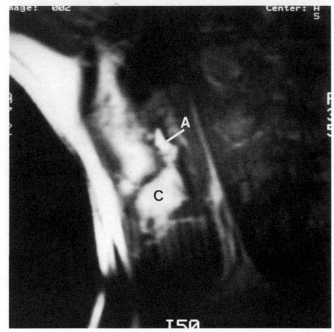

FIG. 11-21 **A,** MRI 1.5 Tesla T1W sagittal image, just off midline, shows the true cord and false cord separated by the dark air-filled ventricle *(arrow). Arrowhead,* Preepiglottic fat; *E,* epiglottis. **B,** More lateral scan shows the cricoid *(C)* and arytenoid *(A).*

cricoid cartilage. The preepiglottic fat is clearly seen on T1W images.

The coronal view represents the ideal orientation for evaluation of the upper margin of the true cord (Fig. 11-22). The ventricle may not be seen, because the patient cannot maintain any particular breathing maneuver during the entire time required for the imaging sequence. The thyroarytenoid muscle represents the bulk of the true cord, and on T1W images, it can be seen contrasted against the high

signal intensity fat of the false cord, which is immediately above it. Although slips of the thyroarytenoid muscle invariably extend up into the false cord level of the paraglottic space, these are very thin, and for practical purposes the upper margin of the true vocal cord is considered to be the upper margin of this muscle. Anteriorly the petiole and the fat of the preepiglottic space are also visible just above the anterior commissure, whereas posteriorly the arytenoids again are seen on the cricoid. The subglottic region is seen on the same images as the true cord.

The axial images represent slices perpendicular to the inner surface of the thyroid and cricoid cartilage, allowing assessment of cartilaginous erosion. Again the appearance of the cartilage is quite variable, depending on the degree of ossification. Ossified cartilage with fat in the medullary space has a high signal intensity on T1W sequences and darkens on T2W sequences. By comparison, the nonossified cartilage tends to be dark on both sequences. If fast spin-echo imaging is used, fat suppression is important if the darkening of the fat is to be diagnostically useful. The ossified cartilage cortex is black on the MR images.

The cord level can be identified with axial MRI in much the same way as it was with CT. The airway is narrow. A T1W scan through the false cord level shows the high signal intensity of fat in the paraglottic area, whereas a scan at the true cord level shows the paraglottic region to be filled with the lower signal intensity of muscle.

The carotid artery, jugular vein, and jugular lymph nodes are seen on all scan orientations. The nodes are often the same shape as the vessels on the axial projection, but they can usually be differentiated from the vessels on the basis of various flow phenomena. On coronal and sagittal views, the nodes often are more obvious because they are still ovoid in shape, whereas the vessels are more linear.

ULTRASONOGRAPHY, NUCLEAR MEDICINE, AND ANGIOGRAPHY

Ultrasonography has significant limitations in the larynx. The proximity of the larynx to the skin surface allows the use of very high-resolution, high-frequency 5 to 10 mHz probes.[17] However, when ossified, the cartilage reflects most of the sound, thus limiting the ultrasonic access into the larynx. The cystic nature of a laryngocele can be determined, and vocal cord mobility can be assessed but has very limited applicability because the cords are almost always accessible to direct visualization. Perichondritis or tumor extension through the thyroid cartilage has been evaluated with ultrasound, but most centers use CT or MRI in this evaluation.[18] More experience with ultrasound may increase its future applicability.

Because the cartilage is not ossified in the pediatric patient, ultrasound can access the inner larynx.[19] Still the acoustic shadowing of the airway limits the ability to evaluate the posterior larynx, especially the cricoid. Mobility of the cords can be assessed, and invasion into the larynx by

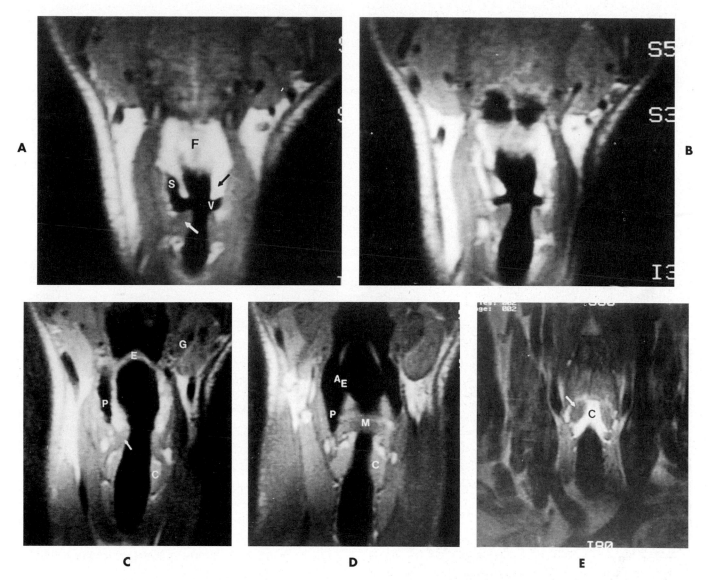

FIG. 11-22   Coronal MRI 1.5 Tesla T1W seen from front to back. **A,** Anterior scan shows the muscle intensity *(white arrow)* of the thyroarytenoid muscle at the level of the cord. The paraglottic space at the level of the false cord shows bright fat intensity *(black arrow)*. *V,* Ventricle; *S,* saccule of the ventricle; *F,* preepiglottic fat. **B,** Slightly more posterior scan. **C,** More posterior to **B.** *Arrow,* Posterior thyroarytenoid muscle; *P,* pyriform sinus; *E,* epiglottis; *C,* cricoid; *G,* submandibular gland. **D,** Posterior to **C.** *C,* Cricoid lamina; *M,* interarytenoid muscle; *AE,* aryepiglottic fold; *P,* pyriform sinus. **E,** Posterior larynx shows the posterior cricoid *(C)*. The muscle intensity to either side *(arrow)* represents the posterior cricoarytenoid muscle. (From Curtin HD. Imaging of the larynx: current concepts. Radiology 1989; 713:1-11.)

lesions such as lymphangiomas can be appreciated. Prenatal ultrasound is not compromised by air because the larynx, trachea, and bronchi are filled with fluid.[20] Thus, prenatal ultrasound has been used to predict laryngeal and tracheal atresia.

Nuclear medicine is seldom used specifically for pathologic conditions of the larynx. Increased uptake in inflam-matory arthropathies or relapsing polychondritis occasionally has been mentioned in the literature.[5]

Arteriography can demonstrate the blood supply to the larynx. A primary glomus (paraganglioma) tumor or other vascular lesion can be evaluated by arteriography, but this is seldom necessary.[21]

References

1. Maguire GH. The larynx: simplified radiological examination using heavy filtration and high voltage. Radiology 1966; 87:102-110.
2. Maguire GH, Beigue RA. Selective filtration: a practical approach to high kilovoltage radiography. Radiology 1965; 85:345-351.
3. Doust DB, Ting YM. Xeroradiography of the larynx. Radiology 1974; 110:727-731.
4. Momose KJ, MacMillan AS. Roentgenologic investigation of the larynx and trachea. RCNA 1978; 16:321-332.
5. Noyek A, et al. The larynx. In: Bergeron RT, Osborne AG, Som PM, eds. Head and neck imaging: excluding the brain. St Louis, Mo: The CV Mosby Co, 1983; 402-490.
6. Powers WE, McGee HH, Seaman WB. The contrast examination of larynx and pharynx. Radiology 1957; 68:169-172.
7. Mancuso AA, Hanafee WN. Computed tomography and magnetic resonance of the head and neck. 2nd Edition. Baltimore, Md: Williams & Wilkins, 1985; 241-357.
8. Mafee MF, Schild JA, Valvassori GE, et al. Computed tomography of the larynx: correlation with anatomic and pathologic studies in cases of laryngeal carcinomas. Radiology 1983; 147:123-127.
9. Castelijns JA, Gerritsen GJ, Kaiser MC, et al. Invasion of laryngeal cartilage by cancer: comparison of CT and MR imaging. Radiology 1987; 166:199-206.
10. Castelijns JA, Kiaser MC, Valk J, et al. MR imaging of laryngeal cancer. JCAT 1987; 11(1):134-140.
11. Hanafee WN. Hypopharynx and larynx. In: Valvassori GE, et al. Head and neck imaging. New York, NY: Thieme Medical Publishers Inc, 1988; 311-338.
12. Lufkin RB, Hanafee WN. Application of surface coil to MR anatomy of the larynx. AJR 1985; 145:483-492.
13. Lufkin RB, Hanafee WN, Worthan D, et al. Larynx and hypopharynx: MR imaging with surface coils. Radiology 1986; 158:747-754.
14. McArdle CB, Bailey BJ, Amparo EG. Surface coil magnetic resonance imaging of the normal larynx. Arch Otolaryngol Head Neck Surg 1986; 112:616-622.
15. Stark DD, Moss AA, Gamsu G, et al. Magnetic resonance imaging of the neck. I. Normal anatomy. Radiology 1984; 150:447-452.
16. Castelijns JA, Gerritsen GJ, Kiaser MC, et al. MRI of normal or cancerous laryngeal cartilage: histopathologic correlation, Laryngoscope 1987; 97:1085-1093.
17. Raghavendra BN, Horii SC, Reede DL, et al. Sonographic anatomy of the larynx, with particular reference to the vocal cords. J Ultrasound Med 1987; 6:225-230.
18. Rothberg R, Noyek AM, Freeman JL, et al. Thyroid cartilage imaging with diagnostic ultrasound: correlative studies. Arch Otolaryngol Head Neck Surg 1986; 112:503-515.
19. Garel C, Contencin P, Polonovski JM, et al. Laryngeal ultrasonography in infants and children: a new way of investigating: normal and pathological findings. Int J Pediatr Otorhinolaryngol 1992; 23:107-115.
20. Isaacson G, Birnholz JC. Human fetal upper respiratory tract function as revealed by ultrasonography. Ann Otol Rhinol Laryngol 1991; 100:743-747.
21. Konowitz PM, Lawson W, Som PM, et al. Laryngeal paraganglioma: update on diagnosis and treatment. Laryngoscope 1988; 98:40-49.

SECTION THREE
PATHOLOGIC CONDITIONS

Congenital, inflammatory, neoplastic, and traumatic abnormalities all affect the larynx.[1,2] Imaging has a definite place in evaluating and diagnosing these lesions. Typically the clinician has a good idea of the basic clinical problem and seeks the radiologist's help to determine the extent of the particular pathologic condition. Because most modern imaging has been directed toward evaluation of neoplasms, this chapter begins with and emphasizes tumors. The evaluation of congenital, traumatic, and inflammatory lesions then follows. Some pathologic conditions are not evaluated by radiology often, but they are included here for completeness.

SQUAMOUS CELL CARCINOMA
General Considerations

Most laryngeal tumors are malignant, and the vast majority of these neoplasms are squamous cell carcinomas (SCCa).[1,2] The diagnosis is seldom in doubt because the larynx is accessible to direct visualization, and these cancers arise on the mucosal surfaces. There is an association of these cancers with both alchohol use and tobacco smoking.

Without the help of imaging, the laryngoscopist may be able to obtain all the information needed for treatment planning. However, the endoscopist has a problem defining the deep extent of a lesion relative to precise landmarks that determine whether the patient is a candidate for speech conservation surgery or radiotherapy. Often a tumor can cross the acceptable limits of a conservation operation by growing deeply through the paraglottic space, completely undetected by the laryngoscopist. A good approach to imaging of the larynx is to concentrate on the specific anatomic landmarks that make a difference in surgical planning. These landmarks are stressed in this chapter.

Clinically, tumors are staged by the TNM classification developed by the American Joint Committee on Cancer.[3] This is a clinically based classification that at present does not take into account the contribution of imaging. Nonetheless the radiologist should be aware of this classification system, which is presented in Box 11-1.

Several points regarding the relationship of radiology and endoscopy must be emphasized. First, whenever possible, CT or MRI should be done before biopsy. This avoids any imaging confusion stemming from the local trauma of

▼

BOX 11-1
TUMOR STAGING BY TNM* CLASSIFICATION

Primary Tumor

TX	Primary tumor cannot be assessed
TO	No evidence of primary tumor
Tis	Carcinoma in situ

Supraglottis

T1	Tumor limited to one subsite of supraglottis, with normal vocal cord mobility
T2	Tumor invades more than one subsite of supraglottis or glottis, with normal vocal cord mobility
T3	Tumor limited to larynx, with vocal cord fixation or invades postcricoid area, medial wall of pyriform sinus, or preepiglottic tissues
T4	Tumor invades through thyroid cartilage or extends to other tissues beyond the larynx (e.g., to oropharynx, soft tissue of neck)

Glottis

T1	Tumor limited to vocal cord(s) (may involve anterior or posterior commissues), with normal mobility T1a Tumor limited to one vocal cord T1b Tumor involves both vocal cords
T2	Tumor extends to supraglottis or subglottis or with impaired vocal cord mobility
T3	Tumor limited to the larynx, with vocal cord mobility
T4	Tumor invades through thyroid cartilage or extends to other tissues beyond the larynx (e.g., oropharynx, soft tissues of the neck)

Subglottis

T1	Tumor limited to the subglottis
T2	Tumor extends to vocal cord(s), with normal or impaired mobility
T3	Tumor limited to larynx, with vocal cord fixation
T4	Tumor invades through cricoid or thyroid cartilage or extends to other tissues beyond the larynx (e.g., oropharynx, soft tissues of the neck)

Regional Lymph Nodes

Larynx

NX	Regional lymph nodes cannot be assessed
NO	No regional lymph node metastasis
N1	Metastasis in a single ipsilateral lymph node, 3 cm or less in greatest dimension
N2	Metastasis in a single ipsilateral lymph node, more than 3 cm but less than 6 cm in greatest dimension, or in multiple ipsilateral lymph nodes, none more than 6 cm in greatest dimension, or in bilateral or contralateral lymph nodes, none more than 6 cm in greatest dimension N2a Metastasis in a single ipsilateral lymph node, more than 6 cm in greatest dimension N2b Metastasis in multiple ipsilateral lymph nodes, none more than 6 cm in greatest dimension N2c Metastasis in bilateral or contralateral lymph nodes, none more than 6 cm in greatest dimension
N3	Metastasis in a lymph node more than 6 cm in greatest dimension

Distant Metastasis

MX	Presence of distant metastasis cannot be assessed

From American Joint Committee on Cancer. Manual for staging of cancer. 3rd Edition. Philadelphia, Pa: JB Lippincott, Co, 1988.
*T, Primary tumor; N, regional lymph nodes; M, metastasis.

the biopsy. Usually the diagnosis is strongly suspected by the clinician after mirror examination, and the clinician can help the radiologist best by initially localizing the lesion. Second the mucosal surfaces are in the realm of the endoscopist, and the radiologist should never perform MRI or CT as a substitute for direct clinical visualization of the lesion. Because small but clinically obvious mucosal lesions may go undetected on CT and MRI, it is impossible to exclude cancer of the larynx based only on imaging.

Voice Conservation Therapy

Voice conservation therapy includes any treatment other than a total laryngectomy. Such treatment primarily includes partial laryngectomy and radiation therapy. The most common voice conservation operations are the (horizontal) supraglottic laryngectomy and the vertical hemilaryngectomy. The supraglottic laryngectomy is done for supraglottic carcinoma, whereas the vertical hemilaryngectomy is done for a lesion isolated to the true vocal cord. These procedures are described in the appropriate sections that follow. The anatomic landmarks used to determine the feasibility of each of these standard partial laryngectomies are also emphasized in the sections dealing with tumors of specific areas within the larynx. Recently, larger segments of the larynx have been removed in the so-called extended, or near-total, laryngectomies, but the discussion here stresses the more standard procedures.[4]

Speech conservation surgery allows the patient to maintain the capability of speech, using the residual portion of the larynx. However, in addition to vocalization the larynx serves two more critical functions: (1) maintenance of a patent airway and (2) protection of the airway from aspiration. After most speech conservation surgery, the patient has to go through a retraining period, learning to swallow without aspiration. To accomplish this, the patient must have both the desire to go through this retraining phase and an adequate pulmonary reserve. Invariably, some degree of aspiration will occur after surgery until the patient learns again to swallow effectively.

Radiation therapy also has the ability to preserve voice function. The imaging approach is similar to that for a partial laryngeal resection. In particular the size or bulk of the tumor is an important factor to the radiation therapist. The volume and depth of penetration also has a predictive value in these tumors.[5,6] In general, radiation therapy is more successful for superficial lesions than it is for deeply invasive tumors. Because of patient preference or medical contraindications to surgery, radiation still may be used in some extensive lesions.

In general, and more specifically when imaging a patient who is planning to recieve radiation therapy, the radiologist must include an evaluation of any tumor invasion of the laryngeal cartilages. If the only treatment is to be irradiation, this information is important and reflects the controversy regarding the effect of laryngeal cartilage tumor invasion on patient prognosis. Previously, cartilage invasion had been considered a contraindication to a radiation therapy cure. However, with modern imaging, more subtle cartilage involvement can be seen than was previously possible, and the significance of this early invasion on prognosis after radiation therapy has yet to be determined.[7]

Only recently have studies appeared in the literature correlating imaging findings with radiation therapy outcome. Initial results have found higher recurrence rates with larger supraglottic lesions. In one study, bulk was not as important in true cord lesions, but the patient numbers were small. Castelijns et al. compared recurrence rates with the involvement of cartilage as shown by MR.[8] Higher recurrence rates were seen in those patients with cartilage abnormality than in those without cartilage invasion. This is an important concept because outcome was compared directly with an imaging finding without exact histologic verification. The patient numbers in all of these studies are small, making definite conclusions somewhat premature. However, if absolute determinations are to be made, these preliminary studies do provide a rationale for further investigations.

If a tumor does recur after radiation therapy, a salvage total laryngectomy can be performed. This treatment sequence does, however, give a slightly lower overall survival than if a total laryngectomy is done at initial diagnosis.

Cartilage Involvement

The laryngeal cartilages should be assessed during the imaging evaluation of any tumor of the larynx. This evaluation is therefore discussed before the specific regions of the larynx are considered. In actual practice a tumor confined to the supraglottic larynx very rarely invades the cartilage. Cartilage invasion is much more of a problem in tumors of the true cord and hypopharynx.

Tumor invasion of the cricoid or thyroid cartilage is considered a negative factor in the prognosis of radiation therapy, and it obviates the standard partial laryngeal resection. Thus cartilage involvement is an important consideration in a patient whether the treatment is radiation therapy or any surgery short of a total laryngectomy.

The epiglottis is not crucial structure to consider because it is an elastic yellow cartilage, which represents a poor barrier to tumor extension. Supraglottic resection still can be done if the epiglottis is involved, and the epiglottis is removed with all supraglottic laryngectomy specimens. Similarly, minimum involvement of the vocal process of the arytenoid does not necessarily exclude a partial resection.

The mineralization of the cartilages is not uniform and is frequently asymmetric. By the age that most patients develop carcinoma, much of both the cricoid and the thyroid cartilages is ossified. It is believed that the ossification follows the line of attachment of the muscles to these cartilages. Thus the thyroid cartilage usually ossifies from the inferior margin superiorly and from the posterior margin anteriorly. Small islands of ossified and nonossified cartilage are frequently seen in the thyroid cartilage's broad, flat alar surfaces. The cricoid cartilage usually ossifies on the top, the back of the lamina, and then along the upper margin of the cricoid arch. The following three possible normal substances can be present in these laryngeal cartilages: cortical bone, marrow, and nonossified cartilage.

With CT a tumor usually has the same attenuation as nonossified cartilage (soft-tissue density) so that minimal cartilage involvement can be very difficult to assess (Fig. 11-23). Gross destruction of course can be determined, and the only truly reliable CT sign of such cartilage destruction is the demonstration of tumor on the opposite side of the cartilage from the primary lesion.

Sclerosis seen on CT is a reactive phenomenon and does not mean actual invasion of the cartilage (Fig. 11-24). A tumor close to the perichondrium can cause sclerosis within the cartilage without tumor cells actually being in the area of the sclerosis. This may be related to the inflammatory response, which is frequently identified at the margin of a squamous cell carcinoma. More experience is needed to clarify this relationship.

On MRI the most reliable sign is still demonstration of a tumor on the outer side of the cartilage but some new evidence suggests that lesser degrees of tumor involvement may be detectable. Early reports indicate that MRI offers an advantage over CT in cartilage evaluation because of the variability in the appearance of both normal and abnormal cartilage afforded by different pulse sequences.[9-11]

MRI shows the cortex of ossified cartilage as a black signal void. Fatty marrow is bright on T1W sequences but darkens on T2W sequences (with fast spin-echo sequences, fat suppression must be added to achieve this effect). The nonmineralized cartilage is relatively dark on T1W images and remains dark on the T2W images. The nonmineralized cartilage is not as black as cortical bone, but it is much darker than the fat.

Tumor is intermediate in intensity or relatively dark on T1W sequences. Thus a segment of cartilage that is relatively dark on a T1W image may represent either tumor or nonmineralized cartilage, and the T2W scans are used to distinguish between the two possibilities (Figs. 11-25 to 11-27).

According to Castelijns et al., a tumor (squamous cell carcinoma) "brightens" on a T2W sequence, whereas the nonmineralized cartilage does not.[9-11] On T2W images the involved and uninvolved cartilage may actually look the same. The tumor is relatively bright, and a fatty medullary area may "retain" a significant amount of signal because of its proximity to the surface coil. The important finding is the change in appearance, with relative brightening between the T1W and T2W images, that suggests the presence of tumor. The use of fast spin-echo with fat suppression has not only allowed highly detailed T2W images, but with fat suppression, the difference between tumor and the fat-containing medullary space accentuates on the T2W images.

Castelijns et al. actually used a midfield strength unit and an earlier echo because of the diminishing signal on the later echo images. Still, they demonstrated the tumor involvement as relative brightening compared with the appearance

on the T1W image. Again, nonmineralized cartilage remained dark. Early experience using highfield units and later echoes are encouraging. More experience is needed for verification, but if reliable, this finding certainly will be diagnostically helpful.

Gadolinium also increases the signal of the tumor. Limited experience has been promising in that, by using T1W, fat-suppressed images, one may be able to define early cartilage invasion (Fig. 11-26). Again, more experience is necessary before a final conclusion can be made. High-quality T2W fast spin-echo images may give the same information as postgadolinium, fat-suppressed images and therefore obviate the need for the contrast study.

The specificity of the high T2W signal intensity has been questioned because the inflammatory changes that frequently accompany squamous cell carcinoma also give a relatively high T2W signal. High T2W signal also can be present with "red" marrow, which may occasionally be found in the thyroid cartilage. Currently, if the cartilage has "normal" signal, one can feel confident that the cartilage is not invaded. If the signal is high on T2W sequences or if the cartilage enhances, the cartilage is probably abnormal. If the tumor abuts the questionable area, suspicion increases that the cartilage is invaded by tumor.

The significance of the inflammatory response is not known. It is possible that the inflammatory edema may carry viable tumor cells and, if this is the case, the inflammatory tissue would have to be treated as tumor and included in the resection or in the port of radiation therapy. This is just a hypothesis, and certainly more experience is needed before an absolute statement can be made. Usually with cases that are questionable, there has been some other factor that tips the decision toward more radical treatment.

Nodal Metastasis

Nodal metastasis is common with supraglottic tumors and is rare with glottic tumors, but it should be considered during the assessment of any tumor arising at any site within the larynx.

The clinical presence or pathologic detection of metastatic lymph nodes is accompanied by a lowered rate of survival.[12] More ominous, is the presence of tumor extension through the capsule of a node, or so-called extracapsular spread. Detection of large nodes by palpation is reliable, but detection of smaller nodes or deeply situated nodes is not. There are many false positives and false negatives. Clinically occult nodes exist, and although imaging is more sensitive than palpation, small positive nodes still go undetected on imaging. These nodes are found histologically. The precise significance of CT- or MRI-detected nonpalpable lymphadenopathy relative to survival remains unresolved.

Currently, treatment of nodes is controversial.[13] Most discussions are based on studies that compare the size and site of origin of a lesion, the histologic findings, and the presence of palpable nodes with the rate of recurrence or survival. Physician bias has a definite impact on treatment tech-

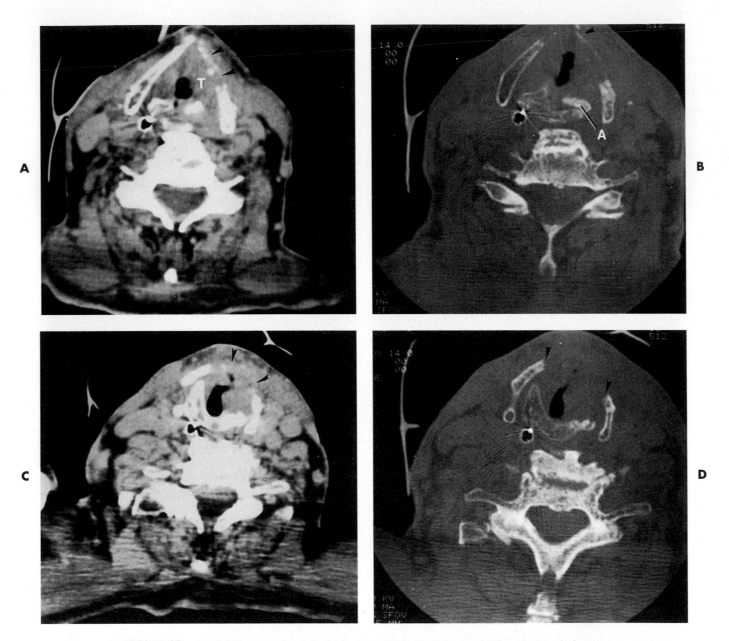

FIG. 11-23   Axial CT scans of a transglottic tumor with cartilage destruction. **A,** Level close to the ventricle shows the tumor *(T).* There is definite demineralization of the thyroid ala *(arrowheads)* but no significant thickening of the strap muscles on the outer surface of the thyroid. **B,** Bone algorithm shows the demineralization of the cartilage, which is strongly indicative of tumor invasion. There actually has been slight buckling *(arrowhead)* of the thyroid ala because of the weakening of the cartilage. The arytenoid *(A)* is sclerotic. **C,** Scan through the cricoid shows tumor within the ring of the cricoid and, at this level, tumor extending outside of the larynx *(arrowheads).* **D,** Bone algorithm showing destruction of the thyroid cartilage *(arrowheads).*

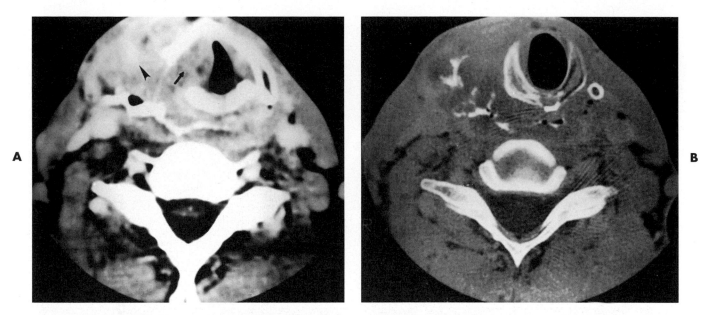

FIG. 11-24   Axial CT scans show extensive pharyngeal tumor invading the larynx. **A,** Tumor of the pyriform sinus extending into the true cord level *(arrow)* and laterally *(arrowhead).* **B,** Lower level shows marked sclerosis of the cartilage on the involved side. The uninvolved side is normal. Tumor did not extend into the cartilage. The sclerotic reaction was definitely free of tumor histologically.

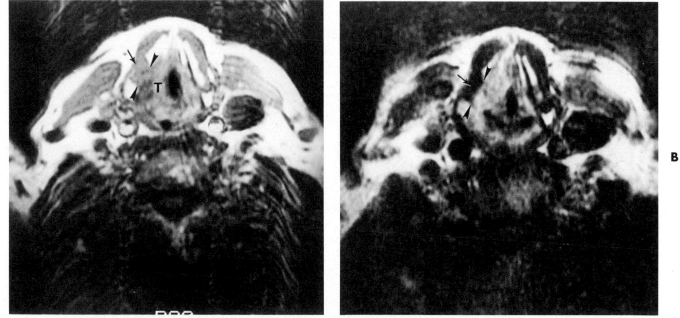

FIG. 11-25   Axial MR shows tumor against nonossified cartilage. **A,** T1W image shows that tumor *(T)* and nonossified cartilage *(arrow)* both have intermediate signal intensity and the tumor-cartilage junction between arrowheads cannot be defined. **B,** T2W image shows brightening of the tumor. The nonossified cartilage does not brighten *(arrow).* The margin between tumor and cartilage is now clearly defined (between *arrowheads*).

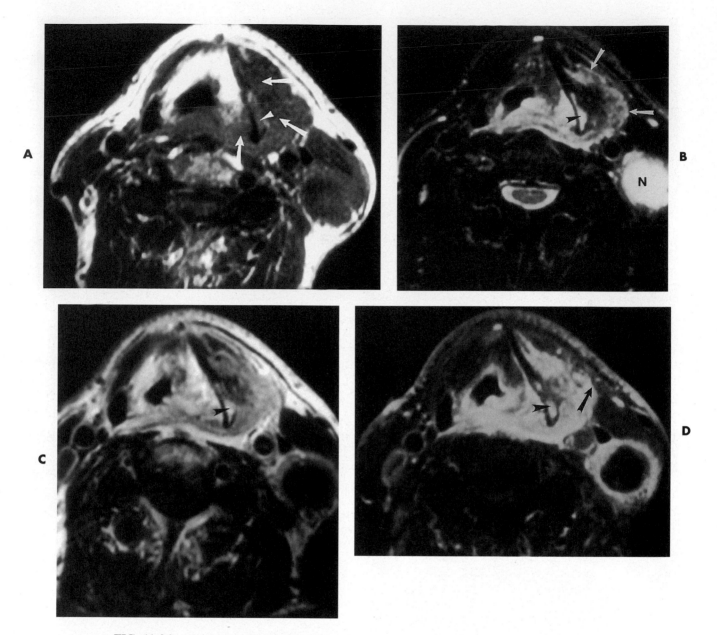

FIG. 11-26   Carcinoma of the pyriform sinus invading the posterior thyroid cartilage and extending along the outer surface. **A,** Axial T1W image without contrast. The tumor *(arrows)* is poorly seen relative to the strap muscles. Note the intermediate signal intensity *(arrowhead)* of the posterior thyroid cartilage. **B,** T2W image fast spin-echo with fat suppression. The margins of the tumor *(arrows)* can be seen more distinctly. Note the high signal *(arrowhead)* within the posterior thyroid cartilage, indicating that it is abnormal. Note the abnormal node *(N)*. **C,** Postcontrast without fat suppression T1W image shows enhancement within the cartilage (compare with the T1W image) and enhancement of the tumor. Enhancing thyroid cartilage *(arrowhead)*. **D,** Postcontrast T1W image with fat suppression. The margin of the tumor, relative to the muscle *(arrow),* is clearly defined. Because fat suppression is used, the high signal within the thyroid cartilage *(arrowhead)* is not fat and is thus presumed to be abnormal. Again, notice the metastatic node.

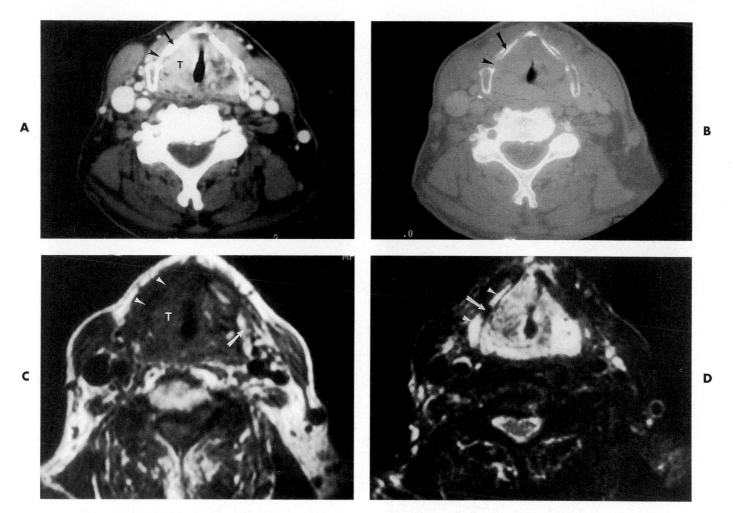

FIG. 11-27   Carcinoma of the larynx, invading the thyroid cartilage. **A,** Axial CT of the larynx shows a tumor *(T)*. On the soft-tissue window the cartilage is unremarkable. Notice the nonossified cartilage *(arrowhead)* and the ossified cartilage *(arrow)*. **B,** Bone algorithm shows no definite abnormality. Again, both nonossified *(arrowhead)* and ossified *(arrow)* cartilage can be identified. **C,** MR T1W image shows tumor *(T)*. The thyroid cartilage *(arrowheads)* on the side of the tumor has intermediate signal, suggesting tumor involvement. On the opposite side there is fat in the medullary cavity of the cartilage *(arrow)*. **D,** Axial T2W image with fat suppression shows definite increase in signal *(arrowheads)* in the involved thyroid cartilage. Note that there is relative sparing of the nonossified portion *(arrow)* of the cartilage.

nique, and if seen at two different centers, surgery or radiation may be recommended for the same lesion.

Although the importance of the CT or MR detection of lymphadenopathy cannot be precisely determined at this time, the evaluation does appear to be worth doing. Accumulated experience certainly has an impact on physician bias, and it is hoped that randomized studies will clarify the question. Further comments are found in the section dealing with specific regions of the larynx, and in Chapter 15.

Further Workup in Squamous Cell Carcinoma

A patient with squamous cell cancer of the larynx, especially of the supraglottic larynx, has a relatively high chance (10%

to 20%) of having or developing a second primary malignancy.[14] This may be the result of the common exposure of certain areas to cigarette smoke or ethanol. The regions most likely involved are the oral cavity, larynx, pharynx, lung, esophagus, and, less often, the stomach (Fig. 11-28).

A barium swallow examination can be performed to search for second primary lesions in a patient diagnosed with a squamous cell carcinoma of the larynx. A truly negative barium swallow examination is a very reliable test. Any area of mucosal irregularity, diminished pliability or distensibility should be evaluated by endoscopy and biopsy.

A chest radiograph is a good survey examination to evaluate for a second primary in the lung or the rare pulmonary metastasis. Some clinicians prefer the higher sensitivity of

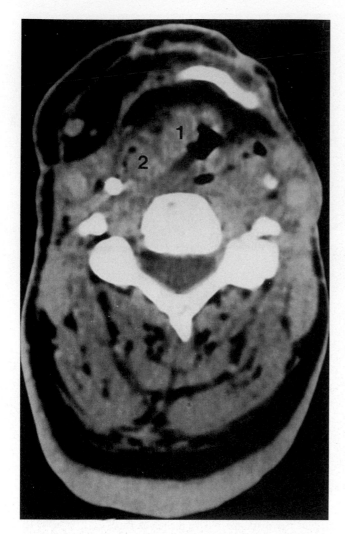

FIG. 11-28 Axial CT shows multiple primaries. Patient with previous floor of the mouth cancer and radical neck dissection now with three separate primaries in the pharynx-larynx. Scan through the supraglottic level shows an endolaryngeal lesion *(1)* and a lesion of the pyriform sinus *(2)*. These lesions were not directly connected. The patient also had a lesion of the opposite subglottic region.

the chest CT study for the preoperative assessment of their patients with head and neck carcinoma.

SITE-SPECIFIC EVALUATION

As stated in the anatomy section, the larynx is subdivided into the supraglottic, glottic, and subglottic areas. This classification is based on embryologic derivation, lymphatic drainage of the mucosa, and the clinical behavior of laryngeal tumors. The division is important to surgical statistics, but for our purposes the glottic and subglottic lesions can be discussed together. Because of the proximity of the hypopharynx and pyriform sinuses to the larynx, the discussion of carcinoma of one region necessitates discussion of

carcinoma of the other; therefore hypopharyngeal carcinoma is covered as well.

Supraglottic Larynx

The speech conservation surgery related to the supraglottic larynx is the supraglottic laryngectomy (refer to Box 11-2).[15-17] Essentially all of the larynx above the ventricle is removed (Fig. 11-29). A horizontal cut is made through the upper thyroid cartilage. The soft-tissue incision line is along the ventricle and just above the anterior commissure. The incision moves upward over the aryepiglottic fold just anterior to the arytenoid before passing along the medial wall of the pyriform sinus to complete the resection. The hyoid may or may not be removed.

Because the false cords are not directly used in vocalization, these tumors do not cause early hoarseness and are discovered somewhat later than are tumors arising from the true vocal cords. Therefore supraglottic tumors are usually larger than tumors of the true cord. Patients with a supraglottic cancer are not usually hoarse unless there is significant tumor extension onto the arytenoids or down into the true cord.

The supraglottic larynx may be subdivided into the suprahyoid and infrahyoid regions. Many tumors involve both regions, but some are small enough to be localized to only one area.

Suprahyoid lesions include those of the free margin of the epiglottis. Small tumors in this area can be resected without removing the entire supraglottic larynx. Management of the base of the tongue is often a clinical problem because these lesions tend to extend anteriorly into the tongue (Fig. 11-30). The criteria for a supraglottic laryngectomy can be expanded to include lesions that extend less than 2 cm into the tongue base. However, unless the lesion is very small, the true size of these lesions is difficult for the

---

▼

BOX 11-2
CONTRAINDICATIONS TO SUPRAGLOTTIC LARYNGECTOMY

1. Tumor extension onto the cricoid cartilage
2. Bilateral arytenoid involvement
3. Arytenoid fixation
4. Extension onto the glottis or impaired vocal cord mobility
5. Thyroid cartilage invasion
6. Involvement of the apex of the pyriform sinus or postcricoid region
7. Involvement of the base of the tongue more than 1 cm posteriorly to the circumvallate papillae

From Lawson W, Biller HF, Suen JY. Cancer of the larynx. In: Suen JY, Myers E, eds. Cancer of the head and neck. New York, NY: Churchill Livingstone Inc, 1989; 533-591.

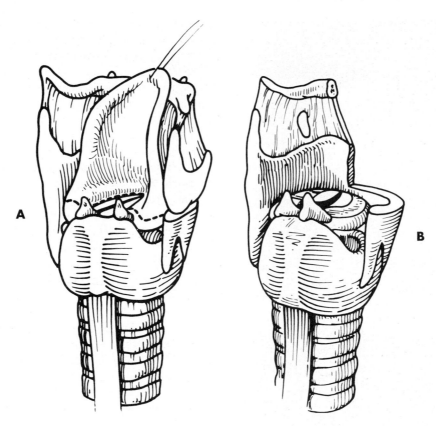

FIG. 11-29 Diagram from the right posterior side of a supraglottic laryngectomy. **A,** Diagram shows the incision through the ventricle (the mucosa over the arytenoid has been removed for illustration). **B,** Diagram shows the postsurgical state. (From Curtin HD. Imaging of the larynx: current concepts. Radiology 1989; 173:1-11.)

endoscopist to appreciate. The lesion may indeed be the tip of an "iceberg," with the tumor extending deeply into the tongue base or the infrahyoid larynx.

The suprahyoid supraglottic larynx is seen well on axial CT and MRI. The lesion can extend laterally along the pharyngoepiglottic folds to reach the pharyngeal wall or along the glossoepiglottic fold in the floor of the valleculae to reach the tongue base. The extension into the tongue base is best seen on MRI, especially on sagittal views (Fig.11-30).[18] In the region of the valleculae the normal lingual tonsil is situated, and at times this normal tissue can be difficult to differentiate from a tumor. This tissue may bulge into the valleculae, but it normally does not extend into the floor or the posterior wall of the valleculae. If mucosal fullness is seen in these areas, tumor should be suspected. Imaging can identify deeper, caudad tumor extension into the infrahyoid larynx and the preepiglottic fat. These areas are well seen on either CT or MRI.

The infrahyoid supraglottic larynx is bordered by the easily visualized aryepiglottic (AE) folds. Lesions at the margin of the AE fold can spill over onto the pharyngeal wall. Anterior extension from midline lesions is into the preepiglottic fat (Fig. 11-31). On gross inspection of the cartilage itself, the appearance of the epiglottis has been

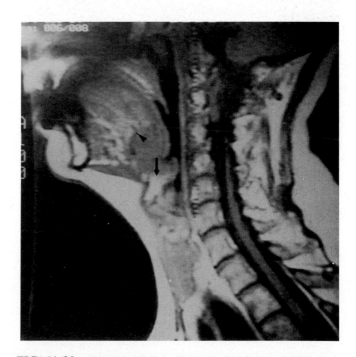

FIG. 11-30 Carcinoma of the free margin of the epiglottis, valleculae, and base of tongue. Sagittal scan shows the margins of the lesion within the tongue *(arrowhead)* and with the fat-filled high signal intensity of the preepiglottic space *(arrow).*

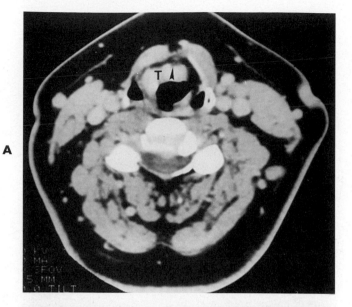

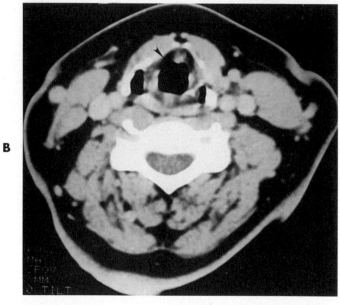

FIG. 11-31 Supraglottic carcinoma (rare adenocarcinoma) **A,** Axial CT superior scan shows the tumor *(T)* as it extends *(arrowhead)* into the preepiglottic fat. **B,** Slightly lower scan shows no tumor. This scan is still at the level of the supraglottic larynx, well above the true cord as evidenced by the paraglottic fat *(arrowhead).*

likened to a sieve. Thus the epiglottis is a poor barrier to tumor spread. Lesions extending into the preepiglottic fat replace the characteristic fat density on CT or the high signal intensity of fat on T1W MRI. The fact that the lesion has entered the preepiglottic fat does not preclude a supraglottic laryngectomy, but it does modify the surgical approach.

Because the resection line of supraglottic resection is through the ventricles, the key to the feasibility of a supraglottic laryngectomy is the inferior tumor extension. The

ventricle, arytenoids, and the anterior commissure are the critical landmarks. The most important of these, from the radiologist's perspective, is the ventricle.

The ventricle is seen in cross section in the coronal plane. Thus the coronal plane can be helpful when determining the relationship of the lower or leading edge of the tumor to the ventricle. Because the slitlike ventricle is actually in the axial plane, it is poorly seen on axial scans. As previously described, the appearance of the arytenoid cartilage and the soft tissues in the paraglottic space can help determine the level of the ventricle.

The arytenoid actually spans the ventricle. The upper arytenoid is at the level of the false cord, and the vocal process is at the level of the true cord. As stated previously, the false cord is composed predominantly of fat, whereas the cord level is marked by the thyroarytenoid muscle. Thus the change from fat to muscle density marks the transition across the ventricle.

If the supraglottic laryngectomy is feasible, on axial scans the radiologist should be able to show a scan without tumor between the scan showing the caudal margin of the tumor and the scan showing the upper margin of the normal true cord (Figs. 11-31, 11-32). On the other hand, if the lesion is seen both above and below the ventricle, it is transglottic (crosses the ventricle) and a supraglottic resection is not possible because the surgical line would go through the ventricle and the tumor (Fig. 11-33).

The greatest diagnostic challenge relates to those cases in which the tumor is very close to the ventricle. Definition of the inferior tumor boundary in these cases can be very difficult.

The tumor can cross the ventricle either by growing along the mucosa or by following the paraglottic space. Mucosal extension may be identified by the endoscopist, unless the view is blocked by the bulk of the tumor. Paraglottic extension is hidden from view and can be detected only with imaging.

Tumor extends laterally into the paraglottic fat by penetrating the quadrangular membrane. Once into the paraglottic fat, the neoplasm can grow caudally and approach the ventricle. The tumor can then grow around the lateral extent of the ventricle and into the lateral edge of the thyroarytenoid muscle (Fig. 11-34). This totally submucosal growth can be completely deep to the mucosa and thus can go undetected on endoscopy. If there is enough growth to actually invade the thyroarytenoid muscle, the cord becomes "fixed" and the invasion can be clinically suspected. However, more limited invasion can cross the ventricle without causing cord fixation, and such disease can be detected only at imaging. Thus the superolateral margin of the thyroarytenoid muscle becomes a key imaging landmark.

The MRI coronal plane gives a perfect cross-section of the ventricle and the thyroarytenoid muscle. Normally a small amount of fat can be seen "tucking" into the upper outer margin of the muscle (Fig. 11-35). The invading tumor

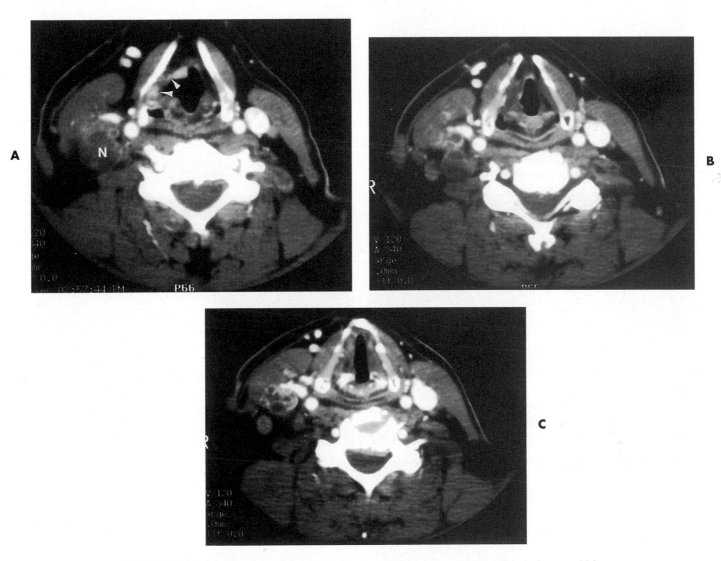

FIG. 11-32   Axial CT of a supraglottic tumor not crossing the ventricle. This lesion would be amendable to a supraglottic resection. **A,** Ulcerated lesion *(arrowheads)* extends into the paraglottic fat from the supraglottic larynx. Note the metastatic node *(N).* **B,** Slightly lower scan shows the paraglottic fat has now returned to normal, indicating that the lesion remains above this level. **C,** Axial scan through the cord is normal.

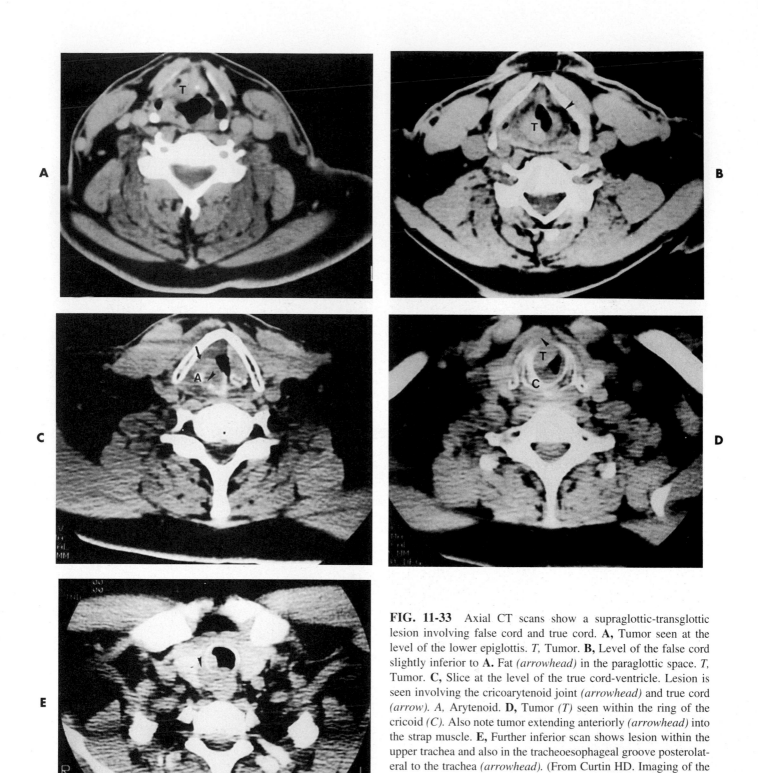

FIG. 11-33 Axial CT scans show a supraglottic-transglottic lesion involving false cord and true cord. **A,** Tumor seen at the level of the lower epiglottis. *T,* Tumor. **B,** Level of the false cord slightly inferior to **A.** Fat *(arrowhead)* in the paraglottic space. *T,* Tumor. **C,** Slice at the level of the true cord-ventricle. Lesion is seen involving the cricoarytenoid joint *(arrowhead)* and true cord *(arrow)*. *A,* Arytenoid. **D,** Tumor *(T)* seen within the ring of the cricoid *(C)*. Also note tumor extending anteriorly *(arrowhead)* into the strap muscle. **E,** Further inferior scan shows lesion within the upper trachea and also in the tracheoesophageal groove posterolateral to the trachea *(arrowhead)*. (From Curtin HD. Imaging of the larynx: current concepts. Radiology 1989; 173:1-11.)

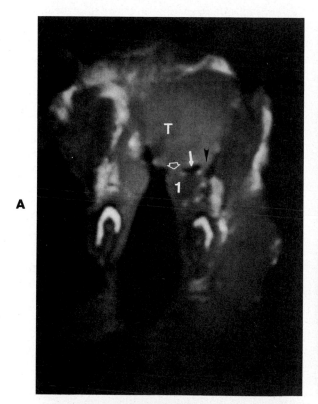

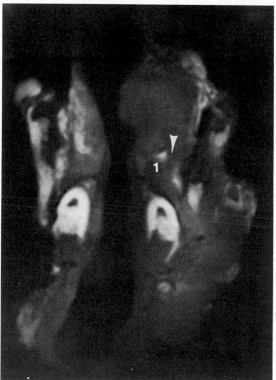

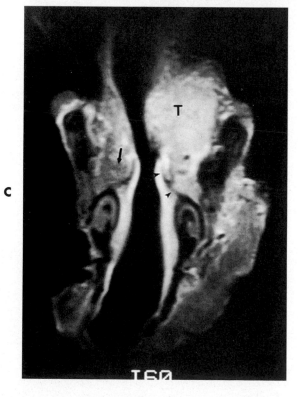

FIG. 11-34   MRI of a total laryngectomy specimen. Supraglottic lesion extending just lateral to the ventricle into the upper margin of the true cord. 1.5 Tesla T1W scan. **A,** Tumor *(T)* with the lower margin at the lateral aspect *(arrowhead)* of the ventricle *(arrow).* The tumor is not crossing the ventricle at the open arrow but has merely fallen onto the upper surface. It could be separated easily. *1,* Thyroarytenoid muscle. **B,** Slightly posterior scan shows tumor extension *(arrowhead)* into the lateral aspect of the thyroarytenoid muscle *(1).* **C,** T2W image shows the tumor *(T)* with relatively increased signal intensity compared with the normal thyroarytenoid muscle opposite side *(arrow).* There is some brightening of the thyroarytenoid muscle on the abnormal side. This was not tumor involvement histologically. This high signal represents an inflammatory reaction to tumor. Conus elasticus *(arrowheads)* is well seen. (From Curtin HD. Imaging of the larynx: current concepts. Radiology 1989; 173:1-11.)

will obliterate this fat and eventually will appear to "pry" the muscle away from the thyroid cartilage (Fig. 11-36). If this fat is intact, this is good evidence that the tumor has not crossed into the cord.

The ventricle is localized in the axial plane by the transition from the fat of the supraglottic larynx to the muscle of the glottic level. If thin scans are used, the small "crease" of fat at the upper outer margin of the thyroarytenoid muscle may be identified, and any tumor may be identified prying its way into this level (Figs. 11-36 to 11-38). This phenomenon is easier to appreciate on MR because the difference between the appearance of muscle and that of tumor is more definite (Fig. 11-39).

MRI signal characteristics, using multiple sequences, help define the relationship of the tumor to the ventricle and the thyroarytenoid muscle. A tumor has approximately the same CT appearance as muscle and has approximately the same signal intensity as muscle on T1W images. However, on T2W images the tumor has a relatively higher signal intensity than normal muscle. Tumor also tends to enhance more than muscle after the administration of gadolinium. These factors are useful in regard to the upper margin of the thyroarytenoid muscle. Relative brightening of the muscle may indicate tumor invasion, but caution must be exercised. Other pathologic processes such as edema may cause such brightening (Figs. 11-34, 11-40). Squamous cell carcinoma is associated with an inflammatory response along the mar-

gin of the tumor, and this gives a high signal on T2W images. Thus the abnormal signal may extend beyond the actual limit of the tumor. The significance of the inflammatory response is unknown. This inflammation may have a protective effect, giving a better therapeutic response. However, it is unknown whether or not the inflamed area should be treated as tumor and thus removed. More experience is needed to evaluate this aspect of laryngeal MRI. Currently, it is very likely that a muscle of normal signal intensity is uninvolved, and one that is bright in signal intensity must be considered abnormal but not necessarily involved by a tumor.

In the midline a lesion growing down along the laryngeal surface of the epiglottis extends toward the anterior commissure rather than the ventricle (Figs. 11-41, 11-42). The anterior commissure is described more extensively in the section on glottic carcinoma. If a supraglottic laryngectomy is to be done for a midline lesion, there should be a 2 to 3 mm separation between the caudal margin of the tumor and the anterior commissure. If assessing this region with axial scan orientation, the radiologist must be very careful to make the scan parallel to the ventricle. If the scan is oblique to the ventricular line, the scan orientation almost always slopes downward from anterior to posterior relative to the long axis of the larynx. This results because the head is usually propped up slightly for patient comfort, angling the larynx out of the plane parallel to the tabletop. In this angle of

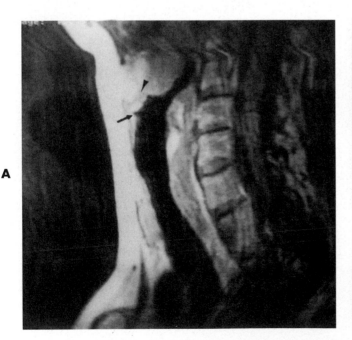
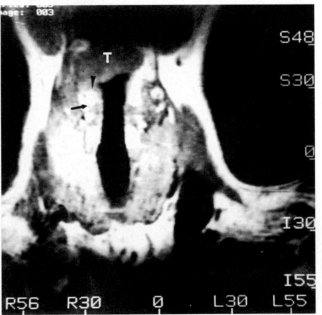

FIG. 11-35 Supraglottic tumor that does not reach the ventricle. A supraglottic laryngectomy is allowed. **A,** Sagittal T1W image. The lower margin *(arrowhead)* is separated clearly from the anterior commissure *(arrow)*. **B,** Coronal T1W image. The lower margin of the tumor *(arrowhead)* is separated by the high-intensity fat of the paraglottic space from the upper margin *(arrow)* of the thyroarytenoid muscle. *T,* Tumor.

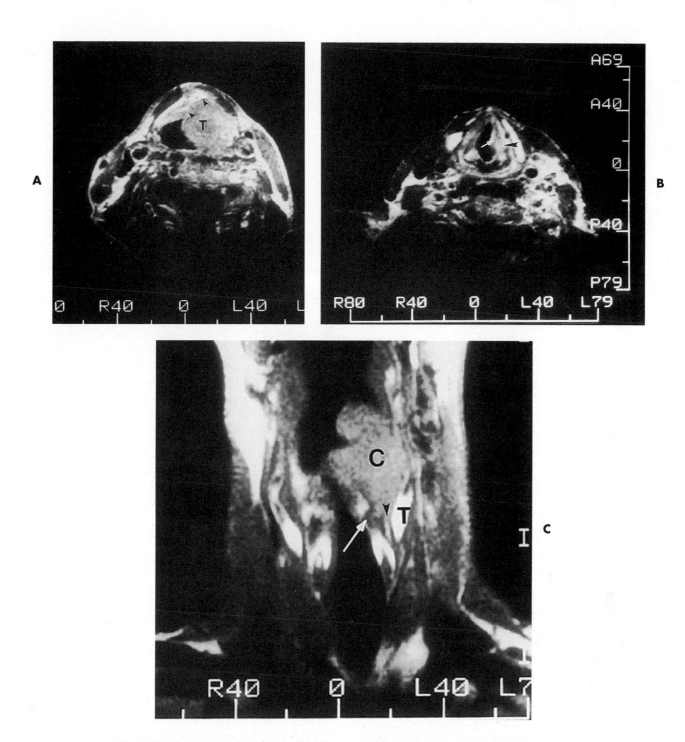

FIG. 11-36 Supraglottic carcinoma crossing the ventricle via the paraglottic space. **A,** Axial T1W image postcontrast. The tumor *(T)* is seen in the supraglottic larynx. Even with contrast the margin *(arrowheads)* relative to the preepiglottic fat is clearly defined. **B,** Lower scan through the level of the cord. The tumor *(arrowhead)* is extending into the lateral portion of the thyroarytenoid muscle *(arrow).* This indicates that the lesion has crossed the ventricle into the true cord. **C,** Coronal image shows the carcinoma *(C)* following the paraglottic space around the ventricle. A very small amount of tumor *(arrowhead)* is squeezing between the thyroid cartilage *(T)* and the thyroarytenoid muscle *(arrow).* The upper edge of the muscle would indicate the level of the ventricle.

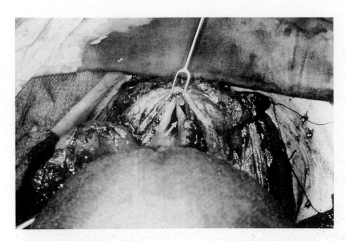

FIG. 11-37 Supraglottic laryngectomy leaving tumor that was unsuspected passing along the paraglottic space. The mucosa of the true cords *(arrow)* is normal. A small amount of tumor *(arrowhead)* has been left because the incision was taken through the ventricle. Compare with Fig. 11-36, *B.* Note the characteristic cut through the thyroid cartilage done as part of the supraglottic resection. (Courtesy Dr. James Boyd.)

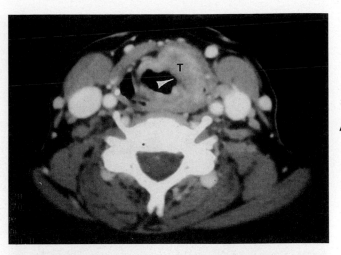

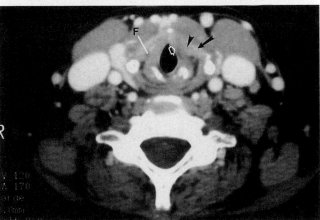

FIG. 11-38 Supraglottic tumor extending beyond the ventricle via paraglottic pathways. **A,** Axial scan through a supraglottic lesion invading anteriorly and laterally. *T,* Tumor; *arrowhead* ulceration. **B,** Scan through the level of the cord shows a small amount of tumor *(arrowhead)* obliterating the fat between the thyroid cartilage *(arrow)* and the thyroarytenoid muscle *(open arrow).* This scan would be just below the level of the ventricle. Compare with fat *(F)* at the outer edge of the muscle on the opposite side.

obliquity the anterior false cord level is imaged on the same scan as the posterior segment of the true cord, thus making possible a miscalculation of the closeness of the tumor to the anterior commissure.

MRI can show the fat on either side of the petiole, and MRI can provide sagittal scans. On a sagittal image the presence of air against the lower epiglottis is a reliable sign that excludes tumor extension to the anterior commissure (Fig. 11-35). However, partial volume artifact can result from the anterior true cords or false cords pressing against each other. This eliminates air from the anterior commisure region and can give a false-positive impression that tumor has reached the anterior commissure. Thus the presence of air in this region is a more reliable sign than the presence of soft tissue.

In the posterior supraglottic larynx the arytenoids are almost always assessed by direct visualization. If the upper level of one arytenoid is minimally involved by tumor, this one arytenoid can be removed surgically. However, involvement of the interarytenoid area is considered to be a contraindication to supraglottic resection because the surgeon would have to remove both arytenoids to attain a clear tumor margin, and the patient would have no true cords with which to phonate. Thus primary lesions of the interarytenoid area, even though small, are almost always treated by total laryngectomy (Figs. 11-43, 11-44). The interarytenoid region is not usually a diagnostic problem for the radiologist because this area is so clearly seen at endoscopy.

Involvement of the thyroid cartilage is also a contraindication to supraglottic resection. This topic is discussed previously in this chapter. However, it is extremely unusual for

a supraglottic tumor to involve the cartilage unless the tumor has crossed the ventricle.

Lymph node involvement is common in supraglottic carcinoma. Nodal involvement is most common in those lesions of the aryepiglottic fold and epiglottis (margin) that also involve the contiguous tongue and pharynx.[13] The incidence of nodal disease gradually diminishes with tumors that involve the margins of the larynx without contiguous spread and is lowest with those small tumors that are isolated to the more central supraglottic larynx. Deeper extension into the preepiglottic and paraglottic spaces is generally associated with a higher incidence of lymph node metastasis.

The lymphatic drainage of the supraglottic larynx is to the upper jugular chain, and bilateral nodal involvement is common, especially if the lesion crosses the midline. Therefore at least these upper nodes must be imaged, usu-

Text continued on p. 651.

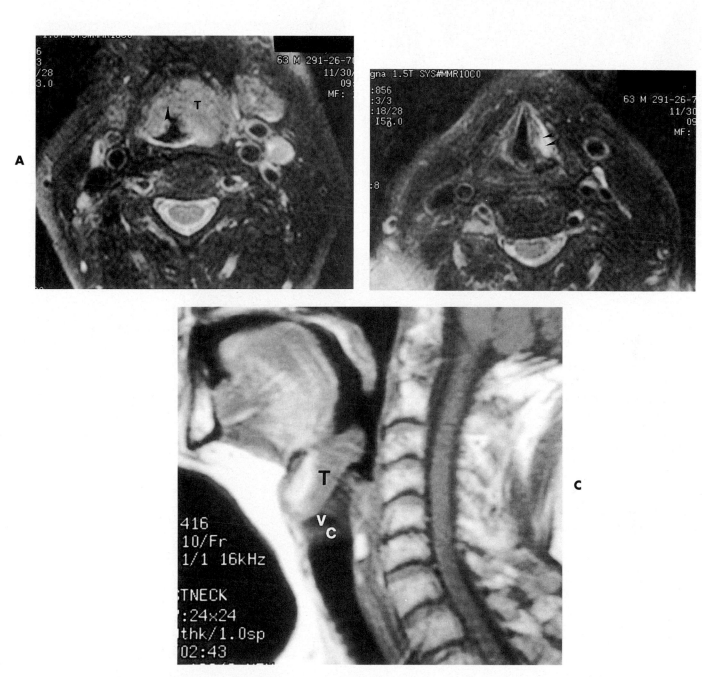

FIG. 11-39 Supraglottic tumor following the paraglottic space around the ventricle into the true cord. **A,** Fast spin-echo T2W image shows the bulk of the supraglottic tumor. Though the tumor *(T)* is predominantly on the left side, there is extension across the midline to the opposite side *(arrowhead)*. **B,** Lower scan through the level of the thyroarytenoid muscle. High signal *(arrowheads)* indicates abnormality along the lateral aspect of the thyroarytenoid muscle *(arrow)*. **C,** Sagittal T1W image shows the bulk of the tumor *(T)* extending down toward the anterior commissure. In this image the ventricle *(V)* and the true cord *(C)* can be visualized.

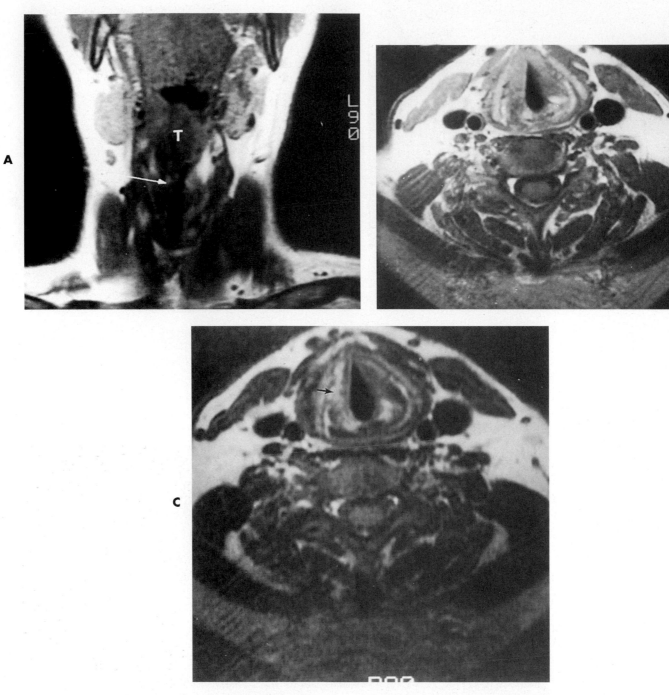

FIG. 11-40   Supraglottic tumor without extension into the true cord but with relative brightening of the atrophic cord on T2W image. **A,** Coronal image shows a supraglottic tumor. The lower margin of the tumor cannot be defined clearly on a T1W image. *T,* Tumor; *arrow;* approximate level of the upper margin of the cord. **B,** Axial T1W. The level of the true cord is fairly symmetrical. **C,** Axial (long TR sequence). There is brightening of the lateral aspect of the true cord *(arrow)* suggesting tumor invasion. Histology showed edema and atrophy but no evidence of tumor extension.

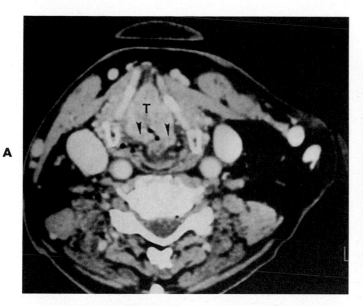

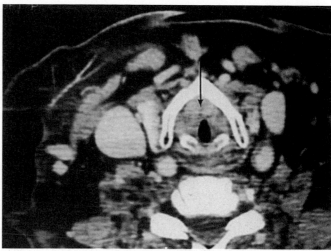

A

B

FIG. 11-41 Axial CT scans **A,** Supraglottic tumor extending to the anterior commissure. Supraglottic tumor *(T)* crosses the midline and involves both aryepiglottic folds *(arrowheads).* **B,** More inferior scan at the level of the true cord shows involvement of the anterior commissure *(arrow).*

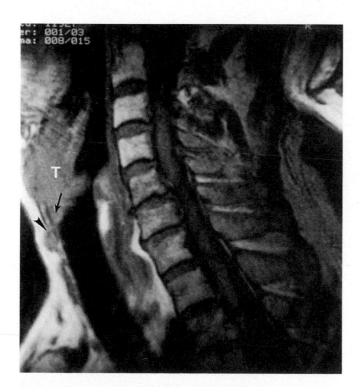

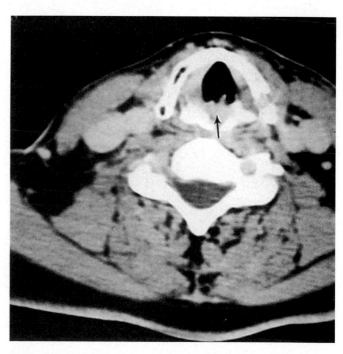

FIG. 11-42 Supraglottic tumor *(T)* with extension to the anterior commissure *(arrow).* Submucosal extension through the cricothyroid membrane involves the region of the Delphian node *(arrowhead).* Sagittal T1 weighted image. 1.5 Tesla.

FIG. 11-43 Axial CT shows tumor at the inter-arytenoid area *(arrow).*

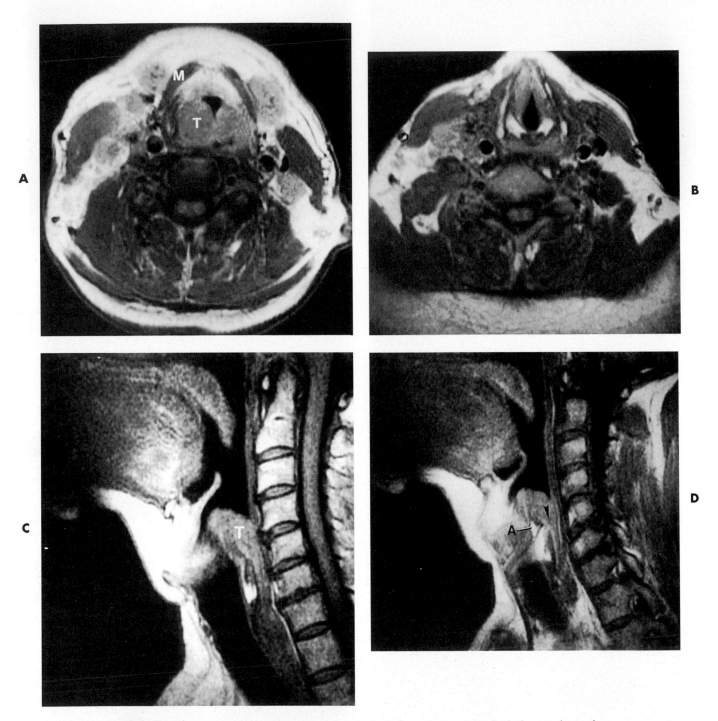

FIG. 11-44   Interarytenoid tumor .35 Telsa. **A,** Scan through the supraglottic larynx shows the tumor *(T)*. *M,* Strap muscle. **B,** Level of the cricoid, tumor is no longer seen. **C,** Sagittal *(near midline)* T1W image shows the tumor *(T)* just superior to the cricoid. **D,** Slightly lateral scan shows the tumor extending behind *(arrowhead)* the arytenoid *(A)*. Lower margin of the tumor is at the level of the upper margin of the cricoid lamina. (Courtesy Dr. Robert Lufkin.)

ally by extended axial scans. With MRI, coronal or sagittal imaging also visualizes these nodes.

Glottic and Infraglottic Regions

The region inferior to the ventricle is divided into the glottic and subglottic, or infraglottic, levels. The division is localized by a plane that is parallel to but 1 cm caudal to an axial plane that goes through the apex of each ventricle. Almost all of the tumors are squamous cell carcinomas associated with smoking. Unlike supraglottic lesions, tumors of the true cord usually present clinically at a fairly early stage because of their interference with normal vocalization. Patients usually become hoarse with a very small lesion of the true cord. If only the subglottic area is involved by tumor and the free margin of the true cord is uninvolved, the patient may not have hoarseness. Fortunately, these lesions are rare.

The speech conservation surgical procedure applicable in this region is the vertical hemilaryngectomy.[15,19,20] The resection removes one false cord, one true cord, and the intervening ventricle, as well as most of the ipsilateral thyroid ala (Fig. 11-45). The outer perichondrium of the thyroid ala is retained. If the tumor is close to or minimally involves the vocal process of the arytenoid, this process can be resected, leaving most of the arytenoid. However, slightly greater involvement necessitates removal of the arytenoid. If there is deep tumor extension, especially involving the cricoarytenoid joint, the procedure is not performed. Similarly, if the lesion is deeply invasive with total fixation of a cord, a vertical hemilaryngectomy is not done. Significant cartilage invasion is also considered a contraindication to this procedure.

With a glottic tumor, the key points for assessment are the inferior tumor extension, the anterior commissure, the arytenoid, the thyroid cartilage, and the paraglottic space at the level of the ventricle (Box 11-3). Nodes are less of a problem than they are with supraglottic carcinoma, but they should be sought in the paratracheal and lower jugular areas.

The most important of these concerns is inferior tumor extent. If the lesion reaches the upper margin of the cricoid, a routine vertical hemilaryngectomy cannot be done. Some surgeons have resected the upper margin of the cartilage, and work is being done on "near-total" laryngectomies. However, the cricoid is the structural foundation of the larynx, and reconstruction of a usable larynx after partial removal of the cricoid is difficult. If the cricoid is involved with tumor, a total laryngectomy must be performed.

The conus elasticus is thought to play an important role relating to the inferior growth of a true cord tumor (Fig. 11-6). This membrane represents the lower boundary of the paraglottic space and extends from the free edge of the true vocal cord to the upper margin of the cricoid cartilage. The membrane affects tumor extension in two situations. A mucosal true cord tumor that has grown caudally is separated from the deeper soft tissues and cartilage by the thick ligamentous conus. Cricoid invasion may be spared. However, caudal to the conus a tumor invading the mucosa can immediately invade the cricoid cartilage. Alternatively, if a tumor has extended deep to the mucosa into the true cord and then grows caudally, the conus elasticus becomes a barrier to inferior growth and directs the tumor laterally, often resulting in no clinically detected subglottic mass.

The key imaging concept is the demonstration of whether or not the tumor has reached the upper margin of the cricoid.

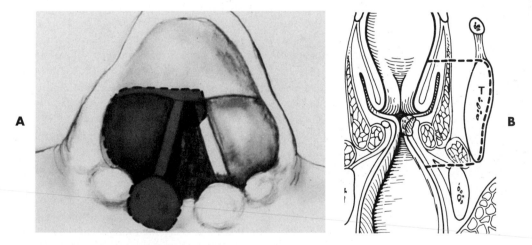

FIG. 11-45 Vertical hemilaryngectomy. **A,** View from above. Diagram of tissue removed in a vertical hemilaryngectomy involving the true cord and the false cord. One arytenoid can be resected. **B,** Coronal diagram showing the tissue resected in a vertical hemilaryngectomy. Note that the outer perichondrium of the thyroid cartilage *(T)* is retained. (**A** from Curtin HD. Imaging of the larynx: current concepts. Radiology 1989; 173:1-11.)

▼

BOX 11-3
CONTRAINDICATIONS TO VERTICAL FRONTOLATERAL HEMILARYNGECTOMY

1. Tumor extension from the ipsilateral vocal cord across the anterior commissure to involve more than one third of the contralateral vocal cord
2. Extension subglottically greater than 10 mm anteriorly and more than 5 mm posterolaterally
3. This technique can still be used if the vocal process and anterior surface of the arytenoid are involved, but involvement of the cricoarytenoid joint, interarytenoid area, opposite arytenoid, or rostrum of the cricoid is a contraindication
4. Extension across the ventricle to the false cord
5. Thyroid cartilage invasion
6. Impaired vocal cord mobility is a relative contraindication

From Lawson W, Biller HF, Suen JY. Cancer of the larynx. In: Suen JY, Myers E, eds. Cancer of the head and neck. New York, NY: Churchill Livingstone Inc, 1989; 533-591.

Inferior extension is easily assessed on axial or coronal scans (Figs. 11-46 to 11-48).

Because of the cricoid's shape, the extent of tolerable inferior growth varies from anterior to posterior. Anteriorly, 1 cm of inferior extension is acceptable. More posteriorly, only 0.5 cm is allowed before the cartilage margin is reached. The cartilage is easily recognizable on axial scans, and if the lesion extends "into the ring," a total laryngectomy is usually necessary. The cricoid also is easily identified on coronal MRI, and tumor extending along its inner cortex is an ominous sign.

Although inferior tumor extension is the most important information sought by the radiologist, other findings also can alter surgical planning. The true vocal cords converge anteriorly, reaching the thyroid cartilage at the anterior commissure. At this midline point, there is only mucosa between the airway and the thyroid cartilage, and a lesion at this position can easily involve the cartilage early in the course of the disease. If air is seen against the inner lamina of the thyroid cartilage, tumor is fairly reliably excluded. The finding of "tissue" against the cartilage is less reliable, as earlier described, because the cords may come together either physiologically or as a result of edema, obliterating the airway.

Even if the lesion crosses the anterior commissure, an extended vertical hemilaryngectomy may be done as long as the posterior half of one true cord is free of tumor and the cartilage is not eroded. The surgeon alters the cut through the thyroid cartilage, depending on the segment of the opposite cord that must be resected.

If possible, superficial tumor extension along the cord or across the anterior commissure is best evaluated by direct clinical visualization. Some estimate can be made on imaging. However, if the finding is crucial in deciding the feasi-

bility of voice-sparing surgery, confirmation by direct inspection is necessary, even though the anterior commissure may at times be difficult to directly visualize.

In the proximity of the anterior commissure the radiologist's attention is once again directed toward a search for deep tumor extension. Cartilage invasion may be assessed by CT or MRI, as previously discussed. Demonstration of the tumor anterior to the cartilage is reliable evidence of cartilage invasion. Many times the anterior tumor growth is through the cricothyroid membrane, just below the inferior margin of the thyroid cartilage (Fig. 11-49). In some cases both the thyroid cartilage and the cricothyroid membrane are involved. This anterior extension can be undetectable on clinical examination.

The area just anterior to the cricothyroid membrane contains the so-called Delphian node. Some authors have described lymphatic extension from the anterior commissure region and the subglottis to this node. However, in many cases this area is involved by direct extension of tumor.

If a vertical hemilaryngectomy is to be performed, the tumor cannot involve an entire arytenoid cartilage. However, as previously discussed, just the vocal process can be involved. If a large portion of the arytenoid is involved, the lesion will touch or be in close proximity to the cricoid cartilage, and a standard resection cannot be performed.

The degree of arytenoid involvement is usually assessed by endoscopy. However, deep extension to the region of the cricoarytenoid joint may be submucosal and thus is best established by CT or MRI.

Superior extension of a glottic tumor brings the tumor into the false cord (Fig. 11-50), and currently, significant extension to the false cord disallows a vertical hemilaryngectomy. Presumably, significant supraglottic tumor requires a supraglottic resection, which cannot be combined easily with a vertical hemilaryngectomy.

Lymph node involvement is seldom a problem with a true cord lesion. However, if the lesion extends significantly below the cord or is primarily in the infraglottic area, nodal involvement can occur in the paratracheal and pretracheal areas. These nodes in turn drain to the lower jugular or upper mediastinal nodes. Thus the lower neck should be examined if significant subglottic tumor is present.

Pharynx

The lower pharynx (hypopharynx, laryngopharynx) has rather simple lateral and posterior walls and a more complex anterior wall formed by the pyriform sinuses, postcricoid area, and the posterior wall of the upper larynx. The superior limit of the hypopharynx is the hyoid bone or valleculae, and the inferior margin is the lower edge of the cricopharyngeus, where the pharynx meets the esophagus.

The pyriform sinus invaginates between the thyroid cartilage and the aryepiglottic fold. As such, the paraglottic space of the larynx is just anterior to the pyriform sinus mucosa. A lesion of the anterior wall of the pyriform sinus extending through the mucosa involves the paraglottic space

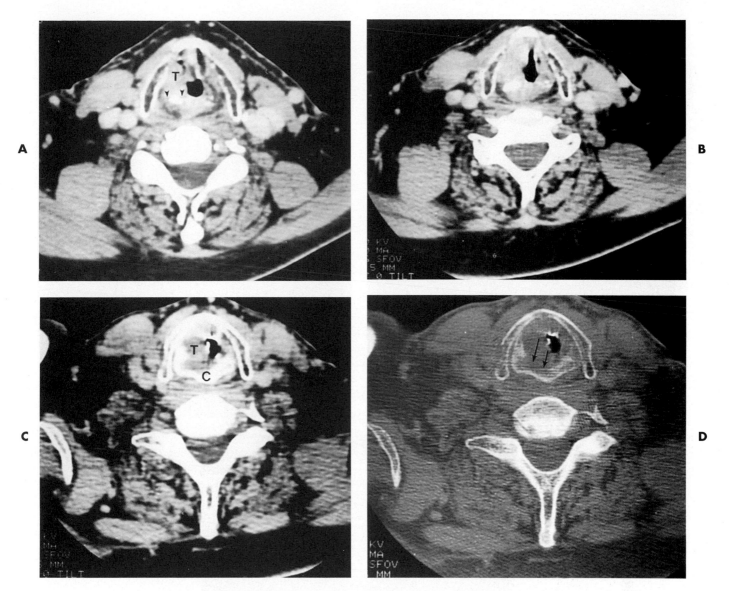

FIG. 11-46   Axial CT scans show a predominantly glottic tumor with extension into the false cord and subglottic extension. **A,** Supraglottic level shows tumor *(T)* with involvement of the anterior surface of the upper arytenoid *(arrowheads).* **B,** Lower scan shows the tumor at approximately the level of the ventricle. **C,** Inferior scan through the level of the cricoid shows tumor *(T)* within the ring. *C,* Cricoid. **D,** Bone algorithm shows loss of the cortical margin of the inner surface of the cricoid *(arrows).*

at the level of the false cord (Figs. 11-51, 11-52). On CT or MRI the lesion can be seen extending between the thyroid and arytenoid cartilages through the "thyroarytenoid gap." The tumor may then extend further inferiorly into the vocal cord via the paraglottic pathway. Primary tumors of the lower false cord and ventricle can extend through the thyroarytenoid gap toward the pharyngeal mucosa, but they usually do not ulcerate this mucosa.

The apex of the pyriform sinus extends deeply into the thyroarytenoid gap and thus is very close to the cricoid cartilage. Lesions of the pyriform apex usually require a total laryngectomy for complete resection. If a lesion is confined

to the upper lateral aspect of the aryepiglottic fold or the upper pyriform sinus, a partial pharyngectomy can be done in combination with a supraglottic laryngectomy (Fig. 11-53).

The involvement of the pyriform apex can be visualized on axial CT or MRI as obliteration of the fat within, or a widening of, the thyroarytenoid gap (Figs. 11-51, 11-52, 11-54). A pharyngogram done with thicker barium or propyliodone (Dionosil) will coat the mucosal surface and help define the margin of a pyriform lesion. As with a laryngogram, the patient puffs out the cheeks (modified Valsalva's maneuver) to distend the pyriform apex. Unlike the laryngogram, no anesthetic or aspiration of contrast is necessary.

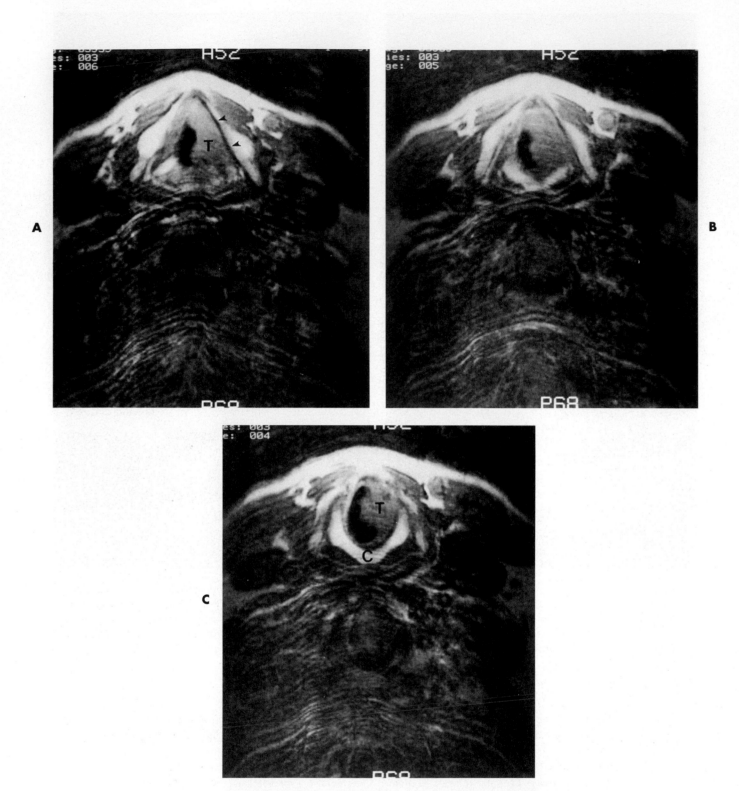

FIG. 11-47 Tumor of the cord with subglottic extension. **A,** Axial scan shows tumor *(T)* at the level of the cord. Note that the cortical line of the thyroid cartilage is intact *(arrowheads).* **B,** Inferior scan shows tumor at the subglottic level. **C,** Inferior scan shows tumor *(T)* definitely within the cricoid ring *(C).*

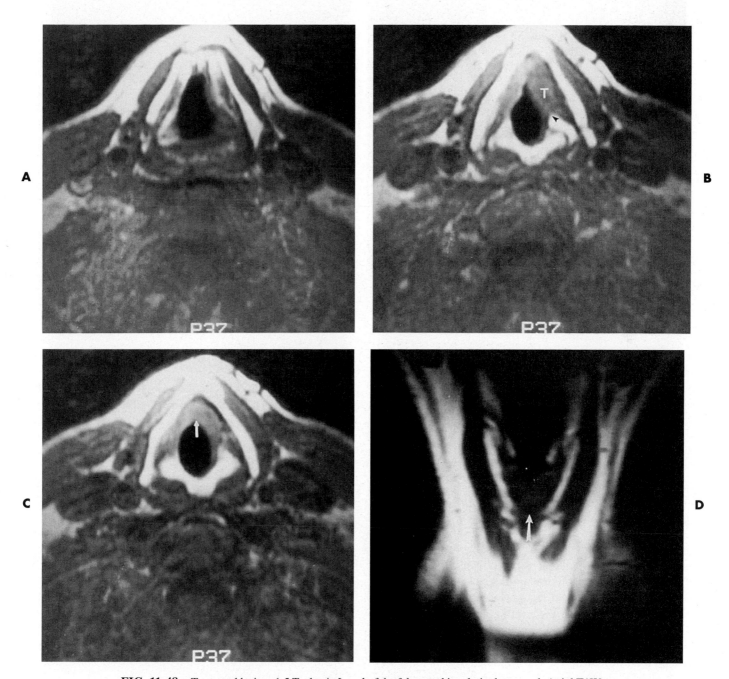

FIG. 11-48   True cord lesion. 1.5 Tesla. **A,** Level of the false cord is relatively normal. Axial T1W. **B,** Tumor *(T)* at the level of the true cord. *Arrowhead,* vocal process. **C,** Level of the lower true cord. The tumor crosses midline *(arrow).* **D,** Coronal image shows increased tissue *(arrow)* beneath the anterior commissure. *Continued*

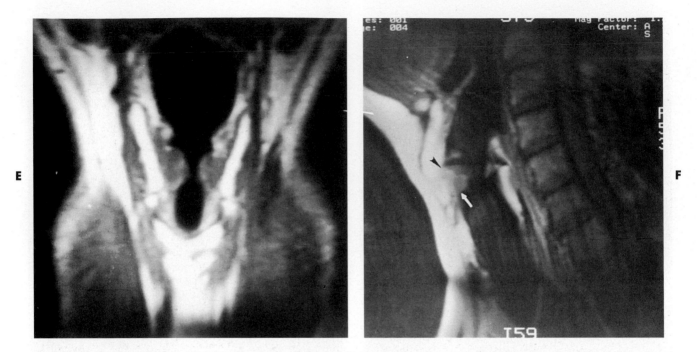

FIG. 11-48, cont'd E, Slightly posterior scan shows only slight thickening of the right true cord. **F,** Sagittal T1W image shows small amount of tumor *(arrow)* immediately inferior to the anterior commissure *(arrowhead).* Evaluation of tumor in this anterior part of the cord can be unreliable because of partial volume artifact.

Most radiologists now prefer to use either CT or MR to determine the inferior tumor margin. With the high resolution scans now available, the mucosal tumor extent can be defined nicely at the same time that the deeper tumor extension is mapped.

The postcricoid region is the anterior segment of the hypopharynx at the level of the posterior cricoid lamina. A lesion in this location necessitates a total laryngectomy because the resection must include the cricoid. Once a tumor is established in this area, the primary surgical concern becomes the lower extent of the lesion, relative to the pharyngoesophageal junction (the cricopharyngeus). This definition of the lower tumor margin helps clinicians decide whether the surgical wound can be closed primarily or alternatively if reconstruction (e.g., with a jejunal interposition) will be necessary.

The definition of the lower tumor margin also can be made on a barium swallow. The cricopharyngeus muscle is almost always identified, so the relationship to the advancing edge of the tumor can be assessed. On axial CT or MRI the level of the cricopharyngeus muscle is approximated by be the lower margin of the cricoid cartilage (Fig. 11-19). Because the cricopharyngeus muscle stretches from one side of the cricoid to the other, the gullet at this level has a band-like or oval appearance. By comparison the esophagus attaches to a midline raphe and has a round, cross-sectional appearance. Thus this important transition zone usually can

be identified at imaging. Lack of esophageal involvement by a tumor is suggested on axial images if the thickness of the pharyngeal wall at the lower margin of the cricoid cartilage returns to normal. However, minimum submucosal tumor spread into the esophagus will go undetected on these images, and often, biopsy is the only way to accurately determine this caudal tumor extent. The sagittal MRI may occasionally help with visualization of the lower margin of the lesion (Fig. 11-55).

The actual mucosal surface in the postcricoid region can be difficult to evaluate on barium swallow because of the normal irregularity of the anterior wall. Most often this irregularity is caused by a prominent venous plexus and an element of mucosal redundancy. The fluoroscopist should attempt to make a judgment regarding the pliability of this surface. However, the pliability of the anterior wall of the postcricoid area is more difficult to assess than the pliability of the lateral or posterior pharyngeal walls. This can be a diagnostic problem because this area is relatively "blind" to the endoscopist; the endoscope seems to "pop" through the muscular ring into the cervical esophagus and so does not afford the clinician a good look at this important area.

The inferior pharyngeal constrictor and the stylopharyngeus muscles act as a relative barrier to tumor spread, attaching to the lateral aspect of the thyroid cartilage. This allows a tumor to "wrap around" the larynx because a lateral pharyngeal wall tumor extends along the outer surface of the

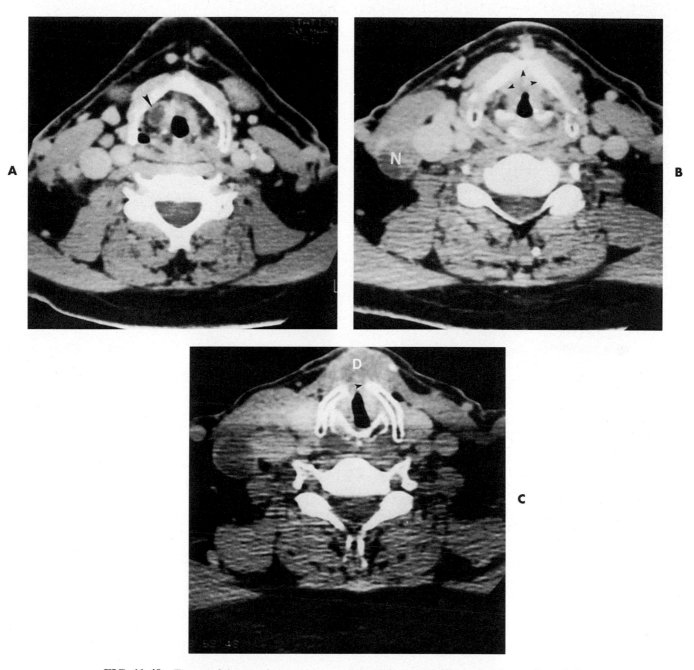

FIG. 11-49 Tumor of the anterior commissure and anterior ventricles. **A,** Axial scan through the supraglottic larynx shows a small saccular cyst (laryngocele) as the tumor obstructs the ventricle. *Arrowhead,* saccular cyst. **B,** Axial scan at level of the anterior commissure and ventricle shows the tumor crossing the midline but no definite erosion of the thyroid cartilage. *Arrowheads,* tumor margins; *N,* node. **C,** Scan through the level of the cricothyroid a membrane shows a very small mass within the airway but shows a large tumor mass in the region of the delphian node *(D).* There is some erosion of the thyroid cartilage *(arrowhead),* but most of the tumor extends through the cricothyroid membrane. (**C** from Curtin HD. Imaging of the larynx: current concepts. Radiology 1989; 173:1-11.)

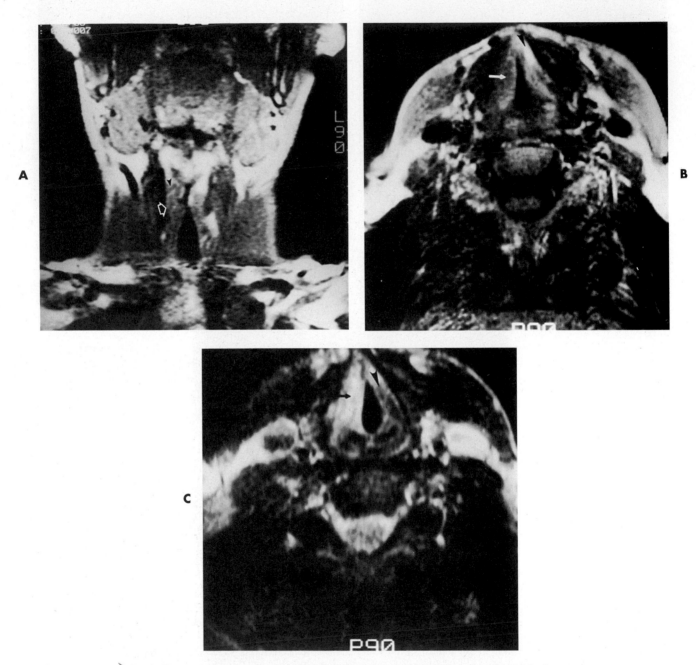

FIG. 11-50   Tumor of the ventricle involving the upper margin of the true cord and the lower margin of the false cord.1.5 Tesla. **A,** Coronal image. Tumor extends around the ventricle involving the false cord *(arrowhead)* and the upper margin of the true cord *(open arrow)*. T1W. **B,** Axial T1W image with tumor at the level of the false cord *(arrow)*. Normal fat indicating false cord level *(arrowhead)*. **C,** T2W image shows brightening of the involved cord *(arrow)*. Note the normal intermediate signal intensity of the thyroarytenoid muscle on the normal side *(arrowhead)*.

thyroid cartilage. This extension may occur before there is actual erosion of the cartilage. (Fig. 11-52).

Direct lateral tumor extention from the lateral wall of the hypopharynx brings the tumor to the carotid artery (Fig. 11-51). Any involvement of this artery is an important and ominous finding. Neither ultrasound nor MRI has proven reliable in identifying tumor fixation to the artery, and the best the radiologist can do is to report the degree to which the tumor encircles the artery.

Direct posterior tumor extension involves the posterior pharyngeal wall and brings the tumor to the prevertebral fascia and muscles, and fixation of this fascia worsens the prognosis and limits the surgical resectability. If the lesion is ulcerative, there often is fascial invasion; however, if the tumor is predominantly exophytic, the fascia may not be involved. This can be assessed on lateral fluoroscopy during a barium swallow, because a lesion that is not fixed to the fascia can slide up and down, relative to the spine, as the barium passes (Fig. 11-56). In these cases, on MRI a high T2W signal intensity or enhancement after gadolinium must be considered abnormal.

Lymphatic spread from pharyngeal lesions initially reaches the high jugular nodes, which are seen easily on axial images. Occasionally, a lesion arising in the lower pharynx can spread superiorly to the high lateral retropharyngeal nodes (nodes of Rouviere), which are immediately beneath the skull base. These areas should be carefully evaluated both at the time of initial diagnosis and on follow-up examinations.

OTHER MALIGNANT TUMORS

Squamous cell carcinoma accounts for 95% of malignancies of the larynx. However, other benign and malignant lesions do occur.[1,2] Although the pathologic diagnosis is still made by endoscopy and biopsy, the radiologist may be able to direct the clinician toward a diagnosis other than squamous cell carcinoma. This is especially true when the lesion is completely submucosal.

Other carcinomas arising in the larynx include adenocarcinoma (1%), arising in the minor salivary glands, verrucous carcinoma, and anaplastic carcinoma.[1]

Adenocarcinoma (Fig. 11-31) has the same subtypes as salivary gland neoplasms elsewhere in the body. Adenoid cystic carcinoma is slightly more common in the subglottic larynx, and mucoepidermoid and adenocarcinoma (not otherwise specified) are more common in the supraglottic larynx. Other subtypes of adenocarcinomas are rare.

Verrucous carcinoma refers to a primarily exophytic tumor that is wartlike and not very invasive. This lesion almost never metastasizes. The appearance of the tumor at endoscopy is very characteristic.

Anaplastic carcinoma, similar to oat cell carcinoma in the lung, is another rare carcinoma of the larynx. The prognosis is poor.

Spindle cell carcinoma is a rare lesion that is composed of a squamous cell carcinoma and a spindle cell stroma. There is a difference of opinion as to whether this is a peculiar kind of squamous cell carcinoma or a combination of squamous cell carcinoma and sarcoma.[1] Either or both components can metastasize. Other names for this lesion occasionally found in the literature are pseudosarcoma, carcinosarcoma, pleomorphic carcinoma, polypoid sarcoma, and pseudosarcomatous squamous cell carcinoma. The basic controversy depends on the definition of the cell of derivation and the potential of the spindle cell stroma. Does the spindle cell develop directly from the squamous cell? Is the spindle cell truly of mesenchymal origin? A third theory holds that the spindle cell stroma is a reactive phenomenon.

Any type of sarcoma can be found in the larynx. As a group, sarcomas make up only 0.3% to 1% of all laryngeal malignancies. Although in rare cases they can be large or fungating, they are primarily submucosal. Usually the masses are somewhat nonspecific on imaging, but a smooth mucosal covering should direct the radiologist away from a diagnosis of squamous cell carcinoma.

Special mention should be made of chondrosarcoma because the calcifications (often ringlike) can indicate a specific radiographic diagnosis. These calcifications may be suggested on MRI but are more obvious on CT (Figs. 11-57, 11-58). The origin of the lesion in the cartilage usually is easily identified by an obvious defect in either the cricoid or the thyroid cartilage. The cartilage may be expanded, particularly in low-grade lesions (Fig. 11-59). This pattern of cartilage abnormality usually is easily differentiated from the destruction associated with squamous cell carcinoma.

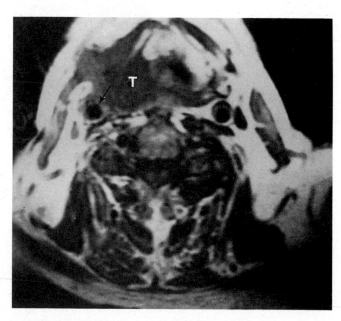

FIG. 11-51 MRI of the tumor of the pyriform sinus extending into the larynx. Level of a supraglottic tumor *(T)*. The tumor touches the carotid artery *(arrow)*.

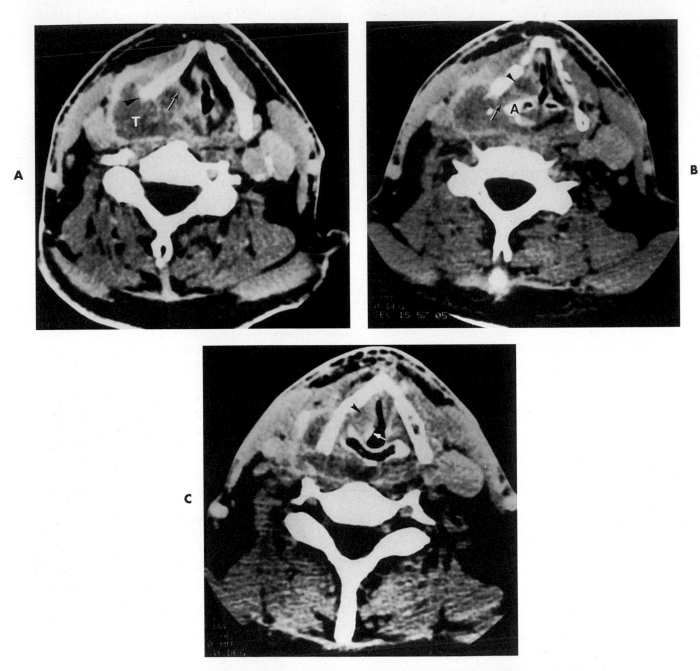

FIG. 11-52   CT of the pyriform sinus tumor invading the larynx and eroding the thyroid cartilage. **A,** Tumor *(T)* extending into the paraglottic fat *(arrow)*. There is erosion of the posterior margin of the thyroid cartilage *(arrowhead)* and tumor extending along the outer aspect of the thyroid cartilage. This phenomenon is due to the attachment of the pharyngeal muscle to the outer cortex of the thyroid cartilage rather than to the posterior margin. **B,** Lower scan still with tumor in the thyroarytenoid gap *(arrow)* and paraglottic space *(arrowhead)*. Again note the erosion of the thyroid cartilage. *A,* Arytenoid. **C,** Lower scan showing tumor in the paraglottic space at the level of the true cord *(arrowhead)* widening the cord. Vocal process *(short white arrow)*.

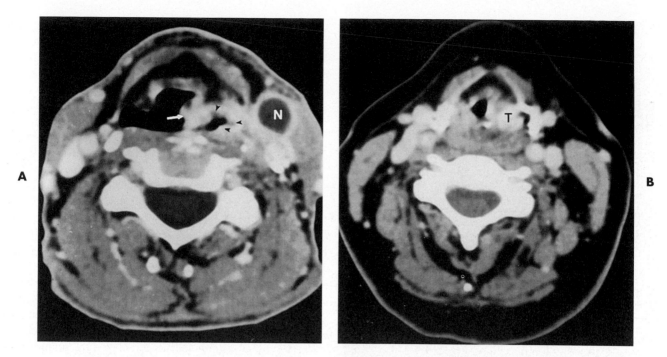

FIG. 11-53 CT of a pharyngeal tumor limited to the level of the supraglottic larynx. **A,** The lesion *(arrowheads)* extends around the lateral wall of the pharynx onto the posterior wall. The aryepiglottic fold *(arrow)* is involved. Typical appearance of a metastatic node *(N)*. **B,** Lower margin of the tumor *(T)* is seen on the axial scan at the level of the supraglottic fat. The scan immediately inferior to this was normal.

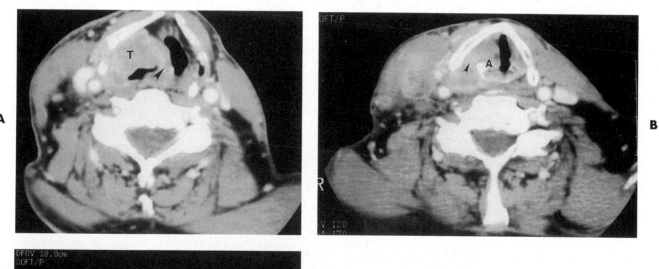

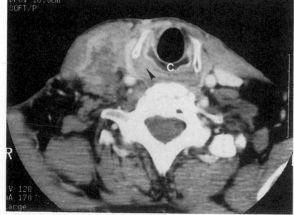

FIG. 11-54 Axial CT shows a pyriform sinus tumor extending through the thyroarytenoid gap into the paraglottic space. **A,** Large tumor *(T)* involving the pyriform sinus. The lesion extends along the aryepiglottic fold *(arrowhead)*. **B,** Lower scan shows the tumor in the lower pyriform sinus. Note how the tumor *(arrowhead)* squeezes between the thyroid cartilage and the arytenoid *(A)*. This is at the level of the true cord. **C,** Slightly inferior scan shows continued asymmetry as the tumor *(arrowhead)* extends slightly into the postcricoid region. *C,* Cricoid. At this level the tumor is contiguous with the cricoid cartilage.

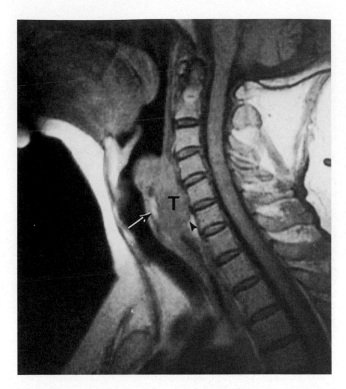

FIG. 11-55 MRI of postcricoid tumor. Sagittal view shows the tumor *(T)*. The inferior margin *(arrowhead)* is best defined in this sagittal view. Bright signal is fat in the medullary cavity of the cricoid lamina *(arrow)*.

Separation of benign from malignant chondroid lesions is usually impossible based on imaging characteristics. However, most of these tumors behave in a low-grade manner. Even after histologic examination of the entire specimen, differentiation of benign and malignant tumors can be difficult. Despite its fairly good prognosis, if a low-grade tumor has extensive cricoid involvement, a total laryngectomy is usually considered.

Rare primary and metastatic melanomas have been found in the supraglottic larynx and true cord.[1] Other rare primary tumors involving the larynx include lymphoma, plasmacytoma, and fibrous histiocytoma.

Secondary involvement of the larynx by other than direct tumor extension is rare. Rare metastases from melanomas, renal cell cancers, and breast and lung primaries have been reported, as has involvement by leukemia and lymphoma. No characteristic imaging appearances have been described.[1,21]

BENIGN TUMORS

Benign lesions of the larynx include vocal cord nodules, juvenile papillomatosis, and a variety of nonepithelial tumors.

Vocal cord nodules (nonneoplastic) represent a stromal reaction that occurs in patients with a history of vocal abuse. The nodules may be an incidental imaging finding, but they usually are clinically diagnosed, with imaging considered unnecessary (Fig. 11-60). Vocal cord nodules occur on the free margin of the true vocal cord.

Papillomas, although benign and noninvasive, tend to recur after therapy.[1] The wartlike lesions, most often multiple, occur most often in children. Any part of the larynx can be affected, and involvement of the trachea and bronchial tree can occur in severe cases, especially if there is a history of tracheostomy. Currently the laser is used to excise the papillomas in children; however, regrowth can be so rapid that many children require repeat procedures every few weeks. Most cases eventually go into remission, but some cases persist into adulthood. Although these lesions are benign, deaths have occurred secondary to pneumonia or airway compromise. The high correlation between children with juvenile papillomatosis and mothers with genital warts suggests a viral etiology. Papillomas do occur in adults, usually men; however in this cases the papillomas are less often multiple.

On plain films and tomography the multiple nodules can be seen impinging on the airway (Fig. 11-61). Chest films are used to evaluate possible pulmonary involvement, which usually is seen as small nodules, that may may cavitate.

Benign nonepithelial or mesenchymal tumors include hemangiomas, neural tumors, lipomas, leiomyomas, rhabdomyomas, chondromas, and a few other rare lesions.[1,2] Of these, lipomas have a characteristic appearance both on CT and MRI because of their high fat content (Fig. 11-62).[22] Chondromas often can be identified by the mineralized matrix and the relationship to the laryngeal cartilage. The lesion cannot be reliably established as benign or malignant unless there is a very aggressive appearance.

Hemangiomas deserve special mention. Hemangiomas are more common in adults than in children, but the pediatric type is more likely to cause airway obstruction and so has received more attention.[23]

Hemangiomas in adults are usually localized (Fig. 11-63) and tend to be glottic or supraglottic. They enhance on CT, and on MRI they have a fairly high T2W signal intensity.

Hemangiomas of the young can occur anywhere in the larynx but have a predilection for the subglottic area (Figs. 11-64 to 11-66). Those hemangiomas arising in the subglottic area are a major clinical problem because even though the hemangioma is expected to regress, airway compromise can force intervention. In a typical pediatric hemangioma the infant has partial airway obstruction within the first 6 to 12 months of life. Because any inflammation further compromises an already narrowed subglottic area, these patients may present as recurrent croup. Because of venous engorgement, crying also exacerbates the problem. The diagnosis may be suggested by radiography but is usually made by endoscopy, when a compressible red or blue mass is seen. Topical epinephrine may cause the lesion to diminish in size. Tracheostomy may be necessary while waiting for the tumor to diminish in size. Steroid therapy and surgery have been tried; however, currently, laser excision or reduction is used because of the lower associated operative bleeding. Eventual tracheal stenosis is not uncommon, especially after surgery. The laryngeal lesion is often associated with cutaneous or soft-tissue hemangiomas.

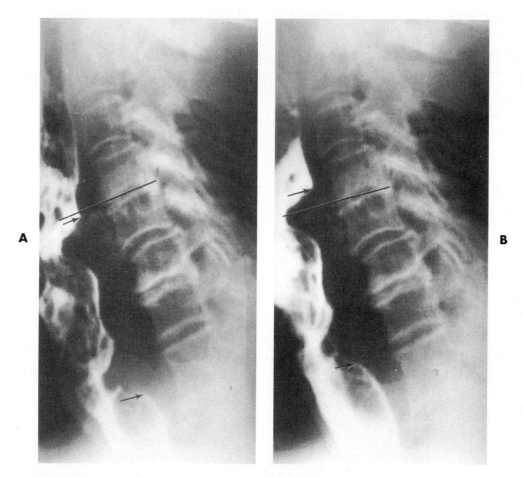

FIG. 11-56 Exophytic lesion of the posterior wall of the pharynx. The lesion is not fixed to the prevertebral fascia. Compare the position of the upper and lower margin of the lesion *(arrows)* with the cervical spine interspace C-4 to C-5. **A,** At rest. **B,** During swallowing.

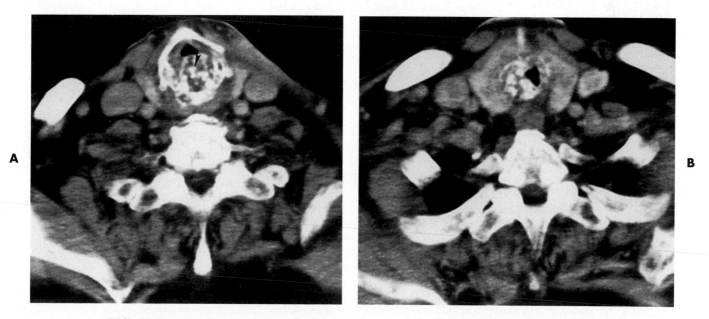

FIG. 11-57 Chondrosarcoma of the larynx. **A,** CT shows definite ringlike calcifications *(arrowhead)* within the tumor mass. **B,** Inferior extension shows similar calcifications.

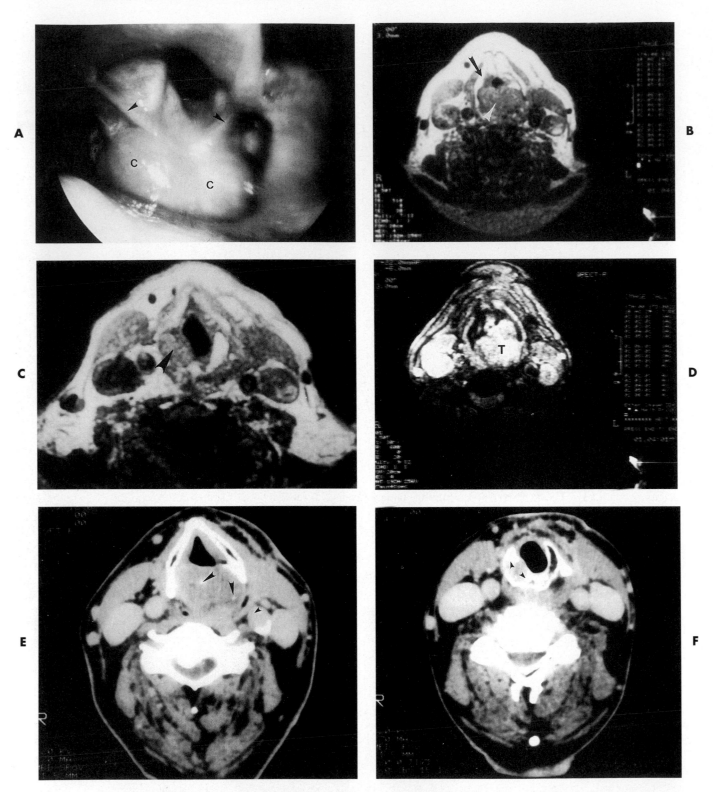

FIG. 11-58   Chondrosarcoma of the larynx. **A,** Endoscopic view shows a large bulge in the region of the cricoid *(C)*. Note that the mucosa is intact and is not ulcerated. *Arrowheads,* AE folds. **B,** T1W image shows the large submucosal mass *(arrowhead)*. Note its position in the posterior larynx. There is no abnormality in the paraglottic fat *(arrow)*. **C,** Slightly lower than **B**. Axial image through the cricoid cartilage shows a well-defined defect *(arrowhead)*. The sharp margin would be unusual in invasion from squamous carcinoma. This indicates the origin within the cricoid cartilage. **D,** T2W axial image shows the tumor *(T)* to have high signal characteristic of chondrosarcoma. **E,** Axial CT shows a large mass with small punctate calcification *(arrowheads)*. This suggests the chondroid nature of the lesion. **F,** Axial scan through the cricoid shows the sharp margin of the lesion *(arrowheads)* as it abuts the normal cartilage.

The most common radiographic appearance of a pediatric hemangioma is a localized bulge or concentric narrowing of the airway just below the true cords. This can be appreciated on CT or MRI with axial, coronal, or sagittal planes. On MRI the lesion has high signal intensity on T2W images (Fig. 11-66). On CT or MRI the lesion enhances with contrast. Conventional tomography also can show the airway well, and the actual airway configuration can be easily appreciated on plain films done in several projections. Occasionally, phleboliths may be seen in a larger hemangioma, either with CT or with plain film (usually in somewhat older patients). Hemangiomas of the extralaryngeal neck rarely extend into the larynx.

Paragangliomas (glomus tumors) have been reported in the larynx, usually in a supraglottic location (Fig. 11-67).[24] These lesions enhance on CT, and as might be expected from their vascular nature, tend to bleed if biopsied. Like hemangiomas, they have intermediate signal intensity on T1W images and high T2W signal intensity.

Schwannomas can occur as isolated submucosal tumors in the larynx. In neurofibromatosis, isolated lesions can occur; however, a plexiform more infiltrative lesion also can diffusely involve the paraglottic structures (Fig. 11-68).[25,26]

Granular cell tumor is a benign lesion of unknown origin that involves the mucosal membranes of the head and neck.[1] Most theories implicate either a Schwann cell or a more primitive mesenchymal cell origin. The larynx can be involved, and the most common site is the true cord. The epithelium over the granular cell tumor may be hyperplastic and thus mimic squamous cell carcinoma at direct inspection. Biopsy establishes the diagnosis. The age of occurrence is usually 35 to 45 years, which is younger than the usual age of squamous cell carcinoma.

CYSTS AND LARYNGOCELES

A variety of cystic structures can occur in or around the larynx. Mucous retention cysts can occur along any mucosal surface, but they are most common in the supraglottic larynx. An obstructed laryngocele can occur, often associated with an obstructing lesion in the ipsilateral laryngeal ventricle. Because the thyroglossal duct passes along the outer margin of the larynx, these cysts commonly occur adjacent to the larynx. Only rarely does a thyroglossal duct cyst actually involve the larynx.

Mucosal cysts can arise anyplace in the larynx that contains submucosal glands.[1,27] Thus only the free margin of the true cord is spared, and virtually any other location within the larynx is a possible site of cyst development. These cysts are superficial and submucosal, and they protrude into the airway. Symptoms depend on the size and location of the cyst and include dysphagia and respiratory distress. Deep extension is not seen. Vallecular cysts are seen anterior to the epiglottis (Fig. 11-69). These cysts often occur in children.

The saccule, or appendix, of the ventricle is a tubular structure that normally extends cranially into the paraglottic

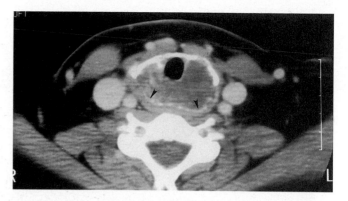

FIG. 11-59 Low-grade chondrosarcoma of the cricoid. The low-grade chondrosarcoma expands the cricoid cartilage. The cortex has been remodeled outward *(arrowheads)*, leaving the general shape of the original cartilage.

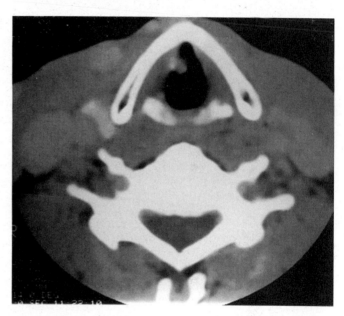

FIG. 11-60 Axial CT shows a polyp of the right true cord. Incidental finding.

region of the false cord (Fig. 11-70). The saccule lumen communicates with the anterior ventricle, and normally the saccule does not produce a noticeable submucosal supraglottic mass. However, if the saccule enlarges so that it does produce a submucosal mass, it is called a *laryngocele* or *saccular cyst*.[28,29] If the saccule remains air-filled, many authors refer to it as a laryngocele. However, if the saccular lumen fills with secretions, it is referred to as a *saccular cyst*, or a *laryngeal mucocele*. Although a saccular cyst can result from inflammatory mucosal swelling, an obstructing lesion in the ventricle always must be sought.

A laryngocele is referred to as being internal, mixed or combined, or external in type. An internal laryngocele remains totally within the larynx, producing a submucosal supraglottic mass. A combined or mixed laryngocele pro-

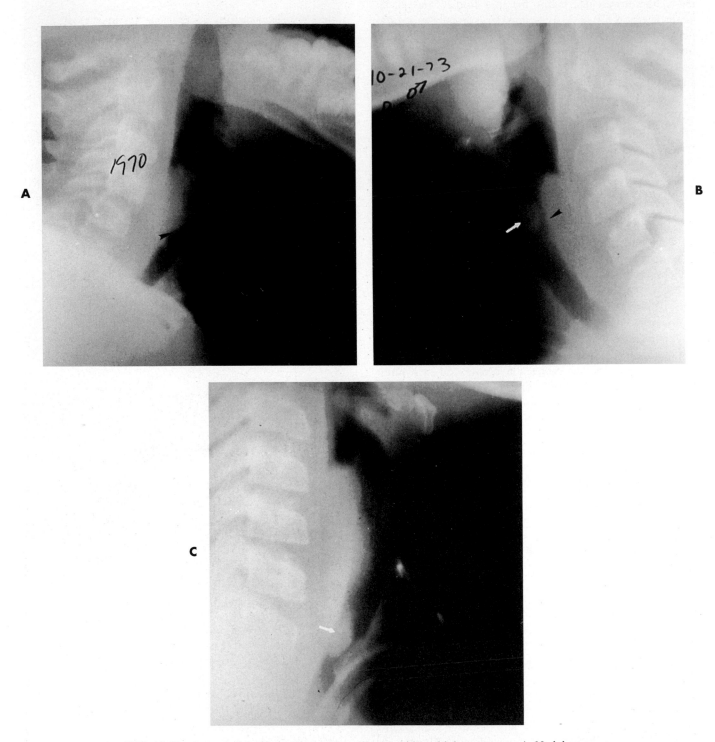

FIG. 11-61   Lateral plain films of juvenile papillomas with multiple treatments. **A,** Nodular tumor mass completely obstructing the larynx. Note the slight nodularity of the inferior margin of the tumor *(arrowhead).* **B,** Later study shows small airway *(arrowhead)* with nodular mass in the anterior larynx *(arrow).* **C,** Later film in adolescent showing good laryngeal airway but nodular mass just above the tracheostomy. *Arrow,* mass.

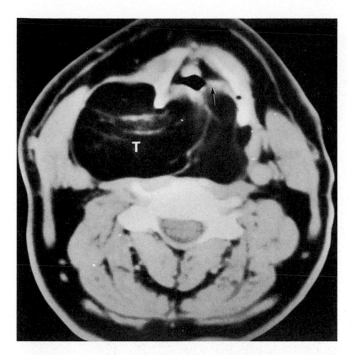

FIG. 11-62 Axial CT shows lipoma in the soft tissues of the neck and retropharyngeal space. Large tumor extending posterior to the larynx, displacing the larynx anteriorly. Note how the fat appears to "bulge" into the supraglottic-paraglottic space *(arrow)*. The lesion at this level is actually retropharyngeal, with pharyngeal lumen going between the tumor and the larynx. The anterior wall of the pyriform sinus is being pushed anteriorly, compressing the paraglottic fat but not invading. *T*, Tumor.

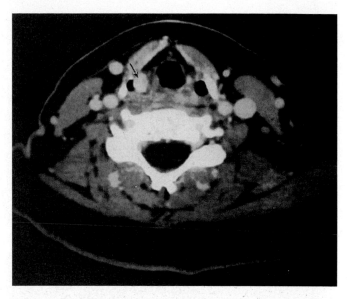

FIG. 11-63 Axial CT of a hemangioma of the pyriform sinus shows enhancement of the small lesion attached to the medial wall of the pyriform sinus just below the aryepiglottic fold. *Arrow*, tumor.

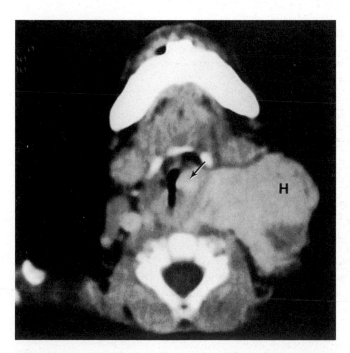

FIG. 11-64 Axial CT of a child with large hemangioma *(H)*, involving the soft tissues of the neck with involvement of the aryepiglottic fold and supraglottic paraglottic space *(arrow)*.

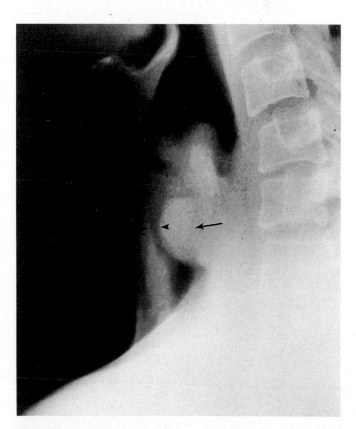

FIG. 11-65 Lateral plain film of large subglottic hemangioma protruding from the posterior wall with significant narrowing of the airway *(arrowheads)*. *Arrow*, hemangioma. This is an older patient than is typical for the infantile type of hemangioma.

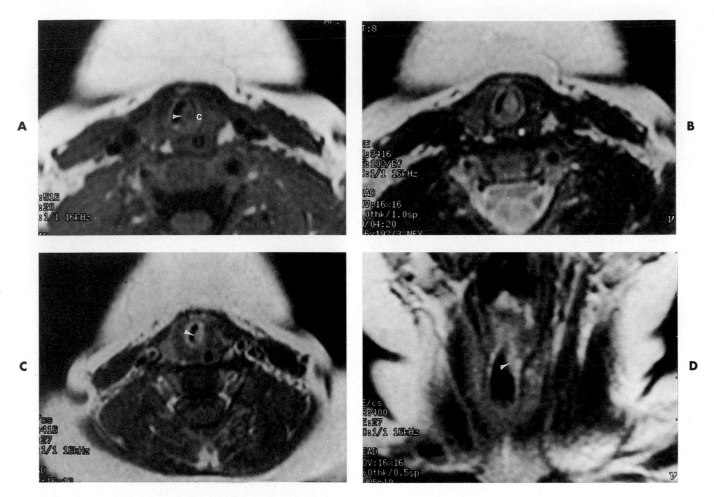

FIG. 11-66   Subglottic hemangioma MR. **A,** Axial T1W image shows a small bulge *(arrowhead)* at the level of the cricoid cartilage. *C,* Cricoid ring. **B,** T2W image shows high signal in the abnormality characteristic of the hemangioma. **C,** Postcontrast T1W image shows enhancement of the hemangioma *(arrowhead)* and the mucosa. **D,** Coronal image shows the enhancing lesion *(arrowhead)* in the subglottic angle. The lesion is limited to the mucosal area.

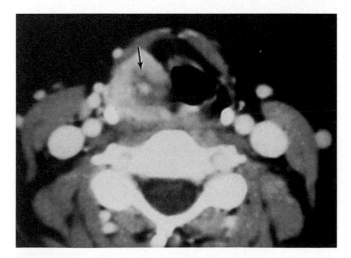

FIG. 11-67   Axial CT of paraganglioma of the supraglottic larynx and pyriform sinus shows enhancing mass in the aryepiglottic fold and pyriform sinus *(arrow)*. (Courtesy Dr. Peter Som)

trudes through the thyrohyoid membrane, producing both an intralaryngeal and extralaryngeal mass. The term *external laryngocele* refers to a combined laryngocele that produces little if any supraglottic mass. However, this is a poor term because any laryngocele that has an external component must also have an internal component, whether or not it produces an intralaryngeal mass.

A laryngocele can be diagnosed on CT, MRI, plain films, and tomography (Figs. 11-71 to 11-75). The internal consistency of the fluid-filled cysts may vary somewhat, depending on their protein content; however, this is only apparent on MRI or CT. On CT or MRI the supraglottic mass can be followed down through the paraglottic area of the false cord to the level of the ventricle. It should be noted that a normal air-filled ventricular appendix can often be seen on axial imaging, and this should not be called a laryngocele unless there is deformity of the ipsilateral supraglottic margin.

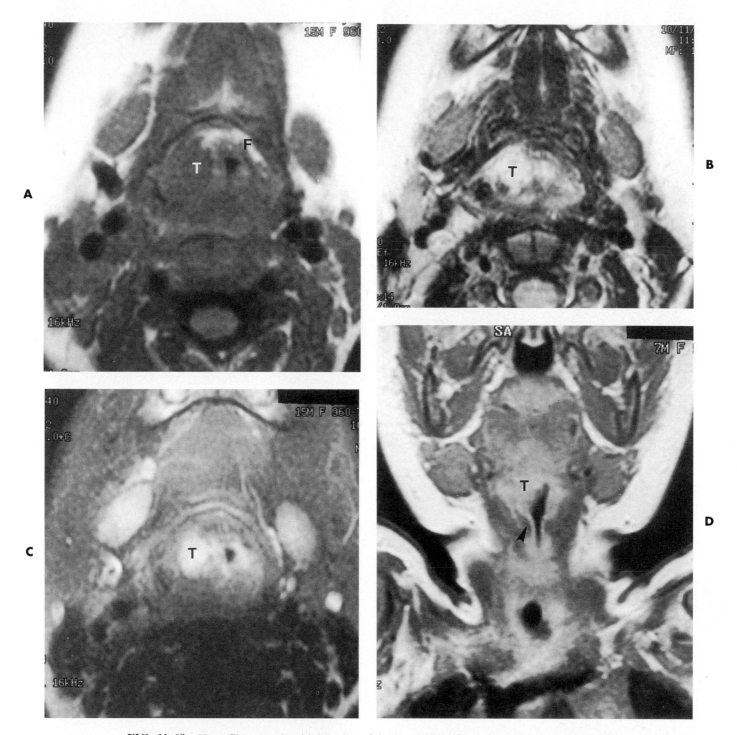

FIG. 11-68 Neurofibromatosis with invasion of the larynx. Plexiform neurofibroma patient with neurofibromatosis. **A,** T1W image through the supraglottic larynx. The tumor *(T)* extends anteriorly in the paraglottic fat. Note the normal paraglottic fat *(F)* on the opposite side. **B,** T2W image (fast spin-echo) shows the high signal of the tumor *(T)*. **C,** Postconstrast T1W image with fat suppression. The tumor *(T)* enhances significantly. Compare with the enhancing mucosa. **D,** Coronal T1W image with contrast. No fat suppression. The tumor *(T)* is seen in the paraglottic space. Note the normal thyroarytenoid muscle *(arrowhead)* at the cord level.

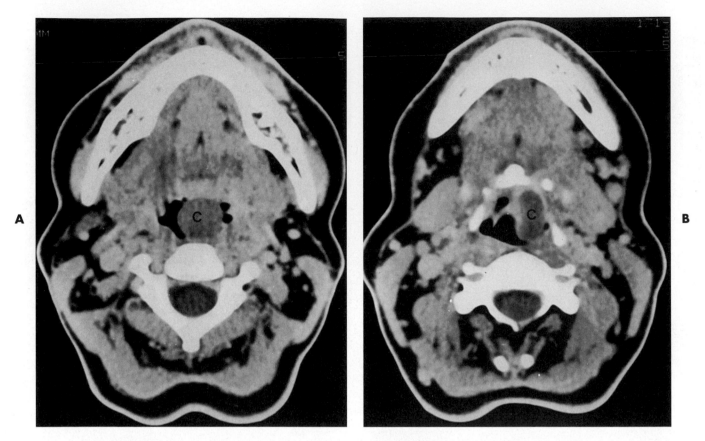

FIG. 11-69 **A,** Vallecular cyst on CT. Midline cyst *(C)* seen at the level of the base of the tongue. **B,** Slightly lower level shows the origin of the cyst in the left valleculae, deforming the epiglottis. *C,* Cyst.

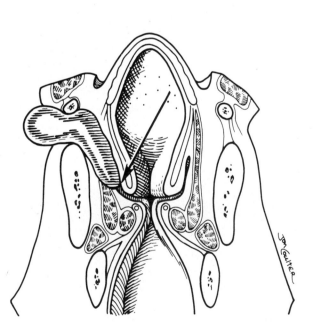

FIG. 11-70 Diagram showing a laryngocele protruding between hyoid and thyroid cartilage. The laryngocele is caused by a relative obstruction *(arrow)* at the level of the ventricle.

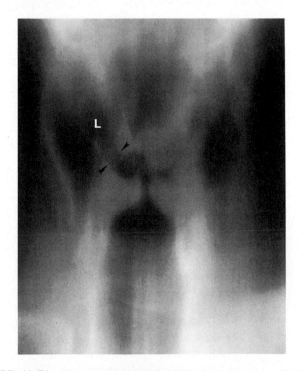

FIG. 11-71 Laryngocele. Modified Valsalva maneuver with distention of the laryngocele *(L)* and widening of the communication with the ventricles *(arrowheads).*

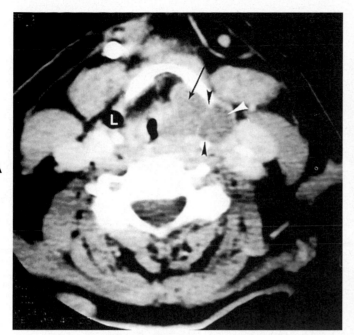 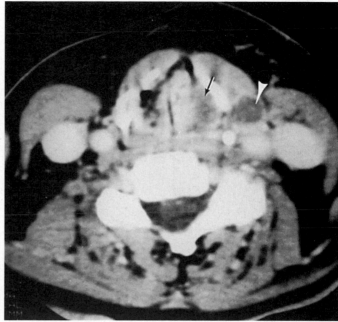

FIG. 11-72   Axial CT of a laryngocele (saccular cyst). **A,** There is both an internal *(arrow)* and external *(white arrowhead)* component. The position of the thyrohyoid membrane is signified by black arrowheads. A small air-filled external laryngocele *(L)* is seen on the opposite side. **B,** Lower scan through the supraglottic larynx shows the abnormality in the paraglottic space *(arrow)* and the external component *(arrowhead)*.

A laryngocele, although always benign, can be associated with a malignancy in the region of the ventricle (Figs. 11-73, 11-74, 11-76). The tumor obstructs the outflow of the saccule, causing either trapping of air or more commonly retention of mucous secretions. The ventricular area should be closely examined in patients with a laryngocele or saccular cyst. However, imaging cannot completely "exclude" a carcinoma, and endoscopy should always be performed.

The term *laryngopyocele* refers to an infected laryngocele (Figs. 11-77, 11-78) and enlargement can cause airway compromise and swelling in the lateral neck.

Treatment of a symptomatic laryngocele is surgical. A tracheostomy is often performed because of concern that even minor postoperative swelling or bleeding can compromise the airway.

Although thyroglossal duct cysts are discussed in several other chapters in this book, they are briefly mentioned here (Fig. 11-79). At the level of the larynx, a thyroglossal duct cyst has a charcteristic location just off midline, insinuated between the strap muscles and the anterior thyroid ala. These cysts are easily distinguished from a laryngocele because of their more anterior location outside the larynx and because they do not have an intralaryngeal component. Rarely, on imaging a thyroglossal duct cyst appears to protrude into the larynx through the superior thyroid notch. However, in these cases the cyst actually is only displacing the thyrohyoid membrane posteriorly into the larynx. There have been a few reports of long-standing large thyroglossal duct cysts that have caused dcossification of the thyroid cartilage and bulged into the larnyx, presenting clinically as a submucosal mass. Treatment was excision, without having to resect any of the larynx.

INFECTION AND INFLAMMATION

Infections that may come to the attention of the radiologist are usually those of childhood, including epiglottitis or croup. Tuberculosis or other granulomatous diseases are rare, as is perichondritis or infection of the laryngeal cartilages, which is ususally associated with prior radiation therapy.[30] Previously, perichondritis and abscesses were caused by typhoid fever, measles, scarlet fever, erysipelas, anthrax, and mycoses.[31] Occasionally, infections of the soft tissues of the neck can involve the larynx secondarily, as can other inflammatory processes such as arthritis and collagen vascular disease.[30]

Croup

Croup refers to an inflammation of the subglottic larynx with greater or lesser involvement of the trachea and bronchi. Occurring in young children (6 months to 3 years of age), croup is usually caused by type 1 parainfluenza

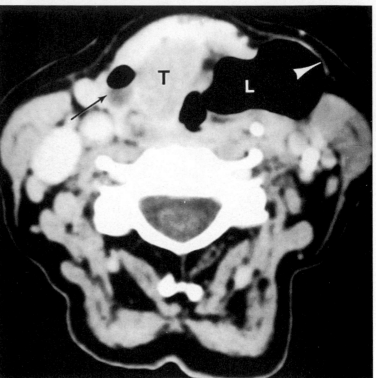

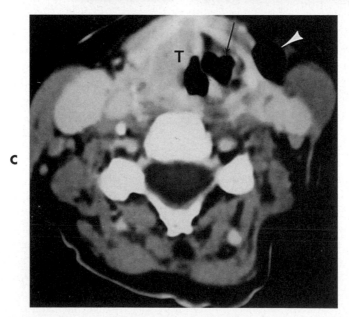

FIG. 11-73   Bilateral laryngocele with large supraglottic tumor on one side. **A,** Scout view shows the dilated air-filled sac *(arrow)*. **B,** Axial scan through the upper larynx shows the air-filled laryngocele *(L)* on the left protruding through the thyrohyoid membrane. The lateral aspect of the laryngocele *(arrowhead)* caused a significant bulge in the neck. Tumor fills the opposite supraglottis *(T)*. The smaller laryngocele *(arrow)* is seen on the side of the tumor with an air-fluid level. **C,** Lower scan shows the tumor *(T)*, intralaryngeal segment (paraglottic space) of the laryngocele *(arrow)*, and the external component *(arrowhead)*.

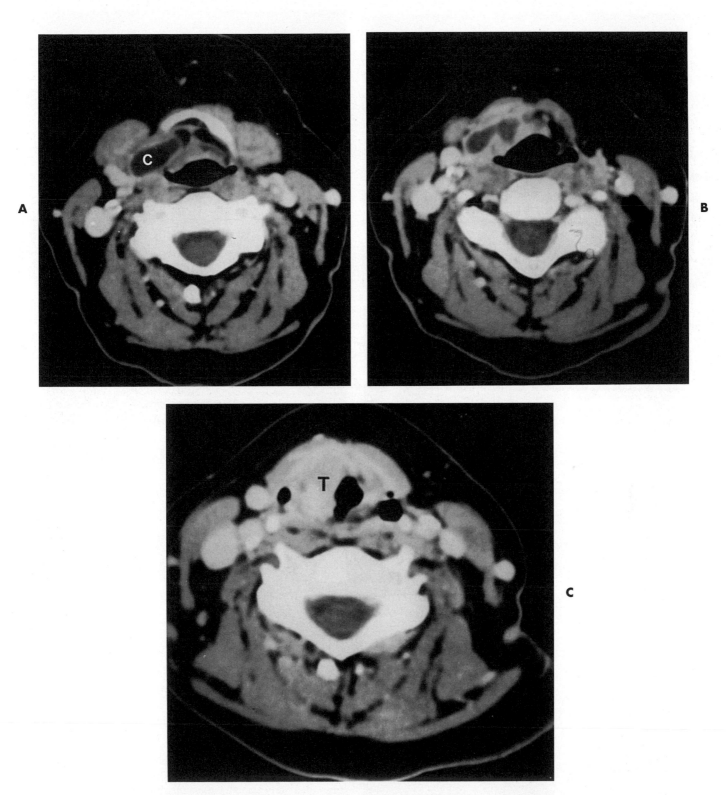

FIG. 11-74   Saccular cyst (laryngocele) with tumor of the lower false cord on CT. **A,** CT scan through the supraglottic larynx shows the saccular cyst *(C)* with smooth margins. **B,** Slightly lower scan shows the bilobular nature of the internal and external component. **C,** Lower scan through the lower false cord shows the tumor *(T)*.

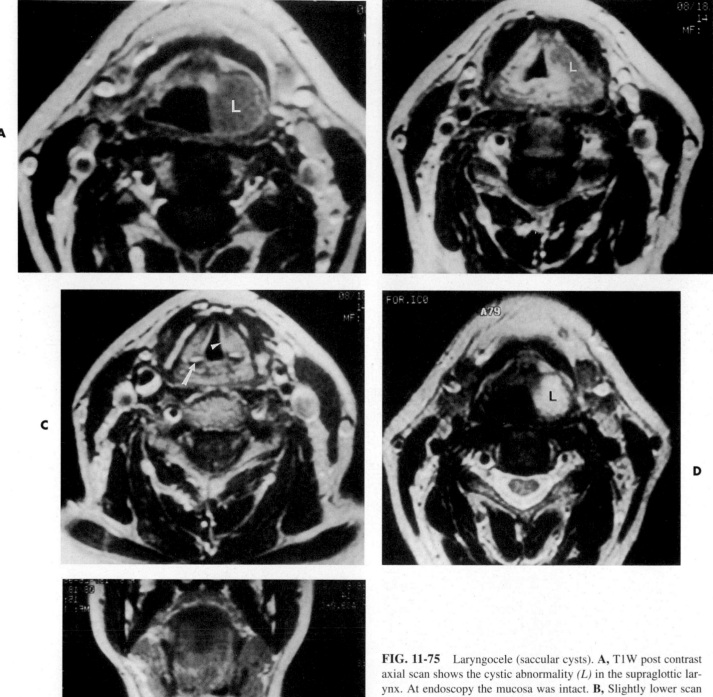

FIG. 11-75 Laryngocele (saccular cysts). **A,** T1W post contrast axial scan shows the cystic abnormality *(L)* in the supraglottic larynx. At endoscopy the mucosa was intact. **B,** Slightly lower scan shows laryngocele *(L)* filling the paraglottic space at the supraglottic level. **C,** T1W image postcontrast. Axial image at the level of the cord shows no abnormality. *Arrowhead,* Vocal ligament; *arrow,* arytenoid. **D,** T2W image shows the high signal in the laryngocele *(L)*. **E,** Coronal T1W postcontrast shows the laryngocele with a fairly smooth outline *(arrowhead)*.

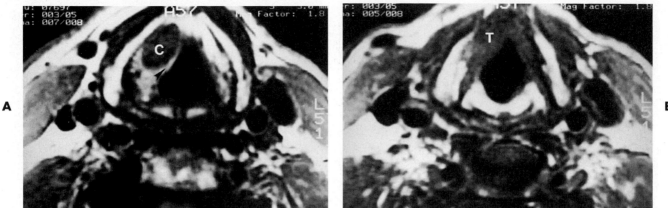

FIG. 11-76 A, Saccular cyst (laryngocele). Well-defined cyst *(C)* fills the supraglottic larynx. Note the definite separation *(arrowhead)* from the mucosa. **B,** Scan inferior to **A** shows a tumor at the level of the ventricle and true cord. *T,* Tumor.

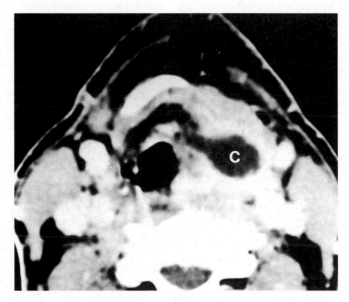

FIG. 11-77 Laryngopyocele with contrast-enhanced CT shows the saccular cyst *(C).* There is irregular enhancement of the inflamed wall.

virus, but many other organisms occasionally have been implicated. Croup produces a barking cough and stridor. The edema involves the mucosa of the subglottic larynx. Because this tissue is looser in children than in adults, the swollen mucosa can impinge upon the airway. This is usually appreciated best on the frontal film as the "wine bottle" or "steeple-shaped" airway, with loss of the subglottic arch (Fig. 11-80). If the film is taken on inspiration, there may be ballooning of the pharynx, including the pyriform sinuses. In expiration the trachea and subglottis may be distended. Usually, however, the diagnosis is made clinically, and the factors that determine more extensive treatment such as intubation or even tracheostomy are clinical rather than

radiographic. Plain films are used to confirm the diagnosis and to exclude a foreign body.

Epiglottitis or Supraglottitis

Epiglottitis or supraglottitis occurs in a slightly older age group than croup and is caused by *Haemophilus influenzae.* A sore throat and inability to swallow are the key clinical features, along with airway compromise. The epiglottis is swollen and has a typical "cherry red" appearance.

The lateral radiograph is characteristic and reflects the extent of the abnormality. The epiglottis is thickened, losing its normal sharp curvilinear shape (Fig. 11-81). The epiglottis blends into the aryepiglottic folds, which are also

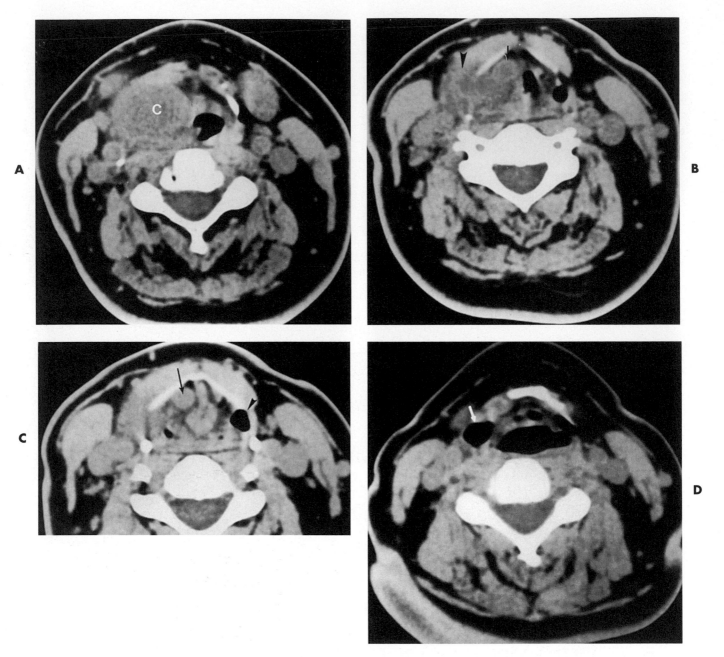

FIG. 11-78   Laryngopyocele, pre- and posttreatment, nonenhanced CT scans. **A,** Supraglottic slice shows a large mass representing the laryngopyocele *(C)*. **B,** Slightly lower scan shows both internal components *(arrow)* and external components *(arrowhead)*. **C,** Slightly lower scan through the false cord level shows the "neck" of the laryngocele *(arrow)* extending through the paraglottic fat. Note the small air-filled laryngocele *(arrowhead)* on the opposite side. **D,** Postantibiotic treatment (no surgery). The mass has resolved and there is air in the laryngocele *(arrow)*.

enlarged. In severe cases the arytenoid prominence may be swollen. The radiograph is taken to document the disease and to exclude foreign bodies. Because epiglottitis can advance quickly to severe airway compromise, manipulation is minimized, including attempts at direct visualization of the enlarged epiglottis. The patient must never be out of an environment where an emergency tracheostomy can be performed. Radiographs are usually done either in the emer-

gency room or even the operating room. In most institutions the child is not submitted to the risk of transportation to the radiology department. Therapy includes intubation or even tracheostomy, as well as administration of antibiotics. Decannulization is usually possible within 24 to 36 hours.

Adult epiglottitis or supraglottitis does occur, but it usually is not as life-threatening as it is in the pediatric patient. Rarely, emphysematous epiglottitis has been reported (Fig. 11-82).[32]

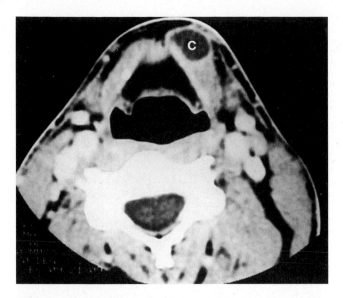

FIG. 11-79 Thyroglossal duct cyst *(C)*. On axial CT. Note that the fat within the larynx is normal. The paraglottic level would be normal as well.

Tuberculosis and Other Granulomatous Lesions

Today, tuberculosis of the larynx is rare. However, in the past it was more common and was associated with pulmonary tuberculosis. Clinically, edema is present early. With more severe involvement, ulceration and necrosis occur, producing a multinodular, irregularly enlarged epiglottis that can be seen on plain films (Fig. 11-83). The cricoarytenoid joint can be involved, causing fixation. Perichondritis can also occur.

Rhinoscleroma (Fig. 11-84), Wegener's granulomatosis, malignant midline or polymorphic reticulosis, pemphigus, leprosy, syphilis, and numerous mycotic infections, all have been noted to rarely involve the larynx. Involvement can be localized to the larynx or in association with pharyngeal involvement (Fig. 11-85). The recent increase in immuno-compromised patients has again made some of these rare infections more of a diagnostic consideration.

Sarcoid can cause diffuse laryngeal thickening, small nodular lesions, or localized infiltrative lesions. No radiographic finding is specific, and the patient usually has other systemic manifestations of this disease.

Neck Infection

Soft-tissue infection arising in the neck rarely involves the larynx (Fig. 11-86). The findings in the larynx reflect the area of involvement, and usually the soft tissues contiguous to the larynx show obvious inflammatory change.

Rheumatoid and Collagen Vascular Disease

The cricoarytenoid and cricothyroid joints are true synovial joints and can be affected by rheumatoid disease.[33] Swelling of the cricoarytenoid joint may cause hoarseness. Later sequelae include joint fixation. On CT this can be identified

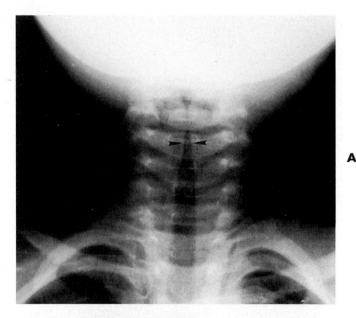

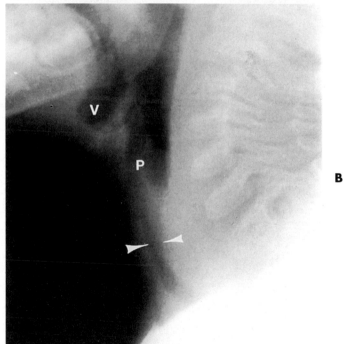

FIG. 11-80 Croup. **A,** Frontal film shows narrowing of the airway between arrowheads just beneath the cord. This is the so-called steeple or winebottle sign. **B,** Lateral film shows dilatation of the pyriform sinuses *(P)* and the valleculae *(V)* with narrowing (between *arrowheads*) of the subglottic larynx.

by irregular sclerosis or erosions in the region of the cricoarytenoid joint. The soft tissues close to the arytenoid may be swollen.

On conventional tomography or fluoroscopy, fixation of the arytenoid can be suggested when the cord does not move as well as the opposite cord, but the immobile cord does not show the typical findings of vocal cord paralysis.

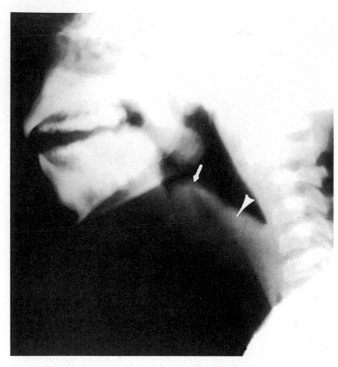

FIG. 11-81 Lateral plain film of epiglottitis showing thickening of the epiglottis *(arrow)* and prominence of the arytenoid *(arrowhead).*

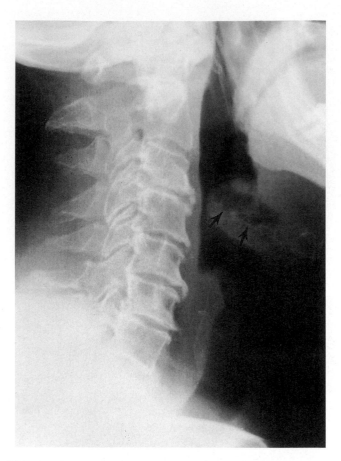

FIG. 11-82 Emphysematous epiglottitis lateral plain film. There is enlargement of the epiglottis, but there is also air seen within the soft tissues *(arrow).* (Courtesy Dr. William Nemzek.)

Relapsing polychondritis is a rare, nonsuppurative inflammatory condition affecting various cartilages.[34] The cause is unknown. The ear cartilages, nasal cartilages, and joint cartilages can be involved. Airway involvement is present in about half of the patients afflicted, often being present as significant airway compromise. The laryngeal cartilages can be involved, and generalized laryngeal edema can occur. Sclerosis and enlargement of the cartilage can be present. Diffuse calcification of the involved areas may also be present. One report showed considerable calcification in the region of the arytenoid. Radionuclide bone scans can be positive over the involved region of the larynx and over other affected areas of the body.[35]

TRAUMA

Vehicular accidents account for most of the significant trauma to the larynx and upper trachea, with the larynx being crushed against the spine.[36] In children the larynx is higher in position relative to the mandible and is thus relatively protected; however, in the adult the lower position of the larynx makes it vulnerable to trauma.

In many circumstances the radiologic examination cannot be performed acutely because of airway compromise.

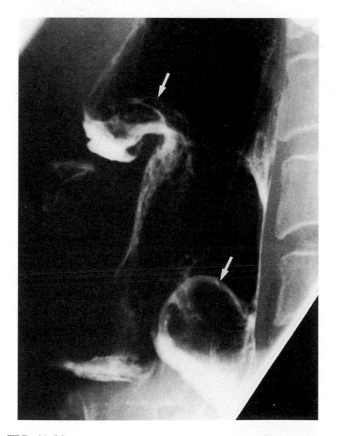

FIG. 11-83 Laryngeal tuberculosis. Lateral view of laryngogram shows nodular, thickened epiglottis *(upper arrow).* The arytenoid mucosa is edematous *(lower arrow).* (Courtesy Dr. Peter Som.)

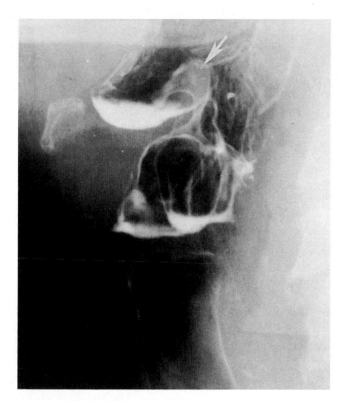

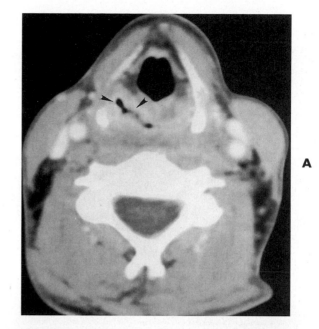

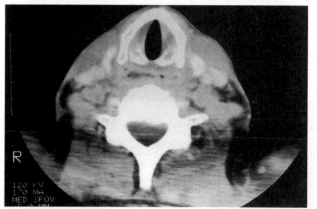

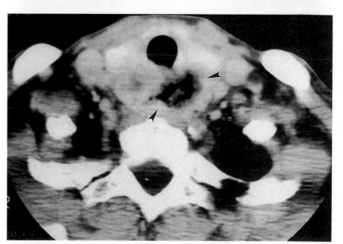

FIG. 11-84 Lateral laryngogram shows rhinoscleroma (Klebsiella rhinoscleromatis). There is polypoid thickening of the epiglottis *(arrow)*. (Courtesy Dr. Peter Som.)

However, early definitive surgical intervention is associated with better results, and the diagnostic evaluation should not be substantially delayed.

If the cartilage is well calcified, fractures can be seen on plain radiographs. CT usually gives better visualization.[37] Of particular interest should be the presence of any cartilage fragments that impinge on the airway or perforate the mucosa. When there is significant airway compromise, endoscopy is done to assess for any mucosal tears. If the airway is perforated, air can be seen in the adjacent soft tissues and is visible on plain films and CT. A hematoma may appear either as a mass or as an obliteration of the normal fat density in the upper larynx (Fig. 11-87).

Fractures of the larynx can involve the thyroid cartilage, cricoid cartilage, or both.[38] Thyroid cartilage fractures are either vertical or horizontal. Vertical fractures result from the splaying of the thyroid cartilage as it is pushed against the spine. A horizontal fracture usually crosses both thyroid alae, and there is usually coexistent supraglottic soft-tissue injury (Fig. 11-88). The superior fragments of the thyroid cartilage can be displaced posteriorly, and the thyroepiglottic ligament or petiole of the epiglottis may be torn, resulting in a dislocated or avulsed epiglottis. (Fig. 11-89).[39] The hyoid bone also may be fractured. Vertical factures of the thyroid cartilage are best appreciated on CT (Fig. 11-90). Horizontal fractures are in the plane of the axial CT scan and may be difficult to demonstrate on these images.

FIG. 11-85 Moniliasis esophagitis and pharyngitis in a patient with AIDS. **A,** CT scan through the supraglottic larynx shows thickening of the pyriform sinus wall *(arrowheads)*. This appearance is the same as carcinoma. **B,** Scan through the level of the true cords shows the abnormality extending into the postcricoid area. The pattern suggests a spreading hypopharyngeal carcinoma. **C,** Thickening of the esophageal wall *(arrowheads)* and extension into the soft tissue in the cervical esophagus.

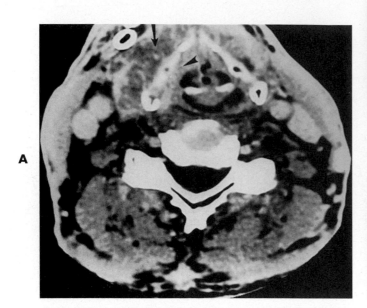
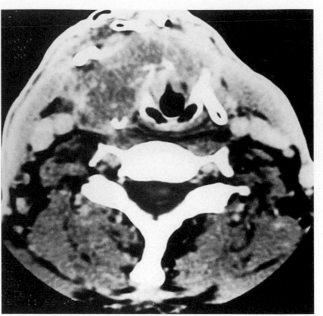

FIG. 11-86 Axial CT scans **A,** Infection of the soft tissues of the neck showing obscuration of the fat plane *(arrow)* and extension into the paraglottic fat of the larynx *(arrowhead)*. The drains in the neck are from decompression of an abscess. **B,** Level of the cricoid showing considerable soft-tissue thickening impinging on the airway.

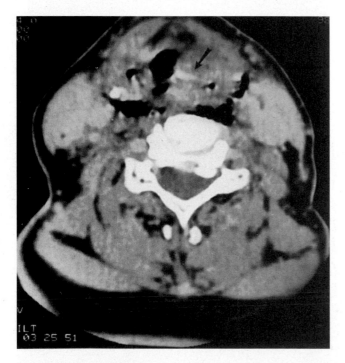

FIG. 11-87 Vehicular injury. Axial CT of a hematoma of the larynx and laceration of the pharynx. There is a hematoma *(arrow)* of the aryepiglottic fold. The gas in the soft tissues is from laceration of the pharyngeal wall.

Occasionally, on axial CT a patient has an asymmetrical curvature to the thyroid cartilage, with one side bowing inward, often creating a submucosal fullness on that side. Although there is no immediate history of trauma, careful questioning often reveals a history of minor trauma to the larynx. Most authors believe that such an appearance on CT represents the late sequellae of old trauma.

Cricoid fractures cause collapse of the normal cricoid ring (Fig. 11-91). Almost always there is more than one fracture, usually with both sides of the cricoid ring being broken to create an anterior and a posterior fragment. The anterior fragment is pushed posteriorly and impinges on the airway, and the free end of a fragment may perforate the mucosa. The fractures may be difficult to appreciate in younger patients because the arch of the cricoid cartilage is not as well calcified; however, usually the cartilage is dense enough that it can be seen on CT (Fig. 11-92). A key finding is the shape of the airway and the presence of subglottic swelling. At the level of the cricoid the normal subglottic airway is slightly oval. A subtle fracture with minimal displacement causes the airway to have a rounder appearance. Edema causes increased soft tissue between the cartilage and the air column. If these important fractures are to be detected, familiarity with the normal appearance of the subglottic area is crucial.

Fractures of the cricoid usually require surgical intervention, repositioning the fragments with suture or stent placement.

Laryngotracheal separation is a complete tear of the trachea, and because of the loss of the airway, it is usually fatal (Fig. 11-93). Plain radiographs may show the malalignment of an incomplete separation. Few of these cases get as far as the radiology department, and those that do usually have already had a tracheostomy.

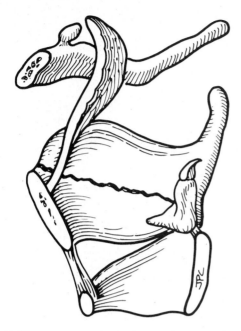

FIG. 11-88   Diagram of a horizontal fracture crossing the thyroid cartilage. These fractures often can involve the petiole and lower epiglottis, causing dislocation of the upper epiglottis.

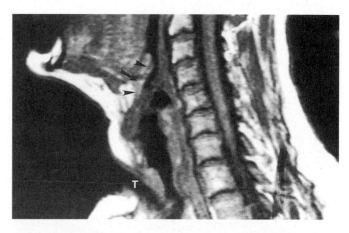

FIG. 11-89   Avulsion of the epiglottic sagittal MR. In this midline scan the area of low signal, representing the epiglottis *(arrowheads),* is not straight but rather bends abruptly in this patient with a fracture avulsion of the epiglottic cartilage. The point of angulation *(arrow)* is thought to represent a site of fracture. *T,* Tracheostomy. (Courtesy Duda JJ Jr, Lewin JS, Eliachar I. MR evaluation of epiglottic avulsion. AJNR (In Press).)

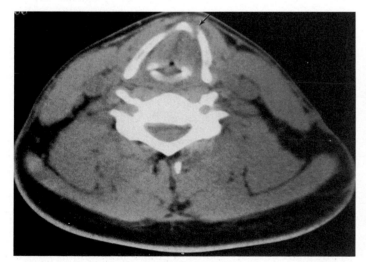

FIG. 11-90   Axial CT longitudinal (vertical fracture of the larynx) scan showing the defect in the ala *(arrow).*

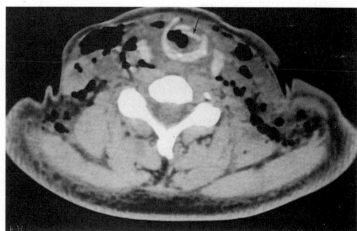

FIG. 11-91   Axial CT shows fracture of the cricoid with posterior positioning of the fragments *(arrow)* into the airway.

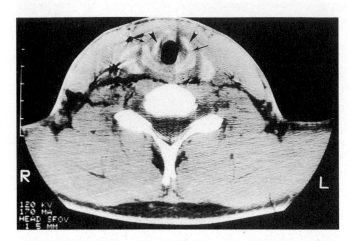

FIG. 11-92   Axial CT shows fracture of the cricoid. The anterior arch of the cricoid has been fractured and pushed posteriorly. Several fragments *(arrowheads)* are noted as the ring collapses inward. The airway is narrowed, but no piece of the cartilage appears to be projected through the mucosa. The position of the fractures is shown in the lateral portion of the arch *(arrows)*.

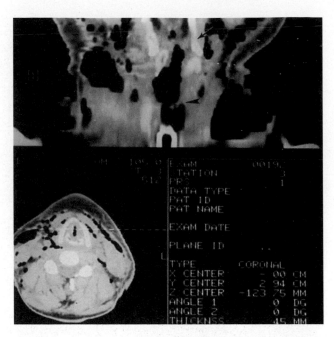

FIG. 11-93   Coronal reformat of a horizontal fracture of the thyroid cartilage *(arrow)* and laryngotracheal partial separation. Note the lack of alignment of the trachea *(arrowhead)*. This finding can be mimicked on reformatted CT slices by movement of the patient during the exam.

Arytenoid dislocation results in an abnormal position of the arytenoid relative to the cricoid cartilage (Fig. 11-94). Often there is an associated fracture of one of the larger laryngeal cartilages, but some dislocations have been reported with fairly minimal trauma to the side of the neck. Minimal dislocations probably can be missed at imaging, but in these cases the radiologist should comment on the position of the arytenoid cartilage relative to the articular tubercle on the upper margin of the cricoid.

A dislocation of the cricothyroid joint is seen as a malalignment of the thyroid and cricoid cartilages (Fig. 11-95). The thyroid cartilage may be rotated to one side, while the cricoid retains a normal orientation. These dislocations usually result from more severe trauma, and usually, cartilage fractures are also present. Before diagnosing a dislocation of the cricothyroid joint, it is important to follow the inferior horn of the thyroid cartilage to its articulation with the cricoid. Even slight obliquity of the scan can cause an apparent widening of the space between these two cartilages, and this effect should not be mistaken for a fracture.

Foreign bodies may be the result of trauma but are more commonly the result of ingestion or aspiration. The pyriform sinus is a common location for a foreign body, and most foreign bodies that enter the larynx do not stay in the larynx, but continue into the trachea or bronchi.

Burn injury of the larynx can result from the inhalation or ingestion of hot material.[40] The supraglottic larynx is most likely to be involved, and generalized edema can occur. Several cases of ingestion of hot foreign substances have been related to "melting" crack cocaine. Small bits of steel wool heated to melt the cocaine can cause a more localized burn in the pyriform sinus or aryepiglottic fold (Fig. 11-96). The imaging findings can mimic tumor, creating diagnostic problems if the pertinent history is withheld.

CONGENITAL LESIONS

Radiology can be helpful in assessing congenital laryngeal anomalies. Plain radiographs or conventional tomography can give an assessment of the size of the airway or the length of a stenosis. CT in the axial plane provides a good cross-sectional view of the airway, allows an estimate of the length of a stenosis to be made, and characterizes the tissues deep to the mucosal surface. Spiral CT can acquire an entire set of images quickly and allows multiplanar reformations to better characterize the length of the abnormality.

Embryology

An outpouching, or bud, initially extends from the primitive pharynx to form the respiratory system. The cells on either side of the entrance to this respiratory diverticulum pinch together to form the tracheoesophageal septum, isolating the trachea from the developing foregut. The cartilages form from the mesenchyme on either side of the primitive respi-

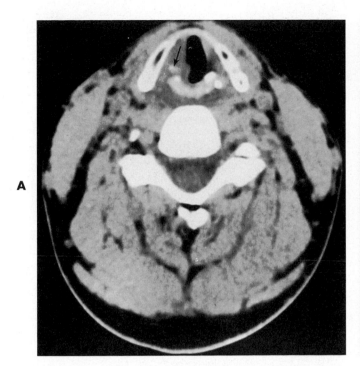

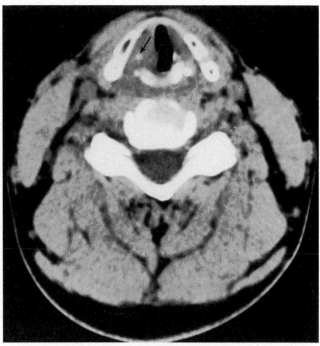

FIG. 11-94 Axial CT scans. **A,** Arytenoid dislocation shows the arytenoid anteriorly displaced *(arrow)*. **B,** Slightly lower scan again shows the abnormal position of the arytenoid *(arrow)*.

ratory passage, and the components from each side fuse to form the cricoid and thyroid cartilages. Congenital abnormalities are related to problems of the development process or simply delays in normal maturation.[41-43]

Laryngomalacia

Laryngomalacia represents delayed development of the laryngeal support system.[44] The structures are present but are not firm enough to keep the larynx open. The supraglottic larynx is affected, and the epiglottis may be floppy, or the entire supraglottic larynx may collapse. The infant outgrows the abnormality as the cartilages mature; however, a tracheostomy may be needed to maintain an airway until this laryngeal maturation is completed.

Subglottic Stenosis

Subglottic stenosis is a narrowing of the subglottic larynx, from the true cord down to the lower cricoid.[44-46] The patient normally outgrows this soft-tissue stenosis, but a tracheostomy may be needed before this maturation is completed. Plain radiographs can demonstrate the narrowing.

Less commonly, a rare cricoid abnormality can occur in which the cricoid shape is elliptical rather than round. This elongated shape narrows the airway.[46] No radiologic cases of the abnormality have been described; however, because the cricoid is not calcified at this age, imaging is unlikely to be helpful. Because of the hard consistency of the subglottic wall, the diagnosis is suggested by endoscopy.

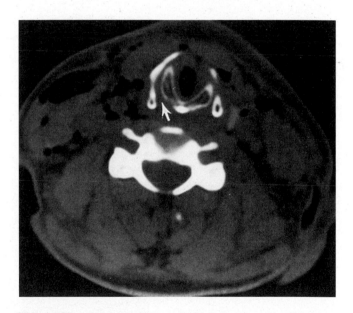

FIG. 11-95 Axial CT shows cricothyroid separation. The cricoid is rotated relative to the thyroid with widening of the space *(arrow)* between the lower thyroid and the cricoid. Compare with the opposite side.

Webs and Atresia

Small webs can be seen at any level of the larynx, but they are usually at the level of the true cords.[44] Subglottic webs may be associated with cricoid abnormalities. Webs are seldom evaluated radiographically, but radiographs may be done to exclude other abnormalities. Atresia of the larynx is

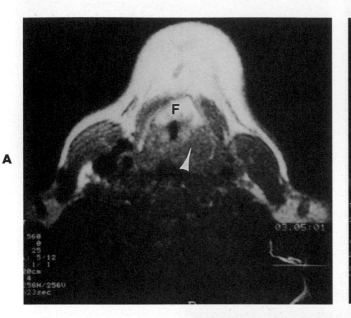
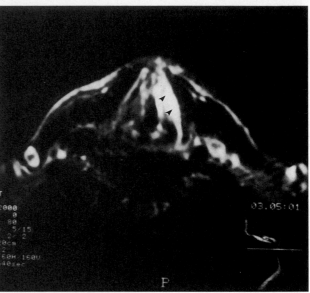
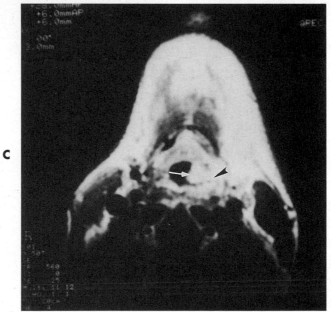

FIG. 11-96   Crack cocaine burn of the larynx. **A,** Axial T1W image shows abnormal tissue in the supraglottic larynx *(arrowhead).* This was relatively bright on the T2W images (not shown). *F,* Normal preepiglottic fat. **B,** T2W image at the level of the cord shows the abnormal signal *(arrowheads)* extending along the paraglottic space into the lateral edge of the true cord mimicing paraglottic extension of tumor. This was edema extending from the burn. **C,** Postgadolinium shows enhancement of the aryepiglottic fold *(arrow)* and the wall of the upper pyriform sinus *(arrowhead).* (From Snyderman C, Weissman JL, Tabor E, et al. Crack cocaine burns of the larynx. Arch Otolaryngol Head Neck Surg 1991; 17(7):792-795.)

a failure of complete recanalization, and no airway exists through the larynx (Fig. 11-97). The trachea, however, is present, and a tracheostomy at birth is life-saving.

There have been reports of laryngeal or tracheal atresia diagnosed prenatally using ultrasound.[47,48] Fluids are secreted into the lungs and cannot pass out of the bronchial tree unless there is a coexisting tracheoesophageal communication. Without such a communication, the bronchial tree enlarges and the lungs become distended with fluid. The enlarged lungs are echogenic because of the small fluid-filled spaces present. A tracheostomy done at birth is crucial

if there is to be any hope of survival; however, in most instances the anomaly is fatal.

Clefts

Laryngotracheal clefts are exceedingly rare and are presumed to be the result of failure of complete fusion of the tracheoesophageal septum as it grows to separate the trachea from the esophagus.[44,49,50] The cricoid cartilage, which results from a fusion of cells from the mesenchyma on either side of the airway, may also be affected. Although an isolated cleft of the larynx does occasionally occur, frequently

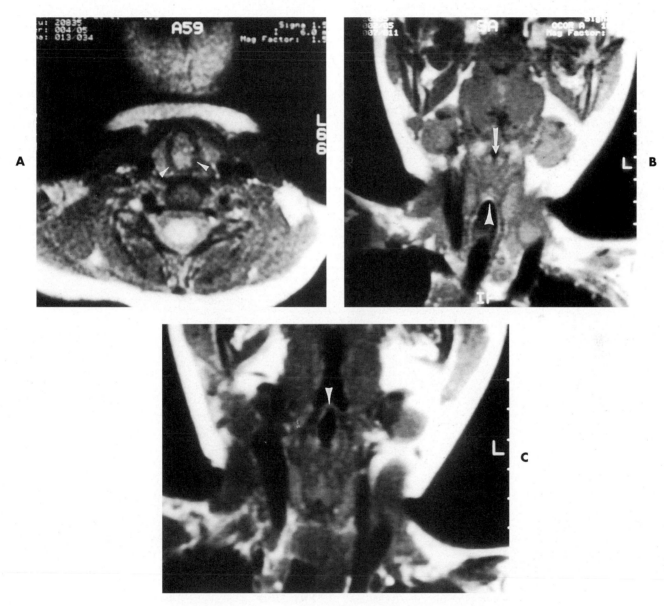

FIG. 11-97   Congenital atresia of the larynx. Patient was born with a complete atresia of the larynx. Emergency tracheostomy done at birth. **A,** Proton-density image suggests that the cricoid *(arrowheads)* is intact. **B,** Coronal T1W image shows that the airway *(arrowhead)* extends up to the subglottic area. Some air *(arrow)* is seen in the vestibule of the larynx. It is impossible to be definite regarding the length of the stenosis without distention of the vestibule of the larynx. **C,** Coronal T1W image shows the epiglottis *(arrowhead)*.

a laryngeal cleft is associated with a tracheal cleft. The child aspirates and may have multiple pneumonias (Fig. 11-98).[51]

Subglottic Hemangiomas

Subglottic hemangiomas were mentioned in the preceding section on benign tumors, but they are included here because they are as much vascular malformations as they are tumors. The lesion usually can be seen as a subglottic narrowing on a lateral neck radiograph. Therapy is conservative, but tracheostomy may be necessary.

Other Anomalies

Other rare anomalies such as a bifid epiglottis or duplication anomalies have been reported.

STENOSIS

Stenosis of the larynx or upper trachea can be either a congenital anomaly, a sequela of trauma, or the result of therapy. The most common stenosis results from prolonged intubation (Figs. 11-99, 11-100). The position of the stenosis secondary to such prolonged intubation or a tracheostomy is characteristic, but stenosis secondary to trauma is more vari-

able. Ingestion of corrosive materials usually causes strictures of the posterior supraglottic larynx. Plain films or conventional tomograms are still good methods for assessing the length of the stenosis or the extent of a "granuloma" (Fig. 11-101). Two projections are used, usually frontal and lateral. Alternatively, spiral CT can be used.

CT in the axial plane offers a cross section of the airway, and this allows characterization of the stenosis. Soft-tissue scars and granulomas can significantly compromise the airway without any change in the cartilage, or the cartilage can collapse and be displaced into the airway, creating a "hard" stenosis (Figs. 11-102, 11-103). This has obvious implications in planning therapy. If the cartilage is not involved, simply lysing of the soft tissues may be adequate therapy. However, if the cartilage itself is impinging on the airway, a more extensive reconstruction will be necessary. Although these problems primarily relate to the trachea rather than the larynx, a traumatically displaced fragment of the anterior cricoid can cause significant narrowing of the subglottic area.

Conventional CT has been limited to the axial plane. However, spiral CT by very rapidly scanning the neck provides excellent-quality reformatted images. A reformatted image can be chosen in the coronal plane, or it can be

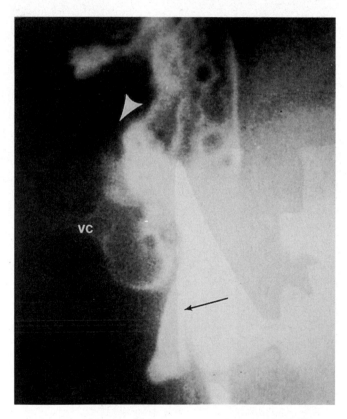

FIG. 11-98 Laryngeal cleft at the level of the cricoid. Barium swallow. Contrast is seen entering the lumen of the trachea via a defect on the posterior wall *(arrow)* at the level of the cricoid. *VC,* Vocal cord level. Normal entrance to the larynx *(arrowhead).* (From Ravich WJ, Donner MW, Kashima H, et al. The swallowing center, concepts and procedures. Gastrointest Radiol July 1985; 10(3):255-261.)

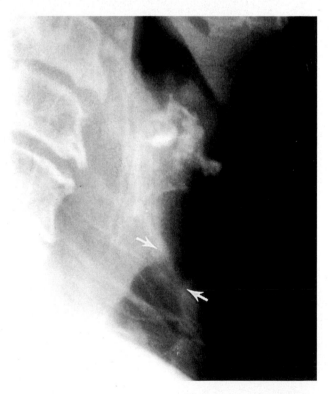

FIG. 11-99 Lateral plain film of tracheal stenosis characteristic of tracheostomy site *(arrows).*

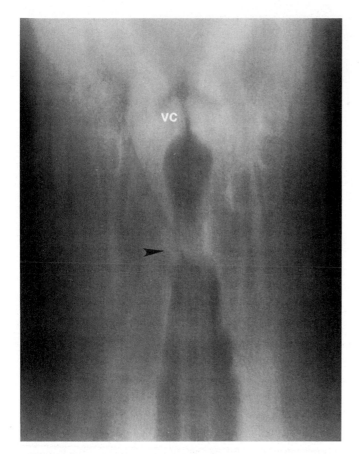

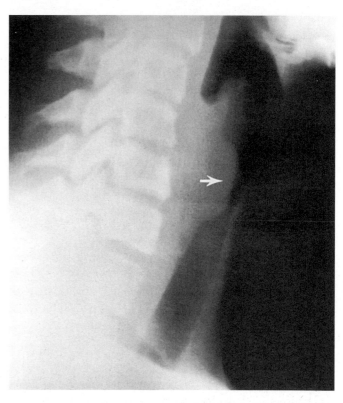

FIG. 11-100   Coronal tomogram showing a narrowing of the tracheal lumen *(arrowhead)* just below the cricoid. *VC,* Vocal cord. A narrowing resulting from prolonged intubation would be lower in position.

FIG. 11-101   Lateral plain film shows granuloma of the posterior wall of the upper trachea *(arrow).*

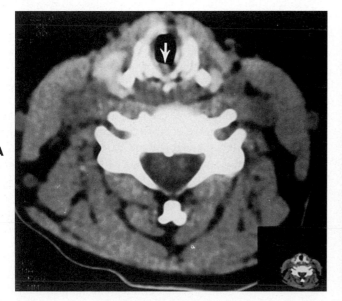

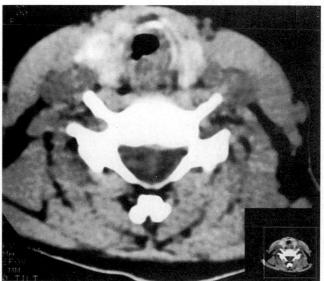

FIG. 11-102   A, Axial CT shows slight soft-tissue thickening *(arrow)* within the cricoid cartilage. **B,** Slightly lower scan gives good estimation of the size of the airway and the thickening within the tracheal ring. The actual distance between the lumen and the cartilage can be defined.

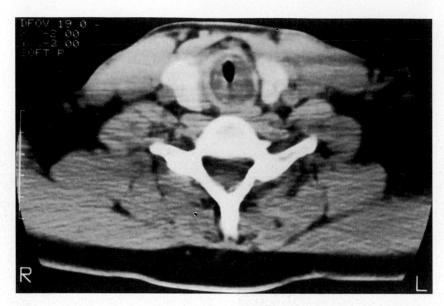

FIG. 11-103   Axial CT of severe narrowing of the trachea by granulation tissue at the level of the thyroid shows an intact ring with soft tissue filling the space between the ring and the airway. No portion of the tracheal ring has been pushed into the lumen.

slightly obliqued to pass exactly through the airway. Thus the vertical exent of a stenosis can be defined at the same time that the character of the wall is examined. MR can also provide good multiplanar images, but it docs not show the calcified cartilages as well as CT. However, MR has proven useful in the examination of lower tracheal narrowing and in the evaluation of various vascular rings.

VOCAL CORD PARALYSIS

Vocal cord paralysis can be categorized as either a superior laryngeal nerve deficit, a recurrent laryngeal nerve deficit, or a total vagal nerve deficit.

Superior Nerve

The only muscle innervated by the superior laryngeal nerve is the cricothyroid muscle, which extends between the cricoid and thyroid cartilages. Contraction of the normal muscles pulls the anterior cricoid ring up toward the lower margin of the thyroid cartilage. This rotates the upper cricoid lamina, and thus the arytenoid, posteriorly, putting tension on the true vocal cords. Contraction of one muscle rotates the posterior cricoid to the contralateral, paralyzed side. At laryngoscopy, the posterior larynx (arytenoid) is deviated toward the side of the nerve abnormality.

With this history, the radiologist should examine the neck for a lesion along the course of the vagus nerve (X), which passes through the pars nervosa of the jugular foramen and follows the carotid artery to the level of the larynx. The imaging findings in the larynx itself are usually normal.

Recurrent Nerve

More commonly, one encounters a paralysis of the recurrent laryngeal nerve.[52] All of the laryngeal muscles other than the cricothyroid are innervated by this nerve. The classic findings of recurrent laryngeal palsy can be identified on plain films, tomography, and CT (Figs. 11-104 to 11-106).

Most of the findings are secondary to atrophy of the thyroarytenoid muscle. As the muscle atrophies, the cord becomes thinner and more pointed, with loss of the subglottic arch. As the muscle diminishes in size, the ventricle enlarges. The pyriform sinus also enlarges on the ipsilateral side. The changes in the shape of the cord are best appreciated by tomography. Different maneuvers show the lack of motion of the paralyzed cord and normal motion of the contralateral side.

CT shows the enlarged ventricle as a large air-filled structure, which may extend almost to the thyroid cartilage. The arytenoid may be seen in a more anteromedial position than normal, and soft-tissue fullness paralleling the vocal cord may be seen in the immediate subglottic region, reflecting the loss of muscle tone and the flattening of the subglottic arch. There also may be mild dilatation of the ipsilateral pyriform sinus and vallecula.

When studying an abnormality of the recurrent laryngeal nerve, the radiologist must examine the pathway of the vagus and recurrent laryngeal nerves. The vagus nerve exits the skull base in the jugular foramen and then runs in the posterolateral portion of the carotid sheath. On the left side the recurrent nerve leaves the sheath and passes anterior to the arotic arch, curving under the arch, and then ascending

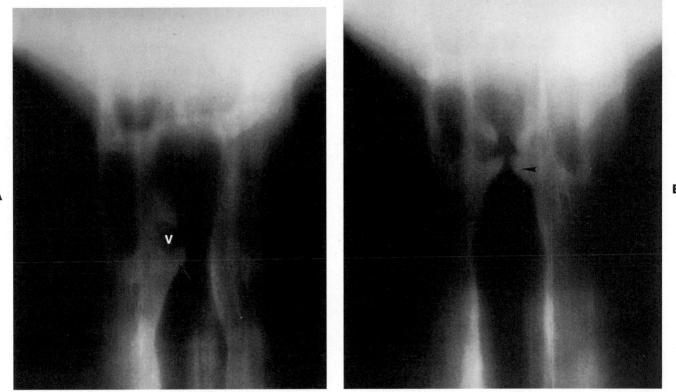

FIG. 11-104   A, Coronal tomogram. Right cord paralysis, inspiration. The true cord on the affected side remains in the paramedian position and is more pointed than usual *(arrow).* The ventricle *(V)* is enlarged. **B,** Phonation. There is no change in the affected cord or ventricle. The normal cord now moves to midline *(arrowhead).* Compare the size of the ventricle on the paralysed side with that on the opposite side.

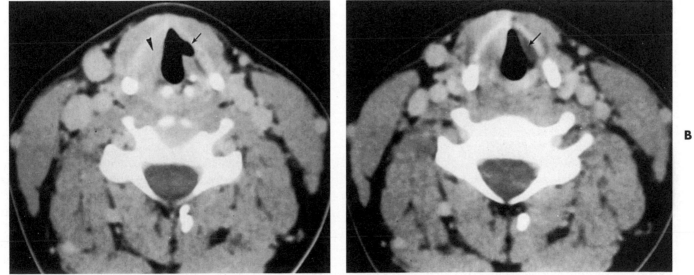

FIG. 11-105   Vocal cord paralysis. **A,** Level of the cord shows dilated ventricle *(arrow).* Thyroarytenoid muscle on the opposite side *(arrowhead)* is of the normal size. **B,** Inferior scan again shows decreased size of the thyroarytenoid muscle with decreased density *(arrow)* compared with the opposite side.

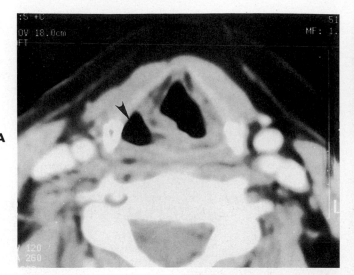
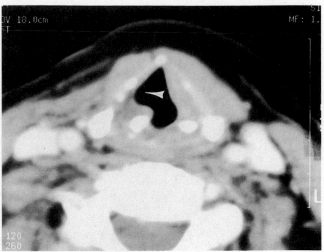
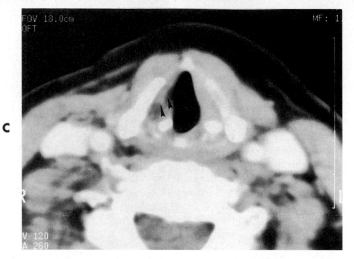

FIG. 11-106 Vocal cord paralysis. **A,** Scan through the supraglottic larynx shows dilated pyriform sinus *(arrowhead).* **B,** Slightly more inferior scan shows enlarged ventricle *(arrowhead).* **C,** Lower scan shows fatty infiltration *(arrowheads)* of the thyroarytenoid muscle. Compare with the normal muscular density on the opposite side.

in the tracheoesophageal groove to enter the larynx near the cricothyroid junction. On the right side the nerve curves around the right subclavian artery, passing anteriorly and under it, to then ascend in the tracheoesophageal groove to the larynx.

Adductor Paralysis

Rare cases of adductor paralysis have been described. This paralysis affects the muscles that bring the cords together but spares the posterior cricoarytenoid muscle. This muscle stretches from the posterior surface of the cricoid to the lateral aspect of the muscular process of the arytenoid. It is the only muscle that rotates the cord outward. Because the posterior cricoarytenoid muscle is unopposed, the cord remains in a lateral position (Fig. 11-107). The lesion must affect only certain fibers of the recurrent laryngeal nerve while sparing others. The cause of this abnormality is poorly understood, although an intracranial etiology has been postulated.[53]

MISCELLANEOUS

Amyloid can affect the larynx and produce nodules or small deposits deep to the mucosal surface.[54] The findings on CT may be mistaken for a tumor (Fig. 11-108).

Diverticula of the pharynx are herniations of mucosa through dehiscences in the muscular constrictors. These have been noted in patients who play wind instruments. Most are just above or below the hyoid bone, extending from the valleculae to the upper pyriform sinus (Figs. 11-109, 11-110). The diverticula are usually incidental findings on barium swallow examinations.

A Zenker's diverticulum is an outpouching of pharyngeal mucosa through the inferior constrictor muscles. Most of the diverticula herniate through Killian's dehiscence, which is the weak area in the pharyngeal wall located in the gap between the uppermost cricopharyngeus and the inferiormost oblique fibers of the inferior pharyngeal constrictors. Although the actual dehiscence or entrance to the diverticu-

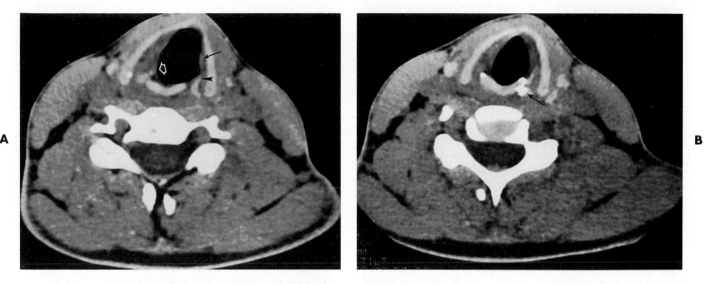

FIG. 11-107   Axial CT scans. **A,** Adductor paralysis. Left side shows almost no thyroarytenoid muscle *(arrow)*. The vocal process *(arrowhead)* is pulled laterally as the posterior cricoarytenoid muscle rotates the arytenoid laterally and posteriorly. Compare the position of the vocal process on the normal side *(open arrow)*. **B,** Slightly lower scan shows a portion of the arytenoid pulled posteriorly and downward *(arrow)* overlapping the posterior surface of the cricoid.

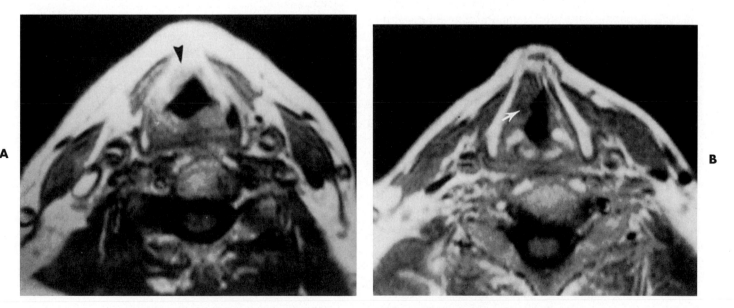

FIG. 11-108   **A,** Submucosal amyloid. Axial scan through the supraglottis shows thickening of the lateral epiglottis with soft tissue extending minimally *(arrowhead)* into the preepiglottic fat (.35 Tesla). **B,** Minor thickening of the true cord *(arrow)*. (**A** courtesy Dr. William Hanafee.)

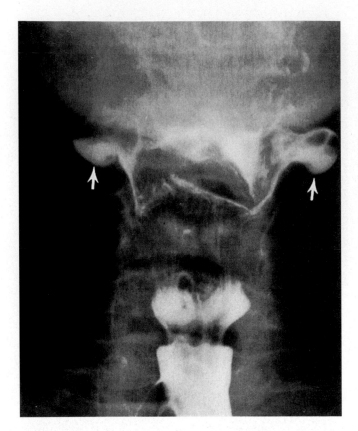

FIG. 11-109   Barium swallow, pharyngeal diverticula. There is a small outpouching extending through the pharyngeal wall.

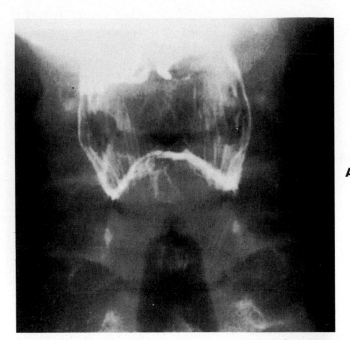

A

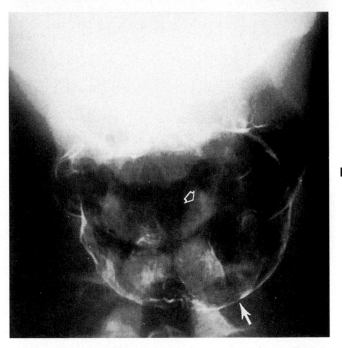

B

FIG. 11-110   Barium swallow, ballooning of the pharynx in a trumpet player. **A,** At rest the striated appearance of the pharynx is due to redundancy of the mucosa. **B,** On Valsalva there is gross distention of the pharynx with bilateral ballooning. Lower margin of the pyriform *(arrow). Open arrow,* AE fold.

lum is in the midline, the diverticulum usually protrudes to the left side. The neck or the anterior wall of the diverticulum is well appreciated on a barium swallow, using oblique, frontal, and lateral projections (Fig. 11-111). Although a Zenker's diverticulum can occasionally be seen on CT (Fig. 11-112), it is easier to diagnose on a barium swallow.

A second weak point in the wall of the pharygoesophageal junction occurs laterally between the cricopharyngeus and esophageal musculature, through the so-called Killian-Jamieson area at the margin of the cricoid. Such herniations have been reported but are rare.

When there is a Zenker's diverticulum, the cricopharyngeus is usually prominent. The cricopharyngeus may also be prominent without a diverticulum (Fig. 11-113). Failure of the muscle to relax during swallowing can cause dysphagia. Occasionally a small collection of barium can be seen just above this muscle after the barium column has passed. This residual contrast is thought by some to represent a "primordial Zenker's diverticulum." However, this theory may not be correct because few of these cases go on to develop classical Zenker's diverticulum.

Failure of relaxation of the cricopharyngeus has been associated with gastric reflux and other abnormal motility problems in the esophagus, as well as with neurologic conditions affecting the medulla.

Benign Cartilage Changes

Cartilage is a changeable tissue and can be remodeled by pressure or eroded by malignancy. Pressure, capable of causing such remodelling, can be the result of prominent osteophytes of the spine, benign tumors, or rarely an enlarged thyroid gland (Figs. 11-114, 11-115).

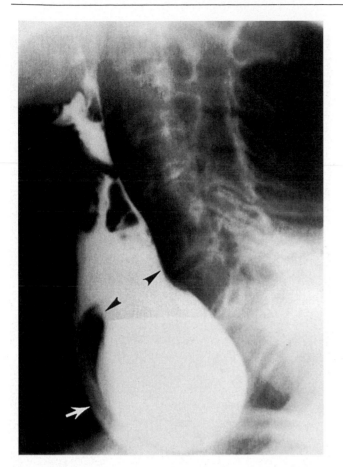

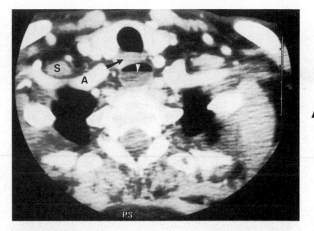

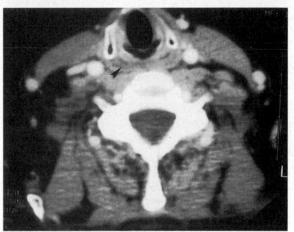

FIG. 11-111   Zenker's diverticulum, Lateral film shows a large diverticulum with a wide entrance *(arrowheads)* and the barium column of the true esophagus continuing anterior to the diverticulum *(arrow)*. The level of the persistent cricopharyngeus is at the level of the anterior arrowhead. This diverticulum was somewhat unusual because of its midline rather than its left-sided position.

FIG. 11-112   Zenker's diverticulum, Axial CT scans. **A,** An air-fluid level *(arrowhead)* is seen within the diverticulum. The actual esophagus *(arrow)* is seen just anteriorly. *A,* Subclavian artery; *S,* anterior scalene. **B,** More superior scan shows the intact pharyngeal wall *(arrowhead)* at the level close to the cricopharyngeus muscle. The abnormality (not shown) actually extends through the various fibers of the muscle.

Occasionally an ala of the thyroid cartilage can bow medially. As described earlier, this may be the result of old trauma. However, many times there is no history of any trauma to explain the finding. The abnormal shape may cause a bulge in the wall of the larynx that endoscopically mimics a submucosal mass. On CT or MRI the lack of obliteration of the paraglottic fat excludes the possibility of tumor (Fig. 11-116).

Osteophytes of the Spine

Large osteophytes arising from the anterior cervical spine can occasionally cause dysphagia.[55] These osteophytes can cause a significant mass effect on the posterior pharyngeal wall or even rarely interfere with the normal movement of the larynx during swallowing. Most often, such osteophytes are seen and the patient has no symptoms related to the area. However, if there is any cause of limitation of laryngeal movement (prior surgery, irradiation, tumor infiltration, neurologic deficit), these osteophytes can become symptomatic,

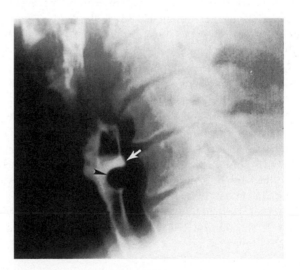

FIG. 11-113   Lateral barium swallow, slightly prominent persistent cricopharyngeus *(arrowhead)*. There is a small collection of barium *(arrow)* just above the muscle band. This is sometimes referred to as a primordial Zenker's.

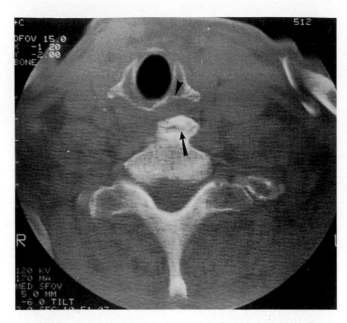

FIG. 11-114 Axial CT, osteophyte *(arrow)* causing erosion *(arrowhead)* of the cricoid.

presumably refecting the combined effects of the limited laryngeal movement and the posterior retropharyngeal mass.

Carotid Position

Frequently the carotid artery deviates medially between the pharynx and spine (Fig. 11-117). Although not likely to cause symptoms, the unusual position should be mentioned, especially in patients for whom surgery is contemplated.

Postsurgical Changes

The appearance of the neck after surgery varies, depending on the procedure performed. However, there are certain general postoperative appearances in the larynx and neck. Radiation changes are also fairly characteristic.

After a total laryngectomy, the normal laryngeal landmarks are no longer present. But, as the fascial layers are disrupted during the surgery, the gullet, or pharyngoesophageal remnant, may migrate anteriorly and should not be mistaken for an airway. The esophagus may actually protrude between the lobes of the thyroid gland, mimicking the trachea (Fig. 11-118). The tracheostomy is usually seen just above the sternal notch, thus identifying the actual airway.

A radical neck dissection removes the sternocleidomastoid muscle and jugular vein, as well as the surrounding nodes.[56] The thyroid gland may assume a rounder shape because of the disruption of the bordering fascial layers, and because the thyroid no longer has a characteristic shape, the appearance may also mimic a tumor recurrence. The gland may also mimic a blood vessel because of the intrinsic high iodine content of the normally functioning thyroid tissue.

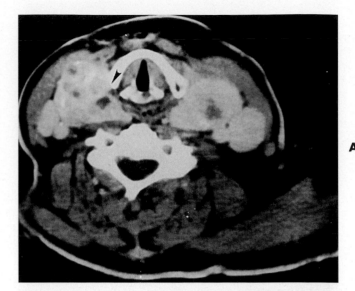

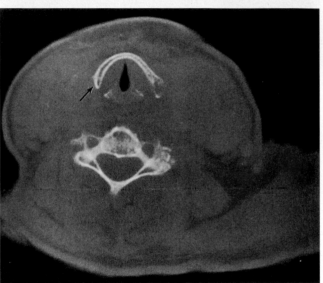

FIG. 11-115 Axial CT scans. **A,** Large multinodular goiter–causing shortening and remodeling of the lateral aspect of the thyroid ala *(arrowhead)*. **B,** Bone algorithm showing the intact cortical line of the remodeled cartilage *(arrow)*.

The various modifications of neck dissections are described in Chapter 22.

The normal laryngeal structures are obviously missing on a barium swallow done after total laryngectomy.[57] At surgical closure, the mucosa is pulled together, often causing a ridge to form just posterior to the tongue base. This ridge can occasionally mimic an epiglottis (Fig. 11-119). This is also the area where most postoperative fistulas occur.

Often, a contrast swallow is performed 7 to 10 days after laryngectomy, before the patient is allowed to eat. Barium can be used, but if a fistula into the soft tissues is present, the residual barium can interfere with follow-up studies. If

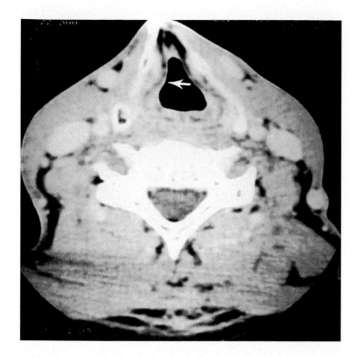

FIG. 11-116 Axial CT, asymmetrical shape of the thyroid causing a slight bulge in the supraglottic larynx *(arrow),* which could be confused with a submucosal tumor.

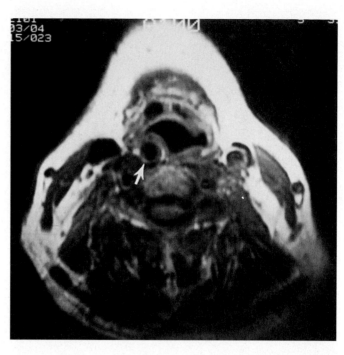

FIG. 11-117 Axial T1W MR shows a tortuous carotid artery *(arrow)* causing a submucosal "mass" of the pharyngeal wall at the level of the epiglottis.

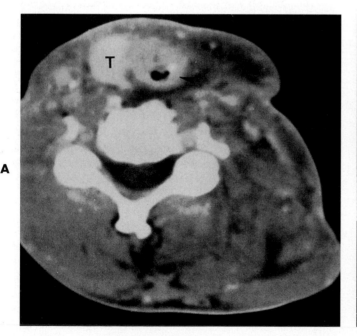

A

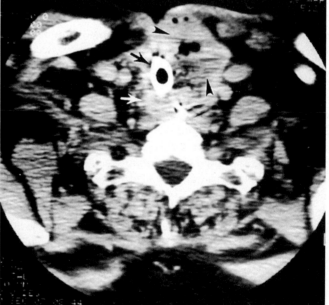

B

FIG. 11-118 Axial CT scans. **A,** Postoperative laryngectomy and bilateral radical neck dissection. The esophagus has migrated anteriorly *(arrowhead)* to lie in the usual position of the trachea next to the thyroid gland *(T).* The sternocleidomastoid and jugular veins have been removed. **B,** Lower scan. The tracheostomy tube is seen documenting the position of the airway *(black arrow).* The esophagus is seen immediately posteriorly *(white arrow).* Note the large stomal recurrence *(arrowheads).*

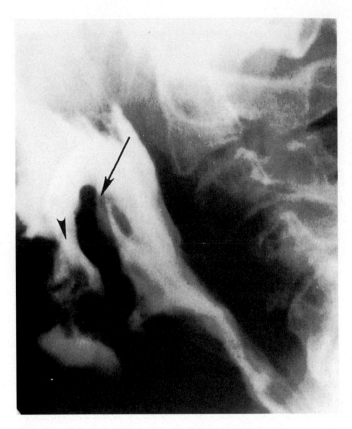

FIG. 11-119 Lateral barium swallow, post laryngectomy with fistula *(arrowhead)* extending to a collection in the soft tissues anteriorly. Note the "pseudoepiglottis" *(arrow)* caused by the drawing up of mucosal folds at the closure.

there is no concern that a fistula passes directly into the trachea, meglumine diatrizoate (Gastrografin) can be used with careful fluoroscopic control to exclude any communication with the airway. If significant aspiration occurs, the hypertonic Gastrografin can cause pulmonary edema. Care must be taken even if there is a sinus tract to the skin, because Gastrografin can tract along the surgical dressing and then go into the tracheal stoma. Before choosing a contrast material, the radiologist should determine whether the surgeon has purposely created a fistula or placed a valve between the trachea and esophagus. If a valve has been placed, a small amount of contrast material may pass into the trachea, and Gastrografin should not be used. Propyliodone (Dionosil) can also be used in questionable cases when connections between the trachea and esophagus are suspected.

In a supraglottic laryngectomy, all of the normal laryngeal structures above the true vocal cords are removed. The hyoid may or may not be included in the resection. A CT scan through the true cords usually appears relatively normal, and the arytenoids usually remain (in rare cases one arytenoid may be removed) (Figs. 11-120, 11-121). Although a large portion of the thyroid cartilage is removed, at the level of the cord the cartilage should look normal.

After a supraglottic laryngectomy, in the early postoperative period, some aspiration is almost always present. Because of this, if a contrast swallow is done, Gastrografin

should not be used. A barium swallow shows absence of the epiglottis and supraglottic structures, and usually some barium coats the vocal cords. A follow-up examination should be done after the patient has been trained in the various maneuvers used to help prevent aspiration.

Vertical hemilaryngectomy removes the true and false cords on one side of the larynx. The vertical hemilaryngectomy may also be extended to take the anterior portion of the opposite cord. The soft tissue on the resected side of the larynx may be flat, or a soft-tissue fullness may be present near the level of the true cord, representing either an attempted reconstruction of the cord (Figs. 11-122, 11-123) or a reaction of operated side's mucosa to the trauma resulting from the functioning contralateral cord hitting against it. In some cases a strap muscle (sternohyoid) may be passed across the larynx and attached to the arytenoid, thus providing bulk against which the opposite cord can appose. In this instance the muscle outside the larynx is abnormal, and excess tissue is present at the level of the cord on the resected side.

The amount of thyroid cartilage resected depends on the extent of the lesion. The resection always extends to midline and often extends a variable distance along the opposite side. The outer perichondrium is left intact, and some regeneration of the thyroid ala often occurs. One arytenoid may be removed if the tumor reaches the vocal process. The cricoid usually remains intact, although some surgeons remove the upper portion of this cartilage if the tumor margin warrants such a resection.

The variability of the postoperative appearance is greater with the vertical hemilaryngectomy than it is with the supraglottic partial laryngectomy. Still, some imaging comments can be made regarding the possibility of deep recurrence, especially if a baseline scan is available.

Reconstruction of a pharyngeal defect can be done by a primary closure of the remaining soft tissues, a jejunal interposition, or various flaps (e.g., the deltopectoral flap). On imaging the jejunal interposition can have a tortuous appearance through the neck, but usually it is in the midline.[58] A flap reconstruction alters the imaging appearance on the side of the neck.[56] This topic is discussed in Chapter 21.

Radiation Changes

Radiation is used to treat many laryngeal lesions, either as isolated therapy or in conjunction with surgery. If laryngeal irradiation has been given, the resulting mucosal changes can confuse the postoperative imaging assessment of possible tumor recurrence.[59,60]

Relatively low doses of radiation can cause mucositis and throat pain. Higher doses result in deeper edema and fibrosis and can be associated with perichondritis and chondronecrosis. Almost all patients receiving 60 Gy to 65 Gy will have definable changes in the soft tissues of the larynx. Clinically the epiglottis thickens and the arytenoids swell, often before the course of radiation is complete. Although gradual improvement is probable, some degree of change persists because of fibrosis and damage to the microvasculature.[61]

Text continued on p. 705

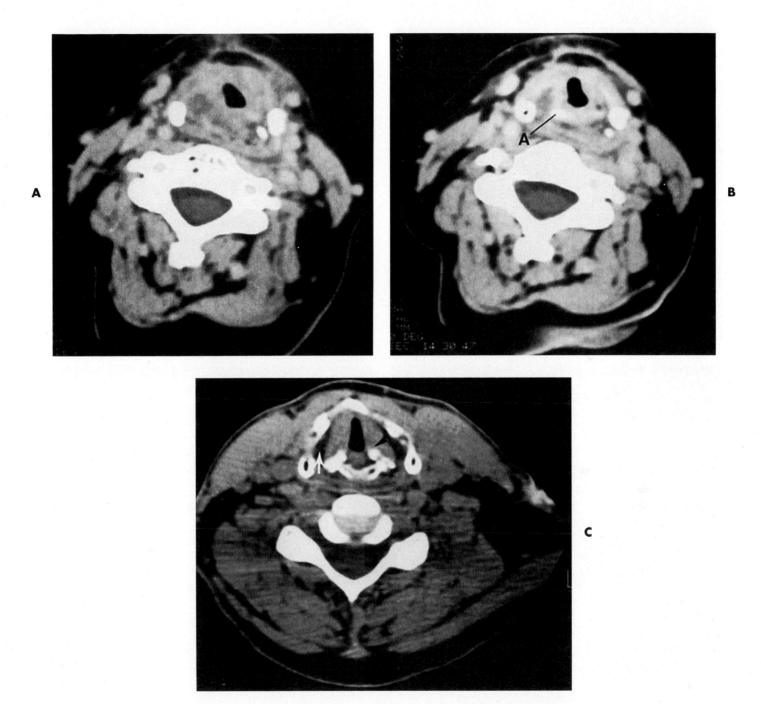

FIG. 11-120 Supraglottic laryngectomy, axial CT scans. **A,** Supraglottic level. There is no evidence of epiglottis or paraglottic space. **B,** At the level of the upper arytenoid *(A)* most of the thyroid cartilage has been resected. **C,** At the level of the true cord the thyroid cartilage is present. There is actually prominence of the paraglottic fat *(arrow)* at the lateral margin of the thyroarytenoid muscle. *Arrowhead,* Vocal process.

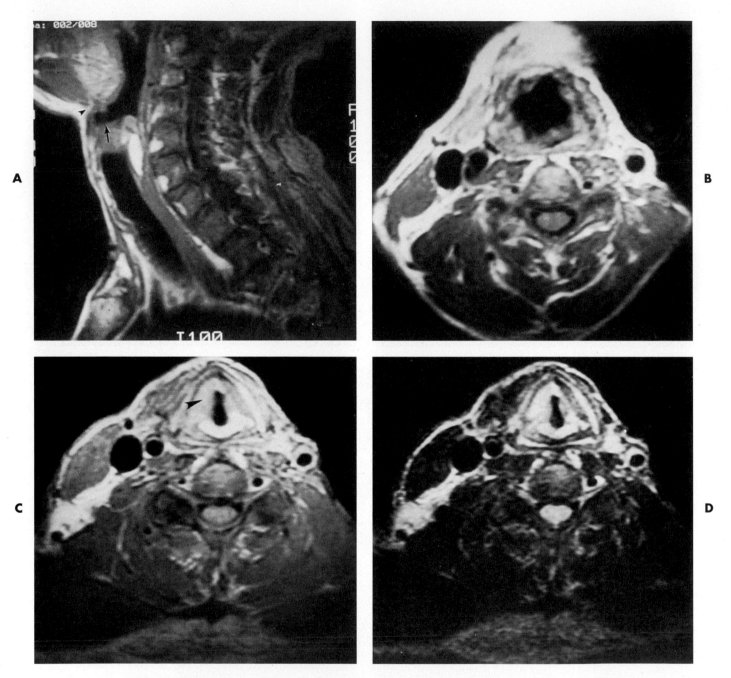

FIG. 11-121   MRI of supraglottic laryngectomy with recurrence at the cord level. **A,** Sagittal T1W image shows the absence of supraglottic structures including the epiglottis. The upper margin of the larynx has taken on a rather square appearance *(arrow)*. The larynx has been sutured to the base of the tongue and mylohyoid *(arrowhead)*. **B,** Axial T1W scan, supraglottic level, shows the irregular appearance of the supraglottic defect above the cord. **C,** Scan shows thickening of the involved cord *(arrowhead)*. **D,** T2W scan shows brightening of the involved cord. This could be from tumor or from edema. In this case it represented recurrence.

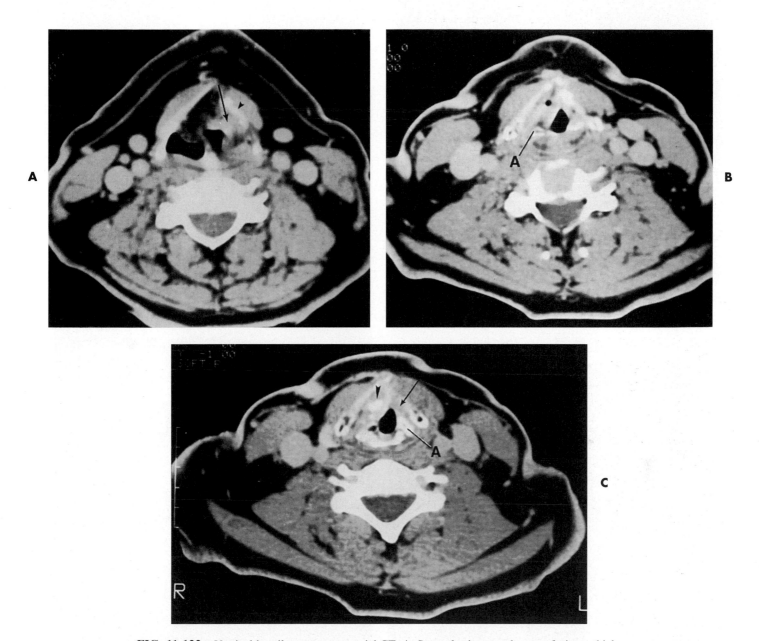

FIG. 11-122   Vertical hemilaryngectomy, axial CT. **A,** Supraglottic scan shows soft-tissue thickening of the supraglottic fat *(arrow)* caused by the resection. The thyroid ala *(arrowhead)* has partially regenerated from the residual perichondrium. **B,** Lower scan through the upper arytenoid *(A)* again shows the loss of tissue on the affected side. **C,** Scan through the level of the true cord shows loss of tissue *(arrow)*. The arytenoid *(A)* has been retained. Teflon has been injected into the normal cord *(arrowhead)* to add bulk, bringing the cord across midline.

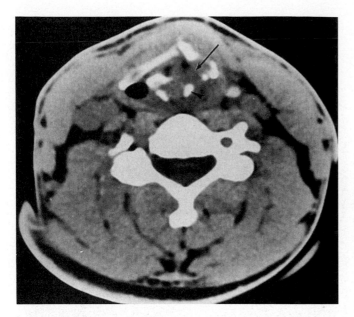

FIG. 11-123 Axial CT, vertical hemilaryngectomy shows loss of soft tissue on the left side of the larynx *(arrow)*. The arytenoid has been removed. The small calcification is the upper margin of the cricoid *(arrowhead)*. Note the irregularity of the resected thyroid cartilage with partial calcification from the retained perichondrium.

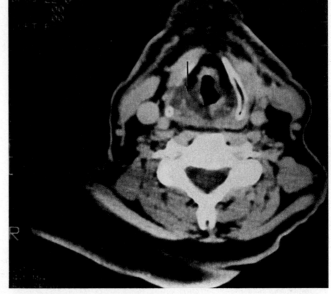

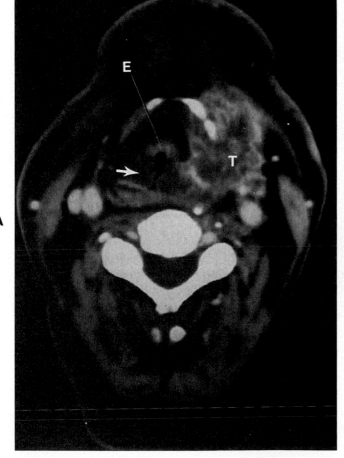

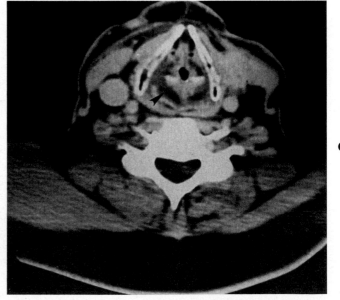

FIG. 11-124 **A,** CT of postradiation tumor recurrence *(T)*. Note the swelling of the aryepiglottic fold *(arrow)* and apparent thickening of the epiglottic cartilage *(E)*. **B,** Lower scan shows increased streaky density and thickening of the wall of the pyriform *(arrow)*. Note also the streaky lymphedema ("dirty fat") in the fat anterior to the larynx. **C,** Scan through the upper arytenoid shows continued swelling in the soft tissues *(arrowhead)* posterior to the arytenoid.

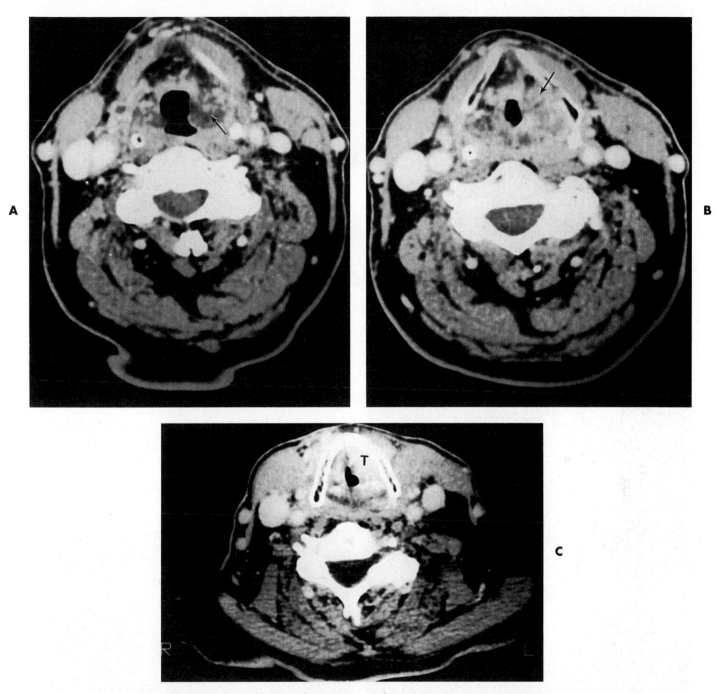

FIG. 11-125 Axial CT, postradiation recurrent lesion of the true cord. **A,** Supraglottic scan shows spotty densities throughout the preepiglottic fat and thickening of the aryepiglottic fold *(arrow).* **B,** Slightly lower level again shows "spotty" densities throughout the paraglottic fat *(arrow)* representing postradiation change. **C,** Lower scan shows tumor *(T)* at the level of the ventricle.

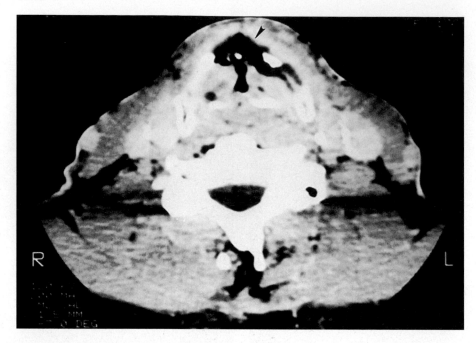

FIG. 11-126   Necrosis and perichondritis of the thyroid cartilage postradiation. Axial CT scan shows necrosis of the anterior thyroid cartilage *(arrowhead)* with gas in the soft tissue.

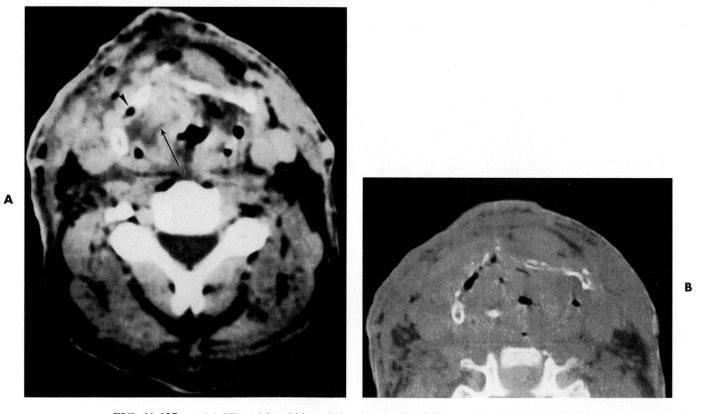

FIG. 11-127   Axial CT, perichondritis and chondronecrosis of the thyroid cartilage postradiation therapy. **A,** Significant soft-tissue swelling of the wall of the larynx *(arrow)*. There are gas bubbles within the thyroid cartilage *(arrowhead)*. **B,** Bone algorithm shows partial collapse of the thyroid cartilage because of demineralization and chondronecrosis.

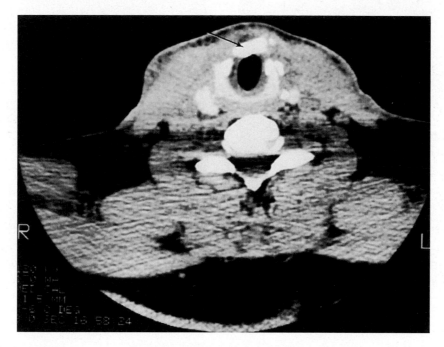

FIG. 11-128   Axial CT, cartilaginous graft *(arrow)* placed in the anterior arch of the cricoid to support and maintain the lumen of the airway.

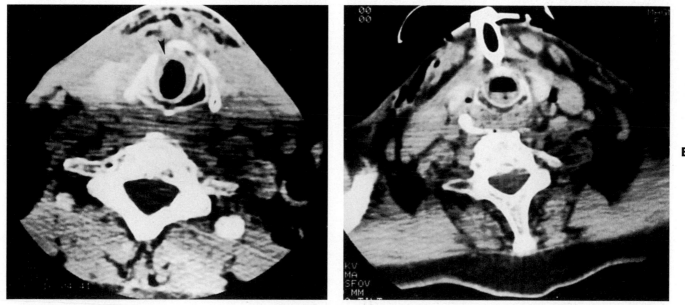

FIG. 11-129   **A,** Tracheostomy tube. Axial CT scan through the cricoid shows swelling in the subglottic region *(arrowhead)* caused by recent tracheostomy placement. This can mimic tumor. **B,** Scan through the cricoid shows the extratracheal portion of the tracheostomy tube and an air-fluid level in the trachea.

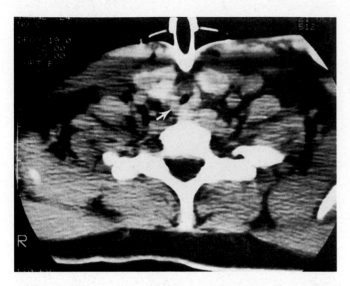

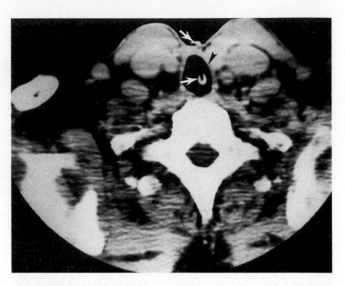

FIG. 11-130   Axial CT scan through the lower neck and tracheostomy tube. The air-filled structure represents the esophagus *(arrow)* in this patient post laryngectomy. The airway and actual trachea would not be found until a more inferior scan.

FIG. 11-131   Axial CT, Blom-Singer valve used to pass air from the tracheostomy site into the esophagus. The tube *(arrows)* is too small to be a tracheostomy tube. The apparent airway *(arrowhead)* is actually a gas-filled esophagus. The airway would be seen on a lower scan. If the air-filled structure were the airway, one would expect to show the esophagus just posteriorly.

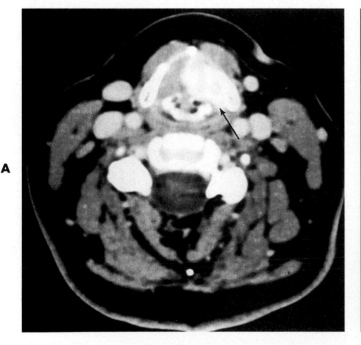

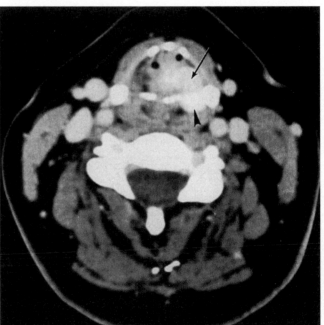

FIG. 11-132   Axial CT **A,** Radiopaque teflon injected into the cord. Note the small amount of teflon *(arrow)* squeezing between the thyroid cartilage and the arytenoid. **B,** Supraglottic scan. The radiopaque teflon *(arrow)* again squeezes between the thyroid cartilage and the upper arytenoid *(arrowhead)*. This amount of teflon is more than is usually seen in a routine injection.

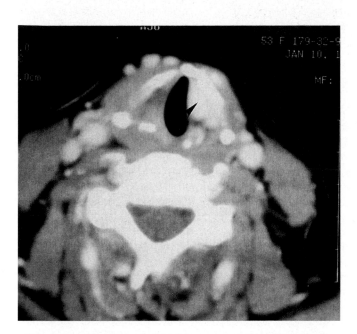

FIG. 11-133   Teflon injection, true cord. CT shows the increased density *(arrowhead)* of the teflon. Note how this pushes the mucosal surface toward midline so that the cords can abut during phonation.

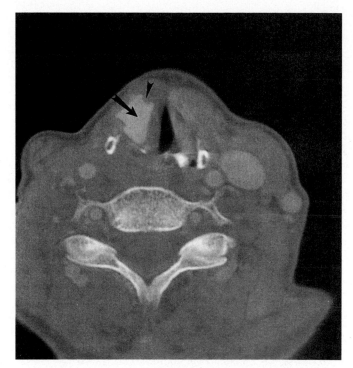

FIG. 11-134   Axial CT, silastic stent for vocal cord paralysis. The preshaped silastic stent *(arrow)* is used to add bulk to the paralyzed cord. The notches seen in the anterior *(arrowhead)* and posterior edges are to stabilize the stent in the surgical opening in the thyroid cartilage.

CT shows thickening of the epiglottis and prominence of the soft tissues in the aryepiglottic folds, false cords, and around the arytenoids (Figs. 11-124, 11-125). There is a streaky, increased attenuation in the preepiglottic and paraglottic spaces (dirty fat). The true vocal cords and subglottic larynx are usually fairly normal in appearance.

Perichondritis and chondronecrosis are much more significant clinical problems. Perichondritis is an inflammation or infection of the cartilages, and high doses of radiation can cause necrosis and collapse of the cartilages. In addition, radiated tissue is less resistent to infection, and deep biopsy of an irradiated larynx (looking for a recurrent tumor) may be associated with a perichondritis. The CT findings are usually superimposed on the changes previously mentioned. Perichondritis causes considerable edema around the cartilage, and at times gas bubbles can be seen (Fig. 11-126). The cartilage may collapse and fragment, assuming unusual angles on the axial scans (Fig. 11-127).

Radiation may lead to collapse of a cartilage invaded by a tumor. This is not necessarily a perichondritis or radiochondronecrosis. In these instances the tumor had replaced the cartilage and actually become part of its support structure. As the tumor regresses, this support structure is lost, and the eroded cartilage collapses.

Stents, Tubes, and Teflon

Stents or bone grafts are most often seen in the anterior arch of the cricoid (Fig. 11-128). They are placed in an effort to maintain or improve the cricoid lumen as part of the treatment of laryngeal stenosis.

Tracheostomy tubes and speaking tubes are seen in the lower neck (Figs. 11-129, 11-130). A tracheostomy tube is usually placed at the level of the midcervical trachea, but if the tracheostomy was done as an emergency procedure, it usually is at the cricothyroid membrane. Secretions can accumulate above the tracheostomy, and there can be some mucosal swelling. This may be difficult to differentiate from a tumor, especially in the immediate subglottic area (Fig. 11-129); however, the secretions are usually of a lower attenuation than a recurrent tumor, which is usually of a similar density to muscle.

The various valves used to force air from the trachea to the esophagus for use in esophageal speech are seen in the lower neck. These are most often noted on CT or barium swallow examinations. They are much smaller than a tracheostomy tube and occasionally can be aspirated into the lung (Fig. 11-131).

Teflon can be injected into the paraglottic space just lateral to the true cord (Figs. 11-132, 11-133). This is done to add bulk to a paralyzed cord so that the cords can better appose and thereby improve voice quality. The procedure has also been performed to build up the resected side of a vertical hemilaryngectomy. The teflon is radiopaque and can easily be seen on CT. More recently, some otolaryngologists have used plastic preformed prostheses and other materials to add bulk to the cord (Fig. 11-134).[62,63]

References

1. Barnes L, Gnepp DR. Disease of the larynx, hypopharynx, and esophagus. In: Barnes L, ed. Surgical pathology of the head and neck. New York, NY: Marcel Dekker Inc, 1985; 141-226.
2. Batsakis JG. Tumors of the head and neck: clinical pathological consideration. 2nd Edition. Baltimore Md: Williams & Wilkins, 1979.
3. American Joint Committee on Cancer. Manual for staging of cancer. 3rd Edition. Philadelphia, Pa: JB Lippincott Co, 1988.
4. Vega MF, Scola Bartolome. Surgical treatment of locally advanced laryngeal carcioma. In: Johnson JT, Didolkar MS, eds. Head and neck cancer. Vol. III. New York, NY: Elsevier Science Publishing Co Inc, 1993; 289-296.
5. Lee WR, Mancuso AA, Saleh EM, et al. Can pretreatment computed tomography findings predict local control in T3 squamous cell carcinoma of the glottic larynx treated with radiotherapy alone? Int J Radiation Oncology Biol Phys 1993; 25:683-687.
6. Freeman DE, Mancuso AA, Parsons JT, et al. Irradiation alone for supraglottic carcinoma: can CT findings predict treatment results? Int J Radiation Oncol Biol Phys 1990; 19:485-490.
7. Million RR. The myth regarding bone or cartilage involvement by cancer and the likelihood of cure by radiotherapy. Head Neck 1989; 11:30-40.
8. Castelijns JA, van den Brekel MWM, Smit EMT, et al. Predictive value of MRI-dependent and non-MRI-dependent parameters for recurrence of laryngeal cancer after radiation therapy. (In press.)
9. Castelijns JA, Kaiser MC, Valk K, et al. MR imaging of laryngeal cancer. JCAT 1987; 11(1):134-140.
10. Castelijns JA, Gerritsen GJ, Kaiser MC, et al. Invasion of laryngeal cartilage by cancer: comparison of CT and MR imaging. Radiology 1987; 166:199-206.
11. Castelijns JA, Gerritsen GJ, Kaiser MC, et al. MRI of normal or cancerous laryngeal cartilage: histopathologic correlation. Laryngoscope 1987; 97:1085-1093.
12. Johnson JT. A surgeon looks at cervical lymph nodes. Radiology 1990; 175:607-610.
13. Johnson J. The role of neck and mediastinal dissection. In: Fried MP, ed. The larynx: a multidisciplinary approach. Boston, Mass: Little, Brown & Co, 1988; 543-556.
14. Wagenfeld DJH, Harwood AR, Bryce DP, et al. Second primary respiratory tract malignant neoplasms in supraglottic carcinoma. Arch Otolaryngol 1981; 107:135-138.
15. Lawson W, Biller HF, Suen JY. Cancer of the larynx. In: Suen JY, Myers EN, eds. Cancer of the head and neck. New York, NY: Churchill Livingstone, 1989; 533-591.
16. Lawson W, Biller HF. Supraglottic cancer. In: Bailey BJ, Biller HF, eds. Surgery of the larynx. Philadelphia, Pa: WB Saunders Co, 1985; 243-256.
17. Thawley SE, Sessions DG. Surgical therapy of supraglottic tumors. In: Thawley SE, Panje WR, eds. Comprehensive management of head and neck tumors. Philadelphia, Pa: WB Saunders Co, 1987; 959-990.
18. Lufkin RB, Larsson SG, Hanafee WN. Work in progress: NMR anatomy of the larynx and tongue base. Radiology 1983; 148:173-177.
19. Bailey BJ. Glottic carcinoma. In: Bailey BJ, Biller HF, eds. Surgery of the larynx. Philadelphia, Pa: WB Saunders Co, 1985; 257-278.
20. Lawson W, Biller HF. Glottic and subglottic tumors. In: Thawley SE, Panje WR, eds. Comprehensive management of head and neck tumors. Philadelphia, Pa: WB Saunders Co, 1987; 991-1015.
21. Batsakis JG, Luna MA, Byers RM. Metastases to the larynx. Head Neck Surg 1985; 7:458-462.
22. Johnson J, Curtin HD. Deep neck lipoma. Ann Otol Rhinol Laryngol 1987; 96:472-473.
23. Jones SR, Myers EN, Barnes EL. Benign neoplasms of the larynx. In: Fried MP, ed. The larynx: a multidisciplinary approach. Boston, Mass: Little, Brown & Co, 1988; 401-420.
24. Konowitz PM, Lawson W, Som PM, et al. Laryngeal paraganglioma: update on diagnosis and treatment. Laryngoscope 1988; 98:40-49.
25. Stines J, Rodde A, Carolus JM, et al. CT findings of laryngeal involvement in von Recklinghausen disease. JCAT 1987; 11(1):141-143.
26. Supance JS, Queneue DJ, Crissman J. Endolaryngeal neurofibroma. Otolaryngol Head Neck Surg 1980; 88:74-79.
27. Henderson LH, Denneny JC III, Teichgraeber J. Airway obstructing epiglottic cyst. Ann Otol Rhinol Laryngol 1985; 94:473-475.
28. Glazer HS, Mauro MA, Aronberg DJ, et al. Computed tomography of laryngoceles. AJR 1983; 140:549-552.
29. Hubbard C. Laryngocele: a study of five cases with reference to radiologic features. Clin Radiol 1987; 38:639-643.
30. Michel JL, Weinstein L. Laryngeal infections. In: Fried MP, ed. The larynx: a multidisciplinary approach Boston, Mass: Little, Brown & Co, 1988; 237-247.
31. Souliere CR, Kirchner JA. Laryngeal perichondritis and abscess. Arch Otolaryngol 1985; 111:481-484.
32. Nemzek WR, Katzberg RW, Van Slyke MA, et al. A reappraisal of

laringe por asta de toro. An Otorrinolaringol Ibero Am 1990; 17(1):77-84.

37. Schaefer SD. Use of CT scanning in the management of the acutely injured larynx. Otolaryngol Clin North Am 1991; 24(1):31-36.

38. Biller HF, Lawson W. Management of acute laryngeal trauma. In: Bailey BJ, Biller HF, eds. Surgery of the larynx. Philadelphia, Pa: WB Saunders Co, 1985; 149-154.

39. Duda JJ Jr, Lewin JS, Eliachar I. MR evaluation of epiglottic avulsion. AJNR.

40. Snyderman C, Weissman JL, Tabor E, et al. Crack cocaine burns of the larynx. Arch Otolaryngol Head Neck Surg 1991; 17(7):792-795.

41. Love JT. Embryology and anatomy. In: Bluestone CD, Stool SE, eds. Pediatric otolaryngology. Philadelphia, Pa: WB Saunders Co, 1983; 1135-1140.

42. Tucker JA. Developmental anatomy of the larynx. In: Bailey B, Biller HF, eds. Surgery of the larynx. Philadelphia, Pa: WB Saunders Co, 1985; 3-14.

43. Sanudo JR, Domenech-Mateu JM. The laryngeal primordium and epithelial lamina. A new interpretation. J Anat 1990; 171:207-222.

44. Cotton R, Reilly JS. Congenital malformations of the larynx. In: Bluestone CD, Stool SE, eds. Pediatric otolaryngology. Philadelphia, Pa: WB Saunders Co, 1983; 1215-1224.

45. McMillan WG, Duvall AJ. Congenital subglottic stenosis. Arch Otolaryngol 1968; 87:272-274.

46. Schlesinger AE, Tucker GF. Elliptical cricoid cartilage: a unique type of congenital subglottic stenosis. AJR 1986; 146:1133-1136.

47. Weston MJ, Porter HJ, Berry PJ, et al. Ultrasonographic prenatal diagnosis of upper respiratory tract atresia. J Ultrasound Med 1992; 11:673-675.

48. Dolkart LA, Reimers FT, Wertheimer IS, et al. Prenatal diagnosis of laryngeal atresia. J Ultrasound Med 1992; 11:496-498.

49. Garel C, Hassan M, Hertz-Pannier L, et al. Contribution of MR in the diagnosis of "occult" posterior laryngeal cleft. Int J Pediatr Otorhinolaryngol 1992; 24:177-181.

50. Wilkinson AG, Mackenzie S, Hendry GM. Complete laryngotracheoesophageal cleft: CT diagnosis and associated abnormalities. Clin Radiol 1990; 41(6):437-438.

51. Ravich WJ, Donner MW, Kashima H. The swallowing center: concepts and procedures. Gastrointest Radiol 1985; 10(3):255-261.

52. Farooq P. Recurrent laryngeal nerve paralysis: laryngographic and computed tomography study. Radiology 1983; 148:149-151.

53. Levine HL, Tucker HM. Surgical management of the paralyzed larynx. In: Bailey BJ, Biller HF, eds. Surgery of the larynx. Philadelphia, Pa: WB Saunders Co, 1985; 117-134.

54. McAlpine JC, Fuller AP. Localized laryngeal amyloidosis: a report of a case with a review of the literature. J Laryngol 1964; 78:296-303.

55. Deutsch EC, Schlid JA, Mafee MF. Dysphagia and Forrestier's disease. Arch Otolaryngol 1985; 111:400-403.

56. Som PM, Biller HF. Computed tomography of the neck in the postoperative patient: radical neck dissection and the myocutaneous flap. Radiology 1983; 148:157-161.

57. Niemeyer JH, Balfe DM, Hayden RE. Neck evaluation with barium-enhanced radiographs and CT scans after supraglottic subtotal laryngectomy. Radiology 1987; 162:493-498.

58. Williford ME, Rice RP, Kelvin FM, et al. Revascularized jejunal graft replacing the cervical esophagus: radiographic evaluation. AJR 1985; 145:533-536.

59. Mukherji SK, Mancuso AA, Kotzur IM, et al. Radiologic appearance of the irradiated larynx. Part I. Expected changes. Radiology 1994; 193:141-148.

60. Mukherji SK, Mancuso AA, Kotzur IM, et al. Radiologic appearance of the irradiated larynx. Part II. Primary site response. Radiology 1994; 193:149-154.

61. Perez CA, Marks JE. Radiation therapy for carcinoma of the larynx. In: Bailey BJ, Biller HF, eds. Surgery of the larynx. Philadelphia, Pa: WB Saunders Co, 1985; 417-434.

62. Orlandi RR, Sercarz JA, Calcaterra TC. Custom silastic keel for anterior laryngeal reconstruction. Laryngoscope 1994; 104(9):1167-1169.

63. Cummings CW, Purcell LL, Flint PW. Hydroxylapatite laryngeal implants for medication. Preliminary report. Ann Otol Rhinol Laryngol 1993; 102(11):843-851.

Index